Stroke Recovery and Rehabilitation

Stroke Recovery and Rehabilitation

Edited By

JOEL STEIN, MD
Simon Baruch Professor of Physical Medicine and Rehabilitation and Chair,
Department of Rehabilitation Medicine
Columbia University College of Physicians and Surgeons

Professor and Chief, Division of Rehabilitation Medicine
Weill Cornell Medical College

Physiatrist-in-Chief, Department of Rehabilitation Medicine
NewYork Presbyterian Hospital
New York, New York

RICHARD L. HARVEY, MD
Associate Professor, Department of Physical Medicine and Rehabilitation
Northwestern University Feinberg School of Medicine

Wesley and Suzanne Dixon Stroke Chair and Medical Director,
    Stroke Rehabilitation Program
The Rehabilitation Institute of Chicago
Chicago, Illinois

RICHARD F. MACKO, MD
Professor, Departments of Neurology, Medicine/Gerontology,
    and Physical Therapy and Rehabilitation Science
University of Maryland School of Medicine

Director, Baltimore Veterans Affairs Center of Excellence in Exercise and Robotics
Veterans Affairs Maryland Health Care System
Baltimore, Maryland

CAROLEE J. WINSTEIN, PhD, PT, FAPTA
Professor and Director of Research, Division of Biokinesiology and Physical Therapy
University of Southern California School of Dentistry
Los Angeles, California

RICHARD D. ZOROWITZ, MD
Associate Professor, Department of Physical Medicine and Rehabilitation
The Johns Hopkins School of Medicine

Chairman, Department of Physical Medicine and Rehabilitation
Johns Hopkins Bayview Medical Center
Baltimore, Maryland

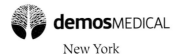

demosMEDICAL
New York

Acquisitions Editor: R. Craig Percy
Cover Design:
Copyediting, Indexing, and Composition: Publication Services, Inc.
Printer:

Visit our website at www.demosmedpub.com

Medicine is an ever-changing science. Research and clinical experience are continually expanding our knowledge, in particular our understanding of proper treatment and drug therapy. The authors, editors, and publisher have made every effort to ensure that all information in this book is in accordance with the state of knowledge at the time of production of the book. Nevertheless, the authors, editors, and publisher are not responsible for errors or omissions or for any consequences from application of the information in this book and make no warranty, express or implied, with respect to the contents of the publication. Every reader should examine carefully the package inserts accompanying each drug and should carefully check whether the dosage schedules mentioned therein or the contraindications stated by the manufacturer differ from the statements made in this book. Such examination is particularly important with drugs that are either rarely used or have been newly released on the market.

Library of Congress Cataloging-in-Publication Data

Stroke recovery and rehabilitation / edited by Joel Stein ... [et al.].
   p. ; cm.
   Includes bibliographical references and index.
   ISBN-13: 978-1-933864-12-9 (hardcover : alk. paper)
   ISBN-10: 1-933864-12-5 (hardcover : alk. paper)
   1. Cerebrovascular disease—Patients—Rehabilitation. I. Stein, Joel, M.D.
   [DNLM: 1. Stroke—rehabilitation. 2. Stroke—complications. 3. Stroke—therapy. WL 355 S9213437 2009]
   RC388.5.S8543 2009
   616.8′106—dc22

                              2008041361

Special discounts on bulk quantities of Demos Medical Publishing books are available to corporations, professional associations, pharmaceutical companies, health care organizations, and other qualifying groups. For details, please contact:

Special Sales Department
Demos Medical Publishing
386 Park Avenue South, Suite 301
New York, NY 10016
Phone: 800–532–8663 or 212–683–0072
Fax: 212–683–0118
Email: orderdept@demosmedpub.com

Made in the United States of America
08 09 10 11   5 4 3 2 1

Contents

VI OTHER REHABILITATION THERAPEUTICS

VII STROKE CARE SYSTEMS AND OUTCOMES

VIII PSYCHOSOCIAL AND COMMUNITY REINTEGRATION

Preface

The 1990s were declared the decade of the brain by the National Institutes of Health. It was during this decade that neuroscience and clinical rehabilitation research began to converge into a new science of neurorehabilitation. The knowledge gleaned from the last 20 years has led to the clear understanding that optimizing functional recovery from stroke is contingent on relatively intense and challenging targeted motor and cognitive relearning of functional skills. This relearning results in measurable cortical neuroplastic changes. This consensus represents a paradigm shift for rehabilitation clinicians who had for the most part previously focused on the neurodevelopmental process of carefully normalizing trunk and limb movement, teaching one-handed techniques, and educating patients on the use of adaptive equipment.

If there had been a standard comprehensive text on stroke rehabilitation, these changes in our conception of rehabilitation and recovery would most certainly require that it be updated. In fact, no such text has been previously assembled that included the basic neuroscience and anatomy of stroke, the physiology of neural recovery after focal injury, or clinical rehabilitation interventions for stroke based on randomized clinical trials. This text was written to fulfill that need: providing the reader with a multidisciplinary and international perspective. The chapters are written by basic scientists and clinicians from a variety of fields including biomedical engineering, neurology, physical medicine and rehabilitation, psychology, neuroscience, physical therapy, occupational therapy, speech and language pathology, neuroradiology, optometry, orthotics, and rehabilitation nursing. The intent was to provide a practical clinical guide to evidence-based stroke rehabilitation built on a foundation of basic neurophysiology and neuroscience.

We would like to thank the authors of this text for taking the time away from their busy clinical schedules, grant writing, and other academic responsibilities to write these chapters. We also would like to thank the editorial staff at Demos Medical Publishing for their patience, encouragement, and support. We hope that this text on stroke recovery and rehabilitation becomes a valuable reference for academicians and clinicians alike, and for all disciplines who have the pleasure of helping survivors of stroke achieve their maximum potential.

Joel Stein
Richard D. Zorowitz
Richard L. Harvey
Richard F. Macko
Carolee J. Winstein

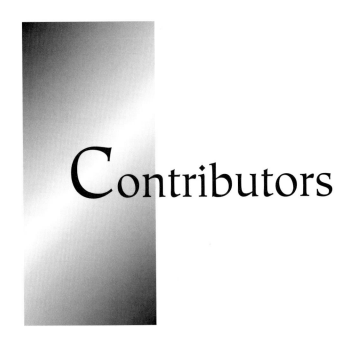

Contributors

Craig S. Anderson, PhD, FRACP, FAFPHM
Director
Department of Neurological and Mental Health
The George Institute for International Health
Sydney, Australia

Tamilyn Bakas, DNS, RN, FAHA, FAAN
Associate Professor
Department of Adult Health
Indiana University School of Nursing
Indianapolis, Indiana

Carol Bartlett, MSW
Manager
Department of Care Coordination
National Rehabilitation Hospital
Washington, DC

Derrick A. Bennett, MSc, PhD, CStat
Senior Biostatistitician
Clinical Trial Service Unit
University of Oxford
Oxford, England

Randie M. Black-Shaffer, MD, MA
Director
Stroke Program
Spaulding Rehabilitaion Hospital
Assistant Professor
Department of Physical Medicine and Rehabilitation
Harvard Medical School
Boston, Massachusetts

Lynne C. Brady Wagner, MA
Director
Stroke Rehabilitation Program
Spaulding Rehabilitation Hospital
Boston, Massachusetts

Bambi Roberts Brewer, PhD
Assistant Professor
Department of Rehabilitation Science and
    Technology
University of Pittsburgh
Pittsburgh, Pennsylvania

Carlo Caltagirone, MD
Scientific Director
Department of Clinical and Behavioral Neurology
IRCLS Santa Lucia Foundation
Department of Neuroscience
University of Rome Tor Vergata
Rome, Italy

John Chae, MD
Associate Professor
Department of Physical Medicine and
    Rehabilitation
MetroHealth Medical Center
Department of Biomedical Engineering
Case Western Reserve University
Cleveland, Ohio

Leora R. Cherney, PhD
Director
Center for Aphasia Research
Rehabilitation Institute of Chicago
Chicago, Illinois

J. Quentin Clemens, MD, MSCI
Associate Professor
Department of Urology
University of Michigan Medical Center
Ann Arbor, Michigan

Brendan E. Conroy, MD, FAAPM&R
Medical Director, Stroke Recovery Program
Department of Medical Affairs
National Rehabilitation Hospital
Washington, DC

Rory A. Cooper, PhD
Director
Department of Human Engineering Research
    Laboratories
Veterans Affairs Center of Excellence in Wheelchairs
    and Associated Rehabilitation
Veterans Affairs Pittsburgh Healthcare System
Pittsburgh, Pennsylvania

Rosemarie Cooper, MPT, ATP
Assistant Professor
Department of Rehabilitation Sciences and Technology
School of Health and Rehabilitation Sciences
University of Pittsburgh
Pittsburgh, Pennsylvania

Steven C. Cramer, MD, MMSc
Associate Professor
Departments of Neurology and Anatomy and
    Neurobiology
University of California
Irvine, California

David Martin Crandell, MD
Instructor
Department of Physical Medicine and Rehabilitation
Harvard Medical School
Boston, Massachusetts

Florence A. Denby, MS, APRN, BN, CRRN
Nurse Practitioner
Department of Physical Medicine and Rehabilitation
Rehabilitation Institute of Chicago
Chicago, Illinois

Francine Dumas, MSc, PT
Research Associate
Department of Rehabilitation
Laval University
Center for Interdisciplinary Research in Rehabilitation
    and Social Integration
Rehabilitation Institute of Quebec City
Quebec, Canada

Sylvia A. Duraski, ARPN BC, MS, BSN
Nurse Practitioner
Department of Physical Medicine and Rehabilitation
Rehabilitation Institute of Chicago
Chicago, Illinois

Anne Epstein, PhD
Assistant Professor
Department of Medicine
University of Colorado
Denver, Colorado

Susan E. Fasoli, ScD
Occupational Therapy Manager
Department of Rehabilitation Services
Newton Wellesley Hospital
Newton, Massachussetts
Instructor
Department of Physical Medicine and Rehabilitation
Harvard Medical School
Boston, Massachusetts

Stephania Fatone, PhD, BPO (Hons)
Research Assistant Professor
Department of Medicine
Northwestern University
Chicago, Illinois

Valery L. Feigin, PhD
Senior Research Fellow
Department of Clinical Trials Research Unit
University of Auckland
Auckland, New Zealand

Hillel M. Finestone, BSc, MDCM, FRCPC
Medical Director Stroke Rehabilitation
Department of Physical Medicine and Rehabilitation
Elisabeth Bruyere Health Centre
Associate Professor
University of Ottawa
Ottawa, Ontario, Canada

Norine Foley, MSc, BASc, RD
Research Associate
Stroke Rehabilitation and Assistive Technologies,
    Aging and Geriatric Care Program
Lawson Health Research Institute
Parkwood Hospital
Ontario, Canada

Gerard E. Francisco, MD
Co-Director
Department of Brain Injury and Stroke Program
The Institute for Rehabilitation Research
Memorial Hermann Hospital
Clinical Associate Professor
Department of Physical Medicine and Rehabilitation
University of Texas Health Science Center
Houston, Texas

Karen L. Furie, MD, MPH
Director
Stroke Service
Massachusetts General Hospital
Boston, Massachusetts

Arthur M. Gershkoff, MD
Clinical Director
Department of Stroke Rehabilitation
Moss Rehab Hospital
Elkins Park, Pennsylvania
Assistant Professor
Department of Rehabilitation Medicine
Thomas Jefferson University
Philadelphia, Pennsylvania

Judith E. Goldstein, OD
Assistant Professor
Departments of Opthalmology and Physical Medicine
  and Rehabilitation
The Johns Hopkins University
Baltimore, Maryland

Marlis Gonzalez-Fernandez, MD, PhD
Assistant Professor
Department of Physical Medicine and Rehabilitation
Johns Hopkins University School of Medicine
Baltimore, Maryland

Eric F. Grabowski, MD, DSci
Associate Professor
Department of Pediatrics (Hematology/Oncology)
Massachusetts General Hospital
Harvard Medical School
Boston, Massachusetts

Steven M. Greenberg, MD, PhD
Co-Director, Neurology Clinical Trials
Assistant Professor
Department of Neurology
Stroke Research Center
Massachusetts General Hospital
Boston, Massachusetts

Linda S. Green-Finestone, PhD, RD
Adjunct Professor
Department of Physical Medicine and Rehabilitation
University of Ottawa
Nutritional Epidemiologist
Centre for Chronic Disease Prevention and Control
Public Health Agency of Canada
Ottawa, Canada

Charlene Hafer-Macko, MD
Associate Professor
Department of Neurology
University of Maryland School of Medicine
Baltimore Veterans Affairs Medical Center
Baltimore, Maryland

Richard L. Harvey, MD
Associate Professor
Department of Physical Medicine and Rehabilitation
Northwestern University Feinberg School of Medicine
Wesley and Suzanne Dixon Stroke Chair and Medical
  Director
Stroke Rehabilitation Program
The Rehabilitation Institute of Chicago
Chicago, Illinois

Kenneth M. Heilman, MD
Distinguished Professor
Department of Neurology and Health Psychology
University of Florida College of Medicine
Gainesville, Florida

Katya Hill, PhD, CCC-SLP
Associate Professor
Department of Communication Science and Disorders
University of Pittsburgh
Pittsburgh, Pennsylvania

Neville Hogan, PhD
Professor
Department of Mechanical Engineering, Brain and
  Cognitive Sciences
Massachusetts Institute of Technology
Cambridge, Massachusetts

Richard Hughes, PT, MS, NCS
Physical Therapist
Partners Home Care
Beverly, Massachusetts

Frederick M. Ivey, PhD
Assistant Professor
Department of Medicine
University of Maryland School of Medicine
Baltimore, Maryland

Alan M. Jette, PT, MPH, PhD
Director, Health and Disability Research Institute
Department of Health Policy and Management
Boston University School of Public Health
Boston, Massachusetts

Robin M. Jones, MD, BA
Associate Professor of Neurology
Department of Neurology
Harvard Medical School
Massachusetts General Hospital
Boston, Massachusetts

Lalit Kalra, MBBS, MD, PhD, FRCP
Professor
Department of Stroke Medicine
King's College London School of Medicine
London, United Kingdom

Patricia Karg, MS
Assistant Professor
Department of Rehabilitation Science and
Technology
University of Pittsburgh
Pittsburgh, Pennsylvania

Amol Karmarkar, MS, BS
Graduate Student Researcher
Department of Human Engineering Research
Laboratories
Veterans Affairs Center of Excellence in Wheelchairs
and Associated Rehabilitation
Veterans Affairs Pittsburgh Healthcare System
Pittsburgh, Pennsylvania

Steven A. Kautz, PhD
Biomedical Engineer
Department of Brain Rehabilitation Research
Malcolm Randall Veterans Affairs Medical Center
Gainesville, Florida

Kristi L. Kirschner, MD
Professor
Departments of Physical Medicine and Rehabilitation
and Medical Humanities and Bioethics
Northwestern University Feinberg School of Medicine
Chicago, Illinois

Andrew M. Kramer, MD
Peter W. Shaughnessy Professor of Medicine
Head of the Division of Health Care Policy and
Research
Department of Medicine
University of Colorado
Denver, Colorado

Hermano Igo Krebs, PhD
Principal Research Scientist
Department of Mechanical Engineering
Massachusetts Institute of Technology
Cambridge, Massachusetts

Amy Karas Lane, BS
Clinical Instructor
Department of Rehabilitation Science and Technology
University of Pittsburgh
Pittsburgh, Pennsylvania

Peter Langhorne, PhD, FRCP
Professor
Academic Section of Geriatric Medicine
University of Glasgow
Glasgow, Scotland

Douglas J. Lanska, MD, MS, MSPH, FAAN
Staff Neurologist
Department of Medicine Service
Veterans Affairs Medical Center
Tomah, Wisconsin
Professor
Department of Neurology
University of Wisconsin School of Medicine and Public
Health
Madison, Wisconsin

Nancy K. Latham, PhD, PT
Research Assistant Professor
Department of Health and Disability Research
Boston University School of Public Health
Boston, Massachusetts

Carlene M. M. Lawes, MBCHB, MPH, FAFPHM
Research Fellow
Clinical Trials Research Unit
Department of Medicine
University of Auckland
Auckland, New Zealand

Marion Levine, MEd, CRC
Vocational Rehabilitation Coordinator
Physical and Occupational Therapy
National Rehabilitation Hospital
Washington, DC

Roger Little, MS
Rehabilitation Engineer
Department of Rehabilitation Science and Technology
University of Pittsburgh
Pittsburgh, Pennsylvania

Chiung-ju Liu, PhD, OT
Assistant Professor
Department of Occupational Therapy
School of Health and Rehabilitation Sciences
Indiana University
Indianapolis, Indiana

Andreas R. Luft, MD
Professor of Neurology and Clinical
Neurorehabilitation
Department of Neurology
University of Zurich
Zurich, Switzerland

Richard F. Macko, MD
Professor
Departments of Neurology, Medicine/Gerontology,
and Physical Therapy and Rehabilitation Science
University of Maryland School of Medicine
Director
Baltimore Veterans Affairs Center of Excellence in
Exercise and Robotics
Veterans Affairs Maryland Health Care System
Baltimore, Maryland

Francine Malouin, PhD
Professor Emeritus
Department of Rehabilitation
Laval University
Center for Interdisciplinary Research in Rehabilitation
    and Social Integration
Rehabilitation Institute of Quebec City
Quebec, Canada

Katherine M. Martinez, MA, BS, NCS
Instructor
Department of Physical Therapy and Human
    Movement Services
Northwestern University Feinberg School of
    Medicine
Chicago, Illinois

Koichiro Matsuo, DDS, PhD
Associate Professor
Department of Special Care Dentistry
Matsumoto Dental University
Nagano, Japan

William Alvin McElveen, MD
Medical Director
Primary Stroke Center
Blake Medical Center
Bradenton, Florida

John R. McGuire, MD
Associate Professor
Department of Physical Medicine and Rehabilitation
Medical College of Wisconsin
Milwaukee, Wisconsin

Stephanie McHughen, BSc
Departments of Neurology and Anatomy and
    Neurobiology
University of California
Irvine, California

Kathleen Michael, PhD, RN, CRRN
Assistant Professor
Department of Organizational Systems and Adult
    Health
University of Maryland School of Nursing
Baltimore, Maryland

Fatemeh Milani, MD, FAAPM&R, FABEM
Chair, Division of Rehabilitation Medicine
Department of Medical Affairs
National Rehabilitation Hospital
Washington, DC

Denise M. Monahan, MS, CCC-SLP
Senior Speech Language Pathologist
Department of Rehabilitation Services
Good Samaritan Hospital
Baltimore, Maryland

Govind Mukundan, MD
Fellow
Department of Neuroradiology
Massachusetts General Hospital
Boston, Massachusetts

Sara J. Mulroy, PhD, PT
Director
Department of Pathokinesiology Laboratory
Rancho Los Amigos National Rehabilitation Center
Downey, California

Donna L. Nimec, MD, MS
Director of Pediatric Rehabilitation
Department of Physical Medicine and Rehabilitation
Spaulding Rehabilitation Hospital
Boston, Massachusetts

Randolph J. Nudo, PhD
Director
Landon Center on Aging
University of Kansas Medical Center
Kansas City, Kansas

Jeffrey B. Palmer, MD
Lawrence Cardinal Sheehan Professor and Chair
Department of Physical Medicine and Rehabilitation
Johns Hopkins University School of Medicine
Baltimore, Maryland

Tamra L. Pelleschi, BS, OTR/L
Faculty
School of Health and Rehabilitation Sciences
Center for Assistive and Rehabilitative Technology
Johnstown, Pennsylvania

Sandra M. Pinzon, MD
Resident
Department of Medicine (Neurology)
Albert Einstein Medical Center
Thomas Jefferson University
Philadelphia, Pennsylvania

Carol L. Richards, PhD, DU, PT, FCAHS
Professor
Department of Rehabilitation
Laval University
Director
Center for Interdisciplinary Research in Rehabilitation
    and Social Integration
Rehabilitation Institute of Quebec City
Quebec, Canada

Mark W. Rogers, BSPT, MS, PhD, FAPTA
Professor and Vice Chair for Research
Department of Physical Therapy and Rehabilitation
    Science
University of Maryland School of Medicine
Baltimore, Maryland

Anthony George Rudd, MB, BChir, FRCP (Lond)
Stroke Unit
Guy's and St. Thomas' NHS Foundation Trust
St. Thomas' Hospital
London, England

Katherine Salter, BA
Research Associate
Stroke Rehabilitation and Assistive Technologies,
 Aging and Geriatric Care Program
Lawson Health Research Institute
Parkwood Hospital
Ontario, Canada

Pamela W. Schaefer, MD
Director of Fellowship Program
Department of Neuroradiology
Massachusetts General Hospital
Boston, Massachusetts

Timothy Schallert, PhD
Professor
Departments of Psychology and Neurobiology
Institute for Neuroscience
University of Texas at Austin
Austin, Texas
Professor
Department of Neurosurgery
University of Michigan
Ann Arbor, Michigan

Jill See, PT, MPT
Departments of Neurology and Anatomy and
 Neurobiology
University of California
Irvine, California

Monika V. Shah, DO
Assistant Professor
Department of Physical Medicine and
 Rehabilitation
Baylor College of Medicine
Director
Brain Injury and Stroke Program
The Institute for Rehabilitation Research
Memorial Hermann Hospital
Houston, Texas

Marianne Shaughnessy, PhD, MSN
Associate Director Education and Evaluation
Geriatric Research Education and Clinical Center
Baltimore Veterans Affairs Medical Center
Baltimore, Maryland

Lynne R. Sheffler, MD
Senior Instructor
Department of Physical Medicine and Rehabilitation
Case Western Reserve University
Department of Physical Medicine and Rehabilitation
MetroHealth Medical Center
Cleveland, Ohio

Samuel C. Shiflett, PhD
Research Associate
Department of Psychology
University of Arizona
Tucson, Arizona

Steven L. Small, PhD, MD
Professor
Department of Neurology and Psychology
The University of Chicago
Chicago, Illinois

David Solomon, MD, PhD
Assistant Professor
Departments of Neurology and Otolaryngology
Johns Hopkins University
Baltimore, Maryland

Gianfranco Spalletta, MD, PhD
Head
Department of Neuropsychiatry
IRCCS Santa Lucia Foundation
Rome, Italy

Joel Stein, MD
Professor and Chair
Department of Rehabilitation Medicine
Columbia University College of Physicians and Surgeons
Professor and Chair
Division of Rehabilitation Medicine
Weill Cornell Medical College
Physiatrist-in-Chief
Department of Rehabilitation Medicine
New York Presbyterian Hospital
New York, New York

Katherine J. Sullivan, PhD, PT, FAHA
Associate Professor of Clinical Physical Therapy
Division of Biokinesiology and Physical Therapy
University of Southern California
Los Angeles, California

Robert W. Teasell, BSc, MD, FRCPC
Professor and Chair
Department of Physical Medicine and Rehabilitation
University of Western Ontario
Ontario, Canada

Karen Tyner, MSW, LICSW
Outpatient Social Worker
National Rehabilitation Hospital
Washington, DC

Carolee J. Winstein, PhD, PT, FAPTA
Professor and Director of Research
Division of Biokinesiology and Physical Therapy
University of Southern California School of Dentistry
Los Angeles, California

Steven L. Wolf, PhD, PT, FAPTA
Professor
Department of Rehabilitation Medicine
Emory University School of Medicine
Atlanta, Georgia

David Tzehsia Yu, MD
Department of Physical Medicine and Rehabilitation
Virginia Mason Medical Center
Seattle, Washington

Richard D. Zorowitz, MD
Associate Professor
Department of Physical Medicine and Rehabilitation
The Johns Hopkins School of Medicine
Chairman
Department of Physical Medicine and Rehabilitation
Johns Hopkins Bayview Medical Center
Baltimore, Maryland

I

INTRODUCTION

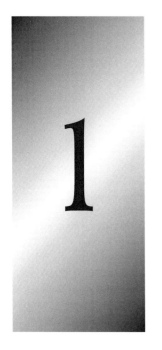

1

The Historical Origins of Stroke Rehabilitation

Douglas J. Lanska

Physical medicine and rehabilitation (PM&R) is a relatively young specialty that developed during the twentieth century, with significant growth and development stimulated by two world wars and by increasingly severe epidemics of paralytic poliomyelitis during the first half of the twentieth century (1–4). During and after each of the world wars, many soldiers returned with serious injuries and severe disabilities, and physicians and therapists were needed to treat and manage their chronic disabling conditions. This was particularly true after World War II, when the availability of antibiotics and improved surgical techniques allowed more injured soldiers to survive, albeit with significant disabilities. Similarly, over the same time period, increasingly severe epidemics of polio, frequent industrial accidents, and escalating motor vehicle accidents as a result of increased availability of automobiles and higher-speed roadways added greatly to the burden of impairment and disability among the civilian population. Thus, events in the first half of the twentieth century necessitated the development of new restorative treatment programs incorporating new physical and rehabilitative techniques, and the establishment of training programs for the physicians and therapists to administer the treatments.

Nevertheless, with the exception of a relatively few scattered physical medicine physicians, it was not demonstrated until the second half of the twentieth century that specialists in rehabilitation medicine could profitably direct their energies exclusively, or even preferentially, to rehabilitation outside of the unprecedented and unsustainable circumstances of wartime military programs. Also largely missing until the second half of the twentieth century were separate departments in academic and non-academic medical centers devoted to the specialty, established training programs in physical medicine and rehabilitation, a sufficient number of physical medicine and rehabilitation practitioners, separate dedicated facilities for provision of rehabilitation services (e.g., dedicated wards in hospitals or separate rehabilitation centers), forums for the interchange of ideas (e.g., texts, journals, and professional societies), recognition by professional colleagues and the public that rehabilitation medicine specialists provided a needed service, and supportive legislation that would provide financial mechanisms to develop and provide such resources (5).

WORLD WAR I AND ITS AFTERMATH: BEGINNINGS OF PHYSICAL MEDICINE AND VOCATIONAL REHABILITATION

During much of the nineteenth century, physicians who employed physical modalities or advocated treatment with fresh air, water, exercise, and dietary modification were at risk of being labeled as quacks by other members of the medical profession. However, near the turn of the century, orthopedic surgeons in particular began using selected physical treatments—massage, exercise, hydrotherapy—as part of special programs to augment medical care and convalescence within hospitals under physician direction.

During World War I (1914–1918), physical and occupational therapy became increasingly important adjuncts to surgical practice, particularly in the treatment of orthopedic casualties, as surgeons realized that surgery alone was insufficient to achieve maximum return of function, and as empirical experience indicated that physical methods were useful adjuncts in the medical care and convalescence of wounded and disabled soldiers (4). In particular, with active U.S. involvement in the war beginning in 1917, Colonel Joel E. Goldthrait, Chief Surgeon in the Orthopedic Medical Corp of the American Expeditionary Forces, and Colonel E. G. Brackett in the Home Service enthusiastically supported a role for physical therapists in the rehabilitation of orthopedic casualties (6, 7). Late in 1917, a program of Women's Auxiliary Medical Aides was established in the Surgeon General's Office, but by April 1918 this was transferred to the Division of Physical Reconstruction and renamed "Reconstruction Aides" (6). Major (later Lieutenant Colonel) Frank B. Granger, MD, was named as director of the Physiotherapy Service of the Reconstruction Division for the Army, and under his command the reconstruction aid program was directed by Chief Aide Marguerite Sanderson (formerly from Dr. Goldthwait's office in Boston) (6, 8). Training programs for the reconstruction aides were established at Walter Reed General Hospital, headed by therapist Mary McMillan, later at Reed College in Portland, Oregon (initially taught also by McMillan during a leave of absence from Walter Reed), and eventually at 13 other programs across the country (6, 9, 10).

Colonel Frank C. Billings, Chief of the Division of Physical Reconstruction in the Medical Department of the United States Army, established separate sections for education, therapy, and clinical work. Military physicians in "reconstruction hospitals" then began treating wounded and disabled soldiers with occupational therapy (then called bedside occupations and curative workshops) and "physiotherapy" (a term indicating use of various physical methods in treatment, including heat, exercise, hydrotherapy, electrotherapy, and massage) (7). By the end of the war, therapy was provided by nearly 800 women volunteers (physical educators or nurses) trained as "reconstruction aides" under the Reconstruction Aide Program (4, 6, 10–12).

Some individuals criticized the prolonged bedside therapeutic activities provided by female reconstruction aides because they were felt to promote dependence and invalidism (13, 14). However, in 1918 Billings described the work of the reconstruction aides and clearly distinguished it as superior to the types of "diversional" tasks previously employed:

> [Ward work] has consisted frequently of work not so purposeful in its character, but rather as diversional in character, in the form of knitting, in the form of basket weaving, etc. But the work which the Surgeon-General utilizes as curative in character in the general hospital for these soldiers is more purposeful than knitting, basket weaving and the like. In other words, it is of the kind and character of curative work that will look toward the training of the soldier for employment after his discharge from the Army. (15)

By the end of the war, physical reconstruction services were available in 35 general hospitals and 18 base hospitals across the country (4, 16), and nearly 50,000 veterans (or about 40% of the 125,000 disabled during the war) had been treated at these facilities (17).

In 1923, Dr. F.B. Granger, who had been instrumental in developing the program for reconstruction aides in the United States, and who was the first physician specializing in physical medicine to become a member of the AMA Council on Physical Therapy (9), summarized how physical therapy originated (18):

> With the onset of the World War the urgent need of hastening the return of the wounded to the front lines, or rehabilitating them sufficiently so that they could be given non-combatant duty, thus presumably relieving an able-bodied man, forced the unification of [the separate treatment modalities]. The Surgeon General of the United States Army, at one stroke, completed their amalgamation when he defined physiotherapy as "Physical measures such as are employed under physiotherapy, including hydro, electro, mechano therapy, active exercises, indoor and outdoor games, and passive exercises in the form of massage." Thus was born modern physiotherapy. (18)

Following the war, Elliot Brackett, a Harvard-trained orthopedic surgeon, promoted the establishment of hospitals "devoted to the medical care of all men who should be returned, also planned and equipped to reinstate the disabled soldier in the industrial world and allow him to become an independent wage earner" (17). Unfortunately, interest in rehabilitative services in the military had waned after the war.

THE 1920s: BEGINNINGS OF PROFESSIONAL ORGANIZATIONS AND FORMAL TRAINING PROGRAMS

Physical Medicine

The 1920s and 1930s saw the beginnings of professional organizational development for the nascent field of physical medicine and rehabilitation. So-called "physical therapy physicians" (i.e., physicians practicing early forms of physical medicine) began efforts to organize themselves and vied for a voice in the American Medical Association. Specifically, in 1923 the American College of Radiology and Physiotherapy was founded as a professional organization of physicians who used physical methods to diagnose and treat illness and disability. Samuel B. Childs, MD, a radiologist from Denver, was elected as the first president. Very soon, however, radiologists separated and developed their own organizations, so that by 1925 the organization became the American Congress of Physical Therapy. Subsequent developments included the assimilation in 1933 of the American Physical Therapy Association (whose membership was comprised solely of physicians), and various changes in the name of the organization initially intended to clarify the distinction between physicians and non-physician therapists using physical methods in treatment (until the present name of the American Congress of Rehabilitation Medicine was selected in 1966).

Specialty physical medicine journals also developed during this period, corresponding to the increasing professional orientation of a small group of physicians to this new area of specialization. The journal *Radiology* began publication in 1920 under the editorship of Albert F. Tyler, MD, and in 1926 was renamed the *Archives of Physical Therapy, X-ray, Radium* to reflect its expanded focus. Subsequent name changes in the journal reflected an early shift away from radiology, a later distinction between physician and non-physician therapists utilizing physical methods in treatment, and ultimately a broadening emphasis on rehabilitation (until the present name of the *Archives of Physical Medicine and Rehabilitation* was selected in 1952).

Most physicians who practiced physical medicine in this era used this as an adjunct to their regular general medical practices, but starting in the mid-1920s, some physicians began devoting their careers to this area and were recognized with academic faculty appointments. The first of these was John Stanley Coulter, MD, who joined the faculty of Northwestern University Medical School in Chicago in 1926 as the first full-time academic physician specializing in physical medicine. He initiated the first continuing teaching program in physical medicine in the form of 3- to 6-month and later 12-month courses. He became chairman of the AMA Council on Physical Therapy (19). For the next two decades, he was a key leader in the development of educational programs for the practice of physical medicine, and also in the development of professional organizations for physical medicine.

Physical Therapy

Formal training for allied health professionals in civilian practice was not available until 1918, when the Mayo Clinic initiated a training program in physiotherapy (20). In 1920, Lieutenant Colonel Hard D. Corbusier wrote to former reconstruction aide Mary McMillan, proposing the formation of a professional society of physical therapists to "advertise to all the physicians and surgeons of the country the importance of treatment by physical means and to elevate and standardize the work and place it on a more substantial basis" (6). In 1921, McMillan organized a group of nearly 300 former reconstruction aides to form the American Women's Physical Therapeutic Association, with Mary McMillan elected as the first president. The first issue of the association's official publication, *The P.T. Review*, was published in March 1921, and the same year McMillan published *Massage and Therapeutic Exercise*, the first textbook written by a physical therapist (10, 21). The organization was renamed the American Physiotherapy Association in 1922, and in 1930 the organization was incorporated to establish educational standards for physical therapists, to support regulation of physical therapy practice, and to cooperate with the medical profession to establish a central registry of physical therapists (10, 22).

Occupational Therapy

In 1914, George Edward Barton—a disabled architect who had benefited from care he received at a convalescent hospital—introduced the term *occupational therapy* at a meeting in Boston of the Massachesetts State Board of Insanity (23) and subsequently founded Consolation House in Clifton Springs, New York, where he provided vocational assistance and workshop activities to other disabled people (14, 23–25). In 1917, Barton organized the first meeting of the National Society for the Promotion of Occupational Therapy at Clifton Springs for "the advancement of occupation as a therapeutic measure, the study of the effects of occupation upon the human being, and the dissemination of scientific knowledge on this subject" (26). In addition to Barton, the founding members included Dr. William Rush Dunton, Jr., a Maryland psychiatrist who was responsible for the occupations program at the Sheppard and Pratt Institute, and who had written monographs and articles on using occupational activities as therapy, including one of the first textbooks on occupational therapy, *Occupational Therapy—A Manual for Nurses* (27, 28); Eleanor Clarke Slagle, who worked with Dunton at Johns Hopkins in Baltimore, and who developed a regimented treatment program ("habit training") for chronic schizophrenic patients; Susan Cox Johnson, director of occupations for the New York State Department of Public Charities; Thomas Kidner, an architect who was the vocational secretary of the Canadian Military Hospitals Commission; Isabel Newton, who was Barton's secretary; and Susan Tracy, a nurse who was a training school superintendent and instructor of occupational therapy courses for nursing students, including the first such course (in 1911) at a general hospital, the Massachusetts General Hospital Training School for Nurses (14, 23–25, 29, 30). Barton became the first president (23). The organization was renamed the American Occupational Therapy Association in 1923 (23). The *Maryland Psychiatric Quarterly*, edited by Dunton, became the official organ of the National Society for the Promotion of Occupational Therapy, until 1922 when the *Archives of Occupational Therapy* was first published as the official publication of the organization (14, 23).

In 1929, Colonel James A. Mattison described the purposes of occupational therapy as employed at the National Home for Disabled Volunteer Soldiers:

> One of the principal aims of occupational therapy is to create morale, and to provide every opportunity for the coordination of all hospital efforts toward returning the patient to community life and economic usefulness. (31)

The first textbook in the United States concerning occupational therapy that was written primarily by occupational therapists was *Principles of Occupational Therapy*, edited by Helen S. Willard and Clare S. Spackman, and first published in 1947 (32).

Speech Therapy

Speech therapy had eighteenth- and nineteenth-century antecedents, particularly in the practical treatment approaches of the elocutionists (i.e., focused on improving speaking, orating, or singing); the beginnings of aphasiology with Paul Broca, Karl Wernicke, and others; and the various "methods" for treating various speech impediments, and for treating mispronunciation and articulatory disturbances among the deaf (33, 34). Professional organization development for speech therapy in the United States began with the founding of the American Speech and Hearing Association in 1925 as the American Academy of Speech Correction (34–36). In 1927, a nomenclature committee of the American Speech Correction Association outlined and described the conditions treated by "speech correctionists" under seven major categories: dysarthria, dyslalia, dyslogia, dysphasia, dysphemia, dysphonia, and dysrhythmia (34, 37).

PROFILE OF FRANK KRUSEN (1898–1973): "THE FATHER OF PHYSICAL MEDICINE"

Frank Hammond Krusen (1898–1973) has been widely regarded as "the father of physical medicine," and particularly during the 1930s and 1940s was influential in the development of this field in the United States and internationally (38). Krusen graduated from Jefferson Medical College in Philadelphia in 1921, but his planned surgical career was interrupted when he developed pulmonary tuberculosis in 1924. During his convalescence at a sanitarium, he became interested in physical medicine. In particular, his own experiences and observations at this time helped Krusen realize that physical deconditioning increased dependence on institutional living and eroded self esteem. He believed that self-assurance and independence could be restored in disabled patients with appropriate physical reconditioning, vocational rehabilitation, and reintegration into non-institutional society (39). From this point forward, Krusen worked to develop physical medicine into a scientifically based and accepted medical specialty.

Upon his return to Philadelphia in 1926, Krusen was appointed as associate dean at Temple Medical School, where in 1929 he started the first academic department of physical medicine in the United States (39–41). In 1930, Krusen published an undergraduate curriculum in physical medicine (42). At the invitation of Dr. William J. Mayo, Krusen moved to the Mayo Clinic in Rochester, Minnesota in 1935, where he founded the department of physical medicine (1935), developed the first three-year residency program in physical medicine (1936), and developed a school of physical therapy (1938) (19, 20, 40). In 1941, he was promoted to professor. In 1942, during World War II, he helped train a large cadre of medical officers from the U.S. Armed Forces with 90-day intensive courses in physical medicine at the Mayo Graduate School of Medicine with the trainees being labeled as "90-day wonders" (3, 16). Krusen's influence was tremendous as judged by his own contributions, as well as by the number and quality of his trainees, and the roles and contributions that they subsequently made to the further development of the specialty (43).

In addition to his role in the development of clinical practice and training programs in physical medicine, Krusen was an organizational leader for the specialty during the late 1930s and through the 1940s. In 1937, with William Bierman and John S. Coulter, Krusen established the American Registry of Physical Therapy Technicians to credential physical therapists (who were conferred the title of "registered physical therapist" upon passing the certifying examination) (3, 39). In 1938, with a small group of other pioneering physical medicine physicians, Krusen and Coulter founded the Society of Physical Therapy Physicians (later named the American Academy of Physical Medicine and Rehabilitation) "to develop physical therapy as a formally recognized specialty," and Krusen was elected its first president (39). In 1941, Krusen wrote the first widely-used textbook of physical medicine, *Physical Medicine: The Employment of*

Physical Agents for Diagnosis and Therapy (44). Subsequently Krusen played critical organizational roles in the founding and initial leadership of the Baruch Committee on Physical Medicine (1943), the American Board of Physical Medicine and Rehabilitation (1947), and the International Federation of Physical Medicine (1952).

In 1938, Krusen proposed the term "physiatrist" to designate the physician specializing in physical medicine, and Krusen further proposed that "physiatrist" should be pronounced with the accent on the third syllable (fiz ē at´ rist) to minimize confusion with "psychiatrist." The name "physiatrist" was derived from the Greek words "physics" (physical phenomena) and "iatreia" (healer or physician) (16). Later, in 1946, the AMA Council on Physical Medicine voted to support the terms "physiatrist" and "physiatry" (12). In 1961, Arthur Watkins proposed "physiatrics" as a new name for the specialty of PM&R based on Krusen's 1938 proposal, and Watkins further proposed changing the name of the American Academy of Physical Medicine and Rehabilitation to the American Academy of Physiatrics (45). However, Krusen supported maintaining the existing name of the organization because otherwise "the rest of the world wouldn't recognize us" (45).

Beginning in the late 1930s, Krusen, in conjunction with more than a dozen other "physical therapy physicians," repetitively petitioned the American Medical Association for specialty status and an examining board for physical medicine, but controversies over certification, financing, and whether physical medicine and rehabilitation should be an independent specialty or a subspecialty delayed successful resolution for over a decade. Ultimately, with Krusen's leadership, the American Board of Physical Medicine and Rehabilitation was founded in 1947 and Krusen served as its first chairman (from 1947 to 1951) (40, 41).

From 1943 to 1951, Krusen served as a critical leader of the Baruch Committee on Physical Medicine (later the Baruch Committee on Physical Medicine and Rehabilitation), an activity which greatly fostered the development of physical medicine in the United States (3, 19, 40, 46). The Baruch Committee was established by financier/philanthropist Bernard Baruch in honor of his father, Simon Baruch, MD, to advance physical medicine through education, clinical care, and research. Dr. Ray Lyman Wilbur was the initial Chairman of the Committee, and with whom Krusen served on the Administrative Board; Krusen was also selected as the chairman of both the Scientific Advisory Committee and the Committee on Physical Rehabilitation (3). The Baruch Committee soon recommended the establishment of teaching and research centers for physical medicine, fellowships and residencies in PM&R, promotion of teaching and research in physical medicine and rehabilitation in medical schools, and development of the American Board of Physical Medicine and Rehabilitation (3, 47). Through the remainder of the 1940s until disbanding in 1951, the Committee provided grant funds for fellowships, and for teaching and research programs in physical medicine at universities and medical schools. The legacy of the Baruch Committee included a marked increase in the number of medical schools teaching physical medicine and rehabilitation, a marked increase in the number of residencies in physical medicine and rehabilitation, and more than thirty Baruch Fellows who went on to become department heads in medical schools, the military, or Veterans Administration hospitals (3).

POLIO EPIDEMICS EXPANDED THE NEED AND ROLE FOR PHYSICAL MEDICINE AND REHABILITATION AMONG CIVILIANS

Although unrecognized at the time, the growing epidemics of paralytic poliomyelitis beginning in the 1890s and occurring throughout the first half of the twentieth century were partly an unanticipated consequence of improved sanitation. Hygienic advances delayed exposure to polioviruses from early infancy (when protection against paralytic disease was afforded by maternal antibodies) to later in childhood or adulthood, at which time paralytic manifestations were much more likely, a phenomenon expressed memorably by John Modlin: "Polio . . . was the unanticipated consequence of the invention of the flush toilet and the adoption of the use of toilet paper" (48).

The first major epidemic of poliomyelitis in the United States, and the one that brought polio into national consciousness, occurred in 1916: nationwide there were 27,000 cases, with 6,000 deaths, almost all under five years of age; and a large number of the survivors were left with lifelong disabilities, and often deformities. Although there was considerable variability from year to year, subsequent annual summer epidemics were less severe, until progressively increasing during the 1940s and early 1950s, with the worst epidemic in 1952 causing nearly 58,000 cases of paralytic poliomyelitis. As increasing numbers of older children and adults became affected during the 1930s and afterwards, the original label of "infantile paralysis" was replaced by either the medical term "poliomyelitis" or the shorter term "polio." Because mortality was high, and because survivors were often left with severe paralysis and resulting disability, these epidemics caused widespread anxiety and fear, particularly during the summer months (49). These polio epidemics also led to major advances in respiratory management and physical therapy (50–52), and further established the role of physiatrists in the management of neuromuscular diseases, especially limb and respiratory muscle weakness, contractures, and gait disorders.

The "Iron Lung"

Following the early epidemics of poliomyelitis in the United States, Philip A. Drinker (1894–1972) and Louis Agassiz Shaw at Harvard University designed an electrically powered tank respirator to facilitate the breathing of patients paralyzed by poliomyelitis (53). This "iron lung" was the first practical means of respiratory support, and Drinker and Charles McKhann soon demonstrated the potential of artificial respiration, using the iron lung in an 8-year-old girl with poliomyelitis who had developed respiratory failure and coma (54, 55). Manufacture of these "iron lungs" began in the early 1930s and expanded in the 1940s and early 1950s, until replaced in the late 1950s and early 1960s by more sophisticated ventilation devices. The iron lung required intensive nursing care and respiratory therapy, and a supporting hospital infrastructure. While the iron lung saved thousands of lives, many patients who would otherwise have died survived with severe disabilities requiring considerable physical therapy, orthotics, and adaptive equipment.

"Sister" Kenny: An outspoken nurse challenges the orthodox treatment of polio

From the 1920s through at least the early 1940s, the orthodox treatment for polio consisted largely of absolute immobilization of affected limbs though splinting or use of plaster casts (often for many months), and subsequent (often permanent) orthopedic braces, leading to disuse atrophy, joint contractures, and lifelong disability (10, 56–58). However, since 1911, an unregistered independent nurse practitioner named Elizabeth Kenny (1880–1952) had been treating patients with poliomyelitis using an alternative approach she developed empirically in a sparsely populated back-country area of Australia in ignorance of the prevailing orthodox treatments (59–61). Later when she came to prominence, Kenny employed the title of "Sister," an honorific designation for a head nurse in the British system which she earned during her military service in the Australian Army Nurse Corps during World War I (61–63). "Sister" Kenny's approach to the treatment of poliomyelitis utilized physical methods (e.g., the labor-intensive application of moist warm wraps of heavy woolen cloth for muscle spasms, aggressive use of passive range of motion, and massage), avoidance of immobilization and bracing, strong encouragement of functional independence, as well as early mobilization and prompt return to normal activities, coupled with confident optimism for improvement (59, 60, 62, 64–66). Kenny later criticized the immobilization approach then in vogue, claiming that it prolonged muscle spasms, promoted joint stiffness, and prevented restoration of normal muscle action:

> My reasons for the condemnation of the principles of immobilization as generally accepted are as follows: 1. Immobilization prevents the treatment of the disease, that is, the symptoms of the disease, in the acute stage. 2. It prolongs the condition of muscle spasm and prevents its treatment. 3. It prevents the treatment for the restoration of coordination of muscle action, a serious error. 4. It promotes the condition of stiffness which according to all reports prevents satisfactory treatment for the symptoms that brought about the condition (muscle spasm) or the development of muscle power be reeducation, or re-awakening of impulse. (65)

During the 1930s, ten Sister Kenny Clinics were established in eastern Australia, initially as "Muscle Re-Education Centres" (59). However, Kenny was not accepted by orthodox medicine in Australia, was denounced by an Australian Royal Commission in the late 1930s, and was widely criticized by orthopedic surgeons and other physicians, who charged that she understood neither the pathophysiology of the disease nor the physiology of muscle (59, 60). Nevertheless, her approach was empirically successful and she developed a large popular following. In 1939, the Queensland government—in spite of the unpopular conclusions of its own Royal Commission—ordered the Kenny treatment be made available in the Queensland public hospital system (59, 60).

Kenny came to the United States in 1940, where her ideas were initially ignored or resisted until tested by Dr Wallace Cole, chief of orthopedic surgery at the University of Minnesota Medical School, and Dr. Miland Knapp, a surgeon who chaired the school's department of physical therapy (67). The Kenny methods were eventually found to reduce length of hospital stay, greatly diminish contracture formation, and improve functional recovery (67–70). As a result, with encouragement from the American Medical Association and initial funding from the National Foundation for Infantile Paralysis and other donors, a well-regarded and very successful Sister Kenny Institute (later known as the Sister Kenny Rehabilitation Institute) was established in Minneapolis in early 1942 and developed a strong affiliation with the University of Minnesota Medical School, with rotating residents and various specialist staff including physiatrists, orthopedic surgeons, neurologists, and others (Figure 1-1) (10, 51, 59, 61, 63). The Kenny methods were widely adopted in the United States and elsewhere in the 1940s (though not in Australia), and were taught to physical therapists and physicians at training satellites around the country. Although the controversial Kenny had her detractors, she also had numerous supporters, including Frank Krusen of the Mayo Clinic. Kenny's approach represented a significant advance in the care of

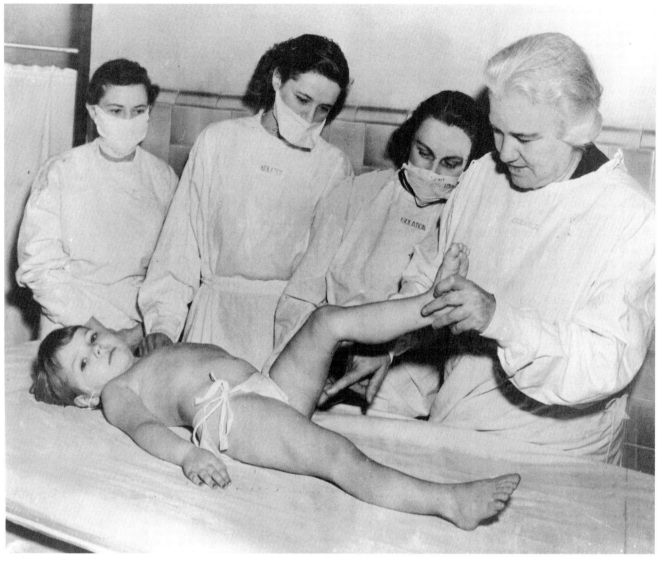

FIGURE 1-1

"Sister" Elizabeth Kenny (1880–1952), shown here demonstrating therapy techniques at the Sister Kenny Institute in Minneapolis, Minnesota, c. 1942. (Courtesy of the Minnesota Historical Society, St. Paul, Minnesota.)

paralyzed patients, and helped foster the growth of physical therapy and physical medicine (6, 51, 72).

In retrospect there is no denying that Sister Kenny's ideas and techniques marked a turning point, even an about-face, in the aftercare of paralytic poliomyelitis. By determination and sheer willpower she helped to raise the treatment of paralyzed patients out of the slough into which it had sunk in the 1930s. The system which prevailed before her advent, i.e., prolonged immobilization of affected limbs which in some instances led to a certain amount of calculated neglect, militated against involving the patient in early efforts to aid return of muscle function. It also eliminated the element of continued encouragement, which [is] so important as a psychological asset to rehabilitation. There was little use in exhorting a patient to exert himself physically if he was in a plaster cast. (71)

FDR, the National Foundation for Infantile Paralysis, and the March of Dimes

Franklin Delano Roosevelt (1882–1945), the most famous victim of polio, contracted the disease in the summer of 1921 and was permanently paralyzed from the waist down (58). Despite his disability, Roosevelt was later elected to the first of four terms as President of the United States in 1932 (58). From the time he became disabled, Roosevelt played an important role in the development of rehabilitation medicine, helped remove some of the social stigma from physical disability, provided inspiration and hope, promoted the idea that polio victims could become "normal" again (even if partly because of careful media management limiting the public's knowledge of the extent of his disability), and provided a mechanism for wide-spread supportive social action and philanthropy. In 1926, Roosevelt purchased a spa in Warm Springs, Georgia to help facilitate his personal rehabilitation. By 1927, Roosevelt founded the Georgia Warm Springs Foundation, which helped develop physical therapy and rehabilitation approaches for polio victims (51). In 1937, the Foundation was reorganized as the National Foundation for Infantile Paralysis (and officially incorporated in 1938), under the direction of Roosevelt's former law partner, D. Basil O'Connor (1892–1972). Under O'Connor's effective organizational leadership, the National Foundation began an unprecedented, innovative, and highly successful fundraising campaign utilizing an annual "President's Birthday Ball" with President Roosevelt and a variety of celebrities promoting the event, print advertisements with images of happy children ("poster children") in wheelchairs or braces and crutches asking for financial support, as well as public appeals to send dimes directly to the White House to help find a cure for polio; this latter campaign was labeled the "The March of Dimes" by entertainer Eddie Cantor (1892–1964) as a play on the words of "The March of Time" newsreel series (73–77). The first March of Dimes appeal in 1938—during the severe 1937 to 1938 recession following closely on the heels of the Great Depression of 1929 to 1934—generated extraordinary interest and raised an unprecedented $268,000 (the equivalent of over $3.4 million in year 2007 currency); see Figure 1-2 (77–79). A stunned President Roosevelt commented on the eve of his birthday:

> During the past few days bags of mail have been coming, literally by the truck load, to the White House. Yesterday between forty and fifty thousand letters came to the mail room of the White House. Today an even greater number—how many I cannot tell you, for we can only estimate the actual count by counting the mail bags. In all the envelopes are dimes and quarters and even dollar bills—gifts from grownups and children—mostly from children who want to help other children to get well. Literally, by the countless thousands, they are pouring in, and I have figured that if the White House Staff and I were to work on nothing else for two or three months to come we could not possibly thank the donors. Therefore . . . I must take this opportunity . . . to thank all who have aided and cooperated in the splendid work we are doing. (77)

The public's fear of contracting the disease, appeals to altruism with heartbreaking stories of afflicted children,

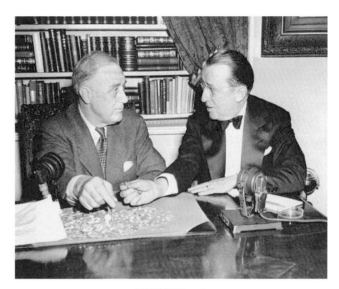

FIGURE 1-2

President Franklin Delano Roosevelt (1882–1945) and former law partner Basil O'Connor (1892–1972) shown counting dimes at the White House, c. 1938.

requests from admired role models (movie stars and politicians), and hope that the disease would soon be conquered were all used so effectively in the campaigns that the nonprofit National Foundation became the largest private charity in history. The National Foundation led the "first large-scale, nationwide biomedical initiative" by a charitable organization (76), and as a result was instrumental in subsidizing the hospital and rehabilitation costs of polio patients, funding basic and applied research concerning the causes and prevention of polio in the 1940s and early 1950s, training nurses and physical therapists in rehabilitation, sponsoring pilot programs to improve the teaching of rehabilitation medicine in medical schools in the early 1950s, and ultimately underwriting the Salk Vaccine Field Trial in 1954 (6, 73, 74, 76). The National Foundation officially changed its name to the March of Dimes in 1979 (after the threat of polio in the United States had passed) (76).

The Salk Vaccine Field Trial of 1954 and Aftermath

Karl Landsteiner (1868–1943) and his assistant Erwin Popper demonstrated that poliomyelitis was transmitted by a virus as early as 1908 (71, 80, 81). By 1948, David Bodian (1910–1992) and colleagues at Johns Hopkins University, and John Paul (1893–1971) and James Trask (?–1942) at Yale University independently showed that there were three strains of poliovirus (rather than one) as defined by cross-protection within the same group—a finding confirmed by the more extensive work of the Committee on Typing of the National Foundation for

Infantile Paralysis in 1951 (of which Jonas Salk was a participant) (71, 81–86). In 1949, John Enders (1897–1985), along with Thomas Weller (1915–) and Frederick Robbins (1916–2003), working at Harvard Medical School and Children's Medical Center in Boston, first cultivated the poliovirus in (non-nervous) tissue culture, for which they were later awarded the 1954 Nobel Prize in Physiology or Medicine (87–91). Also by 1954, several researchers, including Dorothy Horstman at Yale, had demonstrated that there was a period of viremia preceding neurologic involvement (92, 93). These important advances made possible the development by Jonas Salk (1914–1995) of an inactivated trivalent poliovirus vaccine, which was tested in 1954 in a huge clinical trial funded by the National Foundation for Infantile Paralysis (75, 94–97). The 1954 Field Trial of the Salk vaccine was the largest public health experiment ever, involving 1.8 million children who were labeled "Polio Pioneers" and were inoculated with either vaccine or placebo, or were simply observed (71, 73, 94, 98, 99). On April 12, 1955 at a press conference in Ann Arbor, Michigan, epidemiologist and virologist Thomas Francis Jr. (1900–1969), who had conducted the field trial, declared that the Salk inactivated polio vaccine was both safe and effective (94, 99, 100). That same afternoon, an advisory committee to the Laboratory of Biologics Control, the federal agency that was responsible for licensing biologic products, recommended that vaccine licenses be granted to five pharmaceutical companies: Eli Lilly, Parke-Davis, Wyeth, Pitman-Moore, and Cutter Laboratories. However, shortly thereafter, unforeseen manufacturing difficulties with clumping of material and inadequate formaldehyde inactivation of virus during large-scale processing resulted in a huge outbreak of iatrogenic paralytic poliomyelitis (the so-called "Cutter Incident") with muscle weakness developing in 70,000 people, of whom 164 developed severe paralysis and ten died (101–105). The litigation that followed (particularly Gottsdanker v. Cutter Laboratories, 1957) led to new legal interpretations (i.e., the doctrine of liability without fault) and ultimately the development of the National Vaccine Injury Compensation Program in 1986 (104, 105). While these legal issues dragged on for decades, the manufacturing problems were soon corrected, and with wide-scale immunization using the Salk vaccine, rates of paralytic poliomyelitis plummeted.

In 1957, Albert Sabin (1908–1993), utilizing the time-consuming process of infecting monkeys with poliovirus, developed a trivalent live attenuated polio vaccine that was then tested in Russia, endorsed by the American Medical Association in 1961 even before American field trials were begun, and ultimately licensed in the United States in 1963. The Sabin vaccine soon became the polio vaccine of choice, because it (1) was less costly, (2) required minimal training to administer, (3) prevented the disease carrier state, and (4) helped prevent the spread of wild poliovirus. However, by this time rates of polio in the United States had dropped to 50–100 cases per year—down from tens of thousands per year—so the Sabin vaccine had relatively limited impact on overall polio incidence in the United States, but did have an important role around the world. By the early 1970s, remaining incident cases of paralytic poliomyelitis in the United States were almost exclusively either imported cases or caused by the vaccine itself. The Sabin oral polio vaccine was discontinued in the United States in 2000, because the continued risk of vaccine-related polio outweighed the potential benefits of a live-virus vaccine.

PROFILE OF HOWARD RUSK (1901–1989): THE FATHER OF COMPREHENSIVE REHABILITATION MEDICINE

Origins of Comprehensive Rehabilitation during World War II

In 1942, Howard Rusk (Figure 1-3) left his well-established private internal medicine practice in St. Louis to join the

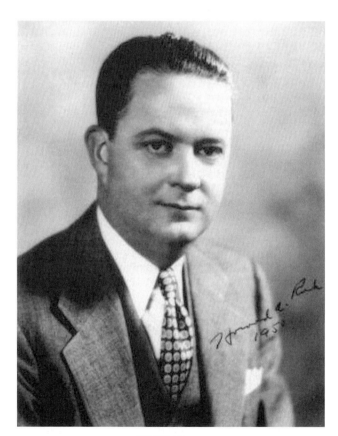

FIGURE 1-3

Dr. Howard A. Rusk (1901–1989), the father of comprehensive rehabilitation medicine (Courtesy of the National Library of Medicine)

Army Air Corps. As Chief of Medical Services at the 1,000-bed hospital at Jefferson Barracks in St. Louis, Rusk observed both a high degree of boredom among the patients, and a high rate of readmission because patients were not physically fit enough to return to active duty in their units after hospital discharge, even though they were no longer in need of acute hospitalization (49, 106–108). Rusk therefore sought to engage the patients in mental and physical restorative and training activities that would utilize their time efficiently, increase their fitness, and decrease the rate of recidivism. Rusk's approach to rehabilitation emphasized treating the entire person, including their emotional, psychological, and social needs, and not just the illness or a specific disability. By 1943, seven special "convalescent hospitals" were established in the Army Air Corps, with multidisciplinary staffs comprising

> medical and surgical specialists, but also physical therapists, educators, athletic trainers [later called "corrective therapists" and still later called "kinesiotherapists"], occupational therapists, social service workers, personal counselors, and vocational guidance advisors—all of whom worked as a team to meet on an individual basis, the needs of the "whole man." . . . a broad program of rehabilitation was put into operation at each convalescent hospital, with the result that each hospital became part school, gymnasium, machine shop, psychiatric clinic, vocational guidance center, and town hall. (46)

Rusk's efforts were soon recognized by generals David Grant and Henry (Hap) Arnold, whereupon Rusk was sent to Washington DC in 1943 to set up similar programs for all 253 Army Air Corps hospitals (106, 109). Rusk's novel Convalescent Training Program was highly effective in decreasing hospital readmissions, saving man-hours, and giving injured and disabled soldiers hope and purpose.

> Despite such success, many of us felt our program was grossly inadequate. The feeling became intensified when wounded boys from the battlefields began being packed into our hospitals by the planeload. Suddenly we were faced by men with broken bodies and, all too often, broken spirits. We concluded that our program was a schoolboy project in the context of what needed to be done for the severely wounded—the amputees (the double, triple, and quadruple amputees), the paraplegics and quadriplegics, the blind, the deaf, the disfigured, the emotionally disturbed. These men would need complete rehabilitation, whatever that might be—I wasn't sure. Just exactly what could be done for them? . . . It was horrible to realize that there was no precedent for rehabilitation programs on a large scale in the military. And as far as I knew, there was no extensive civilian programs either. (106)

Later, similar programs, loosely modeled after Rusk's Convalescent Training Program, were adopted by all branches of the service at the instigation of Bernard Baruch and the subsequent request of President Franklin Delano Roosevelt to Secretary of War Henry Stimson. Rusk had sought Baruch's assistance, and the letter drafted by Baruch for the President's signature became *de facto* military policy and gave official standing to rehabilitation medicine:

> My dear Mr. Secretary, I'm deeply concerned about our casualties returning from overseas, as I know you are. I would like you to see that no one is discharged from service until he has had the full benefit of hospitalization, which will include not only medical care but resocialization, psychological adjustment and rehabilitation. I would like you to see that this is put in operation as soon as possible. (106)

Because of the limited rehabilitation programs available prior to World War II, and the widely held expectation at the time that disabled people could not be productive, people with strokes or other brain and spinal cord injuries received at best custodial care and often died within a short time.

> I recall someone asking me how paraplegics had lived up to that time. The answer was, except in extremely rare cases, they usually died—their life expectancy in those days was often less than a year. They got terrible bedsores, developed kidney and bladder problems, and simply lay in bed, waiting for death. It was almost the same with strokes. The old wives' tale was that you had one stroke, and then you sat around waiting for a second one, or a third one, or however many it took to kill you. If you had any kind of brain injury affecting your locomotive functions, everyone assumed your life was finished. (106)

Rusk's experience with the rehabilitation of wounded soldiers during World War II helped usher in the concept of comprehensive rehabilitation, with both utilitarian and humanitarian aims.

> The modern concept of "the treatment of the whole man" [developed by Rusk, himself] did not develop . . . until World War II, when rehabilitation got its biggest impetus because so many wounded survived—but survived with severe disabilities. (47)

One of our most immediate frustrations in early 1943 was that if we discharged these wounded and disabled veterans from the service—which we had to do since they could no longer function as soldiers—we were turning them over to the Veterans Administration, which at that time was like sending them into limbo. The V.A. had no program for them. They would simply lie around getting custodial care, with nothing to do, bored to distraction, helpless, hopeless, waiting for some kind of infection or disease to carry them off. Gradually the concept of rehabilitation came to me as I found out how much really could be done for these men. In the beginning, I knew only that everything possible should be done to return them to physical and mental health. This meant finding ways for them to function despite their disabilities. First, I had to remember that this was the Air Force, that we were fighting a desperate war, and that we needed all the manpower we could find. It was immediately important, then, to make these men in some way able again. Our initial aim had to be to send them back to duty in the best possible condition and in the shortest time. If they could no longer do their previous jobs, we should help them choose jobs they could do, and then retrain them. This approach would be beneficial to the Air Force and it seemed the best for the boys themselves, too. (106)

The development of comprehensive rehabilitation in the military during World War II was truly novel and the outcomes were unprecedented:

We discovered we had saved at least forty million man-hours of duty time, and that we had gotten more sick or injured men back on duty than any branch of service had done during any way in history. More important, we had prepared thousands of boys for useful roles in civilian life after the war who might otherwise have wasted away for years in veterans hospitals. And by proving the value of rehabilitation, we had made certain that the Veterans Administration, after this war, would actually rehabilitate its disabled men rather than letting them languish in bed, or die for lack of understanding and a program. It is worth noting that of the four hundred men who became paraplegics in World War I, a third died in France, another third died within six weeks thereafter, and of the remaining third, 90 percent were dead within a year. In World War II there were 2,500 American service-connected combat paraplegics, and three fourths of them were alive twenty years later. I might add parenthetically that of these survivors, 1,400 were holding down jobs. (106)

Rusk earned a Distinguished Service Medal for his work in the U.S. military, and retired as a Brigadier General in the U.S. Air Force Reserve.

Later, in retrospect, he was struck by the irony of having such progress made in the field of rehabilitation medicine as a result of a brutal war:

It is paradoxical that through war, a concerted effort to annihilate man, we have learned more and better ways to preserve him. (46)

Change in Management of Disability after Stroke

As an internist prior to World War II, Rusk had been frustrated with the options available for treating patients disabled by stroke, and felt his own knowledge was woefully inadequate. Rethinking his prior management, and discussing his career options with several former patients who had suffered from stroke, reinforced Rusk's belief in the concept of comprehensive rehabilitation and gave him the determination to abandon his previous internal medicine practice and seek opportunities to develop this concept for civilian patients.

There was so little you could do to help a stroke victim in those days that, like many other doctors, I had developed a technique in dealing with them that did no more than pacify them. I had scores of them in my practice, people who were partially paralyzed, and who, therefore, sat home all day, no longer considered fit to work, and with nothing to do but think about their condition. They would want to see me periodically for checkups, but I wanted to see them as seldom as possible. I didn't realize it at the time, but in front of such patients I was overcome by a feeling of insecurity. Deep down inside I felt guilty because I didn't know how to help them. Whenever they came into the office they wanted to talk. They would talk for an hour if you let them, while thirty other people sat in the waiting room. So I would go through the routine of taking their blood pressure . . . and prescribe a little meaningless change in their medication that would make them feel that at least something was being done. Then I'd hurry out of the room while the nurse came in to dismiss them. I didn't want to talk to them because I really didn't know what to say, and I'm sure that's always been true of most doctors everyplace . . . If [a patient] was paralyzed . . . or disabled in some other way, there was virtually no one to whom you could send him. You could get him maybe a "nickel's worth" of physical therapy, and that was about all. Such reminiscences reinforced my determination to throw my energies into rehabilitation. (106)

Moreover, by this time Rusk had an entirely different view of the rehabilitation potential of patients following a stroke, emphasizing what could be done, focusing on remaining abilities, and utilizing simple techniques and equipment, to minimize contractures and other secondary impairments, and to maximize function:

There are a number of simple progressive procedures in the rehabilitation of the hemiplegic who suffers from one of the commonest disabilities seen in general practice. In the early stages of treatment, the following procedures should be instituted to prevent deformities: (1) footboard or posterior leg splint to prevent foot drop; (2) sandbags to prevent outward rotation of the affected leg; (3) a pillow in the axilla to prevent adduction of the shoulder, and (4) quadriceps setting to maintain muscle strength. All of these procedures are relatively simple and require no special equipment. Their use, however, will prevent crippling anatomic deformities and hasten the rehabilitation of the patient.

The next procedure indicated is the institution of pulley therapy. This can be done simply with a small pulley attached to a goose neck pipe over the head of the bed, the ordinary clothes line rope being used with a 1 inch (2.5 cm) webbing for the hand loop. With the stretching and passive exercise provided by pulley therapy, the range of motion can be increased and adhesions prevented. Pulley therapy has the advantage over the usual stretching exercises that are done passively, for the patient, knowing his own pain threshold, will proceed to fully tolerated motion much more quickly . . .

[Ambulation] should be started by: (1) the practice of balance in the standing position, progressing to parallel bars; (2) the teaching of a heel and toe gait to minimize clonus and to reestablish normal walking habits stressing reciprocal motion, and (3) a short leg brace, which will be needed in approximately half of all cases to correct foot drop. All of the equipment for training in ambulation is simple and readily obtained by the general practitioner. If parallel bars are not available, two kitchen chairs may be substituted. In the advanced stages of retraining, ambulation is continued with (1) instruction in crutch walking, starting usually with the alternate four point gait, and (2) teaching elevation, stressing climbing steps, curbs, stairs and ramps. Concurrently with the training in ambulation, attention should be given to retraining in the activities of self care and daily living . . . With such a program, many of the complications usually following apoplexy can be avoided and a great deal of time and ability salvaged. (110)

Not only did Rusk feel that such approaches were extremely helpful, he felt strongly that *failure* to provide rehabilitation to patients was a form of medical negligence:

The physician who fails to see that those patients under his care receive the full benefits of modern methods of medical rehabilitation and retraining is in the same category as the physician who still persists in using dietary restriction alone in the management of diabetes, when insulin is available, for medical care is not complete until the patient has been trained to live and work with what he has left. (110)

Rusk later explained the potential for rehabilitation of stroke patients to colleagues at a meeting of the American College of Physicians in Boston:

I'm talking about the two million people in this country who have suffered strokes and are now sitting around, waiting to die because no one is helping them to live. I'd like to tell you today about a few simple things you can do for many of these people, right in your offices, or in the home or bedside. I told them how to prevent painful hips by sandbagging the patient's leg. I told them how to sandbag a shoulder so it wouldn't become what we call "frozen" and require several weeks of painful therapy and stretching to get it back to normal. I took out some props and showed them how they could make an exercise device for arms and shoulders for stroke victims simply by using a window pulley and six or eight feet of clothesline. I pointed out that a patient could help himself more with this device than a therapist could help him because, by doing it himself, he could sense the pain threshold and therefore stretch farther than a therapist would dare to try. I talked about aphasia, the speech difficulty stroke victims suffer, which seems to me one of the most frustrating problems of all. It's like not being able to say an old friend's name, multiplied to infinity. As I talked, this time I noticed there was absolute silence in the hall, and instead of seeing people leave, I noticed that more people kept arriving until, by the end of my presentation, they were standing in the aisles. (106)

While such information generated considerable interest, referral options were extremely limited because of the lack of comprehensive rehabilitation programs across the country.

Program for Civilian Rehabilitation

After World War II, Rusk began efforts to establish a program for civilian rehabilitation, based in large part upon what he had learned in the military. He initially intended to open a rehabilitation institute in St. Louis, where he had practiced internal medicine for 16 years prior to his military service, but colleagues there were not supportive.

I can't say the idea was well received. The orthopedists, in particular, said, "We're doing all that anyway," and it was true that they had adopted some good methods of therapy. But they failed to see my point: the whole person needed rehabilitation, not just the part of him that had been damaged. They had no concept of the emotional problems which follow disability, or the problems of job placement, or the other fundamentals behind our philosophy. (106)

In 1945, Rusk joined the staff at New York University Medical School, and several wards in Bellevue and Goldwater Hospitals were designated for rehabilitation, although initially the beds were also simultaneously utilized by other services. The previously separate programs for physical and occupational therapy were combined into a new Department of Rehabilitation Medicine (3), and Rusk hired George Deaver, MD, from New York's

Institute of Crippled and Disabled as the Medical Director (3, 47). Deaver had been a pioneer in rehabilitating the severely handicapped, including those with spinal cord injury, cerebral palsy, muscular dystrophy, multiple sclerosis, and rheumatoid arthritis. "At a time when these patients were being rejected and discarded as permanently disabled, Deaver was accepting of them and patiently working with them to achieve the best possible outcomes through rehabilitation" (3). Deaver made unprecedented progress in rehabilitating those with spinal cord injury to independence in self care, crutch or brace-assisted ambulation, or wheelchair living (3, 47): according to Rusk, "It was he who first taught paraplegics how to walk" (47). Deaver had also developed tools and techniques for assessing activities of daily living (as a guide for independent living capability), crutch walking, and prevocational evaluation (3, 47). By 1947, Rusk and Deaver had established the "first comprehensive, total medical rehabilitation program in any community hospital" in the United States at Bellevue Hospital in New York (110).

Despite Rusk's enthusiasm and his previous successes, his initial civilian efforts were nevertheless regarded skeptically by colleagues:

> Many people, even in the medical profession, considered it foolish to spend money or effort on such a "frilly boondoggle." It wasn't that they disapproved of getting disabled people onto their feet and back into the mainstream of life; it was just that they didn't think it was possible. (106)

Nevertheless, Rusk persevered and gained the support of prominent philanthropists, including Bernard M. Baruch, Louis J. Horowitz, and Bernard and Alva Gimbel. In 1950, Rusk founded the Institute of Physical Medicine and Rehabilitation at New York University Medical Center. The institute opened its doors in 1951, but was initially derided as "Rusk's Folly" by former colleagues in St. Louis (109). Renamed the Howard A. Rusk Institute of Rehabilitation Medicine in 1984, two years after Rusk's retirement in 1982, the institute is now the largest university-affiliated center for treatment of civilians with disabilities and for research and training in rehabilitation medicine (111).

Promoting Rehabilitation Medicine

Rusk worked tirelessly, promoting the nascent field of rehabilitation and increasing public awareness of the need for rehabilitation in the spectrum of medical practice in numerous speeches and consultations across the country and around the world, in a weekly column on health issues for *The New York Times* (which Rusk continued until 1971), though influential private sector and government contacts, and through the establishment of

rehabilitation training programs which helped expand the message through various disciples. In 1955, Rusk founded the World Rehabilitation Fund to provide technical assistance for the development of rehabilitation programs in underdeveloped countries, as well as funding for education and training programs on prosthetics around the world, and grants for foreign physicians to study rehabilitation in the United States: "Its basic aim was to sponsor international projects which would help the handicapped and create a better understanding of them and their problems" (106). Rusk also authored several books, including *New Hope for the Handicapped* (1949) and *Living with a Disability* (1953), both with his colleague, Eugene (Jack) Taylor; served as the senior author of *Rehabilitation Medicine* (1958); and wrote his acclaimed autobiography, *A World to Care For* (1972), which summarized the development of his concepts of comprehensive rehabilitation.

In his autobiography, Rusk explained why he got such satisfaction from working with disabled people:

> You don't get fine china by putting clay in the sun. You have to put the clay through the white heat of the kiln if you want to make porcelain. Heat breaks some pieces. Life breaks some people. Disability breaks some people. But once the clay goes through the white-hot fire and comes out whole, it can never be clay again; once a person overcomes a disability through his own courage, determination and hard work, he has a depth of spirit you and I know little about . . . Rehabilitation is one branch of medicine in which the patient has more power than the doctor in setting the limits and possibilities. The doctor can tell the patient what to do, but only the patient himself can decide how much he's going to do. In making these decisions, patients are constantly teaching us doctors new things about rehabilitation by proving that they can do more than we had presumed possible. (106)

Rusk promoted these ideas to medical students as well:

> When I lecture to medical students, it's the brightest day of the year for me. They're so delighted to leave the basic sciences behind for an hour, so eager to heal. I always tell them: "If you can get the same satisfaction out of taking an old hemiplegic out of a wet bed, teaching him to walk, to speak so he can be understood, to take care of himself, getting him to the point where he can live a non-institutional life, perhaps getting him a job, and get the same satisfaction as from making some fancy diagnosis of an arcane disease that you may see once in a lifetime, then you'll make a good doctor. Like it or not, if you go into general medicine, 80% of your patients will have either a chronic or a psychosomatic sickness." (109)

Rusk emphasized that physical disability could be accommodated, and that through vocational rehabilitation many disabled people could live productive lives and be valuable members of the workforce:

> When you work with a handicapped person, you've got to think of his abilities more than his disabilities. You've got to remember that our society doesn't pay for physical strength. We now have machines to do the heavy labor. Our society really pays for just two things, the skill of your hands and what you have in your head. (106)

> The disabled, if properly placed and trained, are good workers with a better production rate, lower accident and absentee rates and a labor turnover 10 times less than normal workers. (111)

In 1955, Rusk received a Christmas card from Adlai Stevenson, containing what has been attributed to be the personal prayer of an unknown Confederate soldier in the Civil War (47):

I asked God for strength, that I might achieve
    I was made weak that I might learn humbly to obey . . .
I asked for health, that I might do greater things
    I was given infirmity, that I might do better things . . .
I asked for riches, that I might be happy
    I was given poverty, that I might be wise . . .
I asked for power, that I might have the praise of men
    I was given weakness, that I might feel the need of God . . .
I asked for all things, that I might enjoy life
    I was given life, that I might enjoy all things . . .
I got nothing that I asked for
    —but everything I had hoped for
Almost despite myself, my unspoken prayers were answered.
    I am among all men, most richly blessed!

Rusk's disabled patients found personal meaning in this prayer, as did their families, so much so that the father of one young patient had the prayer cast in bronze. The prayer that the boy's father cast in bronze now hangs on the wall in the lobby of the institute Rusk founded (47). The prayer continues to be widely reproduced, and is sometimes referred to as the "Prayer of the Disabled."

Rusk closed his autobiography with a quote from Louis Pasteur, emphasizing the patient's role in rehabilitation, and in Pasteur's particular case, his successful rehabilitation following a serious stroke:

> Ultimately, the success of all rehabilitation depends on the patient himself . . . I can never forget a philosophical quotation that serves as a constant reminder of this truth: "I hold the unconquerable belief that science and peace will triumph over ignorance and war, that nations will come together not to destroy but to construct, and that the future belongs to those who accomplish most for suffering humanity." Those words were spoken by the great nineteenth-century scientist Louis Pasteur. Few people know that he suffered a serious stroke when he was in his forties . . . He

rehabilitated himself—working to the age of seventy-three—and many of his greatest scientific achievements came after his stroke. Pasteur's words express what anyone working in this field must feel. To believe in rehabilitation is to believe in humanity. (106)

Rusk never stopped promoting the concept of rehabilitation. As he noted in 1969:

> We who have dedicated our lives to rehabilitation medicine must be not only practitioners but teachers, crusaders, and zealots. The stakes are high, not only for the welfare of the disabled, but also for the future of world understanding . . . If we have the courage and strength and the spirit, this program of rehabilitation medicine will never die but will continue to grow and flourish for the benefit of all mankind. (46)

Rusk received many awards and honors, including three Lasker Awards, the first an Albert Lasker Public Service Award in 1952 "for his pioneering work in the service of the physically disabled and as distinguished rehabilitation mentor to the world," the second an Albert Lasker Award given by the International Society for the Rehabilitation of the Disabled in 1957, and the third an Albert Lasker Medical Journalism Special Award "for his editorial leadership in advancing medical research and public health programs in his weekly columns in the New York Times" in 1959 (112, 113). In 1966, Rusk was recognized by the American Congress of Physical Medicine and Rehabilitation with a gold medal bearing the inscription: "Physician, teacher, author, inspiration to patients and disciples and a prime mover in the development and spread of medical rehabilitation throughout the world" (112).

In 1981, in the "Year of the Disabled," Rusk—then 80—was nominated for the Nobel Peace Prize. At that time, a reporter for the American Medical Association interviewed Rusk, who was still actively promoting comprehensive rehabilitation.

> Although some people, Ronald Reagan among them, call Howard Rusk "The Father of Rehabilitation Medicine," he declines that honor. "Minnesota's Dr. Frank Krusen deserves that title," he says. "He was far ahead of me. He succeeded in getting the AMA to recognize physical medicine as a specialty when most doctors made no bones about brushing it off as a 'social service boondoggle.'" Rusk will admit, however, to being "father, midwife, and pediatrician" to the modern concept of rehabilitation, the radical who argues that physicians should treat the "whole person. Not just the ring finger or toe." . . . Before World War II, physiatrists were concerned almost exclusively with physical and electrical modalities of treating neuromusculoskeletal disease. Under Howard Rusk, rehabilitation medicine has blossomed into a multidisciplinary, in-hospital training program. (109)

Despite Rusk's statement to the contrary, many of his colleagues continued to apply that label to him (3), and to this day the Association of Academic Physiatrists continues to label Rusk the "Father of Rehabilitation Medicine" (and Krusen as the "Father of Physical Medicine") (12).

As the acknowledged father of comprehensive rehabilitation medicine, it is worthwhile recounting Rusk's fully formulated definition of rehabilitation:

> Rehabilitation is the restoration of the handicapped to the fullest physical, mental, social, and economic usefulness of which they are capable. Frequently, it has been called "the third phase of medicine"— following preventive medicine, and curative medicine (and surgery). In contrast to "convalescence, wherein the patient is left alone to rest while time and nature do their cures," medical rehabilitation is a dynamic concept—an active program. The first objective of medical rehabilitation is to eliminate the disability, if that is possible; the second is to reduce or alleviate the disability to the greatest possible degree; and the third, to retrain the person with a residual physical disability "to live and to work within the limits of his disability, but to the hilt of his capabilities." (47)

At the time of renaming of the Institute of Rehabilitation Medicine the Rusk Institute in 1984, Rusk noted that he used "the phenomenon of hope" to train people "not just within the limits of their ability, but up to the heights of their latent ability—to help them live the very best lives possible with what is left" (111). Rusk's framework and focus on treating the "whole person" has been the basis of subsequent programs and developments in the field, and has been incorporated into definitions of the field used by major rehabilitation organizations (12).

EVOLVING CONCEPTS OF DISABILITY AND REHABILITATION SINCE THE 1960S

There have been three fundamentally different approaches to modeling disability: the medical model, the social model, and more recently various bio-psycho-social models that incorporate features of both the medical and social frameworks (114–117).

The medical model of disability

> views disability as a feature of the person, directly caused by disease, trauma or other health condition, which requires medical care provided in the form of individual treatment by professionals. Disability, on this model, calls for medical or other treatment or intervention, to "correct" the problem with the individual. (117)

This medical framework was the foundation of many of the disability-related programs in the United States until the Americans with Disabilities Act in 1990 (116):

> The [medical] model defines disabling conditions as principally the product of physical and mental impairments that constrain performance. Influenced by this view, health and social agencies provide a mix of services that, for the most part, categorize affected individuals as permanently ill and incapable of meeting their own needs. Therefore, the problems that disability-related programs seek to address are often viewed as inherent to the individual and as independent of society. (116)

People with disabilities, however, have championed the "demedicalization" of disability, and have argued for recognition that disability is in large measure the result of a social environment that does not address the needs of those with physical or mental limitations.

> The independent-living and disability-rights movements blame adherence to the medical model for the creation of disability-related programs that foster dependence rather than personal autonomy. Members of these movements correctly argue that disability is the result of a dynamic process involving complex interactions among biological, behavioral, psychological, social, and environmental factors. (116)

The social model of disability, in contrast, "sees disability as a socially-created problem and not at all an attribute of an individual" (114, 117). Within this framework, "disability demands a political response, since the problem is created by an unaccommodating physical environment brought about by attitudes and other features of the social environment" (117). Particularly since the 1970s, there has been greater awareness of the social and environmental contributors to disability, facilitated in part by the advocacy of disability rights groups and by court cases and protest actions initiated by disabled individuals seeking basic civil and human rights (118). These actions helped bring about greater societal acceptance of disability, a shift in the federal government's official objectives to include equal opportunity, independent living, integration, and full participation for all citizens (i.e., a shift "from charity to rights"), as well as the most comprehensive disability rights legislation in history, the Americans with Disabilities Act (ADA) of 1990 (118). The ADA included provisions prohibiting employers from discriminating against a disabled person in hiring or promotion if the individual is otherwise qualified for the job; mandating that businesses make "reasonable accommodations" for disabled workers, including job restructuring and modification if required; mandating that federal, state, and local governments and programs be accessible; mandating that public transportation be accessible to handicapped people; and mandating that privately operated public accommodations (e.g., restaurants, hotels, and retail stores) make "reasonable modifications" to ensure accessibility.

The medical and social models both have value, and both can encourage communication among professionals across different disciplines, facilitate understanding of patients' problems, and help guide efforts to improve functioning of people with disability. Since the 1960s and 1970s, models of disability and rehabilitation have been developed and refined that integrate aspects of both the medical and social frameworks into more balanced bio-psycho-social models (114–117, 119–125). These models specifically acknowledge that "whether a person performs a socially expected activity depends not simply on the characteristics of the person but also on the larger context of social and physical environments" (116). As a result, such models help to "set the rehabilitation agenda clearly in a social context while still recognizing that disease has an important influence on patients' levels of physical activity and social participation and on the process of rehabilitation" (126). Such models also extend "the boundaries of rehabilitation—from the few conditions where recovery is expected to any condition in which someone experiences disability or handicap secondary to (or as part of) illness" (126).

Unfortunately, the terminology employed in these models has changed over the years, making comparisons difficult and hampering understanding. The term "disability" has variably referred to dysfunction at the level of the person, dysfunction due to an inadequate social and physical environment, or an entire spectrum of dysfunction affecting organs and organ systems, the person, and the person's interaction with his or her social and physical environment. In the United States and other countries there has been a movement away from using the word "handicap" (116, 127).

The World Health Organization's Impairments-Disabilities-Handicaps Framework (1980)

In 1980, the World Health Organization (WHO) introduced the *International Classification of Impairments, Disabilities, and Handicaps (ICIDH)*—a tool for the classification of the *consequences* of disease as a complementary framework for the *International Classification of Diseases (ICD)* (123, 128). ICIDH defined the terms impairment, disability, and handicap, and provided a preliminary classification and grading scale for each based on a conceptual framework developed initially in the 1970s by Dr. Philip Wood of the University of Manchester Medical School in Manchester, England (123, 128). Impairment was considered to represent "exteriorization" of a pathological state (disease), that is, an organ-level disturbance evident through symptoms or signs. Disability was considered "objectification" of impairment, a person-level restriction or lack of ability to perform a normal activity such as personal care or walking. Handicap was considered to represent "socialization" of a disability

or impairment: a social disadvantage for an individual that limits or prevents fulfillment of a normal social role such as self-sufficiency. Under this framework, **disease → impairment → disability → handicap.**

ICIDH listed the goals for intervention as they pertain to disability:

1. *Prevention*
2. *Enhancement* (e.g., when activities can be performed unaided but only with difficulty)
3. *Supplementation* (e.g., when activities can be performed only with aid, including the assistance of others)
4. *Substitution* (i.e., when certain activities cannot be performed even with aid) (123).

Under this framework, rehabilitation focuses on the latter three categories (i.e., enhancement, supplementation, and substitution) to minimize handicap.

In many ways, the initial WHO formulation relied heavily on a medical model of disability (116, 117), even though it recognized that social factors were inherent in what it called "handicap" (123). This approach resulted in charges that ICIDH promoted the "medicalization" of disability, and failed to adequately address the major impact of social and environmental factors (116, 122).

The Institute of Medicine's "Disabling Process" Framework (1991)

In a 1991 report of the Institute of Medicine (IOM) titled *Disability in America*, the components of the "disabling process" were refined from those initially described by Saad Nagi of Ohio State University in the 1960s (116, 120–122). Under this framework, the disabling process has four major components: pathology, impairment, functional limitation, and disability, with the usual (although not universal) progression being: **pathology → impairment → functional limitation → disability.**

There are exceptions to this typical progression:

Although [the model] seems to indicate a unidirectional progression from pathology to impairment to functional limitation to disability, and although a stepwise progression often occurs, progression from one stage to another is not always the case. An individual with a disabling condition might skip over components of the model, for example, when the public's attitude toward a disfiguring impairment causes no functional limitation but imposes a disability by affecting social interaction. Also, the effects of specific stages in the model can be moderated by such interventions as assistive devices. Similarly, environmental modification (e.g., elimination of physical obstacles and barriers) is an important form of disability prevention . . . (116)

There are clearly overlaps and differences between the IOM model and the earlier WHO model (123). In the IOM model, *pathology* concerns the abnormal interruption or interference of normal bodily structures or processes due to factors (e.g., disease, infection, trauma, genetic defect, etc.) operating at the molecular, cellular, or tissue level. *Impairment* concerns the loss or abnormality of a mental, physiological, or biochemical function at the organ or organ systems level. A *functional limitation* is the impaired ability or inability to perform a specific task at the level of the whole organism, such as walking or climbing a flight of stairs. A *disability* is a limitation in performing roles and tasks expected of an individual within a social and physical environment: an abnormal gap between the individual's capabilities and the environmental and societal demands.

In the IOM model, the amount of disability a person experiences is directly linked to the "quality of the surrounding environment—for example, whether appropriate and adequate care is accessible and whether a social support network is in place" (119). Thus a major focus of rehabilitation is minimizing disability by physical and social environmental modifications so that an individual can participate fully in society.

Although to some degree a mixed bio-psycho-social model, the IOM framework is based heavily on a social model of disability:

> Disability is the expression of a physical or mental limitation in a social context—the gap between a person's capabilities and the demands of the environment. People with such functional limitations are not inherently disabled, that is, incapable of carrying out their personal, familial, and social responsibilities. It is the interaction of their physical and mental limitations with social and environmental factors that determines whether they have a disability. Most disability is thus preventable. (116)

Further, the IOM report correctly emphasized that disability prevention can be directed at any of the stages of the disabling process. Even at the disability stage, "efforts can focus on reversal of disability, restoration of function, or prevention of complications (secondary conditions) that can greatly exacerbate existing limitations or lead to new ones" (116). However, the focus of disability prevention was placed heavily on social and environmental modification:

> . . . although disability can be prevented by improving the functional capacity of the individual—the traditional aim of rehabilitation—this is not the only or perhaps even the most effective method. Disability can be prevented by changing societal attitudes that now restrict employment opportunities for persons with functional limitations, by modifying the buildings in which the people work, or by providing accessible modes of transportation (all of which are components of the Americans with Disabilities Act). (116)

The Institute of Medicine's "Enabling-Disabling Process" Framework (1997)

In 1997, the IOM published a report titled *Enabling America* as a follow-up and revision of its previous *Disability in America* report from 1991 (116, 119). The 1997 report revised the earlier "Disabling Process" Model to formally recognize that the focus of rehabilitative efforts is to assist the individual in reversing the disabling process through an "enabling process" (119):

> *rehabilitation* is the process by which physical, sensory, and mental capacities are restored or developed in (and for) people with disabling conditions—reversing what has been called the disabling process, and may therefore be called the *enabling process*. This is achieved not only through functional changes in the person (e.g., development of compensatory muscular strength, use of prosthetic limbs, and treatment of posttraumatic behavioral disturbances) but also through changes in the physical and social environments that surround them (e.g., reductions in architectural and attitudinal barriers). (119)

A person without disability is considered to be "fully integrated into society" and has access to social opportunities (e.g., education, employment, parenthood, etc.) and physical space, whereas a person with a potentially disabling condition has increased needs that can manifest as a true disability if the social and physical environment are inadequate for these needs. The enabling (or rehabilitative) process attempts to counteract the disabling process by functional restoration and environmental modification.

The World Health Organization's Functioning-Disability-Health Framework (2001)

The initial version of ICIDH promulgated by the WHO in 1980 was widely adopted around the world and was very influential in stimulating research as well as discussion of the best framework for considering disability. Beginning in 1995, ICIDH underwent an exhaustive revision process with comments from more than 80 countries, field tests in 42 countries, and input from scientists, disability groups, and other non-governmental organizations. The culmination of this revision process was the publication of the *International Classification of Functioning, Disability and Health* (ICF) in 2001 (124, 125).

In a shift from the previous WHO formulation, ICF emphasized health and functioning, rather than disability:

> Previously, disability began where health ended; once you were disabled, you were in a separate category. We want to get away from this kind of thinking . . . This is a radical shift. From emphasizing people's disabilities, we now focus on their level of health. ICF puts the notions of "health" and "disability" in a new light. It acknowledges that every human being can experience a decrement in health and thereby experience some disability. ICF thus "mainstreams" the experience of disability and recognizes it as a universal human experience. By shifting the focus from cause to impact it places all health conditions on an equal footing allowing them to be compared using a common metric—the ruler of health and disability. (117)

"Functioning" in the ICF framework is specifically structured around two broad components: (1) body functions and structure; and (2) activities and participation (i.e., involvement in a life situation). Further, participation can be viewed from either a performance perspective (i.e., what an individual does in the current environment) or a capacity perspective (i.e., what an individual can do in an optimized environment). The discrepancy between capacity and performance, the capacity-performance gap, suggests what could be changed in the current environment to improve performance (129).

ICF is based on a bio-psycho-social model that integrates medical and social frameworks of disability from earlier models:

> Disability is always an interaction between features of the person and features of the overall context in which the person lives, but some aspects of disability are almost entirely internal to the person, while another aspect is almost entirely external. In other words, both medical and social responses are appropriate to the problems associated with disability; we cannot wholly reject either kind of intervention . . . [In] ICF disability and functioning are viewed as outcomes of interactions between health conditions (diseases, disorders and injuries) and contextual factors. Among the contextual factors are external environmental factors (for example, social attitudes, architectural characteristics, legal and social structures, as well as climate, terrain, and so forth); and internal personal factors . . . (117)

Health conditions (i.e., diseases, disorders, and injuries) lead to impairments (i.e., problems in body functions and structure) that may be associated with activity limitations (i.e., difficulties in executing activities), and/or participation restrictions (i.e., problems with involvement in life situations). Thus a stroke (a health condition) can cause hemiparesis (an impairment), which is associated with impaired mobility (an activity limitation), and which may cause inability to use mass transit, find a job, and so on (participation restrictions). Under this framework, the impairments, activity limitations, and participation restrictions are different categories subsumed under a broad umbrella of "disability." This spectrum of disability is dependent upon further interactions with the underlying health condition, and also with contextual factors, including environmental and personal factors. The ICF framework can also be linked to different treatment, rehabilitation, and social/environmental interventions and prevention approaches (117).

EVOLUTION OF STROKE REHABILITATION

In the late nineteenth century and early twentieth century, most medical investigations concerning stroke dealt with clinical phenomenology, pathology, clinical-pathologic correlation, and pathophysiology. At this time, very little was attempted as far as retraining or rehabilitation of stroke victims. Although a few scattered prophets of rehabilitation concepts can retrospectively be identified during this time period, they made relatively little impact and their proposed treatments were at best haphazardly employed (130, 131).

Some of the antecedents of rehabilitation available in the early twentieth century included, for example, the tedious repetition of reading, spelling, and repeated words for aphasia; passive movement of severely paralyzed limbs or programs of exercises for less severe paralysis; various orthotic and assistive devices such as splints to prevent contractures, light braces for support, canes (Figure 1-4) (132–136), crutches (Figure 1-5) (132–136), and wheelchairs; attempts to use electrical stimulation to facilitate recovery or prevent muscle wasting; and various surgical procedures to try to limit contractures or spasticity (130, 131). Even in the 1950s, as noted by Barrow and Metts (1986), the prevailing attitude was one of therapeutic nihilism born of hopelessness, compounded by a lack of resources and trained staff:

> As late as the mid '50s, the attitude of both doctors and families of patients with a completed stroke was one of hopelessness. The patients were placed in a nursing home or in a back room, usually at complete bedrest, and they were waited on and pampered as invalids. Under these conditions, the patients usually deteriorated rapidly and complications of decubitus ulcers, muscle spasms, atrophy, and infections were frequent. Other factors of importance at this time were the lack of physical therapy departments in the hospitals . . . and the unavailability of outpatient physical therapy resources. Even the rehabilitation facilities such as Warm Springs, Georgia, had little activity in the field of stroke rehabilitation. (131)

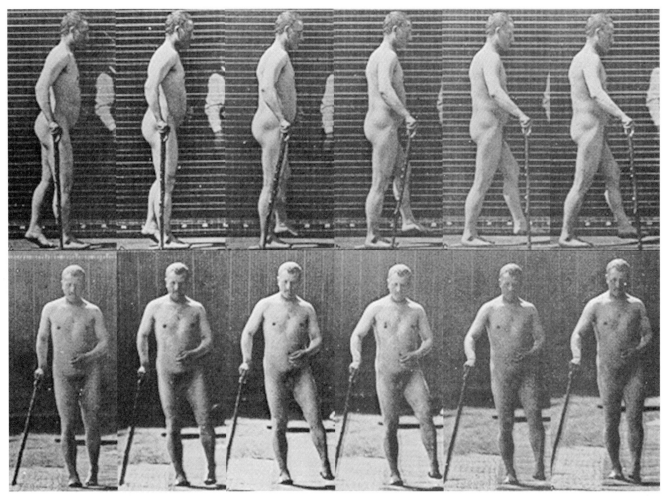

FIGURE 1-4

In the late 1870s and 1880s, prior to the development of movie cameras or projectors, American photographer Eadweard Muybridge (1830–1904) photographed sequential images of people and animals in motion, using arrays of sequentially triggered single-image cameras. In 1885, Philadelphia neurologist Francis Dercum (1856–1931) collaborated with Muybridge at the University of Pennsylvania. This figure shows sequential images of lateral and frontal views from a portion of Muybridge's "Plate 552. Spastic, walking with cane" (*From Ref. 134*). This sequence shows a man with a dense spastic left hemiparesis with the arm held in a flexed posture. As noted by Dercum, "the paralyzed leg is quite stiff, little or no flexion taking place at the knee . . ." Circumduction of the left leg (seen especially on the frontal views) is quite prominent, with the leg first swinging outward during forward motion and then returning toward the midline in an arc. Notice as well, the equinovarus deformity, or as Dercum commented, "the exaggeration of the normal tendency of bringing the outer edge of the foot to the ground in advance of the sole." *From Refs. 132, 133, and 134.*

Rehabilitation of stroke victims was not systemically developed until the second half of the twentieth century (130, 131). In the 1970s and 1980s, the stroke rehabilitation team approach began to develop and spread; stroke units, sometimes combining a seamless transition between acute care and rehabilitation, were developed in larger hospitals in urban areas; and outpatient rehabilitation resources were developed including services provided by health departments, visiting nurse associations, free-standing day care centers, and hospital-associated and independent physical therapy practices (131). The 1970s and 1980s also saw the beginning of an explosion in stroke rehabilitation research, with an escalation in the use of randomized trials of stroke rehabilitation therapies increasing particularly since the 1990s (Figure 1-6) (137). Although spontaneous recovery accounts for most of the improvement in functional ability following stroke (138), a growing body of evidence since the 1990s supports a modest marginal but clinically important benefit of stroke rehabilitation, generally for patients with at most moderate disability (139–144).

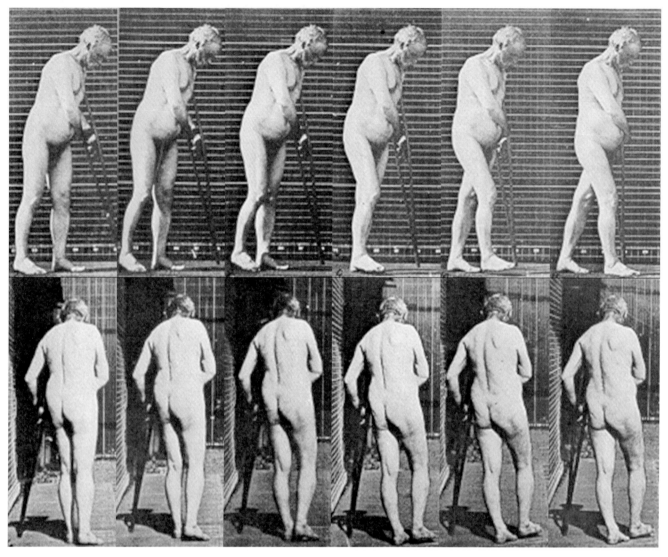

FIGURE 1-5

Sequential images of lateral and posterior views from a portion of Muybridge's "Plate 547. Spastic, walking with crutch" taken in 1885 (*Ref. 134*). This shows an elderly man with a dense spastic right hemiparesis with the arm held in a flexed posture while using a crutch to walk. As noted by Dercum, "the paralyzed leg is quite stiff, little or no flexion taking place at the knee . . . [The foot is] raised from the ground by the enormous swaying of the trunk toward the sound side, to which additional support is given to receive the sway by means of the crutch." See the legend for Figure 1-4, for further details. *From Refs. 132, 133, and 134.*

Organized inpatient multidisciplinary stroke rehabilitation

Since the 1970s, and particularly since the 1990s, it has become clear that organized inpatient multidisciplinary rehabilitation in the post-acute period provides clinically important benefits (139–144). Most data supporting the clinical benefits of inpatient stroke rehabilitation is based on studies of comprehensive stroke units (that provide acute stroke care and rehabilitation) or rehabilitation stroke units (dedicated to rehabilitative care of post-acute patients with stroke), rather than the more common mixed rehabilitation units (that provide stroke

rehabilitation in a mixed rehabilitation setting) (143). Stroke patients who receive inpatient rehabilitation provided by a coordinated multidisciplinary team are more likely to recover the ability to perform activities of daily living, more likely to return to the community, and less likely to die—results that are fairly robust in different meta-analyses and across recent controlled trials (141, 145–152). A Danish population-based study comparing two communities—one where care was provided in a dedicated comprehensive stroke unit with both acute care and rehabilitation care, and the other in which care was provided on general medical and neurologic

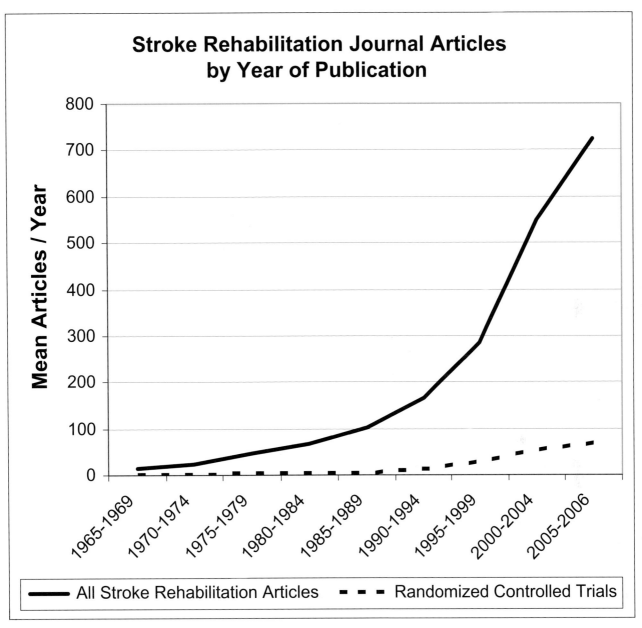

FIGURE 1-6

Stroke rehabilitation journal articles by year of publication. Both the total number of journal articles and the number of journal articles reporting the results of randomized clinical trials show exponential growth, although the rate of growth is greater for randomized trials of stroke rehabilitation since the 1970s [evident on semi-log plots, or on regression analyses of log (mean articles/year) against time; unpublished analyses not shown].

wards—found that stroke unit care reduced the length of hospital stay by 30%, reduced the risk of discharge to nursing home by 40%, and reduced the relative risk of death by 50% (141). In a systematic review of nine trials recruiting 1,437 patients, Langhorne and Duncan found that for every 100 patients who receive organized inpatient multidisciplinary rehabilitation, 5 more returned home in an independent state compared to those who do not receive such care (142). Functional, independence, and

survival benefits to those who underwent early multidisciplinary stroke rehabilitation after stroke are sustained even five to ten years after stroke (153–157). Patients with moderate or severe strokes appear to benefit most (151).

Even where evidence supports a clinical benefit of stroke rehabilitation, it has generally been unclear which specific factors, including which therapies or combinations of therapies, amongst the entire package of individualized treatments for a given patient are most important for providing benefit (143, 158–160). Although data supporting the value of individual team members in the multidisciplinary team is limited, most authorities and clinical care guidelines have advocated a broad team composition, including physicians, nurses, physical therapists, occupational therapists, speech therapists, and social workers (141). Although available studies are limited, the intensity of rehabilitation services is a modest predictor of recovery among stroke patients (152, 161–165), as is particularly an early start to intensive treatment (159, 160). It has also been unclear to what extent findings of randomized clinical trials could be generalized to the routine clinical setting: limited available data suggests that the routine clinical rehabilitation setting can reproduce the benefits of stroke rehabilitation units in controlled trials and meta-analyses, but the magnitude of benefit is smaller outside of the formalized experimental setting (166). Inpatient rehabilitation is also expensive, and the limited available cost-benefit analyses have not strongly supported the cost-effectiveness of inpatient stroke rehabilitation overall (167–169), making it imperative to carefully select patients who will benefit most from such intensive care (170), and also to identify the least expensive care settings that will provide maximum clinical benefit for individual patients (171).

Clinical Pathways

Integrated care pathways have not been shown to improve the outcome of inpatient stroke rehabilitation (172–179). In fact, care pathways for rehabilitation programs have most often resulted simply in decreased patient satisfaction (172–175, 179), and some studies have actually reported slower recovery and lower quality of life among patients receiving rehabilitation as part of an integrated care pathway as opposed to conventional multidisciplinary rehabilitative care (172, 176). As noted by Teasell, "This apparent paradox may signify the importance of using evidence or guidelines to assist rehabilitation clinicians in individualizing the rehab of stroke patients as opposed to a 'one size fits all' approach" (179). Furthermore, despite potential benefits, many clinical pathway programs for acute or rehabilitation care of stroke fail because of inadequate planning and implementation (174, 175). Effective implementation of such programs requires strong administrative and medical staff leadership, active participation of all clinical disciplines involved in the rehabilitative care of patients on the pathway, provision of regular feedback to clinicians, sufficient resources, improved and often more detailed documentation, incorporation of the entire rehabilitation period of care into the pathways, integration with ongoing quality and utilization management programs, and periodic evaluation and modification (174, 175).

Specific Therapies

Based on expert opinion and limited controlled trial data, physical therapy is modestly beneficial for stroke patients (160, 165, 180, 181). However, there continues to be considerable variation in the beliefs (182) and treatment approaches (183, 184) of physical therapists concerning the treatment of stroke patients, in part a function of the treatment approach in vogue when the physical therapists were trained (185). Particularly since the 1950s, several different physical therapy approaches have been developed and applied to the treatment of stroke patients (140, 181–195). Some physical therapists advocate and apply Bobath's "neuro-developmental" approach (188), the "motor re-learning programme" of Carr and Sheperd (189), Brunnström's approach utilizing abnormal synergies (187), or various others. Controlled trial data as yet are inconsistent, and no clearly better approach has been identified from among available approaches for the physical therapy of stroke patients (181, 184). Progressive resistance exercises several times a week can help improve strength and functional abilities in patients with adequate motor control (139, 196). The intensity of therapy initiated early seems to be important in maximizing the degree of functional improvement (162–165).

Based on the results of systematic reviews, comprehensive occupational therapy is modestly beneficial in improving activities of daily living and social participation among stroke patients (197, 198), although there is limited or insufficient evidence supporting many specific occupational therapy interventions, including provision of splints for decreasing muscle tone (197, 199). Even when provided in the community, systematic reviews indicate that occupational therapy can improve basic activities of daily living, as well as domestic and leisure skills (197, 198). Different task-oriented practice strategies can be helpful especially if intensive training in specific skills is provided (139, 162–164, 197). Constraint-induced-movement therapy—based on the idea that "learned non-use" of a weak arm develops because of the greater effort required to use it—seeks to encourage use of the weak arm and promote helpful cerebral plasticity (139, 200); this approach can be helpful in increasing the amount and efficiency of use of the weak arm in the relatively small subset of patients with fairly good motor control to begin with (139, 201–203).

Available data from randomized controlled trials concerning the efficacy of speech therapy in stroke rehabilitation is limited and not entirely consistent (204), with some trials supporting a modest benefit within the first three to six months after stroke (161, 205, 206), and others finding lesser or no significant benefit for most patients (207–209). A greater intensity of therapy in the first several months post-stroke seems to be an important factor in the degree of improvement (161, 204, 210).

Early Supported Discharge

In most countries into the 1990s, stroke patients were treated initially in the hospital, followed by a variable period of inpatient rehabilitation, but rehabilitation frequently stopped after discharge home (211). In some countries, early supported discharge (ESD) approaches have been developed since the 1990s that shorten the period of acute hospital stay and provide rehabilitation services beginning in the hospital and continuing for the first few weeks at home. Proponents have claimed that this approach is not only less costly, but can also improve care by providing "seamless service" spanning inpatient and home care environments, but until recently there was limited data to evaluate such claims (211). Single-blind randomized controlled trials have been reported from the United Kingdom, Scandinavia, Australia, and Canada (212–225). While some studies of ESD have not identified significant benefits of this approach (214), others have reported similar efficacy compared with traditional inpatient rehabilitation along with significant cost savings (213, 225); reductions in total hospitalization (of approximately 50%) (218, 219, 221); reduction in use of inpatient rehabilitation beds (212), improved patient satisfaction (215, 218, 221); less caregiver stress (222); and in some cases, improved performance of activities of daily living (216, 219, 220, 223), and longer sustained non-institutional care (216). In one well-designed study from Norway, stroke patients who received ESD rehabilitation services spent less time in hospital, and were also more likely to be independent and to be living at home after one year (216). As suggested by Langhorne, presumably "the ESD service has improved the patient's ability to regain normal activities despite residual impairment. In particular, the patient's own home is probably the best place to relearn the skills needed to function in that environment" (211). A home environment for rehabilitation may also facilitate having patients with moderate neurologic impairments take greater responsibility and exercise greater influence over their own rehabilitation (224). A systematic review of the economic costs of different settings of rehabilitation care found "'moderate' evidence that ESD services provide care at modestly lower total costs than usual care for stroke patients with mild or moderate disability" (167).

Outpatient Rehabilitation

The role of outpatient rehabilitation services (i.e., therapy-based rehabilitation services targeted at stroke patients living at home) has only recently been studied in any detail, and the results remain less certain than traditional inpatient multidisciplinary stroke rehabilitation (226–230). This is complicated by differences in the types of community-based rehabilitation provided, the setting in which such care is provided (day hospital versus the home), and different clinical circumstances for which this approach is used instead of traditional inpatient rehabilitation (229, 230). Several studies have evaluated use of day hospital rehabilitation care with inconsistent results compared with either inpatient multidisciplinary care or home care (231–233). Costs are generally higher for day hospital rehabilitation than for home care (231, 233), but not universally so (232). Functional outcomes for day hospital rehabilitation are generally similar to rehabilitation provided in other settings (231, 232), although one study reported better functional outcomes with day hospital rehabilitation than with home care (233). Nevertheless, preliminary results suggest that some therapy-based rehabilitation services provided in the home can result in greater ability to perform activities of daily living and reduce risk of deterioration in ability compared with conventional care (i.e., normal practice or no routine intervention) (226–230). Other studies have indicated no benefit for some outpatient services that were not primarily therapy-based, including use of an outreach nursing support program (234, 235). Further studies are needed to define the most appropriate level of service delivery, the most effective services and interventions, and the cost-effectiveness compared with other approaches (226). At present there is "insufficient" evidence concerning the economic costs of community-based rehabilitation (167).

Caregiver Training

Family involvement in support of the post-stroke patient has long been recognized as a strong independent predictor of discharge to home as opposed to an institution (170). Because the degree of family involvement can sometimes be influenced by the rehabilitation team, family and caregiver training has been a major target of therapeutic intervention, and has been increasingly recognized as a predictor of functional outcome as well (170). Caregiver training during the rehabilitation of stroke patients can reduce the cost of care and improve the overall quality of life among caregivers, even as long as a year post-stroke (236, 237). Problem-solving training, including an in-home visit and subsequent telephone contacts by a trained nurse, may also be useful for family caregivers of stroke survivors even after discharge from rehabilitation (238). Caregiver training and education may help caregivers be better prepared to deal with issues, facilitate development of caregiver problem-solving skills, lessen caregiver stress and depression, minimize secondary complications among the patients, and facilitate patient motor tasks that promote functional improvements and lessen the risk of further functional declines (e.g., safe swallowing, and walking for exercise) (139, 238).

Gaps in Theoretical Foundations and Practical Implementation Remain

The development of stroke rehabilitation concepts is still limited, with recognition in the field that many of the therapeutic approaches currently employed have at best limited benefit in a select subgroup of patients, that much of the theoretical justification for different rehabilitation models and approaches remains speculative, and that there is no overall foundation of an accepted "theory of rehabilitation" that could help to prevent fragmentation and division, provide coherence, focus research and development in this area, and facilitate competition for limited research funding (139, 143, 239, 240). Moreover, because rehabilitation interventions are typically multidisciplinary, multifaceted, and customized to the individual patient's needs and goals, they are in practice difficult to standardize, and therefore difficult to measure and compare (139, 143, 239). Available treatment studies are further complicated by the heterogeneity of impairments and disabilities of the patients studied, poor descriptions of the specific treatments administered, inadequate controls, lack of blinding, small sample sizes, and insensitive outcome measures (139).

Current expert consensus has strongly supported the importance of integrating rehabilitation into systems of care to ensure that all patients who could potentially benefit from appropriate stroke care and rehabilitation are provided with the appropriate treatment in a time frame that will maximize recovery and minimize disability (152). According to the American Stroke Association's Task Force on the Development of Stroke Systems:

> Stroke rehabilitation involves a combined and coordinated use of medical, social, educational, and vocational measures for retraining individuals to reach their maximal physical, psychological, social, vocational, and avocational potential. Specifically, stroke rehabilitation programs are provided to optimize neurologic recovery, teach compensatory strategies for residual deficits, teach activities of daily living (ADLs) and skills required for community living, and provide psychosocial and medical interventions to manage depression. The team provides patient and family education about the medical management of poststroke complications and secondary stroke prevention . . . Practice guidelines for rehabilitation are well established in this area, although patients often do not receive a level of care that is consistent with these guidelines . . . The intensity of rehabilitation services often is a critical determinant in the recovery of stroke patients. The use of coordinated, multidisciplinary stroke rehabilitation teams has been shown to diminish mortality rates for stroke patients. In addition, stroke patients who receive care in an inpatient rehabilitation facility are more likely to return to the community and to recover their ability to perform ADLs . . . Building stroke systems throughout the United States is the critical next step in improving patient outcomes in the prevention, treatment, and rehabilitation of stroke. The current fragmented approach to stroke care in most regions of the United States provides inadequate linkages and coordination among the fundamental components of stroke care. (152)

Practice guidelines are now available for stroke rehabilitation (241–243), but in many cases patients do not receive care consistent with the guidelines (143, 152, 244, 245). Further, there are sociodemographic inequalities in the use of rehabilitation services, suggesting inappropriate underuse among certain populations (246).

Even when patients receive inpatient stroke rehabilitation, they spend only a small amount of their inpatient stay participating in potentially rehabilitative activities, and this low intensity of therapy is less likely to produce beneficial outcomes (139, 143, 228, 247). In an observational behavioral mapping study of five stroke units, patients had therapist contact during only 5% of the day, participated in minimal or moderate therapeutic activity for less than 13% of the therapeutic day (8 AM to 5 PM), and were resting in bed 53% of the time and alone 60% of the time (248). Poor participation in therapeutic activities is common during inpatient rehabilitation, and is associated with longer lengths of inpatient stay and lower degrees of improvement in functional performance (249). In addition, formal therapy is typically stopped when there are no evident qualitative gains in function after several weeks of treatment for financial or policy reasons, even though, as Dobkin notes: "A plateau in recovery . . . does not necessarily imply a diminished capacity for further gains in physical speed or precision or in learning a new task" (139).

Furthermore, despite modern treatment and multidisciplinary rehabilitation, perhaps half of patients with stroke are ultimately discharged to home with serious, persistent neurologic impairments, functional limitations, and often disability resulting from inadequate environmental supports (250). Stroke survivors (whether residing at home or in institutional care environments) are prone to multiple secondary conditions that further erode health, including social isolation, depression, physical inactivity, painful joint contractures, deep venous thromboses and pulmonary emboli, decubitus ulcers, incontinence, aspiration pneumonia, inadequate nutrition, falls, hip fractures, and seizures. Such patients are often frail and susceptible to aggravation of existing disease or development of new illness, with resulting functional decline, high resource utilization, high rates of rehospitalization, significant added morbidity, and a high risk of death within the first year after stroke onset. Indeed, in the United States, approximately one-fifth of stroke patients die in the first month after stroke, a quarter within 2 months, and a third within 6 months (251). Patients and caregivers can benefit from a close liaison between inpatient and community care programs, and also from continuing professional support and counseling after discharge following a stroke (250).

Further studies are needed to define the most appropriate level of service delivery for stroke rehabilitation, the most effective services and interventions among the "complex packages of care" that comprise current rehabilitation programs, and the most cost-effective of the different types of stroke rehabilitation services available (143, 226).

References

1. Aldes JH. Rehabilitation—past, present and future. *Am Correct Ther J* 1967; 21:148–154.
2. Cavalier W. The history of rehabilitation. *Am Arch Rehabil Ther* 1986; 34:23–32.
3. Kottke FJ, Knapp ME. The development of physiatry before 1950. *Arch Phys Med Rehabil* 1988; 69 Special Number:4–14.
4. Eldar R, Jelić M. The association of rehabilitation and war. *Disabil Rehabil* 2003; 25:1019–1023.
5. Lanska DJ. The role of technology in neurologic specialization in America. *Neurology* 1997; 48:1722–1727.
6. Beard G. Foundations for growth: A review of the first forty years in terms of education, practice, and research. *Phys Ther Prev* 1961; 41:843–861.
7. Gutman SA. Influence of the U.S. military and occupational therapy reconstruction aides in World War I on the development of occupational therapy. *Am J Occup Ther* 1995; 49:256–262.
8. Strickland BA. Physical medicine in the Army. *Arch Phys Med Rehabil* 1947; 28:229–236.
9. Coulter JS. History and development of physical medicine. *Arch Phys Med Rehabil* 1947; 28:600–602.
10. Moffat MM. This history of physical therapy practice in the United States. *J Phys Ther Educ* 2003; 17:15–25.
11. Low JF. The reconstruction aides. *Am J Occup Ther* 1992; 46:45–48.
12. Association of Academic Physiatrists. *The History of Physiatry (An overview)*. http://www.physiatry.org/Field_history.cfm [Accessed 11-15-2006].
13. Sexton FH. Vocational rehabilitation of soldiers suffering from nervous diseases. *Mental Hygiene* 1918; 2:265–276.
14. Low JF. Historical and social foundation for practice. In: CA Trombly (Editor). *Occupational Therapy for Physical Dysfunction*. Fourth edition. Baltimore: Williams & Wilkins, 1995:3–14.
15. Billings F. Chairman's address—The national program for the reconstruction and rehabilitation of disabled soldiers. *JAMA* 1918; 70:1924–1925.
16. Dillingham TR. Physiatry, physical medicine, and rehabilitation: Historical development and military roles. *Phys Med Rehabil Clin North Am* 2002; 13:1–16
17. Surgeon General's Office. United States Army Medical Services. *Medical Department of the United States Army in the World War*. Volume 1. Washington, D.C.: Government Printing Office, 1923.
18. Granger FB. The development of physiotherapy. [Excerpted from the June 1923 issue of Physiotherapy Review]. *Phys Ther* 1923/1976; 56:13–14.
19. Krusen FH. Historical development in physical medicine and rehabilitation during the last forty years. *Arch Phys Med Rehabil* 1969; 50: 1–5.
20. Nelson CW. Physiotherapy and physical therapy at Mayo. *Mayo Clin Proc* 1995; 70:516.
21. McMillan M. *Massage and Therapeutic Exercise*. Philadelphia: W.B. Saunders Company, 1921.
22. Vogel EE. The beginnings of modern physiotherapy. *Phys Ther* 1976; 56:15–22.
23. Hopkins HL. An historical perspective on occupational therapy. Hopkins HL, Smith HD (Editors). *Willard and Spackman's Occupational Therapy*. Seventh Edition. Philadelphia: J.B. Lippincott Company, 1988:16–37.
24. Peloquin SM. Occupational therapy service: Individual and collective understandings of the founders. *Am J Occup Ther* 1991; 45:352–60, 733–744.
25. Pasquinelli S. History and trends in treatment methods. In: Pedretti LW (Editor). *Occupational Therapy: Practice Skills for Physical Dysfunction*. St. Louis, MO: Mosby, 1996:13–21.
26. National Society for the Promotion of Occupational Therapy. *Constitution*. Baltimore: Sheppard Hospital Press, 1917:1.
27. Dunton WR Jr. *Occupational Therapy—A Manual for Nurses*. Philadelphia: W.B. Saunders, 1915.
28. Dunton WR Jr. History of occupational therapy. *The Modern Hospital* 1917; 8:380–382.
29. Licht S. The founding and founders of the American Occupational Therapy Association. *Am J Occup Ther* 1967; 21:269–277.
30. Bing RK. Eleanor Clarke Slagle Lectureship—1981. Occupational therapy revisited: A paraphrastic journey. *Am J Occup Ther* 1981; 35:499–518.
31. Mattison JS. The program of occupational therapy at the National Home for Disabled Volunteer Soldiers. *Occup Ther Rehabil* 1929; 8:77–81.
32. Willard HS, Spackman CS (Editors). *Principles of Occupational Therapy*. Philadelphia: JB Lippincott, 1947.
33. Rockey D. John Thelwell and the origins of British speech therapy. *Med Hist* 1979; 23:156–175.
34. Duchan JF. *Getting here: a short history of speech pathology in America*. February 24, 2006. http://www.acsu.buffalo.edu/~duchan/new_history/overview.html [Accessed 9-26-06],
35. Paden E. *History of the American Speech and Hearing Association 1925–1958*. Washington, D.C.: American Speech and Hearing Association, 1970.
36. van Riper C. An earlier history of ASHA. *ASHA* 1981; 23:855–858.
37. Anonymous. Association news. *Quart J Speech* 1927; 13:311–317.
38. Stillwell GK. In memoriam: Frank H. Krusen, M.D. *Arch Phys Med Rehabil* 1973; 54:493–495.
39. Opitz JL, Folz TJ, Gelfman R, Peters DJ. The history of physical medicine and rehabilitation as recorded in the diary of Dr. Frank Krusen: Part 1. Gathering momentum (the years before 1942). *Arch Phys Med Rehabil*. 1997; 78:442–445.
40. Eckman J. Frank H. Krusen, M.D.: Pathmaker in physical medicine and rehabilitation. *Lancet* 1967; 87:140–142.

41. Anonymous. Special award: Frank H. Krusen, M.D. *Arch Phys Med Rehabil* 1970; 51:670–672.
42. Krusen FH. The teaching of physical therapeutics to undergraduate medical students. *J Assoc Am Med Coll* 1930; 5:152–158.
43. McCahill W. In memoriam: Frank H. Krusen, M.D.: 1898–1973. *J Rehabil* 1974; 40:30.
44. Krusen FH. *Physical Medicine: The Employment of Physical Agents for Diagnosis and Therapy*. Philadelphia: WB Saunders, 1941.
45. Johnson EW. Struggle for identity: The turbulent 1960s. *Arch Phys Med Rehabil* 1988; 69:20–25.
46. Rusk HA. The growth and development of rehabilitation medicine. *Arch Phys Med Rehabil* 1969; 50:463–466.
47. Rusk HA. Howard Rusk on rehabilitation: Cardiac cases, cancer patients, chronic obstructive lung diseases, lower limb orthotics. *Med Times* 1977; 105:64–75.
48. Modlin JF. Book reviews: *Polio: An American Story; [and] Living with Polio: The Epidemic and its Survivors*. *N Engl J Med* 2005; 353:2308–2310.
49. Wilson DK. A crippling fear: Experiencing polio in the era of FDR. *Bull Hist Med* 1998; 72:464–495.
50. Moffat MM. Three quarters of a century of healing the generations. *Phys Ther* 1996; 76:1242–1252.
51. Neumann DA. Polio: Its impact on the people of the United States and the emerging profession of physical therapy. *J Orthop Sports Phys Ther* 2004; 34:479–492.
52. American Physical Therapy Association. *A Historical Perspective*. http://www.apta.org [Accessed 9-26-06].
53. Drinker P, Shaw LA. An apparatus for the prolonged administration of artificial respiration: I. A design for adults and children. *J Clin Invest* 1929; 7:229.
54. Drinker PA, McKhann CF. The use of a new apparatus for the prolonged administration of artificial respiration: I. A fatal case of poliomyelitis. *JAMA* 1929; 92:1658–1660.
55. Drinker PA, McKhann CF III. The iron lung: First practical means of respiratory support. *JAMA* 1986; 255:1476–1480.
56. Lovett RW. Fatigue and exercise in the treatment of infantile paralysis. *JAMA* 1917; 69:168–176.
57. Irwin CE. Early orthopedic care in poliomyelitis. *JAMA* 1941; 117:280–283.
58. Ditunno JF Jr, Herbison GJ. Franklin D. Roosevelt: Diagnosis, clinical course, and rehabilitation from poliomyelitis. *Am J Phys Med Rehabil* 2002; 81:557–566.
59. Wilson J. The Sister Kenny Clinics: What endures? *Aust J Adv Nurs* 1986; 3:13–21.
60. Wilson J. Sister Elizabeth Kenney's trial by Royal Commission. *Hist Nurs Soc J* 1992–3; 4:91–99.
61. Sister Kenney Rehabilitation Institute. *History*. 2007. http://www.allina.com/ahs/ski.nsf/page/history [Accessed 2-28-07].
62. Swaim MW. A dogma upended from down under: Sister Elizabeth Kenny's polio treatment. *NC Med J* 1998; 59:256–260.
63. Sister Kenney Rehabilitation Institute. *About Sister Kenny Rehabilitation Institute*. 2007. http://www.allina.com/ahs/ski.nsf/page/aboutus [Accessed 2-28-07].
64. Kenny E. *Infantile Paralysis and Cerebral Diplegia: Methods Used in the Restoration of Function*. Sydney: Angus and Robertson, 1937.
65. Kenney E. *The Treatment of Infantile Paralsis in the Acute Stage*. Minneapolis: Bruce, 1941.
66. Kenney E. Kenny concept of the disease infantile paralysis. *Physiother Rev* 1943; 23:1–7.
67. Cole W, Knapp M. The Kenny treatment of infantile paralysis: A preliminary report. *JAMA* 1941; 116:2577.
68. Daly MI, Greenbaum J, Reilly ET, Weiss AM, Stimson P. The early treatment of poliomyelitis with an evaluation of the Sister Kenny treatment. *JAMA* 1942; 118:1433–1477.
69. Pohl J. The Kenny treatment of anterior poliomyelitis: Report of the first cases treated in America. *JAMA* 1942; 118:1428–1433.
70. Pohl J. The Kenny concept and treatment of infantile paralysis: Report of 5 year study of cases treated and supervised by Kenny. *Lancet* 1945; 65:265–271.
71. Paul JR. *A history of poliomyelitis*. New Haven, CT and London: Yale University Press, 1971.
72. Raymond CA. Polio survivors spurred rehabilitation advances. *JAMA* 1986; 255:1403–1404.
73. Smith JS. *Patenting the sun: polio and the Salk vaccine: the dramatic story behind one of the greatest achievements of modern science*. New York: William Morrow and Company, 1990.
74. Helfand WH, Lazarus J, Theerman P. ". . . So others may walk": The March of Dimes. *Am J Public Health* 2001; 91:1190.
75. Oschinsky DM. *Polio: an American story: the crusade that mobilized the nation against the 20ᵗʰ century's most feared disease*. Oxford and New York: Oxford University Press, 2005.
76. March of Dimes. *About Us: United to Beat Polio*. 2007. http://www.marchofdimes.com/aboutus/789_821.asp [Accessed 2-27-07].
77. March of Dimes. *Heroes of the March of Dimes: Eddie Cantor and the Origin of the March of Dimes*. 2007. http://www.marchofdimes.com/aboutus/20311_22634.asp [Accessed 2-27-07].
78. U.S. Department of Labor, Bureau of Labor Statistics. *Consumer Price Index: All Urban Consumers (CPI-U): U.S. City Average: All Items*. February 21, 2007. ftp://ftp.bls.gov/pub/special.requests/cpi/cpiai.txt [Accessed 2-28-07].

79. U.S. Department of Labor, Bureau of Labor Statistics. *CPI Inflation Calculator.* http://data.bls.gov [Accessed 2-28-07].

80. Landsteiner K, Popper E. Übertragung der Poliomyelitis acuta auf Affen. *Z Immunitätsforsch exp Ther.* 1909; 2:377–390.

81. Eggers HJ. Milestones in early poliomyelitis research (1840–1949). *J Virol* 1999; 73:4533–4535.

82. Bodian D. Differentiation of types of poliomyelitis viruses. I. Reinfection experiments in monkeys (second attacks). *Am J Hyg* 1949; 49:200–224.

83. Bodian D, Morgan IM, Howe HA. Differentiation of types of poliomyelitis viruses. III. The grouping of fourteen strains into three basic immunological types. *Am J Hyg* 1949; 49:234–245.

84. The Committee on Typing of the National Foundation for Infantile Paralysis. Immunologic classification of poliomyelitis viruses. *Am J Hyg.* 1951; 54:191–274.

85. Nathanson N. David Bodian's contribution to the development of poliovirus vaccine. *Am J Epidemiol* 2005; 161:207–212.

86. Fee E, Parry M. Biographical memoirs: David Bodian: 15 May 1910–18 September 1992. *Proc Am Phil Soc* 2006; 150:167–172.

87. Enders JF, Weller TH, Robbins FC. Cultivation of the Lansing strain of poliomyelitis virus in cultures of various human embryonic tissues. *Science* 1949; 109:85–87.

88. Enders JF, Robbins FC, Weller TH. The cultivation of the poliomyelitis viruses in tissue culture: Nobel Lecture, December 11, 1954. In *Nobel Lectures, Physiology or Medicine 1942–1962.* Amsterdam: Elsevier Publishing Company, 1964. http://nobelprizes.org/nobel_prizes/medicine/laureates/1954/enders-robbins-weller-lecture.pdf [Accessed 1-16-2007].

89. Zetterström R, Lagercrantz H. J.F. Enders (1897–1985), T.H. Weller (1915–) and F.C. Robbins (1916–2003): a simplified method for the multiplication of poliomyelitis virus. Dreams of eradicating a terrifying disease. *Acta Paediatr.* 2006; 95:1026–1028.

90. Rosen FS. Conquering polio: Isolation of poliovirus—John Enders and the Nobel Prize. *N Engl J Med* 2004; 351:1481–1483.

91. Lepow ML. Conquering polio: Advances in virology—Weller and Robbins. *N Engl J Med* 2004; 351:1483–1485.

92. Bodian D, Paffenbarger R. Poliomyelitis infections in households: Frequency of viremia and specific antibody response. *Am J Hyg* 1954; 60:83.

93. Horstmann DM, McCollum RW, Mascola AD. Viremia in human poliomyelitis. *J Exp Med* 1954; 99:355–369.

94. Francis T Jr. *Evaluation of the 1954 field trial of poliomyelitis vaccine.* Ann Arbor, MI: Edwards Brothers/National Foundation for Infantile Paralysis, 1957.

95. Meldrum M. "A calculated risk": The Salk polio vaccine field trials of 1954. *BMJ* 1998; 317:1233–1236.

96. Monto AS. Francis field trial of inactivated poliomyelitis vaccine: Background and lessons for today. *Epidemiol Rev* 1999; 21:7–23.

97. Katz SL. Conquering polio: From culture to vaccine—Salk and Sabin. *N Engl J Med* 2004; 351:1485–1487.

98. Gould T. *A Summer Plague: Polio and Its Survivors.* New Haven, Connecticut and London: Yale University Press, 1995.

99. Markel H. April 12, 1955—Tommy Francis and the Salk Vaccine. *N Engl J Med* 2005; 352:1408–1409.

100. Francis T Jr, Korns RF, Voight RB, et al. *An evaluation of the 1954 poliomyelitis vaccine trials: Summary report.* Ann Arbor, MI: University of Michigan, 1955.

101. Nathanson N, Langmuir AD. The Cutter incident: Poliomyelitis following formaldehyde-inactivated poliovirus vaccination in the United States during the spring of 1955. I. Background. *Am J Hyg* 1963; 78:16–28.

102. Nathanson N, Langmuir AD. The Cutter incident: Poliomyelitis following formaldehyde-inactivated poliovirus vaccination in the United States during the spring of 1955. II. Relationship of poliomyelitis to Cutter vaccine. *Am J Hyg* 1963; 78:29–60.

103. Hinman AR, Thacker SB. Invited commentary on "The Cutter incident: Poliomyelitis following formaldehyde-inactivated poliovirus vaccination in the United States during the spring of 1955. II. Relationship of poliomyelitis to Cutter vaccine." *Am J Epidemiol* 1995; 142:107–140.

104. Offit PA. The Cutter incident, 50 years later. *N Engl J Med* 2005; 352:1411–1412.

105. Offit PA. *The Cutter Incident: How America's First Polio Vaccine Led to the Growing Vaccine Crisis.* New Haven, CT: Yale University Press, 2005.

106. Rusk HA. *A World to Care For: The Autobiography of Howard A. Rusk, M.D.* New York, Random House: 1972.

107. Rusk Institute. *Rusk Institute of Rehabilitation Medicine: A Guide to the Records.* http://archives.med.nyu.edu/collections/findingaids/rusk.html. [Accessed 11-16-2006].

108. University of Missouri. Western Historical Manuscript Collection-Columbia. *Rusk, Howard A. (1901–1989), Papers, 1937–1991 (C3981).* http://www.umsystem.edu/whmc/invent/3981.html. [Accessed 11-15-2006].

109. Yanes-Hoffman N. Howard Rusk, MD: An equal chance. *JAMA* 1981; 246:1503–1510.

110. Rusk HA. Rehabilitation. *JAMA* 1949; 140:286–292.

111. Robertson N. Institute Rusk founded named for him at last. *New York Times,* November 9, 1984.

112. Anonymous. Special award: Howard A. Rusk, M.D. *Arch Phys Med Rehabil* 1966; 47:48–49.

113. Lasker Foundation. *Former Winners, 1952: Albert Lasker Public Service Award.* http://www.laskerfoundation.org/awards/library/1952public.shtml. [Accessed 2-15-2007].

114. Bickenbach JE, Chatterji S, Badley EM, Ustun TB. Models of disablement, universalism and the International Classification of Impairments, Disabilities and Handicaps. *Soc Sci Med* 1999; 48:1173–1187.

115. Mausner J, Kramer S. *Mausner & Bahn Epidemiology—An Introductory Text.* Second Edition. Philadelphia: W.B. Saunders Co., 1985:9–21.

116. Pope AM, Tarlov AR (Editors). *Disability in America: Toward a National Agenda for Prevention.* Washington, D.C.: National Academy Press, 1991.

117. World Health Organization. *Towards a Common Language for Functioning, Disability and Health: ICF.* Geneva: World Health Organization, 2002.

118. National Council on Disability. *On the Threshold of Independence.* Washington, D.C.: National Council on Disability, 1988.

119. Brandt EN Jr., Pope AM (Eds.). Committee on Assessing Rehabilitation Science and Engineering, Division of Health Sciences Policy, Institute of Medicine. *Enabling America: Assessing the Role of Rehabilitation Science and Engineering.* Washington, D.C., National Academy Press, 1997.

120. Nagi SZ. A study in the evaluation of disability and rehabilitation potential: Concepts, methods, and procedures. *Am J Public Health* 1964; 54:1568–1579.

121. Nagi SZ. *Disability and Rehabilitation.* Columbus: Ohio State University Press, 1969.

122. Nagi SZ. Disability concepts revisited: Implications for prevention. Appendix A. In: Pope AM, Tarlov AR (Editors). *Disability in America: Toward a National Agenda for Prevention.* Washington, D.C.: National Academy Press, 1991: 309–327.

123. World Health Organization. *International Classification of Impairments, Disabilities, and Handicaps: A Manual of Classification Relating to the Consequences of Disease.* Geneva: World Health Organization, 1980.

124. World Health Organization. *International Classification of Functioning and Disability, ICIDH-2. Beta-2 draft, Full Version.* Geneva: World Health Organization, 1999.

125. World Health Organization. *International Classification of Functioning, Disability and Health, ICF.* Geneva: World Health Organization, 2001.

126. Wade DT, de Jong BA. Recent advances in rehabilitation. *BMJ* 2000; 320:1385–1388.

127. Susser M. Disease, illness, sickness: Impairment, disability and handicap. *Psychol Med* 1990; 20:471–473.

128. Badley EM. The ICIDH: Format, application in different settings, and distinction between disability and handicap. *Int Disabil Studies* 1987; 9:3.

129. Young NL, Williams JI, Yoshida KK, et al. The context of measuring disability: Does it matter whether capability or performance is measured? *J Clin Epidemiol* 1996; 49:1097–1101.

130. Licht S. Stroke: A history of its rehabilitation: Walter J. Zeiter Lecture. *Arch Phys Med Rehabil* 1973:54:10–18.

131. Barrow JG, Metts JC. The historical background of stroke prevention, treatment, and rehabilitation in Georgia. *J Med Assoc Ga* 1986; 75:78–81.

132. Dercum FX. The walk and some of its phases in disease: Together with other studies based on the Muybrodge investigation. *Trans Coll Phys Phil* 1888; 17:308–388.

133. Dercum FX. A study of some normal and abnormal movements: Photographed by Muybridge. In: University of Pennsylvania. *Animal Locomotion. The Muybridge Work at the University of Pennsylvania: The Method and the Result.* Philadelphia: J.B. Lippincott Co., 1888:103–133.

134. Muybridge E. *Muybridge's Complete Human and Animal Locomotion: All 781 Plates from the 1887 Animal Locomotion.* Volume II. Abnormal Movements, Males & Females (Nude & Semi-Nude). New York, Dover Publications, 1979: 1081–1139.

135. Lanska DJ. American contributions to the development of medical motion pictures for recording neurologic disorders. *Neurology* 2001; 56 (Suppl. 3):A87–A88.

136. Lanska DJ, Renda J. The Muybridge-Dercum collaboration for motion picture recording of neurologic disorders. *Neurology* 2004; 62 (Suppl. 5):A199.

137. Tate DG, Findley T Jr., Dijkers M, et al. Randomized clinical trials in medical rehabilitation research. *Am J Phys Mede Rehabil* 1999; 78:486–499.

138. Lind KA. Synthesis of studies on stroke rehabilitation. *J Chron Dis* 1982; 35:133–149.

139. Dobkin BH. Rehabilitation after stroke. *N Engl J Med* 2005; 352:1677–1684.

140. Fraser HW, Ersoy Y, Bowman E, et al. The development of stroke services: Entering the new millennium. *Scot Med J* 1999; 44:166–170.

141. Jorgensen HS, Nakayama H, Raaschou HO, et al. The effect of a stroke unit: Reductions in mortality, discharge rate to nursing home, length of hospital stay, and cost. *Stroke* 1995; 26:1178–1182.

142. Langhorne P, Duncan P. Does the organization of postacute stroke care really matter? *Stroke* 2001; 32:268–274.

143. Langhorne P, Legg L. Evidence behind stroke rehabilitation. *J Neurol Neurosurg Psychiatry* 2003; 73 (Suppl. IV):iv18–iv21.

144. Lehmann JF, DeLateur BJ, Fowler RS Jr, et al. Stroke: Does rehabilitation affect outcome? *Arch Phys Med Rehabil.* 1975; 56:375–382.

145. Dennis M, Langhorne P. So stroke units save lives? Where do we go from here? *BMJ* 1994; 309:1273–1277.

146. Evans A, Perez I, Harraf F, et al. Can differences in management processes explain different outcomes between stroke unit and stroke-team care? *Lancet* 2001; 358:1586–1592.

147. Kramer AM, Steiner JF, Schlenker RE, et al. Outcomes and costs after hip fracture and stroke: A comparison of rehabilitation settings. *JAMA* 1997; 277:396–404.

148. Langhorne P, Dennis MS, Williams BO. Stroke units: Their role in acute stroke management. *Vasc Med Rev* 1995; 6:33–44.

149. Langhorne P, Wagenaar R, Partridge C. Physiotherapy after stroke: More is better? *Physiother Res Int* 1996; 1:75–88.

150. Ottenbacher KJ, Jarnell S. The results of clinical trials in stroke rehabilitation research. *Arch Neurol* 1993; 50:37–44.

151. Rønning OM, Guldvog B. Outcome of subacute stroke rehabilitation: A randomized controlled trial. *Stroke* 1998; 29:779–784.

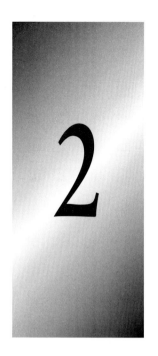

Epidemiology of Stroke*

Valery L. Feigin
Carlene M.M. Lawes
Derrick A. Bennett
Richard D. Zorowitz
Craig S. Anderson

S troke is a major non-communicable disease of increasing socioeconomic importance in aging populations. According to the World Health Organization (WHO) Global Burden of Disease report, stroke was the second leading cause of mortality worldwide in 1990 and the third leading cause of mortality in developed countries (1), causing approximately 4.4 million deaths worldwide.(2) The most recent estimates showed that in 2002, the number of deaths due to stroke reached 5.51 million (3) worldwide, with two-thirds of these deaths occurring in developing countries (4). Stroke also is a major cause of long-term disability (5), and has an enormous emotional and socioeconomic impact on patients, families, and health services. The lifetime cost of stroke per patient is estimated at between $US18,538 and $US228,038.(6) By the year 2020, stroke, along with

coronary artery disease, is expected to be the leading cause of lost healthy life years (7).

Stroke mortality data from many countries generally show that mortality rates have declined over recent decades, most notably in Japan, North America, and Western Europe (1, 8). The contributions of changes in incidence and improved survival to the downward trend in stroke mortality have not been quantified adequately, chiefly because of the difficulties involved in measuring the incidence of stroke accurately. Data from the WHO Monitoring Trends and Determinants in Cardiovascular Disease (MONICA) Stroke Project (9) showed a general tendency of declining mortality and incidence from stroke in people aged 35 to 64 years. This study also reported large geographical differences in both mortality and case-fatality. Substantial geographic variation in the incidence of stroke was also reported for older people in a review of the literature in 1992 (10), while similar between-country age-specific rates for men (11), and little geographic variation in rates, were reported in subsequent reviews of population-based studies (12, 13). Most reviews in this area, while providing important information, have been confined largely to limited age groups within a population (10–15), or included studies with different designs (e.g. population-based studies, hospital-based studies, official mortality statistic studies) (15–18). There are few recent reviews with respect to prevalence of stroke (17, 18), and no reviews

*This chapter has been modified and is an updated version of an article which originally appeared in *Lancet Neurology*. The book editors and publisher express their thanks to the original authors for their gracious help in allowing us to use their work. *From*: Feigin VL, Lawes CM, Bennett DA, Anderson CS. Stroke epidemiology: a review of population-based studies of incidence, prevalence, and case-fatality in the late 20th century. *Lancet Neurol.* 2003 Jan;2(1):43–53.

TABLE 2-1

Characteristics of Population-based Studies Included in the Analysis of Stroke Incidence, Mortality and Case-fatality (≥1990)

STUDY POPULATION, REFERENCE	YEAR(S) OF DATA COLLECTION	DURATION OF STUDY (YEARS)	POPULATION SIZE	AGE RANGE OF POPULATION STUDIED	TOTAL NO. OF INCIDENT STROKES
Melbourne, Australia[25]	1996–1997	1	133816	All	276
Perth, Australia[32]	1995–1996	1	136095*	All	213*
Fredenksberg, Denmark:[42]	1989–1990	1	85611	All	262
South London, UK[26]	1995–1996	2	234533	All	612
Espoo-Kauniainen, Finland[39]	1989–1991	2	134804	≥25*	594
Martinique, French West Indies[27]	1998–1999	1	381364	All	580
Oyabe, Japan[40]	1987–1991	4	170312	≥25	701
Erlangen, Germany[22,33]	1994–1998	2	101450	All	354
Arcadia, Greece[23]	1993–1995	2	80774	≥18	555
Belluno, Italy[28]	1992–1993	1	211389	All	474
L'Aquila, Italy[24]	1994	1	297838	All	819
Auckland, New Zealand[29]	1991–1992	1	945369	≥15*	1305
Inherred, Norway[30]	1994–1996	2	69295	≥15	432
Novosibirsk, Russia[31]	1992	1	158234	All	366
Uzhgorod, West Ukraine[37]	1999–2000	1	125482	All	352

*Additional data were provided by corresponding author of the publication. IS stands for ischemic stroke, PICH – for primary intracerebral hemorrhage, SAH – for subarachnoid hemorrhage, UND – for undetermined pathological type of stroke.

have been published on the incidence of ischemic stroke subtypes.

With these limitations in mind, and the evidence of changing stroke epidemiology (11), the aim of this chapter is to analyze published population-based studies from predominantly developed Western countries of the incidence, prevalence, mortality, and case-fatality of stroke from 1990 onwards, and to review secular trends in incidence and case-fatality.

METHODOLOGY OF DATA COMPILATION

Data for this chapter were identified by searches of MED-LINE (1966 to August 2002), and references from relevant articles. Different subsets of studies were potentially eligible for different parts of this review. The search terms "population-based", "community-based", "community", "epidemiology", "epidemiological", "incidence", "prevalence", "attack rates", "survey", "surveillance",

CRUDE INCIDENCE FOR TOTAL STROKES AND 95% CI	HOSPITAL ADMISSION RATE	CT/MRI OR AUTOPSY RATE	TIMING OF CT/MRI AFTER STROKE	TYPES OF STROKE BY AGE-SEX GROUPS, AS DETERMINED BY CT/MRI/AUTOPSY FINDINGS (CEREBRAL ANGIOGRAPHY OR CSF FOR SAH)
2.1 (1.8, 2.3)	Not reported	91%	28 days	Age-sex specific rates for IS, PICH, SAH, UND
1.6 (1.4, 1.8)*	88%	78%	Not reported	Age-sex specific rates for IS and IS subtypes, PICH, SAH, UND
3.1 (2.7, 3.4)	Not reported	74%	Not reported	Total rates for IS, PICH, SAH, UND
1.3 (1.2, 1.4)	84%	88%	30 days	Total rates for IS, PICH, SAH, UND
2.2 (2.0, 2.4)	86%	62%	Not reported	Age-sex specific rates for total strokes & SAH
1.6 (1.5, 1.8)	94%	93%	30 days	Age-sex specific rates for total strokes, total rates for IS, PICH, SAH, UND
4.1 (3.8, 4.4)	41%	Not reported	Not reported	Age-sex specific rates for total strokes
1.3 (1.2, 1.4)	95%	96%	Between 3–14 days	Age-sex specific rates for IS and IS subtypes, PICH, SAH, UND
3.4 (3.1, 3.7)	90%	82%	7 days	Age-sex specific rates for IS, PICH, SAH, UND, total rates for IS subtypes
2.2 (2.0, 2.4)	92%	90%	30 days	Age-sex specific rates for IS, PICH, SAH, UND
2.8 (2.6, 2.9)	92%	89%	7 days	Age-sex specific rates for IS, PICH, SAH, UND
1.4 (1.3, 1.5)	73%	41%	30 days	Age-sex specific rates for total strokes and SAH
3.1 (2.8, 3.4)	87%	88%	21 days	Age-sex specific rates for IS, PICH, SAH, UND
2.3 (2.1, 2.5)	60%	46%	28 days	Age-sex specific rates for total strokes
2.8 (2.5, 3.1)	66%	41%	Not reported	Age-sex specific rates for total strokes

"mortality", "morbidity", "fatality", "case-fatality", "stroke", "isch(a)emic stroke", "intracerebral", "intra-parenchymal", "subarachnoid", "h(a)emorrhage", and "trends" were used.

Eligibility criteria for studies of stroke incidence, prevalence, mortality, and case-fatality were as follows: (1) complete, population-based case ascertainment, based on multiple overlapping sources of information (hospitals, outpatient clinics, death certificates); (2) standard WHO definition of stroke as "rapidly developed signs of focal (or global) disturbance of cerebral function lasting longer than 24 hours (unless interrupted by death), with no apparent nonvascular cause" (19); (3) first-ever-in-a-lifetime stroke cases reported (for incidence studies only); (4) data collection over whole years in 1990 or later periods (earlier studies were included only if data for 1990 or a later period of data collection were reported); (5) no upper age limit for the population studied; (6) availability of raw numbers sufficient to calculate the rates in question (if not all raw numbers were available in an otherwise eligible publication, a corresponding author of the publication was contacted for missing data); (7) prospective study design; and (8) presentation of data in the mid-decade age bands. These eligibility criteria (except 4 and 5) were largely based on "ideal" criteria suggested by Sudlow and Warlow (20) for comparable stroke incidence studies. Only papers published in English were reviewed. Analysis of stroke incidence and case-fatality was confined to first-ever-in-a-lifetime strokes. Stroke prevalence studies that reported only rates associated with disability or impairment were excluded. If several studies reported the same population over different periods of time, the latest study was used for stroke incidence/prevalence analyses, and all studies were used for the analysis of trends.

Stroke subtype-specific analyses were confined to those population-based studies where computed tomography (CT), magnetic-resonance imaging (MRI), or autopsy findings were available for at least 70% of stroke cases. Strokes were classified into four major types: ischemic stroke (IS), primary intracerebral hemorrhage (PICH), subarachnoid hemorrhage (SAH), and undetermined stroke (UND). IS was diagnosed if CT/MRI within 30 days of stroke showed infarct or no relevant lesion, and/or autopsy showed IS. PICH was diagnosed if CT/MRI and/or autopsy showed PICH. Acceptable criteria for diagnosis of SAH included a clinical picture that was supported by characteristic cerebrospinal fluid (CSF) and/or autopsy/CT/cerebral angiography findings. Patients who fulfilled the WHO criteria for stroke, but for whom neither a CT/MRI nor an autopsy (a cerebral angiography or CSF examination for cases suspected of SAH) was performed, were classified as patients with UND stroke. These criteria (except for UND) are based on standard definitions suggested by Sudlow and Warlow (12) for comparing pathological stroke subtypes. Ischemic strokes (IS) were categorized into four groups, whenever possible, from the original publication: large artery disease (LAD), cardioembolic (CE), small artery disease (SAD) (including lacunar strokes), and other (including boundary strokes).

There was no time limit for studies of time trends in stroke incidence, mortality, and case-fatality. Eligibility criteria were as follows: (1) criteria for comparable studies of stroke incidence suggested by Sudlow and Warlow (20), including WHO definition of stroke, availability of first-ever-in-a-lifetime stroke data, complete, community-based case-ascertainment, and prospective study design; (2) data collection over a period of several years (continuously or periodically for at least one whole calendar year each period) in one and the same catchment area; (3) no upper age limit for the population studied; and (4) availability of age-standardized

incidence/mortality data for time periods compared. Only papers published in English were reviewed.

The incidence of first-ever-in-a-lifetime stroke was calculated per 1,000 person-years. Mortality rates were calculated in the same fashion, with the numerator consisting of all fatalities occurring within one month of the onset of a new stroke. Since stroke case-fatality (the proportion of fatal strokes in all first-ever-in-a-lifetime strokes) at 28 days and at one month are very similar, these figures were presented under the combined heading 'one month case-fatality rates'. The prevalence rate was expressed as the number of patients with self-reported stroke per 1,000 of the population. Incidence (first-ever-in-a-lifetime stroke only) and prevalence were computed by age, sex, and stroke subtype. Age standardization of incidence and prevalence figures was performed using the direct method, with weights from the Segi 1996 world population (21) as the standard population. Age-standardized incidence for those aged over 55, and prevalence for those aged over 65, and their corresponding 95% confidence intervals (CIs) were plotted for each study to facilitate comparison. These age cutoffs were necessary to maximize the number of studies that were included in the age-standardized comparisons. Wider age ranges would have resulted in several studies being excluded, as they did not provide disaggregated data for younger age groups. However, the older age groups still included the majority of stroke events in all studies. Only published age-standardized rates were compared for time trends in stroke incidence.

STROKE INCIDENCE

Fifteen population-based stroke incidence studies were identified and included in the analysis (Table 2-1 and Figure 2-1). These studies covered a population of 3,266,366 in 13 countries, with 4,398,158 person-years of observation. The mean frequency of hospital admission was 81%, ranging from 41% in Japan to 94.6% in Germany. In 10 out of the 15 studies, the information on timing of CT/MRI after stroke onset was not reported. In three studies (22–24), CT/MRI was done within two weeks after stroke onset, and in the other seven studies (25–31) this timing was within 28 to 30 days. Overall, diagnosis of major stroke subtypes was established by CT/MRI or autopsy in 76% of cases (range 41% to 95.5%; and in 10 of the 15 studies this figure was over 70%). Mean age at onset was reported in 9 (60%) studies, and among male patients was 69.8 years (range 60.8 in Uzhgorod, Ukraine to 75.3 in Innherred, Norway), and among female patients mean age at onset was 74.8 years (range 66.6 in Uzhgorod, Ukraine to 78.0 in Perth, Australia).

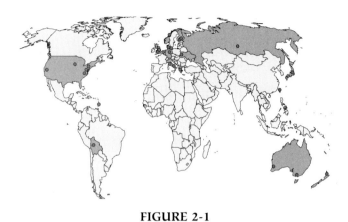

FIGURE 2-1

The fifteen population-based stroke incidence studies included in this chapter's data, covering a population of 3,266,366 in 13 countries, with 4,398,158 person-years of observation.

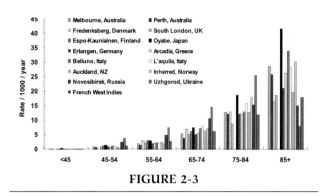

FIGURE 2-3

The age-specific rates of stroke increased progressively with each decade of life. For example, the rate of total stroke for those aged less than 45 years ranged from 0.1 to 0.3 per 1,000 person-years, while in those aged 75 to 84 years the range was 12.0 to 20.0 per 1,000 person-years in most studies.

Figure 2-2 shows the proportional frequency of stroke subtypes in the 10 studies (4,578 strokes) that provided these data. The proportion of IS ranged from 67.3% to 80.5%, with PICH (6.5– 19.6%), SAH (0.8–7.0%), and undetermined stroke (UND) (2.0–14.5%) following. Data on ischemic stroke subtypes were available for studies from Australia (32) and Germany (33). An IS subtype was determined for all strokes in one study (32), but only two-thirds of IS in the other (33), making comparison difficult. LAD constituted 68.0% and 13.4%, CE 17.8% and 26.9%, SAD 9.7% and 22.6%, other and undetermined types of IS, 4.6% and 37.1% respectively in the two studies.

The age-specific rates of stroke increased progressively with each decade of life (Figure 2-3). For example, the rate of total stroke for those aged less than 45 years ranged from 0.1 to 0.3 per 1,000 person-years, while

in those aged 75–84 years the range was 12.0 to 20.0 per 1,000 person-years in most studies. The highest age-specific rates occurred in Oyabe (Japan), Novosibirsk (Russia) and Uzhgorod (Ukraine).

The age-standardized incidence of total stroke for people aged 55 years or more ranged from 4.2 (Perth, Australia) to 11.7 (Uzhgorod, Ukraine) per 1,000 person-years (Figure 2-4), but in 12 of the 15 studies they ranged from 4.2 to 6.5 per 1,000 person-years. The age-standardized rates of total stroke in people aged 55 years or more were not significantly different between study populations, with the exception of Ukraine, Russia, and Japan, where rates were the highest. Fewer studies provided data on stroke subtype, but age-standardized rates per 1,000 person-years for IS ranged from 3.4 (Perth, Australia) to 5.2 (L'Aquila, Italy), for PICH 0.3 (Perth, Australia) to 1.2 (L'Aquila, Italy), and for SAH 0.03 (Fredenksberg, Denmark) to 0.2 (Inherred, Norway) per 1,000 person-years.

With a few exceptions, the incidence of all strokes combined, age-specific incidence, and proportions of stroke subtypes exhibit rather modest geographical variation between the studies included in the analyses, as compared to that observed in the MONICA Project (50, 51). Highest stroke incidence in Russia and Ukraine can be readily attributed to well-known social and economic changes that occurred in these countries over the last decade, including changes in medical care, access to vascular prevention strategies among those at high risk, and the prevalence of risk factors. Reasons for the relatively high stroke incidence in Japan compared to other developed countries are not clear, but can be related to genetic and environmental (e.g. diet, prevalence of cardiovascular risk factors, etc.) parameters. Contributing factors to the four- to seven-fold geographical differences observed in the incidence of IS and PICH may be attributed to the

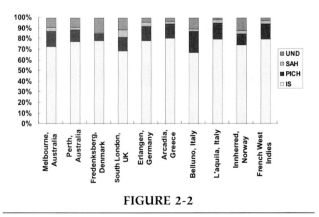

FIGURE 2-2

The proportional frequency of stroke subtypes in 10 studies (4,578 strokes). The proportion of IS ranged from 67.3% to 80.5%, with PICH (6.5–19.6%), SAH (0.8–7.0%), and undetermined stroke (UND) (2.0–14.5%).

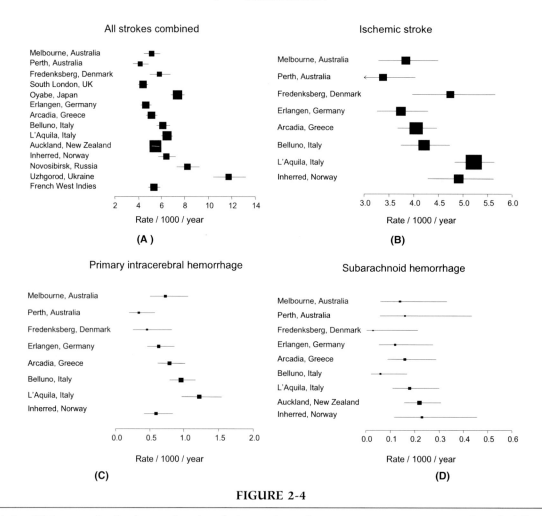

FIGURE 2-4

Stroke statistics. (A) Age-standardized rates of total stroke in people aged 55 years or more were not significantly different between study populations, with the exception of Ukraine, Russia, and Japan, where rates were the highest. (B) Ischemic stroke data. (C) Primary intracerebral hemorrhage data. (D) Subarachnoid hemorrhage data.

Only studies where a CT/MRI or an autopsy was performed in no less than 70% of cases were included in the analyses of stroke subtypes. All stroke subtype analyses were based on cases classified by either CT/MRI/autopsy findings for IS and PICH, or cerebrospinal fluid examination and/or cerebral angiography for SAH.

different proportions and timing of CT/MRI investigations in the studies analyzed. Recent features in stroke incidence and outcome include a leveling off of previous potential geographical differences in stroke incidence and prevalence, and trends towards stabilizing, or increasing rates, especially in the elderly population. The relative between-country similarity in rates is not too surprising, given the homogeneity of the populations studied (predominantly Caucasians, with the exception of the Japanese population) and the restricted time period for data collection (from 1990 onwards). In the Oyabe Study (Japan) (40), the proportion of intracerebral hemorrhage in 1987–1991 was reported to be relatively high (16.4%), as compared to the 1977–1981 period, and that of other studies included in the analysis. Since no information on the documentation of stroke subtypes

by neuroimaging techniques was provided in the publication, no reliable comparisons could be made with other studies. Early total and subtype-specific stroke case-fatality also was similar between the study populations, with the exception of Japan (low rates) and Italy (high rates). A combination of LAD and CE strokes constituted the largest proportion of ISs, which is in line with results of a population-based stroke incidence study in Rochester, Minnesota, United States performed in 1985–1989 (52).

While there are no substantial geographical variations in the incidence of SAH (65) and of all types of stroke combined (12, 13), contradictory findings were observed in the WHO MONICA Project (50, 51). This project found large geographical differences in the incidence and case-fatality of total strokes, and of SAH specifically.

However, studies analyzed in the MONICA Project were performed in the late 1980s, and were restricted to people aged between 25–64 (51) or 35–64 (50) years. However, this review of stroke incidence studies includes more countries (13) than that in the WHO MONICA Project (11 countries) (50). Compared to recent reviews of stroke incidence (10–13), this review is based upon larger numbers of comparable population-based studies performed from 1990 onwards, and covers over three million people of all ages and over four million person-years of observation.

Although more studies in the 1990s, subsequent to the reviews by Sudlow and Warlow (12, 13), reviewed stroke epidemiology for the 1980s, the methodology proposed for undertaking stroke incidence studies has not been updated substantially. In particular, few studies identified stroke incidence according to defined pathological types. However, unlike the previous review by Sudlow and Warlow (12), this methodology extracts data largely from published papers. Unfortunately, three recent population-based stroke incidence studies were excluded from the analysis because they did not meet the inclusion criteria: a study in Sweden (44) was restricted to people aged up to 74 years; a study in Poland (45) did not include SAH, and did not provide age-specific rates for other stroke subtypes; and a study in Portugal (46) was published in the abstract format only, and did not provide age-specific data required for our analysis. Comparable age-standardized rates could not be calculated for a study in Finland (39) because no rates were given for people aged 75 to 84 and 85+ years in the publication. A study in West Indies (27) did not provide age-specific data for stroke subtypes.

Complexities of Measuring the Incidence of Stroke

Stroke should be studied in a population-wide context, because a large proportion of the burden of care for stroke is borne by health services outside the hospital sector and by families of affected patients (72). Assessing the need for prevention strategies and health services, and of geographical and secular trends, is most sensitively achieved with standardized population-based registries, as analysis limited to hospital cases, or varying criteria and definitions, may distort results. However, studying stroke in such a manner is particularly challenging (20), and therefore relatively uncommon in comparison to other study designs, particularly in developing countries where resources and the necessary research infrastructure are limited. Since a major challenge is to ensure accurate case-ascertainment, many population-based stroke registries have been limited to people under the age of 75 years, despite excluding over half of all strokes in the population under

investigation. Tilling et al. (73) used advanced capture-recapture methods to check for completeness of case ascertainment in the South London stroke register. They found that a variety of demographic and stroke severity variables were associated with case identification, and that a capture-recapture model without covariates underestimated the age-standardized incidence rates by as much as 12%. This approach was not used in the other studies reviewed in this chapter, so it is possible that age-standardized rates reported in publications are underestimates.

Only limited data for contemporary health planning can be extracted from stroke incidence studies prior to 1990, as they are either outdated, incomplete, or failed to reliably distinguish stroke subtypes. There is also evidence of inaccuracy of official stroke mortality statistics (74, 50, 75–81). High-quality population-based stroke incidence studies provide accurate data on the occurrence of first-ever-in-a-lifetime stroke, which are important for risk estimates and for comparison between different populations. Information on the occurrence of recurrent stroke is invaluable for estimates of the totality of the burden of stroke in a community, for health care planning, and as an indicator of the effectiveness of secondary stroke prevention programs. Increasing demand for more specific stroke care planning (e.g. accurate resource allocation for carrying out carotid endarterectomy, antithrombotic treatment, aneurysm surgery, etc.) require more detailed information, not just on the major stroke subtypes, but also on ischemic stroke subtypes.

Criteria by which the quality of population-based studies of stroke could be judged were published by Malmgren et al. (82) in 1987, and later updated by Bonita (1995) (83), and Sudlow and Warlow (1996) (20). These remain relevant for all incidence studies, at least in relatively affluent developed countries that have the ability to verify the diagnosis by CT/MRI in at least 80% of cases, and classify IS into subtypes (e.g. LAD, CE, and SAD including lacunar strokes). Other issues to consider are a large sample size to ensure sufficient number of incident strokes per year, and the presentation of age-specific data on first-ever-in-a-lifetime and recurrent stroke in the oldest age groups (≥85 years).

These above-mentioned criteria are not practical for stroke studies undertaken in developing countries, where most strokes occur and resources are limited. To address the problem of accurate and comparable data in these countries, a stepwise approach to increasing detail in the data to be collected for stroke surveillance has recently been proposed by the WHO (71). This flexible and sustainable system includes three steps: standard (hospital-based case-ascertainment for calculating hospital admission due to stroke), expanded population coverage (ascertainment of death certificates or verbal autopsy in the whole community to calculate mortality rates), and comprehensive population-based (additional ascertainment of non-fatal events to calculate incidence and case-fatality in the community). These steps could provide vital, but missing, basic epidemiological estimates of the burden of stroke in many countries around the world.

STROKE PREVALENCE

Nine prevalence studies that met eligibility criteria were identified (Table 2-2 and Figure 2-5). Overall, 8,788 strokes were reported, with age-specific prevalence increasing with advancing age. The age-standardized prevalence for people aged 65 years or more ranged from 46.1 (four regions, United States) to 72.3 (L'Aquila, Italy) per 1,000 population, but ranged from 58.8 (Auckland, New Zealand) to 92.6 (L'Aquila, Italy) per 1,000 population for men, and from 32.2 (four regions, United States) to 48.3 (L'Aquila, Italy) per 1,000 population for women. No strokes were detected among 213 screened adults aged 20–96 in Indonesia. Overall, there was no significant difference in age-standardized prevalence between selected populations in people aged 65 years or more, except in L'Aquila, Italy, which reported the highest figures. Only three studies (34–36) reported both total and disability/impairment associated frequencies of stroke, with the proportion of disability/impairment associated with stroke varying

from 55% in Auckland, New Zealand (36) to 77% in Yorkshire, United Kingdom (35).

Studies performed before 1990 have suggested that the worldwide prevalence of stroke, in all age groups of the population combined, varied between 4 and 20 per 1,000 population (41, 53–62). Since 1990, the range of crude prevalence showed far less geographical difference (5 to 10 per 1,000), with the exception of a rural population of Bolivia, where the prevalence of stroke is as low as 1.7 per 1,000, and Kitava, Indonesia, where no strokes were detected at all. However, in the study in Bolivia, only patients with stroke-related disability were included. In the Indonesian study, only 213 subjects older than 20 years were screened, and the refusal rate in the older age group was 63%. The minimal variation in age-specific and age-standardized prevalence of stroke across the populations is consistent with the relative geographical similarity in stroke incidence and case-fatality. Similar results were found in another review of stroke prevalence studies (63). The relatively high prevalence of stroke in L'Aquila, Italy, could be related to inclusion of minor strokes in the study (64). In only three of the studies analyzed, prevalence of stroke-related disability was reported (34–36), and suggested that about half to three-quarters of prevalent cases had stroke-related disability.

Several recent stroke prevalence studies were not included in this analysis because they did not meet the inclusion criteria. For example, a study from Tanzania was restricted to hemiplegic stroke patients with residual

---

TABLE 2-2
Characteristics of Population-based Stroke Prevalence Studies Included in the Analysis (≥1990)

Study, Reference	Year(s) of Data Collection	Age Range of Population (Years)	Total No. of Stroke Patients	Observed Crude Rate/1,000 Within the Screened Age Group with 95% CI Where Available		
				Men	Women	Total
Auckland, NZ[55]	1991–1992	≥ 15	7491*	10.7	9.7	10.2
Rotterdam, NL[103]	1990–1993	≥ 55	352	5.0 (4.2; 5.8)	4.3 (3.7; 4.9)	NR
Cordillera, Bolivia[70]	1994	All	16	2.5	1.0	1.7 (0.9–2.5)
4 Regions, USA[104]	1989–1990	≥ 65	246**	6.8	3.2	4.7
Yorkshire, UK[35]	1991	≥ 55	415	5.0 (4.3; 5.8)§	4.4 (3.9; 5.1)§	4.7 (4.3; 5.2)
Newcastle, UK[34]	1993	≥ 45	116	Not reported	Not reported	4.7 (4.6; 4.9)
Kitava, Papua New Guinea[105]	1990	20–96	0	0	0	0
Taiwan, China[106]	1994	≥ 35	71	6.37	5.53	5.95
L'Aquila, Italy[64]	1992	≥ 65	80	9.6 (6.9–12.3)	5.5 (3.6–7.3)	7.3 (5.7–8.8)

*Auckland figures are extrapolations to the entire NZ population, as per original publication. **Calculated from the publication cited; NR – not reported. §No age-specific numbers of stroke or population at risk reported.

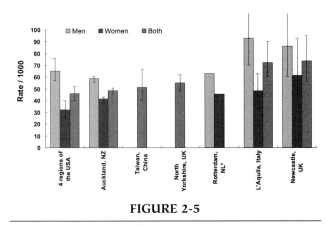

FIGURE 2-5

Stroke prevalence data. There was no significant difference in age-standardized prevalence between selected populations in people aged 65 years or more, except L'Aquila, Italy which reported the highest figures. See text for details.

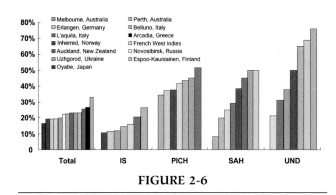

FIGURE 2-6

Stroke case-fatality data. In 13 of 15 selected studies that reported either age-specific or total case-fatality within 1 month of stroke onset, 1,608 of 7,021 total strokes were fatal (22.9%). Case-fatality of total strokes varied little between the populations, with the exception of Oyabe, Japan (17%) and Belluno, Italy (33%).

impairment/disability only (47). Data from a study in Calcutta (48) were not presented in the mid-decade age bands, thus preventing calculation of age-adjusted rates comparable with other studies included in this analysis. In a study from Bengal (49), age-specific data were not reported for people over 61 years of age.

Complexities of Measuring the Prevalence of Stroke

Prevalence of stroke may be determined by cross-sectional surveys, cohort studies, or by indirect calculations from incidence studies that have followed up cases at uniform time intervals after stroke onset (36, 63). International comparisons of stroke prevalence are fraught with difficulties (36), because of the relatively low occurrence of stroke in some countries, wide between-country variations in the population age structure, and few prevalence studies including people in the oldest age groups who are at greatest risk of the disease. Further difficulties include measurement bias, poor verification of stroke subtypes, and resource expenses. Although the prevalence of stroke-related disability is important for health care planning (36, 62), these estimates may not be reliable because of overlapping disabilities caused by co-morbid disorders which often accompany stroke in older people (13).

Suggested criteria for stroke prevalence studies include using the WHO definition of stroke, and a population-based study design of a large, well-defined, and stable population. The choice of study design may vary (e.g., a door-to-door survey may be the design of choice for an elderly population with restricted mobility.) Data should be presented by gender in standard age bands for cases aged ≥85 years.

Self-reported stroke and medically confirmed stroke should be reported, with 95% confidence intervals around prevalence data.

STROKE CASE-FATALITY

In 13 of 15 selected studies which reported either age-specific or total case-fatality within one month of stroke onset (Figure 2-6), 1,608 of 7,021 total strokes were fatal (22.9%). As shown in Figure 2-6, case-fatality of total strokes varied little between the populations, with the exception of Oyabe, Japan (17%) and Belluno, Italy (33%). Age-specific data on stroke case-fatality within 1 month of stroke onset were available in four studies (29, 31, 32, 37), thus allowing calculation of one-month mortality rates. In these studies, age- and sex-specific annual mortality rates increased progressively with age.

TIME TRENDS IN STROKE INCIDENCE AND MORTALITY

Eight population-based studies (29, 32, 38–43) that evaluated secular trends in stroke incidence in a given population are listed in Table 2-3. Overall, these studies yielded 9,121,218 person-years of observation, constituting 13,461 new stroke cases. In five of the eight studies, all age-groups of the population were covered by a stroke registry, while in three studies, the population was restricted to the range 15 or 25 years of age and above. The period of observation varied from seven (Perth, Australia) (32) to 34 years (Rochester, MN, United

TABLE 2-3

Characteristics of Selected Population-based Studies on Time Trends in Stroke Incidence, Mortality and Case-fatality

Study Population, Reference	Age Range	Total Number of Incident Strokes	Total Number of Person-Years	Years Included	Changes in Stroke Incidence	Changes in Stroke Mortality	Changes in Stroke Case-Fatality
Rochester, MN, USA[41]	All	2521	1,665,257*	1955 to 1979 1970s to 1980s	↓ 38% ↑ 19%	NR	At 1 month and 12 month
Fredenksberg, Denmark[42]	All	927	378,240	1972–74 to 1989–90	↑ 15%	NR	NR
Espoo-Kauniainen, Finland[39]	All	1093	769,508	1972–73 to 1978–80 1978–80 to 1989–91	↓ 28% ↑ 9%	} ↓ 46%	} ↓ 33%
Oyabe, Japan[40]	≥25	2068	460,026*	1977–81 to 1982–86 1982–86 to 1987–91 1982–86 to 1987–91	↓ 25–30% ↓ 9% in men ↑ 2% in women	} ↓ NR	} ↓ 26%
Auckland, New Zealand[29]	≥15	1776	1,774,833	1981–82 to 1991–92	↓ 9% in men ↑ 9% in women	} ↓ NR	} ↓ 16%
Copenhagen County, Denmark[38]	≥25	1206	2,121,600	1982 to 1991	↓ 3%	↓ 2%	NR
Novosibirsk, Russia[43]	All	3406	1,683,754*	1982 to 1988 1988 to 1992	↓ 30% ↑ 8%	NR	} ↓ 24%
Perth, Australia[32]	All	464	268,000	1989–90 to 1995–96	↓ 27%	↓ 35%	↑ 5%

Abbreviations: n = number of cases, NR = not reported, (no change in rates, (increase in rates, (decrease in rates. *Estimated from the publication cited

States) (41). All studies provided age-standardized rates for time periods.

While the studies covered different time periods, several common themes were evident. Most of the studies demonstrated a decline in stroke incidence, through the late 1970s or early 1980s (29, 38–41, 43). However, in several studies, this decline appears to have reached a plateau or even reversed into the late 1980s and early 1990s (29, 39–41, 43). There were exceptions, though, with a continued decline in rates being reported in Perth, Australia (32) between 1989–1990 and 1995–1996, and in males in Oyabe, Japan (40) between 1982–1986 and 1987–1991. Data from Fredenksberg, Denmark (42) reported a net increase in incidence, but this study compared rates over a broad time period (1972–1974 to 1989–1990).

Of the few population-based studies that reported time trend data for stroke mortality, the consistent finding was that of a decrease in rates from the 1970s through the 1990s (29, 32, 38–40). Four studies recorded declines in case-fatality between the early 1970s and early 1990s (29, 39, 40, 43), and two reported no change (32, 41).

Evaluating the Time Trends of Stroke

In five of the eight selected studies on stroke incidence time trends, a decrease in stroke incidence to the mid-1980s, and an increase in rates in the late 1980s or early 1990s was observed, especially in the elderly. Even in Japan, a country with the most marked decrease in stroke incidence in 1977–1986 , there was an increase in stroke incidence in women and in people aged over 85 years (40). Although no changes in overall stroke incidence were observed in Auckland, New Zealand for the period 1981–1992, there was an increase in rates in women (29). The only study that showed a decrease of stroke incidence in the mid-1990s as compared to the late 1980s was the study in Perth, Australia (32). It is possible that variations in competing risks (exposures) for diseases across countries might explain the different secular trends in incidence. The changing pattern of stroke incidence over time could be attributed to changing patterns of exposures to, or control of causative risk factors for, stroke (including socioeconomic and environmental factors) in these populations, changing completeness of case ascertainment (e.g. better identification of minor strokes from neuroimaging and diagnostic awareness), birth-cohort or period-cohort effects (e.g. changes in fetal or early childhood health many years ago), or all of these.

Most studies have found a decrease or no change in early stroke case-fatality over the last 20–30 years. Official stroke mortality data from over two dozen countries (8, 84) showed that, in general, these figures have declined for several decades, most notably in Japan,

North America, and Western Europe. In many industrialized countries, stroke mortality has been falling since the early 1950s, but the rate of this decline has decelerated recently (85–87). The contributions of changes in incidence and improved survival to the downward trends in stroke mortality have not been quantified adequately, chiefly because of the difficulties involved in measuring the incidence of stroke accurately (20, 72). Several studies have suggested that declining case-fatality is a major contributor to the declining stroke mortality (88), but these data were not population-based (89–91). Population-based data on trends in stroke mortality and case-fatality are scarce, so it is not possible to assess whether the trends in stroke incidence are associated with similar trends in stroke mortality. Only two studies (32, 38) thus far have found such correlation. Interestingly, the fall in stroke incidence and mortality was associated with no change in stroke case-fatality in one study (32), and an increase in case-fatality in another (38). The most likely explanation for the commonly observed recent increase in stroke incidence is rapid aging of the population. Whether the observed continuous decrease in the incidence and mortality rates from myocardial infarction (92–101) contributed to the changing pattern of stroke incidence remains to be studied. Even less about stroke time trends is known in developing countries.

ADVANTAGES AND LIMITATIONS

Since the publication of two reviews of stroke incidence in various countries in 1997 (12) and 1998 (13), 17 new population-based studies (nine new stroke incidence studies published since 1990 and eight new studies on secular trends in stroke incidence) and nine stroke prevalence studies have not been critically reviewed. In addition, all population age groups have been analyzed, the incidence and case-fatality of major stroke subtypes (including IS subtypes) have been reviewed, and the age-standardized estimates in the elderly population have been calculated without an upper age limit.

There are several limitations to these analyses. The studies of stroke incidence, case-fatality, and prevalence identified in this overview predominantly have been based on Caucasian populations in Western countries. In addition, these studies may not be entirely representative of the countries where they were carried out, due to within-country variations in stroke rates (25, 50, 66), including different rates in various ethnic groups (26, 67–69). No population-based stroke studies have been identified from developing countries, except a prevalence study in Bolivia (70). This precludes generalization of these data to developing countries, where three-quarters of all stroke deaths occur, and where the increasing burden of stroke is likely to be (71). In addition, the absence of time trend studies of stroke incidence in the late 1990s limits our ability to project reliably trends in stroke attack rates and outcome beyond the year 2000.

RESEARCH FRONTIERS

Despite numerous epidemiological studies performed to date, there remain several unresolved issues. First, there is an issue of increasing importance relating to stroke epidemiology in the developing world. While the studies included in this chapter provide some insights into the burden and time trends of stroke in predominantly Western countries, they do not address the burden of stroke in developing regions. Most stroke deaths occur in these regions, and could potentially increase. More stroke data on these regions, using the "best possible" stroke studies (such as a WHO stepwise surveillance system), will contribute to a greater understanding of stroke epidemiology and appropriate measures for stroke health care planning and prevention strategies.

Second, the reasons for changes in stroke incidence (first-ever-in-a-lifetime and recurrent stroke incidence) and mortality rates worldwide and nationwide over time need to be studied more closely. This would help to determine how much emphasis should be placed on secondary stroke prevention compared with primary prevention. In this respect, the necessity of high-quality comparable stroke studies in different parts of the world, including studies in developing countries and various ethnic/race groups of the population, cannot be overestimated. These studies would also allow more meaningful estimates of the worldwide burden of stroke.

Third, monitoring secular trends in the incidence and outcomes (natural history) of stroke in the same populations, together with determining the contribution of changes in stroke risk factors, would help to develop models for predicting future trends in stroke incidence and outcomes. This could lead to the development of best practices for its control, and a means to monitor the progress of prevention and management programs.

Fourth, the identification of differences and similarities of stroke incidence in different populations and its changes over time can also improve our knowledge of stroke etiology. An acceptable alternative to continuous monitoring of such time trends, which is expensive and impractical in most populations, is a performance of population-based incidence studies in the same population once every decade. Monitoring prevalence of stroke risk factors in the same populations can be achieved through risk factors surveillance systems, which could be initially implemented for major risk factors, and then for disease events (102).

Fifth, there is a need for more stroke prevalence studies in different parts of the world. In this respect, a door-to-door survey may be the design of choice. This method is simple, efficient, and can be implemented in many different settings around the world. A consensus for measurements that best reflect a prevalence of stroke-related disability should be developed to facilitate better health care planning.

Sixth, given the continuous aging of the population, particular attention should be given to covering all age groups, including people over 85 years old, the fastest growing segment of populations.

Finally, further attention should be given to verification of stroke subtypes, including ischemic stroke subtypes, because management and prevention strategies for different stroke subtypes vary. Improvement in the quality of routinely available stroke mortality data is also important.

CONCLUSION

A number of important conclusions may be drawn from this review of stroke epidemiology literature. Among areas with population-based studies, the overall age-standardized incidence of stroke in people aged ≥55 years ranged from 4.2 to 11.7 per 1,000 person-years. The proportion ranges of stroke subtypes is as follows: ischemic stroke 67% to 81%; primary intracerebral hemorrhage 7% to 20%; subarachnoid hemorrhage 1% to 7%; and undetermined pathological type of stroke 2% to 15%. Stroke incidence, prevalence, stroke-subtype structure, one month case-fatality, and mortality rates show modest geographical variations, with the exception of Ukraine, Russia, and Japan, where incidence rates are highest, and L'Aquila, Italy, where prevalence rates are highest. The average age of patients affected by stroke is 70 years in men and 75 years in women. More than half of all strokes occur in people over 75 years of age. The age-standardized prevalence rate of stroke in people aged ≥65 years ranges from 46 to 72 per 1,000 population Overall case-fatality within 1 month of stroke onset is approximately 23%, and is higher for intracerebral hemorrhage (42%) and subarachnoid hemorrhage (32%) than for ischemic stroke (16%). Overall, there is a trend towards stabilizing or increasing stroke incidence, especially in the elderly population. Finally, inferences from these data are limited to predominantly Caucasian populations in the developed counties.

Untangling the puzzle of trends in the impact of stroke is a matter of pressing importance. Stroke is a leading cause of disability in the community; and the elderly, the most stroke-prone age group, constitute the fastest-growing segment of the population. Data on trends in the cause-specific incidence of stroke provide important local feedback on public health measures, while patterns of case-fatality and outcome bear a closer relationship to acute treatment and rehabilitation. Both sets of data are required for effective planning of services, both in scope and scale, as they will inevitably come under increasing pressure from restructuring populations and adverse lifestyle changes.

References

1. Sarti C, Rastenyte D, Cepaitis Z, Tuomilehto J. International trends in mortality from stroke, 1968 to 1994. *Stroke* 2000; **31**(7):1588–1601.

2. Murray CJL, Lopez AD. Mortality by cause for eight regions of the world: Global Burden of Disease Study. *Lancet* 1997; **349**:1269–1276.

3. *The World Health Report 2004*. Geneva: World Health Organization, 2000.

4. *The World Health Report 2004*. Geneva: World Health Organization, 1998.

5. Foulkes MA, Wolf PA, Price TR, Mohr JP, Hier DB. The Stroke Data Bank: Design, methods, and baseline characteristics. *Stroke* 1988; **19**(5):547–554.

6. Payne KA, Huybrechts KF, Caro JJ, Green TJ, Klittich WS. Long term cost-of-illness in stroke: An international review *PharmacoEconomics* 2002; **20**(12): 813–825.

7. WHO. *The World Health Report 2000: Health Systems—Improving Performance*. Geneva: WHO, 2000.

8. Bonita R, Stewart A, Beaglehole R. International trends in stroke mortality: 1970–1985. *Stroke* 1990; **21**(7):989–992.

9. Thorvaldsen P, Kuulasmaa K, Rajakangas AM, Rastenyte D, Sarti C, Wilhelmsen L. Stroke trends in the WHO MONICA project. *Stroke* 1997; **28**(3):500–506.

10. Bonita R. Epidemiology of stroke. *Lancet* 1992; **339**(8789):342–344.

11. Bonita R, Beaglehole R, Asplund K. The worldwide problem of stroke. *Current Opinion in Neurology* 1994; **7**(1):5–10.

12. Sudlow CL, Warlow CP. Comparable studies of the incidence of stroke and its pathological types: Results from an international collaboration. International Stroke Incidence Collaboration. *Stroke* 1997; **28**(3):491–499.

13. Warlow CP. Epidemiology of stroke. *Lancet* 1998; **352 Suppl** 3:SIII1–SIII4.

14. Khaw KT. Epidemiology of stroke. *Journal of Neurology, Neurosurgery & Psychiatry* 1996; **61**(4):333–338.

15. Posner JD, Gorman KM, Woldow A. Stroke in the elderly: I. Epidemiology. *Journal of the American Geriatrics Society* 1984; **32**(2):95–102.

16. Kurtzke JF. Epidemiology of stroke: Methods and trends. *Health Reports* 1994; **6**(1):13–21.

17. Mas JL, Zuber M. Epidemiology of stroke. *Journal of Neuroradiology Journal de Neuroradiologie* 1993; **20**(2):85–101.

18. Viriyavejakul A. Stroke in Asia: An epidemiological consideration. *Clinical Neuropharmacology* 1990; **13 Suppl** 3:S26–S33.

19. Hatano S. Experience from a multicentre stroke register: A preliminary report. *Bulletin of the World Health Organization* 1976; **54**(5):541–553.

20. Sudlow CLM, Warlow CP. Comparing stroke incidence worldwide : What makes studies comparable? *Stroke* 1996; **27**(3):550–558.

21. Ahmad OB, Boschi-Pinto C, Murray CJL, Lozano R, Inoue M. Age standardization of rates: A new WHO world standard. 2001. Geneva, Switzerland, WHO. *GPE Discussion Paper Series: No. 31. EIP/GPE/EBD <http://www3.who.int/whosis/discussion_papers/htm/paper31.htm>*.

22. Kolominsky-Rabas PL, Weber M, Gefeller O, Neundoerfer B, Heuschmann PU. Epidemiology of ischemic stroke subtypes according to TOAST criteria: Incidence, recurrence, and long-term survival in ischemic stroke subtypes: A population-based study. *Stroke* 2001; **32**(12):2735–2740.

23. Vemmos KN, Bots ML, Tsibouris PK, Zis VP, Grobbee DE, Stranjalis GS, et al. Stroke incidence and case fatality in southern Greece: The Arcadia stroke registry. *Stroke* 1999; **30**(2):363–370.

24. Carolei A, Marini C, Di Napoli M, Di Gianfilippo G, Santalucia P, Baldassarre M, et al. High stroke incidence in the prospective community-based L'Aquila registry (1994–1998). First year's results. *Stroke* 1997; **28**(12):2500–2506.

25. Thrift AG, Dewey HM, Macdonell RAL, McNeil JJ, Donnan GA. Incidence of the major stroke subtypes: Initial findings from the North East Melbourne Stroke Incidence Study (NEMESIS). *Stroke* 2001; **32**(8):1732–1738.

26. Stewart JA, Dundas R, Howard RS, Rudd AG, Wolfe CDA. Ethnic differences in incidence of stroke: Prospective study with stroke register. *BMJ* 1999; **318**(7189):967–971.

27. Smadja D, Cabre P, May F, Fanon JL, Rene-Corail P, Riocreux C, et al. ERMANCIA: Epidemiology of stroke in Martinique, French West Indies: Part I: Methodology, incidence, and 30-day case fatality rate. *Stroke* 2001; **32**(12):2741–2747.

28. Lauria G, Gentile M, Fassetta G, Casetta I, Agnoli F, Andreotta G, et al. Incidence and prognosis of stroke in the Belluno Province, Italy: First-year results of a community-based study. *Stroke* 1995; **26**(10):1787–1793.

29. Bonita R, Broad JB, Beaglehole R. Changes in stroke incidence and case-fatality in Auckland, New Zealand, 1981–91. *Lancet* 1993; **342**(8885):1470–1473.

30. Ellekjaer H, Holmen J, Indredavik B, Terent A. Epidemiology of stroke in Innherred, Norway, 1994 to 1996. Incidence and 30-day case-fatality rate. *Stroke* 1997; **28**(11):2180–2184.

31. Feigin VL, Wiebers DO, Nikitin YP, O'Fallon WM, Whisnant JP. Stroke epidemiology in Novosibirsk, Russia: A population-based study. *Mayo Clinic Proceedings* 1995; **70**:847–852.

32. Jamrozik K, Broadhurst RJ, Lai N, Hankey GJ, Burvill PW, Anderson CS. Trends in the incidence, severity, and short-term outcome of stroke in Perth, Western Australia. *Stroke* 1999; **30**(10):2105–2111.

33. Kolominsky-Rabas PL, Sarti C, Heuschmann PU, Graf C, Siemonsen S, Neundoerfer B, et al. A prospective community-based study of stroke in Germany: The Erlangen Stroke Project (ESPro) : Incidence and case fatality at 1, 3, and 12 months. *Stroke* 1998; **29**(12):2501–2506.

34. O'Mahony PG, Thomson RG, Dobson R, Rodgers H, James OF. The prevalence of stroke and associated disability. *Journal of Public Health Medicine* 1999; **21**(2):166–171.

35. Geddes JM, Fear J, Tennant A, Pickering A, Hillman M, Chamberlain MA. Prevalence of self reported stroke in a population in northern England. *Journal of Epidemiology & Community Health* 1996; **50**(2):140–143.

36. Bonita R, Solomon N, Broad JB. Prevalence of stroke and stroke-related disability: Estimates from the Auckland Stroke Studies. *Stroke* 1997; **28**(10):1898–1902.

37. Mihalka L, Smolanka V, Bulecza B, Mulesa S, Bereczki D. A Ppopulation study of stroke in west Ukraine: Incidence, stroke services, and 30-day case fatality. *Stroke* 2001; **32**(10):2227–2231.

38. Thorvaldsen P, Davidsen M, Bronnum-Hansen H, Schroll M. Stable stroke occurrence despite incidence reduction in an aging population: Stroke trends in the Danish Monitoring Trends and Determinants in Cardiovascular Disease (MONICA) population. *Stroke* 1999; **30**(12):2529–2534.

39. Numminen H, Kotila M, Waltimo O, Aho K, Kaste M. Declining incidence and mortality rates of stroke in Finland from 1972 to 1991: Results of three population-based stroke registers. *Stroke* 1996; **27**(9):1487–1491.

40. Morikawa Y, Nakagawa H, Naruse Y, Nishijo M, Miura K, Tabata M, et al. Trends in stroke incidence and acute case fatality in a Japanese rural area: The Oyabe Study. *Stroke* 2000; **31**(7):1583–1587.

41. Brown RD, Whisnant JP, Sicks JD, O'Fallon WM, Wiebers DO. Stroke incidence, prevalence, and survival: Secular trends in Rochester, Minnesota, through 1989. *Stroke* 1996; **27**(3):373–380.

42. Jorgensen HS, Plesner AM, Hubbe P, Larsen K. Marked increase of stroke incidence in men between 1972 and 1990 in Frederiksberg, Denmark. *Stroke* 1992; **23**(12):1701–1704.

43. Feigin VL, Wiebers DO, Whisnant JP, O'Fallon WM. Stroke incidence and 30-day case-fatality rates in Novosibirsk, Russia, 1982 through 1992. *Stroke* 1995; **26**:924–929.

44. Stegmayr B, Asplund K, Wester PO. Trends in incidence, case-fatality rate, and severity of stroke in northern Sweden, 1985–1991. *Stroke* 1994; **25**(9):1738–1745.

45. Czlonkowska A, Ryglewicz D, Weissbein T, Baranska-Gieruszczak M, Hier DB. A prospective community-based study of stroke in Warsaw, Poland. *Stroke* 1994; **25**(3):547–551.

46. Rodrigues M, Noronha MM, Vieira-Dias M, I ourenço S, Santos-Bento M, Fernandes H, Stroke incidence and case-fatality in Portugal: Pop-basis 2000 study, final results. *Cerebrovascular Diseases* 2002; **13**((suppl 3)):47. (Abstract)

47. Walker RW, McLarty DG, Masuki G, Kitange HM, Whiting D, Moshi AF, et al. Age specific prevalence of impairment and disability relating to hemiplegic stroke in the Hai District of northern Tanzania. Adult Morbidity and Mortality Project. *Journal of Neurology, Neurosurgery & Psychiatry* 2000; **68**(6):744–749.

48. Banerjee TK, Mukherjee CS, Sarkhel A. Stroke in the urban population of Calcutta—an epidemiological study. *Neuroepidemiology* 2001; **20**(3):201–207.

49. Das SK, Sanyal K. Neuroepidemiology of major neurological disorders in rural Bengal. *Neurology India* 1996; **44**:47–58.

50. Thorvaldsen P, Asplund K, Kuulasmaa K, Rajakangas A-M, Schroll M. Stroke incidence, case fatality, and mortality in the WHO MONICA Project. *Stroke* 1995; **26**(3):361–367.

51. Ingall T, Asplund K, Mahonen M, Bonita R. A multinational comparison of subarachnoid hemorrhage epidemiology in the WHO MONICA Stroke Study. *Stroke* 2000; **31**(5):1054–1061.

52. Petty GW, Brown RDJ, Whisnant JP, Sicks JD, O'Fallon WM, Wiebers DO. Ischemic stroke subtypes: A population-based study of incidence and risk factors. *Stroke* 1999; **30**(12):2513–2516.

53. Aho K, Reunanen A, Aromaa A, Knekt P, Maatela J. Prevalence of stroke in Finland. *Stroke* 1986; **17**(4):681–686.

54. Bharucha NE, Bharucha EP, Bharucha AE, Bhise AV, Schoenberg BS. Prevalence of stroke in the Parsi community of Bombay. *Stroke* 1988; **19**(1):60–62.

55. Christie D. Prevalence of stroke and its sequelae. *Medical Journal of Australia* 1981; **2**(4):182–184.

56. Hu HH, Chu FL, Chiang BN, Lan CF, Sheng WY, Lo YK, et al. Prevalence of stroke in Taiwan. *Stroke* 1989; **20**(7):858–863.

57. Li SC, Schoenberg BS, Wang CC, Cheng XM, Bolis CL, Wang KJ. Cerebrovascular disease in the People's Republic of China: Epidemiologic and clinical features. *Neurology* 1985; **35**(12):1708–1713.

58. Paschalis C, Polychronopoulos P, Makris N, Kondakis X, Papapetropoulos T. Prevalence rate of cerebrovascular disease in the rural population of northwest Peloponnese, Greece. A direct epidemiological study. *European Neurology* 1989; **29**(4):186–188.

59. Razdan S, Koul RL, Motta A, Kaul S. Cerebrovascular disease in rural Kashmir, India. *Stroke* 1989; **20**(12):1691–1693.

60. Sørensen SP, Boysen G, Jensen G, Schnohr P. Prevalence of stroke in a district of Copenhagen the Copenhagen City Heart Study. *Acta Neurologica Scandinavica* 1982; **66**(1):68–81.

61. Urakami K, Igo M, Takahashi K. An epidemiologic study of cerebrovascular disease in western Japan: With special reference to transient ischemic attacks. *Stroke* 1987; **18**(2):396–401.

62. Wyller TB, Bautz-Holter E, Holmen J. Prevalence of stroke and stroke-related disability in Northen Trondelag County, Norway. *Cerebrovascular Diseases* 1994; **4**:421–427.

63. Terént A. Stroke morbidity. In: Whisnant JP, ed. *Stroke: Populations, Cohorts and Clinical Trials*. Oxford: Butterworth-Heinemann; 1993:37–58.

64. Prencipe M, Ferretti C, Casini AR, Santini M, Giubilei F, Culasso F. Stroke, disability, and dementia: Results of a population survey. *Stroke* 1997; **28**(3):531–536.

65. Linn FHH, Rinkel GJE, Algra A, van Gijn J. Incidence of subarachnoid hemorrhage: Role of region, year, and rate of computed tomography: A meta-analysis. *Stroke* 1996; 27(4):625–629.

66. Tuomilehto J, Sarti C, Narva EV, Salmi K, Sivenius J, Kaarsalo E, et al. The FINMONICA Stroke Register. Community-based stroke registration and analysis of stroke incidence in Finland, 1983–1985. *American Journal of Epidemiology* 1992; 135(11):1259–1270.

67. Okwumabua JO, Martin B, Clayton-Davis J, Pearson CM. Stroke Belt initiative: the Tennessee experience. *Journal of Health Care for the Poor & Underserved* 1997; 8(3):292–299.

68. Sacco RL, Boden-Albala B, Gan R, Chen X, Kargman DE, Shea S, et al. Stroke incidence among white, black, and Hispanic residents of an urban community: the Northern Manhattan Stroke Study. *American Journal of Epidemiology* 1998; 147(3):259–268.

69. Bonita R, Broad JB, Beaglehole R. Ethnic differences in stroke incidence and case fatality in Auckland, New Zealand. *Stroke* 1997; 28(4):758–761.

70. Nicoletti A, Sofia V, Giuffrida S, Bartoloni A, Bartalesi F, Bartolo MLL, et al. Prevalence of stroke: A door-to-door survey in rural Bolivia. *Stroke* 2000; 31(4):882–885.

71. Truelsen T, Bonita R, Jamrozik K. Surveillance of stroke: A global perspective. *International Journal of Epidemiology* 2001; 30(Suppl):S11–S16.

72. Bonita R, Beaglehole R. Monitoring stroke. An international challenge [editorial]. *Stroke* 1995; 26(4):541–542.

73. Tilling K, Sterne JA, Wolfe CD. Estimation of the incidence of stroke using a capture-recapture model including covariates. *International Journal of Epidemiology* 2001; 30(6):1351–1359.

74. Asplund K, Bonita R, Kuulasmaa K, Rajakangas AM, Schaedlich H, Suzuki K, et al. Multinational comparisons of stroke epidemiology. Evaluation of case ascertainment in the WHO MONICA Stroke Study. World Health Organization Monitoring Trends and Determinants in Cardiovascular Disease. *Stroke* 1995; 26(3):355–360.

75. Schottenfeld D, Eaton M, Sommers SC, Alonso DR, Wilkinson C. The autopsy as a measure of accuracy of the death certificate. *Bulletin of the New York Academy of Medicine* 1982; 58(9):778–794.

76. Cameron HM, McGoogan E. A prospective study of 1152 hospital autopsies: II. Analysis of inaccuracies in clinical diagnoses and their significance. *Journal of Pathology* 1981; 133(4):285–300.

77. Britton M. Diagnostic errors discovered at autopsy. *Acta Medica Scandinavica* 1974; 196(3):203–210.

78. Bamford J, Sandercock P, Dennis M, Warlow C, Jones L, McPherson K, et al. A prospective study of acute cerebrovascular disease in the community: The Oxfordshire Community Stroke Project 1981–86. 1. Methodology, demography and incident cases of first-ever stroke. *Journal of Neurology, Neurosurgery & Psychiatry* 1988; 51(11):1373–1380.

79. Alter M, Sobel E, McCoy RL, Francis ME, Shofer F, Levitt LP, et al. Stroke in the Lehigh Valley: Incidence based on a community-wide hospital register. *Neuroepidemiology* 1985; 4(1):1–15.

80. Sarti C, Tuomilehto J, Sivenius J, Kaarsalo E, Narva EV, Salmi K, et al. Stroke mortality and case-fatality rates in three geographic areas of Finland from 1983 to 1986. *Stroke* 1993; 24(8):1140–1147.

81. Stegmayr B, Asplund K. Measuring stroke in the population: quality of routine statistics in comparison with a population-based stroke registry. *Neuroepidemiology* 1992; 11(4–6):204–213.

82. Malmgren R, Warlow C, Bamford J, Sandercock P. Geographical and secular trends in stroke incidence. *Lancet* 1987; 2(8569):1196–1200.

83. Bonita R, Broad JB, Anderson NE, Beaglehole R. Approaches to the problems of measuring the incidence of stroke: The Auckland Stroke Study, 1991–1992. *International Journal of Epidemiology* 1995; 24(3):535–542.

84. Thom TJ. Stroke mortality trends. An international perspective. *Annals of Epidemiology* 1993; 3(5):509–518.

85. Stroke: a looming epidemic? *Australian Family Physician* 1997; 26:1137–1143.

86. Reitsma JB, Limburg M, Kleijnen J, Bonsel GJ, Tijssen JG. Epidemiology of stroke in The Netherlands from 1972 to 1994: The end of the decline in stroke mortality. *Neuroepidemiology* 1998; 17(3):121–131.

87. Gillum RF, Sempos CT. The end of the long-term decline in stroke mortality in the United States? *Stroke* 1997; 28(8):1527–1529.

88. Ahmed OI, Orchard TJ, Sharma R, Mitchell H, Talbot E. Declining mortality from stroke in Allegheny County, Pennsylvania. Trends in case fatality and severity of disease, 1971–1980. *Stroke* 1988; 19(2):181–184.

89. Fang J, Alderman MH, Tu JV. Trend of stroke hospitalization, United States, 1988–1997. Editorial comment. *Stroke* 2001; 32(10):2221–2226.

90. Hong Y, Bots ML, Pan X, Hofman A, Grobbee DE, Chen H. Stroke incidence and mortality in rural and urban Shanghai from 1984 through 1991. Findings from a community-based registry. *Stroke* 1994; 25(6):1165–1169.

91. Howard G, Craven TE, Sanders L, Evans GW. Relationship of hospitalized stroke rate and in-hospital mortality to the decline in US stroke mortality. *Neuroepidemiology* 1991; 10(5–6):251–259.

92. Heidenreich PA, McClellan M. Trends in treatment and outcomes for acute myocardial infarction: 1975–1995. *American Journal of Medicine* 2001; 110(3):165–174.

93. Rosen M, Alfredsson L, Hammar N, Kahan T, Spetz CL, Ysberg AS. Attack rate, mortality and case fatality for acute myocardial infarction in Sweden during 1987–95. Results from the national AMI register in Sweden. *Journal of Internal Medicine* 2000; 248(2):159–164.

94. Bata IR, Gregor RD, Eastwood BJ, Wolf HK. Trends in the incidence of acute myocardial infarction between 1984 and 1993—The Halifax County MONICA Project. *Canadian Journal of Cardiology* 2000; 16(5):589–595.

95. Spencer FA, Meyer TE, Goldberg RJ, Yarzebski J, Hatton M, Lessard D, et al. Twenty year trends (1975–1995) in the incidence, in-hospital and long-term death rates associated with heart failure complicating acute myocardial infarction: A community-wide perspective. *Journal of the American College of Cardiology* 1999; 34(5):1378–1387.

96. Kirchhoff M, Davidsen M, Bronnum-Hansen H, Hansen B, Schnack H, Eriksen, et al. Incidence of myocardial infarction in the Danish MONICA population 1982–1991. *International Journal of Epidemiology* 1999; 28(2):211–218.

97. Goldberg RJ, Yarzebski J, Lessard D, Gore JM. A two-decades (1975 to 1995) long experience in the incidence, in-hospital and long-term case-fatality rates of acute myocardial infarction: A community-wide perspective. *Journal of the American College of Cardiology* 1999; 33(6):1533–1539.

98. Volmink JA, Newton JN, Hicks NR, Sleight P, Fowler GH, Neil HA. Coronary event and case fatality rates in an English population: Results of the Oxford myocardial infarction incidence study. The Oxford Myocardial Infarction Incidence Study Group. *Heart* 1998; 80(1):40–44.

99. Rosamond WD, Chambless LE, Folsom AR, Cooper LS, Conwill DE, Clegg L, et al. Trends in the incidence of myocardial infarction and in mortality due to coronary heart disease, 1987 to 1994. *NEJM* 1998; 339(13):861–867.

100. Brophy JM. The epidemiology of acute myocardial infarction and ischemic heart disease in Canada: Data from 1976 to 1991. *Canadian Journal of Cardiology* 1997; 13(5):474–478.

101. Immonen-Raiha P, Arstila M, Tuomilehto J, Haikio M, Mononen A, Vuorenmaa, et al. 21 year trends in incidence of myocardial infarction and mortality from coronary disease in middle-age. *European Heart Journal* 1996; 17(10):1495–1502.

102. Beaglehole R. Global cardiovascular disease prevention: Time to get serious. *Lancet* 2001; 358(9282):661–663.

103. Bots ML, Looman SJ, Koudstaal PJ, Hofman A, Hoes AW, Grobbee DE. Prevalence of stroke in the general population: The Rotterdam Study. *Stroke* 1996; 27(9):1499–1501.

104. Mittelmark MB, Psaty BM, Rautaharju PM, Fried LP, Borhani NO, Tracy RP, et al. Prevalence of cardiovascular diseases among older adults. The Cardiovascular Health Study. *American Journal of Epidemiology* 1993; 137(3):311–317.

105. Lindeberg S, Lundh B. Apparent absence of stroke and ischemic heart disease in a traditional Melanesian island: A clinical study in Kitava. *Journal of Internal Medicine* 1993; 233(3):269–275.

106. Huang ZS, Chiang TL, Lee TK. Stroke prevalence in Taiwan : Findings from the 1994 National Health Interview Survey. *Stroke* 1997; 28(8):1579–1584.

3 Pathophysiology and Management of Acute Stroke

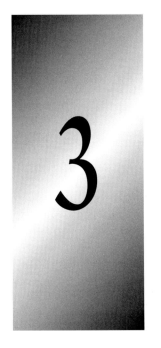

William Alvin McElveen
Richard F. Macko

S troke is the third leading cause of death in the United States, and the most common medical cause of disability. Each year 780,000 Americans have a new or recurrent stroke—a number that will double in upcoming decades as our population advances in age. This condition is therefore the most significant neurologic condition managed in the hospital setting. With the advent of tissue plasminogen activator (rt-PA) for the acute treatment of stroke in 1996, the management of stroke changed dramatically. The move toward treatment algorithms based on evidence-based medicine has also altered the care of the stroke patient. Several states have adopted legislative Stroke Acts which require emergency medical personnel to transport stroke victims to the nearest certified stroke center. The Joint Commission has developed certification criteria for Primary Stroke Centers based on the evidence published in the medical literature. With the advent of specialized stroke centers, the inclusion of guideline-driven acute stroke care, including early rehabilitation, is an important component in the total management of the stroke patient. Acute care rehabilitation issues address prevention of common post-stroke complications such as deep venous thrombosis; emphasize early mobilization, assessment, and management of dysphagia and nutritional status, cognitive

and communication deficits, incontinence, and preventative skin care; and initiate interactive rehabilitation education including the family and caregivers. Hence multiple rehabilitation modalities must be initiated during the acute care period, and continuity of care plans established to optimize long-term functional and health outcomes for the stroke survivor. This chapter focuses primarily on the medical management of acute ischemic stroke and provides a brief introduction to major rehabilitation issues that are commonly encountered during early stroke care.

STROKE RECOGNITION

Rapid recognition of the signs and symptoms of stroke, and timely access to stroke centers, are crucial to optimizing the acute care for stroke. Too often, patients develop signs of stroke and wait hours before seeking care, believing that the deficits will go away if they wait long enough. Community awareness forums have been successful in this endeavor. A study by Feldman in 1993 showed the median time to presentation to emergency departments from onset of symptoms was 13 hours (1). Only 42% of patients presented within 24 hours. During the course of the National Institutes of Health Tissue Plasminogen Activator Pilot Study, public education and awareness campaigns were conducted to encourage early hospital arrival. Following this campaign, the mean time from symptom onset to hospital arrival declined significantly (3.2 hours vs. 1.5 hours). The use of 911 increased from 39% in the first quartile of the study to 60% in the fourth quartile. The five most common symptoms of stroke include

1. Sudden numbness or weakness of face, arm, or leg, especially on one side of the body
2. Sudden confusion, trouble speaking or understanding
3. Sudden trouble seeing in one or both eyes
4. Sudden trouble walking, dizziness, loss of balance or coordination
5. Sudden severe headache with no known cause

Public education as to the significance of these symptoms and the importance of early evaluation is the goal of any comprehensive stroke program.

Emergency medicine system protocols are also critical in the early treatment of stroke. Proper training of paramedics allows these frontline personnel to obtain crucial information from family or bystanders. This includes obtaining history regarding time of onset and medications the patient might be taking. This historical information, as well as physical findings such as aphasia, motor deficit, and vital signs, can be called to the hospital emergency department so that a stroke alert protocol can be activated, saving significant time in treatment.

THE ISCHEMIC PENUMBRA

Following thrombotic occlusion of a cerebral vessel leading to stroke, there is an area of the ischemic core brain region in which blood flow has dropped below a critical level, and which is destined for cell death producing cerebral infarction. A surrounding area of ischemic tissue may also exist that is physiologically silent, but not immediately destined for cell death. It is believed that restoration of cerebral blood flow to this area can result in preventing further cerebral infarction. Although not available in all medical centers, the mismatch of diffusion and perfusion on MRI scan may help to indicate that a patient could benefit from thrombolytic therapy. While the precise duration of brain tissue viability for the penumbra has been debated and may vary between patients contingent on numerous pathophysiologic mechanisms, most clinical and animal studies indicate a decremental temporal profile for tissue survival that is on the order of hours. Hence, "time is brain," and the more rapidly that cerebral perfusion can be restored, the better the neurologic outcome.

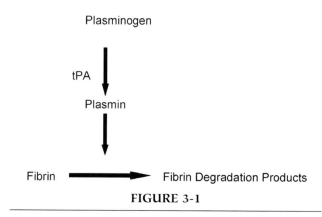

FIGURE 3-1

Diagram showing the site of action of recombinant tPA to activate plasmin, which mediates fibrinolysis.

TISSUE PLASMINOGEN ACTIVATOR

Recombinant tissue plasminogen activator is a serine protease which converts plasminogen to plasmin, a fibrinolytic enzyme (Figure 3-1). Upon administration, recombinant t-PA increases plasmin enzymatic activity, resulting in fibrinolysis. It is used to treat the stroke in the acute stage to restore flow to the ischemic area. This should be administered as quickly as feasible, by protocol standards within a three-hour time period to restore blood supply and optimize recovery.

Tissue plasminogen activator (rt-PA) was approved by the FDA in 1996 for the treatment of acute stroke based of findings of the NINDS stroke trial in 1995 (2). This double-blind placebo-controlled trial demonstrated that patients treated with rt-PA within three hours of symptom onset had a 30% greater likelihood of having minimal to no disability 90 days following treatment, compared to a placebo-treated group. There was a 6.4% risk of symptomatic intracerebral hemorrhage in the rt-PA treated group, compared to 0.6% in the placebo group. However, even considering the risk of bleeding, the mortality at 90 days was 21% in the placebo group, and only 17% in the rt-PA group. Subsequent analyses have shown these findings with rt-PA in the NINDS trial hold up for improved outcomes at the one-year time point (3). The benefits of early thrombolytic therapy are corroborated by the results of two European Cooperative Stroke Studies, as well as clinical experience, substantiating the effectiveness of rt-PA when used according to the guidelines of the clinical trials (4).

EMERGENCY DEPARTMENT MANAGEMENT OF STROKE

Because of the importance of rapid intervention in treating patients with ischemic stroke, it is important that hospitals develop order sheets outlining the protocols to be followed when the stroke patient arrives. If the patient is transported by emergency medical service, the hospital can institute the protocol immediately. Several criteria should be established in the emergency department, including timely interpretation of studies and the availability of neurosurgical intervention should the patient develop symptomatic intracranial hemorrhage. The standardized protocols also insure that key elements of inpatient management, evidence-based strategies for secondary stroke prevention, and early rehabilitation are systematically implemented.

The CT scan should be performed as soon as possible to exclude a hemorrhagic stroke. The CT scan may also demonstrate subtle early signs of infarction. Although the presence of these signs is associated with a poor outcome, this does not preclude the use of rt-PA unless there is evidence of hemorrhage. The scans are generally performed without contrast unless there is reason to suspect tumor.

Evaluation of the patient should also include the NIH stroke scale. Training for this, as well as certification for performing the evaluation, can be obtained through several mechanisms such as the American Stroke Association website. Initially utilized in research trials, this 15-item scale has proven valuable in quantifying the deficits of the stroke patient, which is useful when discussing the patient's condition with the treating primary medical team, and for continuity of rehabilitation care. The NIHSS scale is shown in Figure 3-2.

If it is determined that a patient's symptoms have been present less than three hours, there are other criteria that must be considered to determine if a patient is to be considered for rt-PA administration. These are listed in Figure 3-3.

The consideration of rapidly improving symptoms as they relate to thrombolytic therapy decision making has been somewhat problematic. Improvement over the baseline NIH score is not considered rapid improvement if the patient continues to have a significant deficit. A good rule of thumb has been to assume the patient is not going to show further improvement in their condition. Is the deficit mild enough that the patient can continue to function at a high level? Even mild weakness might be devastating to an individual whose occupation depends on fine motor movements, hence, rt-PA could be a consideration in such patients, even with a low NIHSS value. Barber, et al. noted that one-third of patients deemed to have mild stroke symptoms that excluded them from tPA treatment either died or were left in a dependent state (5).

Further considerations relevant to management in the acute stroke setting include evaluation of glucose and systemic antithrombotic status, and blood pressure. In the acute stroke setting, glucose is important to determine, as hypoglycemia can be associated with focal neurologic deficits, while patients with hyperglycemia have a less favorable prognosis. Partial thromboplastin time

(PTT), international normalized ratio for prothrombin time (INR), and platelet count should be obtained to prevent the use of thrombolytic therapy in patients with coagulation defects. By obtaining the lab values soon after the patient arrives in the emergency department, the determination of these values may be obtained without delaying treatment. A majority of acute stroke patients have elevated blood pressure at the time of admission and across the initial days post-stroke, which must be carefully managed (see below):

After rt-PA is administered, the patient should be monitored for at least 24 hours in an intensive care facility. The present recommendations are to keep systolic blood pressure below 185mm and diastolic below 110mm. Labetolol or nicardipine are the recommended agents to lower blood pressure. The lower limits for blood pressure should be a diastolic of 60 mm. Serial neurologic examinations are requisite, with appropriate clinical pathways for emergent management of complications such as symptomatic intra-cranial hemorrhage.

INPATIENT CARE

Overview

The care of stroke patients is divided into phases of emergency management, acute inpatient care, and rehabilitation and long-term care. In practice, the principles of care for these phases overlap, and the management provided across these periods determines the quality and continuity of ongoing care that affects stroke outcomes. The continued management of patients who have completed rt-PA, or those who were not candidates for the medication, is key to achieving optimal improvement in stroke outcomes. This is underscored by the results of randomized and prospective studies of dedicated stroke units in which these focused care teams produce better outcomes for survival and independent living (6)—findings which have been translated into clinical practice with similar positive results (7).

Among the issues that are central to inpatient care are ongoing neurologic assessment to detect any signs or symptoms of clinical deterioration that may alter clinical pathways, management of blood pressure, blood glucose, fluid balance, anticoagulation or antiplatelet therapy, and initiation of appropriate secondary stroke prevention. Early rehabilitation includes prevention of common post-stroke complications, assessment for therapy needs with initiation of early mobilization, and comprehensive treatment plans, which should involve the family, caregivers, and plans for continuity of care.

Neurologic Assessment

Comprehensive neurologic assessments are crucial, both to optimize general inpatient medical management, and

DATE/TIME:									
Level of Consciousness	0 Alert 1 Drowsy 2 Stuperous 3 Coma								
LOC	0 Answers Both Correctly 1 Answers One (1) Correctly 2 Incorrect								
LOC	0 Obeys Both Correctly 1 Obeys One (1) Correctly 2 Incorrect								
Best Gaze	0 Normal 1 Partial Gaze Palsy 2 Forced Deviation								
Visual	0 No Visual Loss 1 Partial Hemianopia 2 Complete Hemianopia 3 Bilateral Hemianopia Blind								
Facial Palsy	0 Normal 1 Minor 2 Partial 3 Complete								
Motor Arm	0 No Drift 1 Drift 2 Some Effort Against Gravity 3 Limb Falls 4 No Movement	R	L	R	L	R	L	R	L
Motor Leg	0 No Drift 1 Drift 2 Some Effort Against Gravity 3 Limb Falls 4 No Movement	R	L	R	L	R.	L	R	L
Limb Ataxia	0 Absent + = Present 1 One (1) Limb - = Absent 2 Two (2) Limbs Score →	R U L Total:	L	R U L Total:	L	R U L Total:	L	R U L Total:	L
Sensory	0 Normal 1 Mild to Moderate Loss 2 Severe to Total Loss								
Best Language	0 Normal 1 Mild to Moderate Aphasia 2 Severe Aphasia 3 Mute								
Dysarthria	0 Normal 1 Mild to Moderate 2 Severe								
Extinction/ Inattention	0 Normal 1 Partial Neglect 2 Complete Neglect								
Total / Initial:									

FIGURE 3-2

The NIH Stroke Scale.

for planning of rehabilitation care. In the emergency care setting, emphasis is placed on the NIHSS as a standardized assessment instrument in the decision tree for thrombolytic therapy. The NIHSS also provides some guidance for determining prognosis of patients even at the time of admission. Schlegel, et al. have described the utility of the NIH stroke scale in predicting post-hospital disposition. An NIHSS that was 5 or less is most strongly associated with discharge home. An NIHSS between 6 and 13 was correlated with transfer to a rehabilitation unit, while an NIHSS greater than 13 predicted discharge to a long term nursing facility. This information can be useful in early planning for post-hospital care options. Hence, consensus recommendations are to document an NIHSS within 24 hours of admission and at the time of discharge from acute

If any of the following are answered YES, Patient may NOT receive tPA.

☐ Yes ☐ No Stroke symptom onset more than 3 hours (Last time patient was known to be without stroke symptoms)
☐ Yes ☐ No Age 18 or younger
☐ Yes ☐ No Comatose or unresponsive
☐ Yes ☐ No Stroke symptoms clearing spontaneously. Stroke symptoms minor and isolated.
☐ Yes ☐ No Intracranial/Subarachnoid hemorrhage (SAH). Clinical history suggestive of SAH even if CT negative
☐ Yes ☐ No Active internal bleeding or acute trauma (fracture) on examination
☐ Yes ☐ No INR greater than 1.7
☐ Yes ☐ No Platelet count less than 100,000
☐ Yes ☐ No Glucose less than 50
☐ Yes ☐ No HTN uncontrolled despite medication with systolic BP greater than 185 or diastolic BP greater than 110

History of:

☐ Yes ☐ No Active malignancy
☐ Yes ☐ No Recent MI or pericarditis within the past 3 months
☐ Yes ☐ No Recent arterial puncture at noncompressible site within previous 7 days (such as subclavian)
☐ Yes ☐ No Lumbar puncture within 3 days
☐ Yes ☐ No History of GI or urinary hemorrhage within 21 days
☐ Yes ☐ No Pregnancy, lactation, or childbirth within 30 days
☐ Yes ☐ No History of intracranial hemorrhage
☐ Yes ☐ No Major surgery or serious trauma within in last 14 days
☐ Yes ☐ No Seizure with postictal residual neurologic impairment .
☐ Yes ☐ No Major ischemic stroke or head trauma within the last 3 months
☐ Yes ☐ No Heparin within 48 hrs with PTT greater than upper limits of normal
☐ Yes ☐ No Known AV malformation or aneurysm
☐ Yes ☐ No Known bleeding disorder

FIGURE 3-3

Clinical criterion that must be considered when determining eligibility for rt-PA therapy.

inpatient hospitalization, as well as the repeated assessments that are used according to clinical pathways in the event that rt-PA is administered.

The NIHSS does have limitations with respect to inpatient stroke care and evaluating comprehensive rehabilitation needs. For example, elements of brainstem dysfunction are not well reflected. Palatal weakness is not scored on this scale, but a lesion associated with dysphagia can be quite disabling and increase aspiration risk, thereby altering management plans and nutritional planning. The NIHSS does not assess distal weakness, which in the upper extremity is typically greater than proximal weakness; a factor which could influence therapy plans. Hence, proximal limb function should be documented during all assessments. NIHSS was also not developed as a neurocognitive screening instrument. Further assessment and appropriate standardized instruments should be used to comprehensively evaluate mental status and screen for neuropsychologic syndromes such as neglect, depression, and impaired executive function, that can markedly alter rehabilitation planning and recovery profiles (see Chapters 13, 14, and 29). Clinical pathways for inpatient stroke care should also trigger early assessment by occupational and physical therapists as appropriate, as well as standing swallow and communication assessment by speech

and language professionals, as outlined in the following sections.

Dysphagia, Aspiration Risk, and Nutritional Management

One of the major dangers following stroke is aspiration, which may be silent, resulting in aspiration pneumonia. Dysphagia occurs in nearly half of hospitalized stroke patients and strongly predisposes to risk for aspiration pneumonia. Notably, the presence of a gag reflex is not indicative of safety in swallowing. Therefore, patients should be kept NPO until a bedside evaluation can be performed. Speech and language therapists play a significant role in this evaluation, and a videoflouroscopy swallowing study is recommended if bedside screening reveals abnormalities. If the patient is deemed to be at aspiration risk, a dysphagia therapy program should be provided, optimally in consultation with a speech/language professional, as this has been shown to reduce pneumonia in the acute phase of stroke. Individuals at high risk for aspiration pneumonia may require nasogastric feeding tubes or percutaneous endoscopic gastrostomy (PEG). There is controversy regarding which is safer and more effective. While prior reviews provided some initial suggestions that PEG might be more efficacious (8), emerging evidence based on meta-analyses of 15 prospective studies suggests nasogastric tubes are not associated with higher death rates, as previously believed (9). Hence, best clinical judgment must be used, until the results of further clinical research are available. Dysphagia also identifies individuals that are inherently at greater risk for developing malnutrition, which is reported in 15% of stroke cases at the time of initial presentation, and doubles to 30% across the first week of hospitalization (10). Since malnutrition is linked to poorer clinical outcomes, ongoing monitoring of nutritional as well as hydration and electrolyte status becomes an important component of clinical pathways for stroke, particularly individuals with dysphagia and compromised oral intake (11).

Blood Pressure, Fluid, and Glucose Management

Blood pressure management in the acute stroke patient is not the same as for the general population. Cerebral autoregulation in the normal state results in a steady cerebral blood flow for mean arterial pressures between 60 mm and 160 mm. However, autoregulation may be lost in the acute stroke setting, and as a result, decreasing blood pressure decreases cerebral blood flow. Unless there is a cardiac, renal, or other medical reason that the pressure needs to be lowered, the current recommendation is to treat the blood pressure only above 220 over 120. Agents such as sublingual nifedipine that lower the blood pressure quickly should be avoided. A reasonable decrease in blood pressure would be 15% over 24 hours. For patients who have pre-existing hypertension, it is generally agreed that antihypertensive medications should be restarted at 24 hours if they are neurologically stable, unless a specific contraindication to restarting treatment is known.

Hypotonic and glucose-containing intravenous fluids are not recommended in the acute setting of cerebral infarction. Cytotoxic edema resulting from cellular membrane disruption with resulting swelling of the cell body develops with infarct. The use of these solutions can increase the cellular damage with influx of water into the cell. Normal saline is therefore generally utilized in these patients.

In addition to hypoglycemia, numerous studies have shown that patients with sustained glucose greater than 140 have less favorable stroke outcomes than those with lower glucose values. Hyperglycemia after acute ischemic stroke has been shown to predict higher mortality and worse 90-day clinical outcomes for individuals with and without pre-existing history of Type 2 Diabetes Mellitus (12), and appears to blunt the beneficial effect of early recanalization that accompanies rt-PA therapy (13). The glucose levels should be monitored, and if greater than 140 to 180, treated with insulin similar to management in other medical intensive care conditions.

Antithrombotic Therapy

The use of anticoagulation in acute stroke is controversial. The present clinical recommendations are to avoid anticoagulation in the acute phase of stroke. Present data does not indicate that the use of heparin or heparinoids in the acute management of stroke results in a decrease in the risk of early recurrence of stroke. However, there is an increased risk of conversion to a hemorrhagic stroke with the use of anticoagulation in acute stroke. An example of this is seen in Figure 3-4. This recommendation is also for strokes felt to be of cardioembolic origin, such as atrial fibrillation. No subgroup or arterial distribution has been identified in which anticoagulation has demonstrated a significant benefit, when also considering the risk of bleeding. Anticoagulation should not be utilized within 24 hours of rt-PA administration.

Aspirin is the only antiplatelet agent studied showing benefit in the acute management of stroke. Two large trials have been performed. When the results of the Chinese Acute Stroke Trial and the International Stroke Trial were combined, a modest benefit was obtained. This led to a recommendation of instituting aspirin at a dose of 325 mg within the first 48 hours after stroke. The use of aspirin is not recommended within 24 hours of rt-PA administration. A 2007 study compared clopidogrel plus aspirin to aspirin alone given within 24 hours of onset of stroke symptoms (14). There was a 7% recurrent stroke incidence in the combined group, compared to 11% in the aspirin group. However, this did not reach statistical significance. Other trials such as the MATCH trial have indicated there is twice the risk of significant

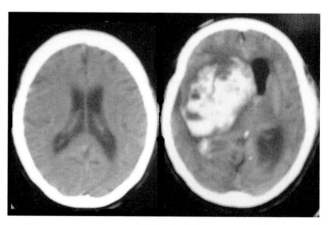

FIGURE 3-4

Patient presents at 10 AM with left hemiparesis, and scan on left is obtained. Heparin was started. At 4PM patient becomes obtunded, and scan on right is obtained.

bleeding complication when using aspirin plus clopido-grel compared to clopidogrel alone. Hence, combinations of antithrombotic agents are generally not recommended for long-term secondary stroke prevention, as they are linked to increased bleeding risks (15).

Evaluating and Managing Neurologic Deterioration

Between 15% and 30% of individuals with acute ischemic stroke experience neurologic deterioration during the acute hospitalization period, and this portends a much poorer prognosis (16). Factors linked to stroke-in-evolution early on tend to be neurovascular, including cerebrovascular thrombus in progression, recurrent stroke, brain swelling, or hemorrhagic transformation (17). A number of other potentially modifiable systemic and medical factors must be considered. These include evaluation of cardiopulmonary and fluid status, glucose and electrolyte status, assessment for infection, metabolic and toxic abnormalities, as well as consideration of medication side effects. Neurologic factors beyond recurrent or progressing stroke that can mediate clinical deterioration in the acute hospital setting include brain swelling with mass effect, herniation syndromes, hemorrhagic transformation of ischemic stroke, and seizures, including subclinical variants that are difficult to diagnose without electroencephalography, and can greatly compromise stroke outcomes. Any neurologic deterioration or signs of fluctuating mental status should trigger rapid assessment for possible etiologies of worsening (16).

Infection.   Infection is known to be a prothrombotic trigger mechanism in as many as 25–33% of ischemic strokes, and has long been recognized as an etiology for clinical worsening in the setting of acute stroke (18–20). Therefore, survey for infection is recommended at the time of initial stroke presentation, and comprehensive infection evaluation should be conducted if clinical deterioration occurs. Aspiration pneumonia and urinary tract infections are the most prevalent, and must be treated aggressively. Since acute infection is linked to a prothombotic state, and elevated temperature can accelerate neuro-excitotoxicity, both fever and infection must be aggressively treated in the acute stroke setting to protect the brain from further ischemic damage.

Seizures.   Change in mental status, particularly episodic, should trigger evaluation for seizures. Incidence of seizures is reported at 9% for ischemic stroke (21). By contrast, seizures are reported in one-third of intracranial hemorrhage cases, and clinical studies suggest that over half of these are electrographic only, that is not accompanied by clinical signs or symptoms of seizure (22). Specifically, continuous EEG recording has revealed seizures in up to 36% of lobar intracranial hemorrhage, and contrary to conventional thinking, seizures including those that are non-convulsive are reported in 21% of subcortical intracranial hemorrhage cases, and these are linked to increased hemispheric mass effect and poorer outcomes (23). Although beyond the scope of this chapter, this illustrates that the acute clinical management of intracerebral hemorrhage, particularly management of hypertension, differs significantly from care protocols for acute ischemic stroke. The reader is referred to consensus recommendations for management of intracerebral hemorrhage for further details (24). Regardless, seizures increase cerebral metabolic demands and intracranial pressure; generalized seizures can increase body temperature. All of these factors can potentially worsen neurologic status and extend brain infarction in individuals with ischemic or hemorrhagic stroke, conditions in which cerebral auto-regulation is already impaired. Hence, seizures must be treated emergently in the setting of stroke. Likewise, suspicion of subclinical seizures warrants bedside electroecenphelography and monitoring, along with rapid and aggressive anticonvulsant therapy, if diagnosed.

Management of Malignant Cerebral Edema.   The management of malignant cerebral edema in large territorial middle cerebral infarctions has historically proven problematic. Massive brain edema with supratentorial cerebral infarction typically presents within the first five days, including one-third of cases within less than 24 hours, and portends a poor prognosis, with fatality approaching 80% regardless of medical management (25, 26). Randomized controlled trials now provide evidence-based recommendations for decision making regarding decompressive surgery for those cases manifesting malignant middle cerebral artery infarction within 48 hours of stroke onset. Pooled analyses from three randomized clinical trials in Europe show decompressive surgery at less than 48 hours is more effective to produce a favorable one-year outcome for the primary outcome defined as Modified Rankin Score of 4 or less when compared to usual care 75% vs. 24% (27). To place this in perspective, a modified Rankin of 4 indicates moderately severe deficits: unable to walk or attend to activities of daily living (ADLs) without assistance (28). Secondary outcomes in favor of decompressive surgery over best medical care included lower fatality rates (78% vs. 29%) and doubling of chances to recover to a Modified Rankin Score of 3 or less by one year; a score of 3 indicates moderate disability, able to walk without assistance. Notably, chances of surviving with severe disability (Score 5, bedridden, incontinent, constant nursing) were not different for decompressive surgery vs. usual medical care (4% vs. 5%). Note that these favorable outcomes for decompressive surgery come from studies that employ strict eligibility and exclusion requirements, including NIHSS greater than 15 in the setting of 50 or greater territorial MCA infarction, and with no space occupying hemorrhagic lesions, fixed dilated pupils, or other major illnesses that could affect outcomes. These factors must be taken into consideration when making decisions regarding early decompressive surgery.

Early Rehabilitation Care and Mobilization

Consensus recommendations support early mobilization in appropriate medically stable subjects (29). While medical instability can limit the scope of rehabilitation early on, there are numerous physiological reasons for early care emphasizing mobility, including prevention of deep venous thrombosis, pressure ulcers, autonomic deconditioning, skin and lung infections, contracture formation, and muscular wasting. Muscular wasting can be rapid and devastating to functional recovery, particularly in frail elderly subjects. For those patients incapable of volitional muscle activation due to altered consciousness or severe motor deficits, early range of motion exercises and/or appropriate splinting as indicated to reduce contracture development, along with change of body positioning and other strategies to minimize skin pressure and friction, are recommended to minimize common post-stroke complications of contractures and pressure ulcers, respectively. For those cardiopulmonary stable individuals with higher neurologic function, resumption with appropriate supervision and training of basic mobility, self-care, and socialization skills is fundamental to early comprehensive rehabilitation care (29). Involvement of family and caregivers, including structured written materials mapping rehabilitation plans and issues, is strongly recommended.

Prevention of Deep Venous Thrombosis.   Patients with stroke frequently have deficits that impair their ability to ambulate safely, or even cause them to be confined to bed. This immobilization, along with elements of the prothtombotic state that are associated with acute ischemic stroke, increase the risk for deep venous thrombosis and associated pulmonary embolism. Therefore, measures should be taken to prevent this complication. Consensus recommendations strongly support the use of subcutaneous low-dose unfractionated heparin or low molecular weight heparin or heparinoids (30). Some evidence exists that the latter may have greater efficacy. For example, a study by Sherman and Alpers indicated a 43% improvement in venous thromboembolism with patients treated with the heparinoid enoxaparin given 40 mg subcutaneously q day, compared to subcutaneous unfractionated heparin (31). This is consistent with meta-analyses that conclude both unfractionated heparin and low molecular weight heparin/heparinoids are partially effective to reduce deep venous thrombosis, but some evidence suggests low molecular weight heparinoids may be more

effective (32). As previously stated, heparin should not be used during the initial 24 hours post-thrombolytic therapy. Intermittent pneumatic compression devices (or elastic stockings) have been recommended to help prevent deep vein thrombosis in patients with contraindications to anticoagulants, and for individuals presenting with acute intracranial hemorrhage; stable patients with intracranial hemorrhage may be switched over to low dose subcutaneous heparin as early as the second day post event (29). Aspirin may provide some mild benefit (33), and is safe to use in combination with low dose heparin (29). Regardless of the medical coverage, early mobilization (preferably in collaboration with physical therapy consultation) and walking is important and can significantly reduce the risk for venous thrombosis (30).

Skin Care and Prevention of Pressure Ulcers.   Pressure ulcers occur in approximately one-tenth of hospitalized stroke patients and one-fourth in nursing homes. Individuals at particular risk are those with greater severity mobility deficits, medical conditions that compromise skin vascular integrity including diabetes and peripheral arterial occlusive disease, individuals with urinary incontinence, and frail elderly with low body mass. Nursing pathways for stroke employ daily skin integrity monitoring, and scheduled care including turning, proper positioning, and appropriate other methodologies to reduce pressure and friction that propagate pressure ulcer formation (30, 33). This includes the use of pressure-relief ankle-foot orthoses as a means to prevent contractures and pressure sore development. Consistent with clinical rehabilitation practice guidelines, early physical therapy assessment and care to optimize recovery of mobilization are also recommended to reduce the longitudinal risk profile for skin breakdown and pressure ulcer development.

Incontinence.   Urinary incontinence is a prevalent early problem after stroke, occurring in about half of hospitalized cases, and decreasing in prevalence to 20% in the chronic post-stroke recovery period. Factors increasing the predisposition to urinary incontinence are similar to those for pressure ulcers: greater stroke severity; diabetes; advanced age. Due to the extremely high prevalence of urinary incontinence (and often fecal incontinence) in individuals with moderate to severe stroke, indwelling catheters are often used during the acute stage. This can facilitate fluid management and reduce risk for skin breakdown. However, continued indwelling catheter usage of more than 48 hours predisposes to infection. During acute stroke hospitalization, assessment for urinary retention should be conducted via catheterization or bladder scan, urinary volume and control assessed, and dysuria documented. Some evidence exists that silver alloy coated catheters may have fewer complications. Regardless, it is optimal to discontinue indwelling catheter use beyond 48 hours, and to employ an individualized bladder training program with prompted voiding training for appropriate cases (30). Similarly, bowel incontinence is common after stroke, and can be associated with increased risk for skin breakdown and infection complications. Patients should be carefully assessed for presence, pattern, and etiology of fecal incontinence, including consideration of mental status and neuromotor control of sphincter function, diarrhea, or constipation with diarrhea around a hardened stool mass, medication, and potential infectious complications that can increase risk for fecal incontinence. Physical therapy to optimize mobility recovery can be useful, as physical activity can influence gastrointestinal transit time. Maintaining skin cleanliness and integrity of the perineal area is crucial, along with attention to dietary fiber content, and implementation of a time-structured regular bowel program and associated medications as clinically indicated.

Cognitive Function and Communication

Global alterations in mental status, as well as a spectrum of specific neuropsychologic syndromes, are highly prevalent during the acute phase of stroke. Approximately one-third of stroke patients have globally altered mental status during their acute hospitalization, which if impaired, can influence all other cognitive and communication assessments, and limit early rehabilitation participation. The first question of the NIHSS categorically documents consciousness level. Those with stupor (or coma), or who fluctuate between drowsiness and stupor, regardless of cardiopulmonary stability, are best managed in a more intensive care setting, with frequent exams documenting the specific stimuli needed to produce arousal. This enables more rapid detection of fluctuating or progressing stroke that triggers emergent evaluation pathways. All patients with adequate alertness require evaluation for visual, motor, and sensory hemineglect syndromes (Chapters 15 and 16), aphasia and, apraxia (Chapter 10), memory deficits and impaired executive function (Chapter 13); all factors that influence acute and longitudinal rehabilitation care pathways.

Some symptoms, such as denial of deficit and hemineglect syndromes, particularly in visual and motor domains, also lead to challenges to the therapist and safety concerns, since the patient may not realize there is a dysfunction. These and other prevalent post-stroke neuropsychologic syndromes (Chapter 27) should optimally be identified during the acute hospitalization period, and their significance explained to caregivers and future rehabilitation providers to optimize continuity of care. Assessment of communication skill including speech, comprehension, repetition, reading, and writing with speech/language therapist consultation is a standard of care discussed in Chapter 10. Early initiation of speech therapy, including visual communication aids, may be

useful to facilitate patients' interaction with staff for routine care, and for socialization with family.

Other elements of neurocognitive health that are often overlooked during the acute hospitalization stage are mood and sleep integrity. Approximately one-third of stroke survivors develop some form of depression, which in many cases can be identified even during acute care hospitalization (Chapter 27). Early recognition and management of depression is requisite to optimizing long-term rehabilitation outcomes. Sleep disordered breathing is also highly prevalent after stroke, particularly during the acute and sub-acute stroke recovery period, where fragmented sleep architecture and/or apnea have been reported in more than half of patients (34, 35). A particular concern is obstructive sleep apnea that is linked to increased stroke risk, prothrombotic state, and may be associated with or exacerbate other neuropsychologic issues such as fatigue, depression, and memory impairment; factors that can complicate rehabilitation and recovery (36, 37). Individuals fitting the profile for sleep disordered breathing may be screened using nocturnal pulse oxymetry, or further evaluated by polysomnography as clinically indicated, as outlined in Chapter 28. Many acute stroke patients have a disturbed sleep-wake cycle, particularly when in intensive care units. Approaches to improving sleep hygiene include transferring the patient from the intensive care unit as soon as possible, and providing a quiet environment with dark during the night and sunlight during the day, to facilitate return of more normal circadian patterns. Selected medications properly timed may be used to facilitate sleep (e.g, trazadone, chloral hydrate), trying to avoid regular use of major sedative-hypnotics and antipsychotics, which can contribute to confused states, particularly in the elderly, and may further alter sleep architecture. Since abnormal sleep architecture is common in acute stroke, and increasing evidence suggests that sleep is critical to memory consolidation, and hence may facilitate sensorimotor recovery in the rehabilitation setting, careful attention to sleep hygiene should be addressed early on (35–37).

In summary, a diversity of neurocognitive, communication deficits, and sleep disturbances can complicate early stroke management and ongoing rehabilitation care. A summary of all cognitive and communication deficits, and neuropsychologic syndromes including depression and sleep disorders that are diagnosed during acute hospitalization, should be discussed with the family and outlined to subsequent care providers to optimize continuity of stroke care.

Disposition and Discharge Planning

Decisions regarding the level of care for ongoing rehabilitation, particularly whether intensive inpatient rehabilitation is needed, should be made by the primary medical or neurologic team in consultation with rehabilitation providers. Three criteria influence the triage decision:

1. The pre-morbid and current functional statuses of the stroke survivors
2. The psychosocial and financial systems to support the stroke survivor in the community
3. The conditions of third-party reimbursement

The first criterion is heavily weighted by the recommendations of the physical, occupational, and speech/language therapists. Consideration must be given as to whether the candidate has adequate physical and neurocognitive capacity to perform basic ADL functions, including mobility with safety using the appropriate assistive device and/or orthosis. For individuals with mobility deficits and elevated fall risk, a home assessment may be recommended to optimize safety and facilitate ADL functionality. Some individuals may require the capacity to maintain their own instrumental ADL functions such as banking, shopping, and cooking for independent functioning. This requires higher levels of communicative and cognitive skills for home management, community living, health management, and the ability to react safely and correctly to emergency situations. Hence, instrumental ADL status must be ascertained prior to discharge, and a follow-up plan for repeated assessment made in the event of discharge to the community.

Psychosocial and financial systems are essential to support the stroke survivor if he or she wishes to return to the community. If the caregivers are ready, willing, and able to assist or supervise the stroke survivor in the community, the stroke survivor may be admitted to an inpatient rehabilitation facility. If the stroke survivor has inadequate support systems to return to the community, it may be prudent to transfer the stroke survivor to a less intensive environment, to give the stroke survivor more time for spontaneous improvement. If the stroke survivor remains at an assisted functional level that cannot be supported in the community, the stroke survivor ultimately will be transferred to a long-term facility.

The final component of the rehabilitation triage decision ultimately rests upon the type of third-party payer policy under which the stroke survivor is covered. While most insurance policies carry contingencies for different levels of rehabilitation care, some may limit the amount of inpatient and/or outpatient coverage per diagnosis. Some may not have provisions for specific levels of rehabilitation. Some may force the stroke survivor to pay for a portion of his or her rehabilitation hospital bills. Some may limit their networks to specific inpatient rehabilitation facilities. In any case, it is imperative for the stroke survivor and his or her caregiver to review his insurance policy to insure proper coverage in the event of a catastrophic event such as stroke. It is equally essential for the case manager to review the policy and confirm benefits before transferring a stroke survivor to an inpatient rehabilitation facility, to insure that the third-party payer will pay for the rehabilitation stay, and to minimize the financial liability on the stroke survivor and caregiver.

A comprehensive rehabilitation follow-up plan should be set in motion before any community discharge. Attention should be given to therapeutic modalities and prevention of post-stroke complications. Other factors such as return to work (Chapter 46), driving (Chapter 43), sexual function (Chapter 45), adaptive equipment (Chapter 34), social adjustments, and planning free-living physical activity and health-promoting exercise are generally managed in the outpatient environment and are dealt with in other chapters (Chapters 24, 42, 44, 47).

STROKE SYNDROMES

Knowledge of the vascular anatomy of the brain and the effects of specific arterial occlusion can be important in determining the location and size of the infarct. This information can be helpful in determining rehabilitation strategies and in formulating decisions for secondary prevention. Chapters 5 and 6 provide detailed clinical and vascular-neuroanatomic descriptions of anterior and posterior circulation stroke syndromes. Following is an abbreviated description of the cerebrovascular supply and some common stroke syndromes.

The posterior portion of the brain is supplied by the basilar artery, and the anterior brain by the bilateral carotid arteries. The internal carotid artery divides into the anterior and middle carotid arteries. Occlusion of the internal carotid artery may be asymptomatic if there is a patent posterior communicating artery supplying adequate collateral circulation to the intracranial carotid branches. If the communicating arteries are not adequate, the symptoms would include contralateral hemiplegia and hemianaesthesia, ipsilateral visual loss if the ophthalmic artery is involved, and aphasia if the dominant hemisphere is affected.

With occlusion of the middle cerebral artery, contralateral hemiparesis and hemianaesthesia, hemianopsia with involvement of the optic tracts, and aphasia with dominant hemispheric lesions are seen. The hemiparesis affects face and arm more than leg. In non-dominant hemispheric infarction, denial syndromes may be seen. If the lesion is in the main trunk of the middle cerebral artery, edema can result in coma.

Occlusion of the anterior carotid artery causes hemiplegia and sensory loss contralateral to the side of occlusion, affecting the lower extremity to a greater degree than the upper extremity. Mental confusion may also be associated with this lesion.

The basilar artery derives from the right and left vertebral artery and supplies the brainstem and cerebellum. It usually terminates to form the posterior cerebral arteries; however, in some individuals there may be a persistent fetal circulation, with origin of the posterior cerebral artery from the middle cerebral artery via the posterior communicating artery. Occlusion of the basilar artery may cause dizziness, coma, diplopia, pinpoint pupils (pons involvement), hemiplegia or quadriplegia, headache, dysphagia, mutism, or ataxia, depending on the degree and location of the occlusion.

The superior cerebellar arteries branch from the top of the basilar artery. Occlusion of this artery results in ataxia ipsilateral to the lesion, with hemianaesthesia contralateral to the lesion. The anterior inferior cerebellar artery branches from the basilar artery at the level of the pons. Symptoms of anterior inferior cerebellar artery (AICA) infarction include sudden hearing loss and vertigo, ipsilateral facial anesthesia or paralysis, Horner's syndrome, contralateral body anesthesia, or ataxia. The posterior inferior cerebellar artery branches from the vertebral artery. Occlusion of this artery is known as the Wallenberg Syndrome. Symptoms include ipsilateral facial sensory loss, Horner's syndrome, and ataxia, as well as contralateral sensory loss and weakness. Ipsilateral paresis of the palate and tongue are seen.

Symptoms of occlusion of the posterior cerebral artery are dependent on the branch involved. The calcarine branch occlusion leads to contralateral hemianopsia. Infarct of the posterior occipital artery may cause a thalamic syndrome with contralateral sensory loss, later leading to dysesthesia and pain.

Determination of the location of the infarct explains the symptoms the patient is experiencing. This in turn is beneficial in planning the rehabilitation program for the patient.

TRANSIENT CEREBRAL ISCHEMIA OR MILD STROKE SYMPTOMS

Transient ischemic attacks (TIA) were previously defined as stroke symptoms that subsided within 24 hours. With the advent of rt-PA treatment requiring treatment within three hours, that definition has been modified. Indeed, MRI studies with diffusion weighted imaging have indicated that over half of the patients whose symptoms lasted more than 60 minutes actually have areas of infarction despite resolution of symptoms. Although the clinical symptoms in TIA have subsided, it is important that the patient be thoroughly evaluated. Emerging guidelines for evaluation and acute medical management of TIA are now moving toward paralleling those of acute ischemic stroke (37). This approach toward the rapid management of TIA is being driven by an increasing recognition that many clinical events formerly classified as TIAs do indeed result in structural damage to the brain, and because the cerebrovascular event rate following TIA is dangerously high (37, 38). Hence, TIA should be considered a medical emergency, with an imperative to optimize comprehensive secondary prevention strategies immediately. While Chapter 22 details the secondary prevention of ischemic stroke, the following section provides a brief review of selected preventative medicine strategies in the setting of acute TIA.

Following a TIA, meta-analyses of 11 prospective studies suggest that the risk for recurrent stroke is 3.5%, 8%, and 9.2% at 2, 30, and 90 days post-TIA, respectively (38). Twenty-one percent of these strokes are fatal, with another 64% resulting in disability. The TIA therefore offers an opportunity to intervene and prevent a significant number of strokes. Indeed, studies from Paris and Oxfordshire, United Kingdom, have indicated that early evaluation and management may decrease the risk of stroke in the 90-day period by as much as 80% (40). Notably, the mean time to comprehensive clinical evaluation in the EXPRESS prospective study of stroke prevention following TIA was less than 1 day, underscoring the importance of rapid care (40).

Some potential risk factors for TIA include hypertension that increases both small (lacunar) and large vessel arterial atherothrombotic risk, atrial fibrillation and selected other cardiac arrhythmias, extra-cranial carotid and intracranial large vessel stenosis, cardiomyopathy, hyperlipidemia, vasculitis, cigarette smoking, hypercoaguable states, diabetes, syphilis, elevated C-reactive protein, and elevated homocystine levels. A timely evaluation of these risk factors is recommended in TIA and acute stroke patients.

The blood pressure may be transiently elevated following a TIA or stroke, and often decreases spontaneously. However, in sustained hypertension, the risk of stroke in the patient with a diastolic blood pressure of 105 is four times that of a diastolic of 90. If the diastolic is 84, the risk is half that of diastolic of 90. Therefore, close control of blood pressure can decrease the stroke risk significantly.

Atrial fibrillation may produce a cardioembolic source of cerebral ischemia. This risk increases with age and comorbid conditions such as congestive heart failure, hypertension, and diabetes. The use of warfarin decreases this risk by 68%. Aspirin decreases the risk slightly, but is significantly less effective than warfarin. There is no data to support the use of combination therapy with warfarin and aspirin or other platelet agents, which increases the risk for bleeding complications.

Carotid stenosis should be evaluated for stenotic lesions in symptomatic patients. Carotid ultrasound may be used for screening patients with a sensitivity of approximately 85%, compared to digital arteriography. In combination with MR angiography, the sensitivity of detecting carotid stenosis improves to close to 100%. CT angiography is also helpful in assessing carotid lesions with a sensitivity of 88–98%, depending on the study. If a question remains regarding the lesion, catheter arteriography may be necessary. These studies are also needed to evaluate for less frequent conditions such as arterial dissection.

In patients with carotid stenosis greater than 70%, the North American Symptomatic Carotid Endarterectomy Trial indicated that carotid endarterectomy reduced the risk of ipsilateral stroke from 26% to 9%, compared to medical management at two years. There was no significant change between the groups for less severe stenosis. The surgical/arteriographic risk for these procedures was less than 3%. For patients who are at higher risk, the benefits of endarterectomy compared to medical therapy would be less, perhaps indicating that medical management would be preferable. The greatest benefit occurred when surgery was performed within two weeks of symptom onset. See Chapter 23 on secondary prevention of ischemic stroke for more detailed results regarding the carotid endarterectomy trials and their impact on stroke care pathways. For patients with contraindications to surgery, such as prior radiation treatment to the neck or lesions that cannot be approached surgically, carotid stents have been approved to manage the stenosis.

Hyperlipidemia is a risk for cardiovascular disease, and to a lesser degree cerebrovascular disease. The current recommendations call for an LDL value less than 100 in patients who have had cerebral ischemic events. If there are multiple risk factors, an LDL of less than 70 is recommended. The statin agents have been shown to decrease the risk of stroke. This may not be solely on the basis of cholesterol control, as they also have some anti-inflammatory properties. This class of drug also lowers C reactive protein, which is another stroke risk factor.

Cigarette smoking is a major modifiable risk factor. All smokers should receive counseling and education regarding the importance of smoking cessation. Several agents and techniques are available to help patients with this endeavor. These include nicotine patch and gum, hypnosis, and pharmacological agents such as varenicline and bupropion.

The use of antiplatelet agents also decreases the risk of recurrent stroke. Aspirin has been shown to decrease the risk of stroke by 18% compared to placebo. Clopidogrel has a relative risk reduction that is 8% better than aspirin.

Controlled release dipyrimadole plus aspirin has been shown to have a decreased stroke rate that is 23% better than aspirin and 37% better than placebo. The use of antiplatelet agents is therefore of paramount importance in preventing recurrent stroke.

CONCLUSIONS

The efficient acute management of stroke requires emergent and structured protocols for efficient patient management. When the patient has had an ischemic stroke, early treatment can result in improved clinical outcomes. Proper medical management, even in patients who are not candidates for thrombolytic or neuro-interventional procedures, results in better outcomes. Studies have demonstrated a significant decrease in the number of patients with severe disability when treated on a dedicated stroke floor, compared to those treated on a general medical ward. Many hospitals are now developing programs as Primary Stroke Centers, and accreditation for these programs has been established. These programs also stress the early rehabilitation plans for the patient. Evaluation of dysphagia to prevent aspiration, nutritional assessment and planning, early patient mobilization, cognitive and communication assessment and speech/language therapy, and measures to prevent skin breakdown and deep vein thrombosis are important components of these programs.

The timely management of transient cerebral ischemia must be stressed. The admission of the patient for observation to obtain the necessary testing within 24 hours is recommended in most cases. With the high incidence of early stroke after TIA, the use of rt-PA might be facilitated by the admission as well. The development of dedicated clinics that see the patient immediately and institute the evaluation of the TIA patient has been possible in some communities. This approach also allows for the timely evaluation and institution of appropriate treatment, but is not widely available. It is recommended that the patient not be discharged from an emergency department to be evaluated in a few days by his or her primary care physician. With proper care and patient management, the risk of stroke and its devastating effects can be overcome. The institution of timely rehabilitation measures can improve daily living function for the patient.

References

1. Feldman E, Cordon N, Brooks JM. Factors associated with early presentation of acute stroke. *Stroke* 1993; 24:1805–1810.
2. Tissue plasminogen activator for acute ischemic stroke. The National Institute of Neurological Disorders and Stroke rt-PA Stroke Study Group. *N Engl J Med* 1995; 333:1581–1587.
3. Kwiatkowski TG, Libman RB, Frankel M, et al. Effects of tissue plasminogen activator for acute ischemic stroke at one year. National Institute of Neurological Disorders and Stroke Recombinant Tissue Plasminogen Activator Stroke Study Group. *N Engl J Med* 1999; 340:1781–1787.
4. Hacke W, Brott T, Caplan L, et al. Thrombolysis in acute ischemic stroke: Controlled trials and clinical experience. *Neurology* 1999; Suppl 4:S3–14.
5. Barber PA, Zhang J, Demchuk AM, et al. Why are stroke patients excluded from TPA therapy? An analysis of patient eligibility. *Neurology* 2001; 56:1015–1020.

6. Stroke Unit Trialists' Collaboration. Organized inpatient (stroke unit) care for stroke. *Cochrane Database Syst Rev* 2007; (4) CD000197.

7. Seenan P, Long M, Langhorne P. Stroke units in their natural habitat: Systematic review of observational studies. *Stroke* 2007; 38:1886–1892.

8. Bath PM, Bath FJ, Smithard DG. Interventions for dysphagia in acute stroke. *Cochrane database Syst Rev* 2000; CD000323.

9. Foley N, Teasell R, Salter K, et al. Dysphagia treatment post stroke: A systematic review of randomized controlled trials. *Age Ageing* 2008; 37:258–264.

10. Singh I, Vilches A, Narro M. Nutritional support and stroke. *Hosp. Med* 2004; 65:721–730.

11. Yoo SH, Kim JS, Kwon SU, et al. Undernutrition as a predictor of poor clinical outcomes in acute ischemic stroke patients. *Arch Neuro.* 2008; 65:39–43.

12. Stead LG, Gilmore RM, Bellolio MF, et al. Hyperglycemia as an independent predictor of worse outcome in non-diabetic patients presenting with acute ischemic stroke. *Neurocrit Care* 2008; Mar 21 Epub ahead of print.

13. Alvarez-Sabín J, Molina CA, Montaner J, et al. Effects of admission hyperglycemia on stroke outcome in reperfused tissue plasminogen activator-treated patients. *Stroke* 2003; 34:1235–1241.

14. Kennedy J, Hill MD, Ryckborst KJ, et al, FASTER Investigators. Fast assessment of stroke and transient ischaemic attack to prevent early recurrence (FASTER): A randomized controlled pilot trial. *Lancet Neurol* 2007; 6:961–969.

15. Toyoda K, Yasaka M, Iwade K, et al, for the Bleeding with Antithrombotic Therapy (BAT) Study Group. Dual antithrombotic therapy increases severe bleeding events in patients with stroke and cardiovascular disease. A prospective, multicenter, observational study. *Stroke* 2008; Apr 3 Epub ahead of print.

16. Ali LK, Saver JL. The ischemic stroke patient who worsens: New assessment and management approaches. *Rev Neurol Dis* 2007; 4:85–91.

17. Karepov VG, Gur AY, Bova I, et al. Stroke-in-evolution: Infarct-inherent mechanisms versus systemic causes. *Cerebrovasc Dis* 2006; 21:42–46.

18. Macko RF, Ameriso SF, Gruber A, et al. Impairments of the protein C system and fibrinolysis in infection-associated stroke. *Stroke* 1996; 27:2005–2011.

19. Macko RF, Ameriso SF, Barndt R, et al. Precipitants of brain infarction. Roles of preceding infection/inflammation and recent psychological stress. *Stroke* 1996; 27:1999–2004.

20. Kwan J, Hand P. Infection after acute stroke is associated with poor short-term outcome. *Acta Neurol Scand* 2007; 115:331–338.

21. Bladin CF, Alexanrov AV, Bellevance A, et al. Seizures after stroke: A prospective multi-center study. *Arch Neurol* 2000; 57:1617–1622.

22. Claassen J, Jetté N, Chum F, et al. Electrographic seizures and periodic discharges after intracerebral hemorrhage. *Neurology* 2007; 69:1356–1365.

23. Vespa PM, O'Phelan K, Shah M, et al. Acute seizures after intracerebral hemorrhage: A factor in progressive midline shift and outcome. *Neurology* 2003; 60:1441–1446.

24. Broderick J, Connolly S, Feldmann E, et al. American Heart Association/American Stroke Association Stroke Council, American Heart Association/American Stroke Association High Blood Pressure Research Council; Quality of Care and Outcomes in Research Interdisciplinary Working Group. Guidelines for the management of spontaneous intracerebral hemorrhage in adults: 2007 update: A guideline from the American Heart Association/American Stroke Association Stroke Council, High Blood Pressure Research Council,

and the Quality of Care and Outcomes in Research Interdisciplinary Working Group. *Circulation* 2007; 116:e391–413.

25. Qureshi AI, Suarez JI, Yahia AM, et al. Timing of neurologic deterioration in massive middle cerebral artery infarction: A multicenter review. *Crit Care Med* 2003; 31:272–277.

26. Hacke W, Schwab S, Horn M, et al. Malignant middle cerebral artery territory infarction: Clinical course and prognostic signs. *Arch Neurol* 1996; 53:309–315.

27. Vahedi K, Hofmeijer J, Juettler E, et al, and DECIMAL, DESTINY, and HAMLET investigators. Early decompressive surgery in malignant infarction of the middle cerebral artery: A pooled analysis of three randomized controlled trials. *Lancet Neuro.* 2007; 6:215–222.

28. Bonita R, Beaglehole R. Modification of Rankin Scale: Recovery of motor function after stroke. *Stroke* 1988; 19:1497–1500.

29. Albers GW, Amarenco P, Easton D, et al. Antithrombotic and thrombolytic therapy for ischemic stroke: The seventh ACCP conference on antithrombotic and throbolytic therapy. *Chest* 2004; 126:483S–512S.

30. VA Employee Education System in Cooperation with the Offices of Quality and Performance and Patient Care Services and the Department of Defense. VA/DoD Clinical practice guideline for the management of stroke rehabilitation: Guideline summary. *National CPG Council* October 2002. http//www.oqp.med.va.gov/cpg.cpg.ttm or http//www.qmo.amedd.army.mil/.

31. Sherman DG, Albers GW, Bladin C, et al, PREVAIL Investigators. The efficacy and safety of enoxaparin versus unfractionated heparin for the prevention of venous thromboembolism after acute ischaemic stroke (PREVAIL Study): An open-label randomized comparison. *Lancet* 2007; 369:1347–1355.

32. André C, de Freitas GR, Fukujima MM. Prevention of deep venous thrombosis and pulmonary embolism following stroke: A systematic review of published articles. *Eur J. Neuro* 2007; 14:21–32.

33. Schubert V, Héraud J. The effects of pressure and shear on skin microcirculation in elderly stroke patients lying in supine or semi-recumbent positions. *Age Aging* 1994; 23:405–410.

34. Hermann DM, Bassetti CL. Sleep apnea and other sleep-wake disorders in stroke. *Curr Treat Option Neurol* 2003; 5:241–249.

35. Brown DL. Sleep disorders and stroke. *Semin Neurol* 2006; 26:117–122.

36. Bassetti CL. Sleep and stroke. *Semin Neurol* 2005; 25:19–32.

37. Walker MP, Stickgold R, Alsop D, et al. Sleep-dependent motor memory plasticity in the human brain. *Neuroscience* 2005; 133:911–917.

38. Ringleb PA. Guidelines for management of ischaemic stroke and transient ischaemic attack. *Cerebrovasc Dis* 2008; 25(5):457–507.

39. Wu CM, McLaughlin K, Lorenzetti DL, et al. Early risk of stroke after transient ischemic attack: A systematic review and meta-analysis. *Arch Intern Med* 2007; 167(22):2417–2422.

40. Rothwell PM, Giles MF, Chandratheva A, et al. Early use of Existing Preventive Strategies for Stroke (EXPRESS) study. Effect of urgent treatment of transient ischaemic attack and minor stroke on early recurrent stroke (EXPRESS study): A prospective population-based sequential comparison. *Lancet* 2007; 370(9596):1432–1442.

4 Neuroimaging of Acute Stroke

Govind Mukundan
Pamela W. Schaefer

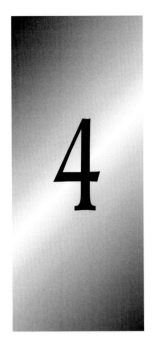

A number of CT and MR techniques are essential for imaging acute stroke patients. Noncontrast CT excludes other causes of acute neurologic deficits and intracranial hemorrhage. CT and MR angiography identify intravascular clot. CTA source images improve the CT detection of acute infarction. Diffusion MRI more precisely estimates the location and age of infarcted core, and perfusion imaging estimates the ischemic penumbra. These new modalities play a critical role in determining which patients should undergo thrombolytic therapy.

Acute stroke imaging is rapidly advancing. Fifteen years ago, state-of-the-art CT and MRI techniques were insensitive in detecting acute stroke, and the diagnosis was usually presumptive. In the 1990s, diffusion-weighted MRI provided the first highly sensitive technique for visualizing acutely ischemic brain tissue. More recently, the development of CT and MR perfusion imaging has allowed the visualization of additional hypoperfused tissue at risk of infarction. The development of CT and MR angiography has allowed highly reliable detection of proximal intravascular clot. Concomitant advances in stroke treatment provide a unique opportunity for imaging to direct and revolutionize stroke triage and management (1).

In this chapter, we review how conventional and advanced CT and MR imaging techniques are used to provide four types of information that are essential to the care of acute stroke patients: (Table 4-1)

1. They establish the diagnosis of ischemic stroke and exclude other potential causes of an acute neurologic deficit.
2. They identify intracranial hemorrhage.
3. They identify the vascular lesion responsible for the ischemic event.
4. They provide additional characterization of brain tissue that may guide stroke therapy by determining the viability of different regions of the brain and distinguishing between irreversibly infarcted tissue and potentially salvageable tissue.

NONCONTRAST COMPUTED TOMOGRAPHY

Computed tomography (CT) is based on the measurement of X-ray beam attenuation through a region of interest, which is proportional to density. Its low cost and accuracy in the detection of intracranial hemorrhage still place it as the first-line diagnostic exam of choice in the emergency room setting in the United States. In addition to excluding hemorrhage, noncontrast CT (NCCT) is obtained primarily to exclude hypodensity in greater than one-third of the middle cerebral artery territory and to exclude other causes of acute neurologic deficits, such as intracranial

TABLE 4-1
Critical Questions in the Imaging Evaluation of Acute Stroke

1. Is there hemorrhage?
2. Is the proximal intravascular thrombus a target for therapy?
3. Is there an infarct (or core) of irreversibly ischemic tissue?
4. Is there severely ischemic, but potentially salvageable, tissue (the penumbra)?

basal cisterns caused by mild swelling; as well as subtle parenchymal hypodensity and hyperdensity within an intracranial vessel such as the MCA from acute thrombus (3). (Figure 4-1, Table 4-2) CT hypodensity is, in general, thought to be secondary to increased total tissue edema. Cytotoxic edema develops within 30 minutes of an acute embolic event caused by failure of Na$^+$K$^+$-ATPase and other ion pumps. Vasogenic edema develops at approximately four to six hours, secondary to disrupted endothelial tight junctions and reperfusion. Because cytotoxic edema results in net shift of water from the extracellular to the intracellular space, not an increase in total water, and CT hypodensity may appear before the onset of vasogenic edema, some authors have proposed that decreased blood volume causes early CT hypodensity (4).

mass lesion, that would preclude the patient from receiving anticoagulation, thrombolytic therapy, or aggressive hypertensive therapy. One large study found that, among patients with symptoms of acute stroke, NCCT achieved sensitivity and specificity of 90 and 99%, respectively, in detecting intracranial hemorrhage (2).

Noncontrast CT findings of acute stroke syndrome are subtle when present and include loss of cortical, basal ganglia or insular grey-white matter differentiation; loss of cortical sulci and reduced sylvian fissure and

Reported sensitivities of NCCT in the detection of acute infarction vary widely in the literature, secondary to dependence on time between symptom onset and imaging, the vascular territory involved, the generation of CT scanner, CT technique, viewing methodology, knowledge of clinical history, and reader experience. In one large retrospective study, in which the mean time from symptom onset to scanning was 2.3 hours and neuroradiologists blinded to clinical history interpreted the scans, the

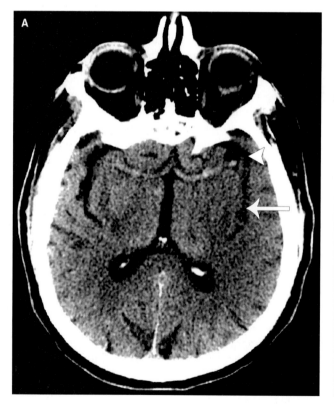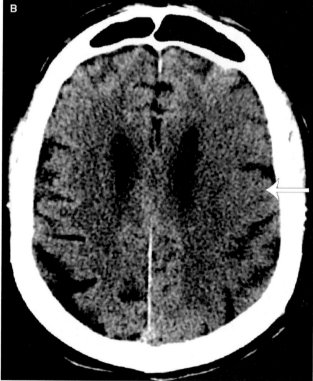

FIGURE 4-1

Early left MCA infarction. Sixty-year-old female with onset of left hemiparesis and aphasia four hours prior to imaging. There is hypodensity, loss of gray-white differentiation, and mild sulcal effacement throughout the visualized MCA territory (yellow arrows). There is hyperdensity in the left MCA stem, consistent with acute thrombus (arrowhead).

TABLE 4-2
NCCT Findings in Acute Ischemic Stroke

IMAGING FINDINGS

Parenchymal hypodensity
Hyperdense vessel sign
Loss of gray white matter differentiation
Mild sulcal effacement
Exclusion criteria for receiving thrombolytic therapy
  Intracranial hemorrhage
  Hypodensity in greater than one-third of the MCA
    territory
Predictors of Intracranial Hemorrhage
  Hypodensity in greater than one-third of the MCA
    territory
  ASPECTS score < 7

sensitivity for detecting acute infarction was 38% (5). The sensitivity improved to 52% when clinical history was provided. In another study of 30 patients, the sensitivity for detection of acute ischemia was 57% using standard windows (window = 40 HU, level = 80 HU) but improved to 71% with narrow windows (window = 36 HU, level = 30 HU) (5). Reported specificities are high, ranging from 89 to 95% (6). In addition, one study found that the hyperdense middle cerebral artery sign was 100% specific for middle cerebral artery occlusion, but only 27% sensitive (7).

The hypodensity in NCCT has a number of important clinical implications. Multiple studies have confirmed that hypodensity on NCCT in the acute stroke setting almost always represents infarcted tissue. One study demonstrated that hypodense tissue on NCCT becomes necrotic with a probability of 97% (8). Hypodensity on NCCT correlates with stroke severity (8). The ECASS study demonstrated that hypodensity in greater than one-third of the MCA territory correlates with an increased risk of hemorrhage following the administration of intravenous TPA; hypodensity in more than one-half of the MCA territory is associated with brain herniation (9).

The Alberta Stroke Program Early CT Score (ASPECTS) represents one effort to improve intra- and interrater reliability, by partially quantifying the extent of hypodensity on NCCT scans (10). In ASPECTS, 10 regions in the MCA territory are assigned a score of zero or one depending on the presence (one) or absence (zero) of hypodensity, and the total number of ischemic regions is subtracted from ten. ASPECTS may be helpful in deciding whether or not thrombolytic therapy should be initiated. One large study found that ASPECTS scores of seven or less, indicating the presence of hypodensity in more than one-third of the MCA territory, are associated

with a substantially increased risk of thrombolysis-related parenchymal hemorrhage (11).

CONVENTIONAL MR IMAGING

T2 and FLAIR images, like NCCT, are capable of detecting parenchymal changes in acute ischemic stroke because of vasogenic edema. However, because there is little vasogenic edema present in the first six hours after stroke onset, parenchymal hyperintensity may be difficult to detect. Furthermore, volume averaging with CSF signal can obscure small lesions. In one study, the sensitivity of T2 weighted images in the first six hours was only 18% (12). Because CSF is hypointense, FLAIR has improved detection of infarctions in brain parenchyma, such as cortex and periventricular white matter, adjacent to CSF. Sensitivity of FLAIR imaging for the detection of parenchymal injury, however, is still as low as 29% in the first six hours (13). Besides parenchymal hyperintensity, other signs of acute stroke on MRI include loss of vascular flow voids on T2 weighted images, arterial hyperintensity on FLAIR images, vascular contrast enhancement caused by slow flow, on gadolinium-enhanced T1 weighted images, intravascular susceptibility (blooming) in the region of the acute thrombus on gradient echo/T2* images, and effacement of sulci, cisterns, and ventricles caused by mild swelling (Table 4-3, Figure 4-4). Gradient echo/T2* images are also highly sensitive for detecting hemorrhage.

MRI DIFFUSION-WEIGHTED IMAGING

Diffusion-weighted imaging is a MR sequence with image contrast dependent on the magnitude of the relative motion or diffusion of water molecules. This property is particularly useful in the setting of acute strokes. Acute ischemia induces a cascade of metabolic and molecular changes that, within minutes, ultimately act to decrease the relative motion of tissue water molecules in the

TABLE 4-3
Appearance of Acute Arterial Infarcts on Conventional MRI

1. T2—loss of *arterial* flow void, +/− subtle parenchymal hyperintensity
2. FLAIR—increased arterial signal +/− subtle parenchymal hyperintensity
3. Gradient echo/T2*—intravascular blooming in the region of the thrombus, and hemorrhage
4. T1 postcontrast—arterial enhancement without parenchymal enhancement

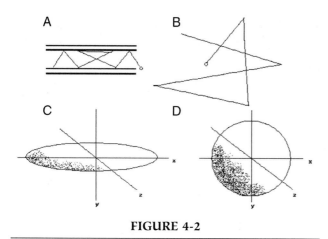

FIGURE 4-2

Anisotropic and isotropic diffusion of water molecules. Diagrammatic path of a water molecule within highly organized tissue such as white matter (A) and the associated three-dimensional representation of diffusion of water molecules in this system (C). Diagrammatic path of water in a nonbounded environment (B) and the associated three-dimensional representation of diffusion of water molecules in this system (D).

affected parenchyma (14, 15). As cytotoxic edema develops, there is a decrease in energy metabolism that leads to failure of Na^+/K^+ ATPase and other ion pumps (14). This results in loss of ionic gradients and net translocation of water from the extracellular to the intracellular compartment, where water movement is relatively more restricted. With cellular swelling, there is also reduction in the extracellular space volume and increased tortuosity of extracellular space pathways (16). In addition, there are significant reductions in intracellular metabolite ADCs that may be caused by increased intracellular viscosity from dissociation of microtubules and fragmentation of other cellular components, increased tortuosity of the intracellular space, and decreased cytoplasmic mobility.

Physical Principles and Diffusion MR Maps

MR is based on the principle of adding energy to the spins of hydrogen atoms in water molecules (referred to as *spins*) and listening to the energy that is emitted back as the spins relax from their higher energy state to a lower basal state. The basic diffusion pulse sequence (Figure 4-3) consists of two equal gradient lobes with a 180-degree refocusing pulse obtained in between (17). The first gradient causes the spins to go out of phase and lose signal. The 180-degree pulse inverts the phase of the spins. The second gradient lobe refocuses the spins. Because the magnitude of the gradient lobes are identical, relatively immobile spins like those in ischemic parenchyma have the gradient-induced phase shifts cancelled out, leaving their initial signal intact. This results in relatively hyperintense signal on the resultant diffusion-weighted MR

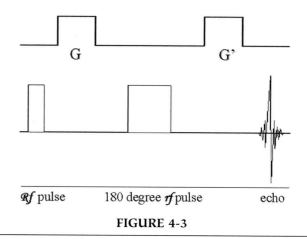

FIGURE 4-3

Fundamental Stejskal-Tanner diffusion MR scheme. During the first gradient lobe (G), the proton spins acquire phase shift. The 180-degree radio frequency (rf) pulse inverts all the spins. The second gradient lobe (G') induces a second refocusing phase shift that is opposite to the first (caused by all spins inverted). Water protons that have not translocated have their phase shifts cancelled and lose no net signal (bright on image). Water protons that have migrated in space result in incomplete refocusing and incomplete cancellation of phase shift leading to loss of signal (dark on image).

image. However, spins with some motion, for example, in normal brain parenchyma, have incomplete cancellation of their accumulated phase proportional to their translocation and have some loss of signal. Thus, normal parenchyma appears relatively hypointense compared to ischemic tissue.

Image Interpretation

Diffusion-weighted images (DWI) and exponential images or apparent diffusion coefficient (ADC) maps should be available for review (Figure 4-4). It is important to understand that the DWI images have T2 contrast as well as contrast caused by differences in diffusion. In order to remove the T2 contrast, the DWI can be divided by the echoplanar T2 image (or b = 0 image) to give an exponential image. Alternatively, an ADC map, whose signal intensity is equal to the magnitude of the apparent diffusion coefficient, can be created. On DW images, regions with decreased diffusion (as in acute ischemia) are hyperintense. Regions with elevated diffusion (as in vasogenic edema) may be hypointense, isointense, or hyperintense, depending on the strength of the diffusion and T2 components. On exponential images, regions with decreased diffusion are hyperintense while lesions with elevated diffusion are hypointense. On ADC maps, regions with decreased diffusion are hypointense, while regions with elevated diffusion are hyperintense. For lesions with decreased diffusion, the DW images have superior lesion conspicuity. However, because hyperintense signal abnormality on DW images

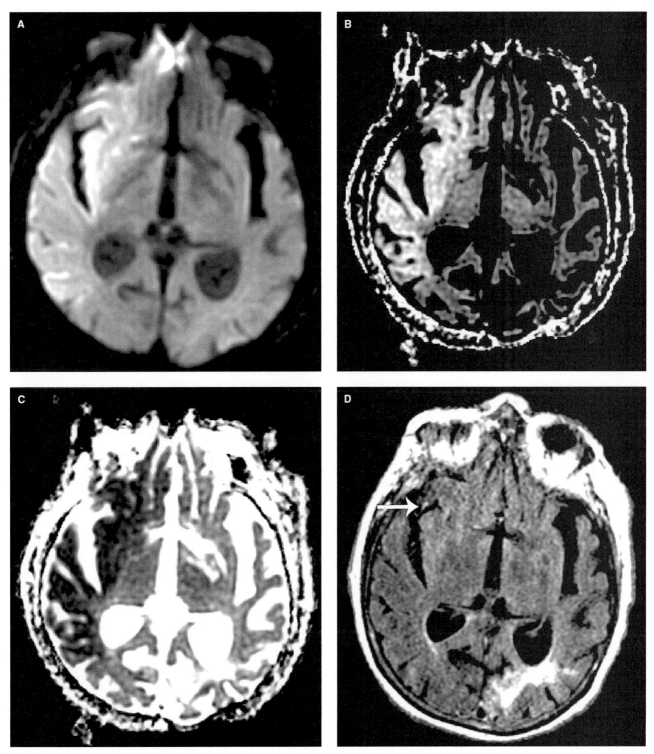

FIGURE 4-4

Diffusion MR images of an 88-year-old female with atrial fibrillation with sudden onset of left hemiparesis, one hour and twenty minutes before imaging. The acute right MCA infarction is hyperintense on DWI (A) and exponential (B) images and hypointense on ADC (C) images. FLAIR (D) and T2-weighted images (E) demonstrate no definite parenchymal abnormality in the region of the acute infarction, but the MCA branches are hyperintense on FLAIR and do not have normal flow voids on T2-weighted images, consistent with slow flow (yellow arrows). There is a chronic left occipital infarction. *(Continued)*

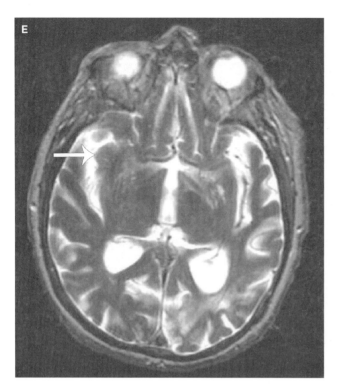

FIGURE 4-4 (Continued)

could result from the T2 component rather than from abnormal diffusion, review of the ADC maps or the exponential images is important.

Regardless of the mechanism, diffusion-weighted images are highly sensitive and specific in the detection of hyperacute and acute stroke (18, 19, 20). Reported sensitivities and specificities are in the greater than 90% range. The rare infarcts not identified on DWI are typically very small lacunar brainstem or deep gray nuclei infarctions. False positive DWI images may occur in patients with a subacute or chronic infarction with T2 shine through. In such cases, a lesion appears hyperintense on the DWI images caused by an increase in the T2 signal. This pitfall is easily avoided by interpreting the DW images in combination with ADC or exponential images (as described above). False positive DWI images can also occur with decreased diffusion caused by ion pump failure (seizures or hypoglycemia), decreased diffusion caused by high viscosity (abscess), decreased diffusion from dense cell packing (some tumors), and decreased diffusion caused by myelin vacuolization (CJD, demyelinative lesions, or diffuse axonal injury). When these lesions are reviewed in combination with routine T1, T2 and gadolinium-enhanced T1-weighted images and clinical history, they can usually readily be differentiated from acute ischemic infarctions.

The DWI lesion is thought to represent tissue that is destined to infarct. Indeed, reversibility (abnormal on

initial DWI but normal on follow-up images) of DWI hyperintense lesions is very rare and usually only seen in the setting of very early reperfusion following intravenous and/or intra-arterial thrombolysis (21). Even with thrombolysis, the amount of DWI abnormal tissue that recovers is usually relatively small and typically involves white matter more often than gray matter. However, judging whether tissue with a diffusion abnormality is normal at follow-up is complicated. Such lesions may appear normal on follow-up DWI, ADC or T2-weighted images, but this may not reflect complete tissue recovery. Kidwell et al. reported a decrease in size from the initial DWI abnormality to the follow-up DWI abnormality immediately after IA thrombolysis in 8/18 patients (21). However, despite the initial apparent recovery, a subsequent increase in DWI lesion volume was observed in five patients. Furthermore, a number of studies have demonstrated that ADCs are significantly higher in DWI reversible tissue compared with DWI abnormal tissue that progresses to infarction. Mean ADCs range from 663 to 732 $\times$ 10^{-6} mm^2/sec in DWI reversible regions, compared with 608 to 650 $\times$ 10^{-6} mm^2/sec in DWI abnormal regions that progress to infarction (21, 22).

The temporal evolution of acute infarcts on DWI imaging is of paramount importance, both from a diagnostic and therapeutic standpoint (Figure 4-5, Table 4-4). The literature reports appreciable reduced diffusion as early as 30 minutes after an ischemic event. The ADC decreases until reaching its nadir at one to four days. This is reflected in marked signal hyperintensity on DWI and exponential images and marked signal hypointensity on ADC maps. Thereafter, with cell membrane disruption and the development of vasogenic edema, the diffusion coefficient begins to rise and returns to baseline at one to two weeks. At this point, a stroke is usually mildly hyperintense from the T2 component on the DWI images and isointense on the ADC images (23). Thereafter, the ADC values continue to rise because of gliosis, cavitation, and increased extracellular water. There is hypointensity, isointensity, or hyperintensity on the DWI images (depending on the strength of the T2 and diffusion components) and increased signal intensity on ADC maps. While multiple variables including patient age, type of infarct, and infarct location can influence the general time course of these ADC changes, it is generally true that infarcts with low ADC and little or no associated abnormality on T2-weighted images are less than approximately six hours in age. Those with lower-than-normal ADC are less than approximately two weeks in age (24, 25).

CT ANGIOGRAPHY

Information about the intracranial and cervical vessels is an important part of the imaging evaluation as the bulk of acute stroke therapy targets intraluminal thrombus.

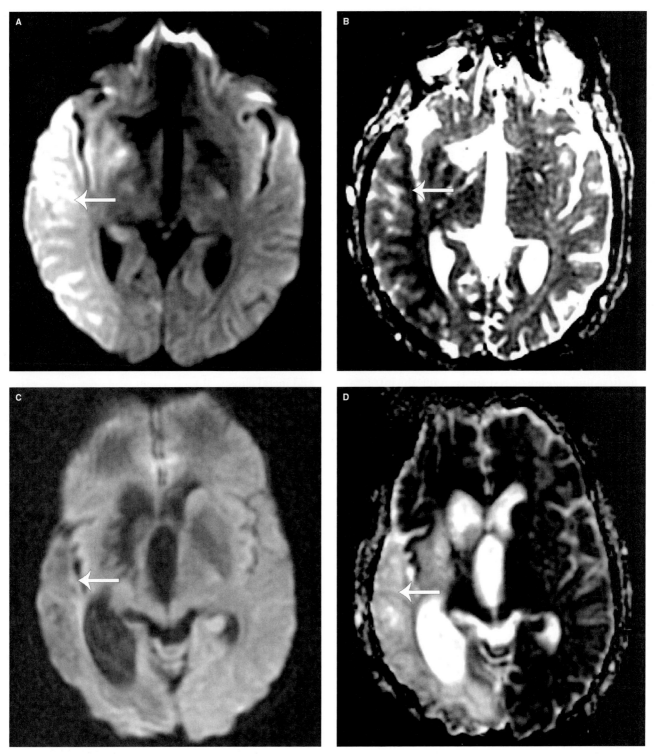

FIGURE 4-5

Evolution of DWI changes in an infarction. Sixty-four-year-old female with sudden onset left facial drop, left-sided weakness, and slurred speech. In the acute stage, the infarction (arrow) is hyperintense on DWI(A) and hypointense on ADC (B) maps from decreased diffusion. In the chronic stage two years later, the infarction is characterized by tissue cavitation and volume loss with associated dilatation of the lateral and third ventricle. There is now more free movement of water molecules with elevated diffusion characterized by decreased signal on the DWI (C) and increase signal on the ADC (D) maps.

TABLE 4-4
Temporal Changes in DWI, ADC, and Exponential Maps

PULSE SEQUENCE	HYPERACUTE (0–6 HOURS)	ACUTE (6–24 HOURS)	EARLY SUBACUTE (1–7 DAYS)	LATE SUBACUTE (1–4 WEEKS)	CHRONIC
Reason for ADC change	Cytotoxic edema	Cytotoxic edema	Cytotoxic edema + smaller vasogenic edema component	Cytotoxic and vasogenic edema	Vasogenic edema and then gliosis and neuronal loss
DWI	Hyperintense	Hyperintense	Hyperintense,	Hyperintense (mostly T2 component)	Isointense to hypointense
ADC	Hypointense	Hypointense	Hypointense	Isointense	Hyperintense
EXP	Hyperintense	Hyperintense	Hyperintense	Isointense	Hypointense

However, thrombolytic therapy carries a significant risk of intracranial hemorrhage. So it is equally important to exclude patients with stroke mechanisms that do not benefit from therapy like lacunar infarcts, or patients with stroke mimics such as seizures.

CTA offers many attractive features that have made it the first-line diagnostic test for imaging the intracranial vasculature in patients with signs and symptoms of acute stroke. CTA is widely available in the emergency setting and is a quick extension of the nonenhanced CT scan. Fast, high-resolution CTA techniques have become possible largely because of the advent of the helical CT scanner and the multidetector design of the scanner array. The helical scanning technology, developed in the 1990s, utilizes a slip ring to allow 360-degree rotation of the tube, scanning the patient with table progression. This results in the acquisition of a three-dimensional helical strip or ribbon of data. The development of multislice or multidetector CT essentially has led to the acquisition of a larger ribbon of data per gantry rotation, allowing larger coverage at higher speeds. Thus, with a single bolus of contrast, high-resolution angiographic images of the major vessels from the arch to the vertex can be obtained within a minute.

Furthermore, required postprocessing can be performed in minutes. For example, three-plane, orthogonal, maximal intensity projection (MIP) images can be reconstructed at the scanner by a technician in less than three minutes. The combination of the source axial images and the three-plane MIPS nearly always allows adequate evaluation of the arterial vasculature for the purposes of triage for thrombolytic therapy. In addition, the speed of CTA makes CTA images relatively resistant to degradation by artifact related to patient motion. CT scanners, unlike MRI scanners, allow for metallic equipment to be brought safely into the scanner room, allowing for easier monitoring of potentially unstable acute stroke patients.

A significant percentage of stroke patients also have cardiac disease that require pacemakers, and they cannot undergoing MR scanning. Also, CTA is less susceptible to other artifacts often encountered in MRA, including susceptibility artifact from calcified atherosclerotic plaque, air (e.g., within the petrous apices and sinuses), and metal clips.

Multiple studies have shown that CTA can detect large vessel intravascular clot with sensitivity and specificity of greater than 95% (26). (Figure 4-6) Thus, CTA plays a critical role in directing acute therapy by detecting occlusion of proximal intracranial arteries that are accessible by endovascular microcatheterization and may be treated by intra-arterial thrombolysis or mechanical clot disruption. Indeed, studies using CTA suggest that proximal occlusions should be treated with intra-arterial rather than, or in addition to, intravenous thrombolysis because intravenous thrombolysis is less effective in treating proximal lesions than in treating distal ones (27, 28). Also, detection of large vessel clots may be important in determining prognosis. One CTA study found that occlusion of a large intracranial artery was one of two factors that independently predicted poor outcome in acute stroke patients. (The other was poor initial neurologic status.) (29).

CTA has a number of other advantages. In the neck, it allows for evaluation for stroke etiology (Figure 4-7). CTA can demonstrate atherosclerotic plaque with thrombus at the internal carotid artery bifurcation. It can differentiate thrombosis from hairline residual lumen, and it can identify dissection. In the head, it allows for the evaluation of collateral circulation and improves the conspicuity of acute ischemia. Assuming a steady state level of contrast during scanning, the CTA source images (CTA-SI) can be considered whole brain perfused blood volume images. These images greatly improve the detection of subtle, early parenchymal ischemic changes compared to NCCT (30). Furthermore, the

CTA-SI lesion size correlates well with the DWI lesion size and may help to identify the infarction core or the tissue that is irreversibly destined for infarction. The CTA-SI may also be important in risk stratification and determining patient prognosis. In one study, CTA-SI increased the utility of the ASPECTS metric in predicting the clinical outcomes of acute stroke patients (31). In another, the degree of hypoattenuation on CTA-SI correlated with the likelihood of hemorrhagic transformation (32).

CTA does have some disadvantages. One of the most significant is the risk of contrast nephropathy (33, 34). This is especially heightened in patients with reduced renal function, diabetes, or both. In addition, a risk of contrast-induced allergic reactions does exist. Although nonionic contrast agents have decreased the overall risk of contrast induced reactions, there is a 0.03% risk of an anaphylactic reaction for nonionic, iodinated contrast agents (35). In addition, CTA imparts a radiation dose, a particularly important fact to consider when imaging children and pregnant women. In addition, multiple CTA examinations can result in a large cumulative dose.

MR ANGIOGRAPHY

MR angiography (MRA) techniques utilized in stroke imaging include noncontrast-enhanced time of flight (TOF) imaging as well as gadolinium-enhanced MRA. The physical principles underlying both techniques are complicated and are beyond the scope of this chapter. Briefly, time of flight techniques utilize a gradient echo sequence that saturates out signal from the stationary spins within a volume of tissue. This is accomplished by multiple radio frequency pulses, followed by dephasing and rephasing gradients. Thus, the only unsaturated spins (signal) are within blood flowing from outside into the volume of interest. Generally, the contrast is proportional to the velocity of flow (37). A saturation band decreases signal from venous flow, which is usually in the opposite direction from the arterial flow. Two-dimensional TOF MRA is generally performed for evaluation of the cervical arterial vasculature with the acquisition of multiple, contiguous, thin slices of tissue. Three-dimensional TOF MRA is usually used to evaluate the intracranial vasculature. This technique, as its name implies, acquires a volume of tissue and, with an

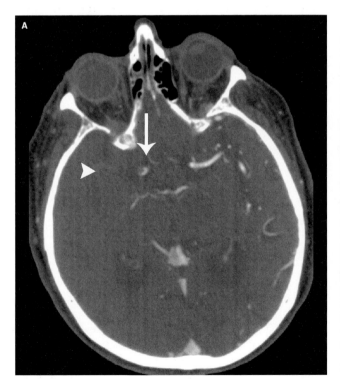
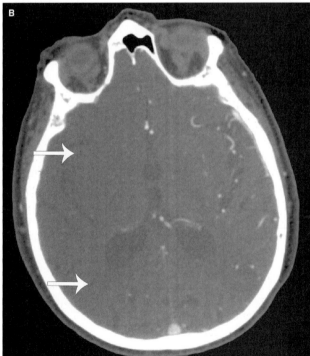

FIGURE 4-6

CTA axial source and maximal intensity projection (MIP) images. Eighty-eight-year-old female with atrial fibrillation and sudden onset of left hemiparesis, one hour and twenty minutes before imaging. Axial CTA source image (A) demonstrates occlusion of the right MCA stem (arrowhead) and distal ICA (arrow head) by thrombus. A and B (also an axial CTA source image) demonstrate no contrast within the right MCA branches, consistent with poor collateral flow (red arrows). *(Continued)*

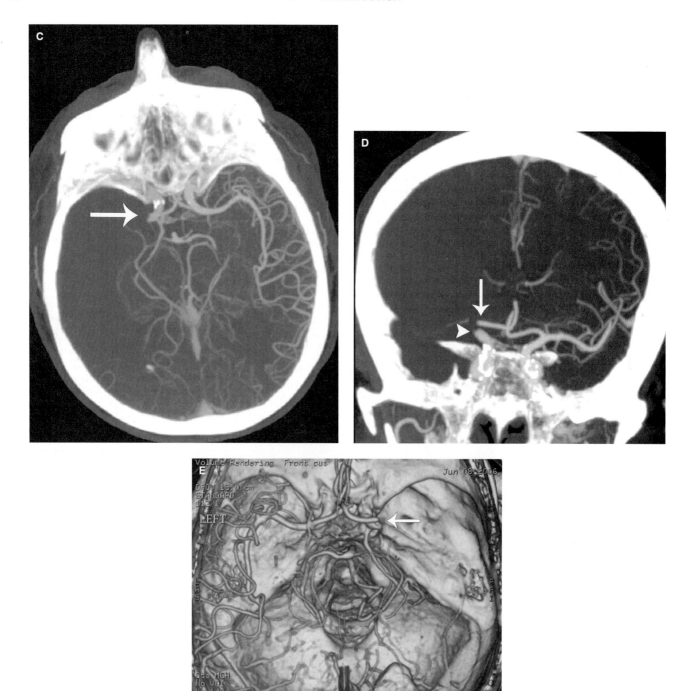

FIGURE 4-6 *(Continued)*

Axial (C) and coronal (D) MIP images also demonstrate occlusion of the distal ICA and proximal MCA as well as of the proximal ACA (arrows). They also demonstrate the poor collateral flow. Volume rendered three-dimensional image from the same CTA data (E). The image is laterally reversed by convention.

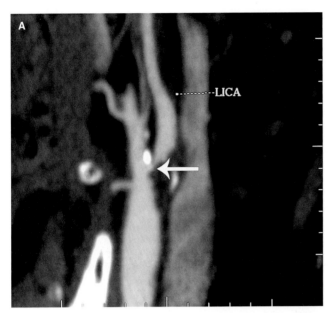

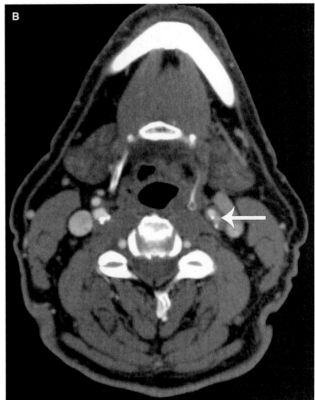

FIGURE 4-7

Sixty-four-year-old male presenting with acute left hemiparesis. CTA, sagittal reformatted (A), and axial source (B) images demonstrate a large hypodense asymmetric plaque at the left carotid bifurcation extending into the proximal left ICA, causing severe stenosis (arrows). This disease was likely the site of the patient's embolus.

additional phase-encoding step, partitions the volume into thin slices. (Figure 4-8).

Three-dimensional TOF MRA provides increased signal to noise ratio and higher spatial resolution versus the two-dimensional TOF technique. However, the volume covered is limited by vascular saturation artifact, thus limiting it largely to the intracranial vasculature. Both techniques, particularly the two-dimensional TOF technique, are susceptible to signal loss from turbulent flow. From a diagnostic standpoint, this tends to cause overestimation of vascular stenoses. A combination of the two techniques called multiple overlapping thin slab acquisition (MOTSA) exists. It allows larger volumes of coverage with decreased saturation effects and increased spatial resolution.

Phase contrast techniques, based on quantitation of the differences in the transverse magnetization between stationary and moving spins, are not typically performed in the evaluation of stroke patients because of the much longer acquisition times that make this technique vulnerable to motion artifact. However, this technique can be used for the evaluation of flow in collateral vessels because, unlike TOF MRA, this technique can measure flow direction.

Contrast-enhanced MRA techniques, based on a short rapid gradient echo sequence, image a bolus of intravenous gadolinium contrast in the arterial phase. The contrast agent shortens the T1 of opacified vessels versus the longer T1 relaxation times of the surrounding soft tissues. This allows for good separation of vessels from surrounding soft tissues on image acquisition (37). Compared to TOF techniques, contrast-enhanced MRA provides coverage of a larger volume with a shorter acquisition time and less vulnerability to patient motion. In addition, this technique generally provides better signal to noise than TOF techniques and has fewer artifacts related to dephasing from turbulence and saturation effects. For these reasons, contrast-enhanced MRA is often used to image the arteries of the neck (Figure 4-9). This can be accomplished in approximately one to two minutes. However, contrast-enhanced MRA has worse spatial resolution compared to noncontrast MRA, making the technique less suitable for imaging the smaller vessels of the head.

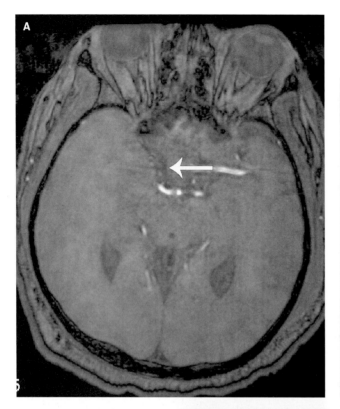

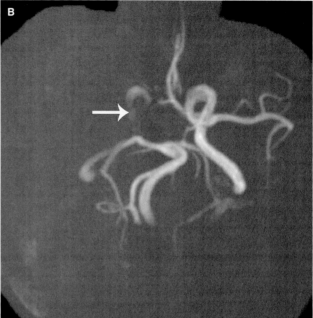

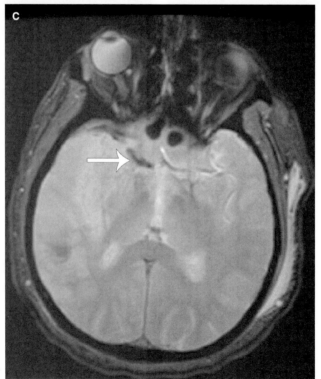

FIGURE 4-8

Sixty-seven-year-old male who had left hemiparesis when he woke up. MRA source (A) and MIP (B) images demonstrate no flow related enhancement within the right MCA stem and poor flow related enhancement within the distal ICA (red arrows). The GRE T2* susceptibility-weighted image (C) demonstrates susceptibility associated with the right MCA thrombus (arrow).

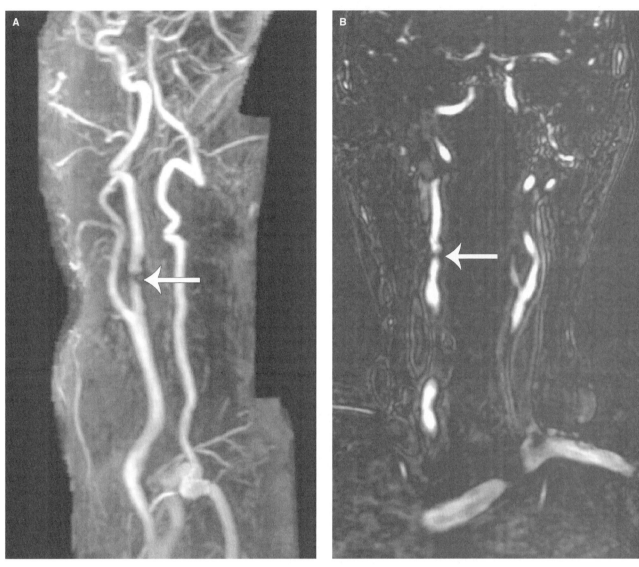

FIGURE 4-9

Gadolinium-enhanced MRA of the neck maximal intensity projection (A) and source (B) images demonstrate a focal severe stenosis of the proximal right Internal carotid artery (arrow).

Multiple studies have demonstrated that contrast-enhanced MRA is highly accurate in differentiating surgical from nonsurgical carotid artery stenoses (38). Other studies have suggested that MRA is also highly accurate in detecting proximal intracranial occlusions (39, 40). However, from a practical standpoint, MRA images of the head and neck are generally inferior to CTA images for scanning acute stroke patients on an emergency basis because motion artifact is a common problem (Table 4-5). Also, compared to CTA, contrast-enhanced MRA images have a narrower window for acquiring images during peak contrast enhancement. Consequently, inadequate arterial enhancement and venous contamination are not uncommon problems. Thus, in the acute stroke practice at the Massachusetts General Hospital, MRA is generally utilized only to evaluate patients with allergies to CT contrast agents, patients with renal failure, and patients such as children and pregnant women who are particularly vulnerable to radiation. However, gadolinium-enhanced MRA techniques cannot be used in patients with renal failure because of the increased risk of developing nephrogenic systemic fibrosis (NSF) (56).

CONVENTIONAL ANGIOGRAPHY

While potentially a front-line diagnostic tool, the risks associated with this invasive procedure, such as stroke, the relatively long preparation time, and relative cost,

TABLE 4-5
CTA and MRA Comparison in the Acute Stroke Setting

	CTA	MRA
Advantages	• Rapid acquisition speed, resulting in decreased motion artifact and greater coverage • Cost and availability: Cheaper physical plant and wider dissemination in the acute setting • Accuracy: Nonflow dependent technique with higher spatial resolution • Can be utilized where MR is contraindicated, e.g., patients with non-MR-compatible implantable devices	• Good for patients with allergic contraindications to iodinated contrast • Can provide velocity and flow direction data
Disadvantages	• Contrast dependent techniques in patients with allergies and renal failure • Radiation dose cumulative effect, especially in repeated imaging	• More susceptible to motion artifact • High cost and less accessibility of equipment • Inferior accuracy • Contrast dependent techniques in patients with renal abnormalities, like nephrogenic systemic fibrosis (NSF) (56)

preclude this modality from most diagnostic acute stroke evaluations. However, catheter-guided therapy using digital subtraction angiography has an important role in acute stroke management. The use of intra-arterial thrombolytic agents, mechanical clot disruption, and clot retrieval for the treatment of acute stroke are discussed in the following chapters.

PERFUSION IMAGING

The circulation of blood through a vascular bed defines tissue perfusion. In the acute stroke setting, perfusion imaging is generally performed with a bolus tracking technique in which a contrast agent is injected rapidly (5–7 cc/sec) into a peripheral intravenous catheter and images are obtained repeatedly as the contrast agent passes through the brain. The technique takes approximately one to two minutes and is performed such that it is sufficient to track the first pass of the contrast bolus through the intracranial vasculature without recirculation effects. The images obtained in the examination are converted by a computer to contrast agent concentration versus time curves. The cerebral blood volume (CBV) is proportional to the area under the curve. The cerebral blood flow (CBF) and mean transit time (MTT) are computed with an arterial input function and deconvolution methodology. Cerebral perfusion parameters are related according to the central volume theorem, that is, MTT = CBV/CBF.

Several variants of MR perfusion exist, broadly employing endogenous and exogenous labeling of blood (Figure 4-10). The primary method is a dynamic susceptibility (T2*) contrast sequence that relies on the decrease in signal caused by magnetic susceptibility effects of gadolinium as it passes through the intracranial vasculature (41). Because blood passes through the brain parenchyma rapidly, the most commonly used sequence is a single-shot gradient echo echo-planar sequence (EPI) capable of multiple slice acquisition from a single repetition time (TR). Approximately 60 images are obtained for each 5-mm brain slice, and the whole brain is covered. The arterial input may be chosen from the ipsilateral or contralateral MCA.

For CT, brain tissue increases and then decreases again in density as an iodine-based contrast agent passes through the brain. Briefly, the technique utilizes a standard cine protocol that obtains approximately 60 sequential images for each scan location over a given volume of coverage (slab). The slab is 2 cm for 16 detector and 4 cm for 64 detector scanners. The volume of the slab is divided into 5-mm thick slices. The arterial input function is usually chosen from the anterior cerebral artery or the top of the internal carotid artery. The venous function, which is required for CT but not for MRI, is usually chosen from the superior sagittal sinus.

A number of studies have demonstrated that lesion volumes on CTperfusion (CBV, CBF, and MTT) maps correlate highly with those obtained from similar MR

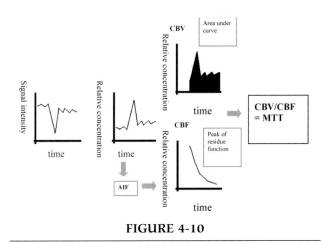

FIGURE 4-10

MR perfusion scheme. For each pixel in each image slice, a graph of signal intensity as a function of time is converted into a change in rate of susceptibility (T2* effect) caused by gadolinium, which is proportional to the gadolinium contrast agent given. This curve can then be used to compute relative cerebral blood volume (CBV), which is proportional to the area under the curve. Using a deconvolution technique, where an arterial input function (AIF), which describes the contrast left in the arteries is used, cerebral blood flow (CBF) can be calculated. CBV/CBF gives mean transit time (MTT).

perfusion maps (42, 43). Compared to MRP, CTP offers wider availability in the acute setting, lower cost, high speed of acquisition, higher spatial resolution, and quantitative perfusion estimates. Also, in patients with contraindications to MR imaging, such as pacemakers, CTP can be readily performed. Compared to CTP, however, MRP offers a larger volume of coverage. This technique also avoids a relatively large dose of radiation. In addition, MRP avoids iodinated contrast-related risks, including contrast allergy and contrast-induced nephropathy, particularly important in older patients at higher risk for stroke syndromes.

CBV, CBF, and MTT relate to acute ischemia as follows. With the onset of acute ischemia, loss of cerebral perfusion pressure (CPP) exceeds the autoregulatory capacity of the cerebral vasculature, and cerebral blood flow (CBF) begins to fall. There is compensatory vasodilatation and capillary recruitment that increases the effective vascular cross-sectional surface area, resulting in a lower blood velocity and an increase in MTT. A decrease in the velocity of blood as it passes through capillaries is adaptive, as it allows time for a greater oxygen extraction fraction (OEF). With modest impairment of blood flow, this mechanism allows for preservation of blood volume and of oxidative metabolism without alteration in electrical function. However, when CPP and, therefore, CBF are sufficiently low, microvascular collapse occurs, and cerebral blood

volume (CBV) falls. OEF reaches a maximum and cannot increase further. Brain tissue ceases to function electrically, resulting in a neurologic deficit. If the oxygen supply falls low enough, the tissue dies. The amount of time it takes for tissue to suffer irreversible damage is inversely related to the severity of the ischemic insult. Tissue that is completely deprived of blood will die within a few minutes, but less severely hypoperfused tissue may survive for many hours and may be saved by therapeutic intervention.

Imaging the Infarct Core and Ischemic Penumbra

In the clinical setting, radiologists and neurologists evaluate the diffusion and perfusion images to determine the infarct core and ischemic penumbra (Table 4-6). Operationally, the DWI images (depicting changes from cytotoxic edema) and the CBV images (depicting changes from capillary collapse) are thought to represent the infarct core or tissue that is frequently near the center of the ischemic lesion, is severely ischemic, is irreversibly damaged, and is unlikely to survive in spite of acute intervention. Indeed, DWI and CBV initial lesion volumes correlate highly with and slightly underestimate final infarct volumes (44). With proximal *emboli:* CBF and MTT lesion volumes are generally much larger than the DWI and CBV lesions, correlate less well with final infarct volume than DWI and CBV, and, on average, greatly overestimate final infarct volume (44, 45). Tissue that appears normal on the DWI and CBV images but abnormal on the CBF and MTT images is thought to represent the ischemic penumbra. The ischemic penumbra

TABLE 4-6
Summary of Perfusion-weighted Parameters and Prediction of Tissue Viability

PARAMETER	INFORMATION
DWI	Infarct core, generally irreversible and highly predictive of final infarct volume
CBV	Infarct core, generally irreversible and highly predictive of final infarct volume
CBF	Yields operational penumbra. For proximal occlusions, CBF is usually much larger than DWI and overestimates final infarct volume
MTT	Yields operational penumbra. For proximal occlusions, MTT is usually much larger than DWI and overestimates final infarct volume

usually surrounds the core where collateral vessels supply some residual perfusion. The penumbra represents tissue that may progress to infarction or may recover, depending on the timing of reperfusion and the degree of collateralization. It is tissue that can potentially be salvaged with reperfusion therapy.

The assumption that the DWI-MTT mismatch (MR perfusion) and the CBV-MTT mismatch (CT perfusion) represent the ischemic penumbra implies that patients with a large mismatch are most likely to benefit from thrombolytic therapy because they have the largest volume of threatened tissue that may be saved by thrombolysis. (Figures 4-11, 4-14, Table 4-7) If these patients cannot be treated with thrombolytic therapy, then they should be treated aggressively with hypertensive therapy. Conversely, patients with little or no diffusion-perfusion mismatch should not receive thrombolytic or other aggressive therapies because their infarctions are unlikely to increase in size and they should be spared the associated risk of hemorrhage. (Figures 4-12, 4-13)

The concept that the mismatch represents the ischemic penumbra and should be used as selection criteria for thrombolysis is supported by studies that demonstrate that patients with larger mismatches demonstrate more lesion growth (46). More importantly, a number of recent studies have validated the concept that the diffusion perfusion mismatch represents the ischemic penumbra. A number of studies have shown that intravenous thrombolysis may be beneficial more than three hours after stroke onset, provided that only patients with a significant diffusion-perfusion mismatch are treated. Ribo et al. found that patients with a significant diffusion-perfusion mismatch could be treated safely and effectively with IV-tPA in the three- to six-hour time period (47). In phase II of the desmoteplase in acute stroke (DIAS) trial, patients with diffusion-perfusion mismatch were treated with desmoteplase up to nine hours after stroke onset and showed better outcomes than patients given placebo, with only a minimal incidence of symptomatic hemorrhage (48). Similar success was achieved in the same time window by the dose escalation study of desmoteplase in acute ischemic stroke (DEDAS) (49). These studies raise the possibility that, one day, imaging-based treatment protocols may allow for intravenous thrombolysis in selected patients well outside of the now-accepted three-hour window and could allow for treatment of a vastly larger number of patients.

A number of investigators have tried to define perfusion parameter thresholds for tissue viability. That is, they have tried to define CBV, CBF, and MTT absolute and relative values that define which ischemic tissue is destined to infarct. One CT perfusion study of 130 patients showed that the perfusion parameter that most accurately describes the infarct core on admission is the absolute CBV with an optimal threshold at 2.0 ml/100 gm. The PCT perfusion parameter that most accurately describes the tissue at risk of infarction in case of persistent arterial occlusion is the relative MTT, with an optimal threshold of 145% (50). Another recent paper demonstrated that ischemic regions with greater than 66% reduction in relative CT-CBF have a greater than 95% positive predictive value for infarction (51). While these studies appear promising, reported thresholds for tissue viability are highly variable as highlighted in an article by Bandera et al., who reviewed multiple articles that addressed CBF thresholds in infarct core and penumbra (52). The reported CBF thresholds for penumbra varied from 14.1 to 35.0 ml/100 gm/minute. The reported CBF thresholds for infarct core varied from 4.8 to 8.4 ml/100 gm/minute.

The variability in perfusion thresholds likely results from a number of different factors. Most importantly, the data obtained represents only a single time point in a dynamic process. One major factor is variability in timing of tissue reperfusion. Jones et al. demonstrated that both severity and duration of CBF reduction up to four hours define an infarction threshold in monkeys (53). The CBF threshold for tissue infarction with reperfusion at two to three hours was 10–12 ml/100 gm/min, while the threshold for tissue infarction with permanent occlusion was 17–18 ml/100 gm/min. Another factor is that normal average cerebral blood flow in human parenchyma varies greatly, from 21.1 to 65.3 ml/100 g/min, depending on age and location in gray matter versus white matter (54, 55). Other factors include variability in methodologies, variability in initial and follow-up imaging times, and variability in postischemic tissue responses.

HEMORRHAGIC TRANSFORMATION OF ACUTE STROKE

Hemorrhagic transformation is a major complication of acute stroke. It is commonly thought that reperfusion into severely ischemic tissue leads to hemorrhagic transformation (Figure 4-15). However, some investigators have shown that it can occur distal to permanently occluded vessels and suggest that collateral flow into ischemic tissue can lead to hemorrhage (57). Furthermore, thrombolytic agents increase the risk of hemorrhage. They are thought to aggravate microvascular damage by activation of the plasminogen-plasmin system with release of metalloproteinases that cause degradation of the basal lamina (58, 59).

CT is considered the gold standard for detecting hemorrhagic transformation. However, T2* sensitive gradient echo MR sequences (GRE) that have increased

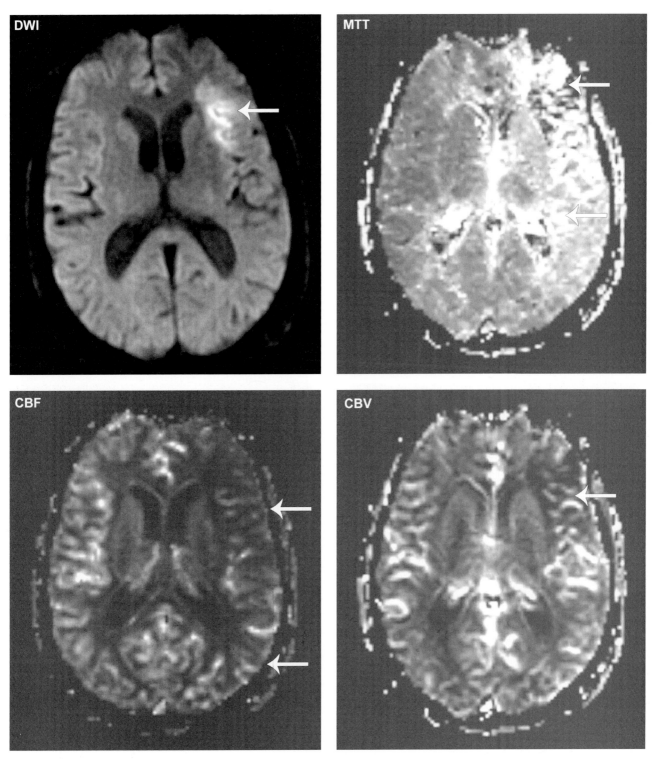

FIGURE 4-11

Sixty-six-year-old male with hypertension with a two-hour history of acute onset of right facial droop and expressive greater than receptive aphasia. The DWI and CBV images demonstrate the infarction core (arrows), involving the left anterior insula and frontal operculum. There is decreased CBF and increased MTT throughout most of the visualized left MCA territory (arrows). These findings are consistent with a large DWI MTT mismatch, suggesting that there is a large amount of tissue at risk of progressing to infarction.

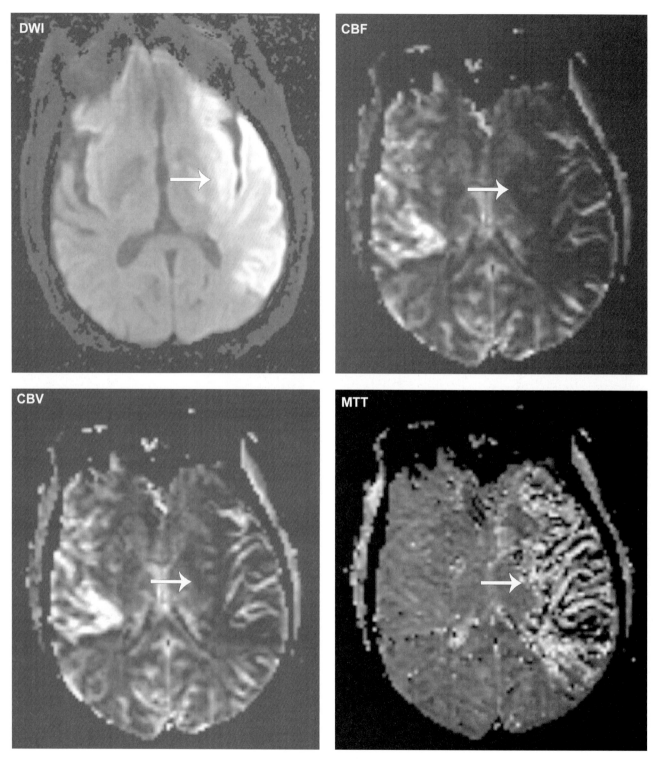

FIGURE 4-12

Seventy-seven-year-old male with sudden onset of right hemiparesis and aphasia, imaged approximately two hours after onset. DWI image demonstrates an acute left MCA infarction (arrow) involving the left frontal and temporal lobes, the insula, the basal ganglia, and the adjacent deep white matter. There is decreased CBF and CBV and increased MTT in the same region. This is an example of a DWI MTT matched infarction without a significant penumbra of ischemic tissue at risk for further infarction.

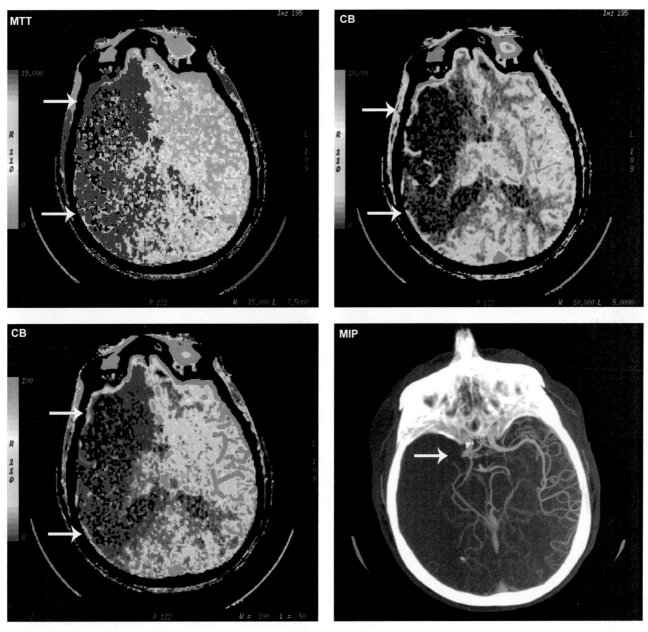

FIGURE 4-13

Eighty-eight-year-old female with atrial fibrillation with sudden onset of left hemiparesis, one hour and twenty minutes before imaging. CT perfusion maps demonstrate markedly decreased CBV throughout the visualized right MCA territory, consistent with infarction core. There is also prolonged MTT and decreased CBF throughout the same region. There is no mismatch between the MTT and CBV images, suggesting that there is no tissue that is at increased risk of further infarction. The CTA MIP image demonstrates occlusion of the right M1 segment of the MCA without significant collateral vasculature.

sensitivity to blood breakdown products because of their paramagnetic properties are as sensitive as CT for the detection of hemorrhage associated with acute stroke (60). Furthermore, following thrombolysis, both contrast extravasation and hemorrhage are hyperdense and may be difficult to differentiate on CT. GRE images can easily differentiate between the two. Hemorrhage has susceptibility effects while iodinated contrast does not.

A number of investigators have reported imaging parameters predictive of hemorrhagic transformation. These parameters are thought to reflect more severe

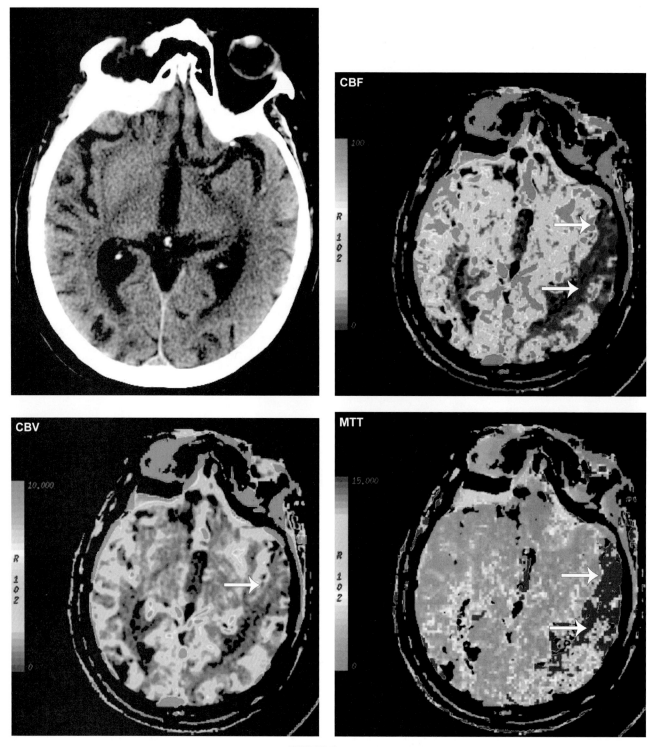

FIGURE 4-14

Seventy-two-year-old female who collapsed and was found to be aphasic 50 minutes prior to imaging. Noncontrast CT image demonstrates no appreciable parenchymal abnormality. There is a small region with decreased CBV in the left anterior temporal lobe (arrow), consistent with infarction core. There is a larger region with decreased CBF and increased MTT in the left anterior temporal lobe (arrows). The mismatch between the CBV and MTT images is thought to represent the penumbra, ischemic but viable tissue at risk for infarction.

TABLE 4-7
DWI and PWI Lesion Volumes and Associated Prediction of Ischemic/Infarct Tissue Behavior

PATTERN	CAUSE	COMMENT
CBF/MTT but no DWI or CBV	Proximal occlusion or critical stenosis with penumbra perfused via collaterals	DWI and CBV abnormalities may develop, depending on collateral supply and timing of reperfusion. Good candidate for reperfusion therapy.
CBF/MTT > DWI/CBV	Proximal occlusion or critical stenosis with penumbra perfused partially by collaterals	Infarct may expand into part or all of the CBF/MTT abnormality, depending on collateral supply and timing of reperfusion. Good candidate for reperfusion therapy.
CBF/MTT = DWI/CBV	Usually, distal occlusions or lacunar infarcts, but can involve proximal occlusions as well	Entire territory has infarcted. No additional tissue at risk and no need for aggressive therapy.
CBF/MTT < DWI/CBV	Proximal, distal, or lacunar infarct	Ischemic tissue has reperfused. No additional tissue at risk and no need for aggressive therapy.
DWI/CBV but no CBF/MTT	Proximal, distal, or lacunar infarct	Ischemic tissue has reperfused. No additional tissue at risk and no need for aggressive therapy. Also, tiny infarcts below resolution of perfusion imaging.

ischemia and breakdown of the blood brain barrier and include:

1. Hypodensity in greater than one-third of the MCA territory on CT (61)
2. Early parenchymal enhancement on gadolinium-enhanced T1-weighted images (62)
3. Larger volume of the initial DWI abnormality (compared to infarctions that do not hemorrhage) (63)
4. A higher percentage of pixels with ADC < 550 × 10^{-6} mm²/sec (compared to infarctions that do not hemorrhage) (64)
5. A more severe decrease in CBV and CBF versus the entire perfusion abnormality (compared to infarctions that do not hemorrhage) (65)
6. At least 126 voxels with cerebral blood volume less than 5% of contralateral normal gray matter in patients who received intravenous tPA (66)
7. Increased T1 permeability (67). Prior microbleeds detected on T2* gradient echo do not signify risk for hemorrhagic transformation following thrombolytic therapy (68).

THE FUTURE: EMERGING TRENDS AND TECHNIQUES

The techniques and modalities employed in imaging acute stroke patients are rapidly evolving. Multidetector CT scanners with larger numbers of detectors promise to shorten scanning time even further and require smaller contrast boluses. New flat-panel CT scanners, now in clinical trials, promise to allow temporal resolution of the contrast bolus. In addition, higher field strength MR magnets coupled with parallel imaging coils promise even faster, higher signal-to-noise ratio MR images and MR angiograms. The physiologic evaluation of the acute stroke patient is moving from a largely subjective to an objective quantitative approach. New sophisticated CT perfusion software allows segmentation of gray and white matter perfusion data.

Imaging of other physiologic parameters, such as blood-brain barrier permeability and sodium concentration, has begun. Permeability can be calculated with gadolinium-enhanced T1-weighted MRI techniques. Increased permeability in the acute infarction core correlates with the risk of hemorrhagic transformation and malignant transformation of middle cerebral artery infarctions (69). Sodium concentration in brain tissue can be calculated with high field strength MR scanners. In the unperturbed state, brain tissue maintains sodium ion homeostasis via energy-dependent mechanisms. This homeostasis is disrupted in ischemia, and there is evidence that tissue sodium concentrations can be used as a tool to predict ischemic tissue viability (70). Optical imaging (near infrared spectroscopy) is being used to study both infarct progression and neuroplasticity following ischemia.

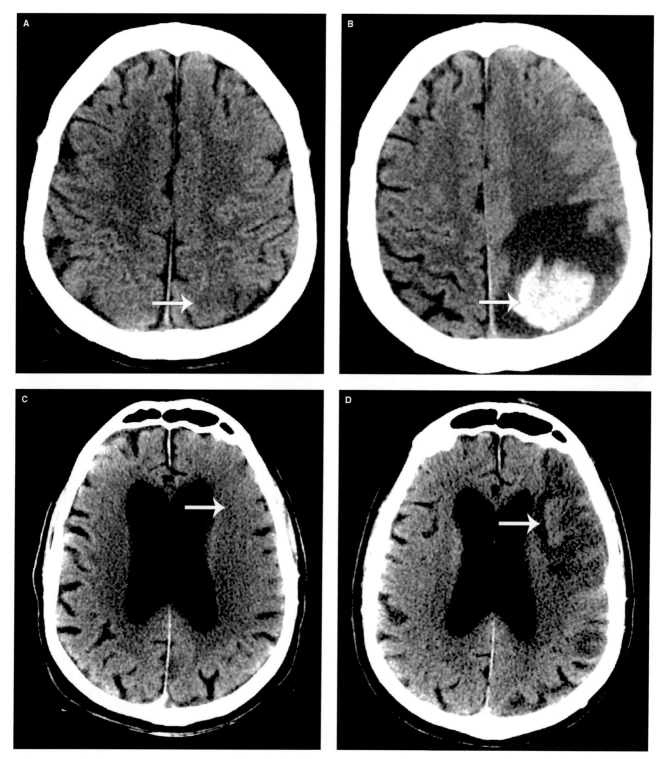

FIGURE 4-15

Hemorrhagic transformation. Fifty-year-old male found down. Initial noncontrast CT examination (A) demonstrates a small infarction within the left parietal region (arrow). On the follow-up study 14 days later (B), there is expansion of the infarction with a relatively large intraparenchymal hemorrhage (arrow). In a second patient with right hemiparesis, initial noncontrast CT (C) demonstrates a left MCA infarction (arrow). On follow-up CT (D), there is petechial hemorrhage within the infarction (arrow).

CONCLUSION

This chapter hopes to inform the reader about the current state of the art and future of acute stroke imaging and its impact on stroke triage. The advent of evaluation of the stroke patient using physiologic stroke parameters, in concert with the advances in stroke therapy, promise better clinical outcomes in the near future.

References

1. American Heart Association. Heart disease and stroke statistics: 2006 update. 2006. Available at www.americanheart.org.
2. Wall SD, Brant-Zawadzki M, Jeffrey RB, Barnes B. High frequency CT findings within 24 hours after cerebral infarction. AJR Am J Roentgenol Feb 1982; 138(2):307–311.
3. Pressman BD, Tourje EJ, Thompson JR. An early CT sign of ischemic infarction: Increased density in a cerebral artery. American Journal of Neuroradiology 1987; 8:645–648.
4. Jaillard A, Hommel M, Baird AE, et al. Significance of early CT signs in acute Stroke: A CT scan-diffusion MRI study. Cerebrovascular Diseases 2002; 13:47–56.
5. Mullins ME, Lev MH, Schellingerhout D, et al. Influence of the availability of clinical history on the noncontrast CT detection of acute stroke. Am J Radiol 2002; 179(1):223–228.
6. Lev MH, Farkas J, Gemmete J, et al. Acute stroke: Improved nonenhanced CT detection-benefits of soft copy interpretation by using variable window width and center level settings. Radiology 213:150–155
7. Leys JP, Pruvo O, Godefroy P, et al. Prevalence and significance of hyperdense middle cerebral artery in acute stroke. Stroke 1992; 23:317–324.
8. Von Kummer R, Meyding-Lamade U, Forsting M, et al. Sensitivity and prognostic value of early CT in occlusion of the middle cerebral artery trunk. Am J Neuroradiol 199415:9–15.
9. Hacke W, Kaste M, Fieschi C, et al. Intravenous thrombolysis with recombinant tissue plasminogen activator for acute hemispheric stroke. J Am Med Assoc 1995; 274:1017–1025.
10. Barber P, Demchuk A, Zhang J, Buchan A. Validity and reliability of a quantitative computed tomography score in predicting outcome of hyperacute stroke before thrombolytic therapy. Lancet 355(9216):1670–1674.
11. Dzialowski H, Coutts SB, Demchuk DM, et al. Extent of early ischemic changes on computed tomography (CT) before thrombolysis: Prognostic value of the Alberta Stroke Program Early CT Score in ECASS II. Stroke 2006; 37(4):973–978.
12. Shimosegawa E, et al. Embolic cerebral infarction: MR findings in the first three hours after onset. Am J Roentgenol 160(5):1077–1082.
13. Perkins CJ, et al. Fluid-attenuated inversion recovery and diffusion and perfusion weighted MRI abnormalities in 117 consecutive patients with stroke symptoms. Stroke 2001; 32(12):2774–2781.
14. Mintorovitch J, et al. Diffusion-weighted magnetic resonance imaging of acute focal cerebral ischemia: Comparison of signal intensity with changes in brain water and Na$^+$, K$^{(+)}$-ATPase activity. J Cereb Blood Flow Metab 1994; 14(2):332–336.
15. Basser PJ, Pierpaoli C. Microstructural and physiological features of tissues elucidated by quantitative-diffusion-tensor MRI. J Magn Reson B 1996; 111(3):209–219.
16. Benveniste H, Hedlund LW, Johnson GA. Mechanism of detection of acute cerebral ischemia in rats by diffusion-weighted magnetic resonance microscopy. Stroke 23(5):746–754.
17. Stejskal E, Tanner J. Spin diffusion measurements: Spin echos in the prescence of time-dependent field gradient. J Chem Phys 1965; 42:288–92.
18. Gonzalez RG, et al. Diffusion-weighted MR imaging: Diagnostic accuracy in patients imaged within six hours of stroke symptoms onset. Radiology 1999; 210(1):155–162.
19. Lovblad Ko, et al. Clinical experience with diffusion-weighted MR in patients with acute stroke. AmJ Neuroradiol 1998; 19(6):1061–1066.
20. Mullins ME, et al. CT and conventional and diffusion-weighted MR imaging in acute stroke: Study in 691 patients at presentation to the emergency department. Radiology 2002; 224(2):353–360.
21. Kidwell CS, et al. Late secondary ischemic injury in patients receiving intraarterial thrombolysis. Ann Neurol 52(6):698–703.
22. Schaefer PW, et al. Predicting cerebral ischemia infarct volume with diffusion and perfusion MR imaging. Am J Neuroradiol 2002; 23(10):1785–1794.
23. Schwamm LH, et al. Time course of lesion development in patients with acute stroke: Serial diffusion and hemodynamic-weighted magnetic resonance imaging. Stroke 1998; 29(11):2268–2276.
24. Copen WA, et al. Ischemic stroke: Effects of etiology and patient age on the time course of the core apparent diffusion coefficient. Radiology 2001; 221(1):27–34.
25. Nagesh V, et al. Time course of ADC changes in ischemic stroke: Beyond the human eye! Stroke 1998; 29(9):1778–1782.
26. Lev MH, et al. CT angiography in the rapid triage of patients with hyperacute stroke to intraarterial thrombolysis: Accuracy in the detection of large vessel thrombus. J Comput Assist Tomogr 2001; 25(4):520–528.
27. Wolpert SM, et al. Neuroradiologic evaluation of patients with acute stroke treated with recombinant tissue plasminogen activator. Am J Neuroradiol 1993; 14(1):3–13.
28. Wildermuth S, et al. Role of CT angiography in patient selection for thrombolytic therapy in acute hemispheric strokes. Stroke 1998; 29(5):935–938.
29. Zivin JA. Factors determining the therapeutic window for stroke. Neurology 50(3):599–603.
30. Schramm P, et al. Comparison of CT and CT angiography source images with diffusion-weighted imaging in patients with acute stroke within six hours after onset. Stroke 33(10):2426–2434.
31. Parsons W, et al. Perfusion computed tomography: Prediction of final infarct extent and stroke outcome. Annals of Neurology 2005; 58(5):672–679.
32. Schwamm LH, et al. Hypoattenuation on CT angiographic source images predicts risk of intracerebral hemorrhage and outcome after intra-arterial reperfusion therapy. American Journal of Neuroradiology 2005; 26:1798–1803.
33. Morcos SK, Thomsen HS, Webb JA. Contrast-media induced nephrotoxicity: Consensus report. Eur Radiol 1999; 9(8):1602–1613.
34. Aspelin P, et al. Nephrotoxic effects in high-risk patients undergoing angiography. N Engl J Med 2003; 348(6):491–499.
35. Cochran ST, Anaphylactoid reactions to radiocontrast media. Curr Allergy Asthma Rep 2005; 5(1):28–31.
36. Murphy KJ, Brunberg JA, Cohan RH. Adverse reactions to gadolinium contrast media: A review of 36 cases. AJR Am J Roentgenol 1996; 167:847–849.
37. Jewells V, Castillo M. MR angiography of the extracranial circulation. Magn Reson Imaging Clin North Am 2003; 11(4): vi, 585–597.
38. Alvarez-Linera J, et al. Prospective evaluation of carotid artery stenosis: Elliptic centric contrast-enhanced MR angiography and spiral CT angiography compared to digital subtraction angiography. Am J Neuroradiology 2003; 24(5):1012–1019.
39. Stock KW, et al. Intracranial arteries: Prospective blinded comparative study of MR angiography and DSA in 50 patients. Radiology 1995; 195(2):451–456.
40. Korogi Y, et al. Intracranial vascular stenoses and occlusion: Diagnostic accuracy of three-dimensional fourier transform, time-of-flight MR angiography. Radiology 193(1):187–193.
41. Rosen BR, Belliveau JW, Vevea JM, Brady TJ. Perfusion imaging with NMR contrast agents. Magn Reson Med 1990; 14:249–265.
42. Eastwood JD, Lev MH, Wintermark M, et al. Correlation of early dynamic CT perfusion imaging with whole-brain MR diffusion and perfusion imaging in acute hemispheric stroke. American Journal of Neuroradiology 2003; 24:1869–1875.
43. Schramm P, Schellinger PD, Klotz E, et al. Comparison of perfusion computed tomography and computed tomography angiography source images with perfusion-weighted imaging and diffusion-weighted imaging in patients with acute stroke of less than six hours' duration. Stroke 2004; 35:1652.
44. Schaefer PW, Hunter GJ, He J, et al. Predicting cerebral ischemic infarct volume with diffusion and perfusion MR imaging. American Journal of Neuroradiology 2002; 23:1785–1794.
45. Karonen JO, et al. Combined perfusion and diffusion-weighted MR imaging in acute ischemic stroke during the first week: A longitudinal study. Radiology 217:886–894.
46. Rordorf G, Koroshetz WJ, Copen WA, et al. Regional ischemia and ischemic injury in patients with acute middle cerebral artery stroke as defined by early diffusion-weighted and perfusion-weighted MRI. Stroke 1998; 29:939–843.
47. Ribo M, Molina CA, Rovira A, et al. Safety and efficacy of intravenous tissue plasminogen activator stroke treatment in the three- to six-hour window using multimodal transcranial doppler/MRI selection protocol. Stroke 2005; 36:602.
48. Hacke W, Albers G, Al-Rawi Y, et al. The desmoteplase in acute ischemic stroke trial (DIAS): A phase II MRI-based nine-hour window acute stroke thrombolysis trial with intravenous desmoteplase. Stroke 2005; 36:66.
49. Furlan AJ, Eyding D, Albers GW, et al. Dose escalation of desmoteplase for acute ischemic stroke (DEDAS) evidence of safety and efficacy three to nine hours after stroke onset. Stroke 2006; 37:1227.
50. Wintermark M, Flanders AE, Velthuis B, et al. Perfusion-CT assessment of infarct core and penumbra receiver operating characteristic curve analysis in 130 patients suspected of acute hemispheric stroke. Stroke 2006; 37:979.
51. Schaefer PW, Roccatagliata L, Ledezma C, et al. First-pass quantitative CT perfusion identifies thresholds for salvageable penumbra in acute stroke patients treated with intra-arterial therapy. American Journal of Neuroradiology 2006; 27:20–25.
52. Bandera E, Botteri M, Minelli C, et al. Cerebral blood flow threshold of ischemic penumbra and infarct core in acute ischemic stroke: A systematic review. Stroke 2006; 37:1334.
53. Jones T, Morawetz R, Crowell R, et al. Thresholds of focal cerebral ischemia in aware monkeys. J Neurosurg 1981; 54:773–782.
54. Lassen N. Normal average cerebral blood flow in younger adults is 50 ml/100 g/min. J Cereb Blood Flow Metab 1985; 5:347–349.
55. Frackowiak R, Lenzi G, Jones T, Heather J. Quantitative measurement of regional cerebral blood flow and oxygen metabolism in man using ^{15}O and positron emission tomography: Theory, procedure, and normal values. J Comput Assist Tomogr 1980; 4:727–736.
56. http://www.fda.gov/cder/drug/infopage/gcca/qa_20061222.htm

57. Ogata J, Yutani C, Imakita M, et al. Hemorrhagic infarct of the brain without a reopening of the occluded arteries in cardioembolic stroke. *Stroke* 1989; 20: 876–883

58. Liotta LA, Goldfarb RH, Brundage R, et al. Effect of Plasminogen Activator (Urokinase), Plasmin, and Thrombin on Glycoprotein and Collagenous Components of Basement Membrane.. *Cancer Research* 1981; 41:4629–4636.

59. Carmeliet P, et al. Urokinase-generated plasmin activates matrix metalloproteinases during aneurysm formation. *Nature Genetics* 1997; 17:439–444.

60. Lin DD, Filippi CG, Steever AB, Zimmerman RD. Detection of intracranial hemorrhage: Comparison between gradient-echo images and b(0) images obtained from diffusion-weighted echo-planar sequences. *AJNR Am J Neuroradiol* 2001; 22:1275–1281.

61. von Kummer R, Allen KL, Holle R, et al. Acute stroke: Usefulness of early CT findings before thrombolytic therapy. *Radiology* 1997; 205:327–333.

62. Vo KD, Santiago F, Lin W, et al. MR imaging enhancement patterns as predictors of hemorrhagic transformation in acute ischemic stroke. *AJNR Am J Neuroradiol* 2003; 24:674–679.

63. Baird A E, et al. Enlargement of human cerebral ischemic lesion volumes measured by diffusion-weighted magnetic resonance imaging. *Annals of Neurology* 2004; 41(5):581–589.

64. Selim M, et al. Predictors of hemorrhagic transformation after intravenous recombinant tissue plasminogen activator: Prognostic value of the initial apparent diffusion coefficient and diffusion-weighted lesion volume. *Stroke* Aug 2002; 33(8):2047–2052.

65. Schaefer PW, Ledezma CJ, Roccatagliata L, Gonzalez RG. Assessing hemorrhagic transformation with diffusion and perfusion MR imaging. *ASNR* 2003.

66. Alsop DC, Makovetskaya E, Kumar S, et al. Markedly reduced apparent blood volume on bolus contrast magnetic resonance imaging as a predictor of hemorrhage after thrombolytic therapy for acute ischemic stroke. *Stroke* 2005; 36:746–750.

67. Kassner A, Roberts T, Taylor K, Silver F, Mikulis D. Prediction of hemorrhage in acute ischemic stroke using permeability MR imaging. *AJNR Am J Neuroradiol* 2005; 26:2213–2217.

68. Ho Sung Kim, Deok Hee Lee, Chang Woo Ryu, et al. Multiple cerebral microbleeds in hyperacute ischemic stroke: Impact on prevalence and severity of early hemorrhagic transformation after thrombolytic treatment. *AJR* 2006; 186:1443–1449.

69. Ding G, Jiang Q, et al. Detection of BBB disruption and hemorrhage by Gd-DTPA enhanced MRI after embolic stroke in rat. Brain Res 2006; 1114(1):195–203.

70. Thulborn KR, Davis D, Snyder J, et al. Sodium MR imaging of acute and subacute atroke for assessment of tissue viability. Neuroimaging Clin N AM 2005; 15(3): xi–xii, 639–53.

5 Cerebral Stroke Syndromes

Richard L. Harvey

The main purpose of the neurologic examination in stroke rehabilitation is to identify impairments that cause functional limitations; the detection of these impairments will determine meaningful therapeutic goals. This contrasts with the neurologic examination performed in acute care, which informs the diagnosis and localizes the injury. In the rehabilitation setting, the lesion location is usually known, such that the neurologic examination focuses on identifying *expected* impairments characteristic of a particular stroke syndrome. Understanding stroke syndromes helps target the examination, which improves the practitioner's efficiency and the accuracy of neurologic assessment.

This chapter will cover the stroke syndromes that occur in brain regions above the tentorium, including the anterior cerebral artery, middle cerebral artery, posterior cerebral artery, and others. In addition, the lacunar syndromes characteristic of infarcts within the territories of subcortical branches originating from these main arteries will be reviewed. The syndromes described are those typical of arterial and branch occlusions rather than hemorrhagic rupture. This chapter is not intended to be an exhaustive review of cerebrovascular and neurologic anatomy, but rather a general anatomical overview that facilitates understanding of common clinical stroke syndromes.

CLINICAL NEUROANATOMY

The two cerebral hemispheres are divided, by convention, into four lobes: frontal, parietal, occipital, and temporal (Figure 5-1).

The frontal lobe is separated from the parietal lobe by the central sulcus. All behavioral motor output, including mobility, object manipulation, directional eye movement, and verbal expression, originate in the frontal lobe, assisted by the basal ganglia and cerebellum. In contrast, processing of all sensory input, including visual, auditory, and somatosensory, is integrated by the thalamus, parietal, occipital, and temporal lobes. However, there is rich neural integration between frontal lobe systems and primary sensory areas. There are also significant interconnections between primary motor cortex and somatosensory cortex, premotor and ventral motor areas, as well as connections from thalamus to motor cortex and motor cortex to basal ganglia, superior and inferior colliculi, and cerebellum.

Cortical Areas of the Frontal Lobe

Primary motor cortex (M1): The primary motor or M1 cortex is located in the precentral gyrus, just anterior to the central sulcus, in both hemispheres. It extends from the medial portion of the frontal lobe at the paracentral

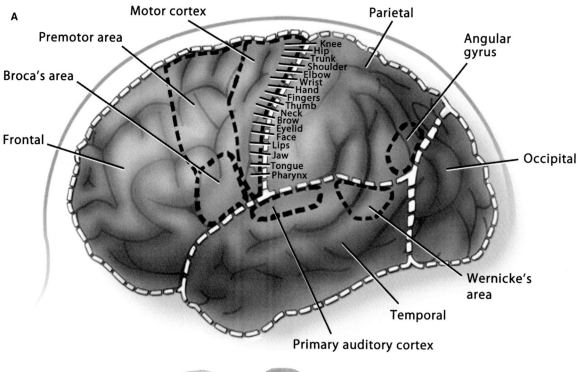

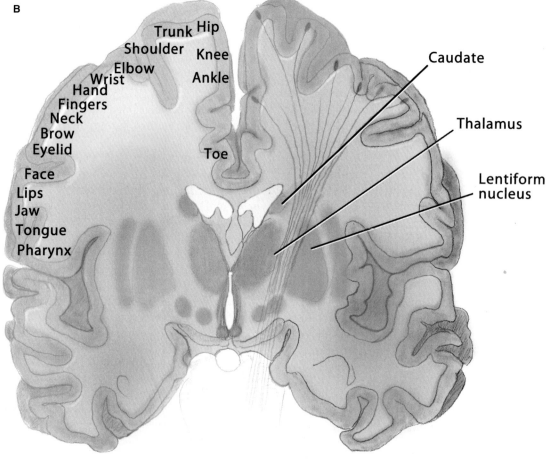

FIGURE 5-1

Cortical and subcortical neuroanatomy of the human brain. 1A. Lobes of the cerebral hemisphere and identified cortical structures. 1B. Coronal view of frontal lobe. 1C. Horizontal view with highlighted language and visual areas and associated tracts.

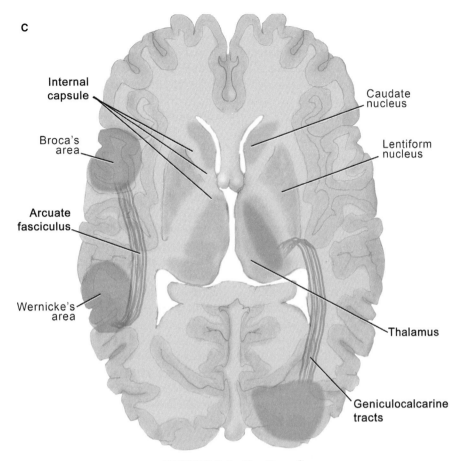

C

Internal capsule

Broca's area

Arcuate fasciculus

Wernicke's area

Caudate nucleus

Lentiform nucleus

Thalamus

Geniculocalcarine tracts

FIGURE 5-1 *(Continued)*

lobule, around the lateral convexity, and into the frontal operculum (the frontal lobe cortical surface tucked within the Sylvian fissure). The motor cortex contains the large pyramidal neurons (Betz cells) that constitute the "upper motor neuron" of the primary motor system and that supply axons for the cortical spinal tract. It is somatotopically organized in the form of the classic "homunculus" described by Penfield, where motor control for the feet is located in medial frontal regions; shoulder, arm, and hand are located along the superior lateral convexity; and face, tongue, and throat are located along the inferior convexity and the operculum (Figure 5-1). Lesions of the M1 cortex result in hemiplegia, often without spastic dystonia.

Broca's area: Named after Paul Broca (1824–1880) (1), Broca's area is one of the two primary cortical language areas. Broca's area is located in the inferior lateral convexity and within the operculum of the dominant (usually left) frontal lobe (2, 3). Interestingly, it is located in the premotor area anterior to M1 cortical representation for face, mouth, tongue, and throat. Thus it makes sense that lesions in this area would result in impaired oral motor communication characterized by nonfluent speech production, apraxic errors, and problems with syntax. However,

lesions in Broca's area often result in mild to moderate loss of auditory comprehension, characterized by failure to understand the syntax of complex sentences. Broca's area is important for facilitating the production of motor activity given on command, especially commands given verbally. Injury to Broca's area results in limb apraxia in both right and left limbs (4).

Frontal eye fields: Although the prefrontal area of the frontal lobe is complex and poorly understood, it is accepted that this area plays an important role in executive decision-making. Within this context, there are cortical areas in the prefrontal area that are important in directional and exploratory eye movements, called the frontal eye fields. Within each hemisphere are located two eye fields. One is known as the "eye field of the dorsomedial frontal cortex," and the other, located dorsolaterally, is the "frontal eye field" (5). A unilateral lesion of either eye field will cause a gaze preference and often head-turning toward the side of the lesion, away from the hemiplegic side. Patients with such lesions will have reduced saccadic gaze and visual pursuit toward the contralateral visual field. Often these symptoms are transient, but they may be long-lasting. In addition, injury to the non-dominant (usually right) prefrontal area impairs exploratory eye movements to the left and contributes to the attentional deficits seen in neurologic neglect syndrome (6). Head- and eye-turning associated with non-dominant prefrontal lesions is often more persistent, whereas these symptoms usually resolve within days to a few weeks with dominant lobe lesions.

Primary Cortical Sensory Areas

Primary somatosensory cortex (S1): The postcentral gyrus is located anteriorly in the parietal lobe, behind the central sulcus, and contains primary somatosensory representation. Like M1 it is somatotopically organized with roughly the same organization anatomically as the primary motor cortex. Lesions in S1 result in loss of two-point discrimination and stereognosis in contralateral body. If subcortical sensory structures such as sensory tracts and thalamus are involved as well, there may also be loss of pain, temperature, and joint position sense.

Primary visual cortex: Located on the medial surface of the occipital lobe, within the longitudinal fissure, is the calcharine or primary visual cortex, a critical structure for vision. Unilateral hemispheric lesions of the visual cortex result in a contralateral homonymous hemianopsia, meaning loss of the half the visual field to an equivalent extent in both eyes. Symptoms of homonymous hemianopsia are not limited to lesion of primary visual cortex and may also occur with lesions involving subcortical structures of the temporal lobes. This is because visual tracts extend from the ventral posterior lateral thalamus, radiate posterolaterally into the temporal lobes, and then arch medially to the occipital cortex (Figure 5-1). Any lesion along this tract will also cause a contralateral homonymous hemianopsia.

Primary auditory cortex: Pure tone recognition is processed in the primary auditory cortex, located on the superior temporal gyrus in the temporal lobe. This is also known as Heschel's gyrus and is more prominent in the dominant hemisphere (7). Auditory cortex is tonotopically organized by sound frequency (8, 9). A lesion to the superior temporal lobe on or near Heschel's gyrus does not result in deafness; however, in the dominant hemisphere such a lesion can cause complex auditory perceptual problems, such as pure word deafness (10).

Cortical Sensory Association Areas

Cortical association areas are local networks connected by extensive reciprocal monosynaptic connections to other cortical areas, as well as to certain subcortical structures. These interconnected local networks make up large-scale networks for distributed processing of neurocognitive activities such as attention, language, and memory. Thus, lesions in association areas can negatively impact complex perceptual, cognitive, and communicative behaviors (6).

Posterior parietal cortex: Located behind the primary somatosensory cortex, the posterolateral parietal area integrates neural information from somatosensory, visual, and auditory cortices in order to construct a cohesive perception of three-dimensional space and the body's position within the surrounding environment (11). Current theory suggests that in humans the non-dominant parietal cortex is oriented to bilateral space, whereas the dominant hemisphere is strongly oriented to the contralateral (usually right) hemispace. As such, lesions in the left parietal cortex usually only cause transient right hemineglect syndrome. In contrast, lesions in the right parietal cortex cause clinically significant left hemineglect syndrome. The neglect syndrome is characterized by reduced recognition of and attention to visual, somatosensory, and auditory stimuli in the contralateral hemispace. In addition, patients with lesion in the right parietal hemisphere have visual perceptual deficits resulting in spatial disorientation. Clinically they are unable to draw figures accurately, cannot use blocks to build a simple structure, and are challenged to orient their clothing to their body while dressing (12). Clinical terms such as *constructional apraxia* and *dressing apraxia* have been applied to this syndrome. However, it is important to note that these problems result from deficits in perception and are not true motor apraxias.

Wernicke's area: Named after Carl Wernicke (1848–1905)(13), Wernicke's area is located posteriorly to Heschel's gyrus in the dominant hemisphere and is a language-association area functioning as a local neural network, situated between the primary auditory and visual cortices. Wernicke's area processes spoken and written symbolic language into meaning and comprehension (2, 3). Along with Broca's area in the frontal operculum, Wernicke's area participates in a larger network for distributed processing of language (6). Lesions in Wernicke's area result in impaired language comprehension and a fluent aphasia mixed with multiple paraphasic errors. Patients with Wernicke's aphasia lack insight about their comprehension deficits, which can complicate care and participation in rehabilitation.

Angular gyrus: Immediately posterior to Wernicke's area, in the posterior superior temporal lobe, is the angular gyrus, which receives visual input from the occipital lobe and the posterior inferior temporal lobe (14). The angular gyrus is an important region for processing written language, such that lesions here can cause alexia (3).

Subcortical Structures

Posterior limb of the internal capsule: Axons that constitute the cortical spinal tract descend from M1 cortex subcortically into the internal capsule. The anterior portion of the posterior limb, beginning at the genu, contains these fibers. This portion of the internal capsule passes between the thalamus and the globus pallidus, into the cerebral peduncle, and then into the midbrain as the ventral crus cerebri (Figure 5-1). The posterior limb of the internal capsule is somatotopically organized with face, hand, arm, and shoulder anterior to trunk, thigh, leg, and foot. Lesions in the internal capsule result in contralateral hemiplegia.

Thalamus: Located between the third ventricle and the posterior limb of the internal capsule, the thalamus functions as a sensory hub for somatosensory, visual, and auditory input (Figure 5-1). Lesions here can result in mild hemiplegia or hemiataxia, sensory deficits, pain syndromes, mild aphasia, and neglect syndrome.

Arcuate fasciculus: Another important structure in the large-scale language network is the arcuate fasciculus, which is a cortical-cortical white matter tract passing reciprocally between Wernicke's and Broca's areas along an arched pathway (6). Lesions along the arcuate fasciculus can cause problems with repetition of language as well as limb apraxia bilaterally (3, 4).

Corpus callosum: The large arch-shaped bundle of white matter connecting the two cerebral hemispheres is the corpus callosum (Figure 5-1). Lesions within this structure can contribute to a disconnection between right and left hemisphere, resulting in various clinical manifestations depending on the location of the lesion.

CEREBROVASCULAR ANATOMY

The Circle of Willis

In his book *Cerebri Anatome*, published in 1664, Thomas Willis provided the first complete description of the cerebral arterial circle, now commonly known as *the circle of Willis* (15). The circle is supplied by three intracranial arteries. The right and left internal carotid arteries supply the circle anteriorly, and the basilar artery provides the posterior supply (Figure 5-2).

The last branch of each internal carotid before entering the circle of Willis is the ophthalmic artery, which

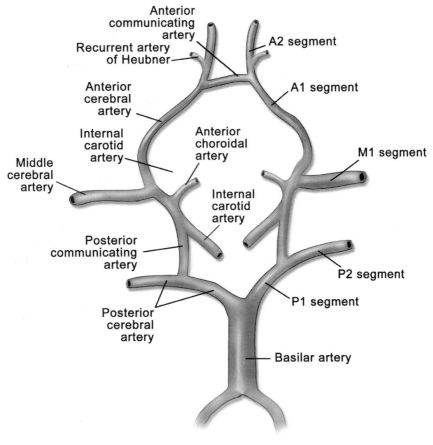

FIGURE 5-2

The circle of Willis and associated branches.

passes into the orbit and supplies the retinal tissue. Small branches of the ophthalmic artery anastomose with branches from the external carotid. After releasing the ophthalmic artery, the internal carotid artery enters the circle of Willis at the point where the posterior communicating artery (PComA) branches posteriorly. The internal carotid then provides a deep perforating cerebral artery, the anterior choroidal artery (AchA), before bifurcating into the middle cerebral artery (MCA) and the anterior cerebral artery (ACA). The basilar artery bifurcates into both posterior cerebral arteries (PCA). The circle is completed by anastomosis of the PComA with the PCA and the anterior communicating artery (AComA) with both ACAs (Figure 5-2).

This "typical" anatomy of the circle is only present in 35% of human specimens. Anatomical variations are numerous, including hypoplastic portions of the circle as well as absent portions, the most common being an absent PComA on one side. In the presence of atherosclerotic disease, the intact circle of Willis can provide important collateral supply of blood flow to the ACA, MCA, PCA, and deep perforating arteries. Another important collateral supply to the circle of Willis, in the presence of atherosclerotic occlusion of an internal carotid, is retrograde blood flow from the external carotid artery through the ophthalmic artery. Finally, leptomeningeal arteries provide another helpful but limited source of collateral blood supply to the cerebral cortex.

The Anterior Choroidal Artery

The last branch of the internal carotid artery before the MCA–ACA bifurcation is the anterior choroidal artery (AChA). It is a major deep perforating artery that supplies the optic tract, globus pallidus, anterior hippocampus, and parts of the thalamus including a branch to the lateral geniculate nucleus (16, 17). In addition, the AChA provides blood supply to the deep white matter of the temporal lobe, including the geniculocalcarine tract and the lower portion of the posterior limb of the internal capsule in the cerebral peduncle. As the AChA's name implies, the terminal branches supply the choroid plexus of the temporal horn.

The Anterior Cerebral Artery

The anterior cerebral artery (ACA) originates from the carotid bifurcation and extends in an anteromedial direction to the anastomosis of the AComA. This portion of the circle of Willis is called the A1 segment. The A2 segment continues after the AComA anastomosis, along the medial frontal lobe within the medial longitudinal fissure between the cerebral hemispheres (Figure 5-3).

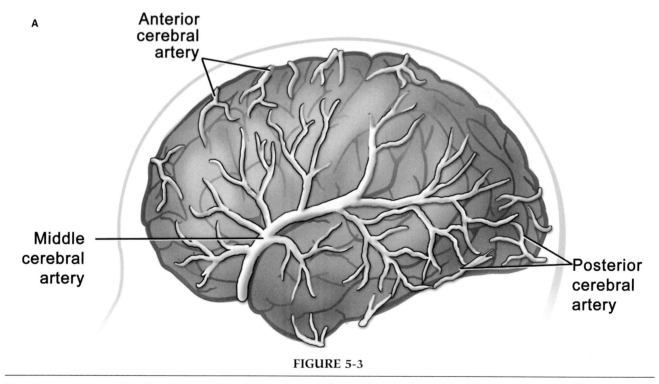

FIGURE 5-3

Vascular supply to cerebral hemisphere of the human brain. (A) Vascular supply to the lateral convexity of the cerebral hemisphere. (B) Vascular supply to the medial portions of the cerebral hemisphere. (C) Distribution of the middle cerebral artery and the subcortical branches of the lenticulostriate arteries.

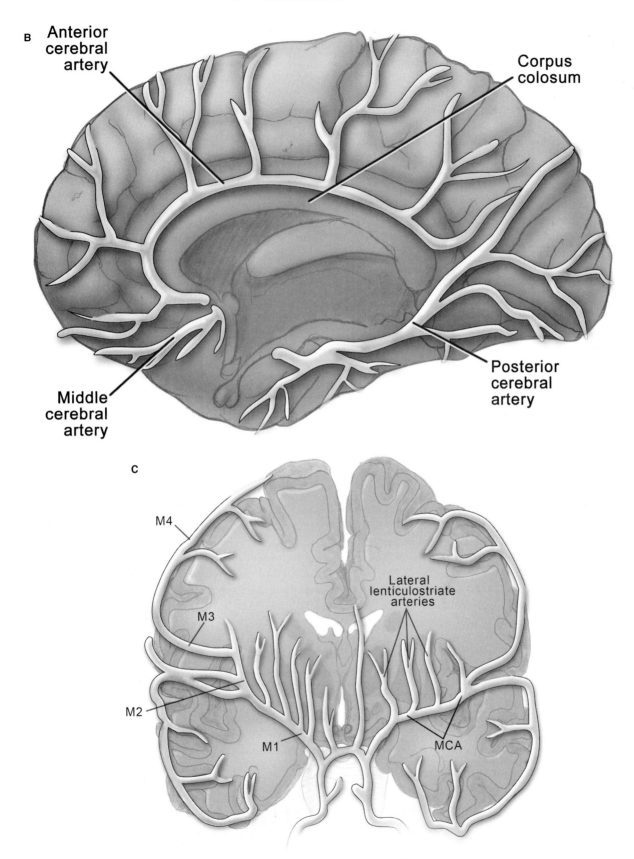

B

Anterior cerebral artery

Corpus colosum

Middle cerebral artery

Posterior cerebral artery

C

M4

M3

M2

M1

Lateral lenticulostriate arteries

MCA

FIGURE 5-3 *(Continued)*

It then passes superiorly and posteriorly around the corpus callosum to supply the medial frontal lobe, the corpus callosum, the cingulate gyrus, the paracentral lobule, and portions of the medial parietal lobe (18). Tributaries from the ACA transverse over the convexity of the cerebral hemisphere and anastomose with tributaries from the MCA in a watershed region.

The recurrent artery of Heubner (RAH) was first described by Johann Otto Leonhard Heubner in 1872 (19). This artery is the largest of a group of deep perforating arteries known as the lenticulostriate, which supply the basal ganglia as well as the intervening internal capsule and other surrounding white matter. The RAH originates from either the proximal A2 segment of the ACA or from anywhere along the A1 segment. Specifically, the RAH supplies the anterior caudate nucleus, the anterior third of the putamen, the tip of the outer segment of the globus pallidus, and the anterior limb of the internal capsule. Within the dominant hemisphere, the RAH supplies subcortical tissue near Broca's area in the frontal operculum.

Middle Cerebral Artery

The middle cerebral artery (MCA) supplies the largest volume of the cerebral hemisphere, including the basal ganglia, the internal capsule, and the visual radiations from the thalamus. The mainstem of the MCA originates from the carotid bifurcation and turns laterally toward the insular cortex. Along this route it supplies a series of lenticulostriate branches to subcortical structures. Once at the insular cortex, deep in the Sylvian fissure, the MCA divides into an upper and lower division. The segment from the carotid bifurcation to the MCA divisions is named M1. The M2 segment constitutes the upper- and lower-division branches within the Sylvian fissure. The M3 segment includes the branches to the opercula, and the M4 are the branches overlying the cerebral convexities (Figure 5-3).

The superior division of the MCA supplies the frontal operculum, the lateral convexity of the frontal lobe, and to a varying extent the parietal lobe. The inferior division of the MCA supplies the temporal operculum, the lateral convexity of the temporal and occipital lobes, and to a varying extent the parietal lobe.

The Posterior Cerebral Artery

The two posterior cerebral arteries (PCAs) divide at the top of the basilar artery and pass posterolaterally toward the medial temporal lobes. The P1 segment constitutes the section from the basilar artery to the branch of the PComA. The PCA then continues as the P2 segment to supply the medial occipital lobe within the longitudinal fissure, the posterior corpus callosum, and the medial

temporal lobes, including portions of the hippocampi. Branch tributaries pass over the convexity of the cerebral hemisphere and anastomose in a watershed region with MCA tributaries. Other tributaries within the longitudinal fissure anastomose with those of the ACA in the region of the medial parietal lobe (Figure 5-3).

CEREBRAL STROKE SYNDROMES

The stroke-related neurologic syndromes associated with major cerebral artery occlusion are predictable when one understands the neuroanatomy and cerebrovascular anatomy described in the first part of this chapter. In the context of cerebrovascular embolism or thrombosis, ischemic infarct can occur in all or a portion of the vascular bed supplied by the artery, depending on whether occlusion is incomplete or total. Immediate or delayed, intrinsically or extrinsically induced thrombolysis may also influence the extent of damage. The presence of atherosclerotic or small-vessel disease can affect the quality of tissue perfusion in watershed regions of major arteries. Thus, patients may experience all the components of a stroke syndrome, but more often only some of the signs and symptoms. Some of the neurologic impairment may be significant, whereas other impairments may be mild.

The following section includes a description of the most common clinical signs and symptoms associated with the major cerebral stroke syndromes. However, it should be understood that individual cases seen in clinical practice may vary somewhat from the classic syndromes. Still, given the history and evidence on imaging of an infarct within a certain vascular distribution, the clinician should look for all signs and symptoms associated with that particular syndrome.

Carotid Artery Syndromes

A thrombus in the common carotid or internal carotid artery is associated with atherosclerotic carotid artery disease. Infarcts can occur from an occlusive carotid thrombus or thromboembolism to distal cerebral arteries (most usually the MCA). Watershed infarcts in the distal MCA distribution can occur, presenting with partial contralateral hemiplegia and a sensory deficit affecting the shoulder more than the hand and leg. Carotid thrombosis often will present with a transient ischemic attack (TIA), which by definition lasts less than 24 hours and usually lasts only minutes. Amaurosis fugax, which is a transient monocular blindness, is a symptom that is peculiar to carotid TIAs. This phenomenon is typically caused by thromboembolism from the carotid to the ophthalmic artery with immediate thrombolysis. Often described as a "curtain dropping over the eye and rising again," amurosis fugax more often presents as a visual obscuration, clouding, or fogginess variably affecting the whole or part of the visual field in one eye. On rare occasions a completed stroke from carotid thrombosis will result in ipsilateral monocular blindness and contralateral hemiplegia.

Anterior Choroidal Artery Syndrome

The anterior choroidal artery syndrome was first described by Foix in 1925 and more thoroughly evaluated by Abbie in 1933 (16, 20). Ischemic injury in the territory of the AChA will cause a contralateral hemiplegia, because of injury to the posterior limb of the internal capsule. Hemianopsia can also occur, which varies depending on what structures are involved. Injury to the optic tract can result in a contralateral hemianopsia and reduced pupillary reaction. A lesion to the geniculocalcarine tract in the medial temporal lobe can also cause a contralateral hemianopsia. If the lateral geniculate nucleus is injured, a contralateral hemianopsia with median horizontal sparing can occur and is diagnostic of an AChA occlusion (21). Visual sparing in the horizontal plane results because a portion of the lateral geniculate is supplied by the lateral choroidal artery. AChA strokes usually cause no language deficit if the infarct is in the dominant hemisphere, but non-dominant injuries may cause a left hemineglect syndrome.

Anterior Cerebral Artery Syndrome

The ACA stroke is an uncommon stroke constituting 3% or fewer of all strokes. Still, patients with ACA stroke present with complex physical and cognitive deficits and usually require comprehensive neurorehabilitation services (22). Patients with a unilateral ACA infarct will present with contralateral hemiplegia worse in the leg and shoulder than in the arm, hand, and face, due to injury to the medial M1 cortex at the paracentral lobule. If facial weakness is noted, it is likely that the recurrent artery of Heubner was occluded as well (19). Sensory loss will be minimal, usually impaired two-point discrimination if present, and in the same distribution as the motor impairment.

Patients with ACA infarcts, whether in the right or left cerebral cortex, will often have limb apraxia that is limited to the left side. This is because the ACA supplies the anterior corpus callosum, which is a main pathway of transcortical interconnectivity between the frontal lobes. Infarcts in either the right or left ACA disconnect the right premotor and M1 cortex from the left language network. This disconnection will result in apraxic errors of the left upper limb when the patient is given a command (4, 14). However, because the left motor cortex is adjacent to Broca's area, ACA strokes do not affect motor performance on command with the right upper limb. These patients usually perform better with the left upper limb if given visual cues to follow.

In cases with injury to the eye fields of the dorsomedial frontal cortex, head and eye deviation ipsilaterally (away from the hemiplegia) is observed (5). Prefrontal lobe injury is also associated with the grasp reflex of the affected hand as well as some paratonia, which is a kind of limb rigidity that becomes more prominent with an increase in effort by the examiner during muscle stretches (force-dependent rigidity). Other "frontal release" signs such as the palmomental or snout reflexes can be seen in some cases.

Medial frontal injury involving supplementary motor area and cingulate gyrus can also result in reduced initiation and, if severe, psychomotor bradykinesia. Patients with ACA stroke may be very slow to respond to questions or commands; however, it should be kept in mind that they are often impulsive and may show no impediment in impulsive actions (such as climbing out of bed in an attempt to get to the restroom). Psychomotor bradykinesia can be severe enough to cause reduced verbal expression or even mutism that may be difficult to differentiate from aphasia (3). Executive cognitive functioning is also impaired with injury to the prefrontal cortex, which can have a negative impact on independent performance of instrumental activities of daily living.

Patients with ACA stroke can present with aphasia when the infarction includes the vascular supply of the left recurrent artery of Heubner (19). This will usually infarct subcortical tissue in the region extending between the supplementary motor area and Broca's area, injuring white-matter portions of the language network (23). This will most commonly cause a transcortical motor aphasia with reduced fluency, some apraxic errors of speech, and intact repetition (2, 3).

Middle Cerebral Artery Syndromes

Mainstem MCA (M1 segment): Occlusion of the MCA within the M1 segment can cause ischemic injury in the entire MCA distribution, which includes most of the lateral convexity of the cerebral hemisphere. In addition, a substantial injury to subcortical structures—including the internal capsule, visual radiations, and thalamocortical white matter—results from hypoperfusion of the lenticulostriate arterial branches off the M1 segment. Large MCA distribution infarcts can produce significant edema and increased intracranial pressure, which can cause contralateral cerebral injury, uncal herniation, and death. Those who survive a large mainstem MCA stroke will have significant neurologic impairment.

A patient with a mainstem MCA infarct will have complete contralateral hemiplegia from injury to the

M1 cortex and the entire internal capsule. Contralateral hemisensory loss or even hemianesthesia can result from substantial injury to the subcortical sensory tracts and the S1 cortex, although the thalamus itself may be spared. Infarct of the ipsilateral frontal eye fields in the lateral prefrontal area will cause head and eye deviation toward the lesion (away from the hemiplegia [5]). Deep infarction to the geniculocalcarine tract causes homonymous hemianopsia in the contralateral visual field.

If the infarct is in the dominant MCA distribution, there will be damage to the language network, including Broca's area, Wernicke's area, the angular gyrus, and the arcuate fasciculus. The patient will have a global aphasia with reduced fluency, severely impaired comprehension, and inability to repeat, read, or write.

A non-dominant MCA stroke will cause severe visual and perceptual deficits with disrupted spatial body orientation, dressing apraxia, and constructional apraxia. Survivors of non-dominant MCA strokes will also have a severe left hemineglect syndrome, contributed in part by reduced left attention (from parietal injury) and reduced exploration (from frontal injury) of the left hemispace. There is severe inattention to the left body as well, such that patients may deny they even have a stroke or stroke-related impairments (anosognosia).

Superior-Division MCA: Occlusion of the MCA at the origin of the superior division results in primarily a cortical infarct of the frontal lobe convexity, sparing the medial frontal lobe and subcortical tissue. Symptoms include a contralateral hemiplegia affecting the arm and hand more than the leg. Sensory deficits are mild, usually loss of two-point discrimination, in the same distribution as the weakness. These patients may have transient head and eye deviation toward the lesion (away from the hemiplegia). Visual fields are usually spared.

When the dominant hemisphere is affected, the patient has Broca's aphasia with decreased fluency of speech, apraxic errors, inability to repeat, and minimally impaired comprehension (2, 3). These patients have bilateral limb apraxia from injury of the frontal-lobe language network (necessary for carrying out motor commands in either upper limb [4]). Patients often struggle to follow motor commands with visual cues as well.

Patients with superior-division MCA strokes in the non-dominant (usually right) hemisphere will have hemineglect syndrome with reduced exploration of left hemispace and mildly reduced attention to left-sided stimuli (11). They often have deficits in visual spatial perception. Oral expression is altered, in that patients may have less prosody in their speech, lacking the normal inflections that emphasize the meaning, importance, or emotional content of a sentence. Aprosodia is seen with non-dominant frontal-lobe injuries (24, 25).

Inferior-division MCA: Occlusion in the inferior division of the MCA results in a primarily cortical infarct of the lateral convexity of the parietal, occipital, and temporal lobes. Patients with infarction in this region have no motor or somatosensory deficits. They may have a partial contralateral hemianopsia because of partial injury to visual radiations in the temporal lobe.

Injury to the dominant hemisphere from an inferior-division MCA stroke will cause a Wernicke's aphasia with fluent speech that is filled with paraphasic errors and poor comprehension of spoken and written language. Patients with non-dominant injuries have a hemineglect syndrome with reduced attention to the left hemispace and perceptual deficits (12). They may also have a *sensory aprosodia*, also known as an affective agnosia, in which the individual has a difficult time comprehending the prosody in another's speech (24–26).

Posterior Cerebral Artery Syndromes

If an occlusion occurs in the proximal PCA (P1) segment, hypoperfusion occurs in the distal PCA and the thalamoperforant arteries supplying the thalamus. This infarct will result in a contralateral sensory syndrome with hypoesthesia, a feeling of heaviness in the limbs, and in some cases dysesthesia (called Déjerine-Roussy syndrome [27]). The PCA distribution stroke will also cause a contralateral homonymous hemianopsia from direct injury to the primary visual cortex in the medial occipital lobe. Injury to the medial temporal lobe and structures of the hippocampus following PCA occlusion have been reported to cause an amnestic disorder in a few cases, but this is not commonly seen with unilateral infarct.

On rare occasions a PCA infarct in the left occipital lobe can result in *alexia without agraphia* (3, 14). These patients are not able to read but can write. The infarct includes the left primary visual cortex, causing a right homonymous hemianopsia. It also includes the posterior corpus callosum, which disconnects the right primary visual cortex from the language network. Thus the patient can see words in the left hemispace but cannot transfer visual images to the language centers. Writing is not affected because there is no disconnection between the language network and motor cortex (14). Patients with this lesion may have some left neglect syndrome as well (28).

Lacunar Stroke Syndromes

The term *lacune* means "little lake" and was coined to describe the pathological appearance of small cavities within brain parenchyma. These cavities are produced by small-branch occlusions of deep perforating vessels such as the lenticulostriate or thalamoperforant arteries. By definition, lacunar infarcts are 1.5 cm or less in the largest diameter, which corresponds to the tissue volume supplied by a deep perforating branch (located in subcortical structures such as the internal capsule, putamen, caudate, thalamus, cerebral white matter, and pons). Lacunar strokes are associated with hypertension and are caused by small-vessel occlusion from lipohylinosis of the vascular intima. C. Miller Fischer reintroduced the term "lacunar stroke" into clinical stroke neurology when he described the lacunar syndromes (29). Although as many as 100 lacunar syndromes have been described, 5 stand out as the most common seen in clinical practice.

One of the most common lacunar syndromes is the *pure sensory stroke* with symptoms of numbness in the face, arm, and leg on one side of the body. There are no associated motor or cognitive deficits. The infarct is usually located in the thalamus. Patients with sensory strokes can develop late or chronic pain syndromes as a result of disruptions of normal sensory tracts. Lesions in other regions of the CNS along sensory pathways may also cause central post-stroke pain syndrome (see Chapter 14).

Pure motor hemiparesis is also common and often will result in some functional limitations that require rehabilitation. The patient will have symptoms of motor loss in the face, arm, and leg, with or without spastic dystonia on one side of the body without associated sensory or cognitive changes. The stroke is located in the posterior limb of the internal capsule or cerebral peduncle, but may also occur in the base of the pons. Prognosis for functional recovery is good because patients lack other symptoms, such as language and visual deficits, and do not have apraxia. Spastic dystonia may complicate the rehabilitation process.

Dysarthria–clumsy hand syndrome, along with *ataxic hemiparesis,* are lacunar syndromes that most commonly occur from lesions in the base of the pons caused by occlusions of the paramedian pontine perforating vessels from the basilar artery. However, dysarthria–clumsy hand syndrome can also present following an infarct at the genu of the internal capsule in the somatotopic regions for face and hand, as well as in other areas of subcortical white matter. These patients will have dysarthria and unilateral facial weakness without language deficits, and a mild hemiparesis of the upper limb on one side of the body. The prognosis for recovery is very good, and the patient will benefit from a course of speech therapy and motor retraining of the upper limb. Patients with ataxic hemiparesis often have a considerable challenge regaining independent gait function because of problems with dynamic balance. But the prognosis is still very good, because the ataxic component often recovers more rapidly than the hemiparesis.

The lesion location for the *sensorimotor stroke* is most likely at the junction of the ventrolateral thalamus and the internal capsule, resulting in sensory loss and motor hemiparesis on one side of the body. Because the vascular supply to thalamus and internal capsule are distinct, the likely explanation is that edema from a thalamic stroke compresses adjacent fibers in the internal capsule, resulting in a mild hemiparesis. This has been described in one pathological case study (30).

RESEARCH FRONTIERS

Historically, our understanding of stroke syndromes came from the careful examination of pathological specimens. Today neuroimaging, especially with magnetic resonance imaging (MRI) and newer digital imaging software, has found a useful role in better defining the anatomical extent of cortical lesions caused by stroke. Techniques such as functional MRI (fMRI [31]) provide the opportunity to study the neuroanatomy following stroke and may further enhance our understanding of the complex relations between clinical behavior, lesion location and altered cortical activity in vivo (see chapter 8).

Large digital-image databases are now being gathered, providing the opportunity to correlate neuroanatomy with genetic and phenotypic variations in normal adult humans (32). No such database currently exists for cases of cerebrovascular lesions, but such an image library would be invaluable. Several small studies have attempted to further characterize the neuroanatomy of language using fMRI and voxel-based lesion-symptom imaging techniques (33, 34). The use of diffusion tensor tractography is helping to increase understanding of the association between white-matter tract lesions and stroke-related behavior (35–37). Such studies will certainly improve our understanding of stroke-related behavior and their neuroanatomical lesions. Even more important, however, are the prospects for better predicting functional outcome and the targeting of candidates for rehabilitation interventions that can improve recovery.

CONCLUSION

Understanding the cerebrovascular and neurologic anatomy of stroke lesions can help the neurorehabilitation clinician perform an efficient neurologic examination and identify clinically meaningful impairments that will impact functional performance. Thus, a clear knowledge of common stroke syndromes becomes a valuable tool for assessing functional limitations and setting realistic rehabilitation goals for the patient with stroke. Future research with modern neuroimaging holds promise for better predicting functional recovery and targeting rehabilitation interventions to achieve optimal outcomes.

References

1. Finger S. Paul Broca (1824–1880). *Journal of Neurology* 2004; 251:769–770.
2. Geshwind N. Aphasia. *New England Journal of Medicine* 1971; 284(12):654–656.
3. Demasio AR, Geshwind N. The neural basis of language. *Annual Reviews in Neuroscience* 1984; 7:127–147.
4. Geshwind N. The apraxias: Neural mechanisms of disorders of learned movement. *American Scientist* 1975; 63(2):188–195.
5. Tehovnik EJ, Sommer MA, Chou IH, et al. Eye fields in the frontal lobes of primates. *Brain Research Reviews* 2000; 32:413–448.
6. Mesulam MM. Large-scale neurocognitive networks and distributed processing for attention, language, and memory. *Annals of Neurology* 1990; 28:597–613.
7. Geshwind N, Levitsky W. Human brain: Left-right asymmetries in temporal speech region. *Science* 1968; 161:186–187.
8. Kilgard MP, Merzenich MM. Distributed representation of spectral and temporal information in rat primary auditory cortex. *Hearing Research* 1999; 134:16–28.
9. Tramo MJ, Cariani PA, Koh CK, et al. Neurophysiology and neuroanatomy of pitch perception: auditory cortex. *Annals New York Academy of Sciences* 2005; 1060: 148–174.
10. Stefanatos GA, Gershkoff A, Madigan S. On pure word deafness, temporal processing, and the left hemisphere. *Journal of the International Neuropsychological Society* 2005; 11(4):456–470.
11. Mesulam MM. Attentional networks, confusional states and neglect syndromes. In Mesulam MM, ed. *Principles of Behavioral and Cognitive Neurology.* New York: Oxford University Press, 2000:174–256.
12. Caplan LR, Kelly M, Kase CS, et al. Infarcts of the inferior division of the right middle cerebral artery: Mirror image of Wernicke's aphasia. *Neurology* 1986; 36:1015–1020.
13. Pillman F. Carl Wernicke (1848–1905). *Journal of Neurology* 2003; 250:1390–1391.
14. Geshwind N. Disconnexion syndromes in animals and man. *Brain* 1965; 88:585–644.
15. Ustun C. Dr. Thomas Willis' famous eponym: The circle of Willis. *Turk J Med Sci.* 2004; 34:271–274.
16. Abbie AA. The clinical significance of the anterior choroidal artery. *Brain* 1933; 56(3): 243–246.
17. Mohr JP, Steinke W, Timsit SG, et al. The anterior choroidal artery does not supply the corona radiata and lateral ventricular wall. *Stroke* 1991; 22:1502–1507.
18. Stafani MA, Schneider FL, Marrone ACH, et al. Anatomic variations of anterior cerebral artery cortical branches. *Clinical Anatomy* 2000; 13:231–236.
19. Loukas M, Louis RG, Childs RS. Anatomical examination of the recurrent artery of Heubner. *Clinical Anatomy* 2006; 19:25–31.
20. Foix C, Chavany JA, Hillemand P, Schiff-Wertheimer S. Obliteration de l'artere choroidienne anterieure: ramollissement de son territoire cerebral: hemiplegie, hemianesthesie, heianopsie. *Bulletin de le Societé d'Ophtalmologie de Paris* 1925; 37:221–223.
21. Helgason C, Caplan LR, Goodwin J, Hedges T. Anterior choroidal artery-territory infarction. Report of cases and review. *Archives of Neurology* 1986; 43:681–686.
22. Critchley M. The anterior cerebral artery, and its syndromes. *Brain.* 1930; 53:120–165.
23. Freedman M, Alexander MP, Naeser MA. Anatomic basis of transcortical motor aphasia. *Neurology* 1984; 34:409–417.
24. Ross ED. Hemispheric specialization for emotions, affective aspects of language and communication and the cognitive control of display behaviors in humans. *Progress in Brain Research* 1996; 107:583–594.
25. Ross ED, Thompson RD, Yenkosky J. Lateralization of affective prosody in brain and the callosal integration of hemispheric language functions. *Brain and Language* 1997; 56:27–54.
26. Darby DG. Sensory aprosodia: A clinical clue to lesions of the inferior division of the right middle cerebral artery? *Neurology* 1993; 43(3):567–572.
27. Bogousslavsky J, Regli F, Uske A. Thalamic infarcts: Clinical syndromes, etiology and prognosis. *Neurology* 1988; 38:837–848.
28. Park KC, Lee BH, Kim EJ, et al. Deafferentation-disconnection neglect induced by posterior cerebral artery infarction. *Neurology* 2006; 66:56–61.
29. Fischer CM. Lacunar strokes and infarcts: a review. *Neurology* 1982; 32:871–876.
30. Mohr JP, Kase CS, Meckler RJ, Fisher CM. Sensorimotor stroke. *Arch Neurol.* 1977; 34:734–741.
31. Calautti C, Baron JC. Functional neuroimaging studies of motor recovery after stroke in adults: a review. *Stroke* 2003; 34:1553–1566.
32. Mazziotta J, Toga A, Evans A, et al. A probablistic atlas and reference system for the human brain: International consortium for brain mapping (ICBM). *Phil. Trans. R. Soc. Lond* 2001; 356:1293–1322.
33. Boatman D, Gordan B, Hart J, et al. Transcortical sensory aphasia: Revisited and revised. *Brain* 2000; 123:1634–1642.
34. Bates E, Wilson SM, Saygin AP, et al. Voxel-based lesion-symptom mapping. *Nature Neuroscience* 2003; 6(5):448–450.
35. Ahn YH, Ahn SH, Kim H, et al. Can stroke patients walk after complete lateral cortical spinal tract injury of the affected hemisphere? *NeuroReport* 2006; 17:987–990.
36. Holodny AI, Gor DM, Watts R, et al. Diffusion-tensor MR tractography of somatotopic organization of corticospinal tracts in the internal capsule: Initial anatomic results in contradistinction to prior reports. *Radiology* 2005; 234:649–653.
37. Holodny AI, Watts R, Korneinko V, et al. Diffusion tensor tractography of the motor white matter tracts in man: current controversies and future directions. Annals of the New York Academy of Sciences 2005; 1064:88–97.

6 Infratentorial Stroke Syndromes

Richard D. Zorowitz

T he infratenorial region, comprising the brain stem and cerebellum, spans the diencephalon and the spinal cord. Despite its small size, the brain stem has the potential to cause neurologic devastation if damaged. It carries fibers that affect motor and sensory function as well as arousal and survival. The brain stem carries fibers that have important modulatory effects on both the cerebral cortex and the spinal cord. While the cerebellum does not contain direct pathways between the cerebrum and spinal cord, it also has the potential to cause neurologic devastation if damaged since it also modulates movement and tone.

This chapter will describe the development of the brain stem and cerebellum. Following this, the neuroanatomy of the brain stem and cerebellum and their organization into columns of afferent and efferent neurons will be discussed. Understanding the organization of the brain stem and cerebellum is essential to understanding the functional correlates of the brain stem. It is these functional correlates that explain the syndromes whose descriptions comprise the remainder of the chapter.

DEVELOPMENT OF THE BRAIN STEM

During development of the nervous system, the *neural tube* gives rise to all of the neurons and glial cells of the central nervous system. The caudal portion of the neural tube develops into the spinal cord, while the rostral portion becomes the brain. The rostral neural tube divides into three vesicles, called the *forebrain*, *midbrain*, and *hindbrain* (Figure 6-1). The forebrain, or *prosencephalon*, ultimately matures to form the *telencephalon* (cerebral hemispheres and lateral ventricles) and the *diencephalon* (thalamus and third ventricle).

Three layers form within the wall of the neural tube. The *neuroepithelial*, or *ventricular* layer, contain the innermost cells that ultimately will line the central canal of the spinal cord and the ventricles of the brain. The *mantle*, or *intermediate* layer, consists of neurons and glial cells that will form the gray matter of the spinal cord. This layer contains the *alar plate*, which gives rise to sensory neuroblasts of the dorsal horn of the spinal cord, and the *basal plate*, which gives rise to motor neuroblasts of the ventral horn of the spinal cord.

The midbrain and hindbrain form the basis of the brain stem. The midbrain, or *mesencephalon*, does not divide, but evolves into the midbrain, cerebral aqueduct, and rostral cerebellum. The *alar plate sensory neuroblasts* form the cell layers of the superior colliculi and the nuclei of the inferior colliculi (1). The *basal plate motor neuroblasts* form the oculomotor (cranial nerve III) and trochlear (cranial nerve IV) nuclei, as well as the Edinger-Westphal (cranial nerve III) nucleus, which give rise to preganglionic parasympathetic fibers. The

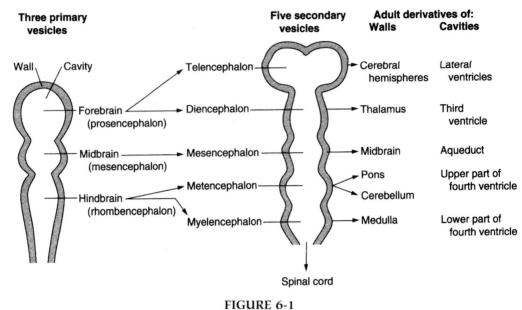

Three primary vesicles   **Five secondary vesicles**   **Adult derivatives of: Walls   Cavities**

FIGURE 6-1

Development of the brain into forebrain, midbrain, and hindbrain. Reprinted with permission from Moore KL. *The Developing Human: Clinically Oriented Embryology.* 4th ed. Philadelphia, PA: W.B. Saunders, 1988: 380.

red nucleus and substantia nigra also originate from the basal plate.

The hindbrain, or *rhombencephalon*, subdivides into two regions: the rostral *metencephalon* and caudal *myelencephalon*. The *metencephalon* matures into the caudal cerebellum, pons, and rostral fourth ventricle. In the pons, the *alar plate sensory neuroblasts* give rise to the spinal and principal sensory trigeminal (cranial nerve V) nuclei and the cochlear and vestibular (cranial nerve VIII) nuclei. The alar plate sensory neuroblasts also form the solitary nucleus, which carries and receives visceral sensation and taste from the facial (cranial nerve VII), glossopharyngeal (cranial nerve IX), vagus (cranial nerve X), and the cranial portion of the accessory (cranial nerve XI) nerves. It also relays information to the cerebellum through the pontine nuclei. The *basal plate motor neuroblasts* form the trigeminal (cranial nerve V), abducens (cranial nerve VI), facial (cranial nerve VII), and superior salivary (cranial nerve VII) nuclei.

The *myelencephalon* ultimately forms the medulla oblongata and caudal fourth ventricle. The *alar plate sensory neuroblasts* of the caudal portion of the medulla oblongata form the nuclei gracilis and cuneatus, inferior olivary (cerebellar relay) nuclei, solitary nucleus, spinal trigeminal (cranial nerve V) nucleus, and cochlear and vestibular (cranial nerve VIII) nuclei. The *basal plate motor neuroblasts* of the medulla oblongata give rise to the hypoglossal (cranial nerve XII) nuclei, nucleus ambiguus (cranial nerves IX, X, and XI), the dorsal motor nucleus of the vagus (cranial nerve X), and the inferior salivatory nucleus of the glossopharyngeal (cranial nerve IX) nerve.

DEVELOPMENT OF THE CEREBELLUM

As stated above, the caudal portion of the cerebellum develops from the metencephalon, and the rostral portion arises from the caudal mesencephalon (2). It is formed by the thickened alar plates of the mantle layer of the neural tube known as *rhombic lips*. Four regions develop from the cerebellar primordium. The *vermis* develops through midline growth. The *cerebellar hemispheres* develop through lateral growth. The *cerebellar cortex* migrates from the ventricles into the marginal zone and forms three layers (molecular, Purkinje cell, and internal granular cell) and four pairs of cerebellar nuclei. The *external granular cell* layer is a germinal cell layer that exists on the surface of the cerebellum between the eighth week of development and the end of the second postnatal year. As the cerebellum grows, *folia* and *fissures* form.

ANATOMY OF THE BRAIN STEM

The brain stem is the lower extension of the brain where it connects to the spinal cord (see Figure 6-2). Neurologic functions located in the brain stem include those necessary for survival (breathing, gastrointestinal function, heart rate, blood pressure) and for arousal and wakefulness. The brain stem also surrounds a narrow passage for the circulation of cerebrospinal fluid. The occlusion of the passage, the *Aqueduct of Sylvius*, often is accompanied by the neurologic complications of hydrocephalus.

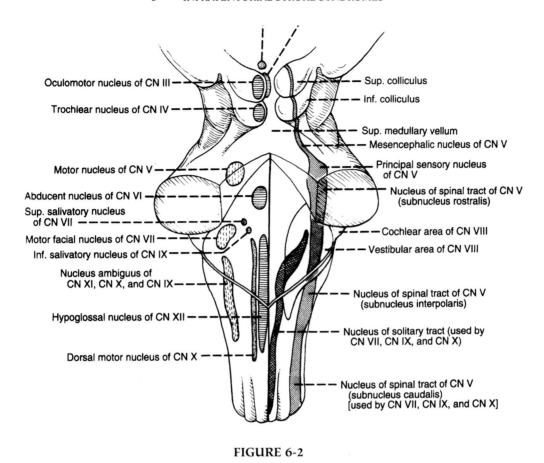

Oculomotor nucleus of CN III

Trochlear nucleus of CN IV

Motor nucleus of CN V

Abducent nucleus of CN VI

Sup. salivatory nucleus of CN VII

Motor facial nucleus of CN VII

Inf. salivatory nucleus of CN IX

Nucleus ambiguus of CN XI, CN X, and CN IX

Hypoglossal nucleus of CN XII

Dorsal motor nucleus of CN X

Sup. colliculus

Inf. colliculus

Sup. medullary vellum

Mesencephalic nucleus of CN V

Principal sensory nucleus of CN V

Nucleus of spinal tract of CN V (subnucleus rostralis)

Cochlear area of CN VIII

Vestibular area of CN VIII

Nucleus of spinal tract of CN V (subnucleus interpolaris)

Nucleus of solitary tract (used by CN VII, CN IX, and CN X)

Nucleus of spinal tract of CN V (subnucleus caudalis) [used by CN VII, CN IX, and CN X]

FIGURE 6-2

Neuroanatomy of the brain stem. Reprinted with permission from Fix, JD. *Neuroanatomy.* 3rd ed. Philadelphia, PA: Lippincott Williams and Wilkins, 2001.

In order to better understand how lesions of the brain stem cause specific neurologic symptoms, it is important to understand the architecture of the brain stem. As the brain stem develops, neuroblasts develop columns that classify the functions of the body into discrete modalities. *General* fibers are found in most spinal nerves, while *special* fibers are found only in specific senses. *Somatic* fibers are found in organs of voluntary movement and sensation, while *visceral* fibers are found in internal organs. *Afferent* fibers travel from the periphery to the central nervous system, while *efferent* fibers travel from the central nervous system to the periphery. Modalities of nerve fibers are classified in Table 6-1. The functional divisions of the cranial nerves are listed by modality in Table 6-2.

As the brain stem develops, the alar plate becomes the sensory (afferent) nerves, while the basal plate becomes the motor (efferent) nerves. The motor nerves are positioned medially, and the sensory nerves are positioned laterally (Figure 6-3). By the time the brain stem is fully developed, the cranial nerve nuclei are organized into seven longitudinal columns (Figure 6-4). The cell columns run roughly parallel to the longitudinal axis of

the brain stem, but are not always continuous. The organization of the cranial nerves into columns is significant for two reasons. First, neurons are organized with similar functions. For example, neurons mediating taste are located in the same position with respect to the midline. Second, different functions are affected when ischemia or hemorrhage damages areas of the brain stem, depending upon whether they are lateral or medial. As a result, one classification scheme of brain stem stroke syndromes is described by its lateral or medial location with respect to the midline.

Structures of the Brain Stem

Midbrain (Figure 6-5): The midbrain is a short, constricted structure that connects the pons and cerebellum with the thalamus and cerebral hemispheres. It consists of three portions: (1) the *cerebral peduncles*, a pair of cylindrical bodies located ventrolaterally; (2) the *corpora quadrigemina*, consisting of four rounded eminences; and (3) the *cerebral aqueduct*, a passage representing the original cavity of the midbrain that connects the third and fourth ventricles. Each cerebral

TABLE 6-1
Modalities of the Cranial Nerves

MODALITY	DEFINITION
General somatic sfferent (GSA)	Arise from cells in spinal ganglia and conduct pain, touch, and temperature from the surface of the body and muscle/tendon/joint sense from deeper structures through posterior roots of the spinal cord
General visceral afferent (GVA)	Arise from viscera through the rami communicantes and posterior roots to spinal cord
General somatic efferent (GSE)	Arise from motor neuron cell bodies in ventral horns of spinal cord gray matter to skeletal muscle (i.e., alpha motor neurons, gamma motor neurons)
General visceral efferent (GVE)	Arise from cells in lateral column or base of the anterior column through anterior roots and white rami communicantes to sympathetic ganglia that conduct motor impulses to smooth muscles of the viscera and vessels and secretory impulses to the glands
Special somatic afferent (SSA)	Arise from nerves of special senses to the central nervous system (e.g., optic nerve, acoustic nerve)
Special visceral afferent (SVA)	Arise from nerves associated with gastrointestinal tract to the central nervous system (e.g., olfactory nerve, facial nerve, glossopharyngeal nerve, vagus nerve)
Special visceral efferent (SVE)	Arise from central nervous system to muscles of pharygeal arches (e.g., trigeminal nerve, facial nerve, glossopharyngeal nerve, vagus nerve, accessory nerve)

Adapted from Composition and central connections of the spinal nerves. In: Gray H. *Anatomy of the Human Body*. Philadelphia: Lea & Febiger, 1918; Bartleby.com, 2000. www.bartleby.com/107/. Accessed on February 10, 2008.

peduncle is divided into a dorsal and ventral part, separated by the *substantia nigra*. The dorsal part is known as the *tegmentum*, and the ventral part is known as the *base* or *crusta*. The major gray matter structures of the tegmentum are the *red nucleus* and the *interpeduncular ganglion*. The major tracts include the *superior cerebellar peduncle*, the *medial longitudinal fasciculus*, and the *medial lemniscus*.

The *red nucleus* is located in the anterior aspect of the tegmentum and the posterior aspect of the subthalamic region. It appears circular in shape and receives fibers from the superior cerebellar peduncle and medial lemniscus. Axons cross the midline and project into the lateral funiculus of the spinal cord as the *rubrospinal tract*, an important part of the pathway from the cerebellum to the lower motor centers.

The *superior cerebellar peduncles* (*brachia conjunctiva*) are two axonal tracts that arise from the dentate nucleus of the cerebellum. The fiber bundles pass rostrally through the dorsal pons to the level of the inferior colliculus. At this point, the fibers decussate, ascend farther, and terminate either in the red nucleus or within the motor, ventral lateral, or ventral anterior nuclei of the thalamus. The majority of fibers that convey signals out of the cerebellum to the brain stem are located in these tracts.

The *medial longitudinal fasciculus* (MLF) carries information about the direction that the eyes should move as well as information about head movement (from cranial nerve VIII). The MLF arises from the vestibular nucleus and is thought to mediate the maintenance of gaze. This is achieved by inputs from several

TABLE 6-2
Functional Anatomy of the Brain Stem

CRANIAL NERVE	MODALITY	STRUCTURE
Olfactory (I)	SVA	Projects directly to telecephalon
Optic (II)	SSA	Projects directly to diencephalon
Oculomotor (III)	GSE	Oculmotor nucleus
	GVE	Edinger-Westphal nucleus
Trochlear (IV)	GSE	Trochlear nucleus
Trigeminal (V)	GSA	Principal sensory and spinal nucleus of V
	GVE	Motor nucleus
Abducens (VI)	GSE	Abducens nerve
Facial (VII)	SVE	Facial nucleus
	GVE	Superior salivary nucleus
	GVA	Solitary nucleus
	SVA	Solitary nucleus
	GSA	Spinal nucleus of V
Vestibular (VIII)	SSA	Vestibular nucleus
Cochlear (VIII)	SSA	Cochlear nucleus
Glossopharyngeal (IX)	SVE	Nucleus ambiguus
	GVE	Inferior salivary nucleus
	SVA	Solitary nucleus
	GVA	Spinal nucleus of V
Vagus (X)	SVE	Nucleus ambiguus
	GVE	Motor nucleus of X
	SVA	Solitary nucleus
	GVA	Solitary nucleus
	GSA	Spinal nucleus of V
Accessory (XI)	SVE	Nucleus ambiguus and accessory nucleus
Hypoglossal (XII)	GSE	Hypoglossal nucleus

Key: GSA: general somatic afferent; GVA: general visceral afferent; GSE: general somatic efferent; GVE: general visceral efferent; SSA: special somatic afferent; SVA: special visceral afferent; SVE: special visceral efferent.

structures: the acoustic (cranial nerve VIII) nerve, which mediates head movements; the flocculus of the cerebellum, which adjusts gain; and head and neck proprioceptors, and foot and ankle muscle spindles, through the fastigial nucleus. It mediates conjugate gaze by carrying electrical signals from the abducens (cranial nerve VI) nuclei, across the midline, and then ascending to the oculomotor (cranial nerve III) and trochlear (cranial nerve IV) nuclei. The MLF also descends into the cervical spinal cord, where it innervates some muscles of the neck.

The vertical gaze center is located in the rostral interstitial nucleus of the MLF, which lies just posterior to the red nucleus. From each vertical gaze center, signals are conducted to the subnuclei of the ocular muscles that control vertical gaze in both eyes. Cells mediating downward eye movements are intermingled in the vertical gaze center, but ischemia of this region may result in selective paralysis of upgaze.

The *medial lemniscus* originates in the nucleus gracilis and cuneatus of the medulla oblongata and crosses to the opposite side in the sensory decussation. It then ascends through the medulla oblongata into the pons and lower portion of the midbrain, where it receives fibers from sensory nuclei of the contralateral cranial nerves. The majority of the fibers, however, enter the ventral lateral nucleus of the thalamus, gives off collaterals, and then terminates in the principal sensory nucleus of the thalamus.

The *corpora quadrigemina* are four rounded structures that form the dorsal aspect of the midbrain.

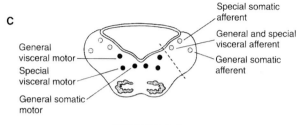

FIGURE 6-3

Positions of the motor and sensory nuclei in the developing brain stem. Sensory nuclei develop from the alar plate, while motor nuclei develop from the basal plate. Reprinted with permission from Kandel ER, Schwartz JH, Jessell TM. *Principles of Neural Science*. 3rd ed. New York: McGraw Hill Professional Neurosciences, 1995: 686.

The corpora quadrigemina are arranged in pairs as the *superior* and *inferior colliculi*. The superior colliculi are associated with the sense of sight, the inferior with that of hearing. The afferent fibers of the superior colliculi largely originate in the retina and are conveyed to the superior colliculi through the superior brachium and lateral geniculate body. Some of the efferent fibers cross the midline to the opposite colliculus, while many ascend

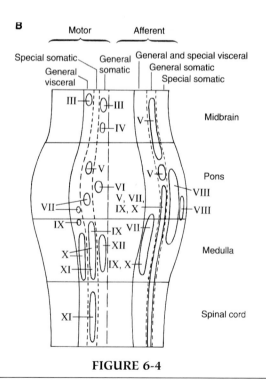

FIGURE 6-4

Columnar organization of the motor and sensory nuclei in the brain stem. Reprinted with permission from Kandel ER, Schwartz JH, Jessell TM. *Principles of Neural Science*. 3rd ed. New York: McGraw Hill Professional Neurosciences, 1995: 688.

through the superior brachium and terminate in the cortex of the occipital lobe.

Pons (Figure 6-6): The pons is a bridge-like structure that links different parts of the brain and relays information from the medulla oblongata to the higher cortical structures of the cerebrum. It contains the ventilatory and horizontal gaze centers. The pons sits in front of the cerebellum and is connected to the cerebellum through the *middle cerebellar peduncle*. The pons consists of two aspects: the ventral surface (pars basilaris pontis) and the dorsal surface (pars dorsalis pontis). The ventral surface of the pons consists of superficial and deep transverse fibers, longitudinal fasciculi, and some small nuclei of gray substance (termed *nuclei pontis*) that give rise to transverse fibers. It is in the nuclei pontis that cortical axons that travel through the internal capsule and cerebral peduncle form synapses with transverse fibers that decussate and pass through the middle peduncle into the cerebellum. The dorsal surface of the pons consists largely of ascending projections of the reticular formation and gray substance from the medulla oblongata. Other significant structures in the pons include the *superior olivary nucleus* and the *paramedian pontine reticular formation*.

The *paramedian pontine reticular formation* (PPRF) is located anterolaterally to the MLF. It receives input from the superior colliculus and from the frontal eye fields. The rostral aspect of the PPRF (rostral interstitial nucleus of the MLF) probably coordinates vertical saccades, while the caudal aspect of the PPRF may generate horizontal saccades. In particular, excitatory burst neurons (EBNs) in the PPRF generate "pulse" movements that initiate a saccade. With respect to horizontal saccades, the "pulse" information is conveyed via axonal fibers to the abducens (cranial nerve VI) nucleus, subsequently initiating horizontal eye movements.

Medulla Oblongata (Figure 6-7): The medulla oblongata extends from the inferior border of the pons to a plane passing transversely between the pyramidal decussation and the first pair of cervical nerves. This plane corresponds with the upper border of the atlas and basilar part of the occipital bone behind and the middle of the odontoid process of the axis in front. The medulla oblongata functions primarily as a relay station for the crossing of motor tracts between the spinal cord and the brain. It also contains the respiratory, vasomotor, and cardiac centers, as well as many mechanisms for controlling some involuntary actions, including coughing, gagging, swallowing, and vomiting. Significant structures in the medulla oblongata include the *olive* and the *inferior cerebellar peduncle*. The *olive* is located lateral to the pyramidal tracts.

The *inferior cerebellar peduncle* is located in the superoposterior portion of the medulla oblongata. It is a thick, rope-like strand that sits between the inferior

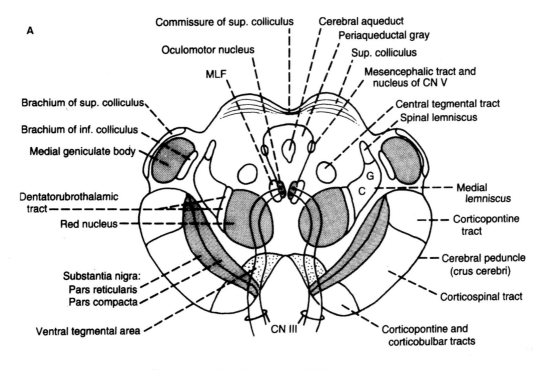

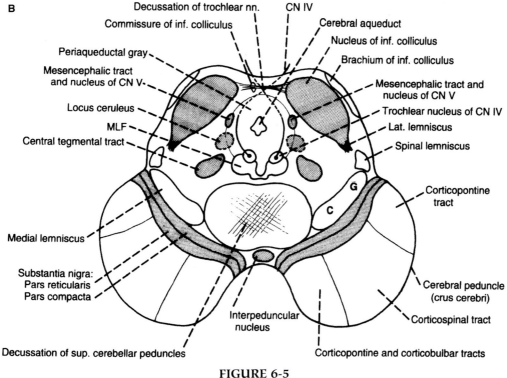

FIGURE 6-5

Clinical neuroanatomy of the midbrain. (A) Midbrain at the level of the superior colliculus. (B) Midbrain at the level of the inferior colliculus. Reprinted with permission from Fix, JD. *Neuroanatomy*. 3rd ed. Philadelphia, PA: Lippincott Williams and Wilkins, 2001.

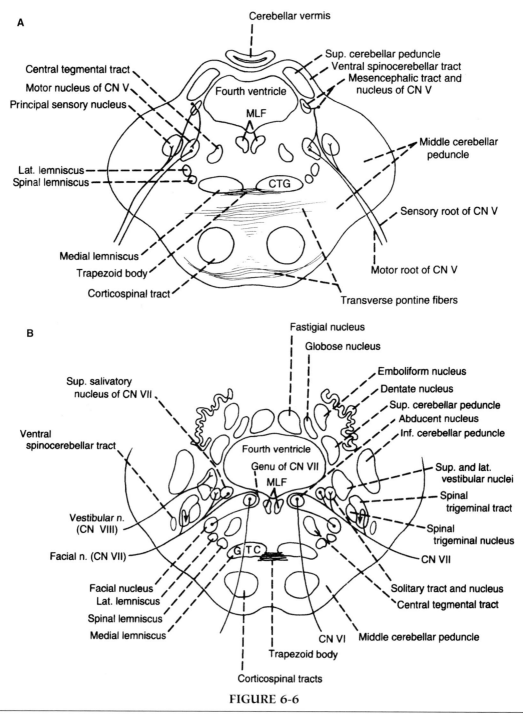

FIGURE 6-6

Clinical neuroanatomy of the pons. (A) Midpontine region. (B) Caudal aspect of the pons. Reprinted with permission from Fix, JD. *Neuroanatomy*. 3rd ed. Philadelphia, PA: Lippincott Williams and Wilkins, 2001.

portion of the fourth ventricle and the glossopharyngeal (cranial nerve IX) and vagus (cranial nerve X) nerve roots. The inferior cerebellar peduncles connect the spinal cord and medulla oblongata with the cerebellum. The inferior cerebellar peduncle carries many types of input and output fibers that mainly integrate proprioceptive sensory input with motor vestibular functions, such as balance and posture maintenance. Proprioceptive information from the body is conveyed to the cerebellum through the posterior spinocerebellar tract. The inferior cerebellar peduncle also carries information directly from Purkinje cells to the vestibular (cranial nerve VIII) nuclei at the junction of the pons and medulla oblongata.

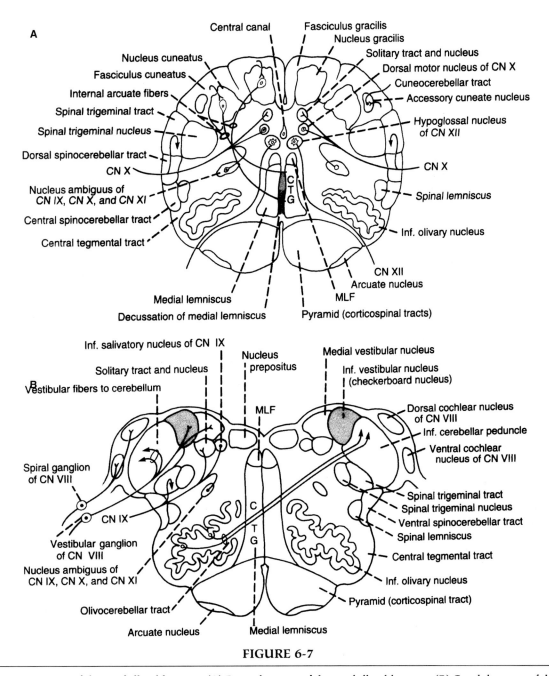

FIGURE 6-7

Clinical neuroanatomy of the medulla oblongata. (A) Rostral aspect of the medulla oblongata. (B) Caudal aspect of the medulla oblongata. Reprinted with permission from Fix, JD. *Neuroanatomy*. 3rd ed. Philadelphia, PA: Lippincott Williams and Wilkins, 2001.

Nuclei: A cranial nerve nucleus is a collection of neurons (gray matter) in the brain stem associated with one or more cranial nerves. Axons carrying information to and from cranial nerves synapse at these nuclei. Ischemic or hemorrhagic lesions of these nuclei usually lead to neurologic deficits that resemble those seen when the nerves with which these nuclei are associated are severed. All cranial nerve nuclei except for the trochlear (cranial nerve IV) nerve supply nerves on the same side of the body.

The *olfactory nerve* (cranial nerve I) arises from spindle-shaped bipolar cells in the surface epithelium of the olfactory region of the nasal cavity. The non-myelinated axons ascend through the cribriform plate to the olfactory bulb. At this point, several fibers, each ending in a tuft of terminal filaments, come into contact with the brush-like end of a single dendrite from a mitral cell, giving rise to the olfactory glomeruli of the bulb. The termination of a number of olfactory fibers in a single glomerulus accounts, in part at least, for the detection by the olfactory organs of very dilute solutions. The olfactory fibers form synapses with dendrites of one or two mitral cells, providing for the summation of stimuli in the mitral cells. The majority of the axons that arise from the mitral cells of the olfactory bulb and courses into the olfactory tract travels through the lateral olfactory stria to the uncus and hippocampal gyrus and terminate in the cortex. Other fibers may pass to the uncus and hippocampal gyrus from the primary olfactory centers in the trigonum and anterior perforated substance. The branches and axons that pass backward terminate partly in the hippocampus, the dentate gyrus, and hippocampal gyrus. Shorter association fibers connect various sections of the gyrus fornicatus (cingulate gyrus, isthmus, and hippocampal gyrus) and these with other regions of the cortex. These gyri constitute the cortical center for smell.

The *optic nerve* (cranial nerve II) consists chiefly of coarse fibers that arise from the ganglionic layer of the retina. They constitute the third neuron in the series composing the visual path and are supposed to convey only visual impressions. A number of fine fibers also pass in the optic nerve from the retina to the primary centers and are supposed to be concerned with pupillary reflexes. In addition, there are a few fibers that pass from the brain to the retina. They reportedly control chemical changes in the retina and the movements of the pigment cells and cones.

In the optic chiasma, the nerves from the medial half of each retina cross to the opposite optic tract, and the nerves from the lateral half of each retina continue in the optic tract of the same side. The crossed fibers occupy the medial side of each optic nerve but are more intermingled in the chiasma and in the optic tract. Most of the fibers of the optic tract terminate in the lateral geniculate body, but some may pass through the superior brachium to the superior colliculus or through the lateral geniculate body to the pulvinar of the thalamus. The superior colliculus receives fibers from the visual sensory cortex in the occipital lobe that pass through the optic radiations.

The *oculomotor nerve* (cranial nerve III) contains somatic motor fibers to the inferior oblique, inferior rectus, superior rectus, levator palpebræ superioris, and medial rectus muscles. In addition, preganglionic sympathetic efferent fibers are carried to the ciliary ganglion. The postganglionic fibers from the ciliary ganglion supply the ciliary muscle and the sphincter of the iris. The axons arise from the nucleus of the oculomotor nerve and traverse the posterior longitudinal bundle, tegmentum, red nucleus, and the medial margin of the substantia nigra to emerge from the oculomotor sulcus on the medial side of the cerebral peduncle.

The nucleus of the oculomotor nerve contains several distinct groups of cells that vary in size and appearance from each other and terminate their axons at separate muscles. It is uncertain which group supplies which muscle. There are seven of these nuclei on either side of the midline and one medial nucleus. The cells of the anterior nuclei are smaller and may give off sympathetic efferent axons. The majority of fibers arise from the nucleus of the same side. However, some may cross to the opposite side and supply the contralateral medial rectus muscle. Since the oculomotor and abducens nuclei are connected by the MLF, this decussation of fibers to the medial rectus may facilitate the conjugate movements of the eyes in which the medial and lateral recti muscles are involved.

The *trochlear nerve* (cranial nerve IV) contains somatic motor fibers only. It supplies the superior oblique muscle of the eye. Its nucleus is a small, oval mass located in the ventral part of the central gray matter of the cerebral aqueduct at the level of the superior aspect of the inferior colliculus. The axons from the nucleus descend in the tegmentum toward the pons but abruptly turn dorsally before reaching it, cross horizontally, and decussate with the nerve of the opposite side. The nerve emerges immediately behind the inferior colliculus. There are no branches from the fibers of the pyramidal tracts to these nuclei. It is thought that the volitional pathway must be an indirect one.

The *trigeminal nerve* (cranial nerve V) contains somatic motor and sensory fibers. The motor fibers arise in the trigeminal motor nucleus and travel ventrolaterally through the pons to supply the muscles of mastication. The sensory fibers arise from the semilunar ganglion and are distributed to the face and anterior two-thirds of the head. The central fibers pass into the pons with the motor root and bifurcate into ascending and descending branches that terminate in the sensory nuclei of the trigeminal.

The sensory nucleus consists of an enlarged upper end, the main sensory nucleus, and a long, more slender portion that descends through the pons and medulla oblongata to become continuous with the dorsal part of the posterior column of the gray matter of the spinal cord. This descending portion consists mainly of substantia gelatinosa and is called the *nucleus of the spinal tract of the trigeminal nerve*. Most of the fibers cross to the trigeminothalamic tract of the opposite side, ascend dorsally to the medial lemniscus, and terminate in a distinct part of the thalamus. The somatic sensory fibers of the vagus, the glossopharyngeal, and the facial nerves probably end in the nucleus of the descending tract of the trigeminal. Their cortical impulses probably are carried up in the central sensory path of the trigeminal.

The *abducens nerve* (cranial nerve VI) contains only somatic motor fibers, which supply the lateral rectus muscle of the eye. The fibers arise from the abducens nucleus, pass ventrally through the pons, and exit from the transverse groove between the caudal edge of the pons and the pyramid. These fibers probably terminate in relation with the MLF, which controls conjugate gaze. The fibers of the MLF originate in the terminal nuclei of the vestibular nerve and give off collateral and terminal neurons to the abducens, trochlear, and oculomotor nuclei. The abducens nucleus also receives collateral and terminal neurons from the tectospinal fasciculus, the reflex auditory center in the inferior colliculus, and other sensory nuclei of the brain stem.

The *facial nerve* (cranial nerve VII) consists of somatic and visceral afferent and efferent fibers. The afferent fibers arise from cells in the geniculate ganglion and often are known as the *nervus intermedius*. There are few somatic afferent fibers. Their purpose is to convey impulses from the middle ear, but their existence and central termination have not been confirmed fully. There also are a few visceral afferent fibers, and their termination is likewise unknown. Taste fibers carry impulses from the anterior two-thirds of the tongue via the *chorda tympani* to the solitary tract and nucleus.

Somatic efferent fibers supply muscles derived from the hyoid arch and originate in the facial nucleus. The facial nucleus consists of a dorsal and ventral region. The dorsal region innervates muscles of the upper face, and the ventral region innervates muscles of the lower face. Impulses are carried from the cerebral cortex through the corticobulbar tract. Interestingly, the dorsal region of the facial nucleus receives bilateral cortical input, while the ventral region receives only contralateral input. The facial nucleus also receives fibers from the superior colliculus and ventral longitudinal bundle for optic reflexes, and it receives fibers from the inferior colliculus through the auditory reflex path. The facial nucleus also receives fibers indirectly from sensory nuclei of the brain stem.

Visceral efferent fibers arise from either the small cells of the facial nucleus or cells in the reticular formation, located dorsomedially to the facial nucleus, known as the *superior salivary nucleus*. These preganglionic fibers synapse at the submaxillary ganglion with postganglionic fibers that innervate the submaxillary and sublingual glands. Other preganglionic fibers travel by way of the great superficial petrosal nerve and the sphenopalatine ganglion.

The *acoustic nerve* (cranial nerve VIII) consists of the *cochlear nerve* and the *vestibular nerve*. The *cochlear nerve*, the nerve of hearing, terminates at the *cochlear nucleus*. The cochlear nucleus consists of a larger dorsal nucleus on the dorsolateral aspect of the inferior peduncle and a ventral nucleus more ventral to the inferior peduncle and medial geniculate body. Most of the axons

continue to ascend beneath the optic tract into the corona radiata and subsequently to the cortex of the superior temporal gyrus.

The *vestibular nerve* mediates the maintenance of bodily equilibrium. Once within the medulla oblongata, it bifurcates into ascending and descending branches. The descending branch terminates in the medial vestibular nucleus, the principal nucleus of the vestibular nerve. The ascending branch passes through the inferior cerebellar peduncle to the contralateral nucleus tecti.

The *glossopharyngeal nerve* (cranial nerve IX) contains somatic and sympathetic afferent, taste, somatic motor, and sympathetic efferent fibers. The afferent fibers arise from the superior ganglion and in the petrosal ganglion. There are few somatic afferent fibers that carry sensory impulses from the external ear, pharynx, and faucial arches. The visceral afferent fibers from the pharynx and middle ear assist with chewing and swallowing. Taste fibers from the tongue combine with fibers from the *nervus intermedius* and terminate in the solitary nucleus. Somatic efferent fibers originate in the nucleus ambiguus and innervate the stylopharyngeus muscle. Visceral efferent fibers originate in the nucleus dorsalis or the inferior salivary nucleus and synapse through the otic ganglion to their termination in the parotid gland.

The *vagus nerve* (cranial nerve X) contains somatic and visceral afferent and efferent fibers as well as taste fibers. There are few somatic afferent fibers that carry impulses from a small area of the skin on the back of the ear and posterior part of the external auditory meatus. The visceral afferent fibers carry impulses from the heart and pancreas, and probably the stomach, esophagus, and respiratory tract, to the *dorsal nucleus of the vagus* and glossopharyngeal nerves. The dorsal nucleus comes into relation with neurons that may carry impulses to the muscles of ventilation, for example, the phrenic nerve and the nerves to the intercostal and levatores costarum muscles. Taste fibers conduct impulses from the epiglottis and larynx through the vagus nerve and join the *solitary tract*, subsequently terminating in the *solitary nucleus*. The solitary nucleus connects with motor centers of the pons, medulla oblongata, and spinal cord to mediate mastication and swallowing. Somatic efferent fibers from the *nucleus ambiguus* innervate voluntary muscles of the pharynx and larynx and receive impulses from the opposite pyramidal tract. Visceral efferent fibers arise from the dorsal nucleus and synapse through sympathetic ganglia to fibers that facilitate the function of the esophagus, stomach, small intestine, gallbladder, and lungs; inhibit the function of the heart; and cause secretion within the stomach and pancreas.

The *accessory nerve* (cranial nerve XI) contains only somatic efferent fibers and consists of spinal and cranial portions. The spinal portion arises from lateral cells in the anterior column of the upper five or six segments of the cervical spinal cord and innervates the trapezius and sternocleidomastoid muscles. The cranial portion originates in the nucleus ambiguus. The fibers travel through the vagus nerve to the laryngeal nerves and supply the muscles of the larynx. The spinal portion receives impulses from the ipsilateral pyramidal tracts, while the cranial portion receives impulses from the opposite pyramidal tract and from the terminal sensory nuclei of the cranial nerves.

The *hypoglossal nerve* (cranial nerve XII) contains only somatic efferent fibers and innervates the muscles of the tongue. Its axons originate in the hypoglossal nucleus and exit the medulla oblongata at the anterolateral sulcus. The hypoglossal nuclei are connected by commissural fibers and dendrites of motor cells that connect the two nuclei. The hypoglossal nucleus receives impulses from the contralateral pyramidal tract.

Tracts (Figure 6-8): The brain stem is the "superhighway" among the cerebrum, cerebellum, and spinal cord. Motor impulses travel from the cerebral cortex to the extremities, while sensory impulses travel in the opposite direction. Motor and sensory signals also are relayed to and from cranial structures through bulbar pathways. Signals to the cerebellum modulate movement and tone. Impulses to and from the autonomic nervous system mediate the function of visceral structures. Overall, three major types of tracts provide the connections among all of these structures: motor, sensory, and extrapyramidal.

Corticospinal (pyramidal) tract: The *corticospinal* tract is also called the *pyramidal* tract because the bundle of corticospinal axons looks like two column-like structures ("pyramids") on the ventral surface of medulla oblongata. The corticospinal tract contains a massive number of motor axons that travel between the cerebral cortex of the brain and the spinal cord. The axons originate in the motor cortex and move closer together as they travel caudally through the cerebral white matter and form part of the posterior limb of the internal capsule. The fibers continue into the brain stem and remain uncrossed until they reach the spinomedullary junction. At this point, approximately 90% of the corticospinal fibers cross over to the contralateral side in the medulla oblongata (pyramidal decussation), forming the *lateral corticospinal tract* of the spinal cord. The remaining 10% of fibers remain ipsilateral, forming the *anterior corticospinal tract.* These fibers cross at the level that they exit the spinal cord, thereby combining with the lateral corticospinal tract axons at the ventral horn of a given spinal cord level to synapse with the second-order neuron. It is not difficult to understand why one side of the brain controls the opposite side of the body.

The *corticobulbar tract* is considered to be a pyramidal tract. The corticobulbar tract carries signals that control motor neurons located in cranial nerve brain nuclei. The neurons in the motor cortex send axons contralaterally to the cranial nuclei of the midbrain (corticomesencephalic tract), pons (corticopontine tract), and medulla oblongata (corticobulbar tract), and decussate when they reach each cranial nucleus.

Spinothalamic tract: The *spinothalamic tract* is a sensory pathway originating in the spinal cord. It transmits information about pain, temperature, itch, and crude touch to the thalamus. The pathway decussates at the spinomedullary junction, below the decussations of the posterior column-medial lemniscus pathway and corticospinal tract.

The cell bodies of neurons that comprise the spinothalamic tract originate primarily in the dorsal horn of the spinal cord. The axons of cells that mediate pain and temperature decussate through the anterior white commissure just above their level of entrance to the spinal cord and travel rostrally in the contralateral spinothalamic tract. The axons of cells that mediate proprioception and vibration travel in the ipsilateral dorsal columns to the nucleus gracilis and nucleus cuneatus within the medulla oblongata, at which time they decussate to the contralateral medial lemniscus. After they enter the brain stem, the sensory axons are positioned more dorsally and ultimately synapse with third-order neurons in the medial dorsal, ventral posterior lateral, and ventral medial posterior nuclei of the thalamus.

Cerebellar tracts (see also the Internal Structures of the Cerebellum subsection in Structures of the Cerebellum section below): The cerebellum is connected to the brain stem through three pathways known as *cerebellar peduncles.* The *superior cerebellar peduncle* connects the cerebellum to the pons and midbrain and contains the *dentatorubrothalamic* and *ventral spinocerebellar* tracts. The *middle cerebellar peduncle* contains contralateral pontocerebellar fibers. The *inferior cerebellar peduncle* connects the medulla oblongata to the cerebellum and contains the ipsilateral *dorsal spinocerebellar* tract.

The cerebellum receives significant input from and gives feedback to the cerebral hemispheres through the *corticopontocerebellar* and *cerebellothalamocortical* tracts. The corticopontocerebellar tracts arise from all lobes of the cerebral hemispheres, most notably the prefrontal area, sensorimotor cortex, and occipital lobes. First-order neurons travel caudally to the ipsilateral pons and synapse with second-order neurons that cross to the contralateral cerebellar hemisphere via the middle cerebellar peduncle. The *cerebellothalamocortical* tract

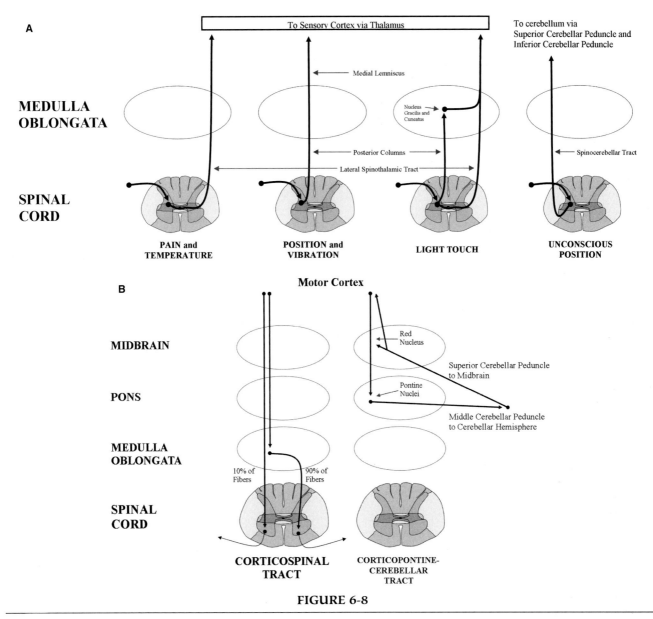

FIGURE 6-8

Schematic diagrams of the brain stem tracts. (A) Brain stem sensory tracts. (B) Brain stem motor tracts.

originates largely from the contralateral dentate nucleus and nucleus interpositus of the cerebellum. The fibers travel through the superior cerebellar peduncle into the contralateral ventral lateral nucleus of the thalamus. They synapse with fibers that ultimately terminate in the contralateral premotor and primary motor cortices (although some fibers may terminate ipsilaterally as well).

Vasculature of the Brain Stem

Vertebral artery: The main blood supply of the brain stem comes from the vertebral artery, the first branch of the subclavian artery (Figure 6-9). The vertebral artery ascends through the foramina in the transverse processes of the upper six cervical vertebrae, winds behind the superior articular process of the atlas, enters the skull through the foramen magnum, and unites at the inferior aspect of the pons with the opposite vertebral artery to form the basilar artery. Dissection of the vertebral artery may occur when sudden torque forces are applied to the vertebrae.

The branches of the vertebral artery are classified by those given off in the neck and those given off within the cranium. Spinal branches enter the vertebral canal through the intervertebral foramina, and each divides into two branches: one supplies the spinal cord and its

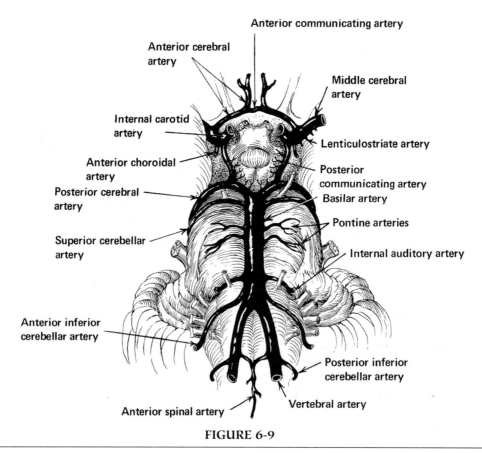

FIGURE 6-9

Vasculature of the brain stem and cerebellum. Reprinted with permission from Chusid, JG. *Correlative Neuroanatomy and Functional Neurology*. 17th ed. Los Altos, CA: Lange Medical Publications, 1979: 47.

membranes; the other divides into an ascending and a descending branch, which forms an anastomotic chain with arteries from above and below to supply the periosteum and bodies of the vertebrae. Muscular branches supply the deep muscles of the neck along with the occipital and deep cervical arteries. The meningeal branch originates opposite the foramen magnum and supplies the falx cerebelli. Medullary branches, known as *bulbar arteries*, are minute vessels that supply blood to the medulla oblongata.

The *posterior spinal arteries* arise at the level of the medulla oblongata and enter the vertebral canal through the intervertebral foramina. Branches from the posterior spinal arteries anastomose around the posterior roots of the spinal nerves and communicate with vessels from the opposite side. An ascending branch near the origin of each posterior spinal artery ends at the side of the fourth ventricle.

The *anterior spinal artery* arises near the union of the vertebral arteries, descends anteriorly to the medulla oblongata, and unites with the opposite artery at the level of the foramen magnum. The single trunk descends anterior to the spinal cord and is reinforced by many small branches which enter through intervertebral foramina

throughout the vertebral canal. The *posterior inferior cerebellar artery* (PICA) is the largest branch of the vertebral artery. In the brain stem, it supplies the medial and inferior vestibular nuclei, inferior cerebellar peduncle, nucleus ambiguus, intra-axial fibers of the glossopharyngeal and vagus nerves, and portions of the spinothalamic tract and spinal trigeminal nucleus and tract. Disruption of the PICA may cause Horner's syndrome since it also supplies a portion of the hypothalamospinal tract to the ciliospinal center of Budge at T1–T2.

Basilar Artery: The basilar artery is named because of its position at the base of the skull. It ascends from its union of the vertebral arteries in the inferior aspect of the pons to the superior border of the pons. At this level, it divides into the two posterior cerebral arteries.

The *pontine branches* come off at right angles from both sides of the basilar artery and supply the pons and adjacent parts of the brain.

The *internal auditory artery* arises near the middle of the artery and accompanies the acoustic nerve through the internal acoustic meatus, where it supplies blood to the internal ear.

The *anterior inferior cerebellar artery* (AICA) supplies the facial nucleus and intra-axial fibers, the spinal trigeminal nucleus and tract, vestibular nuclei, cochlear nuclei, intra-axial fibers of the acoustic nerve, spinothalamic tract, and inferior and middle cerebellar peduncles. In most people, the AICA gives rise to the labyrinthine artery. Disruption of the AICA also may cause Horner's syndrome since it supplies a portion of the hypothalamospinal tract.

The *superior cerebellar artery* (SCA) originates just below the division of the basilar artery. It supplies the rostral and lateral pons as well as the superior cerebellar peduncle and spinothalamic tract.

ANATOMY OF THE CEREBELLUM

The cerebellum comprises the largest part of the hindbrain (Figure 6-10). It is positioned posterior to the pons and medulla oblongata. The cerebellum is characterized by a laminar appearance, with deep, curved fissures that divide it into a number of layers or leaves. Between the central portion of the cerebellum and the brain stem is the cavity of the fourth ventricle. It is not convoluted like the cerebrum, but contains many sulci that vary in depth. The proportional size of the cerebellum to the cerebrum increases from approximately 1:20 in the infant to 1:8 in the adult.

The function of the cerebellum is the coordination of movement necessary in equilibration, locomotion, and prehension. The cerebellum processes impulses that mediate muscle and tendon sense, joint sense, and equilibratory disturbances. The exact functions of its different parts are still not well understood.

Structures of the Cerebellum

Lobes of the Cerebellum: The cerebellum has three sections, one median and two lateral, that are contiguous and similar in structure. The median section is the *vermis*, named for its ring-like bands that form ridges and furrows. The lateral sections are the *hemispheres*. The superior aspect of the vermis is subdivided from anterior to posterior into the *lingula*, the *lobulus centralis*, the *monticulus*, and the *folium vermis*. With the exception of the lingula, each division is contiguous with the corresponding portion of the hemispheres: the *alae*, the *quadrangular lobules*, and the *superior semilunar lobules*.

The inferior aspect of the cerebellum also is divided into the midline *inferior vermis* and the *hemispheres* on either side. The inferior vermis is subdivided from anterior to posterior into the *nodule*, the *uvula*, the *pyramid*, and the *tuber vermis*. The corresponding subdivisions of the hemispheres consist of the *flocculus*, the *tonsilla cerebelli*, the *biventral lobule*, and the *inferior semilunar lobule*, respectively.

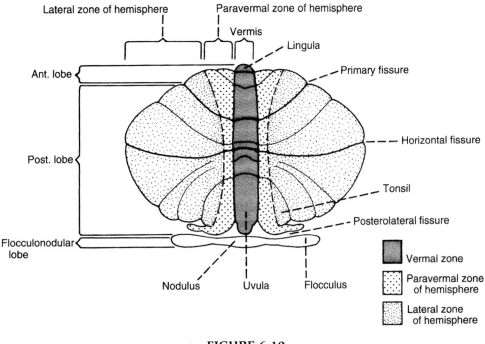

FIGURE 6-10

Schematic neuroanatomy of the cerebellum. Reprinted with permission from Fix, JD. *Neuroanatomy*. 3rd ed. Philadelphia, PA: Lippincott Williams and Wilkins, 2001: 232.

Internal structure of the cerebellum: The cerebellum consists of white and gray matter. In the sagittal plane, the interior consists of a gray mass, the *dentate nucleus*, that sits in the middle of a central stem of white matter. The white matter contains two sets of nerve fibers: the *projection fibers* and the *fibrae propriae*. The projection fibers consist of the three cerebellar peduncles (Figure 6-11,; see also Cerebellar Tracts subsection of the Brain Stem Tracts section above).

The *dentate nucleus* lies slightly medial to the center of the stem of white matter of the hemisphere. It consists of an irregularly folded grayish-yellow lamina that contains white matter. Most of the fibers of the superior peduncle emerge from the anteromedial aspect of the dentate nucleus, where an opening, the *hilus*, is found. It is responsible for the planning, initiation, and control of volitional movement.

The *superior cerebellar peduncles* are largely derived from cells of the dentate nucleus of the cerebellum. They travel rostrally beneath the corpora quadrigemina, decussate ventrally to the sylvian aqueduct, and divide into ascending and descending tracts. The ascending tract terminates in the red nucleus, thalamus, and oculomotor nucleus, while the descending tract appears to terminate in the dorsal aspect of the pons.

The *middle cerebellar peduncles* are comprised entirely of cells that originate in the contralateral pontine nuclei and terminate in the cerebellar cortex. The tracts have three fasciculi. The superior fasciculus distributes nerve fibers to the inferior lobules of the cerebellar hemisphere and to posterolateral margins of the superior surface. The inferior fasciculus distributes nerve fibers to the folia close to the inferior vermis. The deep fasciculus distributes nerve fibers to the upper anterior cerebellar folia and inferior cerebellar peduncles.

The *inferior cerebellar peduncles* consists of a variety of nerve fibers: (1) the *dorsal spinocerebellar tract* that terminates in the superior vermis; (2) the ipsilateral and contralateral nucleus gracilis and nucleus cuneatus; (3) the contralateral olivary nuclei; (4) the ipsilateral and contralateral medullary reticular formation; (5) the vestibular nucleus and tract that terminate partly in the contralateral roof nucleus; (6) contralateral cerebellobulbar tracts from the contralateral roof nucleus and dentate nucleus; and

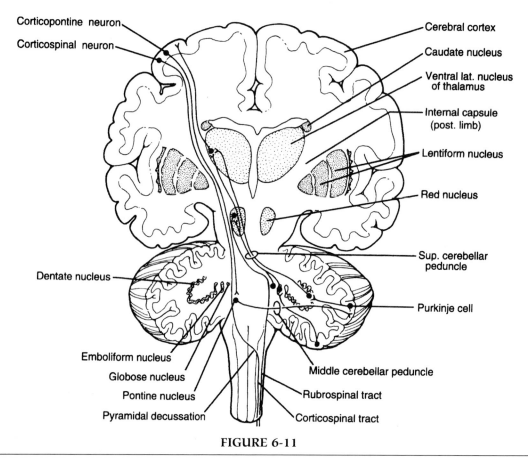

FIGURE 6-11

Connections to the cerebellum. Reprinted with permission from Fix, JD. *Neuroanatomy.* 3rd ed. Philadelphia, PA: Lippincott Williams and Wilkins, 2001: 236.

(7) some nerve fibers from the *ventral spinocerebellar tract* that combine with the dorsal spinocerebellar tract.

The *fibrae propriae* of the cerebellum are of two kinds: (1) *commissural* fibers, which connect the two halves of the cerebellum by a decussation at the anterior and posterior aspects of the vermis; and (2) *arcuate* or *association* fibers, which connect adjacent laminae.

Vasculature of the Cerebellum

The cerebellum receives its vascular supply from branches of the vertebral and basilar arteries (see Figure 6-9). When any of the arteries are disrupted, there is potential for collateral flow from the other cerebellar arteries. In patients with acute basilar artery thrombosis, the neurologic outcome improved after intra-arterial thrombolysis if the basilar artery demonstrated collateral filling and thrombosis of the basilar artery was not proximal (3). Patients with collateral filling of the basilar artery also tolerated their symptoms longer.

The *posterior inferior cerebellar artery* (PICA) traverses the superior portion of the medulla oblongata over the inferior peduncle to the undersurface of the cerebellum. Here it divides into two branches: medial and lateral. The medial branch continues posteriorly to the notch between the two hemispheres of the cerebellum. The lateral branch supplies the undersurface of the cerebellum to its lateral border, where it anastomoses with the anterior inferior cerebellar and superior cerebellar arteries.

The *anterior inferior cerebellar artery* (AICA) travels posteriorly to the anterior portion of the undersurface of the cerebellum. It anastomoses with the posterior inferior cerebellar artery.

The *superior cerebellar artery* (SCA) travels laterally around the cerebral peduncle to the upper surface of the cerebellum and dentate nucleus. It then divides into branches that supply the pia mater and anastomose with the anterior and posterior inferior cerebellar arteries.

MIDBRAIN SYNDROMES

The clinical anatomy of the midbrain is not as complicated as that of the pons or medulla oblongata (Figure 6-12). However, symptoms of midbrain lesions may be quite varied because of the multiplicity of functions for which the midbrain is responsible (Table 6-3). In addition to facial and limb sensory-motor deficits, cranial nerve III and IV lesions may cause oculomotor deficits and Horner's syndrome. Infarcts of the tegmentum may result in upgaze paralysis. Classic lacunar infarcts, such as pure motor stroke and ataxic hemiparesis, can be related to infarcts of the dorsolateral midbrain. Subthalamic infarcts may be associated with unilateral or bilateral ballismus or asterixis. Involvement of the red nucleus causes the

typical resting tremor worsened with movement. Coma or changes in consciousness may occur with bilateral midbrain infarcts, but neuropsychological changes should be suspected because of involvement of the posterior cerebral arteries downstream of the midbrain lesions (4).

Weber Syndrome

Marotte (1853) first described a patient who presented with a cranial nerve III palsy and contralateral hemiplegia. However, Weber (1863) provided the first detailed clinical description of this syndrome. He also attempted to relate the clinical signs and symptoms of the syndrome with vivisection of the human brain in order to answer the question of localization of the lesion. Of note, Weber described clonus of the ankle and flexor spasms of the leg but did not recognize its significance in cerebral infarction. In this article, he also accurately described the clinical findings of the Babinski sign nearly thirty years before Babinski reported the same.

Benedikt Syndrome

The lesion of Benedikt syndrome causes ipsilateral oculomotor paralysis with contralateral tremor and hemiparesis. Patients with this syndrome often have ipsilateral sensory loss. Because the major outflow of the cerebellum traverses the superior cerebellar peduncle (brachium conjunctivum) and red nucleus on its way to the ventral lateral nucleus of the thalamus, patients have a "rubral" tremor, present at rest but amplified with movement. Benedikt (1889) first described the syndrome in a cursory manner in 1874 but spoke of it in more detail during a lecture in Paris. He developed the concept of a primary motor system and coined the term "parallel motor system" for the afferent and efferent pathways of the cerebellum.

Parinaud Syndrome

The lesion of Parinaud syndrome causes paralysis of conjugate upward gaze and convergence. It is often accompanied by paralysis of conjugate downward gaze and pupillary areflexia. Parinaud (1883) concluded that the lesion should be located in the tegmentum of the midbrain. It was many years after his death in 1905 that the actual structure—the superior colliculi—and its connections were identified.

Koerber-Salus-Elschnig Syndrome

This lesion of the periaqueductal gray of the midbrain causes rhythmic retraction of the eyes into the orbit, independent of eye movement. Voluntary eye movements usually amplify the abnormality. Salus (1910) found a cysticercus cyst that localized the lesion very specifically

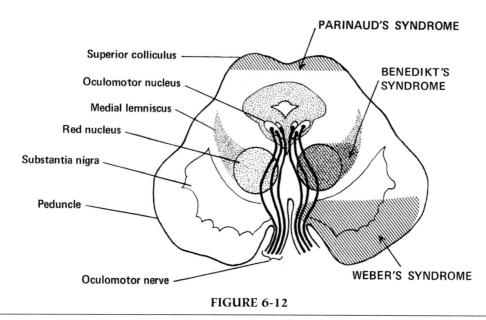

FIGURE 6-12

Midbrain syndromes. Reprinted with permission from Chusid, JG. *Correlative Neuroanatomy and Functional Neurology.* 17th ed. Los Altos, CA: Lange Medical Publications, 1979: 29.

to this region. While Koerber (1903) and Elschnig (1913) share the name of the syndrome, Koerber did not have any brain tissue for neuroanatomic correlation and termed the syndrome "nystagmus retractorius." Elschnig was Salus' teacher, encouraged him to write the case study, and found another case of the syndrome the following year.

PONTINE SYNDROMES

The pons is supplied by three groups of arteries (12). Branches from the basilar artery form the anteromedial and anterolateral groups. Branches from the AICA form the lateral group. Branches from the SCA form the posterior group.

Infarcts of the pons may result in a range of symptoms (Figure 6-13). Cranial nerve VI and medial longitudinal fasciculus lesions may cause oculomotor deficits. Infarcts of the paramedian pontine reticular formation may result in conjugate horizontal gaze paralysis. Classic lacunar infarcts, such as pure motor stroke and ataxic hemiparesis, can be related to infarcts of the basis pontis. Involuntary limb spasm also has been described (13).

Pontine syndromes are classified in two manners. Table 6-4 uses an anatomic scheme, categorizing lesions as superior, midpontine, and inferior; and as medial or lateral. Medial pontine lesions usually affect the corticospinal tract and medial lemniscus, resulting in contralateral hemiparesis and proprioception and vibration. Lateral pontine lesions usually affect the trigeminal sensory nucleus or tract, autonomic fibers, and spinothalamic tract, resulting in ipsilateral loss of facial sensation, ipsilateral Horner's syndrome, and contralateral loss of

pain and temperature. Table 6-5 lists pontine syndromes by eponym.

Millard-Gubler Syndrome

The Millard-Gubler syndrome affects cranial nerve VII and the corticospinal tract, resulting in ipsilateral facial weakness and contralateral hemiparesis. Gubler (1856) described the lesion as invading the medial pons but missing cranial nerve VI because of its slightly anterior course within the pons. He also demonstrated clinical evidence of the decussation of the facial nerve, thereby differentiating between the "central" lower facial droop and the "peripheral" total facial weakness. In contrast, Millard (1856) made no attempt to localize the anatomy of the lesion. His name is attached to Gubler's probably because the manuscripts were published one after the other.

Foville Syndrome

The Foville syndrome consists of conjugate horizontal gaze paralysis in the ipsilateral direction. Cranial nerve VII paralysis results in ipsilateral facial weakness but hemiparesis is contralateral. Foville (1858) is the first to document the presence of a lateral gaze center in the pons. While the hemiparesis usually resolves, the gaze paralysis and facial weakness persist indefinitely.

Raymond Syndrome

The Raymond syndrome consists of ipsilateral cranial nerve VI paralysis with contralateral hemiparesis.

TABLE 6-3
Midbrain Syndromes

SYNDROME	STRUCTURE	SYMPTOM(S)
Weber	III	ipsilateral ptosis, external strabismus, dilated pupil
	corticospinal/corticobulbar tracts	contralateral paresis of lower face, tongue, arm, leg
Benedikt	III	ipsilateral ptosis, external strabismus, dilated pupil
	red nucleus	contralateral coordination deficit (ataxia, dysmetria, dysdiadochokinesia, rubral tremor [coarse resting tremor that increases with movement], psuedo-Parkinson tremor
	corticospinal tract	contralateral paresis of lower face, tongue, arm, leg
	medial lemniscus (sometimes) spinothalamic tract (sometimes)	contralateral touch, proprioception (contralateral pain, temperature)
Claude	III	ipsilateral ptosis, external strabismus, dilated pupil
	red nucleus	contralateral coordination deficit (ataxia, dysmetria, dysdiadochokinesia, rubral tremor [coarse resting tremor that increases with movement], psuedo-Parkinson tremor
Parinaud (dorsal rostral midbrain)	pretectal nuclei (high midbrain tegmentum ventral to superior colliculus)	bilateral upward gaze paralysis
	corticotectal fibers (supranuclear fibers to III)	convergence paralysis, pupillary areflexia
Koerber-Salus-Elschnig (Sylvian aqueduct)	III	ipsilateral ptosis, external strabismus, dilated pupil altered mental status abnormal respiration
Chiray-Foix-Nicolesco (midbrain tegmentum)	upper red nucleus	contralateral coordination deficit (ataxia, dysmetria, dysdiadochokinesia, rubral tremor [coarse resting tremor that increases with movement], psuedo-Parkinson tremor
	corticospinal/corticobulbar tracts	contralateral paresis of lower face, tongue, arm, leg
	spinothalamic tract	contralateral hemisensory deficit
Nothnagel (dorsal midbrain)	III	ipsilateral ptosis, external strabismus, dilated pupil
	brachium conjunctivum	vertical gaze paralysis
	medial longitudinal fasciculus	ipsilateral adduction paresis on attempted horizontal gaze, contralateral monocular nystagmus of abducting eye on attempted horizontal gaze
Akinetic mutism (upper segment of basilar artery)	reticular activating system	absolute mutism tetraplegia with bulbar paralysis except for eyes

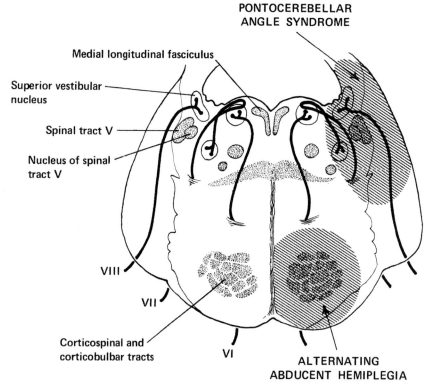

PONTOCEREBELLAR
ANGLE SYNDROME

Medial longitudinal fasciculus

Superior vestibular
nucleus

Spinal tract V

Nucleus of spinal
tract V

VIII

VII

Corticospinal and
corticobulbar tracts

VI

ALTERNATING
ABDUCENT HEMIPLEGIA

FIGURE 6-13

Pontine syndromes. Reprinted with permission from Chusid, JG. *Correlative Neuroanatomy and Functional Neurology.* 17th ed. Los Altos, CA: Lange Medical Publications, 1979: 30.

Raymond (1896) described a patient with right hemiplegia but with aphasia and difficulty recognizing her husband's face (prosopagnosia) (17). The cranial nerve VI paralysis did not occur for another three months. He described this condition as a "special hemiplegia" that was treated with "mercurial packs and high doses of potassium iodide" for "intensive antisyphilitic treatment." With this treatment, the visual disturbances and cognitive impairments resolved, but the hemiplegia resolved only partially.

Locked-in Syndrome

The locked-in syndrome occurs when an occlusion of the basilar artery causes an infarction of the basis pontis bilaterally. The corticospinal and corticobulbar tracts are interrupted, resulting in tetraplegia and paralysis of all cranial nerve muscles except for those controlling eye movements. It is not unusual for the paramedian pontine reticular formation to be affected, such that horizontal eye movements are affected and only vertical eye movements are possible. Since the reticular formation above the caudal pons is spared, patients remain awake and aware. Their only means of communication is systematic eye movements, which can be utilized manually to

respond to questions, or with augmentative communication devices.

MEDULLARY SYNDROMES

The medulla oblongata receives its blood supply from a number of penetrating arteries located in the distal vertebral artery (see Table 6-6 for list medullary symptoms). There also may be variable blood supplies from small branches of the PICA, AICA, or the basilar artery. Typically, a lateral medullary infarct occurs because of occlusion of one or more of these penetrating arteries or more often by occlusion of the vertebral artery (18). The dorsal medulla oblongata receives its blood supply exclusively from the PICA and is usually accompanied by cerebellar infarction (19). The medial medulla oblongata receives its blood supply caudally from penetrating arteries of the anterior spinal artery and rostrally from branches of the vertebral artery (20). Medial infarcts usually affect the corticospinal tracts, causing contralateral hemiparesis. Lateral infarcts usually involve the spinothalamic tracts, resulting in contralateral loss of pain and temperature. Other infarcts may occur as well, but are less common (Figure 6-14).

TABLE 6-4
Pontine Syndromes by Location

SYNDROME	STRUCTURE	SYMPTOM(S)
Medial inferior	VI	ipsilateral horizontal diplopia with nystagmus
	corticospinal tract	contralateral face/arm/leg hemiplegia
	medial lemniscus	contralateral touch/proprioception hemideficit
	paramedian pontine reticular formation	ipsilateral conjugate gaze paralysis
Lateral inferior	vestibular nuclei (VIII)	ipsilateral horizontal/vertical nystagmus, vertigo, nausea, vomiting, oscillopsia
	VII	ipsilateral peripheral facial palsy
	paramedian pontine reticular formation	ipsilateral conjugate gaze paralysis
	VIII	tinnitus, deafness
	middle cerebellar peduncle	ataxia
	V sensory	ipsilateral impaired facial sensation
	spinothalamic tract	contralateral arm/leg pain/temperature deficit
Medial midpontine	middle cerebellar peduncle	ipsilateral ataxia arm/leg and gait
	corticospinal/corticobulbar tracts	contralateral face/arm/leg hemiplegia, eye deviation
	variable medial meniscus	contralateral touch/proprioception deficit
Lateral midpontine	middle cerebral peduncle	ipsilateral limb ataxia
	V motor	ipsilateral mastication muscle paralysis
	V sensory	ipsilateral hemisensory deficit (including corneal reflex)
Medial superior	superior/middle cerebellar peduncle	ipsilateral cerebellar ataxia
	medial longitudinal fasciculus	internuclear ophthalmoplegia
	central tegmental bundle	palate/pharynx/vocal cord/ventilatory apparatus/face/oculomotor apparatus myoclonus
	corticospinal/corticobulbar tracts	contralateral face/arm/leg hemiplegia
	rare medial lemniscus	contralateral touch/proprioception face/arm/leg hemideficit
Lateral superior	superior/middle cerebellar peduncle	ipsilateral arm/leg/gait ataxia
	vestibular nuclei (VIII)	dizziness, nausea, vomiting, horizontal nystagmus
	spinothalamic tract	contralateral face/arm/leg pain/temperature loss
	lateral medial lemniscus	touch/proprioception leg>arm hemideficit
	unknown	conjugate gaze paresis to side of lesion, loss of optokinetic nystagmus, skew deviation, Horner syndrome

Wallenberg (Lateral Medullary) Syndrome

The Wallenberg syndrome probably is one of the best known brain stem syndromes, comprising approximately 2% of all admissions for acute stroke (21). Wallenberg (1895) described this "acute disease of the medulla" with the onset of intense vertigo associated with vomiting. He also listed the presence of dysphonia and dyphagia; ipsilateral facial hemisensory deficit, limb ataxia, and palate and vocal cord paralysis; and contralateral arm and leg hemisensory deficit. Although an ipsilateral Horner's syndrome is present, Wallenberg did not document its presence because his patient had a congenital disease of the eyes. Because of its lateral location, the syndrome does not cause paralysis since the corticospinal tract is a medial structure.

Jackson Syndrome

The Jackson syndrome consists of cranial nerve X, spinal XI, and XII paralysis resulting in ipsilateral weakness

TABLE 6-5
Pontine Syndromes by Eponym

SYNDROME	STRUCTURE	SYMPTOM(S)
Millard-Gubler	VII tract	ipsilateral facial palsy
	corticospinal tract	contralateral arm/leg hemiparesis
Foville	paramedian pontine reticular formation	ipsilateral horizontal gaze palsy
	VII	ipsilateral facial palsy
	corticospinal tract	contralateral arm/leg hemiparesis
Raymond	VI tract	ipsilateral lateral rectus paresis
	corticospinal tract	contralateral arm/leg hemiparesis
Pontocerebellar angle	VIII	early ipsilateral tinnitus, deafness, head tilt/rotation; late hyperacusis
	inferior/middle cerebellar peduncles	ipsilateral intention tremor, dysmetria, ataxic gait, adiadochokinesis
	V spinal tract	ipsilateral facial pain/temperature hemisensory deficit
	VII	ipsilateral facial palsy, taste loss anterior 2/3 tongue
	spinothalamic tract	contralateral arm/leg pain/temperature hemisensory deficit
	occasional XI, XII	ipsilateral trapezius, tongue
Brissaud	VII	ipsilateral facial spasm
	corticospinal tract	contralateral arm/leg hemiparesis
One-and-a-half	paramedian pontine reticular formation	ipsilateral horizontal gaze palsy
	medial longitudinal fasciculus	contralateral internuclear ophthalmoplegia
Locked-in	Bilateral corticospinal/corticobulbar tract	Tetraplegia with facial palsy (except blinking eyes)
	Bilateral paramedian pontine reticular formation	Bilateral horizontal gaze palsy

of the trapezius, sternocleidomastoid, soft palate, and tongue, as well as dysphagia and dysphonia. Jackson (1865) described this syndrome in a patient with tuberculosis throughout the brain stem. The correlative neuroanatomy is not well described, but the eponym remains attributed to him.

CEREBELLAR SYNDROMES

Cerebellar infarcts typically present with the cardinal signs of vertigo, headache, emesis, and gait ataxia (24). However, it was not until the advent of magnetic resonance imaging (MRI) that clinicians could accurately diagnose cerebellar infarcts and correlate them with vascular territories. There is now a better understanding of how to characterize cerebellar infarcts based upon the vascular territories they supply. Table 6-7 reflects one of these classification schemas (25).

RESEARCH FRONTIERS

As the descriptions of the syndromes above demonstrate, the understanding of brain stem and cerebellar syndromes largely came from the vivisection of autopsy specimens. With the advent of MRI, the neuroanatomy of these lesions could be defined better and earlier (26). Techniques such as functional MRI have provided vital information in better understanding the functional anatomy of the auditory system (27), visual system (28), and the cerebellum (29). Diffusion-weighted images (DWIs) with direction-selective gradients have been used to identify both nuclei and white matter tracts within the brain stem (30). Newer high-resolution MRI technology may lead to spatially unbiased localization of lesions, that is, the location of structures on an MRI image equals the expected anatomic location of that structure (31). Diffusion tensor imaging (DTI) currently is the only method available to non-invasively study the three-dimensional structure of

subjects receiving electrical stimulation over the cerebellum to hand movement performance. In better understanding the neuroanatomical correlates of behavior and activity, clinicians more accurately can predict the types of deficits that occur with brain stem and cerebellar strokes. Using this information, more research needs to explore physical and pharmacological interventions that can improve recovery from stroke. Ultimately, clinicians can gain a better understanding of functional outcomes when specific infarcts or hemorrhages occur in these regions.

CONCLUSION

Recognition of signs and symptoms of infratenorial stroke syndromes is essential in the diagnosis and treatment of stroke. Infratentorial strokes affect a wide variety of body systems, and knowledge of combinations of neurologic signs is vital if one is to suspect the presence of a brain stem or cerebellar infarct or hemorrhage. While imaging modalities have vastly improved our ability to visualize previously unvisualizable lesions, the diagnosis of a stroke still begins with a detailed physical examination and knowledge of neuroanatomic correlates. However, more research is needed to better understand the interactions between nuclei and tracts that form the foundation of activity and behavior. With a more detailed knowledge base, clinicians may be able to more effectively diagnose and treat infratenorial strokes with appropriate physical and pharmacological modalities. With more effective and varied treatments, clinicians may be able to improve functional outcomes and quality of life in the future.

References

1. Fix JD. Chapter 4. Development of the nervous system. In: Fix JD. *BRS Neuroanatomy*, 4th ed. Philadelphia, PA: Lippincott Williams and Wilkins, 2007, pp. 59–79.
2. Martin JH. Chapter 3. Development of the nervous system. In: Martin JH. *Neuroanatomy: Text and Atlas.* New York: McGraw Hill, 2003: 69.
3. Cross DT, Moran CJ, Akins PT, et al. Collateral circulation and outcome after basilar artery thrombolysis. *Am J Neuroradiol* 1998; 19:1557–1563.
4. Hommel M, Besson G. Chapter 39. Midbrain Infarcts. In: Bogousslavsky J, Caplan L, eds. *Stroke Syndromes*. 2nd ed. Cambridge, UK: Cambridge University Press, 2001, pp. 512–519.
5. Marotte M. Observation de ramollissement du pédoncle cérébral gauche, avec lésion du nerf oculaire commun. *Union Médicale* 1853; 7:407–408.
6. Weber H. A contribution to the pathology of the crura cerebri. *Medico-Chirurgical Transactions of the Royal Medical and Chirurgical Society* 1863; 46 (Second Series 28):121–139.
7. Benedikt M. Tremor with crossed oculomotor paralysis. *Le bulletin medical* 1889; 3:547–548.
8. Parinaud H. Paralysis of conjugate eye movement. *Archives de neurologie* 1883; 5:145–172.
9. Salus R. Acquired retraction movements of the globe. *Archiv für Augenheilkunde* 1910; 68:61–76.
10. Koerber H. Über drei Fälle von Retraktionsbewegung des Bulbus (Nystagmus retractorius). *Die ophthalmogische Klinik* 1903; 7:65–67.
11. Elschnig A. Nystagmus retractorius, ein cerebrales Herdsymptom. *Medizinische Klinik* 1913; 9: 8–11.
12. Tatu L, Moulin T, Bogousslavsky J, Duvernoy H. Arterial territories of human brain: brain stem and cerebellum. *Neurology* 1996; 47:1125–1135.
13. Kaufman DK, Brown RD, Karnes WE. Involuntary tonic spasms of a limb due to a brain stem lacunar infarction. *Stroke* 1994; 25:217–219.
14. Gubler A. Alternating hemiplegia, a sign of pontine lesion, and documentation of the proof of the facial decussation. *Gazette hebdomadaire de médecine et chirugie* 1856; 3:749–754, 789–792, 811–816.
15. Millard A. Correspondence. *Gazette hebdomadaire de médecine et chirugie* 1856; 3:816–818.
16. Foville AL. Note on a little-known paralysis of the eye muscles, and its relation to the anatomy and physiology of the pons. *Bulletin de la societé anatomique de Paris* 1858; 33:373–405.
17. Raymond F. Concerning a special type of alternating hemiplegia. *Leçons sur les maladies nerveux 1894–1895. Première série.* Paris: Ricklin and Souques, 1896:365–383.
18. Fisher CM, Karnes WE, Kubik CS. Lateral medullary infarction—the pattern of vascular occlusion. *J Neuropath Exp Neurol* 1961; 20:323–379.
19. Escourolle R, Hauw J-J, Der Agopian P, Trelles L. Les infarctes bulbaires. Etude des lésions vasculaires dans 26 observations. *J Neurol Sci* 1976; 28:103–113.
20. Bassetti C, Bogousslavsky J, H Mattle H, Bernasconi A. Medial medullary stroke: report of seven patients and review of the literature. *Neurology* 1997; 48(4):882–890.
21. Norrving B, Cronqvist S. Lateral medullary infarction: prognosis in an unselected series. *Neurology* 1991; 41:244–248.
22. Wallenberg A. Acute disease of the medulla (Embolus to the posterior inferior cerebellar artery?). *Archiv für Psychiatrie* 1895; 24:509–540.
23. Jackson JH. Lecture on hemiplegia. *Clinical Lectures and Reports by the Medical and Surgical Staff of The London Hospital* 1865; 2:297–300, 313–315.
24. Lerich J, Winkler G, Ojemann R. Cerebellar infarction with brain stem compression: diagnosis and surgical treatment. *Arch Neurol* 1970; 22:490–498.
25. Aramenco P, Lévy C, Cohen A, et al. Causes and mechanisms of territorial and nonterritorial cerebellar infarcts in 115 consecutive cases. *Stroke* 1994; 25:105–112.
26. Mäurer J, Mitrovic T, Knollmann FD, et al. In vitro delineation of human brain-stem anatomy using a small resonator: correlation with macroscopic and histological findings. *Neuroradiol* 1996; 38(3):217–220.
27. Lockwood AH, Salvi RJ, Coad ML, et al. The functional anatomy of the normal human auditory system: responses to 0.5 and 4.0 kHz tones at varied intensities. *Cerebral Cortex* 1999; 9(1):65–76.
28. Greenlee MW, Tse PU. *Functional Neuroanatomy of the Human Visual System: A Review of Functional MRI Studies.* Berlin, Germany: Springer Berlin Heidelberg, 2008.
29. Grodd W, Hülsmann E, Ackermann H. Functional MRI localizing in the cerebellum. *Neurosurg Clin N Am* 2005; 16(1):77–99.
30. Fitzek C, Weissmann M, Speckter H, et al. Anatomy of brain-stem white-matter tracts shown by diffusion-weighted imaging. *Neuroradiol* 2001; 43(11):953–960.
31. Diedrichsen J. A spatially unbiased atlas template of the human cerebellum. *Neuroimage* 2006; 33(1):127–138.
32. Nagae-Poetscher LM, Jiang H, Wakana S, et al. High-resolution diffusion tensor imaging of the brain stem at 3 T. *Am J Neuroradiol* 2004; 25:325–1330.
33. Cheng P, Magnotta VA, Wu D, et al. Evaluation of the GTRACT diffusion tensor tractography algorithm: a validation and reliability study. *NeuroImage* 2006; 31(3):1075–1085.

II

NEUROPHYSIOLOGY OF STROKE RECOVERY

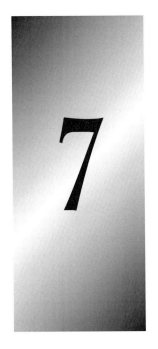

7 The Mechanisms and Neurophysiology of Recovery from Stroke

Randolph J. Nudo

More than two decades have passed since the groundbreaking studies of Michael Merzenich, Jon Kaas, and others, who demonstrated that the neural representations of the hand in the somatosensory cortex are altered by peripheral injury. A once-tenuous notion that functions of the cerebral cortex are alterable in adult mammals has developed into a neuroscientific tenet. The phenomenology of cortical plasticity and the study of its underlying mechanisms have rapidly migrated from the laboratory to the clinic, as new interventional strategies are now conceptualized in relation to their ability to encourage adaptive plasticity.

After injury to the cerebral cortex, as often occurs in stroke, a large portion of the sensory-motor apparatus in the frontal and parietal cortex can be damaged, resulting in deficits in motor function in the contralateral musculature. However, substantial spontaneous recovery occurs in the weeks to months following injury. Understanding how the remaining sensory-motor apparatus can support the recovery of such functions has been a primary goal of much of the recent research in this area. Thus, this chapter will review the basic organization of sensorimotor cortex, the current theoretical models for functional recovery, and our understanding of the ability of spared tissue to be functionally and structurally altered. This review relies most heavily on recent neurophysiological and neuroanatomical data from non-human primate and rodent models, and neuroimaging studies in humans.

ORGANIZATION OF MOTOR CORTEX IN PRIMATES

Since middle cerebral artery strokes often affect the motor cortex, we provide a brief review of the structure and function of cortical areas involved in motor control of skeletal musculature. Motor cortex, defined as the part of the cerebral cortex that requires the least amount of electrical stimulation to evoke movement, is subdivided into several distinct areas (Figure 7-1).

Though each area has been reported to play a somewhat different role in the control of movement, there is considerable overlap in function (1, 2). Further, it is now clear that the motor cortex does not execute motor tasks in isolation. A broad network minimally involving the primary and secondary motor areas, the dorsolateral prefrontal cortex, the posterior parietal cortex, the striatum, and the cerebellum is involved in motor skill acquisition, planning, and execution. Thus, motor behavior is controlled by a distributed network, and it may be overly simplistic to think in terms of compartmentalized units that have mutually exclusive functions (3).

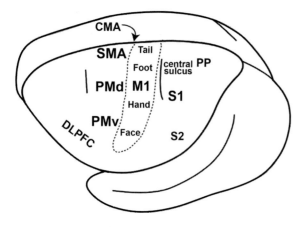

FIGURE 7-1

Motor areas in the frontal cortex of a non-human primate (squirrel monkey). At least 5 separate motor areas can be identified. These include M1, SMA, PMd, PMv, and CMA. This basic arrangement is similar in all primates, though these areas have been divided further in some species. Also, in some primates, the sulci are much deeper (e.g., humans, macaques), and thus, these motor areas are not as accessible. Each motor area contains a separate representation of the forelimb, and some areas contain a complete representation of the skeletal motor apparatus. It has been suggested that each of these motor areas plays a somewhat different role in motor control; though considerable overlap exists. Thus, it is more accurate to consider the cortical motor apparatus as part of a distributed network for control of movement. M1: primary motor cortex; S1: primary somatosensory cortex; PMd: dorsal premotor cortex; PMv: ventral premotor cortex; SMA: supplementary motor area; CMA: cingulate motor areas; DLPFC: dorsolateral prefrontal cortex; PP: posterior parietal cortex; S2: second somatosensory area.

Primary Motor Cortex

The primary motor cortex (M1) is thought to mediate skilled voluntary movements, especially of the distal musculature, since M1 lesions result in disruption of skilled limb use in the contralateral musculature (4–7). The global topography of motor representations in M1 follows an orderly progression from hindlimb medially to forelimb and face laterally (Figure 7-1). M1 is subdivided into a caudal component ($M1_c$), receiving predominantly cutaneous somatosensory information, and a rostral component ($M1_r$), receiving predominantly proprioceptive input (8, 9). Consistent with this parcellation, in non-human primates, differential motor deficits result from small lesions in either $M1_r$ or $M1_c$ (10). Cortical areas that are reciprocally connected with M1 include primary somatosensory areas 3a, 1, 2, the second somatosensory area (S2), the ventral premotor cortex (PMv), the dorsal premotor cortex (PMd), the supplementary motor area

(SMA), cingulate motor areas (CMA), and, to a lesser extent, primary somatosensory area 3b, posterior parietal cortex (PP), and the ventral parietal area PV (11–14).

The corticospinal (CS) neurons provide the cerebral cortex with direct access to spinal cord motoneurons and have been the subject of intense investigation since the mid-1800s. Corticospinal neurons can be found throughout much of frontal and parietal cortex, though the concentration is greatest in M1 (15). A subset of CS neurons, found predominantly in M1, project monosynaptically to motoneurons of the spinal cord, and are thus called corticomotoneuronal (CM) cells. Spike-triggered averaging techniques in awake primates reveal that individual corticomotoneuronal cells can facilitate up to four or five motoneuron pools (16). This provides further evidence of the divergence in the anatomical projections from cortex to spinal cord and challenges the notion that functional organization in motor cortex was based on muscle-specific domains. Direct evidence refuting muscle-specific domains in motor cortex was provided recently with neuronanatomical evidence. Rabies viruses can be used as transneuronal retrograde markers. Injecting the virus into a single muscle results in retrograde transport of the virus to the cell bodies in the spinal cord motoneuron pool. There, the virus replicates and is picked up by terminal arbors that innervate the motoneurons. In turn, the virus is retrogradely transported back to second order neurons in the cerebral cortex, red nucleus, and other locations. At the appropriate survival time, post-mortem analysis reveals the location of corticospinal neurons that contain the virus. Thus, these neurons represent corticomotoneuronal cells that project to the specific motoneuron pool of interest. Combining results of injections into various forelimb muscles of different animals reveals that the cortical neurons that influence the various forelimb muscles are completely interspersed and overlapping (17). Thus, the motor cortex can be viewed as containing a shared neural substrate for motor control of the hand. The highly overlapping and divergent architecture provides an ideal substrate for flexibility in outputs to the spinal cord that can be rearranged based on behavioral demands.

One of the more common methods for demonstrating the functional spatial topography of M1 is via electrical or magnetic stimulation and the observation of evoked movements or electromyographic activity. Current thresholds for evoking movement via either invasive or non-invasive stimulation methods are lowest in M1, coinciding with the location of large numbers of CM cells. Due to these neuroanatomical and neurophysiological differences, M1 is thought to be the cortical motor area most related to movement execution. However, discrete movements of specific joints can also be evoked by stimulation of other motor areas of the frontal cortex, though at somewhat higher current levels. At least seven non-primary motor areas involved in controlling arm movements have been identified in frontal cortex of primates (18). Many of these premotor areas have also been identified in humans based on functional neuroimaging data, though homologies are in some instances not completely clear (14, 15, 19–21).

Dorsal Premotor Cortex

The premotor areas are located anterior to the M1 motor strip in Brodmann's area 6. Based on separate hand representations, different anatomical connectivity, and somewhat different functional attributes, the premotor cortex has been subdivided into a dorsal portion, or dorsal premotor cortex (PMd), and a ventral portion, or ventral premotor cortex (PMv). PMd is located immediately anterior to the M1 representation. The histologically-defined boundary between M1 and PMd is not well defined. For example, using the density of large CS neurons as a guide to the identification of the M1-PMd border yields a gradient, rather than a sharp boundary, with more large CS neurons located in M1. PMd contains a separate representation of the forelimb, hindlimb, and trunk, and is thought to be involved in visually guided tasks since PMd neurons are active during a preparatory motor-set (22) and in relation to visuomotor-association tasks (23). Compared with M1, activity of PMd neurons (and PMv, SMA neurons) is less related to the kinematics of the movement, but more related to aspects of the goal (24) and to movement selection (25). PMd inactivation affects the ability of macaque monkeys to select movements without affecting the spatial organization of the movements selected (26). Neuroimaging studies in humans confirm the role of PMd in visually guided motor tasks (27). Similar to PMv, the PMd hand area has topographically organized, intracortical connections with other frontal motor regions (11, 28, 29) and with the posterior parietal cortex.

Ventral Premotor Cortex

In non-human primates, the ventral premotor cortex (PMv) is located anterior and lateral to the M1 hand representation. In primate species with lissencephalic brains (e.g., prosimian primates, squirrel monkeys, marmoset monkeys) PMv is exposed on a flat sector of cortex, whereas in other primate species (e.g., macaque monkeys, Cebus monkeys) PMv is largely buried in the arcuate sulcus. In general, PMv is thought to be involved in visual- and somatosensory-motor integration for motor control of the upper extremity (30–37). PMv provides prominent inputs to M1, exerting a powerful facilitatory effect, especially during visually guided movements of the hand (38, 39). PMv also has reciprocal, topographically organized connections with other motor areas of the frontal cortex (M1, SMA, PMd, CMA) (11, 19, 28, 29) and with the parietal cortex, much like PMd. However, there are substantial differences between PMd and PMv

in their connections with the parietal cortex. PMd is not strongly connected with somatosensory areas of the anterior parietal lobe but, rather, with medial parietal areas that are more related to visual and visuomotor function (29, 30, 40–42). Most of the parietal inputs to PMv (15% of all inputs) (11) arise from more lateral areas, such as the second somatosensory area (S2) and the parietal ventral area (PV). Relatively few inputs (1.5%) arise from the more medial PP areas that are thought to be most involved in visually guided motor behaviors (11, 43). Human neuroimaging studies have shown somatotopic maps of face and fingers in PMv (44). In addition, activation is increased in PMv of humans during a working memory task requiring a vibrotactile discrimination (45). Thus, while PMv appears to receive polymodal information, its primary inputs are from parietal somatosensory areas. Inactivation of PMv in macaque monkeys has little effect on the ability to reach out and grasp food morsels (37), in contrast to M1 inactivation (6).

Supplementary Motor Area

The supplementary motor area (SMA), sometimes called M2, is located in the medial aspect of Brodmann's area 6, largely extending onto the medial wall. Evidence from neuroanatomical and neurophysiological studies in monkeys and from neuroimaging studies in humans suggest a direct (though not exclusive) involvement of SMA in motor planning, especially in motor sequences and in bimanual motor control (46–48). Like other cortical motor areas, movements of the skeletal musculature can be evoked by stimulation of SMA, and constituent neurons project directly to the spinal cord (15, 49, 50). Several human neuroimaging studies and monkey neurophysiological studies have implicated SMA in movement planning, especially of learned movement sequences (48, 51, 52). Lesions of SMA in macaque monkeys result in deficits in bimanual coordination (53) and in mild impairment in errors made during motor sequence tasks (54). SMA shares connections with PMd, PMv, M1, CMA, areas rostral to SMA, and PP cortex medial to the intraparietal sulcus (41, 55–59). Thus, SMA connections are similar to PMd connections, in that parietal connections are primarily with more medial areas. One exception is that connections between SMA and S2 have been reported in some primate species (55, 56).

Two SMA representations can be differentiated in primate species based on distinct cytoarchitecture, intracortical microstimulation neuronal response properties, and connection patterns. These two areas, located on the medial surface of the cerebral hemispheres, are referred to as SMA-proper (or simply SMA; also called F3) and the pre-SMA (also called F6), situated more rostrally (60). In general, SMA proper is thought to be involved primarily in simple tasks, while pre-SMA is activated during relatively complex tasks (2). SMA and pre-SMA can also be differentiated in human neuroimaging studies; though until recently, reliable distinctions among the motor areas of the medial wall (SMA, pre-SMA, and cingulate motor areas) were rarely possible. New approaches using diffusion tensor imaging may provide significant improvements in differentiating these areas (61).

Differential Processing Streams Between Parietal and Premotor Cortex

To summarize, PMv, PMd, and SMA are strongly connected to parietal areas, though they receive differential input from separate sensorimotor processing streams (Figure 7-2) (32, 42). PMv is strongly interconnected with unimodal somatosensory areas of the anterior parietal lobe and with visual and polymodal areas in the lateral portions of parietal cortex (7b, not shown). In contrast, PMd and SMA receive input primarily from visual and polymodal PP areas medial to the IP sulcus. Thus, except for the possible exception of S2 projections to both PMv and SMA, these premotor areas, PMv, and PMd/SMA appear to be involved in different aspects of motor control of the hand.

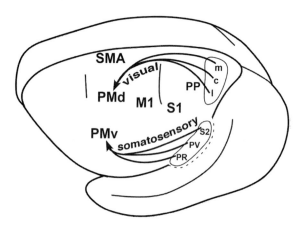

FIGURE 7-2

Sensory streams between parietal cortex and premotor areas of the frontal cortex. Recent tract-tracing results have revealed two distinct processing streams from parietal to premotor areas (11, 29). PMv receives substantial inputs from somatosensory fields PR, PV, and S2, conveying cutaneous and proprioceptive information relayed from S1. In contrast, PMd and SMA receive substantial input from PP cortex (PPm, PPc, PPl), conveying visual and polymodal information. These PP areas are probably homologous to areas 5, 7a, 7ip, 7m, and possibly areas MIP and PO of macaques (29). Thus, it appears that PMv and PMd/SMA process different sets of sensorimotor information and, thus, may have separate roles in motor control of the hand. Not shown in the figure are SMA connections with S2.

Cingulate Motor Areas

At least three cingulate motor areas—CMAd, CMAv, and CMAr—located on the medial wall, project directly to M1, other premotor areas, and directly to the spinal cord. It is thought that many of the functions originally associated with SMA may be mediated by CMA (47). Because it is less accessible for neurophysiological mapping studies and associated focal lesions, it is not a specific focus of this chapter.

Primary Somatosensory Cortex

While not strictly a motor structure, the somatosensory cortex must be considered in the cortical control of movement, especially with respect to potential plasticity mechanisms involved in recovery after M1 lesions. Both primary (S1) and secondary (S2) somatosensory areas contain a large proportion of CS neurons; though most terminate in superficial and intermediate laminae of the spinal cord. Thus, CS neurons originating in somatosensory cortex are thought to be involved primarily in modulating somatosensory inputs to the cord (62). While stimulus-evoked muscle effects can be elicited by ICMS in S1, the effects are much weaker in magnitude and require higher currents (63). However, focal lesions in the S1 hand area result in deficits in motor skill, similar to those produced by M1 lesions (64). Further, neuroimaging studies in humans have demonstrated structural and functional plasticity in S1 after M1 injury (65). Thus, S1 should be included in any comprehensive study of cortical areas contributing to recovery of motor function after M1 injury.

EXPERIENCE-DEPENDENT PLASTICITY IN CEREBRAL CORTEX

Over two decades of experimentation in the cerebral cortex have demonstrated many physiological and anatomical examples of cortical plasticity. Although these phenomena are triggered by many endogenous and exogenous events, one of the most potent modulators of cortical structure and function is behavioral experience (66–71). Emergent properties of each cortical area are shaped by behavioral demands, driven largely by repetition and temporal coincidence. For example, skilled motor activities requiring precise temporal coordination of muscles and joints must be practiced repeatedly. Such repetition is thought to drive the formation of discrete modules where the conjoint activity is represented as a unit (70).

One possible mechanism for mediating functional changes in motor cortex is the modification of synaptic strength of horizontal connections (72). In slice preparations after motor learning, rats have larger amplitude field potentials in the motor cortex contralateral to the trained forelimb (73). Thus, the synaptic strength of horizontal connections in the motor cortex is modifiable and may provide a substrate for altering the topography of motor maps during acquisition of motor skills. Structural alterations also occur in adult animals as a consequence of experience (74). Dendritic and synaptic morphology of motor cortex neurons are altered by specific motor learning tasks (75–79). Plasticity in motor cortex is probably skill- or learning-dependent, rather than strictly use-dependent. Tasks that require the acquisition of new motor skills induce neurophysiologic and neuroanatomic changes in motor cortex, but simple repetitive motion or strength training tasks do not (77, 80, 81).

While the majority of our understanding of the relationship between behavior and motor cortex organization at the cellular and synaptic levels of analysis comes from rodent studies, the use of non-human primates has provided invaluable knowledge. Primates possess several unique advantages over rodents, including differentiated motor and sensory cortices, which can be subdivided into smaller regions similar to human sensorimotor cortical organization (11). This allows for the study of the differential contribution of various subregions to motor learning, and allows for a more direct comparison to human studies. Furthermore, it allows for an understanding of how these subregions are functionally integrated through their extensive network of intracortical connections. In addition, primates possess the ability to perform complex behavioral tasks, especially those that require the use of fine digit manipulation. This digital dexterity is, with few exceptions, unrivaled in the animal kingdom (82) and is ideal for studying the acquisition of motor skills, as well as allowing for a large degree of control and detail in the design of behavioral training and testing paradigms.

The term "motor learning" is not rigidly defined in most experimental models, but instead thought of as a form of procedural learning that encompasses such elements as skill acquisition and motor adaptation. More specific is motor skill learning, itself, which is often described as the modification of the temporal and spatial organization of muscle synergies, which results in smooth, accurate, and consistent movement sequences (83). Functional magnetic imaging studies in humans have led to the hypothesis that motor learning is a two-stage process (84). The first stage is rapid and results in within-session decreases in neural activity. The second, slower stage results in increases and expansion of activity in M1.

While it is evident that numerous brain areas are involved in the production of complex motor movements, the M1 has long been implicated in the acquisition and performance of skilled motor behaviors. While originally believed to be involved in the activation of complex motor reflexes (85), the subsequent advancement of electrophysiological techniques revealed that movements could be elicited through electrical stimulation of the precentral gyrus (86). Based on these early findings, John Hughlings Jackson (1884) hypothesized that movement control was somatotopically organized. This hypothesis was later confirmed when more systematic cortical stimulation studies were used to develop a somatotopic map of the precentral gyrus (87, 88).

The development of the more sophisticated intracortical microstimulation (ICMS) technique in the late 1960s by Asanuma and colleagues allowed for the derivation of much higher spatial resolution maps within M1, which, in turn, revealed a more complex and dynamic cortical map organization, including the presence of columnar organization (89). The ICMS technique typically consists of applying a volley of short-duration cathodal pulses at a high frequency while using very weak currents ($\leq 60 \mu A$), thus allowing for relatively little spread of cortical excitation. This greater spatial resolution revealed that while M1 is somatotopically organized on a macro scale, discrete cortical areas are comprised of a montage of representations of individual muscles and movements, which are repeated and highly overlapping. Based upon ICMS mapping experiments that define movements evoked by the lowest possible current levels, motor map organization resembles a fractured mosaic of movement representations, overlaid over a gross somatotopic representation.

Since the advent of ICMS, numerous studies have expanded our understanding of the relationship between motor maps and motor skill learning. Several general principles of motor map organization have been demonstrated that are thought to underlie the motor cortex's ability to encode motor skills (90). First, as mentioned above, motor maps are fractionated, in that they contain multiple, overlapping representations of movements. Second, adjacent areas within cortical motor maps are highly interconnected via a dense network of intracortical fibers. Third, these maps are extremely dynamic and can be modulated by a number of intrinsic and extrinsic stimuli. Together, these characteristics provide a framework that facilitates the acquisition of novel muscle synergies, at least in part, through changes in the intracortical connectivity of individual movement representations.

However, the dynamic nature of motor maps belies the issue of stable neural connections that must be maintained to respond to environmental demands and to retain acquired motor skills. Within the cortex, this balance is thought to be achieved through interactions of the excitatory and inhibitory connections of pyramidal cells and local inhibitory networks (91–93). This, in turn, requires an internal mechanism that is capable of shifting this balance toward strengthening relevant synaptic connections. Horizontal fiber connections have been shown to arise from excitatory pyramidal neurons and allow for the co-activation of adjacent and non-adjacent cortical columns. In addition to activating excitatory pyramidal cells, they also generate inhibitory responses via the activation of GABAergic interneurons (94). Furthermore, the activity of these horizontal fibers has been shown to be mediated by both long-term potentiation (LTP) and long-term depression (LTD) between distant motor cortical areas (72, 95). LTP and LTD are persistent increases or decreases (respectively) in synaptic strength. These processes are thought to represent the synaptic mechanisms responsible for learning and memory.

While the phenomena of LTP and LTD are now well established from experiments in slice preparations and intact animals, the concept of use-dependent modulation of synaptic strength was postulated much earlier by Hebb in the 1940s. Hebb proposed that synaptic efficacy can be increased by a presynaptic cell's repeated or persistent stimulation of a postsynaptic cell. This concept has taken on many forms and is pervasive in most theories of the synaptic basis of learning and memory. Many contemporary terms still honor Hebb's contribution to this field, such as Hebbian learning, Hebbian cell assemblies, and Hebbian engrams. Hebb's theories are often summarized in the now-common phrase "neurons that fire together, wire together." Specifically with regard to plasticity in cortical networks, alterations in synaptic strength in horizontal fibers provide a mechanism capable of both facilitating the activation of multiple novel muscle synergies that are required for motor skill acquisition, while likewise providing a mechanism, via inhibitory processes, of motor map stability that is required to maintain stable, neural representations in response to irrelevant (i.e., untrained) environmental events.

Utilizing manual dexterity training in combination with ICMS maps has been crucial in demonstrating the dynamic relationship between motor skill learning and cortical map plasticity. The first study to directly examine this relationship used varying behaviorally demanding tasks to selectively activate specific components of motor maps (70). In these tasks, monkeys were rewarded with small, banana-flavored food pellets for performing skilled movements with the hand. In one task, the pellets were placed one at a time into food wells of different diameters. The monkey simply was required to extract the pellet. Large food wells required minimal manual skill. Small food wells required the insertion of only one or two digits and, thus, maximal manual skill. Retrieval from the smaller wells required practice over the course of about 10–12 days for asymptotic performance to be achieved. In a second task, monkeys were required to reach through a narrow tube and rotate a key back and forth, requiring repetitive pronation and supination of the forearm. Post-training ICMS mapping revealed training-induced changes in motor map topography that directly reflected the demands of the particular behavioral task. That is, the pellet-retrieval task resulted in expansion of digit representations, whereas the key-turning task resulted in expansion of wrist and forearm representations.

In addition, an increase in ICMS-evoked multi-joint movements was observed. These movements consisted of simultaneous executions of digit and wrist, or proximal movements at low ICMS thresholds, and were only observed after training on the digit-use intensive manual dexterity task. Both before and after training, thresholds for evoking multi-joint responses were significantly lower than single joint responses. These results imply that behaviorally relevant, simultaneous or sequential movements may become associated in the motor cortex through repeated activation.

A temporal correlation hypothesis has been proposed to explain these phenomena and derives from similar results obtained from studies in somatosensory cortex. For example, digit representations in somatosensory cortex are typically individuated, with sharp boundaries between adjacent digit areas. If two digits are experimentally joined surgically in a so-called digital syndactyly procedure then the representations of those digits become fused, with neurons displaying multi-digit receptive fields that cross the suture line. The hypothesis suggests that as inputs from the two separate digits are made temporally coincident by the syndactyly, the new multi-digit representations appear as an emergent property of the plastic somatosensory cortex. It is possible that this hypothesis is generalizable to motor cortex as well. Thus, muscle and joint synergies used in complex, skilled motor actions may be supported by alterations in local networks within the motor cortex. As skilled tasks become more stereotyped in the timing of sequential joint movements, functional modules emerge in the cortex to link the outputs of different motoneuron pools.

These findings lead to the question of what aspects of motor skill learning drive the observed changes in map representations. It is possible that increased muscle activity alone produced the observed changes in map representations. To address this issue, a group of monkeys were trained exclusively on either the largest or the smallest well in the manual dexterity task described above. The rationale in this design is that the largest well allows for simple multi-digit movements for pellet retrieval, which does not require the subject to develop novel skilled digit movements since simply grasping for food is a normal part of their daily home cage behavior and already part of their behavioral repertoire. Small-well food pellet retrieval, in contrast, requires the monkey to manipulate one or two digits to retrieve the pellet, which is considerably harder, given that squirrel monkeys lack monosynaptic corticospinal projections to motoneurons, which probably limits individuation of digit movements (96). Compared to pre-training maps, monkeys trained on the large-well pellet retrieval did not show an expansion of the digit representation, while those trained on the small well did exhibit an expansion of the digit representation (80). These findings strongly suggest that an increase in motor activity in the absence of motor skill acquisition is insufficient to drive neurophysiological changes in the motor cortex. Similar findings have been found in rodents during examinations of pellet retrieval vs. bar pressing. Rats that learned to retrieve pellets from a rotating platform displayed more distal movements in their motor maps. This expansion was associated with significant synaptogenesis (68, 77).

PLASTICITY IN ADJACENT TISSUE AFTER FOCAL DAMAGE TO M1

Direct evidence that adjacent regions of the cortex might function in a vicarious manner after injury can be traced to studies by Glees and Cole in the early 1950s (97). Monkeys were subjected to focal injury to the thumb representation. When brains were remapped following behavioral recovery, the thumb area reappeared in the adjacent cortical territory. However, using ICMS techniques, somewhat different findings were observed by Nudo et al. in the 1990s. Small, subtotal lesions were made in a portion of the distal forelimb representation (DFL) in squirrel monkeys, and the animals were allowed to recover spontaneously (i.e., without the benefit of rehabilitative training) for several weeks. In contrast to earlier findings, the remaining DFL was reduced in size, giving way to expanded proximal representations (70). However, in animals that underwent rehabilitative training with the impaired limb, the DFL was preserved or expanded (98). In retrospect, it is quite possible that the re-emergence of thumb representations in the early study may have been driven by post-injury behavioral demands.

Recent studies in human stroke patients suggest that the intact, peri-infarct cortex may play a role in neurologic recovery (99–101). Using transcranial magnetic stimulation (TMS) after stroke, it has been shown that the excitability of motor cortex is reduced near the injury, and the cortical representation of the affected muscles is decreased (102, 103). It is likely that this effect occurs from a combination of diaschisis-like phenomena and disuse of the affected limb (104). Further, after several weeks of rehabilitation, motor representations in the injured hemisphere are enlarged relative to the initial post-injury map (103, 105). Also, when goal-directed movement with the impaired hand is encouraged, a significant enlargement of the representation of the paretic limb is produced (106), closely paralleling results in non-human primates.

Neuroanatomical changes also occur in the peri-infarct cortex. After middle cerebral artery occlusion in rats, Stroemer and colleagues examined immunohistochemical correlates of neuronal sprouting in the spared, peri-infarct tissue. Between 3 and 14 days post-infarct, rats demonstrate increased GAP-43 immunoreactivity, suggesting significant neurite outgrowth in the peri-infarct region (107). Then, 14–60 days post-infarct, synaptophysin staining is elevated, signifying increased synaptogenesis (107).

While these experiments provided indirect support for neurite outgrowth and synaptogenesis in the peri-infarct zone after a cortical injury, direct evidence for local axonal sprouting has been obtained more recently in experiments utilizing the so-called rodent cortical barrel field (107). This specialized region of somatosensory cortex in rats and many other species contains a somatosensory representation of the mystacial vibrissae, or simply, whiskers. The advantages of this system are two-fold: First, an individual "barrel" in the rat barrel field represents a single whisker, thus allowing precise experimental manipulation of the inputs to this isolated region. Second, the barrel field, and individual barrels, can be identified in histological stains, allowing for precise identification of the barrel that has been manipulated. In recent studies by Carmichael and colleagues, focal ischemic lesions were made in the rodent barrel-field cortex. A few weeks later, a neuroanatomical tract-tracer was injected into the cortical tissue bordering the infarcted region, and the axonal projections of the labeled neurons were plotted. Rats with small ischemic strokes in barrel cortex had local, axonal projections arising from the peri-infarct cortex that were substantially different in orientation compared with control tissue. This result implies that new intracortical (horizontal) connections are formed in the peri-infarct tissue, at least over short distances of perhaps a millimeter in rats (108). While we are just beginning to understand the molecular events that drive local axonal growth after injury, the picture is now emerging of an evolving peri-infarct environment in which growth inhibition is suppressed for about one month post-infarct. This period is followed by "waves" of growth promotion that may modulate axonal sprouting and, thus, the brain's self-repair processes (109).

Based on the large number of paradigms demonstrating that the adult somatosensory cortex is plastic, it is not surprising that somatosensory organization is altered by cortical injury, as might occur in stroke. After small, ischemic lesions that destroy single-digit representations in S1 of adult monkeys, the destroyed representation re-emerges in the adjacent cortical territory (64). Neuroimaging studies in human stroke survivors suggest that structural plasticity accompanies somatosensory cortical reorganization. Cortical areas that undergo changes in activation response to tactile stimuli show increased cortical thickness (65).

FUNCTIONAL AND STRUCTURAL PLASTICITY IN REMOTE REGIONS AFTER FOCAL DAMAGE TO M1

Primate brains are endowed with a rich intracortical network that allows reciprocal communication among the various sensory and motor areas. Injury to the motor cortex results in a potent disruption of integrated sensorimotor networks, resulting in loss of fine motor control (69). Thus, even focal

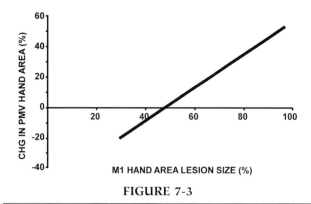

FIGURE 7-3

Relationship between size of lesion in primary motor cortex (M1) hand representation and subsequent change in hand representation in ventral premotor cortex (PMv). The percentages refer to the proportion of the M1 hand representation that was destroyed by an experimental cortical infarct in squirrel monkeys. Note that as lesion sizes exceed 50% of the M1 hand representation, hand representations in PMv expand in a linear fashion (112).

injuries produce widespread and persistent changes in areas that are quite remote from the site of injury. For example, injury to M1 in rats and non-human primates results in upregulation of NMDA receptors and down-regulation of GABA$_A$ receptors throughout the ipsilesional and contralesional hemisphere (110). Therefore it follows that intact, motor areas outside of M1 may also contribute to recovery. As mentioned previously, the frontal cortex contains several areas that contribute to skilled motor behaviors in primates, including PMd, PMv, and SMA. All of these areas possess reciprocal connections with M1, contain numerous corticospinal neurons, and contain complete hand representations. Thus, it is plausible that following an injury to M1, the remaining, intact motor areas play some role in functional recovery, via intracortical connectivity with other cortical regions and/or their direct corticospinal projection pathways.

Experiments by Liu and Rouiller (111) showed in non-human primates that inactivation of the premotor cortex with the GABAergic agonist muscimol following an M1 ischemic lesion reinstated behavioral deficits. This reinstatement was not observed with inactivation of the peri-lesional or contralateral cortex. Thus, it follows that if the premotor cortex is capable of compensating for the loss of motor function following an M1 injury, there should exist physiological changes that accompany this recovery. In adult squirrel monkeys ICMS mapping techniques have characterized representational maps of both M1 and PMv before and after experimental ischemic infarcts that destroyed at least 50% of the M1 hand representation (112). All subjects showed an increased hand representation in

PMv, specifically in digit, wrist, and forearm sites. Further, the amount of PMv expansion was correlated with the amount of the M1 hand representation that was destroyed. In other words, the more complete the M1 hand area lesion, the greater the compensatory reorganization in PMv (Figure 7-3).

Interestingly, when lesions were smaller than 50% of the M1 hand area, the PMv hand representation decreased in size (Figure 7-3). Thus, examining the entire spectrum of M1 infarcts of varying sizes, the linear relationship is maintained. This result occurred despite the fact that some of these subtotal M1 hand area lesions nonetheless destroyed nearly the entire terminal field of PMv-M1 connections. What possible compensatory changes in the neuronal network could account for proportional gains in premotor hand areas but losses with very small lesions? This phenomenon is reminiscent of Lashley's classic description of the relationship between cerebral mass and behavioral change (113, 114). According to this hypothesis, lesion size is generally assumed to be associated with the severity of deficits, while lesion location is related to the specificity of deficits. Lashley also proposed the concept of equipotentiality, suggesting that each portion of a given cortical area is able to encode or produce behavior normally controlled by the entire area. In that vein, after smaller lesions, the surviving M1 tissue could potentially subserve the recovery of function. In that case, reorganization in distant, interconnected cortical areas would be a more "passive" process, resulting from the loss of intracortical connections. This reorganization could be compared to a "sustained diaschisis" of PMv. After larger lesions, reorganization of the adjacent tissue may not suffice for normal motor execution. Thus, learning-associated reorganization would need to take place elsewhere, resulting in greater PMv expansion. Accordingly, in rats, the contralesional cortex is thought to be involved in behavioral recovery only after large lesions (115). Lesion size appears to be a major factor involved in the initiation of some of the vicarious processes that purportedly play a role in recovery from CNS lesions.

Recently, yet another form of post-injury sprouting of cortical projection pathways from PMv was discovered in the injured hemisphere of adult non-human primates. Five months after an ischemic injury to the M1 hand representation, most intracortical connection patterns of the PMv remain intact (116). This is despite the fact that the major intracortical target of PMv is destroyed by this procedure. However, after M1 lesions, monkeys display a remarkable proliferation of novel PMv terminal projections in primary sensory cortex (S1), when compared to uninjured control monkeys, specifically in the hand representations of areas 1 and 2. Likewise, this somatosensory area had a significant increase in the

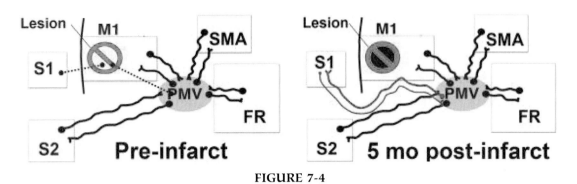

FIGURE 7-4

Rewiring of intracortical connections after M1 infarct. Normally, PMv provides a major input to M1. M1 shares significant connections with S1. Five months after an infarct in M1, novel connections form between PMv and S1 (116). Other intracortical connections of PMv remain unchanged.

number of retrogradely labeled cell bodies, indicating an increase in reciprocal projections from S1 to PMv. In addition, intracortical axonal projections from PMv significantly altered their trajectory near the site of the lesion (Figure 7-4).

This finding is particularly interesting, given the direct intracortical connections between M1 and somatosensory cortex as well as the presence of direct corticospinal projections originating from PMv. One hypothesis is that the post-injury sprouting represents a repair strategy of the sensorimotor cortex to re-engage the motor areas with somatosensory areas. In intact brains, M1 receives input from various regions of the parietal lobe that supply cutaneous and proprioceptive information that is largely segregated in the M1 hand area—cutaneous information arriving in the posterior portion of M1 and proprioceptive information arriving in the more anterior portion. The functional importance of this somatosensory input can be appreciated from studies employing discrete lesions in these subregions in M1. Lesions in the posterior M1 hand area lesions result in behavioral deficits akin to those seen after S1 lesions. These deficits appear to be similar to sensory agnosia, in which the animal reaches for food items but does not appear to know whether the item is actually in the hand. In contrast, anterior M1 hand area lesions result in deficits in metrics of the reach, perhaps indicating the disruption of proprioceptive information in the motor cortex (10). One lesson from these studies is that the motor cortex cannot be considered solely as a motor structure. Deficits result from sensory-motor disconnection, in addition to disruption of motor output. Thus, after M1 injury, there is a substantial reduction of somatosensory input to motor areas. Perhaps the novel connection between PMv and S1 is an attempt by the cortical motor systems to reconnect with somatosensory input.

It is likely that this phenomenon of intracortical sprouting of remote pathways, interconnected with the injured zone, is not a unique event. It is more likely that many structures, both cortical and subcortical, that are normally connected with the injured tissue undergo substantial physiological and anatomical alterations. For instance, each of the other cortical motor areas (PMd, SMA, cingulate motor areas) is likely to change its intracortical connectivity pattern since its targets are destroyed. If so, it follows that the brain with a focal injury is a very different system. It is not simply a normal system with a missing piece. If intracortical reorganization is a predictable process, as we think it is, then we may be able to begin to develop ways of enhancing adaptive, while suppressing maladaptive, connection patterns.

After stroke in humans, widespread changes occur in activation patterns associated with movement of the paretic limb in both the ipsilesional and contralesional hemispheres (117–119). Whether such bilateral activation is adaptive or maladaptive is still a matter of debate, but it appears that, as recovery proceeds, activation of the various regions in the ipsilesional cortex increases (105, 118). Increased ipsilateral activation after stroke is quite widespread, including spared premotor areas (120, 121). In one longitudinal study, increased activation of SMA was correlated with better recovery (122). Stroke survivors with middle cerebral artery strokes that included lateral PM areas had poorer recovery (123), while increased lateral PM activity was associated with better recovery (124). In an experiment analogous to monkey secondary inactivation studies, the ipsilesional PMd of human stroke survivors was inactivated temporarily with low-frequency repetitive TMS. This procedure resulted in reaction-time delays that were not generated by inactivation of the contralesional PMd or the PMd of healthy subjects (125). From the results to date, it is not possible to determine if any one motor area is more important in the recovery of motor abilities after stroke. A likely hypothesis is that the entire cortical and subcortical motor system spared by the injury participates to varying degrees depending upon the extent and location of the injury and behavioral demands. At least some of the functions of the injured region(s) are thus redistributed across the remaining cortical and subcortical motor network.

An example of this can be seen after unilateral cortical lesions in rats where corticostriatal fibers, which primarily connect cortical motor areas with the striatum on the same side of the brain, sprout from the intact cortex on the opposite side of the brain and cross to the opposite striatum (i.e., on the side of the lesion) (126). In other words, unilateral lesions produce novel crossed corticostriatal pathways that originate in areas completely remote from the injured zone. While still speculative, such plasticity in crossed fiber systems may provide one mechanism for the remaining intact hemisphere to participate in recovery by gaining access to the deafferented striatum in the injured hemisphere.

ROLE OF BEHAVIOR IN MODULATING POST-INFARCT RECOVERY

Several new approaches to improving functional recovery after stroke recently have been developed that are based on neuroplasticity mechanisms. Constraint-induced movement therapy encourages use of the impaired limb, and engages it in functional tasks that purportedly drive adaptive plasticity in the intact portions of the ipsilesional hemisphere. Recent clinical trials support the efficacy of this approach over standard and usual care (see Chapter 18) (127). D-amphetamine administration, when combined with behavioral experience, appears to enhance recovery in rodent and non-human primate models, though clinical results have been mixed (128). D-amphetamine is known to induce increased synaptogenesis in the peri-infarct region in rats (see Chapter 10). Cortical electrical stimulation, when combined with rehabilitative training, appears to have a positive effect on recovery in rodents and non-human primates (129, 130). While the mechanism is not well understood, the approach is thought to enhance excitability of the intact regions of the ipsilesional hemisphere. Non-invasive analogs of this approach are now being examined (131). What these approaches have in common is the importance of repetitive behavioral tasks, especially those that have high skill demands. Thus, while pharmacological and device-oriented approaches to increasing cortical excitability and growth of neuronal processes are clearly

beneficial, their effects are modulated and shaped by behavioral experience.

Recent evidence from developmental and injury studies may suggest ways in which behavior may specifically influence neuroanatomical plasticity after injury. First, during development, guidance cues for axonal sprouting are activity-dependent. There are two phases in the maturation of thalamocortical connections. In the first phase, thalamocortical axons are directed to their cortical targets by axonal guidance molecules. This process may involve spontaneous neural activity (132). In the second phase, cortical activity guides axonal sprouting within the cerebral cortex, determining topological connectivity patterns (133). Postnatal axonal branching patterns within cerebral cortex have also been shown to involve sensory related stimulus activity, possibly by initiating molecular retrograde signals such as brain-derived neurotrophic factor (134). After a focal ischemic infarct in rats, synchronous neuronal activity is a signal for post-infarct axonal sprouting to be initiated from the intact cortical hemisphere to peri-infarct cortex and the contralateral dorsal striatum (135). Thus, evidence now supports the importance of cortical activity for axonal sprouting within the developing and adult brain.

The significance of neuroplasticity for rehabilitation is that it provides a mechanistic rationale for understanding therapeutic interventions. Thus, it may be possible to develop more effective recovery protocols if we can elucidate the effects of such interventions on physiological and anatomical plasticity in the injured brain.

As demonstrated by the mapping studies after microinfarcts in non-human primates noted above, it is clear that behavior is one of the most powerful modulators of post-injury recovery. Behavioral interventions to enhance recovery after stroke have become increasingly popular due to the success of task-oriented functional therapeutic interventions, such as constraint-induced movement therapy. Whether such behaviorally driven changes in motor performance are due to reestablishment of original motor programs in spared tissue or due to compensatory use of unimpaired body parts remains a controversial subject. Nonetheless, plastic changes must take place in the spared neuronal substrate, whether the improvement is due to true restoration of function or compensation. Behavioral use clearly plays a role in the contralesional changes that take place in the uninjured cortex of rats following cortical infarction. Other studies have demonstrated that task-specific rehabilitative training is most effective in driving post-injury neuroanatomical changes. Thus, it would appear that CNS injury produces an environment in which the neuronal network is particularly receptive to modulation by specific behavioral manipulations.

References

1. Kakei S, Hoffman DS, Strick PL. Sensorimotor transformations in cortical motor areas. *Neurosci Res* 2003; 46(1):1–10.

2. Picard N, Strick PL. Motor areas of the medial wall: A review of their location and functional activation. *Cereb Cortex* 1996; 6(3):342–353.

3. Nudo RJ. Neurophysiology of motor skill learning. In: Byrne JH, ed. *Learning and Memory—A Comprehensive Reference.* Vol 126. Oxford, UK: Elsevier Ltd., 2007.

4. Passingham RE, Perry VH, Wilkinson F. The long-term effects of removal of sensorimotor cortex in infant and adult rhesus monkeys. *Brain* 1983; 106 (Pt 3):675–705.

5. Phillips CG, Porter R. Corticospinal neurones: Their role in movement. *Monogr Physiol Soc* 1977(34):v–xii, 1–450.

6. Schieber MH, Poliakov AV. Partial inactivation of the primary motor cortex hand area: Effects on individuated finger movements. *J Neurosci* 1998; 18(21):9038–9054.

7. Whishaw IQ, Pellis SM, Gorny BP, Pellis VC. The impairments in reaching and the movements of compensation in rats with motor cortex lesions: An endpoint, videorecording, and movement notation analysis. *Behav Brain Res* 1991; 42(1):77–91.

8. Preuss TM, Stepniewska I, Jain N, Kaas JH. Multiple divisions of macaque precentral motor cortex identified with neurofilament antibody SMI-32. *Brain Res* 1997; 767(1):148–153.

9. Strick PL, Preston JB. Two representations of the hand in area 4 of a primate. II. Somatosensory input organization. *J Neurophysiol* 1982; 48(1):150–159.

10. Friel KM, Barbay S, Frost SB, et al. Dissociation of sensorimotor deficits after rostral versus caudal lesions in the primary motor cortex hand representation. *J Neurophysiol* 2005; 94(2):1312–1324.

11. Dancause N, Barbay S, Frost SB, et al. Ipsilateral connections of the ventral premotor cortex in a new world primate. *J Comp Neurol* 2006; 495(4):374–390.

12. Holsapple JW, Preston JB, Strick PL. The origin of thalamic inputs to the "hand" representation in the primary motor cortex. *J Neurosci* 1991; 11(9):2644–2654.

13. Matelli M, Luppino G, Fogassi L, Rizzolatti G. Thalamic input to inferior area 6 and area 4 in the macaque monkey. *J Comp Neurol* 1989; 280(3):468–488.

14. Stepniewska I, Preuss TM, Kaas JH. Architectonics, somatotopic organization, and ipsilateral cortical connections of the primary motor area (M1) of owl monkeys. *J Comp Neurol* 1993; 330(2):238–271.

15. Nudo RJ, Masterton RB. Descending pathways to the spinal cord, III: Sites of origin of the corticospinal tract. *J Comp Neurol* 1990; 296(4):559–583.

16. Fetz EE, Cheney PD, German DC. Corticomotoneuronal connections of precentral cells detected by postspike averages of EMG activity in behaving monkeys. *Brain Research* 1976; 114(3):505–510.

17. Rathelot JA, Strick PL. Muscle representation in the macaque motor cortex: An anatomical perspective. *Proc Natl Acad Sci U S A* 2006; 103(21):8257–8262.

18. Hoshi E, Tanji J. Distinctions between dorsal and ventral premotor areas: Anatomical connectivity and functional properties. *Curr Opin Neurobiol* 2007:17(2):234–242.

19. Ghosh S, Gattera R. A comparison of the ipsilateral cortical projections to the dorsal and ventral subdivisions of the macaque premotor cortex. *Somatosens Mot Res* 1995; 12(3–4):359–378.

20. Preuss TM, Kaas JH. Parvalbumin-like immunoreactivity of layer V pyramidal cells in the motor and somatosensory cortex of adult primates. *Brain Res* 1996; 712(2):353–357.

21. Takada M, Tokuno H, Nambu A, Inase M. Corticostriatal projections from the somatic motor areas of the frontal cortex in the macaque monkey: Segregation versus overlap of input zones from the primary motor cortex, the supplementary motor area, and the premotor cortex. *Exp Brain Res* 1998; 120(1):114–128.

22. Wise SP, Mauritz KH. Set-related neuronal activity in the premotor cortex of rhesus monkeys: Effects of changes in motor set. *Proc R Soc Lond B Biol Sci* 1985; 223(1232):331–354.

23. Kurata K, Wise SP. Premotor cortex of rhesus monkeys: Set-related activity during two conditional motor tasks. *Exp Brain Res* 1988; 69(2):327–343.

24. Wu W, Hatsopoulos NG. Coordinate system representations of movement direction in the premotor cortex. *Exp Brain Res* 2007; 176(4):652–657.

25. Rushworth MF, Johansen-Berg H, Gobel SM, Devlin JT. The left parietal and premotor cortices: Motor attention and movement. *Neuroimage* 2003; 20 (Suppl 1):S89–100.

26. Kurata K, Hoffman DS. Differential effects of muscimol microinjection into dorsal and ventral aspects of the premotor cortex of monkeys. *J Neurophysiol* 1994; 71(3):1151–1164.

27. Prado J, Clavagnier S, Otzenberger H, et al. Two cortical systems for reaching in central and peripheral vision. *Neuron* 2005; 48(5):849–858.

28. Dum RP, Strick PL. Frontal lobe inputs to the digit representations of the motor areas on the lateral surface of the hemisphere. *J Neurosci* 2005; 25(6):1375–1386.

29. Stepniewska I, Preuss TM, Kaas JH. Ipsilateral cortical connections of dorsal and ventral premotor areas in New World owl monkeys. *J Comp Neurol* 2006; 495(6):691–708.

30. Gentilucci M, Fogassi L, Luppino G, et al. Somatotopic representation in inferior area 6 of the macaque monkey. *Brain Behav Evol* 1989; 33(2–3):118–121.

31. Godschalk M, Lemon RN, Nijs HG, Kuypers HG. Behaviour of neurons in monkey peri-arcuate and precentral cortex before and during visually guided arm and hand movements. *Exp Brain Res* 1981; 44(1):113–116.

32. Hoshi E, Tanji J. Functional specialization in dorsal and ventral premotor areas. *Prog Brain Res* 2004; 143:507–511.

33. Kurata K, Tanji J. Premotor cortex neurons in macaques: Activity before distal and proximal forelimb movements. *J Neurosci* 1986; 6(2):403–411.

34. Murata A, Fadiga L, Fogassi L, et al. Object representation in the ventral premotor cortex (area F5) of the monkey. *J Neurophysiol* 1997; 78(4):2226–2230.

35. Mushiake H, Inase M, Tanji J. Neuronal activity in the primate premotor, supplementary, and precentral motor cortex during visually guided and internally determined sequential movements. *J Neurophysiol* 1991; 66(3):705–718.

36. Rizzolatti G, Matelli M, Pavesi G. Deficits in attention and movement following the removal of postarcuate (area 6) and prearcuate (area 8) cortex in macaque monkeys. *Brain* 1983; 106 (Pt 3):655–673.

37. Schieber MH. Inactivation of the ventral premotor cortex biases the laterality of motoric choices. *Exp Brain Res* 2000; 130(4):497–507.

38. Cerri G, Shimazu H, Maier MA, Lemon RN. Facilitation from ventral premotor cortex of primary motor cortex outputs to macaque hand muscles. *J Neurophysiol* 2003; 90(2):832–842.

39. Shimazu H, Maier MA, Cerri G, et al. Macaque ventral premotor cortex exerts powerful facilitation of motor cortex outputs to upper limb motoneurons. *J Neurosci* 2004; 24(5):1200–1211.

40. Godschalk M, Lemon RN, Kuypers HG, Ronday HK. Cortical afferents and efferents of monkey postarcuate area: An anatomical and electrophysiological study. *Exp Brain Res* 1984; 56(3):410–424.

41. Kurata K. Corticocortical inputs to the dorsal and ventral aspects of the premotor cortex of macaque monkeys. *Neurosci Res* 1991; 12(1):263–280.

42. Tanne-Gariepy J, Rouiller EM, Boussaoud D. Parietal inputs to dorsal versus ventral premotor areas in the macaque monkey: Evidence for largely segregated visuomotor pathways. *Exp Brain Res* 2002; 145(1):91–103.

43. Leichnetz GR. Connections of the medial posterior parietal cortex (area 7m) in the monkey. *Anat Rec* 2001; 263(2):215–236.

44. Huang RS, Sereno MI. Dodecapus: An MR-compatible system for somatosensory stimulation. *Neuroimage* 2007; 34(3):1060–1073.

45. Preuschhof C, Heekeren HR, Taskin B, et al. Neural correlates of vibrotactile working memory in the human brain. *J Neurosci* 2006; 26(51):13231–13239.

46. Padoa-Schioppa C, Li CS, Bizzi E. Neuronal activity in the supplementary motor area of monkeys adapting to a new dynamic environment. *J Neurophysiol* 2004; 91(1):449–473.

47. Picard N, Strick PL. Activation of the supplementary motor area (SMA) during performance of visually guided movements. *Cereb Cortex* 2003; 13(9):977–986.

48. Roland PE, Larsen B, Lassen NA, Skinhoj E. Supplementary motor area and other cortical areas in organization of voluntary movements in man. *J Neurophysiol* 1980; 43(1):118–136.

49. Dum RP, Strick PL. The origin of corticospinal projections from the premotor areas in the frontal lobe. *J Neurosci* 1991; 11(3):667–689.

50. He SQ, Dum RP, Strick PL. Topographic organization of corticospinal projections from the frontal lobe: Motor areas on the lateral surface of the hemisphere. *J Neurosci* 1993; 13(3):952–980.

51. Hikosaka O, Sakai K, Miyauchi S, et al. Activation of human presupplementary motor area in learning of sequential procedures: A functional MRI study. *J Neurophysiol* 1996; 76(1):617–621.

52. Nakamura K, Sakai K, Hikosaka O. Neuronal activity in medial frontal cortex during learning of sequential procedures. *J Neurophysiol* 1998; 80(5):2671–2687.

53. Brinkman C. Lesions in supplementary motor area interfere with a monkey's performance of a bimanual coordination task. *Neurosci Lett* 23 1981; 27(3):267–270.

54. Nakamura K, Sakai K, Hikosaka O. Effects of local inactivation of monkey medial frontal cortex in learning of sequential procedures. *J Neurophysiol* 1999; 82(2):1063–1068.

55. Fang PC, Stepniewska I, Kaas JH. Ipsilateral cortical connections of motor, premotor, frontal eye, and posterior parietal fields in a prosimian primate, Otolemur garnetti. *J Comp Neurol* 2005; 490(3):305–333.

56. Luppino G, Matelli M, Camarda R, Rizzolatti G. Corticocortical connections of area F3 (SMA-proper) and area F6 (pre-SMA) in the macaque monkey. *J Comp Neurol* 1993; 338(1):114–140.

57. Morecraft RJ, Van Hoesen GW. Cingulate input to the primary and supplementary motor cortices in the rhesus monkey: Evidence for somatotopy in areas 24c and 23c. *J Comp Neurol* 1992; 322(4):471–489.

58. Morecraft RJ, Van Hoesen GW. Frontal granular cortex input to the cingulate (M3), supplementary (M2), and primary (M1) motor cortices in the rhesus monkey. *J Comp Neurol* 1993; 337(4):669–689.

59. Tokuno H, Tanji J. Input organization of distal and proximal forelimb areas in the monkey primary motor cortex: A retrograde double labeling study. *J Comp Neurol* 1993; 333(2):199–209.

60. Wu CW, Bichot NP, Kaas JH. Converging evidence from microstimulation, architecture, and connections for multiple motor areas in the frontal and cingulate cortex of prosimian primates. *J Comp Neurol* 2000; 423(1):140–177.

61. Lehericy S, Ducros M, Krainik A, et al. 3-D diffusion tensor axonal tracking shows distinct SMA and pre-SMA projections to the human striatum. *Cereb Cortex* 2004; 14(12):1302–1309.

62. Ralston DD, Ralston HJ III. The terminations of corticospinal tract axons in the macaque monkey. *J Comp Neurol* 1985; 242(3):325–337.

63. Widener GL, Cheney PD. Effects on muscle activity from microstimuli applied to somatosensory and motor cortex during voluntary movement in the monkey. *J Neurophysiol* 1997; 77(5):2446–2465.

64. Xerri C, Merzenich MM, Peterson BE, Jenkins W. Plasticity of primary somatosensory cortex paralleling sensorimotor skill recovery from stroke in adult monkeys. *J Neurophysiol* 1998; 79(4):2119–2148.

65. Schaechter JD, Moore CI, Connell BD, et al. Structural and functional plasticity in the somatosensory cortex of chronic stroke patients. *Brain* 2006; 129(Pt 10):2722–2733.

66. Feldman DE, Brecht M. Map plasticity in somatosensory cortex. *Science* 2005; 310(5749):810–815.

67. Karni A, Meyer G, Rey-Hipolito C, et al. The acquisition of skilled motor performance: Fast and slow experience-driven changes in primary motor cortex. *Proc Natl Acad Sci U S A* 1998; 95(3):861–868.

68. Kleim JA, Barbay S, Nudo RJ. Functional reorganization of the rat motor cortex following motor skill learning. *J Neurophysiol* 1998; 80(6):3321–3325.

69. Nudo RJ. Functional and structural plasticity in motor cortex: Implications for stroke recovery. *Phys Med Rehabil Clin N Am* 2003; 14(1 Suppl):S57–76.

70. Nudo RJ, Milliken GW, Jenkins WM, Merzenich MM. Use-dependent alterations of movement representations in primary motor cortex of adult squirrel monkeys. *J Neurosci* 1996; 16(2):785–807.

71. Pascual-Leone A, Grafman J, Hallett M. Modulation of cortical motor output maps during development of implicit and explicit knowledge. *Science* 1994; 263(5151):1287–1289.

72. Hess G, Donoghue JP. Long-term potentiation of horizontal connections provides a mechanism to reorganize cortical motor maps. *J Neurophysiol* 1994; 71(6):2543–2547.

73. Rioult-Pedotti MS, Friedman D, Hess G, Donoghue JP. Strengthening of horizontal cortical connections following skill learning. *Nat Neurosci* 1998; 1(3):230–234.

74. Diamond MC, Rosenzweig MR, Bennett EL, et al. Effects of environmental enrichment and impoverishment on rat cerebral cortex. *J Neurobiol* 1972; 3(1):47–64.

75. Greenough WT, Larson JR, Withers GS. Effects of unilateral and bilateral training in a reaching task on dendritic branching of neurons in the rat motor-sensory forelimb cortex. *Behav Neural Biol* 1985; 44(2):301–314.

76. Jones TA. Multiple synapse formation in the motor cortex opposite unilateral sensorimotor cortex lesions in adult rats. *J Comp Neurol* 1999; 414(1):57–66.

77. Kleim JA, Barbay S, Cooper NR, et al. Motor learning-dependent synaptogenesis is localized to functionally reorganized motor cortex. *Neurobiol Learn Mem* 2002; 77(1):63–77.

78. Kleim JA, Lussnig E, Schwarz ER, et al. Synaptogenesis and Fos expression in the motor cortex of the adult rat after motor skill learning. *J Neurosci* 1996; 16(14):4529–4535.

79. Withers GS, Greenough WT. Reach training selectively alters dendritic branching in subpopulations of layer II-III pyramids in rat motor-somatosensory forelimb cortex. *Neuropsychologia* 1989; 27(1):61–69.

80. Plautz EJ, Milliken GW, Nudo RJ. Effects of repetitive motor training on movement representations in adult squirrel monkeys: Role of use versus learning. *Neurobiol Learn Mem* 2000; 74(1):27–55.

81. Remple MS, Bruneau RM, VandenBerg PM, et al. Sensitivity of cortical movement representations to motor experience: Evidence that skill learning but not strength training induces cortical reorganization. *Behav Brain Res* 2001; 123(2):133–141.

82. Heffner RS, Masterton RB. The role of the corticospinal tract in the evolution of human digital dexterity. *Brain Behavior and Evolution* 1983; 23(3–4):165–183.

83. Hammond G. Correlates of human handedness in primary motor cortex: A review and hypothesis. *Neuroscience and Biobehavioral Reviews* 2002; 26(3):285–292.

84. Ungerleider LG, Doyon J, Karni A. Imaging brain plasticity during motor skill learning. *Neurobiology of Learning and Memory* 2002; 78(3):553–564.

85. Sherrington C. On the instability of a cortical point. *Proceedings of the Royal Society of London.* 1912; B 85:250–277.

86. Fritsch G, Hitzig E. Uber die elektrische Erregbarkeit des Grosshirns. *Archiv fur Anatomie, Physiologie, und Wissenschaftl. Mediz* 1870; 37:300–332.

87. Penfield W, Rasmussen, T. *The cerebral cortex of man.* New York: Macmillan, 1950.

88. Woolsey CN, Settlage PH, Meyer DR, et al. Patterns of localization in precentral and "supplementary" motor areas and their relation to the concept of a premotor area. *Res Publ Assoc Res Nerv Ment Dis* 1952; 30:238–264.

89. Asanuma H. Recent developments in the study of the columnar arrangement of neurons within the motor cortex. *Physiological Reviews* 1975; 55(2):143–156.

90. Monfils MH, Plautz EJ, Kleim JA. In search of the motor engram: Motor map plasticity as a mechanism for encoding motor experience. *The Neuroscientist* 2005; 11(5):471–483.

91. Aroniadou VA, Keller A. The patterns and synaptic properties of horizontal intracortical connections in the rat motor cortex. *Jl of Neurophysiology* 1993; 70(4):1553–1569.

92. Huntley GW, Jones EG. Relationship of intrinsic connections to forelimb movement representations in monkey motor cortex: A correlative anatomic and physiological study. *J of Neurophysiology* 1991; 66(2):390–413.

93. Lowel S, Singer W. Selection of intrinsic horizontal connections in the visual cortex by correlated neuronal activity. *Science* 1992; 255(5041):209–212.

94. Jones EG. GABAergic neurons and their role in cortical plasticity in primates. *Cerebral Cortex* 1993; 3(5):361–372.

95. Hess G, Donoghue JP. Long-term depression of horizontal connections in rat motor cortex. *European J of Neuroscience* 1996; 8(4):658–665.

96. Lemon RN, Griffiths J. Comparing the function of the corticospinal system in different species: Organizational differences for motor specialization? *Muscle and Nerve* 2005; 32(3):261–279.

97. Glees P, Cole J. Recovery of skilled motor functions after small repeated lesions of motor cortex in macaque. *J of Neurophysiology* 1950; 13:137–148.

98. Nudo RJ, Wise BM, SiFuentes F, Milliken GW. Neural substrates for the effects of rehabilitative training on motor recovery after ischemic infarct. *Science* 1996; 272(5269):1791–1794.

99. Cramer SC, Nelles G, Benson RR, et al. A functional MRI study of subjects recovered from hemiparetic stroke. *Stroke* 1997; 28(12):2518–2527.

100. Jaillard A, Martin CD, Garambois K, et al. Vicarious function within the human primary motor cortex?: A longitudinal fMRI stroke study. *Brain* 2005; 128(Pt 5):1122–1138.

101. Teasell R, Bayona NA, Bitensky J. Plasticity and reorganization of the brain post stroke. *Top Stroke Rehabil* 2005; 12(3):11–26.

102. Butefisch CM, Kleiser R, Seitz RJ. Post-lesional cerebral reorganization: Evidence from functional neuroimaging and transcranial magnetic stimulation. *J Physiol Paris* 2006; 99(4–6):437–454.

103. Traversa R, Cicinelli P, Bassi A, et al. Mapping of motor cortical reorganization after stroke: A brain stimulation study with focal magnetic pulses. *Stroke* 1997; 28(1):110–117.

104. Liepert J, Graef S, Uhde I, et al. Training-induced changes of motor cortex representations in stroke patients. *Acta Neurol Scand* 2000; 101(5):321–326.

105. Carey JR, Kimberley TJ, Lewis SM, et al. Analysis of fMRI and finger tracking training in subjects with chronic stroke. *Brain* 2002; 125(Pt 4):773–788.

106. Liepert J, Miltner WH, Bauder H, et al. Motor cortex plasticity during constraint-induced movement therapy in stroke patients. *Neurosci Lett* 1998; 250(1):5–8.

107. Stroemer RP, Kent TA, Hulsebosch CE. Neocortical neural sprouting, synaptogenesis, and behavioral recovery after neocortical infarction in rats. *Stroke* 1995; 26(11):2135–2144.

108. Carmichael ST. Plasticity of cortical projections after stroke. *Neuroscientist* 2003; 9(1):64–75.

109. Carmichael ST. Cellular and molecular mechanisms of neural repair after stroke: Making waves. *Ann Neurol* 2006; 59(5):735–742.

110. Redecker C, Luhmann HJ, Hagemann G, et al. Differential downregulation of GABAA receptor subunits in widespread brain regions in the freeze-lesion model of focal cortical malformations. *J Neurosci* 2000; 20(13):5045–5053.

111. Liu Y, Rouiller EM. Mechanisms of recovery of dexterity following unilateral lesion of the sensorimotor cortex in adult monkeys. *Experimental Brain Research* 1999; 128(1–2):149–159.

112. Frost SB, Barbay S, Friel KM, et al. Reorganization of remote cortical regions after ischemic brain injury: A potential substrate for stroke recovery. *J of Neurophysiology* 2003; 89(6):3205–3214.

113. Lashley KS. *Brain Mechanisms and Intelligence: A Quantitative Study of Injuries to the Brain.* Chicago: Chicago Press; 1929.

114. Lashley KS. Basic neural mechanisms in behavior. *Physiol Rev* 1930; 37:1–24.

115. Biernaskie J, Szymanska A, Windle V, Corbett D. Bi-hemispheric contribution to functional motor recovery of the affected forelimb following focal ischemic brain injury in rats. *European Jl of Neuroscience* 2005; 21(4):989–999.

116. Dancause N, Barbay S, Frost SB, et al. Extensive cortical rewiring after brain injury. *J Neurosci* 2005; 25(44):10167–10179.

117. Chollet F, DiPiero V, Wise RJ, et al. The functional anatomy of motor recovery after stroke in humans: A study with positron emission tomography. *Ann Neurol* 1991; 29(1):63–71.

118. Nelles G, Spiekramann G, Jueptner M, et al. Evolution of functional reorganization in hemiplegic stroke: A serial positron emission tomographic activation study. *Ann Neurol* 1999; 46(6):901–909.

119. Weiller C, Ramsay SC, Wise RJ, et al. Individual patterns of functional reorganization in the human cerebral cortex after capsular infarction. *Ann Neurol* 1993; 33(2):181–189.

120. Seitz RJ, Kleiser R, Butefisch CM. Reorganization of cerebral circuits in human brain lesion. *Acta Neurochir Suppl* 2005; 93:65–70.

121. Weiller C, Chollet F, Friston KJ, et al. Functional reorganization of the brain in recovery from striatocapsular infarction in man. *Ann Neurol* 1992; 31(5):463–472.

122. Loubinoux I, Carel C, Pariente J, et al. Correlation between cerebral reorganization and motor recovery after subcortical infarcts. *Neuroimage* 2003; 20(4):2166–2180.

123. Miyai I, Suzuki T, Kang J, et al. Middle cerebral artery stroke that includes the premotor cortex reduces mobility outcome. *Stroke* 1999; 30(7):1380–1383.

124. Miyai I, Yagura H, Hatakenaka M, et al. Longitudinal optical imaging study for locomotor recovery after stroke. *Stroke* 2003; 34(12):2866–2870.

125. Fridman EA, Hanakawa T, Chung M, et al. Reorganization of the human ipsilesional premotor cortex after stroke. *Brain* 2004; 127(Pt 4):747–758.

126. Napieralski JA, Butler AK, Chesselet MF. Anatomical and functional evidence for lesion-specific sprouting of corticostriatal input in the adult rat. *J Comp Neurol* 1996; 373(4):484–497.

127. Wolf SL, Winstein CJ, Miller JP, et al. Effect of constraint-induced movement therapy on upper extremity function 3 to 9 months after stroke: The EXCITE randomized clinical trial. *JAMA* 2006; 296(17):2095–2104.

128. Barbay S, Zoubina EV, Dancause N, et al. A single injection of D-amphetamine facilitates improvements in motor training following a focal cortical infarct in squirrel monkeys. *Neurorehabil Neural Repair* 2006; 20(4):455–458.

129. Adkins DL, Campos P, Quach D, et al. Epidural cortical stimulation enhances motor function after sensorimotor cortical infarcts in rats. *Exp Neurol* 2006; 200(2):356–370.

130. Plautz E, Nudo R. Neural plasticity and functional recovery following cortical ischemic injury. *Conf Proc IEEE Eng Med Biol Soc* 2005; 4:4145–4148.

131. Webster BR, Celnik PA, Cohen LG. Noninvasive brain stimulation in stroke rehabilitation. *NeuroRx* 2006; 3(4):474–481.

132. Hanson MG, Landmesser LT. Normal patterns of spontaneous activity are required for correct motor axon guidance and the expression of specific guidance molecules. *Neuron* 2004; 43(5):687–701.

133. Price DJ, Kennedy H, Dehay C, et al. The development of cortical connections. *Eur J Neurosci* 2006; 23(4):910–920.

134. Uesaka N, Ruthazer ES, Yamamoto N. The role of neural activity in cortical axon branching. *Neuroscientist* 2006; 12(2):102–106.

135. Carmichael ST, Chesselet MF. Synchronous neuronal activity is a signal for axonal sprouting after cortical lesions in the adult. *J Neurosci* 2002; 22(14):6062–6070.

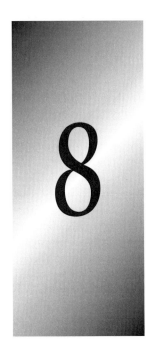

8 Functional Imaging and Stroke Recovery

Stephanie McHughen
Jill See
Steven C. Cramer

INTRODUCTION

Stroke remains a leading cause of death and disability in the United States and many other countries. Stroke can cause deficits in a number of neurologic domains, most commonly in the motor system (1, 2). In most patients, the time when spontaneous behavioral recovery is seen is the first three months following a stroke (3, 4)—though this time period might be longer for neglect, aphasia, and other cognitive areas (5–9). However, for most patients, behavioral restitution during this period of spontaneous recovery is incomplete, and significant impairment and disability remain.

There is a wide range in the severity of enduring deficits after stroke. Many factors have been examined as predictors. For example, severity of initial deficits has been found to be a strong predictor of final behavioral outcome, with some patients having mild-moderate initial stroke deficits and showing an excellent prognosis, but with others having severe baseline stroke deficits and showing a more variable recovery (10). In one study, a relative improvement of the initial motor score of about 20% in the first four weeks after stroke was associated with good outcome (11).

In considering the underlying basis for spontaneous recovery from stroke, attention can be directed at predictors of recovery. A number of other measures have been found to predict the degree of spontaneous recovery after stroke. Age, cognitive impairment, sensory or motor evoked potentials, accompanying neurologic deficits, volume of injury, MRI spectroscopy, features of injury, and location of injury have each been found to have value for predicting recovery and final motor status after stroke (11–24). Such a long list is not surprising, however, given the large number of factors that influence brain function after stroke (Table 8-1) (25). Measures of brain function also can predict behavioral outcome, as well as predict response to intervention, as discussed below.

GENETIC INFLUENCES ON STROKE RECOVERY

One area receiving increased attention in relation to stroke recovery and its influences is genetics. Variance in selected genotypes, particularly in brain-derived neurotrophic factor (BDNF), likely influences a number of recovery-related processes. BDNF is a protein that is found throughout the brain and is necessary for many essential functions, including developmental neuronal differentiation, axon outgrowth, long-term potentiation, synaptic plasticity, and repair (26–28, 29, 30). In adults, BDNF is released in a region-selective, activity-dependent manner, making it a critical regulator of experiential plasticity (31, 32).

TABLE 8-1

Clinical Variables that Likely Modify Brain Function After Stroke

Stroke topography and sites injured
Time post stroke
Age
Hemispheric dominance
Side of brain affected
Depression and psychiatric comorbidities
Injury to other brain network nodes
Infarct volume
Initial stroke deficits
Arterial patency
Medical comorbidities
Pre-stroke disability, social function, experience,
   and education
Type and amount of poststroke therapy
Acute stroke interventions
Medications during stroke recovery period
Final clinical status
Stroke mechanism
Genetics

Each human has two BDNF alleles. A single nucleotide polymorphism producing a valine to methionine amino acid substitution at codon 66 occurs in one of these alleles in approximately 27% of the American population (33). This val66met polymorphism affects intracellular BDNF trafficking and secretion and, therefore, likely impacts significantly upon synaptic plasticity (34, 35).

A number of changes in brain structure and function have been described in human subjects heterozygous for the BDNF val66met polymorphism, such as reduction in hippocampal volume, which is associated with reduced performance on memory tests, as well as decreased volume in the dorsolateral prefrontal cortex and subcortical regions like the caudate nucleus (34, 36–38). These reductions in volume might result from any number of changes to cortical morphology influenced by BDNF, including increased cell death, decreased neurogenesis, or reduced dendritic branching.

Studies using functional magnetic resonance imaging (fMRI) have shown that during tasks that result in hippocampal activation, such as a place recognition task, subjects with the BDNF val66met polymorphism have significantly lower levels of hippocampal activation during both encoding and retrieval when compared to subjects lacking this polymorphism (36). Similarly, Egan et al., using the N-back test, a working memory task, found that subjects with this polymorphism failed to demonstrate normal hippocampal activation, as compared to subjects without the polymorphism (34). In this study, the presence of this polymorphism was also associated with reduced performance on tests of episodic memory.

These data, together with the observation that this polymorphism is associated with lower depolarization-induced but not constitutive BDNF secretion (34), suggest that BDNF genotype might influence cortical function and thus be an important determinant of behavioral recovery after stroke. A recent study of cortical plasticity in healthy subjects provides some support toward this hypothesis (Figure 8-1). Subjects with the BDNF val66met polymorphism in one or both alleles showed significantly impaired short-term experience-dependent motor cortex plasticity, as assessed with transcranial magnetic stimulation (TMS) (39). Given the central role that cortical plasticity has in behavioral recovery after stroke, such effects of the BDNF val66met polymorphism suggest that this gene might have an important influence on stroke recovery.

METHODS FOR EXAMINING SPONTANEOUS BEHAVIORAL RECOVERY FOLLOWING STROKE

Animal Studies

A number of molecular events underlying spontaneous behavioral recovery after stroke have undergone increased study. Available evidence suggests a range of processes, many of which might be related to logical therapeutic targets in humans (30, 40–51). Direct measurement of such events is generally not possible in human subjects, however. In addition, animal models do not completely extrapolate to the human condition (52), as these often rely on quadrapeds, lack the heterogeneity of injury found in human strokes, vary with nature of induced injury (45, 53), have uniform preinfarct behavioral status, lack human stroke risk factors, and study the young and healthy.

Human Brain Mapping

Insights into the basis of spontaneous recovery after stroke are available from human brain mapping studies. Such functional neuroimaging can be a unique source of neurobiologic insights. For example, in subjects with a normal neurologic exam and normal brain anatomy, functional imaging can measure the effects on the brain of genes associated with neurologic disease (54–58). Functional imaging can measure the effects of CNS infection at a time when exam is normal, correlates of cognitive deficits with traumatic brain injury and normal brain anatomy (59), activity of brain motor systems in the setting of complete plegia (60, 61), and variability in cognitive reserve among healthy elderly subjects (62, 63).

Brain mapping data have provided insights into changes arising after stroke, many of which are concordant with repair-related findings in animals (42, 64–70). The

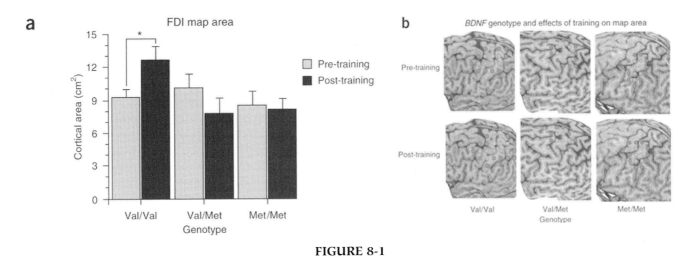

FIGURE 8-1

Changes in motor map area with training. (a) Mean (± SEM) representation area for the right first dorsal interosseus (FDI) muscle (*P < 0.05). (b) Representative motor maps of representations for this muscle from subjects lacking the val66met polymorphism (Val/Val), with the polymorphism on one allele (Val/Met), and with the polymorphism on both alleles (Met/Met), each superimposed onto a composite MRI image of the cortex. Blue dot, location of the site with lowest motor threshold. Green, other sites positive for producing a motor evoked response in right FDI upon TMS of left motor cortex. Red, negative sites. The presence of the val66met polymorphism on one or both alleles, present in 27% of the human population, is associated with reduced measures of experience-dependent cortical plasticity. From Kleim JA, Chan S, Pringle E,et al. Bdnf val66met polymorphism is associated with modified experience-dependent plasticity in human motor cortex. *Nat Neurosci* 2006;9:735–737.

current review considers these data, with an emphasis on fMRI of the motor system. One goal of these studies is to better understand reorganization of brain function to optimize restorative interventions and behavioral recovery, for example, by better predicting outcome, triaging, or defining measures of therapy at the level of the individual patient. This perspective is considered below.

CHANGES IN BRAIN FUNCTION IN RELATION TO RECOVERY OF BEHAVIOR AFTER STROKE

Ample data from studies in animals and humans have shown that the brain has the capacity to change structure and function, in association with behavioral recovery, in the days to weeks following a stroke. Several patterns of altered brain function have been described.

Increased Activation Across a Network

A common pattern described since the first functional imaging study of brain function after stroke (71) is increased activation within multiple nodes that together comprise distributed networks (72–85). This has been reported in numerous brain networks, including those related to motor, language, and attention functions. These studies converge on the conclusion that maintenance of behavioral output after injury to one node of a network is associated with increased activation within surviving

network areas, a finding further substantiated as studies have imaged patients with a broader range of behavioral outcomes (86, 87). In healthy subjects, performance of an increasingly complex task is also associated with increased activation of multiple brain areas comprising a network, and so in this regard, brain function after stroke can be thought of as analogous to perpetually performing in a high complexity setting (88–93).

Additional studies have shed light on these overactivations that are distant from the site of stroke-related injury. Increased activation in distal sites is highest in those with the poorest behavioral outcome (86, 94). However, evidence suggests that this change in brain function is nevertheless important to whatever behavioral recovery does occur spontaneously after stroke. Studies using a virtual lesion (95–99) and neurophysiological (100–102) approaches support the conclusion that the above post-stroke changes in brain function do contribute to motor status, but generally in association with an incomplete restoration of function.

Diaschisis

Other changes can arise in injured areas distant from stroke, including diaschisis. Diaschisis refers to reduced blood flow and metabolism in uninjured brain areas that have rich connections with injured brain areas (22, 103, 104). In some studies, behavioral recovery is related to resolution of diaschisis, that is, restitution of brain activity in uninjured areas that are distant from, but connected to, the site of infarct (105–107).

Reduced Activation in the Injured Zone

Though distant areas often show increased activity after stroke, the injured zone sometimes shows reduced activity, especially if injury is to elegant/eloquent cortex or its efferents (78). For example, a study of subjects who had reached a plateau in motor recovery after paresis-inducing stroke found that primary sensorimotor cortex activation in the stroke-affected hemisphere during affected hand movement was smallest in those with lesser recovery, moderate in those with full recovery, and largest in healthy controls (108). These results are concordant with TMS studies of motor cortex after stroke (109), which show that, after stroke, motor maps are smaller and corticospinal tract integrity is reduced in parallel with the severity of clinical deficits. Similar findings have been described with stroke affecting the language system, where aphasia is accompanied by increased activation in secondary cortical regions and decreased activation in the key dominant hemisphere language regions (81, 82, 110–112).

Displacement of Function and Representational Maps

In some cases, depending on the topography of injury, function can be displaced to neighboring areas (113). A common example of this compensatory event in the motor system is that, after stroke injures motor system elements related to hand movement, hand representation extends ventrally toward the face area. Weiller et al. described a ventral shift in the center of activation during motor task performance in recovered patients whose stroke affected the posterior aspect of the internal capsule (73). Subsequent fMRI studies reported the same finding among a wider range of patients with stroke (78, 87, 108). A shift of the motor cortex hand representation after stroke in the dorsal (114) or posterior (87, 115–119) direction has also been described, suggesting that topographic shifts in cortical representation site might reflect survival of distinct subsets of corticospinal tract fibers. Different patterns of injuries might thus invoke different forms of cortical map plasticity, a consideration that might explain the mosaic of reorganization patterns reported in some group analyses of stroke recovery (94).

Changes in Peri-Infarct Activity

One area that requires further study is the zone of surviving tissue that surrounds a cortical infarct. When examined histologically in animals, this zone shows the greatest levels of growth-related molecular changes after stroke (30, 40–43, 46–49, 51, 113, 120–124). Furthermore, in some cases these specific peri-infarct events can be further amplified by therapeutic intervention, a phenomenon that has been associated with additional behavioral gains (47, 48, 125, 126). Together, these observations suggest that this zone is of particular importance to the return of function after stroke, an assertion supported by human studies that found that the volume of threatened but surviving peri-infarct tissue is directly related to final clinical outcome (127, 128). Functional assessments of this zone in humans, using a range of functional neuroimaging modalities, has specifically noted activation in the peri-infarct region of patients with chronic stroke (74, 83, 112, 116, 129–136). The significance of these observations can be further clarified, for example, by assessing whether the extent of these events is related to behavioral status. One recent fMRI study of patients with cortical stroke did not find a significant correlation between the extent of peri-infarct activation and behavioral outcome after stroke (132). However, this correlation was complicated by the additional observation that the T2*-weighted MRI signal used to measure brain activation with fMRI was itself altered in the peri-infarct zone. This observation complicates interpretation of peri-infarct fMRI data in patients with cortical stroke and suggests that functional neuroimaging methods besides fMRI might be important to best understand the contribution that peri-infarct activity has to behavioral outcome after stroke.

Another finding in subjects with stroke is a reduction in the laterality of brain activity (72–76). For example, a right-hand motor task or language task that activates the left hemisphere in healthy controls will activate relevant regions within both the right and the left hemispheres in patients with a left hemisphere stroke. Indeed, a number of cases have been published where the main sites of brain activation are restricted to the non-stroke hemisphere, contralateral to findings in controls (74, 76, 137–139). This issue has also received considerable attention in the study of normal aging (63) and has also been discussed in a number of other contexts, including epilepsy (140), traumatic brain injury (141), and multiple sclerosis (142). Shift of activation balance toward the contralesional hemisphere is particularly common in the early days to weeks after a stroke (143). Subsequently, the activation balance shifts back toward the stroke-affected hemisphere, more so in patients with better behavioral outcome (81, 86, 87, 143–146).

A shift in hemispheric lateralization might in part reflect changes in the balance of interhemispheric inhibition (147–151). Whatever the underlying mechanism, several lines of evidence do support the assertion that this supranormal contralesional recruitment does indeed contribute to behavioral recovery after stroke (80, 81, 95–97, 152–158).

Changes in Inter-hemispheric Laterality

A number of factors have been found to modify the extent to which stroke is associated with a reduction in the degree of inter-hemispheric laterality. Examples include time after stroke, with laterality increasing toward normal as patients recover (81, 106, 143, 144, 159, 160); hemispheric dominance, with motor task performance with the non-dominant hand being less lateralized than with the dominant hand in both healthy controls and after stroke (74, 108, 161); topography of injury, with reduced laterality being more common with a cortical, as opposed to subcortical, infarct (130, 160); and greater injury and/or deficits, with reduced laterality present with larger infarcts and more severe behavioral deficits (87, 144, 162, 163). Other factors relevant to laterality in normal subjects are also likely important after stroke, with less lateralization present with increasing task complexity (88–93), increasing subject age (63), lower task familiarity (164), and more proximal movement (119, 165, 166). In one study, gender also influenced laterality of brain activation (167). Note that when laterality is reduced and activation shifted toward the hemisphere ipsilateral to movement, the site of activation is different, at least in the motor system. Activation during ipsilateral hand movement differs from that present during movement of the contralateral hand, in that the former, possibly representing premotor cortex activity, is often anterior and ventral (139, 168).

Time is also an important factor in the study of brain function after stroke. Early after stroke, insulted brain areas show reduced function. Intact areas with strong connections to sites of injury sometimes show reduced function as a consequence of diaschisis. Laterality is shifted toward the non-affected hemisphere. Over time, the shift of balance points back toward the affected hemisphere, with reduced activation in the non-stroke hemisphere and increased activation in the stroke-affected hemisphere. Some therapies have demonstrated value in increasing this shift back toward the affected hemisphere (78, 81, 94, 106, 143, 144, 146, 156, 160, 169, 170).

One principle apparent from review of the literature is that changes in brain function after stroke for a given task are related in part to the normal functional anatomy for that task. Thus, swallowing (171), facial movement (87), and gait (172) are more bilaterally organized than distal extremity movements normally, and a shift in hemispheric balance after stroke occurs most often and with greatest clinical gains in these tasks. Similarly, movement of the non-dominant hand is more bilaterally organized than the dominant hand normally, and this too remains true after stroke (108). This principle suggests the hypothesis that behaviors that are more bilaterally organized normally might benefit from a more bilateral approach to therapy. However, elegant and eloquent neocortex functions are generally highly lateralized, that is, localized to the dominant hemisphere, and for these brain regions, the best behavioral outcomes are apparent when this remains true after stroke.

THERAPEUTIC INTERVENTION AND RECOVERY

A number of restorative interventions are under study, including cells, selective serotonin re-uptake inhibitors, catecholaminergics, regional electrical stimulation of brain, genetic manipulations, neuroprosthetics, robotics, imagery-based protocols, and function-oriented physical therapy regimens (48, 49, 126, 173–181). However, none is currently approved therapy for enhancing outcome after CNS injury such as stroke. The maximum value of functional neuroimaging methods such as fMRI will be appreciated when used to improve application of an established restorative intervention.

One case for use of functional neuroimaging to improve application of restorative interventions is made from examining medical practice in non-neural systems. For many body systems, data on the functioning of an organ are used to inform and improve clinical decision-making. Hypothyroidism is optimally treated by serial measures of pituitary-thyroid axis via serum TSH. Treatment of myeloproliferative and other hematological syndromes is dosed based on serial measure of the cell population of interest. Cardiac arrhythmias are sometimes treated by inducing tissue dysfunction and then evaluating the effectiveness of the selected drug. Coronary artery disease is often assessed by stressing the heart with exercise or the sympathomimetic dobutamine. These practices suggest that some form of functional neuroimaging might be useful for patient selection, treatment selection, or treatment dosing when introducing a restorative intervention with the intent of modifying brain function and behavioral status.

Brain Mapping to Guide Post-stroke Therapy

Some studies have already made strides in this regard. One series of studies used fMRI to guide details of decision-making during therapy (179, 182). An fMRI scan was used to identify the centroid of primary motor cortex activation in patients with stroke. This information then guided neurosurgical placement of an investigational epidural cortical stimulation device. Using this approach, patients receiving stimulation plus rehabilitation therapy showed significant greater arm motor gains than patients receiving rehabilitation therapy alone. A similar approach was used in studies that found repetitive TMS to be useful for improving motor function after stroke (178, 183). These studies employed TMS to identify the optimal physiological representation site for hand motor function.

Brain Mapping to Predict Treatment Responses and Outcomes

Several studies have used an assessment of brain function to predict response to a restorative intervention (184–188). For example, Koski et al. (187), using transcranial magnetic stimulation, and Dong et al. (185), using fMRI, have found that changes in brain function early into therapy anticipate final behavioral gains.

A recent study (188) examined the ability of a baseline fMRI to predict trial-related behavioral gains. These patients each underwent baseline clinical and functional MRI assessments, received six weeks of rehabilitation therapy with or without investigational motor cortex stimulation, and then had repeat assessments. Across all patients, several baseline measures showed predictive value for trial-related gains in univariate analyses. However, multiple linear regression modeling found that, when controlling for other factors, only two variables remained significant predictors: degree of motor cortex activation on fMRI (lower motor cortex activation predicted larger gains) and arm motor function (greater arm function predicted larger gains). This study emphasizes that an assessment of brain function can be uniquely informative for clinical decision-making in the setting of restorative therapy after stroke. Interestingly, clinical gains during study participation were paralleled by boosts in motor cortex activity, suggesting that, in some patients, lower baseline cortical activity represents under-use of surviving cortical resources.

Functional Imaging of Treatment-induced Recovery

The principles important to reorganization of brain function during spontaneous recovery from stroke might also operate in the setting of treatment-induced recovery. If true, functional imaging might be a useful tool to help guide patient selection or choice of rehabilitation strategies, for example, by measuring the capacity of residual brain networks to respond to therapeutic challenges. Differences in patients and their patterns of injury are likely associated with divergent responses to rehabilitation therapy. As with spontaneous recovery, functional imaging of therapy-induced recovery might be a unique source of insights. Published studies support this for constraint-induced motor therapy.

Constraint-induced motor therapy is an approach to improving motor function that is effective in producing enduring (189) motor gains in eligible patients in the setting of chronic (181, 189, 190), subacute (191), or acute (192) stroke. A range of functional neuroimaging methods, including EEG, fMRI, and TMS (193–198), has demonstrated changes in brain function that parallel treatment-related motor gains. Changes in brain function after constraint-induced motor therapy include altered motor excitability, a shift in activated brain areas, a change in motor system inter-hemispheric laterality, and an increase in affected hand motor representation area (199, 200). However, studies disagree as to how post-stroke constraint-induced motor therapy affects these measures of brain function. This divergence in findings likely reflects differences in patient characteristics. For example, successful constraint-induced motor therapy was associated with reduced inter-hemispheric laterality in a study of weaker (194), and increased laterality in a study of stronger (198), patients with chronic stroke. Prior to therapy, brain function after stroke differs in relation to behavioral status; this is likely equally true during and after therapy. Understanding these differences might be important to using functional imaging as a tool to guide post-stroke rehabilitation therapy.

Motor Learning and Plasticity

Application of rehabilitation therapies might be improved if based on models of patterns of brain plasticity seen in normal subjects. For example, some authors have drawn a parallel between brain events related to learning and those underlying rehabilitation-based motor gains after stroke (201). Motor learning theory is particularly important to the clinical application of post-stroke therapies, such as constraint-induced motor therapy, given that a goal of these approaches includes improved performance and retention of new motor skills. Studies of motor learning provide insights into the brain events underlying acquisition or refinement of movement skills (202–204), for example, with activity shifting from cortical to subcortical (204–207) or cerebellar (203) areas. Such changes can be short-term (205, 208, 209) or long-term (208, 209), with both measures being potentially important to understanding how structures of the brain motor system store kinematic details induced by motor training. Implicit motor learning is an approach that might be particularly valuable for subjects with stroke, given the frequency with which concomitant deficits could impair explicit learning (210–214), though specific lesions such as of thalamus or basal ganglia might interfere with implicit motor skill acquisition (215).

Future Studies

A recent review (216) examined studies that have employed functional neuroimaging as a biological marker of treatment effects targeting the motor system after stroke. Across 13 studies of 121 patients, conclusions included that motor deficits have been most often studied, in part because of their substantial contribution to overall disability after stroke, and in part because of their relatively high prevalence. Most published studies have focused on patients with good to excellent outcome at baseline since they were more able to perform the motor tasks required to probe brain function. Consequently, less is known about the functional anatomy of therapy-induced recovery processes in the large population of patients with more severe deficits after stroke. Very few studies have used functional imaging to examine treatment effects during the first few months after stroke, when spontaneous behavioral recovery is at its greatest. The effects that many key variables such as lesion site, recovery level, gender, and age have on the performance of functional neuroimaging in this context requires further study. Studies could be improved by incorporating measures of injury and/or physiology

Measuring the function of the brain is likely useful for defining features of therapy. A better understanding of the underlying neurobiologic principles related to therapy-induced behavioral gains will likely improve application of interventions that aim to minimize impairment and reduce disability in patients with stroke.

References

1. Rathore S, Hinn A, Cooper L, et al. Characterization of incident stroke signs and symptoms: Findings from the atherosclerosis risk in communities study. *Stroke* 2002; 33:2718–2721.
2. Gresham G, Duncan P, Stason W, et al. *Post-stroke rehabilitation*. Rockville, MD: U.S. Department of Health and Human Services: Public Health Service, Agency for Health Care Policy and Research, 1995.
3. Nakayama H, Jorgensen H, Raaschou H, Olsen T. Recovery of upper extremity function in stroke patients: The copenhagen stroke study. *Arch Phys Med Rehabil* 1994; 75:394–398.
4. Duncan P, Lai S, Keighley J. Defining post-stroke recovery: Implications for design and interpretation of drug trials. *Neuropharmacology* 2000; 39:835–841.
5. Kertesz A, McCabe P. Recovery patterns and prognosis in aphasia. *Brain* 1977; 100 Pt 1:1–18.
6. Hier D, Mondlock J, Caplan L. Recovery of behavioral abnormalities after right hemisphere stroke. *Neurology* 1983; 33:345–350.
7. Desmond D, Moroney J, Sano M, Stern Y. Recovery of cognitive function after stroke. *Stroke* 1996; 27:1798–1803.
8. Kotila M, Waltimo O, Niemi M, et al. The profile of recovery from stroke and factors influencing outcome. *Stroke* 1984; 15:1039–1044.
9. Wade D, Parker V, Langton Hewer R. Memory disturbance after stroke: Frequency and associated losses. *Int Rehabil Med* 1986; 8:60–64.
10. Jorgensen HS, Nakayama H, Raaschou HO, Olsen TS. Stroke: Neurologic and functional recovery. The Copenhagen Stroke Study. *Phys Med Rehabil Clin N Am* 1999; 10:887–906.
11. Binkofski F, Seitz RJ, Hacklander T, et al. Recovery of motor functions following hemiparetic stroke: A clinical and magnetic resonance-morphometric study. *Cerebrovasc Dis* 2001; 11:273–281.
12. Hinkle JL. Variables explaining functional recovery following motor stroke. *J Neurosci Nurs* 2006; 38:6–12.
13. Tzvetanov P, Milanov I, Rousseff RT, Christova P. Can ssep results predict functional recovery of stroke patients within the "therapeutic window"? *Electromyogr Clin Neurophysiol* 2004; 44:43–49.
14. Tzvetanov P, Rousseff RT, Milanov I. Lower limb ssep changes in stroke-predictive values regarding functional recovery. *Clin Neurol Neurosurg* 2003; 105:121–127.
15. Kwakkel G, Kollen BJ, van der Grond J, Prevo AJ. Probability of regaining dexterity in the flaccid upper limb: Impact of severity of paresis and time since onset in acute stroke. *Stroke* 2003; 34:2181–2186.
16. Trompetto C, Assini A, Buccolieri A, et al. Motor recovery following stroke: A transcranial magnetic stimulation study. *Clin Neurophysiol* 2000; 111:1860–1867.
17. Feys H, Van Hees J, Bruyninckx F, et al. Value of somatosensory and motor-evoked potentials in predicting arm recovery after a stroke. *J Neurol Neurosurg Psychiatry* 2000; 68:323–331.
18. Escudero J, Sancho J, Bautista D, et al. Prognostic value of motor-evoked potential obtained by transcranial magnetic brain stimulation in motor function recovery in patients with acute ischemic stroke. *Stroke* 1998; 29:1854–1859.
19. Watanabe T, Honda Y, Fujii Y, et al. Three-dimensional anisotropy contrast magnetic resonance axonography to predict the prognosis for motor function in patients suffering from stroke. *J Neurosurg* 2001; 94:955–960.
20. Heald A, Bates D, Cartlidge N, et al. Longitudinal study of central motor conduction time following stroke. 2. Central motor conduction measured within 72 h after stroke as a predictor of functional outcome at 12 months. *Brain* 1993; 116:1371–1385.
21. Wenzelburger R, Kopper F, Frenzel A, et al. Hand coordination following capsular stroke. *Brain* 2005; 128:64–74.
22. Binkofski F, Seitz R, Arnold S, et al. Thalamic metabolism and corticospinal tract integrity determine motor recovery in stroke. *Ann Neurol* 1996; 39:460–470.
23. Crafton K, Mark A, Cramer S. Improved understanding of cortical injury by incorporating measures of functional anatomy. *Brain* 2003; 126:1650–1659.
24. Pendlebury S, Blamire A, Lee M, et al. Axonal injury in the internal capsule correlates with motor impairment after stroke. *Stroke* 1999; 30:956–962.
25. Cramer S. Functional imaging in stroke recovery. *Stroke* 2004; 35:2695–2698.
26. Huang EJ, Reichardt LF. Neurotrophins: Roles in neuronal development and function. *Annu Rev Neurosci* 2001; 24:677–736.
27. Bibel M, Barde YA. Neurotrophins: Key regulators of cell fate and cell shape in the vertebrate nervous system. *Genes Dev* 2000; 14:2919–2937.
28. Kang H, Schuman EM. Long-lasting neurotrophin-induced enhancement of synaptic transmission in the adult hippocampus. *Science* 1995; 267:1658–1662.
29. Levine ES, Dreyfus CF, Black IB, Plummer MR. Brain-derived neurotrophic factor rapidly enhances synaptic transmission in hippocampal neurons via postsynaptic tyrosine kinase receptors. *Proc Natl Acad Sci U S A* 1995; 92:8074–8077.
30. Kleim JA, Jones TA, Schallert T. Motor enrichment and the induction of plasticity before or after brain injury. *Neurochem Res* 2003; 28:1757–1769.
31. Ishibashi H, Hihara S, Takahashi M, et al. Tool-use learning induces bdnf expression in a selective portion of monkey anterior parietal cortex. *Brain Res Mol Brain Res* 2002; 102:110–112.
32. Kuipers SD, Bramham CR. Brain-derived neurotrophic factor mechanisms and function in adult synaptic plasticity: New insights and implications for therapy. *Curr Opin Drug Discov Devel* 2006; 9:580–586.
33. Shimizu E, Hashimoto K, Iyo M. Ethnic difference of the bdnf 196g/a (val66met) polymorphism frequencies: The possibility to explain ethnic mental traits. *Am J Med Genet B Neuropsychiatr Genet* 2004; 126:122–123.
34. Egan MF, Kojima M, Callicott JH, et al. The bdnf val66met polymorphism affects activity-dependent secretion of bdnf and human memory and hippocampal function. *Cell* 2003; 112:257–269.
35. Chen ZY, Patel PD, Sant G, et al. Variant brain-derived neurotrophic factor (bdnf) (met66) alters the intracellular trafficking and activity-dependent secretion of wild-type bdnf in neurosecretory cells and cortical neurons. *J Neurosci* 2004; 24:4401–4411.
36. Hariri AR, Goldberg TE, Mattay VS, et al. Brain-derived neurotrophic factor val66met polymorphism affects human memory-related hippocampal activity and predicts memory performance. *J Neurosci* 2003; 23:6690–6694.
37. Pezawas L, Verchinski BA, Mattay VS, et al. The brain-derived neurotrophic factor val66met polymorphism and variation in human cortical morphology. *J Neurosci* 2004; 24:10099–10102.
38. Szeszko PR, Lipsky R, Mentschel C, et al. Brain-derived neurotrophic factor val66met polymorphism and volume of the hippocampal formation. *Mol Psychiatry* 2005; 10:631–636.
39. Kleim JA, Chan S, Pringle E, et al. Bdnf val66met polymorphism is associated with modified experience-dependent plasticity in human motor cortex. *Nat Neurosci* 2006; 9:735–737.
40. Carmichael ST. Plasticity of cortical projections after stroke. *Neuroscientist* 2003; 9:64–75.
41. Carmichael ST, Archibeque I, Luke L, et al. Growth-associated gene expression after stroke: Evidence for a growth-promoting region in peri-infarct cortex. *Exp Neurol* 2005; 193:291–311.
42. Carmichael ST. Cellular and molecular mechanisms of neural repair after stroke: Making waves. *Ann Neurol* 2006; 59:735–742.
43. Nudo R, Plautz E, Frost S. Role of adaptive plasticity in recovery of function after damage to motor cortex. *Muscle Nerve* 2001; 24:1000–1019.
44. Dijkhuizen R, Singhal A, Mandeville J, et al. Correlation between brain reorganization, ischemic damage, and neurologic status after transient focal cerebral ischemia in rats: A functional magnetic resonance imaging study. *J Neurosci* 2003; 23:510–517.

45. Voorhies A, Jones T. The behavioral and dendritic growth effects of focal sensorimotor cortical damage depend on the method of lesion induction. *Behav Brain Res* 2002; 133:237–246.

46. Biernaskie J, Corbett D. Enriched rehabilitative training promotes improved forelimb motor function and enhanced dendritic growth after focal ischemic injury. *J Neurosci* 2001; 21:5272–5280.

47. Kleim J, Bruneau R, VandenBerg P, et al. Motor cortex stimulation enhances motor recovery and reduces peri-infarct dysfunction following ischemic insult. *Neurol Res* 2003; 25:789–793.

48. Stroemer R, Kent T, Hulsebosch C. Enhanced neocortical neural sprouting, synaptogenesis, and behavioral recovery with d-amphetamine therapy after neocortical infarction in rats. *Stroke* 1998; 29:2381–2395.

49. Kawamata T, Dietrich W, Schallert T, et al. Intracisternal basic fibroblast growth factor (bfgf) enhances functional recovery and upregulates the expression of a molecular marker of neuronal sprouting following focal cerebral infarction. *Proc Natl Acad Sci* 1997; 94:8179–8184.

50. Jones T, Schallert T. Overgrowth and pruning of dendrites in adult rats recovering from neocortical damage. *Brain Res* 1992; 581:156–160.

51. Li Y, Chen J, Zhang CL, et al. Gliosis and brain remodeling after treatment of stroke in rats with marrow stromal cells. *Glia* 2005; 49:407–417.

52. Cramer S. Clinical issues in animal models of stroke and rehabilitation. *Ilar J* 2003; 44:83–84.

53. Napieralski JA, Butler AK, Chesselet MF. Anatomical and functional evidence for lesion-specific sprouting of corticostriatal input in the adult rat. *J Comp Neurol* 1996; 373:484–497.

54. Bookheimer S, Strojwas M, Cohen M, et al. Patterns of brain activation in people at risk for alzheimer's disease. *N Engl J Med* 2000; 343:450–456.

55. Phelps M. PET: The merging of biology and imaging into molecular imaging. *J Nucl Med* 2000; 41:661–681.

56. Harris GJ, Codori AM, Lewis RF, et al. Reduced basal ganglia blood flow and volume in pre-symptomatic, gene-tested persons at-risk for Huntington's disease. *Brain* 1999; 122 (Pt 9):1667–1678.

57. Eidelberg D, Moeller J, Antonini A, et al. Functional brain networks in dyt1 dystonia. *Ann Neurol* 1998; 44:303–312.

58. Brooks DJ. The early diagnosis of Parkinson's disease. *Ann Neurol* 1998; 44:S10–S18.

59. Fontaine A, Azouvi P, Remy P, et al. Functional anatomy of neuropsychological deficits after severe traumatic brain injury. *Neurology* 1999; 53:1963–1968.

60. Cramer S, Mark A, Barquist K, et al. Motor cortex activation is preserved in patients with chronic hemiplegic stroke. *Ann Neurol* 2002; 52:607–616.

61. Cramer SC, Lastra L, Lacourse MG, Cohen MJ. Brain motor system function after chronic, complete spinal cord injury. *Brain* 2005; 128:2941–2950.

62. Scarmeas N, Zarahn E, Anderson K, et al. Cognitive reserve modulates functional brain responses during memory tasks: A PET study in healthy young and elderly subjects. *Neuroimage* 2003; 19:1215–1227.

63. Cabeza R. Hemispheric asymmetry reduction in older adults: The Harold model. *Psychol Aging* 2002; 17:85–100.

64. Ziemann U, Hallett M. Hemispheric asymmetry of ipsilateral motor cortex activation during unimanual motor tasks: Further evidence for motor dominance. *Clin Neurophysiol* 2001; 112:107–113.

65. Ward NS, Cohen LG. Mechanisms underlying recovery of motor function after stroke. *Arch Neurol* 2004; 61:1844–1848.

66. Takahashi CD, Der Yeghiaian L, Cramer SC. Stroke recovery and its imaging. *Neuroimaging Clin N Am* 2005; 15:681–695.

67. Rijntjes M, Weiller C. Recovery of motor and language abilities after stroke: The contribution of functional imaging. *Prog Neurobiol* 2002; 66:109–122.

68. Nudo R. Functional and structural plasticity in motor cortex: Implications for stroke recovery. *Phys Med Rehabil Clin N Am* 2003; 14:S57–76.

69. Munoz-Cespedes JM, Rios-Lago M, Paul N, Maestu F. Functional neuroimaging studies of cognitive recovery after acquired brain damage in adults. *Neuropsychol Rev* 2005; 15:169–183.

70. Baron J, Cohen L, Cramer S, et al. Neuroimaging in stroke recovery: A position paper from the first international workshop on neuroimaging and stroke recovery. *Cerebrovasc Dis* 2004; 18:260–267.

71. Brion J-P, Demeurisse G, Capon A. Evidence of cortical reorganization in hemiparetic patients. *Stroke* 1989; 20:1079–1084.

72. Chollet F, DiPiero V, Wise R, et al. The functional anatomy of motor recovery after stroke in humans: A study with positron emission tomography. *Ann Neurol* 1991; 29:63–71.

73. Weiller C, Ramsay S, Wise R,. Individual patterns of functional reorganization in the human cerebral cortex after capsular infarction. *Ann Neurol* 1993; 33:181–189.

74. Cramer S, Nelles G, Benson R,. A functional MRI study of subjects recovered from hemiparetic stroke. *Stroke* 1997; 28:2518–2527.

75. Seitz R, Hoflich P, Binkofski F, et al. Role of the premotor cortex in recovery from middle cerebral artery infarction. *Arch Neurol* 1998; 55:1081–1088.

76. Cao Y, D'Olhaberriague L, Vikingstad E,. Pilot study of functional MRI to assess cerebral activation of motor function after poststroke hemiparesis. *Stroke* 1998; 29:112–122.

77. Calautti C, Leroy F, Guincestre J, et al. Sequential activation brain mapping after subcortical stroke: Changes in hemispheric balance and recovery. *Neuroreport* 2001; 12:3883–3886.

78. Tombari D, Loubinoux I, Pariente J, et al. A longitudinal fMRI study: In recovering and then in clinically stable sub-cortical stroke patients. *Neuroimage* 2004; 23:827–839.

79. Weiller C, Isensee C, Rijntjes M, et al. Recovery from Wernicke's aphasia: A positron emission tomographic study. *Ann Neurol* 1995; 37:723–732.

80. Thulborn K, Carpenter P, Just M. Plasticity of language-related brain function during recovery from stroke. *Stroke* 1999; 30:749–754.

81. Heiss W, Kessler J, Thiel A, et al. Differential capacity of left and right hemispheric areas for compensation of poststroke aphasia. *Ann Neurol* 1999; 45:430–438.

82. Cao Y, Vikingstad E, George K, et al. Cortical language activation in stroke patients recovering from aphasia with functional MRI. *Stroke* 1999; 30:2331–2340.

83. Rosen H, Petersen S, Linenweber M, et al. Neural correlates of recovery from aphasia after damage to left inferior frontal cortex. *Neurology* 2000; 55:1883–1894.

84. Mesulam MM. Large-scale neurocognitive networks and distributed processing for attention, language, and memory. *Ann Neurol* 1990; 28:597–613.

85. Corbetta M, Burton H, Sinclair R, et al. Functional reorganization and stability of somatosensory-motor cortical topography in a tetraplegic subject with late recovery. *Proc Natl Acad Sci U S A* 2002; 99:17066–17071.

86. Ward N, Brown M, Thompson A, Frackowiak R. Neural correlates of outcome after stroke: A cross-sectional fMRI study. *Brain* 2003; 126:1430–1448.

87. Cramer SC, Crafton KR. Somatotopy and movement representation sites following cortical stroke. *Exp Brain Res* 2006; 168:25–32.

88. Just M, Carpenter P, Keller T, et al. Brain activation modulated by sentence comprehension. *Science* 1996; 274:114–116.

89. Sadato N, Campbell G, Ibanez V, et al. Complexity affects regional cerebral blood flow change during sequential finger movements. *J Neurosci* 1996; 16:2691–2700.

90. Baumgaertner A, Weiller C, Buchel C. Event-related fMRI reveals cortical sites involved in contextual sentence integration. *Neuroimage* 2002; 16:736–745.

91. Hummel F, Kirsammer R, Gerloff C. Ipsilateral cortical activation during finger sequences of increasing complexity: Representation of movement difficulty or memory load? *Clin Neurophysiol* 2003; 114:605–613.

92. Wexler B, Fulbright R, Lacadie C, et al. An fMRI study of the human cortical motor system response to increasing functional demands. *Magn Reson Imaging* 1997; 15:385–396.

93. Shibasaki H, Sadato N, Lyshkow H, et al. Both primary motor cortex and supplementary motor area play an important role in complex finger movement. *Brain* 1993; 116:1387–1398.

94. Ward N, Brown M, Thompson A, Frackowiak R. Neural correlates of motor recovery after stroke: A longitudinal fMRI study. *Brain* 2003; 126:2476–2496.

95. Lotze M, Markert J, Sauseng P, et al. The role of multiple contralesional motor areas for complex hand movements after internal capsular lesion. *J Neurosci* 2006; 26:6096–6102.

96. Winhuisen L, Thiel A, Schumacher B, et al. Role of the contralateral inferior frontal gyrus in recovery of language function in poststroke aphasia: A combined repetitive transcranial magnetic stimulation and positron emission tomography study. *Stroke* 2005; 36:1759–1763.

97. Johansen-Berg H, Rushworth M, Bogdanovic M, et al. The role of ipsilateral premotor cortex in hand movement after stroke. *Proc Natl Acad Sci U S A* 2002; 99:14518–14523.

98. Werhahn K, Conforto A, Kadom N, et al. Contribution of the ipsilateral motor cortex to recovery after chronic stroke. *Ann Neurol* 2003; 54:464–472.

99. Fridman E, Hanakawa T, Chung M, et al. Reorganization of the human ipsilesional premotor cortex after stroke. *Brain* 2004; 127:747–758.

100. Butefisch CM, Kleiser R, Korber B, et al. Recruitment of contralesional motor cortex in stroke patients with recovery of hand function. *Neurology* 2005; 64:1067–1069.

101. Serrien DJ, Strens LH, Cassidy MJ,. Functional significance of the ipsilateral hemisphere during movement of the affected hand after stroke. *Exp Neurol* 2004; 190:425–432.

102. Gerloff C, Bushara K, Sailer A, et al. Multimodal imaging of brain reorganization in motor areas of the contralesional hemisphere of well-recovered patients after capsular stroke. *Brain* 2006; 129:791–808.

103. von Monakow C. Diaschisis. Mood, states and mind. In: Pribram K, ed. *Brain and Behavior*. Baltimore: Penguin Books, 1914:26–34.

104. Feeney D, Baron J. Diaschisis. *Stroke* 1986; 17:817–830.

105. Carmichael ST, Tatsukawa K, Katsman D, et al. Evolution of diaschisis in a focal stroke model. *Stroke* 2004; 35:758–763.

106. Nhan H, Barquist K, Bell K, et al. Brain function early after stroke in relation to subsequent recovery. *J Cereb Blood Flow Metab* 2004; 24:756–763.

107. Seitz R, Azari N, Knorr U, et al. The role of diaschisis in stroke recovery. *Stroke* 1999; 30:1844–1850.

108. Zemke A, Heagerty P, Lee C, Cramer S. Motor cortex organization after stroke is related to side of stroke and level of recovery. *Stroke* 2003; 34:E23–E28.

109. Talelli P, Greenwood RJ, Rothwell JC. Arm function after stroke: Neurophysiological correlates and recovery mechanisms assessed by transcranial magnetic stimulation. *Clin Neurophysiol* 2006; 117:1641–1659.

110. Blank S, Bird H, Turkheimer F, Wise R. Speech production after stroke: The role of the right pars opercularis. *Ann Neurol* 2003; 54:310–320.

111. Hillis A, Wityk R, Tuffiash E, et al. Hypoperfusion of Wernicke's area predicts severity of semantic deficit in acute stroke. *Ann Neurol* 2001; 50:561–566.

112. Warburton E, Price C, Swinburn K, Wise R. Mechanisms of recovery from aphasia: Evidence from positron emission tomography studies. *J Neurol Neurosurg Psychiatry* 1999; 66:155–161.

113. Nudo R, Wise B, SiFuentes F, Milliken G. Neural substrates for the effects of rehabilitative training on motor recovery after ischemic infarct. *Science* 1996; 272:1791–1794.

114. Jaillard A, Martin C, Garambois K, et al. Vicarious function within the human primary motor cortex?: A longitudinal fMRI stroke study. *Brain* 2005; 128:1122–1138.

115. Rossini PM, Caltagirone C, Castriota-Scanderbeg A, et al. Hand motor cortical area reorganization in stroke: A study with fMRI, MEG and TCS maps. *Neuroreport* 1998; 9:2141–2146.

116. Cramer S, Moore C, Finklestein S, Rosen B. A pilot study of somatotopic mapping after cortical infarct. *Stroke* 2000; 31:668–671.

117. Pineiro R, Pendlebury S, Johansen-Berg H, Matthews P. Functional MRI detects posterior shifts in primary sensorimotor cortex activation after stroke: Evidence of local adaptive reorganization? *Stroke* 2001; 32:1134–1139.

118. Calautti C, Leroy F, Guincestre J, Baron J. Displacement of primary sensorimotor cortex activation after subcortical stroke: A longitudinal PET study with clinical correlation. *Neuroimage* 2003; 19:1650–1654.

119. Cramer S, Crafton K. Changes in lateralization and somatotopic organization after cortical stroke. *Stroke* 2004; 35:240.

120. Speliotes E, Caday C, Do T, et al. Increased expression of basic fibroblast growth factor (BFGF) following focal cerebral infarction in the rat. *Brain Res Mol Brain Res* 1996; 39:31–42.

121. Witte O, Bidmon H, Schiene K, et al. Functional differentiation of multiple perilesional zones after focal cerebral ischemia. *J Cereb Blood Flow Metab* 2000; 20:1149–1165.

122. Eysel U. Perilesional cortical dysfunction and reorganization. *Adv Neurol* 1997; 73:195–206.

123. Xerri C, Merzenich M, Peterson B, Jenkins W. Plasticity of primary somatosensory cortex paralleling sensorimotor skill recovery from stroke in adult monkeys. *J Neurophysiol* 1998; 79:2119–2148.

124. Cramer S, Chopp M. Recovery recapitulates ontogeny. *Trends Neurosci* 2000; 23:265–271.

125. Plautz E, Barbay S, Frost S, et al. Post-infarct cortical plasticity and behavioral recovery using concurrent cortical stimulation and rehabilitative training: A feasibility study in primates. *Neurol Res* 2003; 25:801–810.

126. Chen J, Li Y, Katakowski M, et al. Intravenous bone marrow stromal cell therapy reduces apoptosis and promotes endogenous cell proliferation after stroke in female rat. *J Neurosci Res* 2003; 73:778–786.

127. Furlan M, Marchal G, Viader F, et al. Spontaneous neurological recovery after stroke and the fate of the ischemic penumbra. *Ann Neurol* 1996; 40:216–226.

128. Heiss W, Grond M, Thiel A, et al. Tissue at risk of infarction rescued by early reperfusion: A positron emission tomography study in systemic recombinant tissue plasminogen activator thrombolysis of acute stroke. *J Cereb Blood Flow Metab* 1998; 18:1298–1307.

129. Binkofski F, Seitz R. Modulation of the bold-response in early recovery from sensorimotor stroke. *Neurology* 2004; 63:1223–1229.

130. Luft A, Waller S, Forrester L, et al. Lesion location alters brain activation in chronically impaired stroke survivors. *Neuroimage* 2004; 21:924–935.

131. Rossini P, Dal Forno G. Integrated technology for evaluation of brain function and neural plasticity. *Phys Med Rehabil Clin N Am* 2004; 15:263–306.

132. Cramer SC, Shah R, Juranek J, et al. Activity in the peri-infarct rim in relation to recovery from stroke. *Stroke* 2006; 37:111–115.

133. Butz M, Gross J, Timmermann L, et al. Perilesional pathological oscillatory activity in the magnetoencephalogram of patients with cortical brain lesions. *Neurosci Lett* 2004; 355:93–96.

134. Hensel S, Rockstroh B, Berg P, et al. Left-hemispheric abnormal EEG activity in relation to impairment and recovery in aphasic patients. *Psychophysiology* 2004; 41:394–400.

135. Demougeot C, Walker P, Beley A, et al. Spectroscopic data following stroke reveal tissue abnormality beyond the region of t2-weighted hyperintensity. *J Neurol Sci* 2002; 199:73–78.

136. Heiss WD, Huber M, Fink GR, et al. Progressive derangement of peri-infarct viable tissue in ischemic stroke. *J Cereb Blood Flow Metab* 1992; 12:193–203.

137. Gold B, Kertesz A. Right hemisphere semantic processing of visual words in an aphasic patient: An fMRI study. *Brain Lang* 2000; 73:456–465.

138. Buckner R, Corbetta M, Schatz J, et al. Preserved speech abilities and compensation following prefrontal damage. *Proc Natl Acad Sci USA* 1996; 93:1249–1253.

139. Cramer S, Finklestein S, Schaechter J, et al. Distinct regions of motor cortex control ipsilateral and contralateral finger movements. *J Neurophysiology* 1999; 81:383–387.

140. Detre J. fMRI: Applications in epilepsy. *Epilepsia* 2004; 45 Suppl 4:26–31.

141. Christodoulou C, DeLuca J, Ricker J, et al. Functional magnetic resonance imaging of working memory impairment after traumatic brain injury. *J Neurol Neurosurg Psychiatry* 2001; 71:161–168.

142. Lee M, Reddy H, Johansen-Berg H, et al. The motor cortex shows adaptive functional changes to brain injury from multiple sclerosis. *Ann Neurol* 2000; 47:606–613.

143. Marshall R, Perera G, Lazar R, et al. Evolution of cortical activation during recovery from corticospinal tract infarction. *Stroke* 2000; 31:656–661.

144. Fujii Y, Nakada T. Cortical reorganization in patients with subcortical hemiparesis: Neural mechanisms of functional recovery and prognostic implication. *J Neurosurg* 2003; 98:64–73.

145. Small S, Hlustik P, Noll D, et al. Cerebellar hemispheric activation ipsilateral to the paretic hand correlates with functional recovery after stroke. *Brain* 2002; 125:1544–1557.

146. Saur D, Lange R, Baumgaertner A, et al. Dynamics of language reorganization after stroke. *Brain* 2006; 129:1371–1384.

147. Shimizu T, Hosaki A, Hino T, et al. Motor cortical disinhibition in the unaffected hemisphere after unilateral cortical stroke. *Brain* 2002; 125:1896–1907.

148. Manganotti P, Patuzzo S, Cortese F, et al. Motor disinhibition in affected and unaffected hemisphere in the early period of recovery after stroke. *Clin Neurophysiol* 2002; 113:936–943.

149. Liepert J, Hamzei F, Weiller C. Motor cortex disinhibition of the unaffected hemisphere after acute stroke. *Muscle Nerve* 2000; 23:1761–1763.

150. Butefisch C, Netz J, Wessling M, et al. Remote changes in cortical excitability after stroke. *Brain* 2003; 126:470–481.

151. Murase N, Duque J, Mazzocchio R, Cohen L. Influence of interhemispheric interactions on motor function in chronic stroke. *Ann Neurol* 2004; 55:400–409.

152. Musso M, Weiller C, Kiebel S,. Training-induced brain plasticity in aphasia. *Brain* 1999; 122 (Pt 9):1781–1790.

153. Cardebat D, Demonet J, De Boissezon X, et al. Behavioral and neurofunctional changes over time in healthy and aphasic subjects: A PET language activation study. *Stroke* 2003; 34:2900–2906.

154. Cappa S, Perani D, Grassi F, et al. A PET follow-up study of recovery after stroke in acute aphasics. *Brain Lang* 1997; 56:55–67.

155. Luft A, McCombe-Waller S, Whitall J, et al. Repetitive bilateral arm training and motor cortex activation in chronic stroke: A randomized controlled trial. *JAMA* 2004; 292:1853–1861.

156. Carey J, Kimberley T, Lewis S, et al. Analysis of fMRI and finger tracking training in subjects with chronic stroke. *Brain* 2002; 125:773–788.

157. You SH, Jang SH, Kim YH, et al. Virtual reality-induced cortical reorganization and associated locomotor recovery in chronic stroke: An experimenter-blind randomized study. *Stroke* 2005; 36:1166–1171.

158. Pariente J, Loubinoux I, Carel C, et al. Fluoxetine modulates motor performance and cerebral activation of patients recovering from stroke. *Ann Neurol* 2001; 50:718–729.

159. Calautti C, Leroy F, Guincestre J, Baron J. Dynamics of motor network overactivation after striatocapsular stroke: A longitudinal PET study using a fixed-performance paradigm. *Stroke* 2001; 32:2534–2542.

160. Feydy A, Carlier R, Roby-Brami A, et al. Longitudinal study of motor recovery after stroke: Recruitment and focusing of brain activation. *Stroke* 2002; 33:1610–1617.

161. Kim S-G, Ashe J, Hendrich K, et al. Functional magnetic resonance imaging of motor cortex: Hemispheric asymmetry and handedness. *Science* 1993; 261:615–617.

162. Turton A, Wroe S, Trepte N, et al. Contralateral and ipsilateral EMG responses to transcranial magnetic stimulation during recovery of arm and hand function after stroke. *Electroenceph Clin Neurophys* 1996; 101:316–328.

163. Netz J, Lammers T, Homberg V. Reorganization of motor output in the non-affected hemisphere after stroke. *Brain* 1997; 120:1579–1586.

164. Lohmann H, Deppe M, Jansen A, et al. Task repetition can affect functional magnetic resonance imaging-based measures of language lateralization and lead to pseudoincreases in bilaterality. *J Cereb Blood Flow Metab* 2004; 24:179–187.

165. Colebatch J, Deiber M-P, Passingham R, et al. Regional cerebral blood flow during voluntary arm and hand movements in human subjects. *J Neurophys* 1991; 65:1392–1401.

166. Cramer S, Nelles G, Schaechter J, et al. A functional MRI study of three motor tasks in the evaluation of stroke recovery. *Neurorehabil Neural Repair* 2001; 15:1–8.

167. Vikingstad EM, George KP, Johnson AF, Cao Y. Cortical language lateralization in right handed normal subjects using functional magnetic resonance imaging. *J Neurol Sci* 2000; 175:17–27.

168. Bucy P, Fulton J. Ipsilateral representation in the motor and premotor cortex of monkeys. *Brain* 1933; 56:318–342.

169. Ward NS, Brown MM, Thompson AJ, Frackowiak RS. Longitudinal changes in cerebral response to proprioceptive input in individual patients after stroke: An fMRI study. *Neurorehabil Neural Repair* 2006; 20:398–405.

170. Carey L, Abbott D, Puce A, et al. Reemergence of activation with poststroke somatosensory recovery: A serial fMRI case study. *Neurology* 2002; 59:749–752.

171. Hamdy S, Aziz Q, Rothwell J, et al. Recovery of swallowing after dysphagic stroke relates to functional reorganization in the intact motor cortex. *Gastroenterology* 1998; 115:1104–1112.

172. Miyai I, Yagura H, Hatakenaka M, et al. Longitudinal optical imaging study for locomotor recovery after stroke. *Stroke* 2003; 34:2866–2870.

173. Bang OY, Lee JS, Lee PH, Lee G. Autologous mesenchymal stem cell transplantation in stroke patients. *Ann Neurol* 2005; 57:874–882.

174. Scheidtmann K, Fries W, Muller F, Koenig E. Effect of levodopa in combination with physiotherapy on functional motor recovery after stroke: A prospective, randomized, double-blind study. *Lancet* 2001; 358:787–790.

175. Ren J, Kaplan P, Charette M, et al. Time window of intracisternal osteogenic protein-1 in enhancing functional recovery after stroke. *Neuropharmacology* 2000; 39:860–865.

176. Walker-Batson D, Smith P, Curtis S, et al. Amphetamine paired with physical therapy accelerates motor recovery after stroke: Further evidence. *Stroke* 1995; 26:2254–2259.

177. Dam M, Tonin P, De Boni A, et al. Effects of fluoxetine and maprotiline on functional recovery in poststroke hemiplegic patients undergoing rehabilitation therapy. *Stroke* 1996; 27:1211–1214.

178. Khedr EM, Ahmed MA, Fathy N, Rothwell JC. Therapeutic trial of repetitive transcranial magnetic stimulation after acute ischemic stroke. *Neurology* 2005; 65:466–468.

179. Brown JA, Lutsep HL, Weinand M, Cramer SC. Motor cortex stimulation for the enhancement of recovery from stroke: A prospective, multicenter safety study. *Neurosurgery* 2006; 58:464–473.

180. Mansur CG, Fregni F, Boggio PS, et al. A sham stimulation-controlled trial of RTMS of the unaffected hemisphere in stroke patients. *Neurology* 2005; 64:1802-1804.

181. Wolf SL, Winstein CJ, Miller JP, et al. Effect of constraint-induced movement therapy on upper extremity function 3 to 9 months after stroke: The excite randomized clinical trial. *JAMA* 2006; 296:2095–2104.

182. Cramer S, Benson R, Himes D, et al. Use of functional MRI to guide decisions in a clinical stroke trial. *Stroke* 2005; 36:e50–e52.

183. Kim YH, You SH, Ko MH, et al. Repetitive transcranial magnetic stimulation-induced corticomotor excitability and associated motor skill acquisition in chronic stroke. *Stroke* 2006; 37:1471–1476.

184. Platz T, Kim I, Engel U, et al. Brain activation pattern as assessed with multi-modal EEG analysis predict motor recovery among stroke patients with mild arm paresis who receive the arm ability training. *Restor Neurol Neurosci* 2002; 20:21–35.

185. Dong Y, Dobkin BH, Cen SY, et al. Motor cortex activation during treatment may predict therapeutic gains in paretic hand function after stroke. *Stroke* 2006; 37:1552–1555.

186. Fritz SL, Light KE, Patterson TS, et al. Active finger extension predicts outcomes after constraint-induced movement therapy for individuals with hemiparesis after stroke. *Stroke* 2005; 36:1172–1177.

187. Koski L, Mernar T, Dobkin B. Immediate and long-term changes in corticomotor output in response to rehabilitation: Correlation with functional improvements in chronic stroke. *Neurorehabil Neural Repair* 2004; 18:230–249.

188. Cramer S, Parrish T, Levy R, et al. An assessment of brain function predicts functional gains in a clinical stroke trial. *Stroke* 2007; 38:520 (abstract).

189. Taub E, Miller N, TA N, et al. Technique to improve chronic motor deficit after stroke. *Arch Phys Med Rehabil* 1993; 74:347–354.

190. Wolf S, Lecraw D, Barton L, Jann, BB. Forced use of hemiplegic upper extremities to reverse the effect of learned nonuse among chronic stroke and head-injured patients. *Exp Neurol* 1989; 104:125–132.

191. Blanton S, Wolf S. An application of upper-extremity constraint-induced movement therapy in a patient with subacute stroke. *Phys Ther* 1999; 79:847–853.

192. Dromerick A, Edwards D, Hahn M. Does the application of constraint-induced movement therapy during acute rehabilitation reduce arm impairment after ischemic stroke? *Stroke* 2000; 31:2984–2988.

193. Kopp B, Kunkel A, Muhlnickel W, et al. Plasticity in the motor system related to therapy-induced improvement of movement after stroke. *Neuroreport* 1999; 10:807–810.

194. Schaechter J, Kraft E, Hilliard T, et al. Motor recovery and cortical reorganization after constraint-induced movement therapy in stroke patients: A preliminary study. *Neurorehabil Neural Repair* 2002; 16:326–338.

195. Liepert J, Miltner W, Bauder H, et al. Motor cortex plasticity during constraint-induced movement therapy in stroke patients. *Neurosci Lett* 1998; 250:5–8.

196. Park SW, Butler AJ, Cavalheiro V, et al. Changes in serial optical topography and TMS during task performance after constraint-induced movement therapy in stroke: A case study. *Neurorehabil Neural Repair* 2004; 18:95–105.

197. Wittenberg G, Chen R, Ishii K, et al. Constraint-induced therapy in stroke: Magnetic-stimulation motor maps and cerebral activation. *Neurorehabil Neural Repair* 2003; 17:48–57.

198. Johansen-Berg H, Dawes H, Guy C, et al. Correlation between motor improvements and altered fMRI activity after rehabilitative therapy. *Brain* 2002; 125:2731–2742.

199. Liepert J. Motor cortex excitability in stroke before and after constraint-induced movement therapy. *Cogn Behav Neurol* 2006; 19:41–47.

200. Seitz R, Butefisch C, Kleiser R, Homberg V. Reorganisation of cerebral circuits in human ischemic brain disease. *Restor Neurol Neurosci* 2004; 22:207–229.

201. Matthews PM, Johansen-Berg H, Reddy H. Non-invasive mapping of brain functions and brain recovery: Applying lessons from cognitive neuroscience to neurorehabilitation. *Restor Neurol Neurosci* 2004; 22:245–260.

202. Frensch PA, Runger D. Implicit learning. *Psychol Sci* 2003; 12:13–18.

203. Ramnani N, Toni I, Josephs O, et al. Learning- and expectation-related changes in the human brain during motor learning. *J Neurophysiol* 2000; 84:3026–3035.

204. Puttemans V, Wenderoth N, Swinnen SP. Changes in brain activation during the acquisition of a multifrequency bimanual coordination task: From the cognitive stage to advanced levels of automaticity. *J Neurosci* 2005; 25:4270–4278.

205. Classen J, Liepert J, Wise SP, et al. Rapid plasticity of human cortical movement representation induced by practice. *J Neurophysiol* 1998; 79:1117–1123.

206. Rauch SL, Whalen PJ, Savage CR, et al. Striatal recruitment during an implicit sequence learning task as measured by functional magnetic resonance imaging. *Hum Brain Mapp* 1997; 5:124–132.

207. Reiss JP, Campbell DW, Leslie WD, et al. The role of the striatum in implicit learning: A functional magnetic resonance imaging study. *Neuroreport* 2005; 16:1291–1295.

208. Karni A, Meyer G, Jezzard P, et al. Functional MRI evidence for adult motor cortex plasticity during motor skill learning. *Nature* 1996; 377:155–158.

209. Floyer-Lea A, Matthews PM. Distinguishable brain activation networks for short- and long-term motor skill learning. *J Neurophysiol* 2005; 94(1):512–518.

210. Pohl PS, McDowd JM, Filion D, et al. Implicit learning of a motor skill after mild and moderate stroke. *Clin Rehabil.* 2006; 20:246–253.

211. Pohl PS, McDowd JM, Filion DL, et al. Implicit learning of a perceptual-motor skill after stroke. *Phys Ther* 2001; 81:1780–1789.

212. Boyd LA, Winstein CJ. Cerebellar stroke impairs temporal but not spatial accuracy during implicit motor learning. *Neurorehabil Neural Repair* 2004; 18:134–143.

213. Orrell AJ, Eves FF, Masters RS. Motor learning of a dynamic balancing task after stroke: Implicit implications for stroke rehabilitation. *Phys Ther* 2006; 86:369–380.

214. Boyd L, Winstein C. Explicit information interferes with implicit motor learning of both continuous and discrete movement tasks after stroke. *J Neurol Phys Ther* 2006; 30:46–57; discussion 58–59.

215. Exner C, Weniger G, Irle E. Implicit and explicit memory after focal thalamic lesions. *Neurology* 2001; 57:2054–2063.

216. Hodics T, Cohen LG, Cramer SC. Functional imaging of intervention effects in stroke motor rehabilitation. *Arch Phys Med Rehabil* 2006; 87:36–42.

9 Physiological Basis of Rehabilitation Therapeutics in Stroke

Andreas R. Luft
Charlene Hafer-Macko
Timothy Schallert

In the past decade, stroke rehabilitation research has shifted its focus from empiric evidence to biological targets. Physiology, especially neurophysiology, has identified a number of targets that can be accessed by rehabilitation interventions. These physiological targets focus upon the potential for neuroplasticity at multiple levels of the central nervous system (CNS), including sensorimotor cortex, subcortical networks, and the spinal cord. Moreover, a synthesis of clinical and animal research suggests that a diversity of biological mechanisms, including alterations in selected neurotransmitter pathways and growth factors that modulate neuroplastic adaptations, may interact to promote recovery. While the evidence based on randomized clinical trials is currently insufficient to generate consensus practice recommendations, increasing experimental evidence supports a rationale for further research combining pharmacotherapeutic strategies with task practice to optimize sensorimotor recovery after stroke. Finally, the biological targets to improve stroke recovery must go beyond the CNS to include skeletal muscle and metabolic function. Following stroke, there are major body composition abnormalities, including structural and metabolic abnormalities in hemiparetic muscle, that can worsen disability, constituting important targets for physical rehabilitation and, potentially, pharmacological therapies. In the following sections, we discuss these biological targets and the interventions designed to interact with them. A focus is maintained on current knowledge in human rehabilitation, followed by a brief overview of some clinical and translational research in animal models that may help to define future research directions. Table 9-1 gives an overview of biological targets and related treatments. The further text focuses on the CNS, spinal cord, and skeletal muscle.

CENTRAL NERVOUS SYSTEM

A stroke damages the central nervous system (CNS). The CNS is therefore the prime target for therapies aiming for cure at the origin of the disease. Two properties in the organization of the CNS theoretically allow for recovery: redundancy and plasticity. Redundancy implies a certain overcapacity of the CNS so that limited tissue loss can immediately be compensated. Plasticity is a double-edged sword. It can be beneficial as well as detrimental if regrowing neurons reach false targets and cause additional motor impairment. Detrimental plasticity is commonly referred to as *maladaptation*. In the following, redundancy and plasticity are discussed.

Studies in patients with brain lesions demonstrate that the CNS has redundancy, albeit limited. The brain's

TABLE 9-1
Biological Targets and Treatment Strategies

BIOLOGICAL TARGET	MECHANISM	TREATMENT STRATEGY
Brain (cognitive systems)	Adaptations in emotional, reward, and other cognitive systems.	Psychological and motivational therapies providing reward and emotional support as well as social and occupational therapy.
	Reorganization of speech and language networks.	Physical therapies combining multiple tasks to train attention and distractability.
Brain (sensorimotor system)	Neuroplasticity in cortical and subcortical motor systems.	Speech and language therapy.
	Motor skill learning.	Repetitive, task-oriented physical and occupational therapy.
Spinal cord	Adaptations in spinal reflex circuits preventing spasticity and maladaptive reflex behaviors.	Classical physical therapies (neurodevelopmental and sensory feedback).
Muscle	Reversal of muscle atrophy and phenotype alterations. (Stroke causes shift to fast muscle fibers.)	Repetitive resistive and aerobic exercise.
	Relief of spasticity.	Botulinum toxin injections.
Cardiorespiratory	Fitness.	Aerobic exercise therapy.

redundancy is not like that of other organs, such as the liver or kidneys, where removal of a part is easily and instantly compensated by the remaining tissue. Within a theoretical neural network, the dropout of a limited number of single cells or cell-to-cell connections can be tolerated without much dysfunction (1). Clinically unnoticed lacunes document this scenario. Because overcapacity declines with age, compensability also decreases.

In contrast to lesions that injure a few cells, territorial lesions that affect entire or large parts of neuronal networks cannot go unnoticed. Compensation for such lesions can only come from parallel networks that provide the same function but are underused in the healthy brain, for example, because their capabilities were replaced by more potent systems during evolution. Such parallel systems could be recruited after failure of the dominant system and may provide slow functional compensation. One example for a parallel system is the rubrospinal system compensating for corticospinal injury (2). However, the number of parallel systems is certainly limited. Another form of redundancy exists between the two hemispheres of the brain. Certain lateralized functions mainly executed by one can be adopted by the other hemisphere. Swallowing is an example (3). Dysphagia typically recovers faster than other impairments caused by interhemispheric compensation.

Plasticity of neurons is an alternative mechanism that enables recovery of function. Plasticity is the reprogramming of neuronal circuits by modifying their firing patterns (synaptic efficacy or weights) and/or architecture. The stimulus for plastic reorganization can occur through the use of damaged circuits, such as through active training (skilled use-dependent plasticity). An alternative stimulus may arise from the stroke lesion itself, for example, through lesion-induced expression of plasticity-related genes (4).

Plastic phenomena have been observed in a variety of different brain regions, including cortical and subcortical areas. Depending on the research methodology used, the phenomena may reflect structural, functional plasticity, or both. After injury to CNS motor areas or their descending tracts, motor recovery is associated with plastic adaptations in motor cortex. Cortical representations of body parts, as determined by stimulating different areas of cortex, reduce in surface area after an infarct. Motor training prevents this shrinkage of cortical maps and can even expand representations in monkeys (5). Well-recovered stroke survivors with descending tract lesions have motor cortical activation patterns that differ substantially from healthy controls (6–9) and change longitudinally over time, reflecting the reorganization of the cortical motor system (10–12). Similar to animal studies, motor cortex stimulation has documented adaptations in the input-output organization of the motor cortex after stroke (13). Areas other than the motor cortices (primary motor cortex, premotor cortex, SMA, and cingulate motor areas), such as somatosensory cortex (14) and temporal and parietal regions, may also contribute to recovery, but they are not established to be as consistently involved in recovery-related plasticity processes (although this may be, in part, because current neurologic assessment methods are insufficiently sensitive). Functional imaging in stroke survivors with different degrees of impairment also suggests a role of the cerebellum. In well-recovered subjects, cerebellar activation during movement of the affected side is stronger than in the impaired (15).

Hence, motor cortices and cerebellum are brain targets that can mediate recovery or functional compensation if properly triggered. This triggering may be a particularly successful approach considering that the lesion itself attracts neuroblasts to migrate from the subventricular zone to cortex (16), which, in turn, could be reprogrammed by active use.

Genetic determination may affect how apt the motor system is to plastic changes. The Val66met polymorphism in the brain-derived neurotrophic factor (BDNF) gene was shown to be associated with reduced reorganization of motor cortex somatotopy after learning (17).

Rehabilitation Training Techniques Targeting CNS

Specific training therapies aim at inducing neuroplastic adaptations in the CNS. Constraint-induced movement therapy (CIMT) is an effective intervention that provides sustained benefits to stroke survivors with long-term disability (18). CIMT combines active training with the paretic arm with constraining the unaffected arm; the latter helps to overcome learned nonuse of the paretic side (19). CIMT is associated with changes in cortical physiology. The representation of the paretic hand in the ipsilesional hemisphere, as determined by transcranial magnetic stimulation (TMS), increases in size after therapy. This increase correlates with improved arm function (20). The enlargement occurs into areas with decreased intracortical inhibition (21), indicating a role for a GABAergic mechanism in this form of plasticity. Plasticity mechanisms may depend on lesion location. A patient with a lesion in a primary motor area or its descending pathways, as defined by an abnormal motor-evoked potential in response to TMS, showed an increased area representation and decreased cortical excitability or increased inhibition. Patients without such lesions show the opposite pattern (22). Functional imaging studies indicate that CIMT can induce plasticity in other brain areas, such as the contralesional primary motor area (reduction of activation), cerebellum, supplementary motor area, and frontal gyri (23–25).

Bilateral arm training (BATRAC) is an effective therapy for most patients (26, 27). Some patients, despite improving their reach, do not gain movement abilities relevant for daily life. Bilaterality and rhythmicity are

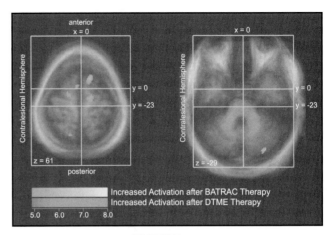

FIGURE 9-1

Bilateral arm training with rhythmic auditory cueing (BATRAC) recruits brain areas in both hemispheres, but mainly in the contralesional hemisphere to the control of the paretic limb. (Red areas represent foci of novel activation after training; used with permission of *JAMA*.)

elements adopted from motor learning techniques that are possibly acting through interhemispheric signaling and movement sequencing. Patients that improve in motor impairment, as measured by the Fugl Meyer score, show increased recruitment of bihemispheric premotor and motor areas (Figure 9-1) (26). In contrast, patients without functional improvement demonstrate no cortical reorganization, suggesting a mechanistic link between recruitment of ipsi- and contralesional motor cortices and improved arm function.

Other upper extremity training regimens also utilize neuroplasticity to improve function. Task-specific training of tracking waveforms with the paretic index finger leads to a shift in the activation of sensorimotor cortices (primary sensory, motor, and premotor cortex) from the contralesional to the ipsilesional side (28). Similar results were obtained by using a home-based, task-oriented training protocol (29). In another study, a task-oriented arm training program led to increases in the activation of ipsilesional primary motor cortex as well as inferior parietal and premotor cortex (30). Activation changes were neither observed in healthy controls undergoing the same training program nor in patients subjected to conventional physiotherapy techniques.

Gait training on a treadmill while facilitating paretic leg movements using somatosensory stimulation produces healthy patterns of cortical activation. These patterns are closer to those of healthy controls during unfacilitated treadmill walking (31). In contrast, unfacilitated treadmill walking in stroke patients is associated with abnormal activation patterns. While this observation provides no evidence for neuroplastic adaptations in the brain, it demonstrates that specific physiotherapy techniques can reverse abnormal brain activation. It is possible that the entraining of normal activation patterns leads to long-term encoding and a persistent functional benefit. A randomized controlled study comparing aerobic treadmill exercise to stretching demonstrated a superiority of the treadmill interventions with respect to walking velocity and fitness. Increases in walking velocity were correlated with recruitment of subcortical brain networks, namely cerebellum-red nucleus circuits (32). This study demonstrated that subcortical networks can be modified by specific interventions that improve ambulation for chronic stroke survivors.

Other Interventions Supporting CNS Plasticity

Cortical stimulation: CNS neuroplasticity can be facilitated by certain adjunct treatments. One of these emerging interventions is cortical stimulation. Stimulation can be delivered transcranially either via a magnetic coil (TMS) or by applying weak, direct current (tDCS). Cortical stimulation alters cortical excitability. For example, applying tDCS to primary motor cortex (anodal stimulation) in the lesioned hemisphere enhanced excitability results in improved use of the paretic arm (33). Also, in association with enhanced cortical excitability is a reduced intracortical inhibition, suggesting changes in GABA and glutamatergic neurotransmission as the likely underlying mechanism (34). Interestingly, downregulation of excitability by applying cathodal stimulation to the contralesional hemisphere also improves arm function (35). This observation indicates that transcallosal interhemispheric signaling is part of the pathophysiology of hemiparesis. Similar results have been shown with repetitive TMS (36–38). Excitability changes that are observed following cortical stimulation are short-lived and only improve motor performance for minutes to hours (33). Daily application in combination with training may provide persistent effects that are greater than those induced by training alone (36), but this remains to be confirmed in larger trials.

Pharmacotherapy: Systemic administration of levodopa in combination with physiotherapy was superior to physiotherapy alone (39). In this trial, the combination treatment was given for three weeks during subacute recovery after a stroke that occurred three weeks to six months prior. Amphetamines have been suggested to provide similar benefits (40), but conflicting evidence has been reported (41). A meta-analysis based on 10 trials acknowledges benefits for motor function, but it found the evidence to be insufficient to allow for definitive conclusions or guidelines (42). The mechanism of action for dopamine and amphetamine is thought to be the enhancement of cortical norepinephrine (especially in the terminals of the hemisphere contralateral to the injury), but direct effects of dopamine have also been suggested (43). Inhibiting norepinephrine reuptake by reboxetine has been shown to enhance learning of a motor skill (44, 45).

Sensitive animal models are necessary to better understand how certain substances affect recovery or learning. Only this knowledge will lead to optimized use by defining the delivery method, the time to use, the duration of treatment, and so forth.

SPINAL CORD

The spinal cord harbors reflex circuits that are inhibited by a pathway from motor cortex to the brain stem ventromedial reticular formation (46). If a stroke injures this pathway, the reflex circuits become hyperactive, leading to upper motor neuron (UMN) signs such as clonus, positive extensor plantar reflexes, and spasticity. However, these symptoms develop over time, suggesting that it is not simply the removal of cortico-reticulospinal signaling that causes symptoms of upper motor neuron syndrome. Instead, slow, plastic changes within the spinal cord must be involved (46). Little is known about these changes that are a deleterious form of spinal plasticity. Potential mechanisms are the sprouting of afferent axons, which, in turn, connect to previously inhibitory synapses, converting them to excitatory synapses or up-regulation of receptor sensitivity as a consequence of denervation (46). Spasticity and muscular hypertonus lead to adaptations in muscle tissue and have biomechanical consequences, such as contractures and impaired posture.

Deleterious plasticity, or *maladaptation*, can occur because neurons lose their targets after injury and then rewire inappropriately. Rewiring may be maladaptive because the patterns of activation that occur during active use are missing. It has been hypothesized that maladaptive rewiring leads to the inability of newly formed synapses to undergo lasting modification of synaptic strength, hence, learning (47). The basis for this hypothesis is that, in the normal state, an oscillating balance exists between learning and recall, that is, between plastic change of synaptic strength or interneuronal connections and their stable maintenance. Studies on the mechanisms of consolidation and reconsolidation after an early recall of stored information are consistent with this idea (48). By destroying part of the neuronal network caused by stroke, this delicate balance is severely disturbed. Maladaptive rewiring leads to a permanent disruption of this balance. As a consequence, the neuronal networks are locked in a stability-plasticity dilemma, which leads to catastrophic forgetting of the information that was previously stored in these networks (47). This forgetting may contribute to motor paralysis in stroke survivors. The classical pathophysiological model of paralysis that emphasizes deefferentiation from the interruption of CNS-muscle pathways probably contributes as well, but it is clearly not the sole explanation for paralysis. The fact that stroke patients demonstrating plegia in neurologic examinations sometimes move their arm subconsciously or automatically when they wake up in the morning underlines this idea.

Rehabilitation Training Techniques Targeting Spinal Cord

Original neurorehabilitative techniques, such as the Bobath neurodevelopmental technique (49), aim at avoiding upper motor neuron syndrome maladaptations at the level of the spinal cord. Whether or not they achieve this goal has not been demonstrated. They may also produce benefits by targeting other elements of the motor system. Proof of clinical efficacy of these techniques comes from experience more than clinical investigation (50, 51).

The spinal cord harbors central pattern generators that produce automated movement, such as stepping, and they are under cortical and subcortical control. In animal models of spinal cord injury, these pattern generators can be modulated by gait training on a treadmill, possibly reflecting spinal plasticity (52). In humans, body weight supported treadmill training (BWSTT) is advocated for spinal cord-injured patients. A randomized controlled trial comparing BWSTT with overground training has shown clinical benefits for both interventions (53). This is expected, assuming that any task—for example, gait-specific training, whether on a treadmill or on the ground—will induce activity-dependent adaptations. In humans, whether these adaptations occur on the spinal level or in the brain remains to be investigated.

Spinal cord networks are specifically targeted by the antispasticity drug, baclofen, applied via continuous intraspinal infusion using an implanted pump. In a controlled double-blinded trial (n = 21), comparing a one-time bolus injection of baclofen versus saline, significant improvements in spasticity were documented in favor of the active drug (54). Responders to the bolus were then offered an implantation of a baclofen pump. At the twelve-month follow-up, spasticity scores were markedly decreased.

SKELETAL MUSCLE

There are a number of skeletal muscle alterations that could propagate disability and increase cardiovascular risk after stroke. These skeletal muscle alterations include muscular atrophy and increased intramuscular adiposity (55), fiber phenotype shift (56), and changes in muscle metabolism that are linked to insulin resistance (57). Stroke leads to profound cardiovascular deconditioning that relate to gait deficit severity and body composition changes. In 26 chronic hemiparetic stroke patients, body composition analysis by dual X-ray absorptiometry (DXA) found hemiparetic thigh lean mass was lower than the nonparetic thigh (8.4 ± 1.9 kg vs. 8.6 ± 1.8, $p < 0.05$) (58). Stepwise regression revealed both hemiparetic thigh lean mass and walking speed were independent and robust predictors of reduced fitness level. In contrast, the NIH stroke scale, modified Ashworth spasticity scale, latency since stroke onset, and percent body fat were not related to the fitness level. In addition, bilateral mid-thigh CT scans confirmed the gross muscular atrophy (20% lower muscle cross-sectional area, $p < 0.0001$) in the hemiparetic, compared to nonparetic thigh in 30 chronic stroke patients (59). The hemiparetic thigh muscle also had 25% higher intramuscular area fat deposition ($p < 0.0001$), a finding strongly associated with insulin resistance (59). These findings suggest that reduced muscle mass is fundamentally related to poor fitness and physical performance capacity after stroke (55, 61).

Skeletal muscle fibers have great adaptive potential. Myosin heavy chain is an important structural and regulatory contractile protein that is expressed in different isoform profiles and, thereby, imparts functional diversity to muscles. Slow (MHC 1) isoform fibers are rich in mitochondria, resistant to fatigue, and less pH-sensitive because of their highly oxidative metabolism (62). Fast twitch fibers have glycolytic metabolism and faster force generation capacity, but they fatigue easily. The structural and functional characteristics of muscle fibers can be modified in response to several physiological and pathological conditions. Muscle phenotype is regulated by hormones, growth factors, changes in load, innervation patterns, aging, hypoxia, electrical stimulation, and exercise. After stroke, skeletal muscle responds to altered use, loading states, and neural activation pattern. The most comprehensive study of muscle pathology reveals a shift to greater fast twitch fiber proportions in hemiparetic leg *vastus lateralis* (VL) based on ATPase staining and a reliance on anaerobic metabolism with rapid lactate generation during isolated hemiparetic limb exercise, in contrast to oxidative metabolism during nonparetic leg exercise (63). These findings are similar to recent studies that find a major shift to fast MHC by routine ATPase staining at pH 4.6 and MHC gel electrophoresis of hemiparetic leg VL muscle biopsies in 13 chronic stroke patients (56). The hemiparetic leg has elevated proportion of fast MHC isoforms ($68 \pm 14\%$, range 46–88% of total MHC) compared to the nonparetic leg ($50 + 13\%$, range 32–76%, $p < 0.005$). These findings that are restricted to the hemiparetic leg suggest that neurologic alterations may be partially responsible for the shift of muscle phenotype. The proportion of fast MHC isoform, only in the hemiparetic limb, strongly negatively relates to self-selected walking speed (r = −0.78, p < 0.005), suggesting modulation of gait deficit severity. The shift to fast MHC after stroke in the hemiparetic leg muscle would be expected to result in a more fatigable muscle fiber type that could be more insulin-resistant. Interestingly, spinal cord injury results in a parallel shift to fast MHC muscle composition, which can be reversed with partial weight suspension treadmill training (64).

Tumor necrosis factor alpha (TNFα) has been implicated with muscular wasting in models of disuse, cachexia, sarcopenia, and insulin resistance. TNFα may cause atrophy and insulin resistance through a number of mechanisms. It inhibits protein synthesis, reduces transcriptional factors regulating myofiber gene expression, induces protein breakdown through activation of ubiquitin proteases and induction of apoptotic cell death, and alters insulin signaling (63–67). TNFα mRNA expression is elevated in hemiparetic VL compared to nonparteic leg of stroke patients and age-matched controls (57). TNFα mRNA levels are 2.8-fold higher in hemiparetic muscle and 1.7-fold higher in nonparetic VL compared with matched controls. The findings of elevated TNFα in both the hemiparetic and nonparetic muscles suggest that systemic as well as local inflammation could augment muscular atrophy and increased insulin resistance after stroke. This inflammatory mediator can negatively impact muscle mass, structural proteins, performance, and metabolism. These secondary biological abnormalities in body composition and skeletal muscle should be considered as potential targets for rehabilitation and therapeutic exercise after stroke.

Rehabilitation Training Techniques Targeting Muscle

In a small trial (n = 32) comparing robot-assisted gait training (Lokomat, Hocoma, Inc., Volketswil, Switzerland) to conventional physiotherapy (training of trunk stability, gait symmetry, and step initiation) in subacute stroke patients, Husemann et al. showed beneficial changes in whole-body composition with robot training (70)—that is, increases in muscle and decrease in fat mass compared to the control group over the four-week intervention. Functional benefits were comparable between groups, but the trial may not have been sufficiently powered to show such differences. These findings indicate that specific physiotherapy interventions can differentially affect body composition, and the benefit for the stroke survivors remains to be assessed.

A systematic meta-analysis covering 21 trials using various strengthening methods—including electrical stimulation, biofeedback, muscle reeducation for very weak acute or chronic stroke survivors, and resistance exercise for weak participants—demonstrated an overall benefit on strength and activity. The benefit was greater in acute than chronic and in weak than very weak subjects. The carryover between strength and activity was comparably low, which was explained by the selection of muscles for strength training. Instead, daily tasks require whole muscle groups. Strength training did not increase spasticity (71).

Spasticity is limiting active training to induce plastic adaptation. It is therefore desirable to relieve spasticity either through physiotherapy or pharmacotherapy. Brashear and colleagues compared botulinum toxin injections into flexor muscles with a placebo in a randomized multicenter trial (72). At four, six, eight, and twelve weeks of follow-up, botulinum toxin was beneficial in improving muscle tone and self-reported disability without producing adverse events. It remains to be investigated whether botulinum toxin, which has a time-limited effect, may enable specific training interventions that recover motor ability and prevent a relapse of spasticity.

SUMMARY

Rehabilitation training approaches for motor recovery after stroke can target all levels of the motor system (Table 9-1). Many patients require psychological and cognitive training targeting higher cognitive and language systems in order to understand and motivate themselves for rehabilitation and to cope with disability and related social stressors. Repetitive and task-oriented training therapies target the brain's motor systems to induce neuroplastic changes that provide recovery of motor function or compensation for disability. These training therapies may be supported by pharmacological, for example, dopamine, or electrical therapies that render the motor cortex more apt to plastic changes. The neural and behavioral effectiveness of physical therapy may depend on its timing, the age of the patient, what psychotherapeutic drugs they are taking, and nutritional factors (73–77). Spinal cord reflex mechanisms are targeted by conventional rehabilitation therapies, but little is known about the ability for lasting changes in the spinal cord after stroke. Maladaptive changes in spinal cord may lead to spasticity, which, together with muscle degeneration after stroke, can be a limiting factor to CNS training therapies. Therefore, measures to reduce spasticity, such as botulinum toxin injections and sensory feedback therapy, may be a prerequisite to further training. Muscle degeneration may be reversed by resistive and nonresistive exercise. Finally, reduced cardiovascular fitness after stroke is limiting any movement effort. Aerobic exercise therapies targeting the cardiovascular and respiratory systems may enhance fitness and provide sufficient energy reserve for enduring daily life activities.

The neuroscience of rehabilitation is just at its beginning. Much needs to be learned about the brain's ability to adapt and recover, including the use of restorative approaches (e.g., via stem cells). Because many therapies already exist and will be expanded in the future, it will be crucial to learn about efficacy, prerequisites for response, treatment intensity, and sequence. Most likely, we will have to tailor the rehabilitative protocol to the individual patient.

References

1. Murre JMJ, Griffioen R, Robertson IH. Self-repairing Neural Networks: A Model for Recovery from Brain Damage. Berlin: Springer, 2003:1164–1171.

2. Lawrence DG, Kuypers HG. The functional organization of the motor system in the monkey. II. The effects of lesions of the descending brainstem pathways. Brain 1968; 91(1):15–36.

3. Hamdy S, Rothwell JC. Gut feelings about recovery after stroke: The organization and reorganization of human swallowing motor cortex. Trends Neurosci 1998; 21(7):278–282.

4. Carmichael ST. Plasticity of cortical projections after stroke. Neuroscientist 9(1):64–75.

5. Nudo RJ, Wise BM, SiFuentes F, Milliken GW. Neural substrates for the effects of rehabilitative training on motor recovery after ischemic infarct. Science 1996; 272(5269):1791–1794.

6. Chollet F, DiPiero V, Wise RJ, et al. The functional anatomy of motor recovery after stroke in humans: A study with positron emission tomography. Ann Neurol 1991; 29(1):63–71.

7. Cramer SC, Nelles G, Benson RR, et al. A functional MRI study of subjects recovered from hemiparetic stroke. Stroke 1997; 28(12):2518–2527.

8. Marshall RS, Perera GM, Lazar RM, et al. Evolution of cortical activation during recovery from corticospinal tract infarction. Stroke 2000; 31(3):656–661.

9. Weiller C, Chollet F, Friston KJ, et al. Functional reorganization of the brain in recovery from striatocapsular infarction in man. Ann Neurol 1992; 31(5):463–472.

10. Calautti C, Baron JC. Functional neuroimaging studies of motor recovery after stroke in adults: A review. Stroke 2003; 34(6):1553–1566.

11. Calautti C, Leroy F, Guincestre JY, Baron JC. Dynamics of motor network overactivation after striatocapsular stroke: A longitudinal PET study using a fixed performance paradigm. Stroke 2001; 32(11):2534–2542.

12. Ward NS, Brown MM, Thompson AJ, Frackowiak RS. Neural correlates of motor recovery after stroke: A longitudinal fMRI study. Brain 2003; 126(11):2476–2496.

13. Butefisch CM, Kleiser R, Seitz RJ. Post-lesional cerebral reorganisation: Evidence from functional neuroimaging and transcranial magnetic stimulation. J Physiol Paris 2006; 99(4–6):437–454.

14. Schaechter JD, Moore CI, Connell BD, et al. Structural and functional plasticity in the somatosensory cortex of chronic stroke patients. Brain 2006; 129(10):2722–2733.

15. Small SL, Hlustik P, Noll DC, et al. Cerebellar hemispheric activation ipsilateral to the paretic hand correlates with functional recovery after stroke. Brain 2002; 125(7):1544–1557.

16. Ohab JJ, Fleming S, Blesch A, Carmichael ST. A neurovascular niche for neurogenesis after stroke. J Neurosci 2006; 26(50):13007–13016.

17. Kleim JA, Chan S, Pringle E, et al. BDNF val66met polymorphism is associated with modified experience-dependent plasticity in human motor cortex. Nat Neurosci 2006; 9(6):735–737.

18. Wolf SL, Winstein CJ, Miller JP, et al. Effect of constraint-induced movement therapy on upper extremity function 3 to 9 months after stroke: The EXCITE randomized clinical trial. JAMA 2006; 296(17):2095–2104.

19. Taub E. Constraint-induced movement therapy and massed practice. Stroke 2000; 31(4):986–988.

20. Liepert J, Bauder H, Miltner WH, et al. Treatment-induced cortical reorganization after stroke in humans. Stroke 2000; 1(6):1210–1216.

21. Liepert J, Haevernick K, Weiller C, Barzel A. The surround inhibition determines therapy-induced cortical reorganization. Neuroimage 2006; 32(3):1216–1220.

22. Hamzei F, Liepert J, Dettmers C, et al. Two different reorganization patterns after rehabilitative therapy: An exploratory study with fMRI and TMS. Neuroimage 2006; 31(2):710–720.

23. Dong Y, Dobkin BH, Cen SY, et al. Motor cortex activation during treatment may predict therapeutic gains in paretic hand function after stroke. Stroke 2006; 37(6):1552–1555.

24. Kim YH, Park JW, Ko MH, et al. Plastic changes of motor network after constraint-induced movement therapy. Yonsei Med J 2004; 45(2):241–246.

25. Szaflarski JP, Page SJ, Kissela BM, et al. Cortical reorganization following modified constraint-induced movement therapy: A study of four patients with chronic stroke. Arch Phys Med Rehabil 2006; 87(8):1052–1058.

26. Luft AR, McCombe-Waller S, Whitall J, et al. Repetitive bilateral arm training and motor cortex activation in chronic stroke: A randomized controlled trial. JAMA 2004; 292(15):1853–1861.

27. Whitall J, McCombe WS, Silver KH, Macko RF. Repetitive bilateral arm training with rhythmic auditory cueing improves motor function in chronic hemiparetic stroke. Stroke 2000; 31(10):2390–2395.

28. Carey JR, Kimberley TJ, Lewis SM, et al. Analysis of fMRI and finger tracking training in subjects with chronic stroke. Brain 2002; 125(4):773–788.

29. Jang SH, Kim YH, Cho SH, et al. Cortical reorganization induced by task-oriented training in chronic hemiplegic stroke patients. Neuroreport 2003; 14(1):137–141.

30. Nelles G, Jentzen W, Jueptner M, et al. Arm training induced brain plasticity in stroke studied with serial positron emission tomography. Neuroimage 2001; 13(6):1146–1154.

31. Miyai I, Yagura H, Oda I, et al. Premotor cortex is involved in restoration of gait in stroke. Ann Neurol 2002; 52(2):188–194.

32. Luft AR, Macko R, Forrester L, et al. Subcortical reorganization induces by aerobic locomotor training in chronic stroke survivors. Stroke 2008, published online 8-28.

33. Hummel F, Celnik P, Giraux P, et al. Effects of noninvasive cortical stimulation on skilled motor function in chronic stroke. Brain 2005; 128(3):490–499.

34. Hummel FC, Cohen LG. Noninvasive brain stimulation: A new strategy to improve neurorehabilitation after stroke? Lancet Neurol 2006; 5(8):708–712.

35. Fregni F, Boggio PS, Mansur CG, et al. Transcranial direct current stimulation of the unaffected hemisphere in stroke patients. Neuroreport 2005; 16(14):1551–1555.

36. Khedr EM, Ahmed MA, Fathy N, Rothwell JC. Therapeutic trial of repetitive transcranial magnetic stimulation after acute ischemic stroke. Neurology 2005; 65(3):466–468.

37. Mansur CG, Fregni F, Boggio PS, et al. A sham stimulation-controlled trial of rTMS of the unaffected hemisphere in stroke patients. Neurology 2005; 64(10):1802–1804.

38. Takeuchi N, Chuma T, Matsuo Y, et al. Repetitive transcranial magnetic stimulation of contralesional primary motor cortex improves hand function after stroke. Stroke 2005; 36(12):2681–7686.

39. Scheidtmann K, Fries W, Muller F, Koenig E. Effect of levodopa in combination with physiotherapy on functional motor recovery after stroke: A prospective, randomised, double-blind study. Lancet 2001; 358(9284):787–790.

40. Crisostomo EA, Duncan PW, Propst M, et al. Evidence that amphetamine with physical therapy promotes recovery of motor function in stroke patients. Ann Neurol 1988; 23(1):94–97.

41. Gladstone DJ, Danells CJ, Armesto A, et al. Physiotherapy coupled with dextroamphetamine for rehabilitation after hemiparetic stroke: A randomized, double-blind, placebo-controlled trial. Stroke 2006; 37(1):179–185.

42. Martinsson L, Hardemark H, Eksborg S. 2007. Amphetamines for improving recovery after stroke. Cochrane Database Syst Rev(1):CD002090.

43. Breitenstein C, Floel A, Korsukewitz C, et al. A shift of paradigm: From noradrenergic to dopaminergic modulation of learning? J Neurol Sci 2006; 248(1–2):42–47.

44. Plewnia C, Bartels M, Cohen L, Gerloff C. Noradrenergic modulation of human cortex excitability by the presynaptic alpha(2)-antagonist yohimbine. Neurosci Lett 2001; 307(1):41–44.

45. Plewnia C, Hoppe J, Cohen LG, Gerloff C. Improved motor skill acquisition after selective stimulation of central norepinephrine. Neurology 2004; 62(11):2124–2126.

46. Sheean G. The pathophysiology of spasticity. Eur J Neurol 2002; 9(1):3–9, 53–61.

47. Krishnan RV. Relearning toward motor recovery in stroke, spinal cord injury, and cerebral palsy: A cognitive neural systems perspective. Int J Neurosci 2006; 116(2):127–140.

48. Nader K, Schafe GE, LeDoux JE. The labile nature of consolidation theory. Nat Rev Neurosci 2000; 1(3):216–219.

49. Bobath B. Adult Hemiplegia: Evaluation and Treatment. London: Heinemann, 1978.

50. Lennon S, Ashburn A. The Bobath concept in stroke rehabilitation: A focus group study of the experienced physiotherapists' perspective. Disabil Rehabil 2000; 22(15):665–674.

51. Paci M. Physiotherapy based on the Bobath concept for adults with post-stroke hemiplegia: A review of effectiveness studies. J Rehabil Med 2003; 35(1):2–7.

52. Pearson KG. Neural adaptation in the generation of rhythmic behavior. Annu Rev Physiol 2000; 62:723–753.

53. Dobkin B, Apple D, Barbeau H, et al. Weight-supported treadmill vs. over-ground training for walking after acute incomplete SCI. Neurology 2006; 66:484–493.

54. Meythaler JM, Guin-Renfroe S, Brunner RC, Hadley MN. Intrathecal baclofen for spastic hypertonia from stroke. Stroke 2001; 32:2099–2109.

55. Ryan AS, Dobrovolny CL, Smith GV, et al. Hemiparetic muscle atrophy and increased intramuscular fat in stroke patients. Arch Phys Med Rehabil 2002; 83(12):1703–1707.

56. De Deyne PG, Hafer-Macko CE, Ivey FM, et al. Muscle molecular phenotype after stroke is associated with gait speed. Muscle Nerve 2004; 30(2):209–215.

57. Hafer-Macko CE, Yu S, Ryan AS, et al. Elevated tumor necrosis factor-alpha in skeletal muscle after stroke. Stroke 2005; 36(9):2021–2023.

58. Ryan AS, Dobrovolny CL, Silver KH, et al. Cardiovascular fitness after stroke: Role of muscle mass and gait deficit severity. *J Stroke Cerebro Disease* 2000; 9:185–191.

59. Ryan AS, Dobrovolny CL, Smith GV, Silver KH, Macko RF. Hemiparetic muscle atrophy and increased intramuscular fat in stroke patients. *Arch Phys Med Rehab* 2002; 83(12):1703–1707.

60. Ryan AS, Nicklas BJ. Age-related changes in fat deposition in mid-thigh muscle in women: Relationships with metabolic cardiovascular disease risk factors. *Int J Obes Relat Metab Disord* 1999; 23:126–132.

61. Patterson SL, Forrester LW, Rodgers MM, Ryan AS, Ivey FM, Sorkin JD, Macko RF. Determinants of walking function after stroke: Differences by deficit severity. *Arch Phys Med Rehab* 2007; 88(1):115–119.

62. Bottinelli R. Functional heterogeneity of mammalian single muscle fibres: Do myosin isoforms tell the whole story? *Pflugers Arch* 2001; 443:6–17.

63. Landin S, Hagenfeldt L, Saltin B, Wahren J. Muscle metabolism during exercise in hemiparetic patients. *Clin Sci Mol Med* 1977; 53(3):257–269.

64. Stewart BG, Tarnopolsky MA, Hicks AL, et al. Treadmill training-induced adaptations in muscle phenotype in persons with incomplete spinal cord injury. *Muscle Nerve* 2004; 30:61–68.

65. Frost RA, Lang CH, Gelato MC. Transient exposure of human myoblasts to tumor necrosis factor-alpha inhibits serum and insulin-like growth factor-I stimulated protein synthesis. *Endocrinology* 1997; 138:4153–4159.

66. Goodman MN. Tumor necrosis factor induces skeletal muscle protein breakdown in rats. *Am J Physiol* 1991; 260:E727–E730.

67. Huey KA, Haddad F, Qin AX, Baldwin KM. Transcriptional regulation of the type I myosin heavy chain gene in denervated rat soleus. *Am J Physiol Cell Physiol* 2003; 284:738–748.

68. Llovera M, Garcia-Martinez C, Agell N, et al. TNF can directly induce the expression of ubiquitin-dependent proteolytic system in rat soleus muscles. *Biochem Biophys Res Commun* 1997; 230:238–241.

69. Saghizadeh M, Ong JM, Garvey WT, et al. The expression of TNF alpha by human muscle: Relationship to insulin resistance. *J Clin Invest* 1996; 97:1111–1116.

70. Husemann B, Muller F, Krewer C, et al. Effects of locomotion training with assistance of a robot-driven gait orthosis in hemiparetic patients after stroke: A randomized controlled pilot study. *Stroke* 2007.

71. Ada L, Dorsch S, Canning CG. Strengthening interventions increase strength and improve activity after stroke: A systematic review. *Aust J Physiother* 2006; 52(4):241–248.

72. Brashear A, Gordon MF, Elovic E, et al. Intramuscular injection of botulinum toxin for the treatment of wrist and finger spasticity after a stroke. *N Engl J Med* 2002; 347(6):395–400.

73. Zhao C, Harikainen S, Schallert T, et al. CNS-active drugs in aging population at high risk of cerebrovascular events: Evidence from preclinical and clinical studies. *Neurosci Biobehav Rev* 2008; 32:56–71.

74. Kleim JA, Jones TA, Schallert T. Motor enrichment and the induction of plasticity before and after brain injury. *Neurochem Res* 2003; 28(11):1757–1769.

75. Grotta JC, Noser EA, Boake C, et al. Constraint induced movement therapy. *Stroke* 2004; 35:2699–2701.

76. Woodlee MT, Schallert T. The impact of motor activity and inactivity on the brain: Implications for the prevention and treatment of nervous system disorders. *Curr Direct Psychol* 2006; 15:203–206.

77. Schallert T, Woodlee MT. Brain-dependent movements and cerebral-spinal connections: Key targets of cellular and behavioral enrichment in CNS injury models. *J Rehab Res Develop* 2003; 40(4):9–18.

III

SPECIFIC NEUROLOGIC IMPAIRMENTS AND THEIR TREATMENT

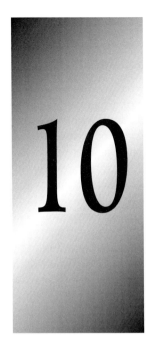

10 Aphasia, Apraxia of Speech, and Dysarthria

Leora R. Cherney
Steven L. Small

S peech and language problems are common sequelae of stroke that significantly impact the daily lives of stroke survivors. Reduced speech and language skills have negative ramifications on the individual's social, vocational, and recreational activities, often leading to social isolation, loneliness, loss of autonomy, restricted activities, role changes, and stigmatization (1–7). Given the importance of communication to the stroke survivor's quality of life, it is essential that rehabilitation professionals recognize and address the speech and language disorders associated with stroke.

Normal speech and language is extraordinarily complex. A number of steps are required, some accomplished sequentially and some in parallel, that incorporate the following: (a) conceptualization of an idea and generation of a communicative goal; (b) formulation of a grammatically structured sequence of verbal symbols (words), each consisting of an interacting set of ordered sounds; (c) selection of a series of neural commands or sensorimotor "programs" that will activate the speech muscles at appropriate coarticulated times, durations, and intensities; and (d) central and peripheral nervous system innervation of muscles of respiration,[1] phonation, resonance, and articulation to produce the intended acoustic signal.

Stroke can disrupt any of the stages of speech and language, resulting in one or more of the disorders of aphasia, apraxia of speech, and dysarthria. Disruption to the initial stage involving the structure and rules of the linguistic message results in *aphasia*. Impairment of the capacity to plan and program sensorimotor commands for the positioning and movement of muscles for the volitional production of speech results in *apraxia of speech*. It can occur without significant weakness or neuromuscular slowness and in the absence of disturbances of conscious thought or language (8). *Dysarthria* results from abnormal neuromuscular execution that affects the speed, strength, range, timing, or accuracy of speech movements. Dysarthria

---

[1]Respiration, by strict definition, refers to the exchange of gases between the bloodstream and the environment, while ventilation refers to the exchange of air between the lungs and the environment. However, it is customary for speech-language pathologists to refer to the breathing muscles of inhalation and exhalation as the muscles of respiration. Therefore, the term *respiration* will be used in this chapter rather than the term *ventilation*.

can affect respiration, phonation, resonance, articulation, and prosody, either singly or in combination.

Although by definition the disorders of aphasia, apraxia of speech, and dysarthria are distinguishable, in practice they often co-occur, making it challenging for even the experienced clinician to distinguish among them. Yet distinguishing aphasia from dysarthria, and both disorders from apraxia of speech, can be important, not only because of the neurologic implications regarding underlying pathology, but also because a specific diagnosis can have implications for selection of the appropriate management techniques and strategies.

This chapter, therefore, is divided into three parts, each of which addresses the primary characteristics of aphasia, apraxia of speech, and dysarthria, as well as assessment suggestions and management strategies. It will become obvious that the section on aphasia is far more detailed than the sections on the other two disorders. There are several reasons for this disparity, including differences in the incidence and prevalence of these disorders following stroke, the severity and persistence of the disorders, and their impact on the stroke survivor. The disparity also reflects our current knowledge of these disorders following stroke. For example, while there is a large body of literature about the characteristics of dysarthria and their assessment and treatment in general, relatively little pertains to dysarthria resulting specifically from stroke. There is far more research on the diagnosis and treatment of dysarthrias that are caused by Parkinson's disease, amyotrophic lateral sclerosis (ALS), and other progressive neuromuscular disorders. By contrast, stroke is the leading cause of aphasia, and most of the literature on aphasia relates to aphasia that is caused by stroke. Furthermore, since vascular lesions are not functionally selective—the same arteries and arterial branches supply brain areas that mediate functions important for all three disorders—the diagnosis and treatment of aphasia often must take into consideration these other disorders concomitantly.

APHASIA

Aphasia has been defined as a multimodality language disorder resulting from damage to brain areas that subserve the formulation and understanding of language and its components (i.e., phonology, syntax, morphology, and semantics). While it is beyond the scope of this chapter to provide a tutorial on language, it is important for those involved in aphasia rehabilitation to have a basic understanding of these different components of language in order to clarify the definition and to provide some basis for the discussion of rehabilitation.

Language Components

Phonology. *Phonology* refers to the linguistically important speech sounds or phonemes of a language and the rules for combining them. It is contrasted with *phonetics*, which is involved with the physical production of these sounds. Each consonant or vowel in a language may take a number of different pronunciations. For example, the letter *c* can sound like *k* or like *s*, and each pronunciation within that language is considered a *phoneme*. Many patients with aphasia have problems at the phonological level of processing. On the production side, they may substitute one phoneme or one syllable (combination of phonemes) for another, and on the comprehension side, patients can misinterpret particular phonemes or syllables, thereby hearing an unintended word and misinterpreting what is being said. Obviously, ascertaining these phonological errors in production is easier than in comprehension.

Syntax and Morphology. *Syntax* (or *grammar*) is the set of rules that governs the structure of sentences in a particular language, while morphology refers to the internal structure of words. In both cases, the structural rules have specific impacts on meaning. In English, for example, the addition of -*ed* to many regular verbs changes their tense, while the addition of -*s* to many regular nouns changes them from singular to plural. Whereas in English, word order plays the most important role in syntactic processing, word order plays less of a role in other languages (e.g., Italian, German), in which affixation or even semantic context are more important (9). This can lead to differences in the manifestations of aphasia across languages.

Syntactic impairments are common in aphasia. Some observers believe that grammatical processing problems are characteristic of patients with damage to the frontal part of the left peri-sylvian region and have called this disorder *agrammatism*. Such patients are more likely to say and understand single meaningful words, called *content words* (e.g., nouns and verbs) than they do the small *function words* (e.g., prepositions, articles). Importantly, the content words of a language form an *open class* (i.e., one in which new items can be added), whereas function words form a *closed class*. Function words do not denote objects, actions, or locations, but rather play a role similar to word affixes and word order in guiding sentence production or interpretation. A less common syndrome, called *paragrammatism*, involves grammatical processing problems and results from damage to the posterior (temporo-parietal) portion of the left peri-sylvian region (10, 11).

Semantics. Semantics is meaning, and conveying meaning in context is the fundamental goal of communication. The study of word meanings is called *lexical semantics*. The study of sentences and their different meanings—conveying entire "thoughts" or statements—is called *sentential semantics*. The meanings of sentences are built up from a combination of the meanings of the individual (content) words in the sentence, the syntactic aspects of word order, function words, word affixes, and the higher linguistic context (i.e., the entire conversation or discourse).

Lexical semantic processing is often disrupted in aphasia. Many patients with stroke cannot find the names of objects and actions that they understand visually and functionally. They may substitute a related but unintended word for the target word. Patients with agrammatism sometimes cannot distinguish the subject from the object of a sentence, particularly if word order is less common (e.g., in a passive sentence) and the subject and object words are both able to perform the actions (e.g., the boy was kicked by the girl). This is a problem of syntax and sentential semantics.

Working Memory. Certainly it is not possible to use language without various types of memories, including memory for words, grammatical rules, affixation rules, and so forth. Separating out language-specific memory from other types of memory is a topic of significant controversy, and one that we will not address here. However, one type of memory is particularly important in the understanding of aphasia, and that is *working memory*, the memory that is required to maintain the partial fragments of what is being heard or said to insure completion of the comprehension or production of the desired word, phrase, or sentence (12). All language computations require this type of very short-term memory, and it is commonly disrupted in aphasia (13, 14).

Language Modalities

Since aphasia is a multimodality disorder of language, it impairs, in varying degrees, the understanding (input) and expression (output) of both oral and written language modalities. Producing and understanding oral speech requires mechanisms for encoding and decoding auditory waveforms and mechanisms for encoding and decoding the words and sentences that constitute the message. Since oral speech is both the phylogenetic and ontogenetic backbone of language—it is learned first and in some cases exclusively—it is thought to be the evolutionary foundation and architectural core of the neural circuits involved in language. Patients with disorders of spoken language production and comprehension usually have concomitant problems in the written modality, reinforcing the ontogenetic coupling of these two neuroanatomical systems.

Consequently, aphasia is defined in terms of impairments in oral expression (speaking) and understanding, and a preponderance of treatment approaches are aimed directly at this form of communication. To the extent that the oral and written modalities share underlying mechanisms, such as lexical retrieval and sentence syntax and semantics, treatment does not need to be modality specific. However, when the language deficit is inextricably entwined with modality-specific problems, such as apraxia of speech, treatment that targets the specific modality might be preferable.

Producing written language requires neural and motor mechanisms for encoding a message in letters and visual words and performing the somatic motor movements to write or type the visual product. Understanding written language requires distinguishing particular visual stimuli as linguistic and then decoding them into letters, words, and sentences. There is also neural circuitry to convert these visual stimuli into phonological forms. Although it has not been completely determined when and how such circuitry is used, it seems to play its most important role in the case of less common (or pretend) words with regular spellings. It can also play a role in certain reading disorders caused by stroke. Disorders of reading and writing are an integral part of the aphasia, suggesting a significant degree of common underlying neural substrate for language processing from the oral and written modalities. When a writing disorder occurs that is disproportionate to the degree of impairment in speaking, it is called *dysgraphia* (or *agraphia*). The analogous reading disorder is called *dyslexia* (or *alexia*).

Anatomy of Language

In 1861 Pierre Paul Broca presented a paper to the Anatomical Society of Paris discussing the autopsy findings on his patient with a language disorder (15). Broca found a large brain lesion in the left inferior frontal region (the frontal "convolutions") and postulated a role for this region in the physiology of language. While neurologists prior to Broca had suspected and even published similar arguments (16), Broca is generally acknowledged as the initiator of the modern study of language and the brain through the method of clinico-pathological correlation (*lesion analysis* or *neuropsychological localization*) (17, 18). Following this work a number of additional papers were published on the brain mechanisms of language, including those by Wernicke (1874), Lichtheim (1884), Grashey (1885), and Freud (1891)(19–22). Their work led to the general notions that (a) the left peri-sylvian region is anatomically responsible for most of the neural mechanisms of language; (b) the codes and processes of the language output channel are anatomically instantiated by structures in and around the opercula of the left inferior frontal gyrus; and (c) the analogous codes and processes for the language input channel are anatomically centered around the posterior aspect of the superior temporal gyrus (20).

Thus, the classical zone of language, as defined by Dejerine in the late 19th and early 20th centuries, was located in the left hemisphere within the distribution of the middle cerebral artery, surrounding the sylvian fissure on the lateral surface of the hemisphere and incorporating portions of the frontal, parietal, and temporal lobes (23). The zone includes Broca's area (in the premotor region of the frontal lobe) anteriorly and Wernicke's area (auditory association cortex in the posterior portion of the superior temporal gyrus) posteriorly. Connecting Wernicke's and Broca's is a subcortical white matter pathway (i.e., the *arcuate fasciculus*, which is a portion of superior longitudinal fasciculus) that passes through the angular gyrus and supramarginal gyrus at the posterior rim of the sylvian fissure, where temporal and parietal lobes come together (23). The location of these critical language areas is illustrated in Figure 10-1.

Since that time, much research has been done within the lesion analysis method, and some of the finer functional structures of these areas have been determined. Most recently, the development of noninvasive in vivo neuroimaging techniques such as computer tomography (CT), positron emission tomography (PET), static and functional magnetic resonance imaging (sMRI and fMRI, respectively), electroencephalography, transcranial magnetic stimulation, and magentoencephalography, has transformed the study of the neurologic basis of language.

In some ways, though, the anatomical localization of function has become more rather than less muddled. For example, one line of research has been to challenge the specific role of the frontal operculum as the seat of language production. One finding was that patients with damage to this region demonstrated certain problems with language comprehension, possibly related to complex grammatical structures (24, 25). The behavioral data have been supplemented by both direct cortical stimulation, demonstrating a role for this region in language comprehension, and by functional neuroimaging (26). Both PET and fMRI have

demonstrated that the frontal operculum is important for a variety of tasks, including verbal working memory and certain motor tasks (27, 28).

In general, increasing evidence is being accrued to challenge the concept that small regions of the brain are specifically responsible for language functions such as comprehension or naming. This is not to say that brain regions do not have specific functions or that there are not neural circuits to perform these classically determined functions. It simply appears that the homomorphic relationship between historically important brain regions and functions has broken down. The same problem holds for other brain regions, such as the thalamus, basal ganglia, and the inferior parietal lobule, and other functions (29).

Current theory therefore rejects the notion of a one-to-one correspondence between specific linguistic structural elements and focal segments of the brain. Rather it recognizes the existence of distributed anatomical circuits, interactivity among regions, and different types of functions (30, 31). It takes into account evidence that multiple complex and overlapping neuronal systems most likely are involved in language processing. As Albert and Helm-Estabrooks explain, the networks include cortical and subcortical components, some of which are near each other providing the basis for regional contributions to language; others are more distant, providing the basis for widely distributed parallel processing of aspects of language (32). All the regional and widely distributed networks are multiply interconnected.

Within the classical zone of language, there is extensive superposition of the neural networks critical to language. These areas of multiple overlap may correspond to what in classical neurology were called the "centers" of language (20). Since these areas likely represent "critical crossroads, points of intersection, or points of integration for processing selected elements of language," a focal lesion in one of these critical locations could potentially result in a predictable aphasia deficit (32).

The Aphasia Syndromes: Assessment and Differential Diagnosis

Over the past 150 years, aphasiologists have developed several taxonomies for distinguishing various aphasia subtypes. These classification systems range from simplistic severity systems to more complex syndrome approaches (33). Perhaps the most widely used classification system is the Boston classification system, so named because it was based on early classical descriptions of aphasia subtypes and brought to the fore in the 1960s by Boston-based aphasiologists, including Geschwind, Benson, Goodglass, and Kaplan (34, 35). This classification system applies the early connectionist descriptions of aphasia subtypes and cortical syndromes and is still in use today by many practitioners.

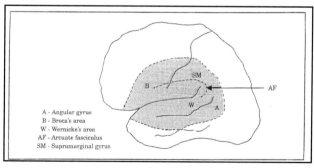

A - Angular gyrus
B - Broca's area
W - Wernicke's area
AF - Arcuate fasciculus
SM - Supramarginal gyrus

FIGURE 10-1

Diagrammatic representation of the cortical areas that are critical for language (32). Reprinted from Helm-Estabrooks N and Albert ML. *Manual of Aphasia and Aphasia Therapy, Second Edition, 2004.* Austin: Pro-Ed with permission.

While there are compelling arguments both for and against classifying in aphasia, the use of some common classification system helps the clinician understand the basic relationships between the aphasia syndrome, various patterns of language impairments, and their source in the central nervous system (36). In addition, it provides a common language for the efficient communication of patient information within and across professional disciplines. Therefore, the assessment and differential diagnosis of the aphasia subtypes is presented first, and cautions about the application of the classification system are discussed in the section following.

Syndrome Classification of Aphasia. Three language behaviors are helpful in classifying aphasia by syndrome: fluency of verbal output, auditory comprehension, and repetition.

Assessment of Fluency: Nonfluent aphasia is characterized by language output that is slow, labored, and effortful. The individual may have difficulty initiating speech, and agility of the articulatory movements is reduced. Phrase length is short, and agrammatism is typically present. In contrast, fluent aphasia is characterized by normal prosody, easy articulation, adequate phrase length, and varied syntax.

Phrase length has been defined as the number of words produced continuously without a significant pause. However, there is variability in aphasia fluency, which is affected by several factors including the emotionality of the topic, memory demands, and vocabulary constraints. To more objectively determine phrase length, using the best average phrase length from three different narrative tasks such as describing a picture, responding to an open ended question (e.g., What happened to you?), and responding to a historical question of emotional significance (e.g., Where were you on September 11, 2001?) has been suggested (32). A best average phrase length of 5 words or less is categorized as "frankly nonfluent," while a best average phrase length of 9 words or more is categorized as "frankly fluent." Patients who are nonfluent usually have a lesion anterior to the central sulcus, and these include Broca's aphasia, transcortical motor aphasia, and global aphasia. Those with fluent aphasia typically have a lesion posterior to the central sulcus. The fluent aphasias include Wernicke's aphasia, conduction aphasia, transcortical sensory aphasia, and anomic aphasia. A third group with a best average phrase length of 6–8 words is called "borderline fluent" and may include individuals with nonfluent aphasia who have demonstrated some degree of recovery as well as individuals with aphasia resulting from subcortical strokes (32).

Assessment of Auditory Comprehension: The second differentiating language behavior is auditory comprehension. Auditory comprehension is poor in individuals with global aphasia, Wernicke's aphasia, and transcortical sensory aphasia. Although auditory comprehension is relatively good in the other types of aphasia, difficulties may occur with understanding more complex information such as multistep commands or a lecture. Therefore, assessment requires several tasks that range in difficulty from the single word to lengthy complex materials. Auditory comprehension is often assessed with questions that require a "yes/no" response. In these cases, it is important to ensure that the person does indeed have a reliable "yes/no" response—either verbal or nonverbal (e.g., nodding their head, thumbs up or down, pointing to the written word *yes* or *no*). Since there is always a 50% chance of getting the response correct, some tests present pairs of questions and both questions need to be correct in order for credit to be given. At the single-word level, comprehension tasks usually include identification of different objects, actions, body parts, colors, and numbers, since word frequency and semantic class influence comprehension. The ability to follow single and multistep commands also should be assessed; however, when responses require body movements or object manipulation, some individuals may fail because of their motor/limb apraxia and not because of their aphasia. At the level of complex, lengthy material, it is important to consider the familiarity of the topic, the context in which the material is presented, and whether the questions or discussion are based on factual or implied and inferential information.

Assessment of Repetition: Repetition is the third language behavior that can assist with the classification of aphasia. In particular, the presence of relatively preserved repetition skills can help identify the transcortical aphasias, while relatively poor repetition skills in an individual with fluent aphasia may help differentiate conduction aphasia from anomic aphasia. Repetition tasks should include words of different semantic categories and frequencies and different syllable length and phonological complexity as well as phrases and sentences of different length and complexity. When making a differential diagnosis, the examiner should consider the relative preservation or disturbance of repetition skills as compared to spontaneous conversational speech. Many problems with repetition appear to relate to limited working memory for different types of linguistic fragments.

Table 10-1 describes each of the classical aphasia syndromes and illustrates how fluency, comprehension, and repetition are differentially impaired in each type of aphasia.

Assessment of Aphasia: Other Considerations. **Word retrieval:** Word-retrieval problems are a core feature of aphasia. However, since they are present in all aphasias, they do not serve to distinguish among aphasia

TABLE 10-1

Characteristics of the Cortical Aphasias

Type of Aphasia	Fluency	Oral Expression: Other Features	Auditory Comprehension	Repetition
Broca's aphasia	Non-fluent. Slow and effortful output. Short phrase length (less than 4 words). Disrupted prosody of speech.	Agrammatism—uses primarily substantive content words (nouns, verbs) with few function words (pronouns, prepositions, articles). Most sentences are simplified. May have an associated apraxia of speech.	Relatively good comprehension except for sentences that involve syntactic complexity.	Poor.
Wernicke's aphasia	Fluent. Well-articulated speech, often produced at an increased rate. Phrase length greater than four words.	Paraphasic errors (sound substitutions). In the severest cases, neologisms may dominate so that output consists of prosodic fluent-sounding jargon. In other cases, speech may be characterized as empty (lack of content words, perseverations).	Poor Do not self-monitor and are often unaware that they are not communicating information.	Poor.
Anomic aphasia	Fluent. Word-finding pauses may interrupt speech flow, but average phrase length is within normal ranges.	Uses grammatically correct sentences. Clear difficulty finding words. May circumlocute or use nonspecific terms (e.g., thing, this, that) when they cannot find the word they want.	Good.	Good.
Conduction aphasia	Quite fluent with normal average phrase length. May be word-finding pauses. Attempts to self-correct phonemic paraphasias may also disrupt the fluency of speech.		Good but may show verbal short-term memory deficits.	Poor. Major deficit is the inability to repeat.

Global aphasia	Nonfluent. Severely impaired.	Stereotypic utterances may be present. They are produced during attempts to verbalize and consist of nonsense syllables or real words, often well articulated with prosodic variation.	Severely impaired.	Severely impaired.
Transcortical motor aphasia	Non-fluent. Slow and effortful output. Short phrase length (less than 4 words). Disrupted prosody of speech.	Impaired initiation of verbal output. Agrammatic.	Relatively good comprehension except for sentences that involve syntactic complexity.	Major characteristic is the good repetition in relation to speech output.
Transcortical sensory aphasia	Fluent. Well-articulated speech, often produced at an increased rate. Phrase length greater than four words.	Paraphasic errors—includes both sound and word substitutions.	Poor auditory comprehension.	Major characteristic is the good repetition.
Mixed nonfluent aphasia	Nonfluent. Verbal output may be limited to stereotypic utterances, but sometimes meaningful speech is produced with articulatory effort.	Phonemic paraphasias and perseverations. Severity lies somewhere between global and Broca's aphasia; may occur as the patient recovers from global aphasia.	Auditory comprehension poor but not as severely impaired as global aphasia.	Poor repetition.

types. Nevertheless, assessment of their severity (which may range from mild difficulty in producing a desired word during conversation to virtual inability to produce the target word in any conditions) and an analysis of the types of naming errors that occur are important for treatment planning. In addition, it is important for the practitioner to ascertain that the word-finding problems are independent of other causes including memory problems, thought disorders, or confusional states (32). There are several ways to assess word retrieval including presentation of objects and pictures for naming or using pictured scenes and free recall tasks such as conversation, explaining directions for a familiar route, or the procedures for completing a familiar task (e.g., making a sandwich), which allow the clinician to observe the naming difficulties in connected language. Generative naming or word-fluency tasks in which the person is asked to name as many items as possible within a particular category (e.g., animals, words starting with a specific letter) may also be used.

Reading and writing: Similarly, virtually all individuals with aphasia display reading and writing problems, although the assessment of reading and writing skills does not contribute to the differential diagnosis of the classical aphasias. Most standardized tests of aphasia include tasks that assess reading comprehension and written expression at different levels of complexity beginning with single letters and moving to word, phrase, sentence, and paragraph levels. In addition, there are tests that are specifically aimed at assessing these skills, and a comprehensive treatment plan for aphasia should address treatment of the reading and writing problems.

Standardized Tests of Aphasia: There are a variety of standardized tests that have been developed specifically for the assessment of aphasia. Table 10-2 lists those that are commonly used in clinical practice and characterizes the language functions that they assess. In addition to these formal tests, clinicians also use informal tasks to assess functional everyday performance; selection of these tasks depends on the individual patient's communication needs and goals.

Cognition: Although aphasia is a language disorder, examination of all domains of cognition is important for successful rehabilitation of the person with aphasia. The ability to maximize the use of residual language, compensate for language deficits, and return to independence depends to a large extent on the integrity of other aspects of cognition, which can be used to assist with communication and other functional activities of daily living. However, accurate assessment of cognitive skills in the presence of aphasia is a challenge since many neuropsychological tests depend on language skills to varying degrees, thereby making them less reliable for use with patients with aphasia. The Mini-Mental State

Examination (36), commonly used in the assessment of dementia, has poor validity with patients with aphasia who, for example, may be fully oriented to place and time, but unable to state or write the month, day, facility name and so forth.

A commonly used test of nonverbal cognitive ability is the Ravens Colored Progressive Matrices (RCPM) (37), a test of visual analogic thinking that uses design patterns and requires a pointing response. In fact, a portion of this test has been integrated into the Western Aphasia Battery (38, 39), which, in addition to yielding an aphasia quotient, also provides a Cognitive quotient (CQ) score. The CQ represents a summary of scores from the RCPM together with constructional, visuospatial, and calculation tasks. In addition, the Cognitive Linguistic Quick Test (40) was designed for individuals with aphasia and provides a screening of the areas of attention, memory, and executive skills.

Classifying Aphasia Syndromes: Cautions. There are as many reasons not to use classification systems in aphasia as there are arguments in favor, and even the authors of this article are not in agreement on this issue. However, using such systems does represent a valuable shorthand, and even if these systems do not have strong validity for neurolinguistic research (41–43), they may have some advantages in the clinical setting.

Even a major proponent of the classification system suggests that clinicians use the system cautiously, stating that syndromes are simply suggestive of a given behavior profile and should not be rigorously applied (33). He lists several limitations, which include the following:

- Syndromes must not be tied firmly to a given site of lesion. As previously described, current theory in aphasia rejects the notion of a one-to-one correspondence between specific linguistic structural elements and focal segments of the brain. Rather, one should understand that specific regions of the brain are an essential or critical element in a widely distributed neural network, and not that a particular language skill that is now deficient resides in a particular part of the brain.
- Syndromes are not static—as a person recovers, he or she may evolve from one syndrome to another, even though the anatomical locus of the lesion does not change.
- Within a given syndrome, individuals with aphasia may exhibit a wide variety of severity and symptoms.
- Not all individuals with aphasia are classifiable. Approximately 80% of individuals with aphasia conform roughly to the aphasia syndrome and anatamoclinical scheme (32). Individual differences

TABLE 10-2
*Commonly Used Standardized Language Tests for Aphasia
Showing the Modalities Assessed*

TEST	AUDITORY COMPREHENSION	ORAL EXPRESSION	READING COMPREHENSION	WRITTEN EXPRESSION
Western aphasia battery—Revised[1]	X	X	X	X
Boston diagnostic aphasia examination—3rd edition[2]	X	X	X	X
Porch index of communicative ability[3]	X	X	X	X
Communication activities of daily living—2nd edition[4]	X	X	X	X
Boston assessment of severe aphasia (BASA)[5]	X	X	X	X
Aphasia diagnostic profiles[6]	X	X	X	X
Psycholinguistic assessments of language processing in aphasia[7]	X	X	X	X
Boston naming test[8]	X			
Revised token test[9]		X		
Reading comprehension battery for aphasia—2nd edition[10]			X	
Discourse comprehension test[11]	X		X	

[1]Kertesz A. *Western Aphasia Battery Revised.* Harcourt Assessment Inc, San Antonio, TX: Harcourt Assessment Inc; 2007.
[2]Goodglass H, Kaplan E, Barresi B. *The Assessment of Aphasia and Related Disorders* 3rd ed . Philadelphia, PA: Lippincott Williams &Wilkins, 2001.
[3]Porch BE. *Porch Index of Communicative Ability.* Palo Alto, CA: Consulting Psychologists Press, 1981.
[4]Holland AL, Frattali CM, Fromm D. *Communication Activities of Daily Living.* 2nd ed. Austin, TX: Pro-Ed, 1998.
[5]Helm-Estabrooks N, Ramsberger G, Nicholas M, Morgan A. *Boston Assessment of Severe Aphasia.* Austin, TX: Pro-Ed, 1989.
[6]Helm-Estabrooks N. *Aphasia Diagnostic Profiles.* Austin,TX: Pro-Ed, 1992.
[7]Kay J, Lesser R, Coltheart M. *PALPA: Psycholinguistic Assessments of Language Processing in Aphasia.* East Sussex, England: Lawrence Erlbaum, 1992.
[8]Kaplan E, Goodglass H, Weintraub S. *Boston Naming Test.* Philadelphia, PA: Lea & Febiger, 2000.
[9]McNeil MR, Prescott TE. *Revised Token Test.* Baltimore, MD: University Park Press, 1978.
[10]LaPointe LL, Horner J. *Reading Comprehension Battery for Aphasia.* 2nd ed. Austin, TX: Pro-Ed, 1998.
[11]Brookshire RH, Nicholas LE. *The Discourse Comprehension Test.* Minneapolis, MN: BRK Publishers, 1993.

in brain structure, lesion size and location, and etiology as well as factors such as age, handedness, prior brain damage, presence of seizures, depression, or other medical or psychiatric disorders all may influence brain-behavior relations. Finally, it should be noted that this connectionist classification scheme was developed to address the cortical aphasias, yet aphasia-producing lesions may not be limited to the cortex. Lesions to the thalamus and anterior and posterior capsular putamen may also result in an aphasia that is not classifiable using the scheme (29, 44).

Yet despite these limitations and cautions, the most common tests of aphasia (Western Aphasia Battery and Boston Diagnostic Aphasia Examination) (40, 45) are based on this schema. Indeed, as Brookshire (41) has observed, "the connectionist model is in many respects a fiction, but it remains a useful one" (p. 176).

Recovery and Prognosis

Individuals with aphasia and their family members frequently want an assessment of prognosis. For the clinician, reliable information regarding factors associated with both positive and negative recovery impact several clinical decisions and actions, including determining prognosis, counseling significant others, and identifying candidates for treatment. Discussions about recovery and prognosis focus on three interrelated key questions: How much recovery can be expected? What is the time course of recovery? Will therapy have an impact on recovery? Additionally, there are many different outcome areas that can be assessed, so another question relates to which particular factors are being referred to in the discussion on prognosis (e.g., improvements in specific language modalities, improvements in communication skills, and improvements in quality of life).

Factors Affecting Prognosis. Basso (1992) has differentiated between neurologic and anagraphic factors, which may serve as indicators of prognosis. Neurologic factors are related to etiology, size and site of lesion, and severity and type of aphasia. In addition, through modern neuroimaging technologies, there has been an increased focus on pathophysiological indicators of recovery, the long-term cerebral changes related to resolving aphasia, and the neurophysiological consequences of therapeutic interventions. Anagraphic factors include personal characteristics such as age, sex, handedness, and health status.

Neurologic factors: One of the difficulties encountered in research on recovery from aphasia and prognosis is that many of these factors are interrelated. For example, site of lesion determines to some extent the type of aphasia; size of lesion and type of aphasia have some implications for severity; and type of aphasia may not be independent of age.

Consider for example the discussion on initial severity of aphasia, lesion size and location, and their impact on recovery. Some researchers have stated that initial aphasia severity is the single most important factor for ultimate language function, a finding that is consistent with earlier findings (47–49). Another basic assumption about recovery from aphasia has been that lesion size exerts a negative influence on recovery (48, 50–56). However, Basso (1992) asserts that while the negative effect of extent of lesion on initial severity of aphasia is unquestionable, once initial severity has been taken

into account, the effect of lesion size on recovery is not clear-cut.

In a series of studies that looked at location and extent of lesion on CT scans and the severity of impairment in different groups of aphasic individuals, Naeser and colleagues indicated that rather than total lesion size, it is the size of the lesion within specific areas that may affect recovery from aphasia (57–59). In their study of 10 patients with Wernicke's aphasia, there was no correlation between total temporoparietal lesion size and severity of auditory comprehension (58). However, a correlation was found between the amount of temporal lobe damage within Wernicke's area and severity of auditory comprehension. If damage was in half or less of Wernicke's area, patients exhibited good comprehension at 6 months post onset. If the lesion involved more than half of Wernicke's area, patients exhibited poor comprehension, even at 1 year post-onset. Furthermore, anterior-inferior temporal lobe extension into the middle temporal gyrus area was associated with particularly poor recovery (58).

Similarly, Kertesz and colleagues correlated outcome measures of aphasia severity and comprehension with lesion extent in 22 patients with Wernicke's aphasia (54). Like Naeser et al., they found that the extent of involvement within specific structures, rather than overall lesion size, contributed to the prediction of language recovery (54, 58). The angular gyrus and the anterior mid-temporal area were important for overall language recovery, while the extent of involvement of angular gyrus contributed most significantly to recovery of auditory comprehension at 1 year.

Time Frame of Recovery. Expectations for recovery include not only the amount of recovery but also the time frame in which recovery can be expected. Historically, recovery was thought to be complete by 3–6 months post stroke. However, more recent research indicates that recovery from aphasia continues throughout the life of the person and that the benefits of rehabilitative intervention also continue throughout this entire period.

Hillis and Heidler have suggested that functional recovery from aphasia involves at least three overlapping stages, which extend over years (60). The acute stage, occurring in the first few days after stroke, involves the recovery of transiently impaired neural tissue in the ischemic penumbra, the area of the brain surrounding the core infarct. Although this area receives sufficient blood to survive, it is not enough to function. Restoration of function occurs only following increased blood flow to this area. The second stage of recovery begins within days of the stroke, continues for weeks, months, or possibly years after onset, and involves reorganization of structure/function relationships. When the reorganization is complete, further recovery (the third stage) depends on establishing new pathways for processing components that were "cut off" by the brain damage as well as learning compensatory strategies to facilitate more effective communication.

Neurophysiology of Recovery and Rehabilitation. Neuroimaging studies are increasingly being used to examine changes in brain activation patterns after left-hemisphere stroke and aphasia. Despite a number of studies, understanding of the complex process of cortical reorganization of language-related brain regions during recovery from aphasia and the effects of therapeutic interventions on brain systems involved in language processing is limited.

A basic issue relates to whether language improvement during recovery and rehabilitation is sustained by left-hemisphere zones spared by the lesion, by recruitment of homologous right-hemisphere regions, or both. Several studies in recovering aphasic patients have reported shifts in activation to homologous right-side territories and have interpreted these as compensatory (61–65). Recently, however, the role of right-hemisphere activation during functional imaging has been questioned, suggesting that it is a maladaptive response reflecting loss of active transcallosal inhibition (66–68).

The apparent contribution of right- and left-hemisphere activity to language recovery may depend on when it is measured following stroke onset. Right-hemisphere activation seems to occur early during recovery (69–71) and may depend on the site of the left-hemisphere lesion (71, 72). Right-hemisphere participation may also be more relevant when there is greater damage to the left-hemisphere language areas (70, 73–75).

Studies that directly assess functional anatomical changes occurring with language therapy are emerging; yet, there remains no consensus even on the most basic question of laterality. Left-side activations have been reported following a positive response to the intervention with melodic intonation therapy (MIT) (66), phonological training via reading aloud (76), repetitive naming of semantically related pictures (77), and memorization of articulatory gestures followed by repetition, reading aloud, and picture naming of a core of words (78). Two of these studies found that post-therapy patterns were consistent with task-dependent activity in healthy adults (76, 78), while one study found increased activity in the perilesional cortex (77). In contrast, others have found increased activity in right homologues of the anterior (79) and posterior (79, 80) language areas with therapy.

Several issues about these imaging studies and the reported alterations in functional activation following therapy deserve comment. First, no study so far has reported more than a few patients at any one time. Second, the neurobiological measures differ across studies. Combining individual differences with task differences leads to a wide variety of possible outcomes. Clearly, many questions remain regarding recovery and the effect of rehabilitation on patterns of language organization. Nevertheless, there is a long history of behavioral treatments for aphasia, which are presented below followed by a discussion of treatment efficacy and outcomes.

Approaches to Aphasia Rehabilitation

Taxonomy of Language Remediation Approaches. There have been several attempts to categorize the numerous treatment techniques and procedures for language remediation in adults with aphasia. For example, a literature review of articles that were published in five major journals and that spanned approximately 20 years (1971–1991) identified six broad models of aphasia treatment, each of which are discussed below (81). More recently, Basso (2003) presented a general taxonomy of approaches to and theoretical underpinnings of aphasia rehabilitation, based on historical trends in the latter half of the twentieth century. Interestingly, her taxonomy closely agrees with the categories identified previously (81). Yet any taxonomy is a simplification—it is not always clear where one approach ends and another begins, so some specific treatments may be consistent with more than one approach. For example, Horner et al. (1994) note that of the articles they reviewed, the majority (21.7%) used a hybrid or multitheoretic approach. Other language therapies may not fit into any of the approaches, particularly when therapies from different countries worldwide are considered (83). Nevertheless, the following six categories serve as an initial guide to the rich and varied treatments for aphasia. Selection of treatments occurs with consideration of patient-specific factors such as type, severity and chronicity of the aphasia, the presence of associated impairments, and the patient's communication environments.

Stimulation-facilitation approach: The stimulation-facilitation approach is a name that is often used synonymously with that of Hildred Schuell, who proposed and supported this approach (84, 85). It is based on the philosophy that in aphasia, language is not lost, but rather cannot be accessed. Aphasia is considered to be uni-dimensional in nature, so individuals with aphasia share many similarities in behavioral impairment and differ only in terms of severity. Therefore, regardless of type of aphasia or site and size of the neurologic lesion, language rehabilitation can be essentially the same for all patients.

Since the auditory modality is of prime importance in language processing and is also a key area of deficit in aphasia, treatment involves repetitive intensive auditory stimulation. The presentation of the auditory stimulation, which is designed to elicit a maximum number of responses, is sometimes paired with stimulation in other modalities. Error responses occur when stimulation is insufficient.

Therefore, they are not corrected but are followed by additional stimulation, which if adequate, is likely to elicit the correct response. While the assumptions underlying this approach have undergone serious argument, the stimulation method has been the predominant approach to treatment in the United States since the 1960s.

Modality model approach: In contrast to the premise that aphasia is uni-dimensional, proponents of the modality model view language as modality bound and aphasia as a modality specific performance deficit involving one or more modalities. The goal of treatment is to remediate the specific input or output modalities, singly or in combination. One way that this can be accomplished is by systematically pairing weak and strong modalities to "de-block" impaired performance. This principle can be applied regardless of the specific modality that is being treated. For example, when confrontation naming is difficult, repetition may be used to help the patient produce the correct response; then immediately after de-blocking has occurred through the use of repetition, the target response may be accessed in the previously inaccessible modality (i.e., confrontation naming) (86).

Luria's functional reorganization approach, which has widely influenced aphasia research and therapy, is consistent with the modality model (81). According to Luria, when brain tissue is destroyed, its original function cannot be restored to its previous form, but it can be performed by means of a partially new neural organization (87, 88). Therapy therefore is directed toward reorganization and transfer of the function to other brain structures or functional systems. With intersystemic organization, new functional systems are created through the use of other undamaged links. With intrasystemic organization, the impaired function is carried out at a different level of the same functional system, either at a lower and more automatic level or at a higher and more voluntary level. Precise identification of which modalities are damaged and which are preserved makes it possible to develop and implement different training procedures.

Processing approach: The processing approach is based on the cognitive neuropsychological models of normal language processes that have been developed for specific language tasks such as reading, spelling, naming, or sentence production (89). These information processing models assume that a complex cognitive function consists of a system of distributed and interconnected modules or mental representations that allow for processing of different types of information in cascade fashion. The representations and processes do not necessarily correspond to locations in the brain, but reflect functional components of a cognitive operation. Rehabilitation begins, for each individual patient, with identifying which cognitive processes and representations underlying the language task are impaired and which processes and representations are intact. For example,

the task of reading words aloud involves the graphemic input lexicon, while repetition of words involves the phonological input lexicon. However, both tasks involve the semantic system and the phonological output lexicon. By comparing performance across tasks, inferences about the integrity of these cognitive processes can be made. Treatment then focuses on either the remediation of the impaired cognitive processes, compensation via the intact cognitive processes, or both. The primary contribution of the processing approach is that it guides the choice of interventions; however, it does not provide direct motivation for specific treatment strategies (89). There are many studies, mostly single case descriptions, in which cognitive analyses have been used to focus treatment, and examples can be found in Hillis (2002).

Non-dominant hemisphere approach: Several treatment approaches are based on the premise that the hemisphere that is non-dominant for language has specific abilities, such as visual-spatial, affective-prosodic, and paralinguistic abilities, that can be used to facilitate communication. Melodic intonation therapy (MIT) is perhaps the best known of these treatment approaches (91–93). MIT is a hierarchically structured program that uses intonation and rhythm to increase the patient's ability to independently produce high-probability phrases and sentences. The steps of MIT range from intoning a melodic line with synchronous left-hand tapping to answering questions using drilled phrases and sentences. MIT may be most appropriate for those with large left-hemisphere lesions whose recovery may depend more on the right than the left hemisphere (94), and some limited evidence for its efficacy has recently emerged (94–96). Other remediation approaches that are consistent with the non-dominant hemisphere mediation model utilize drawing as a communicative function (97) and encourage humor within the therapy session (98).

Linguistic approach: The linguistic (neurolinguistic) approach is based on the principle that language has an internal organization that can be described by a specialized system of rules. In aphasia, there is disruption of lexical-semantic, syntactic, and/or phonologic performance. Treatment therefore focuses on restoring language performance using neurolinguistic principles that are specific for each linguistic impairment. For example, the sentence production program for aphasia systematically trains syntax using a story completion format (99). Selection of syntactic structures was based on a study of agrammatism that identified a hierarchy of difficulty across 14 grammatical constructions with imperative intransitive statements being the easiest and future tense statements the most difficult. Another sentence-production training program, cuing verb treatments, is based on the notion that the verb is the central constituent in sentence structure (100). In this approach, verbs are presented as the central core of the simple active sentence; patients are trained to produce the verb, and in response to a "wh"-question cuing strategy, also specific sentence constituents (usually noun phrases) that are assigned to various thematic roles by the verb (e.g., agent, theme).

Based on aspects of formal linguistic theory and neurolinguistic research, and consistent with Chomsky's conceptual framework, Thompson and colleagues have developed a series of treatment strategies to improve sentence comprehension and production of complex sentences such as "wh"-questions and passives (101–103). Of particular clinical relevance is a finding that has been called the "complexity hypothesis" (104, 105). The hypothesis suggests that there is more generalization of improvements from treated to untreated grammatical forms when treatment begins with more complex structures than when treatment is limited to simple forms. This contrasts with traditional treatment, which typically is hierarchically organized and starts at a simple level and gradually increases in level of difficulty.

A similar finding has been noted in the area of semantics. There is an extensive literature examining recovery of naming in patients with aphasia (106, 107). One form of treatment, called semantic feature analysis, was developed to strengthen the semantic attributes or features of target words (108–112). The treatment involves repeated practice associating the target word with its various defining characteristics (e.g., *robin: has wings, has beak, lays eggs, flies, small, builds nest, lives in trees, bird*). More recently, it has been demonstrated that when the treatment uses target words that are less typical of their category and therefore more complex (e.g. *penguin, ostrich are not typical of birds because they do not fly or live in trees*), generalization of treatment effects is greater than when typical targets are used (113–115). This hypothesis has been called the "semantic complexity hypothesis" and provides further support for the notion that treatment should not necessarily be provided in a hierarchical fashion from easy to more difficult (113–115).

Functional communication approach: In the functional communication or pragmatic approach, therapists are no longer interested only in the accuracy of the linguistic message, but focus on the patient's ability to communicate the intent of the message. Communication involves more than just speaking and understanding, but reflects the application of pragmatic rules and the ability to use language in a context. Therefore, treatment includes compensatory strategies for circumventing communication breakdown as well as strategies for communication breakdown repair. One of the best-known pragmatic approaches is PACE (Promoting Aphasic's Communicative Effectiveness) (116). In the PACE technique, four major treatment principles have been delineated in an attempt to incorporate rules of natural communication into semistructured treatment: the clinician and patient participate equally as senders and receivers of messages; the

interaction incorporates the exchange of new information between clinician and patient; patients freely choose the channels through which they will communicate—words, gestures, drawing or any other communication device; and the clinicians' feedback is based on the patient's success in communicating the message.

Other approaches such as practicing scripted conversations (117–119), ensuring a positive communication environment by training communication partners to use conversational supports (120), extending treatment into natural communication settings including aphasia communication groups (121), and removing environmental barriers to participation in community activities (122) also may be considered "functional" approaches. However, the term "social approach" may better describe some of these treatments since they are *explicitly* designed to improve communication, life participation, and/or personal well being (6, 123–131).

Life Participation Approach to Aphasia. Recently, an umbrella philosophy called the life participation approach to aphasia (LPAA) has fueled even greater interest in the social approaches to the management of aphasia (124). The LPAA is a set of values that guides intervention, assessment, and research. It calls for a broadening and refocusing of clinical practice, suggesting that the focus of aphasia treatment be on "re-engagement in life" for the person with aphasia.

The LPAA has applicability throughout and beyond the period of formal rehabilitation, beginning with initial assessment and intervention and continuing, after hospital discharge, until the person with aphasia no longer elects to have communication support. All those affected by aphasia are regarded as legitimate targets for intervention, including not only the person with aphasia but family members, coworkers, and individuals in the community who may interact with the person with aphasia. According to the LPAA, treatment includes facilitating the achievement of life goals. Therefore, in addition to work on improving and/or compensating for the language impairment, clinicians should be prepared to work on anything in which aphasia is a barrier to life participation, even if the activity is not directly related to communication. This may include targeting environmental factors outside of the individual since a highly supportive environment can lessen the consequences of aphasia on one's life, whatever the lanuage impairment (124).

Biological Approaches to Language Remediation. As we acquire new knowledge about aphasia and brain-behavior relations, additional approaches to treatment that are not easily categorized with the present taxonomy are emerging. For example, Small has advocated for a biological model of aphasia rehabilitation in which the goal of remediation is to alter brain anatomy and physiology so that language function can be restored (132, 133). In order to effect the necessary neural changes, both novel biological treatments and speech-language treatment are necessary. The biological treatment stimulates or repairs the injured brain area, while the language treatments are provided to retrain the new circuitry and integrate it with the preserved, existing tissue.

Pharmacotherapy: Pharmacotherapy is the most frequently used biological therapy for aphasia. To date, the majority of studies have investigated the effects of four groups of neurotransmitters on language deficits in aphasia (134). These include the following: dopamine agonists such as bromocriptine (135–139); dextro-amphetamine and other agents that affect catecholamine systems (140, 141); cholinergic medications such as donepezil, an acetylcholinesterase inhibitor (142, 143); and the nootropic agent, piracetam (144, 145). Following a systematic review of this literature, de Boissezon et al. (2007) concluded that efficacy of each pharamcologic agent remains questionable. However, the majority of the studies concerned the chronic stage of aphasia, and the authors suggest that the adjuvant pharmacologic treatment may best be applied before most neural reorganization has taken place. Indeed, the most efficacious results were evident with amphetamine and piracetam, both of which were investigated with individuals with aphasia between 6 and 12 weeks post-stroke onset. Additionally, treatments were less efficient when given alone than when there was associated speech therapy (134). This finding resonates with Small's suggestion that pharmacologic treatment has promise, but only when accompanied by concommitant language therapy (132, 133).

Any discussion of aphasia and pharmacology must also consider the deleterious effects that some drugs may have on stroke recovery, including aphasia recovery. A retrospective study of medication use during aphasia rehabilitation indicated that over 80% of all patients were taking some medicine at the time of their stroke and that 65% were taking multiple medications (146). Included in this list were such drugs as adrenergic blockers and benzodiazepines, which are known to impede stroke recovery in animal studies. Deleterious effects have been reported for neuroleptics (haloperidol), thiazides, and tricyclic antidepressant agents (146, 147). Therefore drugs that potentially interfere with catecholaminergic or GABAergic function or are thought to delay recovery by empirical study (i.e., the drugs in Table 10-3) should be avoided if possible during aphasia rehabilitation (43).

Cortical stimulation: A relatively new area of investigation is the direct application of stimulation to the cerebral cortex to facilitate brain plasticity and enhance stroke recovery. There are several methods of delivering cortical brain stimulation transcranially—these include direct epidural cortical stimulation (148), repetitive transcranial magnetic stimulation (rTMS) (149, 150), and transcranial

---

TABLE 10-3
Drugs with Potentially Deleterious Effects on Stroke Recovery

Benzodiazepines
Clonidine
Haloperidol
Phenothiazines
Phenytoin
Prazosin

---

direct current stimulation (tDCS) (151, 152), each of which have been applied to the rehabilitation of language after stroke. Results suggest a potential role for cortical stimulation as an adjuvant strategy in aphasia rehabilitation.

There is only one study that assesses the safety and efficacy of direct epidural cortical stimulation in combination with intensive speech-language therapy on individuals with chronic aphasia (148). Eight participants received intensive behavioral therapy using a combination of articulation drills, oral reading, and conversational practice, delivered 3 hours daily for 6 weeks. Four of these participants also underwent fMRI-guided surgical implantation of an epidural stimulation device, which was activated for all therapy sessions. Behavioral data were collected before treatment, immediately after treatment, and at 6 and 12 weeks following the termination of therapy. Imaging data were collected before and after treatment. Results indicated that investigational subjects showed a mean aphasia quotient change of 8.0 points immediately post-therapy and at 6-week follow-up and 12.3 points at 12 weeks. The control group had smaller mean changes of 4.6, 5.5, and 3.6 points, respectively. Similar changes were noted on subjective caregiver ratings of the participants' language and communication skills, with larger changes being noted for the investigational group as compared to the control group at all time points. Functional imaging suggested increased consolidation of activity in interventional subjects. Therefore, while behavioral speech-language therapy improved the nonfluent aphasia, independent of cortical stimulation, the epidural stimulation of the ipsilesional premotor cortex may have augmented this effect. The largest effects between the groups were evident after completion of the therapy. The neural mechanisms underlying these effects were manifested in the brain by decreases in the volume of activity globally and in particular regions. Although the number of patients enrolled in this trial precludes strong conclusions, epidural stimulation could play an adjunctive role in treatment of nonfluent aphasia.

Although further investigation of the effects of direct epidural cortical stimulation is warranted, the clinical applicability of this procedure may be limited by the invasiveness of the procedure, which requires neurosurgical implantation of the electrodes. A less invasive therapy for language remediation in aphasia is repetitive transcranial magnetic stimulation (rTMS) (149, 150). Based on the premise that overactivity of the right-hemisphere language homologues may be maladaptive and interfere with, rather than promote, aphasia recovery, rTMS was applied to the right hemisphere to reduce its cortical excitability. Preliminary results obtained in four individuals with chronic nonfluent aphasia indicated improved picture naming following 10 sessions of rTMS (150).

tDCS may also have potential for clinical use in view of its noninvasive application, ease of administration, and relatively low cost. tDCS is a method of delivering weak polarizing electrical currents to the cortex via two electrodes placed on the scalp: an active electrode placed on the site overlying the cortical target and a reference electrode usually placed over the contralateral supraorbital area. The nature of the effect depends on the polarity of the current. Anodal tDCS has an excitatory effect believed to result from the partial depolarization of superficial cortical axons, while cathodal tDCS induces inhibition via presumed hyperpolarization. Studies on the efficacy of tDCS are emerging (151, 152), and may, in the future, provide promise, especially when linked with intensive language treatment.

Treatment Intensity, Constraint-induced Aphasia Therapy, and Computers. Regardless of the treatment approach, a critical question remains regarding how much treatment is optimal and at what frequency. The question of treatment intensity is of considerable importance in light of recent work in neuroscience demonstrating that the neuroplasticity of the adult brain can be impacted by several experience-dependent principles including intensity of training (153). In addition, a growing literature suggests that, with intensive treatment, individuals with chronic aphasia continue to demonstrate language recovery for years post stroke. For example, Bhogal et al. (2003) conducted a literature review that suggests that intensive speech language therapy delivered over a short period of time (average of 8.8 hours per week for 11.2 weeks) resulted in significant improvements, while lower intensity therapy provided over a longer period of time (average of 2 hours per week over 22.9 weeks) did not result in positive change.

Pulvermuller, Meinzer and their colleagues have spurred increased interest about treatment intensity with their studies of constraint-induced language therapy (CILT) for individuals with aphasia (155–158). Within CILT, training responses are constrained to the verbal modality, that is, forced use of verbal production, in contrast to other aphasia treatment approaches in which the use of all communication modalities is encouraged. In addition, CILT emphasizes the importance of massed practice, and treatment is provided on an intensive schedule, 3 hours

per day for 2 weeks. Despite positive findings reported for CILT, it has been difficult to determine whether the treatment results emanate from the constrained forced language use, the intensity of the treatment schedule, or a combination of these two factors (158–160).

Nevertheless, it is generally agreed that intensity of speech-language therapy is an important component of aphasia intervention (159). However, providing intensive treatment to individuals with chronic aphasia can be costly, and the current healthcare environment in the United States is one that does not typically recognize its value. As a result, clinicians and researchers in the field are left searching for cost-effective ways to deliver aphasia treatment. One method of providing less costly but intensive treatment is via the computer.

A well-documented body of literature supports the positive effects of computerized treatment for aphasia (161–163). While many earlier computer-based therapy programs relied on predefined exercises that were fairly inflexible, more recent programs have been designed to allow specifically for treatment that is interactive and individualized to clients' needs. Two examples of aphasia treatment software that have undergone extensive efficacy research are AphasiaScripts™ (117, 118) and SentenceShaper (164). The AphasiaScripts software program uses an animated agent or virtual therapist that is programmed to produce natural speech with correct movements of the speech articulators. This virtual therapist serves as the conversational partner, while the person with aphasia repetitively practices prerecorded individualized conversational scripts with varying degrees of support and cues that are generated by the computer (117). Similarly, the SentenceShaper assists the person with aphasia practice their self-generated short stories, but without the benefit of a virtual conversational partner (164).

As computer technology becomes more accessible and researchers and clinicians continue to explore the utilization and benefit of computerized treatments in clinical practice, computer treatment will become more commonplace. Yet, computer therapy, even when practiced by individuals with aphasia independently in their homes, does not negate or diminish the importance of the experienced practitioner. The clinician plays a critical role in all aspects of treatment planning and development, while the computer provides the intensive, massed practice required for automatization of the learned narrative or conversational script, a laborious and time-consuming process when provided by a therapist.

Efficacy of Aphasia Treatment

Any discussion about language remediation in adults must also address the basic question of whether aphasia treatment works. One source of confusion surrounding this issue is the concept of remediation versus eradication. At the present time, there is no aphasia therapy that cures aphasia. Yet there is ample evidence that frequent sessions of aphasia therapy over a long period of time can lead to continued improvement.

To date, the historical record of clinical outcomes for treatments of aphasia is extensive (165). Over time, experimental methodologies in the field of aphasia have improved (e.g., measuring the change in communication behavior from pre-test to post-test; controlling for time post-onset; setting clear exclusion and inclusion criteria to establish homogeneous groups; introducing no-treatment control groups or using deferred treatment groups; random assignment; and controls on the type(s), amount, and duration of treatment), so that findings have become less ambiguous and support the conclusion that treatment for aphasia is both efficacious and effective (165). While there are relatively few randomized clinical trials of aphasia treatment (166), over 100 single-subject aphasia treatment studies have appeared in the literature. In addition, meta-analyses applied to the

aphasia treatment literature have concluded that aphasia treatment is effective (167–170). In two of these meta-analyses, based on 21 studies and 55 studies respectively (168, 169), it was also concluded that recovery of treated individuals was, on average, nearly twice as extensive as the recovery of untreated individuals when treatment was begun before 3 months post-onset. Treatment brought about appreciable gains, even when begun after 3 months post onset, and treatment brought about large effects even in individuals with severe aphasia.

Treatment Outcomes. Returning to the question of what constitutes "outcome" in aphasia treatment, Kagan et al. (2008) have developed a framework that serves as a guide for categorizing different measures of outcome. Based on the World Health Organization's International Classification of Functioning, Disability and Health (ICF) (172), the Living with Aphasia: Framework for Outcome Measurement (A-FROM) model is pictured in Figure 10-2. The A-FROM framework consists of the following overlapping domains:

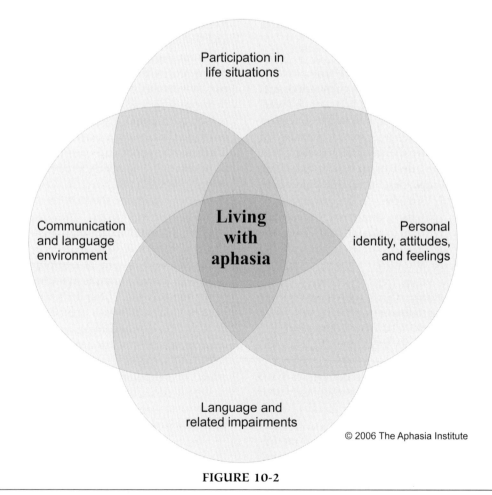

FIGURE 10-2

Living with aphasia: framework for outcome measurement (A-FROM). Reprinted with permission from the Aphasia Institute, Toronto, Canada.

- *The participation domain*: This includes the life situations specific to an individual such as life roles (e.g., mother, teacher); responsibilities (e.g., managing finances, performing a job); relationships (e.g., engaging in conversation, making friends); activities of choice (e.g., leisure and recreation, community participation); and tasks engaged in by an individual (e.g., writing letters, cashing a check—described as "Activities" in the ICF).
- *Language and related impairments domain:* This is the correlate of the "Body Function" domain of the ICF and includes outcomes in the realm of language and cognitive processing such as auditory comprehension (e.g., pointing to pictures named); reading (e.g., matching a written word to a picture); speaking (e.g., word finding, sentence formulation), and writing (e.g., writing the names of objects).
- *Communication and language environment domain:* This is the correlate of ICF "Environmental Context" domain and includes aspects of external context that might facilitate or impede language, communication, or participation of people with aphasia such as physical environment (e.g., signage, lighting, written supports); social environment (e.g., attitudes of people, skills of partners); and political environment (e.g., policies supporting participation).
- *Personal factors/identity domain:* This includes ICF factors such as age, gender, and culture, but expands the ICF domain to include internal factors that vary as a consequence of aphasia such as confidence and personal identity.
- *Living with aphasia domain:* This is a dynamic interaction of four life domains, capturing elements of quality of life (how satisfied someone is with their life).

The A-FROM is not intended to be prescriptive in relation to aphasia intervention, but rather serves as a guide for selecting outcome domains across diverse aphasia interventions (171). The ultimate goal of any intervention is to make a difference to the everyday experiences of individuals with aphasia and their families, and there are multiple ways for clinicians to work toward accomplishing this. Thus, the A-FROM can also serve as a guide for the clinician to use when counseling patients and their families about the goals of rehabilitation and the specific focus of any one or more treatments within the context of the overriding goal of living successfully with aphasia. Although the A-FROM was developed to address specifically the outcomes of those with aphasia, its breadth makes it applicable to any type of communication disorder, including apraxia of speech and dysarthria, which are discussed in the next sections.

APRAXIA OF SPEECH

Apraxia of speech (AOS) is a disorder that is distinguishable at a theoretical level from both aphasia and dysarthria, but remains somewhat controversial at a more practical level. The main problem is that it still has an unclear neurologic and functional basis and has no universally agreed-upon definition (173).

Traditionally, AOS was defined as a disorder of motor programming, "an articulatory disorder resulting from impairment, due to brain damage, of the capacity to program the positioning of speech musculature for the volitional production of phonemes and the sequencing of muscle movements for the production of words" (174). More recently, Van der Merwe (1997) has suggested that AOS is a motor planning disorder rather than a disturbance in the programming of movements for speech. Difficulties arise at an earlier stage of speech processing in which the neural codes for specifying the spatial and temporal characteristics of the output are computed.

Neurologically, both hypotheses assume that specification and programming are mediated by the cortical association areas including the lateral premotor cortex, the supplementary motor area, the prefrontal areas, and the posterior parietal areas. In contrast, some studies have observed AOS from isolated damage to the anterior portion of the insula, concluding that the insula must be damaged in order for AOS to occur (176, 177). These findings are not without dispute since other studies have demonstrated that AOS occurs in the absence of insular damage (178–180), and there may be alternative explanations for the data on the insula (181).

Characteristics of AOS

Despite the debate about AOS, there is general consensus that AOS is a disorder of articulation and prosody of speech. Numerous articulatory characteristics have been specified. For example, based on previous reports (174, 182, 183), Freed (2000) compiled a list of as many as 14 articulatory characteristics that occur most commonly. However, not all patients with AOS display all characteristics. Differences in the manifestation of AOS may be related to the possible existence of AOS subtypes, to various concomitant effects of a coexisting aphasia, or to variability associated with AOS severity.

Nevertheless, there are some core symptoms of AOS that consistently form part of the diagnostic description and these have been identified in a report by the Cochrane collaboration as follows (184):

- Effortful "groping" (that is trial-and-error attempts) at finding the correct articulatory positions for the target phonemes and therefore difficulty producing the correct sounds

- Inconsistent or variable errors (i.e., the same sounds are not always in error, and each attempt at a word could produce a different error)
- More consonant than vowel errors
- Articulatory errors that are characterized by perceived substitutions, distortions, omissions, and repetitions; phonemes and words often approximate the target; they sound similar but are not exactly the same as the target sound or word
- Difficulty in producing consonants that are adjacent to each other (e.g., *str*, *bl*, *kr*, *spl*) resulting in a tendency to insert additional vowels
- Awareness of errors

Prosodically, the rate of connected speech in AOS is usually slower than normal. Equal stress may be placed on the syllables in an utterance. Inappropriate pauses may occur at the start of a word or between syllables. These pauses may result from articulatory groping or because each syllable is being produced individually rather than being produced fluently by blending one syllable into another. The normal variations of pitch and loudness are restricted. In some cases, the altered prosody may lead to the perception of a foreign accent in monolingual speakers (185, 186), although this may not be the only underlying mechanism of foreign accent syndrome (187). There are several explanations for the rate and prosodic abnormalities of AOS. They may be a fundamental feature of the disorder, a simple by-product of the articulation deficits, or they could reflect efforts at compensation for the articulation deficit.

An issue that is commonly discussed is whether AOS always co-occurs with Broca's aphasia or nonfluent aphasia, or whether it is isolable neurologically. Many of the articulatory and prosodic perceptual features of AOS have been confirmed by acoustic and physiologic studies (8). These studies also have provided data supporting the conclusion that many of the features of AOS reflect a phonetic disorder of motor planning and programming rather than deficits that are fundamentally linguistic in character (8, 182).

In addition, Duffy (1995) asserts that most definitions of Broca's aphasia do not give overt recognition to the existence of a motor speech programming disorder, despite the description of poor "articulatory agility" and speech that is slow, labored or effortful, reduced in phrase length, and abnormal in prosody. While these characteristics are consistent with those of AOS, individuals with Broca's aphasia also have grammatical and syntactical errors and problems with word retrieval, as well as problems with auditory comprehension, reading, and writing. Therefore, a reasonable conclusion is that patients with Broca's or nonfluent aphasia usually have AOS, but that the aphasic components of Broca's aphasia include additional deficits that are outside of the definition of AOS (182).

Assessment of AOS

Most clinicians assess AOS with a comprehensive motor speech evaluation (8, 188). This involves assessing muscle strength and tone and speed, range, and accuracy of movements during single and repetitive movements in both nonspeech and speech activities. It also includes specific tasks to assess phonation, articulation, resonance, prosody, and ventilatory support for speech.

Tasks that require the patient to sequence speech sounds are particularly sensitive to the presence of AOS. These tasks include alternating motion rates (repetition of the same sound such as *pa*) and sequential motion rates (repetition of different sounds requiring multiple articulatory positions such as *pa-ta-ka*). Other sensitive tasks include repetition of words of increasing length (e.g., *fan*, *fancy*, *fantastic*), multisyllabic words with complex phonemes combinations, and phrases and sentences. In addition, connected speech is analyzed from reading aloud paragraphs and through spontaneous conversation.

Before making a diagnosis of AOS, it is important to rule out other conditions that may cause movement difficulties similar to AOS. For example, muscle weakness and incoordination can cause slow, labored, or awkward movements. However, in AOS, the abnormal movements affecting speech are more obvious during voluntary movements. The patient may have no difficulty automatically saying *goodbye* when leaving the company of someone but may be unable to say *goodbye* out of context. Similarly, speech may sound quite good during production of automatic sequences such as counting, saying the days of the week, or reciting a familiar poem.

There are only a few published tests for AOS. These include the Apraxia Battery for Adults(189) and the Comprehensive Apraxia Test (190). Neither test provides data that discriminate impairments resulting from apraxia of speech, aphasia, or dysarthria. Therefore, the differential diagnosis is one that the clinician must make based on observations of performance during the assessment tasks.

Treatment of AOS

Most treatments for AOS are behavioral, yet they are diverse in terms of their focus and theoretical underpinnings (191). Four general groups of treatments for AOS have been identified (192, 193). Although these approaches are not mutually exclusive and some treatments use a combination of techniques that cross one or more categories, the availability of a categorization scheme can be helpful for treatment planning.

The most common group of treatments for AOS target improved positioning and movements of the articulators and have been referred to as *articulatory kinematic* treatments (192). In general, these treatments tend to be time-intensive, repetitive, and highly structured, progressing from simple to complex verbal productions of targeted phonemes, words, and phrases. Emphasis is placed on self-monitoring and self-correction, with feedback from the clinician helping to facilitate this.

Several specific strategies are incorporated, to various degrees, into these types of treatments. During imitation, the patient simply watches and listens as the clinician provides a model that the patient then attempts to reproduce. A variation of imitation is called "integral stimulation" in which the patient is instructed to "watch me, listen to me, and say it with me" while the clinician exaggerates the presentation of the stimulus to make it as salient as possible (194, 195). Another strategy is phonetic derivation, the progressive approximation or shaping of the positioning and movement of the articulators using sounds and movements that the patient can already make to teach the placement and movement of sounds that he/she cannot make. For example, patients may be instructed to put their lips together and blow to assist with the production of p and b sounds, thereby using a nonspeech posture to help produce the target speech sounds.

Phonetic placement techniques make use of explicit verbal, written, and graphic descriptions of how a sound is made in combination with physical manipulation of the articulators. An example of a program that includes direct instruction for speech production is PROMPT (Prompts for Restructuring Oral Muscular Phonetic Targets) (196). In PROMPT, the clinician provides a complex combination of auditory, visual, tactile, and kinesthetic cues to the face and neck to represent the various positions of the articulators during speech and to signify various aspects of speech production, including relative timing of speech segments.

Darley et al. (1975) have emphasized the use of phonemic drills involving repeated production, as many as 10–20 times, of the same consonant-vowel combinations. Careful selection of the target sounds is essential. The drills begin with just a single vowel, and consonants are slowly added. The first consonant is typically the m, which is highly visible and often the easiest to produce. The position of the vowel in the word is alternated from the initial position (ma), to the final position (am), and then to the medial position (ama). Different combinations of consonant-vowel syllables that gradually increase in complexity and length are practiced before moving to real words, two-word combinations, and phrases. Similar drills have been described by Dabul and Bollier (1976), who set a criteria for each target combination of 60 one-syllable repetitions or 20 two-syllable repetitions in 15 seconds before moving to combinations at the next level of difficulty (197).

Although treatment may begin at the level of the individual phoneme or speech sound, especially for more severe cases, there is general agreement that, as much as possible, target stimuli be made up of functional words that are immediately useful to the patient (183, 194). To promote generalization of sound production to words, the key word technique involves practicing the target sounds in a core vocabulary, and then expanding the limited number of words into a larger set.

A second group of treatments addresses speech rate and the rhythmic, temporal, or prosodic aspects of speech production (198, 199). In these techniques, an external source of control is applied to the speaker's productions such as finger counting, hand tapping, and/or a metronome. Some studies have also used computer-generated controls of rate and rhythm (200, 201). The underlying premise of these treatments is that AOS is characterized by disruptions in the timing of speech production, although the mechanism responsible for behavioral change is not well understood. Some techniques have also incorporated speech prolongation and reduced rate as part of the rhythm control. The additional slowing of speech production may provide extra time for motor planning and/or programming, as well as for processing of sensory feedback.

A third group of treatments reflects the concept of *intersystemic facilitation/reorganization*. These approaches are based on the premise of using relatively intact systems or modalites to facilitate speech production. Gestural reorganization has been studied most frequently with the gestures serving as a relatively intact nonverbal ability that helps to reorganize speech. In most studies, the gestures are paired with verbalizations during treatment (202). The use of singing in the treatment of AOS may also be considered a form of intersystemic facilitation/reorganization (203).

The final approach to working with AOS involves the use of *alternative and/or augmentative communication* (AAC) methods to substitute for or supplement verbal communication. Selection of the AAC approach needs to be highly individualized and may include one or more of the following: picture and word communication books; writing or drawing; gestures; alphabet supplementation; voice output aids; and informed communication partners. Goals may vary from instruction of a consistent "yes/no" response to conversational practice and role playing in simulated situations (204–206).

As Peach (2004) points out, however, few treatments have been reported where the individual had a pure AOS. Usually, patients tend to have a coexisting /accompanying aphasia. Therefore, selection of treatments must consider the severity of the accompanying aphasia. There are a few treatment programs that have addressed aspects of both the AOS and the aphasia, including melodic intonation therapy (MIT) discussed previously as well as a technique called oral reading for language in aphasia (ORLA) (208). ORLA combines integral stimulation of sentences, multimodality paced choral reading, and rhythmic pointing and has been used successfully with individuals with nonfluent aphasia and AOS (208).

Efficacy of Treatments for AOS

Several recent reviews of treatments for AOS are available (173, 185, 192, 193). A Cochrane review of interventions for apraxia of speech following stroke did not identify any trials that matched their search criteria of randomized controlled trials of nondrug interventions for adults with AOS in which the primary outcome was functional speech at 6 months follow-up (185). Therefore the authors concluded that rehabilitation approaches for AOS following stroke "have yet to be supported or refuted by randomized trials" (185).

In contrast to the Cochrane group, a systematic review of the evidence for treatment of AOS was conducted by a committee of the Academy of Neurologic Communication Disorders and Sciences (ANCDS) using search criteria of "providing data pertinent to the effects of treatment with at least one person with AOS" (192, 193). From a total of 59 data-based treatment reports that met these criteria, the committee concluded that, taken as a whole, individuals with AOS "show gains in measured performance as a result of treatment," even when the AOS is chronic. They acknowledge that study quality was generally weak, with methodological issues relating to insufficient description of the subjects and their AOS, trial design that often lacked experimental control, inclusion of small numbers of subjects, and outcome measures that were not always reliable and valid (209). Yet a growing body of evidence is available to support the articulatory kinematic treatments, and evidence for the other types of treatments for AOS is "promising, but limited" (193).

In conclusion, apraxia of speech is a condition with a range of severities and manifestations. While future research continues to address the question of treatment efficacy, clinicians working with individuals with AOS have a repertoire of different approaches from which to choose and adapt to the unique characteristic and needs of their patients.

DYSARTHRIA

Dysarthria is a collective term for the group of speech disorders that result from paralysis, weakness, or incoordination of the speech musculature following damage to the central or peripheral nervous system (174, 210, 211). The definition of dysarthria includes disturbances of any of the basic components underlying speech production (i.e., respiration, phonation, articulation, resonance, and prosody).

Classifying the Dysarthrias

In clinical practice, the most common approach used to classify the dysarthrias is the perceptual method. Its premise is that each type of dysarthria sounds different and that these perceptual differences can be tied to specific underlying neuropathologies (174, 210, 211). Based on cluster analysis of listener judgments of speech dimensions, six distinctive types of dysarthria—flaccid, spastic, ataxic, hypokinetic, hyperkinetic, and mixed—were identified initially (210, 211). A seventh dysarthria type, unilateral upper motor neuron dysarthria, was later recognized and subsequently described by Duffy (1995). Examples of the perceptual dimensions used to characterize the different dysarthrias are listed in Table 10-4 (212).

Although theoretically a stroke could cause damage to the central and peripheral nervous system resulting in any type of dysarthria, vascular incidents within the central nervous system typically affect certain cortical areas, the cerebellum, or the brainstem. Therefore, the most common dysarthrias following a stroke are unilateral upper motor neuron dysarthria, spastic, ataxic, flaccid, and mixed dysarthrias. Each of these dysarthrias are discussed with an emphasis on the characteristic perceptual features of the disordered speech.

Unilateral upper motor neuron (UUMN) dysarthria: UUMN dysarthria, as its name implies, is caused by unilateral cortical damage involving the upper motor neurons. As a result, there is damage to the lower face, with weakness of the lips and tongue on the opposite side from the lesion. Movements, therefore, are slow and reduced in range of motion, with the main perceptual characteristic of UUMN dysarthria being imprecise consonant production. However, intelligibility of speech is usually only mildly affected. In some patients, the resultant dysarthria is transient. In others, the effects of the dysarthria can be persistent so that referral to speech therapy is appropriate (182).

Effects of UUMN damage on other structures of speech production (velum, pharynx, larynx) are less well understood. Because the upper motor neurons on the unaffected side provide sufficient innervation to the cranial nerves serving the two sides of these structures, they should not be affected. However, there is some individual variability in anatomy that could alter this, and a harsh vocal quality and hypernasality have been noted in some patients.

Spastic dysarthria: Spastic dysarthria occurs from a single stroke in the brainstem or from more than one lesion that causes bilateral upper motor neuron damage affecting both the pyramidal and extrapyramidal systems. The symptoms reflect the combined effects of both systems on the speech muscles. Weakness and spasticity result in slow movement and reduced range and force. The weakness and slowness are most evident in movements of the

TABLE 10-4
Sample Speech Dimensions and Characteristics Rated in the Perceptual Method of Classifying Dysarthria[1]

SPEECH DIMENSIONS	SAMPLE CHARACTERISTICS
Pitch characteristics	Pitch level (decreased, increased), pitch breaks, monopitch, tremor
Loudness	Overall loudness (decreased), monoloudness, excess loudness variation, alternating loudness
Vocal quality	Harsh, hoarse (wet), breathiness (continuous), breathiness (transient), strained/strangled, voice stoppages, hypernasality, hyponasality, nasal emission
Ventilation	Audible inspiration, forced inspiration-expiration, grunt at end of expiration
Prosody	Rate (fast, slow), phrases (short), increased rate in segments of speech, inappropriate silences, short rushes of speech, excess and equal stress
Articulation	Imprecise consonants, distorted vowels, irregular articulatory breakdown
Overall	Intelligibility, bizarreness

[1]Reprinted with permission from Hammen VL. Motor speech problems associated with stroke: the dysarthrias. *Top Stroke Rehabil.* 1994; 1(2):68.

tongue and lips, leading to imprecise consonant production, vowel distortions, and a slow rate of speech. The effect of spasticity on the velum causes incomplete velopharyngeal closure and hypernasality. Spasticity in the laryngeal muscles results in hyperadduction of the vocal folds, which is perceived as a harsh and strained-strangled vocal quality. Because of difficulty forcing subglottic air through hyperadducted vocal folds, the person may speak in short phrases in conversational speech. In addition, the frequent inhalations of air interrupt the normal rhythm of speech. Prosodically, a low pitch as well as monopitch and monoloudness may be present. Spastic dysarthria may be associated with pseudobulbar affect in which uncontrollable laughing or crying accompanies the damage to the upper motor neurons of the brain stem.

Flaccid dysarthria: Flaccid dysarthria results from injury to the lower motor neurons in one or more of the cranial or spinal nerves. It reflects problems in the nuclei, axons, or neuromuscular junctions that make up the motor units of the final common pathway. Weakness, hypotonia, and diminished reflexes are the primary characteristics, and atrophy, fasciculations and fibrillations commonly accompany them.

The effects of flaccid dysarthria on respiration, phonation, articulation, resonance, and prosody vary depending on which cranial nerves are affected. The cranial nerves of speech production are the trigeminal nerve (V), facial nerve (VII), glossopharyngeal nerve (IX), vagus nerve (X), accessory nerve (XI), and hypoglossal nerve (XII). Damage to the facial and hypoglossal nerves most often causes imprecise consonant production, ranging in severity from only mild distortions to complete unintelligibility. Bilateral facial nerve involvement can affect production of bilabial (*p, b, m*) and labiodental (*f, v*) phonemes, as well as consonant and vowels that require lip rounding. Bilateral damage to the hypoglossal nerve likely results in misarticulation of phonemes requiring tongue elevation (e.g., *l, r*). Damage to the trigeminal nerve can also affect articulation because of difficulty elevating the jaw sufficiently to bring the articulators into contact with each other.

Hypernasality is one of the most noticeable signs of flaccid dysarthria, although it is not unique to it. Nasal emission (escape of air through the nasal cavity) may also occur because of incomplete velopharyngeal closure. At the laryngeal level, damage to the recurrent branch of the vagus nerve that provides innervation to almost all of the intrinsic muscles of the larynx leads to incomplete adduction of the vocal folds during phonation and a resulting breathy voice quality.

The spinal nerves are also important because they innervate the muscles of respiration. If the cervical and thoracic spinal nerves responsible for innervating the diaphragm and the intercostal muscles are damaged, then decreased inhalation or impaired control of exhalation during speech leads to reduced subglottic air pressure for speech and, therefore, reduced loudness, shortened phrase lengths, and a strained vocal quality.

Ataxic dysarthria: Ataxic dysarthria is associated with cerebellar damage or damage to the neural pathways that connect the cerebellum to other parts of the central nervous system. Cerebellar damage disrupts the timing, force, range, and direction of movements needed to maintain normal articulation. Articulation deficits are a major problem, with imprecise consonant articulation being the most prevalent speech error. Often, the articulation errors are inconsistent, varying from utterance to utterance and giving the speech the characteristic described as irregular articulatory breakdowns.

Prosodic errors also are prominent in ataxic dysarthria. Many speakers tend to put equal stress on syllables or words that would normally have varied stress patterns. They also tend to put excessive stress on syllables or words that are not normally stressed to any degree, giving the impression that each syllable or word is produced separately. Additionally, ataxic speech is characterized by prolonged phonemes and prolonged intervals between phonemes contributing to an overall slow rate of speech.

Cerebellar damage may cause tremors that affect various body parts, and when the laryngeal or respiratory muscles are involved, the result can be a voice tremor. Cerebellar damage can also cause uncoordinated movements in the respiratory muscles. Exaggerated movements of the respiratory muscles can lead to excessive loudness variations during many speech tasks including conversation.

Mixed dysarthrias: When neurologic damage extends into two or more parts of the motor system, the resulting dysarthria is called a mixed dysarthria. For example, a flaccid-ataxic mixed dysarthria results from involvement of both the lower motor neurons and the cerebellum. A flaccid-spastic mixed dysarthria may result from a brainstem stroke in which the lower and upper motor neurons are in close proximity to each other. The speech characteristics of a mixed dysarthria reflect a combination of the characteristics found in the single or pure dysarthrias, with the location and extent of the neurologic damage determining which characteristics are likely to appear. Thus, the relative prominence of each dysarthria type can vary from patient to patient. For example, in one individual with a flaccid-spastic dysarthria, the flaccid component (e.g., nasal emission) may be much more evident than the spastic component (e.g., strained-strangled voice quality), while the opposite may be apparent in another individual.

Assessment of Dysarthria

Most clinicians assess dysarthria with a comprehensive motor speech evaluation that is similar to the assessment described previously for apraxia of speech (8, 184). The motor speech examination includes tasks designed to describe the speech characteristics and the underlying neuromuscular features that influence speech production. Speech characteristics include those at the levels of respiration, phonation, articulation, resonance, and prosody, while the "salient" features of neuromuscular function include muscle strength, speed, range, accuracy, steadiness, and tone (8, 182).

The oral mechanism (lips, tongue, jaw, velum, pharynx, larynx) is examined at rest and during nonspeech activities to provides confirmatory evidence and information about the size, strength, range, tone, steadiness, speed, and accuracy of orofacial structures and movements. Speech tasks include vowel prolongation during which pitch, loudness, voice quality, and duration are observed. Alternating motion rates for assessing the speed and regularity of rapid repetitive articulatory movements and sequential motion rates for assessing the ability to move quickly from one articulatory position to another are also included in the motor speech assessment.

Contextual speech such as reading aloud a paragraph, retelling a story, or responding in conversation show how well all the components of speech are integrated.

Judgments of speech intelligibility are also made. These may include estimates by the clinician or formal assessment with standard intelligibility tests such as the Frenchay Dysarthria Assessment (213) and the Assessment of Intelligibility of Dysarthric Speech (214).

Many acoustic and physiologic tests are available to study motor speech disorders, and they have the potential to quantify and explain clinical perceptual observations and to increase our understanding of the pathophysiologic underpinnings of dysarthric speech (8). However, they are not yet standard practice, and their use is limited primarily to the research laboratory.

Treatment of Dysarthria

A successful program for the management of dysarthria following a stroke should address both the impairment and the activity/participation limitations imposed by the impairment. Treatment techniques for the impairment focus on improving the physiologic support for speech including respiration, phonation, articulation, and resonance with an emphasis on muscle tone, strength, movement precision, and coordination. Treatment techniques at the level of activity and participation may include modifying speech through compensatory speaking strategies, developing alternative and augmentative means of communication, and controlling the environment and communicative interactions to maximize communication.

Body positioning can influence respiratory support for speech (215, 216). Therefore, postural adjustments, particularly for patients in wheelchairs, may be a simple way to improve respiratory drive for speech. However, improvements in respiratory support are ideally targeted during actual speech production. Some patients may simply need to practice inhaling more deeply or using more force when exhaling during speech. When the number of words produced on a single exhalation of air is limited, chunking utterances into short syntactic units with normal pauses within and between sentences may facilitate production.

At the phonological level, effort closure techniques are exercises that help the vocal folds adduct by providing overall increased muscle contractions in the torso and neck regions (215, 216). Examples of effort closure techniques include pushing or pulling with both hands against the bottom of one's chair or clasping one's hands together and squeezing as hard as possible. Such exercises may improve vocal fold strength, resulting in increased loudness and reduced breathy voice quality (215). In contrast, hyperadduction of the vocal folds is treated with various tension-reducing strategies emphasizing easy onset of phonation such as "yawn-sigh," "chewing," or "chanting" techniques. Various forms of muscle relaxation exercises of the head and neck areas, enhanced with biofeedback, have also been noted in the literature (215).

Consultation with medical staff outside the usual rehabilitation team may be indicated for some patients. For example, if vocal folds are not functioning adequately, an otolaryngologist may determine if injectible substances or thyroplasty surgery might improve laryngeal functioning. When a patient has velopharyngeal weakness, a prosthodontist may fit a prosthetic device such as a palatal lift.

Many clinicians incorporate oral strengthening exercises for muscle weakness of the tongue, lips, and jaw into their treatment program. These oral exercises take the form of moving the articulators in various directions against some sort of resistance, followed by attempts to hold them in their position of maximum range. Strengthening exercises for the velum include various blowing and sucking tasks (217). The value of these strengthening exercises for muscle weakness is controversial, and to date, there are no definitive research studies to support their use in the recovery of speech production.

Strategies to improve intelligibility of speech focus on increasing the precision of articulation, controlling the rate of speech, and improving prosody so that communication sounds more natural. Direct instruction on the correct placement of the articulators during production of a specific sound helps the patient understand how to produce the sound correctly as well as the cause of the sound errors, thereby preventing errors from occurring.

A treatment procedure of overarticulation or exaggerating consonants helps the patient to more fully articulate words, in particular those sounds that are in the middle or at the ends of words. Minimal contrast drills involve practicing words that vary by only one vowel or consonant. The differences between the words may be in the voicing (*park/bark*), the manner of production (*dime/mime*), or the place of production (*sea/she*) (184). Rate control can be accomplished by reciting words and syllables to a metronome or by finger or hand tapping to set the pace of appropriate syllable production (218). Slowing the speaking rate is often helpful because the patient may have more time to achieve articulatory placements. When speakers pause more often to slow down their rate, the listener is also given more time to process what is being said. Problems with intonation, stress, and rhythm contribute to the unnaturalness of speech. Treatment may include pitch range exercise or contrastive stress drills in which words, phrases, and sentences are practiced with different stress patterns each time.

Environmental modification may involve altering the number of listeners, the amount of noise, and the distance between the speaker and listener and improving eye contact. Modifications may also include informing new listeners about speech disorders and how best to communicate and strategies for repairing breakdowns in communication (e.g., repeating utterances, rephrasing, spelling, writing, and answering clarifying questions).

If a speaker remains unable to communicate satisfactorily using speech, augmentative or alternative communication modes should be considered (219). Selection of one or more systems depends on factors such as the motor, sensory, cognitive, and linguistic abilities of the patient. AAC devices may range from simple picture boards or spelling boards to portable amplification systems to high-tech electronic devices.

Efficacy of Dysarthria Treatment

A series of recent systematic reviews have addressed the efficacy of techniques for the management of dysarthria. These reviews have included behavioral procedures for managing respiratory and phonatory dysfunction (216) and velopharyngeal dysfunction (217), behavioral techniques for the treatment of loudness, rate, and prosody (218), and speech supplementation techniques (e.g., indicating the first letter or the topic of the sentences) for those with severe dysarthria (213). However, few of the studies reviewed were specific to patients with stroke. Furthermore, while results from the majority of the studies indicated positive outcomes, many of the studies included very small numbers of subjects.

With this in mind, a Cochrane review of speech and language therapy for dysarthria due to nonprogressive brain damage (stroke) did not identify any randomized controlled trials that met their standards of inclusion (220). The review concluded that "there is no evidence of the quality required to support or refute the effectiveness of speech and language therapy interventions for dysarthrias following non-progressive brain damage."

Yet, as noted by Yorkston, Spenser, and Duffy (2003), "treatments for which there is evidence of effectiveness do not necessarily represent the most appropriate or the most effective treatments that are available; they only represent the treatments for which evidence about treatment effects have been acquired." They further note that there are many techniques and treatments for which there is only expert opinion about effectiveness, or lack thereof.

Future research demonstrating the efficacy and effectiveness of the various treatment approaches for dysarthria using rigorous scientific methodologies is critical. A focus on more homogeneous groups of individuals based on etiology may serve to inform our knowledge base of dysarthria resulting specifically from stroke. An essential question is whether the potential facilitation of speech relearning could have a significant effect on reducing functional limitations and improving quality of life for people with dysarthria. Hopefully, further research will provide clarification and lead to more effective treatments for individuals with dysarthria.

ACKNOWLEDGMENT

Preparation of this manuscript was supported in part by grants H133G040269 and H133G060055 from the National Institute on Disability and Rehabilitation Research, U.S. Department of Education (to LRC) and by grant R01 DC007488 from the National Institute on Deafness and Other Communication Disorders (to SLS).

References

1. Black-Schaffer RM., Osberg JS. Return to work after stroke: Development of a predicitve model. *Arch Phys Med Rehabil* 1990; 71:285–290.
2. Herrmann M, Johannsen-Horback H, Wallesch C. The psychosocial aspects of aphasia. In Lafond D, DeGiovani R, Joannette Y, et al., eds. *Living with Aphasia: Psychosocial Issues*. San Diego, CA: Singular Publishing, 1993:17–36.
3. LeDorze G, Brassard C. A description of the consequences of aphasia on aphasic persons and their relatives and friends based on the WHO model of chronic diseases. *Aphasiology* 1995; 9:239–255.
4. Parr S. Coping with aphasia: Conversations with 20 aphasic people. *Aphasiology* 1994; 8:457–466.
5. Parr S, Byng S, Gilpin S, Ireland S. *Talking about aphasia: Living with loss of language after stroke*. Buckingham, UK: Open University Press, 1997.
6. Sarno MT. Aphasia rehabilitation: psychosocial and ethical considerations. *Aphasiology* 1993; 7:321–334.
7. Sarno MT. Quality of life in aphasia in the first post-stroke year. *Aphasiology* 1997; 11:665–678.
8. Duffy J. *Motor Speech Disorders: Substrates, Differential Diagnosis, and Management*. 2nd ed. St. Louis, MO: Elsevier Mosby, 2005.
9. Bates E, Friederici A, Wulfeck B. Grammatical morphology in aphasia: Evidence from three languages. *Cortex* 1987; 23:545–574.
10. de Bleser R. From agrammatism to paragrammatism: German aphasiological traditions and grammatical disturbances. *Cogn Neuropsychology* 1987; 4:187–256.
11. Kolk H, Heeschen C. Agrammatism, paragrammatism, and the management of language. *Lang Cogn Process* 1992; 7:89–129.
12. Baddeley AD. *Working Memory*. Oxford: Clarendon Press, 1986.
13. Haarman H, Just M, Carpenter P. Aphasic sentence comprehension as a resource deficit: a computational approach. *Brain Lang* 1997:59; 76–120.
14. Just M, Carpenter P. A capacity theory of comprehension: Individual differences in working memory. *Psychol Rev*. 1992:99; 122–149.
15. Broca PP. Nouvelle observation d'aphémie produite par une lesion de la partie postérieure des deuxième et troisième circonvolutions frontales. *Bull Soc Anat Paris* 1861; 6:398–407.
16. Dax M. Lésions de la moitié gauche de l'encéphale coincident avec l'oublie des signes de la pensée. *Gazette Hebdomaire de la Médicine et de Chirurgie* 1865; 33:259.
17. Damasio H, Damasio AR. *Lesion Analysis in Neuropsychology*. New York: Oxford University Press, 1989.
18. Kertesz A. *Localization in Neuropsychology*. New York: Academic Press, 1983:527.
19. Wernicke C. *Der Aphasische Symptomenkomplex*. Breslau:Cohn & Weigert, 1874.
20. Lichtheim, L. Ueber Aphasie. *Deut. Arch. f. klin. Med.* 1884; 36:204–268.
21. Grashey H. On aphasia and its relation to perception (Uber Aphasie und ihre Beziehungen zur Wahrnehmung). *Archiv fur Psychiatrie und Nervenkrankheiten* 1885.
22. Freud S. *On Aphasia: A Critical Study* (E. Stengel, Trans.). London: Imago, 1953 (original pub. 1891).
23. Déjerine J. *Anatomie des centres nerveux*. vol. i–ii. Paris: Rueff et Cie, 1895.
24. Heilman KM, Scholes RJ. The nature of comprehension errors in Broca's, conduction, and Wernicke's aphasics. *Cortex* 1976; 12:258–265.
25. Schwartz MF, Saffran EM, Marin OSM. The word order problem in agrammatism I: Comprehension. *Brain Lang* 1980; 10:249–262.

26. Schäffler L, Luders HO, Dinner DS, et al. Comprehension deficits elicited by electrical stimulation of Broca's area. *Brain* 1993; 116 pt 3:695–715.
27. Cohen JD, Forman SD, Braver TS, et al. Activation of prefrontal cortex in a non-spatial working memory task with functional MRI. *Hum Brain Mapp* 1994; 1:293–304.
28. Fox PT. Broca's area: Motor encoding in somatic space. *Behav Brain Sci* 1995; 18:344–345.
29. Craver CF, Small SL. Subcortical aphasia and the attribution of functional responsibility to parts of distributed brain processes. *Brain Lang* 1997; 58(3):427–435.
30. Damasio AR, Damasio H, Tranel D, Brandt JP. Neural regionalization of knowledge access: Preliminary evidence. *Cold Spring Harbor Symposia on Quantitative Biology LV*. Woodbury, NY: Cold Spring Harbor Laboratory Press, 1990:1039–1047.
31. McClelland JL. *The Case For Interactionism In Language Processing*. Hillsdale, NJ: Lawrence Erlbaum Associates, 1987.
32. Albert ML, Helm Estabrooks N. *Manual of Aphasia and Aphasia Therapy*. Austin, TX: Pro-Ed, 2004.
33. Rao PR. The aphasia syndromes: Localization and classification. *Top Stroke Rehabil* 1994; 1(2):1–13.
34. Benson DF. *Aphasia, Alexia and Agraphia*. New York, NY: Churchill Livingstone, 1979.
35. Goodglass H, Kaplan E. *The assessment of aphasia and related disorders*. Philadelphia, PA: Lea Febiger, 1972.
36. Folstein MF, Folstein SE, McHugh PR. "Mini-mental state." A practical method for grading the cognitive state of patients for the clinician. *J Psychiatr Res* 1975; 12(3):189–198.
37. Raven JC. *Raven's Coloured Progressive Matrices*. San Antonio, TX: The Psychological Corporation, 1995.
38. Kertesz A. *Western Aphasia Battery*. New York, NY: Harcourt Brace Jovanovich, 1982.
39. Kertesz A. *Western Aphasia Battery Revised*. San Antonio, TX: Harcourt Assessment Inc, 2007.
40. Helm-Estabrooks N. *Cognitive Linguistic Quick Test*. San Antonio, TX: Psychological Corp, 2001.
41. Brookshire RH. *Introduction to Neurogenic Communication Disorders*. 6th ed. St. Louis, MO: Mosby, 2003.
42. Small SL. Metaphors and models in the neuropsychiatry of language. *J Nerv Ment Dis* 1994; 182(4):216–219.
43. Small SL. Aphasia rehabilitation. In Lazar RB. ed. *Principles of Neurologic Rehabilitation*. New York, NY: McGraw Hill, 1998:517–552.
44. Crosson B. Subcortical mechanisms in language: Lexical-semantic mechanisms and the thalamus. *Brain Cogn* 1999; 40(2):414–438.
45. Goodglass H, Kaplan E, Barresi B. *The Assessment of Aphasia and Related Disorders*. 3rd ed . Philadelphia, PA: Lippincott Williams & Wilkins, 2001.
46. Basso, A. Prognostic factors in aphasia. *Aphasiology* 1992; 6:337–348.
47. Mark VW, Thomas BE, Berndt RS. Factors associated with improvement in global aphasia. *Aphasiology* 1992; 6(2):121–134.
48. Mazzoni M, Vista M, Pardossi L, et al. Spontaneous evolution of aphasia after ischaemic stroke. *Aphasiology* 1992; 6:387–396.
49. Pederson PM, Jorgensen HS, Nakayama H, et al. Aphasia in acute stroke: Incidence, determinants, and recovery. *Ann Neurol* 1995; 38:659–666.
50. Demeurisse G, Capon A. Language recovery in aphasic stroke patients: Clinical, CT, and CBF studies. *Aphasiology* 1987; 1:301–315.

51. Ferro JM. The influence of infarct location on recovery from global aphasia. *Aphasiology* 1992; 6(4):415–430.

52. Goldenberg G, Spatt J. Influence of size and site of cerebral lesions on spontaneous recovery of aphasia and on success of language therapy. *Brain Lang* 1994; 47:684–698.

53. Kertesz A, Harlock W, Coates R. Computer tomographic localization, lesion size and prognosis in aphasia and nonverbal impairment. *Brain Lang* 1979; 8:34–50.

54. Kertesz A, Lau WK, Polk M. The structural determinants of recovery in Wernicke's aphasia. *Brain Lang* 1993; 44:153–164.

55. Ludlow CL, Rosenberg J, Fair C, et al. Brain lesions associated with nonfluent aphasia fifteen years following penetrating head injury. *Brain* 1986; 109 Pt 1:55–80.

56. Selnes OA, Knopman DS, Niccum N, et al. Computed tomographic scan correlates of auditory comprehension deficits in aphasia: A prospective recovery study. *Ann Neurol* 1983; 5:558–566.

57. Naeser MA, Gaddie A, Palumbo CL, Stiassny-Eder D. Late recovery of auditory comprehension in global aphasia. *Arch Neurol* 1990; 47:425–432.

58. Naeser MA, Helm-Estabrooks N, Haas G, et al. Relationship between lesion extent in 'Wernicke's area' on computed tomographic scan and predicting recovery of comprehension in Wernicke's aphasia. *Arch Neurol* 1987; 44:73–82.

59. Naeser MA, Palumbo C.L, Helm-Estabrooks N, et al. Severe nonfluency in aphasia. *Brain* 1989; 112:1–38.

60. Hillis AE., Heidler J. Mechanisms of early aphasia recovery. *Aphasiology* 2002; 16:885–895.

61. Buckner, RL, Corbetta M, Schatz J, et al. Preserved speech abilities and compensation following prefrontal damage. *Proc Natl Acad Sci U S A* 1996; 93:1249–1253.

62. Cardebat D, Demonet JF, Celsis P, et al. Right temporal compensatory mechanisms in a deep dysphasic patient: a case report with activation study by SPECT. *Neuropsychologia* 1994; 32:97–103.

63. Ohyama M, Senda M, Kitamura S, et al. Role of the nondominant hemisphere and undamaged area during word repetition in post-stroke aphasia. A PET activation study. *Stroke* 1996; 27, 897–903.

64. Thulborn KR, Carpenter PA, Just MA. Plasticity of language-related brain function during recovery from stroke. *Stroke* 1999; 30(4):749–754.

65. Weiller C, Isensee C, Rijntjes M, et al. Recovery from Wernicke's aphasia: A positron emission tomography study. *Ann Neurol* 1995; 37:723–732.

66. Belin P, Van Eeckhout P, Zilbovicious M, et al. Recovery from nonfluent aphasia after melodic intonation therapy: A PET study. *Neurology* 1996; 47:1504–1511.

67. Blank SC, Bird H, Turkheimer F, Wise RJ. Speech production after stroke: The role of the right pars opercularis. *Ann Neurol* 2003; 54:310–320.

68. Rosen HJ, Petersen SE, Linenweber MR, et al. Neural correlates of recovery from aphasia after damage to left inferior frontal cortex. *Neurology*. 2000; 55:1883–1894.

69. Fernandez B, Cardebat D, Demonet JF, et al. Functional MRI follow-up study of language processes in healthy subjects and during recovery in a case of aphasia. *Stroke* 2004; 35:2171–2176.

70. Heiss W-D, Kessler J, Thiel A, et al. Differential capacity of left and right hemispheric areas for compensation of poststroke aphasia. *Ann Neurol* 1999; 45:430–438.

71. Abo M, Senoo A, Watanabe S, et al. Language-related brain function during word repetition in post-stroke aphasics. *Neuroreport* 2004; 15(12):1891–1894.

72. Xu XJ, Zhang MM, Shang DS, et al. Cortical language activation in aphasia: A functional MRI study. *Chin Med J (Engl)* 2004; 117:1011–1016.

73. Cao Y, Vikingstad EM, George KP, et al.. Cortical language activation in stroke patients recovering from aphasia with functional MRI. *Stroke* 1999; 30:2331–2340.

74. Karbe H, Thiel A, Luxenburger GW, et al. Brain plasticity in post-stroke aphasia: What is the contribution of the right hemisphere? *Brain Lang* 1998; 64:215–230.

75. Karbe H, Thiel A, Weber-Luxenburger G, et al. Reorganization of the cerebral cortex in post-stroke aphasia studied with positron emission tomography. *Neurology* 1998; 50:A321.

76. Small SL, Flores DK, Noll DC. Different neural circuits subserve reading before and after therapy for acquired dyslexia. *Brain Lang* 1998; 62:298–308.

77. Cornelissen K, Laine M, Tarkianen A, et al. Adult brain plasticity elicited by anomia treatment. *J Cogn Neurosci* 2003; 15:444–461.

78. Leger A, Demonet J-F, Ruff S, et al. Neural substrates of spoken language rehabilitation in an aphasic patient: An fMRI study. *Neuroimage* 2002; 17:174–183.

79. Thompson CK. Neuroplasticity: Evidence from aphasia. *J Commun Disord* 2000; 33:357–366.

80. Musso M, Weiller C, Kiebel S, et al. Training-induced brain plasticity in aphasia. *Brain* 1999; 122:1781–1790.

81. Horner J, Loverso FL, Rothi, LG. Models of aphasia treatment. In Chapey R, ed. *Language intervention strategies in adult aphasia*. 3rd ed. Baltimore: Williams Wilkins, 1994:135–145.

82. Basso, A. *Aphasia and its therapy*. Oxford: University Press, 2003.

83. Holland AL, Forbes M. *Aphasia treatment. World perspectives*. San Diego, CA: Singular Publishing Group, 1993.

84. Duffy J. R., Coehlo C. A. Schuell's stimulation approach to rehabilitation. In Chapey, R. ed. *Language intervention strategies in aphasia and related neurogenic communication disorders*. 4th ed. Philadelphia, PA: Lippincott Williams & Wilkins, 2001:341–382.

85. Schuell H, Jenkins JJ, Jimenez-Pabon E. *Aphasia in adults*. New York: Harper Row, 1964.

86. Weigl E. The phenomenon of temporary deblocking in aphasia. *Zeitschrift fur Phonetik Sprachwissenschaft und Kommunikationsforschung* 1961; 14: 337–364.

87. Luria, AR. *Restoration of function after brain injury*. Oxford: Pergamon Press, 1963.

88. Luria, AR. *Traumatic aphasia*. The Hague: Mouton, 1970.

89. Hillis AE. Cognitive neuropsychological approaches to rehabilitation of language disorders. In Chapey R, ed . *Language intervention strategies in aphasia and related neurogenic communication disorders*. 4th ed. Philadelphia: Lippincott Williams & Wilkins, 2001:513–523.

90. Hillis AE. *The handbook of adult language disorders: Integrating cognitive neuropsychology, neurology, and rehabilitation*. New York: Psychology Press, 2002.

91. Albert ML, Sparks RW, Helm, NA. Melodic intonation therapy for aphasia. *Arch Neurol* 1973; 29:130–131.

92. Sparks R, Helm N, Albert M. Aphasia rehabilitation resulting from melodic intonation therapy. *Cortex* 1974; 10:303–316.

93. Sparks R, Holland A. Method: melodic intonation therapy for aphasia. *J speech hear disord* 1976; 41:287–297.

94. Schlaug G, Marchina S, Norton A. From singing to speaking: Why singing may lead to recovery of expressive language function in patients with Broca's aphasia. *Music Perception* 2008; 25:315–323.

95. Bonakdarpour B, Eftekharzadeh A, Ashayeri H. Preliminary report on the effects of melodic intonation therapy in the rehabilitation of Persian aphasic patients. *Iranian J Med Sci* 2000; 25:156–160.

96. Wilson SJ, Parsons K, Reutens DC. Preserved singing in aphasia: A case study of the efficacy of the Melodic Intonation Therapy. *Music Perception* 2006; 24:23–36.

97. Lyon JG. Drawing: Its value as a communication aid for adults with aphasia. *Aphasiology* 1995; 9:33–94.

98. Simmons-Mackie N. Just kidding! Humour and therapy for aphasia. In Duchan, JF, Byng S, eds. *Challenging aphasia therapies*. New York: Psychology Press, 2004:101–117.

99. Helm-Estabrooks N, Nicholas M. *Sentence production program for aphasia*. Austin, TX: Pro-Ed, 2000.

100. Loverso FL, Prescott TE, Selinger M. Cuing verbs: A treatment strategy for aphasic adults. *J Rehabil Res* 1986; 25:47–60.

101. Thompson CK. Treatment of underlying forms: A linguistic specific approach for sentence production deficits in agrammatic aphasia. In Chapey R, ed. *Language intervention strategies in aphasia and related neurogenic communication disorders*. 4th ed. Philadelphia: Lippincott, Williams & Wilkins, 2001:605–628.

102. Thompson CK, Shapiro LP. Treating agrammatic aphasia within a linguistic framework: Treatment of Underlying Forms. *Aphasiology* 2005; 19(10–11):1021–1036.

103. Thompson CK, Shapiro LP, Ballard KJ, et al. Training and generalized production of wh- and NP-movement structures in agrammatic aphasia. *J Speech Lang Hear Res* 1997; 40(2):228–44.

104. Thompson CK, Shapiro LP. Complexity in treatment of syntactic deficits. *Am J Speech Lang Pathol* 2007; 16:30–42.

105. Thompson CK, Shapiro LP, Kiran S, Sobecks J. The role of syntactic complexity in treatment of sentence deficits in agrammatic aphasia: The complexity account of treatment efficacy (CATE). *J Speech Lang Hear Res* 2003; 46(3):591–607.

106. Maher LM, Raymer AM. Management of anomia. *Top Stroke Rehabil* 2004; 11(1):10–21.

107. Nickels L. Therapy for naming disorders: Revisiting, revising, and reviewing. *Aphasiology*. 2002; 16(10/11):935–979.

108. Boyle M. Semantic feature analysis treatment for anomia in two fluent aphasia syndromes. *Am J Speech Lang Pathol* 2004; 13(3):236–249.

109. Boyle M, Coehlo C. Application of semantic feature analysis as a treatment for aphasic dysnomia. *Am J Speech Lang Pathol* 1995; 4:94–98.

110. Coelho CA, McHugh RE, Boyle M. Semantic feature analysis as a treatment for aphasic dysnomia: A replication. *Aphasiology* 2000; 14(2):133–142.

111. Drew RL, Thompson CK. Model-based semantic treatment for naming deficits in aphasia. *J Speech Lang Hear Res* 1999; 42(4):972–989.

112. Lowell S, Beeson PM, Holland AL. The efficacy of a semantic cueing procedure on naming performance of adults with aphasia. *Am J Speech Lang Pathol* 1995; 4(4):109–114.

113. Kiran S. Semantic complexity in the treatment of naming deficits. *Am J Speech Lang Pathol* 2007; 16:1–12.

114. Kiran S, Thompson CK. Effect of typicality on online category verification of animate category exemplars in aphasia. *Brain Lang* 2003; 85(3):441–450.

115. Kiran S, Thompson CK. The role of semantic complexity in treatment of naming deficits: Training semantic categories in fluent aphasia by controlling exemplar typicality. *J Speech Lang Hear Res* 2003; 46(4):773–787.

116. Davis G, Wilcox M. *Adult aphasia rehabilitation: Applied pragmatics*. Windsor: NFER-Nelson, 1985.

117. Cherney LR, Halper AS, Holland AL, Cole R. Computerized script training for aphasia: Preliminary results. *Am J Speech Lang Pathol* 2008; 17:19–34.

118. Cherney LR, Halper AS, Holland AL, et al. Improving conversational script production in aphasia with virtual therapist computer treatment software. *Brain Lang* 2007; 103:246–247.

119. Youmans GL, Holland AL, Munoz M, Bourgeois M. Script training and automaticity in two individuals with aphasia. *Aphasiology* 2005; 19:435–450.

120. Kagan A, Black SE, Duchan JF, et al. Training volunteers as conversation partners using "Supported Conversation for Adults with Aphasia" SCA: A controlled trial. *J Speech Lang Hear Res* 2001; 44:624–638.

121. Elman RJ, Bernstein-Ellis E. The efficacy of group communication treatment in adults with chronic aphasia. *J Speech Lang Hear Res* 1998; 42(2):411–419.

122. Lubinski R. Environmental systems approach in adult aphasia. In Chapey R, ed. *Language intervention strategies in aphasia and related neurogenic communication disorders*. 4th ed. Philadelphia: Lippincott Williams & Wilkins, 2001:269–296.

123. Cruice M, Worrall L, Hickson L, Murison R. Finding a focus for quality of life in aphasia: Social and emotional health, and psychological well-being. *Aphasiology* 2003; 17(4):333–354.

124. LPAA Project Group. Life participation approach to aphasia: A statement of values for the future. *ASHA Leader* 2000; 5(3):4–6.

125. Lyon J. Communication use and participation in life for adults with aphasia in natural settings: The scope of the problem. *Am J Speech Lang Pathol* 1992; 1:7–14.

126. Pound C, Parr S, Lindsay J, Woolf C. *Beyond Aphasia: Therapies for Living with Communication Disability*. Bicester, UK: Speechmark, 2000.

127. Sarno MT. Aphasia therapies: Historical perspectives and moral imperatives. In Duchan J, Byng S, eds. *Challenging Aphasia Therapies*. Hove, UK: Psychology Press, 2004:17–31.

128. Simmons-Mackie N. A solution to the discharge dilemma in aphasia: Social approaches to aphasia management. *Aphasiology* 1998; 12:231–239.

129. Simmons-Mackie N. Social approaches to the management of aphasia. In Worrall L, Frattali C, eds. *Neurogenic communication disorders: A functional approach*. New York: Thieme, 2000.

130. Simmons-Mackie N. Social approaches to aphasia intervention. In Chapey R, ed. *Language intervention strategies in aphasia and related neurogenic communication disorders*. 4th ed. Philadelphia: Lippincott, Williams & Wilkins, 2001:246–268.

131. Worrall L. A conceptual framework for a functional approach to acquired neurogenic disorders of communication and swallowing. In Worrall L, Frattali C, eds. *Neurogenic communication disorders: A functional approach*. New York: Thieme, 2000:3–18.

132. Small SL. Biological Approaches to the Treatment of Aphasia. In Hillis A, ed. *Handbook on Adult Language Disorders: Integrating Cognitive Neuropsychology, Neurology, and Rehabilitation*. Philadelphia, PA: Psychology Press, 2002:397–411.

133. Small SL. The biology of aphasia rehabilitation: Pharmacological perspectives. *Aphasiology* 2004; 8 (5/6/7):473–492.

134. de Boisezzon X, Peran P, de Boysson C, Demonet J-F. Pharmacotherapy for aphasia: Myth or reality? *Brain Lang* 2007; 102:114–125.

135. Bragoni M, Altieri M, Di Piero V, et al. Bromocriptine and speech therapy in nonfluent chronic aphasia after stroke. *Neurol Sci* 2000; 21:19–22.

136. Gupta SR, Mlcoch AG. Bromocriptine treatment of nonfluent aphasia. *Arch Phys Med Rehabil* 1992; 73:373–376.

137. Gupta SR, Mlcoch AG, Scolaro MS, et al. Bromocriptine treatment of nonfluent aphasia. *Neurology* 1995; 45:2170–2173.

138. Sabe L, Leiguarda R, Starkstein SE. An open-label trial of bromocriptine in nonfluent aphasia. *Neurology* 1992; 42(8):1637–1638.

139. Sabe L, Salvarezza F, García Cuerva A, et al. A randomized, double-blind, placebo-controlled study of bromocriptine in nonfluent aphasia. *Neurology* 1995; 45(12):2272–2274.

140. Walker-Batson D, Curtis S, Natarajan R, et al. A double-blind, placebo-controlled study of the use of amphetamine in the treatment of aphasia. *Stroke* 2001; 32(9):2093–2098.

141. Walker-Batson D, Devous MD, Curtis S, et al. Response to amphetamine to facilitate recovery from aphasia subsequent to stroke. *Clinical Aphasiology* 1991; 21:137–143.

142. Berthier ML, Green C, Higueras C, et al. A randomized, placebo-controlled study of donepezil in poststroke aphasia. *Neurology* 2006; 67(9):1687–1689.

143. Berthier ML, Hinojosa J, Martin MC, Fernandez I. Open-label study of donepezil in chronic post-stroke aphasia. *Neurology* 2003; 60:1218–1219.

144. Enderby P, Broeckx J, Hospers W, et al. Effect of piracetam on recovery and rehabilitation after stroke: A double-blind placebo-controlled study. *Clin Neuropharmacol* 1994; 17:320–321.

145. Huber W, Willmes K, Poeck K, et al. Piracetam as an adjuvant to language therapy for aphasia: A randomized double-blind placebo controlled pilot study. *Arch Phys Med Rehabil* 1997; 78:245–250.

146. Goldstein LB, Investigators SiASS. Common drugs may influence motor recovery after stroke. *Neurology* 1995; 45:865–871.

147. Porch B, Wyckes J, Feeney DM. Haloperidol, thiazides, and some antihypertensives slow recovery from aphasia abstract. *Annual Meeting of the Society for Neuroscience* 1985; 11:52.

148. Cherney LR, Small SL. Intensive language therapy for nonfluent aphasia with and without surgical implantation of an investigational cortical stimulation device: Preliminary language and imaging results. Platform presentation, Clinical Aphasiology Conference, Phoenix AZ; May 2007.

149. Martin PI, Naeser MA, Theoret H, et al. Transcranial magnetic stimulation as a complementary treatment for aphasia. *Semin Speech Lang* 2004; 25(2):181–191.

150. Naeser MA, Martin PI, Nicholas M, et al. Improved picture naming in chronic aphasia after TMS to part of right Broca's area: An open-protocol study. *Brain Lang* 2005; 93:95–105.

151. Hesse S, Werner C, Schonhardt EM, et al. Combined transcranial direct current stimulation and robot-assisted arm training in subacute stroke patients: A pilot study. *Restore Neurol Neurosci* 2007; 25:9–15.

152. Kang EK, Sohn HM, Oh M-K, et al. Paradoxical facilitatory effect of cathodal transcranial direct current stimulation on post-stroke aphasia. *Arch Phys Med Rehabil* 2007; 88:E8.

153. Kleim JE, Jones TA. Principles of experience-dependent neural plasticity: Implications for rehabilitation after brain damage. *J Speech Lang Hear Res* 2008; 51: S225–S239.

154. Bhogal SK, Teasell R, Speechley M. Intensity of aphasia therapy: Impact on recovery. *Stroke* 2003; 34:987–993.

155. Meinzer M, Djundja D, Barthel G, et al. Long-term stability of improved language functions in chronic aphasia after constraint-induced aphasia therapy. *Stroke* 2005; 36:1462–1466.

156. Meinzer M, Elbert T, Wienbruch C, et al. Intensive language training enhances brain plasticity in chronic aphasia. *BMC Biology* 2004; 2:20.

157. Pulvermuller F, Hauk O, Zohsel K, et al. Therapy-related reorganization of language in both hemispheres of patients with chronic aphasia. *Neuroimage* 2005; 28:481–489.

158. Pulvermuller F, Neininger B, Elbert T, et al. Constraint-induced therapy of chronic aphasia after stroke. *Stroke* 2001; 32:1621–1626.

159. Cherney LR, Patterson J, Raymer A, et al. Evidence-based systematic review: Effects of intensity of treatment and constraint-induced language therapy for individuals with stroke-induced aphasia. *Journal of Speech, Language and Hearing Research* 2008; 51:1282–1299.

160. Maher LM, Kendall D, Swearengin JA, et al. A pilot study of use-dependent learning in the context of constraint induced language therapy. *J Int Neuropsychol Soc* 2006; 12:843–852.

161. Katz RC. Computer applications in aphasia treatment. In Chapey R, ed. *Language Intervention Strategies in Aphasia and Related Neurogenic Communication Disorders*. 4th ed. Philadelphia: Lippincott Williams & Wilkins, 2001:718–741.

162. Loverso FL, Prescott TE, Selinger M. Microcomputer treatment applications in aphasiology. *Aphasiology* 1992; 6:155–162.

163. Petheram B. Computers and aphasia: A means of delivery and a delivery of means. *Aphasiology* 2004; 18:187–191.

164. Linebarger M, McCall D, Virata T, Berndt RS. Widening the temporal window: Processing support in the treatment of aphasic language production. *Brain Lang* 2007; 100(1):53–68.

165. Cherney LR, Robey RR. Aphasia treatment: recovery, prognosis and clinical effectiveness. In Chapey R, ed. *Language Intervention Strategies in Aphasia and Related Neurogenic Communication Disorders*. 4th ed. Philadelphia: Lippincott Williams & Wilkins, 2001:148–172.

166. Greener J, Enderby P, Whurr R. Speech and language therapy for aphasia following stroke. *The Cochrane Database of Systematic Reviews* 2000; 2:CD000424.

167. Greenhouse JB, Fromm D, Iyengar S, et al. The making of a meta-analysis: A quantitative review of the aphasia treatment literature. In Wachter KW, Straf ML, eds. *The Future of Meta-Analysis*. New York: Russell Sage Foundation, 1990.

168. Robey RR. The efficacy of treatment for aphasic persons: A meta-analysis. *Brain Lang* 1994; 47:582–608.

169. Robey RR. A meta-analysis of clinical outcomes in the treatment of aphasia. *J Speech Lang Hear Res* 1998; 41:172–187.

170. Whurr R, Lorch MP, Nye C. A meta-analysis of studies carried out between 1946 and 1988 concerned with the efficacy of speech and language treatment for aphasic patients. *Eur J Disord Commun* 1992; 27:1–17.

171. Kagan A, Simmons-Mackie N, Rowland A, et al. Counting what counts: A framework for capturing real-life outcomes of aphasia intervention. *Aphasiology* 2008; 22:258–280.

172. World Health Organization. *International classification for functioning, disability and health ICF*. Geneva, Switzerland: World Health Organization, 2001.

173. Ballard KJ, Granier JP, Robin DA. Understanding the nature of apraxia of speech: Theory, analysis, and treatment. *Aphasiology* 2000; 14(10):969–995.

174. Darley FL, Aronson AE, Brown JR. *Motor Speech Disorders*. Philadelphia, PA: Saunders, 1975.

175. Van der Merwe A. A theoretical framework for the characterization of pathological speech sensorimotor control. In: McNeil MR, ed. *Clinical Management of Sensorimotor Speech Disorders*. New York: Thieme, 1997:1–25.

176. Dronkers NF. A new region for coordinating speech articulation. *Nature* 1996; 384:159–161.

177. Ogar J, Willock S, Baldo J, ET AL. Clinical and anatomical correlates of apraxia of speech. *Brain Lang* 2006; 97:343–350.

178. Duffau H, Bauchet L, Lehericy S, Capelle L. Functional compensation of the left dominant insula for language. *Neuroreport* 2001; 12(10):2159–2162.

179. McNeil MR, Weismer G, Adams S, Mulligan M. Oral structure nonspeech motor control in normal, dysarthric, aphasic, and apraxic speakers: Isometric force and static position control. *J Speech Hearing Res* 1990; 33:255–268.

180. Riecker A, Ackermann H, Wildgruber D, et al. Articulatory/phonetic sequencing at the level of the anterior perisylvian cortex: A functional magnetic resonance imaging (fMRI) study. *Brain Lang* 2000; 75:259–276.

181. Hillis AE, Work M, Barker PB, et al. Re-examining the brain regions crucial for orchestrating speech articulation. *Brain* 2004; 127:1479–1487.

182. Duffy J. *Motor Speech Disorders: Substrates, Differential Diagnosis, and Management*. St. Louis, MO: Mosby, 1995.

183. Wertz RT, LaPointe LL, Rosenbek JC. *Apraxia of Speech in Adults: The Disorder and its Management*. San Diego, CA: Singular Publishing Group, 1991.

184. West C, Hesketh A, Vail A, Bowen A. Interventions for apraxia of speech following stroke. *The Cochrane Collaboration*, 2007:3.

185. Laures-Gore J, Henson JC, Weismer G, Rambow M. Two cases of foreign accent syndrome: An acoustic-phonetic description. *Clin Linguist Phon* 2006; 20(10):781–790.

186. Roth EJ, Fink K, Cherney LR, Hall KD. Reversion to a previously learned foreign accent after stroke. *Arch Phys Med Rehabil* 1997; 78(5):550–552.

187. Kurowski KM, Blumstein SE, Alexander M. The foreign accent syndrome: A reconsideration. *Brain Lang* 1996; 54(1):1–25.

188. Freed D. *Motor Speech Disorders: Diagnosis and Treatment*. San Diego, CA: Singular Publishing Group, 2000.

189. Dabul B. *Apraxia Battery for Adults*. 2nd edition. Austin, TX: Pro-Ed Inc, 2000.

190. DiSimoni FG. *Comprehensive Apraxia Test*. Dalton, PA: Praxis House, 1989.

191. Wambaugh JL. A summary of treatments for apraxia of speech and review of replicated approaches. *Semin Speech Lang* 2002; 23(4):293–308.

192. Wambaugh JL, Duffy JR, McNeil MR, et al. Treatment guidelines for acquired apraxia of speech: Treatment descriptions and recommendations. *J Med Speech Lang Pathol* 2006; 14(2):xxxv–lxvii.

193. Wambaugh JL, Duffy JR, McNeil MR, et al. Treatment guidelines for acquired apraxia of speech: A synthesis and evaluation of the evidence. *J Med Speech Lang Pathol* 2006; 14(2):xv–xxxiii.

194. Rosenbek JC, Lemme ML, Ahern MB, et al. A treatment for apraxia of speech in adults. *J Speech Hear Disord* 1973; 38:462–472.

195. Wambaugh JL, Kalinyak-Fliszar MM, West JE, Doyle PJ. Effects of treatment for sound errors in apraxia of speech and aphasia. *J Speech Lang Hear Res* 1998; 41:725–743.

196. Square-Storer PA, Hayden DC. PROMPT treatment. In Square-Storer PA, ed. *Acquired Apraxia of Speech in Aphasic Adults.* Hove and London: Lawrence Erlbaum, 1989:190–219.

197. Dabul B, Bollier B. Therapeutic approaches to apraxia. *J Speech Hear Disord* 1976; 41(2):268–276.

198. Tjaden K. Exploration of a treatment technique for prosodic disturbances following stroke. *Clin Linguist Phon* 2000; 14(8):619–641.

199. Wambaugh JL, Martinez AL. Effects of rate and rhythm control treatment on consonant production accuracy in paraxial of speech. *Aphasiology* 2000; 14(8):851–871.

200. Brendel B, Ziegler W, Deger K. The synchronization paradigm in the treatment of apraxia of speech. *J Neuroling* 2000; 13:241–327.

201. Southwood H. The use of prolonged speech in the treatment of apraxia of speech. In Brookshire RH, ed. *Clinical Aphasiology Conference Proceedings.* Minneapolis: BRK, 1987:277–287.

202. Raymer AS, Thompson CK. Effects of verbal plus gestural treatment in a patient with aphasia and severe apraxia of speech. *Clin Aphasiology* 1991; 20:285–298.

203. Keith RL, Aronson AE. Singing as therapy for apraxia of speech and aphasia: Report of a case. *Brain Lang* 1975; 2(4):483–488.

204. Lasker JP, Bedrosian JL. Promoting acceptance of augmentative and alternative communication by adults with acquired communication disorders. *AAC: Augmentative and Alterative Communication* 2001; 17(3):141–153.

205. Rabidoux P, Florance C, McCauslin L. The use of a Handi Voice in the treatment of a severly apractic nonverbal patient. In Brookshire RH, ed. *Clinical Aphasiology Conference Proceedings.* Minneapolis: BRK, 1980:294–301.

206. Yorkston KM, Waugh PF. Use of augmentative communication devices with apractic individuals. In Square-Storer PA, ed. *Acquired Apraxia of Speech in Aphasic Adults.* Hove and London: Lawrence Erlbaum, 1989:267–283.

207. Peach RK. Acquired apraxia of speech: Features, accounts, and treatment. *Top Stroke Rehabil* 2004; 11(1):49–58.

208. Cherney LR. Efficacy of oral reading in the treatment of two patients with chronic Broca's aphasia. *Top Stroke Rehabil* 1995; 2(1):57–67.

209. Wambaugh JL. Treatment guidelines for apraxia of speech: Lessons for future research. *J Med Speech Lang Pathol* 2006; 14(4):317–321.

210. Darley FL, Aronson AE, Brown JR. Differential diagnostic patterns of dysarthria. *J Speech Hear Res* 1969; 12(2):246–69.

211. Darley FL, Aronson AE, Brown JR. Clusters of deviant speech dimensions in the dysarthrias. *J Speech Hear Res* 1969; 12(3):462–496.

212. Hammen VL. Motor speech problems associated with stroke: The dysarthrias. *Top Stroke Rehabil* 1994; 1(2):65–75.

213. Enderby P, Palmer R. *Frenchay Dysarthria Assessment.* 2nd ed. Austin, TX: Pro-Ed, 2008.

214. Yorkston KM, Beukelman DR. *Assessment of Intelligibility of Dysarthric Speech.* Tigard, Oregon: CC Publications, 1981.

215. Spencer KA, Yorkston KM, Duffy JR. Behavioral management of respiratoryventilatory/phonatory dysfunction from dysarthria: A flowchart for guidance in clinical decision making. *J Med Speech Lang Pathol* 2003; 11(2):xxxix–lxi.

216. Yorkston KM, Spencer KA, Duffy JR. Behavioral management of respiratory/phonatory dysfunction from dysarthria: A systematic review of the evidence. *J Med Speech Lang Pathol* 2003; 11(2):xiii–xxxviii.

217. Yorkston KM, Spenser K, Duffy J, et al. Evidence-based practice guidelines for dysarthria: Management of velopharyngeal function. *J Med Speech Lang Pathol* 2001; 9(4):257–274.

218. Yorkston KM, Hakel M, Beukelman DR, Fager S. Evidence for effectiveness of treatment of loudness, rate, or prosody in dysarthria: A systematic review. *J Med Speech Lang Pathol* 2007; 15(2):xi–xxxvi.

219. Hanson EK, Yorkston KM, Beukelman DR. Speech supplementation techniques for dysarthria: A systematic review. *J Med Speech Lang Pathol* 2004; 12(2):ix–xxix.

220. Sellars C, Hughes T., Langhorne P. Speech and language therapy for dysarthria due to non-progressive brain damage. *The Cochrane Collaboration,* 2007; 3.

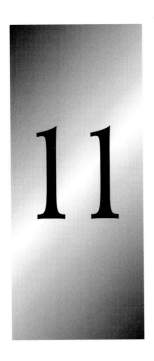

11 Dysphagia

Marlis Gonzalez-Fernandez
Denise M. Monahan
Koichiro Matsuo
Jeffrey B. Palmer

EPIDEMIOLOGY

Swallowing dysfunction, or dysphagia, is common after stroke. The true incidence of dysphagia after acute stroke is unclear, but estimates range from 20–90%, largely dependent on timing and method of ascertainment (1). Conservative estimates of the true incidence report nearly 50% of acute stroke patients experiencing dysphagia within the first few days after stroke (2–4). Dysphagia is associated with development of pneumonia, dehydration, and malnutrition; increased length of stay; and mortality after stroke (5–8). Dysphagia has traditionally been associated with brain stem and bilateral cerebral infarctions (1, 9), but, in recent years, it has been shown to occur in isolated cerebral infarctions as well. The incidence may be as high as 25% for left hemisphere and 15% for right hemisphere lesions (6, 10).

Aspiration Pneumonia

Aspiration, the passage of food or other foreign material through the vocal folds, is common in stroke patients with dysphagia. The risk of aspiration pneumonia is increased threefold in stroke patients with dysphagia and between eleven- and twentyfold in patients with aspiration confirmed by videofluoroscopy (3, 11). Aspiration can sometimes be detected with clinical examination, but silent aspiration, that is, aspiration without cough, occurs in up to two-thirds of stroke patients who aspirate (12). While aspiration on videofluoroscopy is associated with an increased risk of pneumonia, the risk of dehydration and death is similar to the risk of other dysphagic stroke patients (13). The material aspirated is also an important consideration. The effects of the aspirated material depend largely on the amount, bacterial load, acid content, and its physical characteristics (14, 15).

Aspiration of gastric material usually leads to chemical pneumonia with bacterial infection occurring as a complication two to three days after injury or in cases where the pH of the gastric content is higher due to antacids, proton pump inhibitors, or H2-receptor blockers (15). Aspiration of material with a pH greater than 2.5 causes severe lung injury with parechymal inflammation, which can lead to adult respiratory distress syndrome (16). Gastric colonization with gram-negative bacteria has been documented in patients receiving enteral feeding, placing them at risk for combined chemical and bacterial pneumonia after aspiration of gastric contents (17).

Bacterial pneumonia is predominantly related to aspiration of oral flora and upper airway colonization (14, 15), thus multiple organisms can be isolated (18). Good oral care can reduce the risk of pneumonia by reducing the bacterial load (19).

Malnutrition

The prevalence of malnutrition in stroke patients has been reported from 8–34% (20, 21). Malnutrition has also been associated with poor outcomes after stroke, including longer lengths of stay and increased number of complications such as pressure ulcers, falls, tachycardia, and infections (22). Details on nutrition and nutritional interventions after stroke are detailed in Chapter 29.

Recovery of Swallow Function after Stroke

The potential for recovery of swallow function is good. Swallowing dysfunction generally resolves for about half of stroke patients within seven days, and only 11–13% have persistent swallowing dysfunction after six months (23, 24). Prognosis is dependent on many factors related to medical status, dysphagia, and rehabilitation potential. Severity of stroke, recurrent stroke, low serum albumin levels, dependence on tube feedings, need for ultra-thickened liquids, and aspiration documented on a videofluorographic swallowing study (VFSS) have been linked to poor outcomes (25, 26). Advanced age, impaired cognition, and dependence on a wheelchair are also linked to poor outcomes (27). The best outcomes occur when individuals receive early assessment and treatment of dysphagia with a structured, interdisciplinary team approach.

SWALLOWING PHYSIOLOGY

The process of swallowing, or deglutition, is a series of complex volitional and reflexive movements with two critical biomechanical functions:

1. Food passage, propelling the food bolus carried from the oral cavity to the stomach
2. Airway protection, insulating the nasal passages, larynx, and lower respiratory tract from the pharynx during food passage

The main anatomical structures involved include the oral cavity, pharynx, larynx, and esophagus (Figure 11-1).

Swallowing Stages

The swallowing process is classically divided into four stages according to the location of the bolus (28). After ingestion, food is prepared for propulsion to the pharynx (oral preparatory stage). The tongue pushes the bolus through the fauces and into the pharynx (oral propulsive stage). Stereotyped movements of pharyngeal structures move the bolus from the pharynx to the esophagus through the upper esophageal sphincter (pharyngeal stage). Finally, peristalsis and gravity carry the bolus down the esophagus and through the lower esophageal sphincter to the stomach (esophageal stage). According to the traditional model of swallowing, the oral preparatory stage is initiated voluntarily, but, once oral propulsion starts, the rest of the process follows immediately. The total duration of food transit to the esophagus occurs in less than one second in normal adults.

Oral Stage: Differences between Drinking and Eating

While the general sequence of an oral swallow is the same for liquid and solid boluses, there are differences relative to preparation and timing. Once ingested, liquids are collected by the tongue and maintained between the tongue dorsal surface and hard palate surrounded by the upper dental arch until the oral propulsive stage is started (Figure 11-2). Liquids are prevented from leaking into the oropharynx before swallow initiation by a seal made through soft palate and dorsal tongue contact. Although this posterior oral seal is usually effective in young, healthy individuals, it is often incomplete, and some liquid may enter the pharynx before the onset of oral propulsion. In contrast to single liquid boluses, during continuous drinking, for example, as seen during drinking with a straw, the bolus often advances to the level of the valleculae prior to swallow initiation (29).

The oral propulsive stage starts when the tip of the tongue makes contact with the hard palate just behind the upper anterior teeth. The tongue surface moves upward and the tongue-palate contact area expands posteriorly, squeezing the bolus into the pharynx.

Eating solid food is quite different from drinking liquid because the food requires significant processing before it is ready to swallow (30, 31). The process model, a recent development in understanding the physiology of swallowing, incorporates critical aspects of mastication and oral food transport (32, 31). When solid food is placed in the mouth, the tongue shifts backward and then rotates its surface to one side. This movement pulls the food back to the molar region and places it on the occlusal surfaces of the postcanine teeth during stage I transport (Figure 11-3a). Then food particles are reduced in size by mastication and softened with saliva until the consistency of the food is optimized for the swallow (food processing). The movements of the

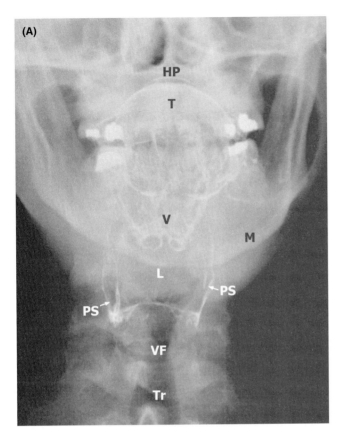 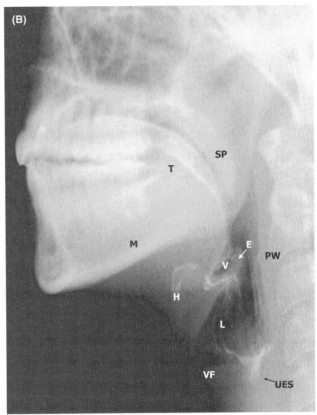

FIGURE 11-1

Videofluorographic image, lateral and AP views. (A) Postero-anterior projection in a videofluorographic image. (B) Lateral projection in a videofluorographic image. CC, Cricoid cartilage; E, Epiglottis; H, Hyoid bone; HP, Hard palate; M, Mandible; PW, posterior pharyngeal wall; L, Laryngeal vestibule; PS, Pyriform sinus; SP, Soft palate; T, Tongue; TB, Tongue base; TC, Thyroid cartilage; Tr, Trachea; UES, Upper esophageal sphincter; V, Valleculae; VF, Vocal folds (Reprinted from *Physical Medicine and Rehabilitation*, Third edition, Randall L. Braddom Ed., Rehabilitation of Patients with Swallowing Disorders, Page 599, © 2007, with permission from Elsevier)

jaw, tongue, cheek, soft palate, and hyoid are rhythmical and linked to each other, spatially and temporally, during food processing (33–36). Processed food particles are placed on the dorsal tongue surface and squeezed back to the pharynx during stage II transport (Figure 11-3b), with a mechanism that is nearly identical to that indicated for the oral propulsive stage described above. Stage II transport occurs intermittently during food processing cycles so that a food bolus may form in the oropharynx and gradually accumulates for several seconds before the pharyngeal swallow. When sufficient food has accumulated, the pharyngeal stage of swallowing is initiated.

Pharyngeal Stage

The location of the bolus at the initiation of pharyngeal swallowing differs between drinking and eating. The bolus is usually maintained in the mouth during discrete liquid swallows, but it can be in the oropharynx during sequential swallows or with solid food (29–31, 37). The leading edge of the bolus is often in the hypopharynx at swallow onset when eating food with mixed consistencies (liquids and solids) (38).

The pharyngeal stage is a rapid sequence of overlapping and nearly synchronous events (39–42) (Figure 11-2c–d):

1. The soft palate elevates and contacts the lateral and posterior wall of the pharynx, closing the nasopharynx.
2. The base (pharyngeal surface) of the tongue retracts, pushing the bolus posteriorly and downward. The pharyngeal wall contracts around the tongue, both from the back and from the sides, squeezing the bolus. The pharyngeal contraction is sequential, beginning at the top of the pharynx and proceeding downward (43). The pharynx also shortens vertically, reducing its volume (44).

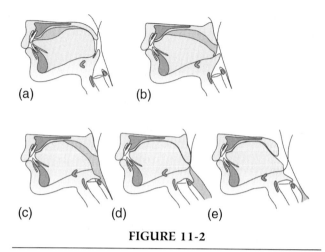

(a)   (b)

(c)   (d)   (e)

FIGURE 11-2

Normal swallowing of a liquid bolus. These drawings are based on an actual videofluorographic sequence recorded in the lateral projection. a) The bolus is held between the anterior surface of the tongue and hard palate, in a swallow-ready position. The tongue presses against the palate both in front of and behind the bolus to prevent spillage. b) The bolus is propelled from the oral cavity to the pharynx through the fauces. The anterior tongue pushes the bolus against hard palate just behind the upper incisor. The posterior tongue drops away from the palate. c) The soft palate elevates closing off the nasopharynx. The area of tongue-palate contact spreads posteriorly, squeezing the bolus backward to the pharynx. The larynx elevates, and the epiglottis tilts downward. d) The upper esophageal sphincter opens. The tongue vbase retracts to contact the pharyngeal wall, which contracts around the bolus, starting superiorly and then progressing downward toward the esophagus. e) The soft palate descends, and the larynx and pharynx reopen. The upper esophageal sphincter returns to its usual closed state after the bolus passes. (Reprinted from Physical Medicine and Rehabilitation, Third edition, Randall L. Braddom Ed., Rehabilitation of Patients with Swallowing Disorders, Page 600, © 2007, with permission from Elsevier)

3. The hyoid bone and larynx are pulled upward and forward by contraction of the suprahyoid muscles and thyrohyoid muscle. The anterior and superior movements of these structures are critical for airway protection and opening of the upper esophageal sphincter (UES) (45).

4. Prior to UES opening, the vocal folds close to seal the glottis (46–48). The arytenoid cartilages tilt forward to contact the base of the epiglottis. The anterior and superior movements of the hyoid and larynx tuck the larynx under the base of the tongue and fold the epiglottis backward to seal the laryngeal vestibule. Downward bolus movement and tongue base retraction also helps epiglottal tilt (49). Breathing ceases briefly during swallowing (deglutitive apnea) for approximately 0.4 to 1.0 seconds (50, 51). Breathing resumes in

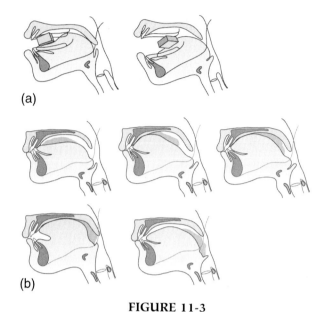

(a)

(b)

FIGURE 11-3

Mechanisms of food transport in a normal subject eating solid food. a) Stage I transport: The tongue carries the bite of food back to the post-canine region and then rotates to place it on the occlusal surfaces. b) Stage II transport: The tongue squeezes the bolus backward along the palate, through the fauces, and into the pharynx. (Reprinted from Physical Medicine and Rehabilitation, Third edition, Randall L. Braddom Ed., Rehabilitation of Patients with Swallowing Disorders, Page 601, © 2007, with permission from Elsevier)

the expiratory phase; this helps prevent inhalation of food.

5. Opening of the UES is essential for the bolus to reach the esophagus. The UES is held closed at rest by tonic contraction of the cricopharyngeus muscle (45, 52). Muscles just above and below the cricopharyngeus may also assist in UES closure. During a swallow, these muscles relax, and the UES opens. Three important factors contribute to this opening:
   • The active relaxation of the cricopharyngeus muscle
   • Contraction of the suprahyoid muscles, which move the hyoid bone and larynx forward, effectively pulling the sphincter open (45)
   • The pressure of the descending bolus (53), which pushes the UES outward, assisting its opening

Esophageal Stage

The bolus transit mechanism in the esophagus is different from that of the pharynx. The cervical esophagus (upper one-third) is mainly composed of striated muscle, but the thoracic esophagus (lower two-thirds) is smooth muscle. Peristalsis is controlled by autonomic nerves. Once the bolus passes the UES and enters the esophagus, a peristaltic wave carries the bolus down to the stomach. Gravity assists peristalsis in the upright position. The lower esophageal sphincter (LES) contracts tonically between swallows to prevent gastroesophageal reflux and relaxes to allow bolus passage into the stomach.

NEURAL CONTROL OF SWALLOWING

Swallowing is a complex process that involves sequential muscle contraction and inhibition of more than 30 muscles (54). The major muscles involved in swallowing and their innervation are detailed in Table 11-1. Similar to respiratory control, swallowing functions are controlled primarily by centers in the brain stem. Although the main center controlling swallowing is in the brain stem, the cerebral cortex and other supratentorial structures also have a role in swallowing control.

Brain Stem: Central Pattern Generator

The swallowing central pattern generator (CPG) generates the sequential pattern of motor activities required for a swallow. The pattern for muscle contraction and inhibition is dependent on three distinct components:

1. The afferent input to the to the CPG in the brain stem (sensory and supramedullary)
2. The efferent output that provides innervation to the swallowing muscles
3. The interneuronal network that integrates afferent and efferent input in the CPG (55)

The CPG is located within the nucleus tractus solitarius (NTS) and the reticular formation surrounding both the NTS and above the nucleus ambiguus (NA) in the rostral and ventrolateral medulla (55, 56). The CPG is organized into two main regions with distinct functions:

1. The dorsal group involved in triggering, shaping, and timing of the sequential swallowing pattern
2. The ventral group that distributes the swallowing drive to the various pools of motor neurons involved in swallowing (56)

Sensory (afferent) input from the mechanoreceptors, chemoreceptors, and thermoreceptors in the oral cavity, pharynx, and larynx to the CPG has been implicated in swallowing initiation, facilitation, and airway protection (1, 57–61). General sensory neurons from the oral cavity synapse in the trigeminal sensory nuclei while those from the pharynx and larynx travel in branches of cranial nerves IX, X, and XI and synapse in the NTS (62).

The ventral CPG premotor neurons have connections with the trigeminal (V), facial (VII), hypoglossal (XII) motor neurons, and the nucleus ambiguus (IX and X) that innervate the swallowing muscles (56). The output from the CPG can be modified by sensory feedback. Motor timing varies with bolus characteristics and other variables (63).

Wallenberg's Syndrome: Disruption of the Swallowing Central Pattern Generator

Disruption of the swallow CPG can result in a severe and long-standing dysphagia associated with aspiration (57, 64). Wallenberg's, or lateral medullary, syndrome results from occlusion of the vertebral,

---

TABLE 11-1
Innervation of Major Muscles Related to Swallowing

CRANIAL NERVE	MUSCLES
Trigeminal nerve (V)	Masticatory muscles Mylohyoid Tensor veli palatini Anterior belly of digastrics
Facial nerve (VII)	Facial muscle Stylohyoid Posterior belly of digastrics
Glossopharyngeal nerve (IX)	Stylopharyngeus
Vagus nerve (X)	Levator veli palatine Palatopharyngeous Salpingopharyngeous Intrinsic laryngeal muscles Cricopharyngeus Pharyngeal constrictors
Hypoglossal nerve (XII)	Intrinsic tongue muscles Hyoglossus Geniohyoid Genioglossus Styloglossus Thyrohyoid

(Reprinted from Physical Medicine and Rehabilitation, Third edition, Randall L. Braddom Ed., Rehabilitation of Patients with Swallowing Disorders, Page 602, © 2007, with permission from Elsevier)

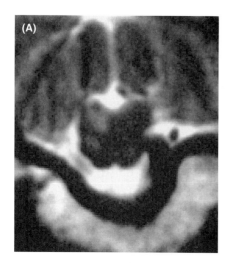
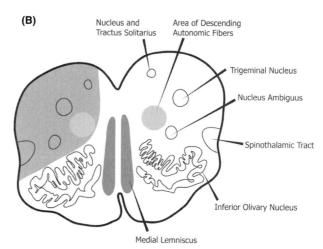

FIGURE 11-4

Lateral medullary syndrome, axial cut through the rostral medulla. (a) MRI (b) Diagram Lateral medullary syndrome causes dysphagia by affecting the NTS and nucleus ambiguus. Other deficits include: Contralateral loss of pain and temperature: Involvement of the spinothalamic tract. Ipsilateral loss of pain and temperature sensation on the face: Involvement of the descending nucleus and tract of V. Ipsilateral Horner's syndrome (ptosis, meiosis, and anhidrosis): Involvement of descending autonomic fibers. Ipsilateral ataxia: Involvement of the inferior cerebellar peduncle (restiform body).

posterior inferior cerebellar, or medullary arteries. Lateral medullary infarction (LMI) can affect the NTS, NA, and motor nuclei of the cranial nerves involved in swallowing (Figure 11-4). Involvement of the NA produces weakness or paralysis of the ipsilateral muscles of the pharynx, larynx, and soft palate. Involvement of the NTS can hamper initiation and coordination of the pharyngeal swallow.

Electrophysiological evidence suggest that, in LMI, swallowing function is affected bilaterally, indicating an acute disconnection syndrome to the contralateral swallowing centers (57). The mechanism for recovery of swallowing after lateral medullary infarction is poorly understood.

Supramedullary Control of Swallowing

Although the swallowing CPG is located in the brain stem, mounting evidence suggests that several supratentorial structures, most prominently the cerebral cortex, have an essential role in swallowing regulation (65–67). Voluntary initiation of swallowing requires integrity of the motor areas of the cerebral cortex (59). Studies using positron emission tomography (PET) have identified multiple, asymmetric loci associated with swallowing, including the right orbitofrontal cortex, left mesial premotor cortex and cingulate, right caudolateral sensorimotor cortex, right anterior insula, bilateral medial cerebellum, and bilateral temporopolar cortices (68). The strongest activation has been seen in the sensorimotor cortices, insula, and cerebellum. Swallowing is represented

asymmetrically in the cortex, and there is no clear right or left laterality (69). Studies in stroke patients have shown that the size of the swallowing area in the unaffected cortex determined the presence or absence of dysphagia (70). The cortical representation of swallowing within the motor and premotor cortex has been shown to be bilateral but markedly asymmetric (71). Using this theoretical framework, one would expect individuals with strokes of the hemisphere with higher swallowing representation to have a predisposition to dysphagia.

Although mechanisms of recovery of swallowing function remain unclear, studies using transcranial magnetic stimulation suggest that recovery of swallowing function after a cortical stroke is associated with compensatory cortical reorganization in the undamaged hemisphere (72). In spite of the obvious contributions of the cerebral cortex, insula, cerebellum, and others to the normal swallowing mechanism, it is still unclear how these areas are integrated with the brain stem to produce functional and voluntary swallowing. It is also unclear why recovery does not occur in some cases of unilateral supratentorial stroke.

Suprabulbar Palsy: Disruption of the Corticobulbar System

Disruption of the corticobulbar system may result in suprabulbar palsy (SBP). Suprabulbar palsy, or pseudobulbar palsy, is a clinical syndrome characterized by dysphagia dysarthria, dysphonia, impairment of voluntary movements of tongue and facial muscles, and emotional lability. The most common cause of SBP is multiple bilateral lacunar infarcts, but it is also associated with amyotrophic lateral sclerosis (ALS), Parkinson's disease, and multiple sclerosis. Swallowing difficulties in these patients are common and range from mild, subclinical findings to severe dysphagia precluding oral feeding.

Studies in SBP patients suggest that the basal ganglia and associated neural pathways play a role in the pathogenesis of dysphagia after stroke and that progressive involvement of the excitatory and inhibitory corticobulbar fibers is responsible for the difficulties that SBP patients experience (73). The swallowing problems in SBP cases are primarily difficulties in triggering a swallow and a dysfunctional cricopharyngeal sphincter that is hyperactive and uncoordinated (73). Slowing of oropharyngeal swallowing and saliva accumulation in the mouth was also associated with extrapyramidal dysfunction.

SWALLOWING IN THE ELDERLY

Because stroke is primarily a disease of the elderly, it is important to consider specific deficits that might be present prior to a brain event that can impact dysphagia outcomes after a stroke.

Dentition generally worsens with age. This is further worsened by the development of oral infections, such as periodontal disease or dental caries. With aging, masticatory muscles weaken, masticatory forces decrease, and speed of jaw motion slows. These factors result in increased mastication time and reduced efficiency (74). Despite the increase in mastication time, the bolus size at the time of swallow onset is larger in the elderly than in the young, primarily because of the decrease in masticatory function. Strength of labial closure and tongue-palate pressure also decreases. Although saliva secretion is stable with aging, disease, atrophy of the salivary glands, or medication side effects can cause xerostomia, or dry mouth, in elderly individuals (75, 76).

The duration of transit from the oral cavity to the pharynx increases with aging (53). The time interval from arrival of the bolus at the pharynx until onset of laryngeal elevation is also extended. Because of this time interval increase, laryngeal penetration is more frequent in the elderly, but aspiration is not (77–79).

Aging also affects UES function. Decreased UES compliance and reduced hyolaryngeal elevation reduce UES opening, resulting in increased hypopharyngeal intrabolus pressure during trans-sphincteric flow (53). The interval from the onset of the oral stage to the UES opening is delayed in the elderly, but the intervals from the onset of pharyngeal stage or from the onset of glottal closure until UES relaxation are not affected by age (61, 53). Aging lowers resting pressure and shortens the length of the UES, but no significant effect is seen on the LES (80).

Aging increases the duration of swallow apnea, but it does not change the typical resumption of breathing in the expiratory phase after a swallow (40, 81, 82).

Dysphagia Rehabilitation

Rehabilitation of dysphagia includes improving overall function, increasing swallowing function by correcting underlying physiologic abnormalities, using compensation for unsafe or inefficient swallowing, and preventing complications such as aspiration pneumonia and malnutrition.

Abnormal Swallowing after Stroke

The specific dysphagia symptoms following stroke depend on the site of the lesion and differ in severity among individuals with the same site of lesion. Deficits may be unilateral or bilateral and may affect sensory and/or motor components of the swallow. Labial weakness can result in an inability to adequately ingest a bolus from a utensil and difficulty containing the bolus in the mouth. Lingual and buccal weakness may result in inadequate bolus formation and propulsion, leading to ineffective oral clearance and piecemeal swallowing. Impaired mandibular and tongue movements result in ineffective mastication of solid foods. Sensory deficits may result in pocketing of oral residue into one or both cheeks or retention of food on the lips and tongue after swallowing.

Pharyngeal dysfunction can result in delayed swallow initiation, ineffective bolus propulsion, and retention of food after swallowing. Velopharyngeal inadequacy can cause nasal regurgitation. Impaired laryngeal elevation, vocal cord dysfunction, or epiglottic inversion result in ineffective airway protection. This places individuals at risk for laryngeal penetration (food material entering the larynx above the level of the vocal cords) or aspiration (food material passing through the vocal cords). An ineffective cough, caused by vocal cord dysmotility, weakness of expiratory muscles, or impaired coordination of glottal adduction with expiration, hampers clearance of aspirated material. Laryngeal sensory impairments can result in silent aspiration in which there is lack of cough response to aspiration. Impaired opening of the UES can result in pharyngeal food retention, placing individuals at risk for aspiration after the swallow. Esophageal dysmotility leads to ineffective esophageal clearance and reflux. Esophageal dysfunction is not typically a problem after stroke, but it should be considered as it may coexist with oral and pharyngeal impairments.

The presence of a tracheostomy tube presents additional challenges. A tracheostomy tube is associated with altered laryngopharyngeal aerodynamics, eliminating the normal post-swallow expiration through the pharynx, reducing laryngeal sensation, and limiting ability to effectively cough and clear aspirated material.

Evaluation of Dysphagia

Early assessment and management of dysphagia reduces pneumonia rates and length of stay and improves overall outcome from stroke (83–85). An interdisciplinary team's involvement in the dysphagia evaluation process is crucial to address the complex needs of the dysphagic individual. This team should include a physician, speech language pathologist, dietician, occupational therapist, nurse, and other subspecialties as needed. Speech language pathologists have substantial training in evaluation and treatment of dysphagia and should be consulted whenever a problem with oral or pharyngeal swallowing is suspected.

Comprehensive assessment of swallow functioning after stroke begins with a thorough medical history. Specific lesion localization may be useful in predicting presence and severity of dysphagia, as a large percentage of brain stem lesions, most prominently lateral medullary infarcts, result in severe dysphagia (10). However, dysphagia can be present in cases with no brain stem involvement, particularly in cases of multiple or bilateral cerebral infarction. Medical history and current medical status need to be considered, including cardiac, pulmonary, neurologic, and nutritional information. Medications, such as barbiturates, benzodiazepines, antihistamines, or antidepressants, may negatively affect physical or neurologic function and limit an individual's participation in the rehabilitation process. A clear description of dysphagia-related symptoms, such as choking or coughing with food or liquids, vomiting, or the sensation of food stuck in throat, provides information regarding possible deficits and indicates the need for further evaluation. The sensation of food sticking in the throat or chest is an important symptom of dysphagia. The sensation of food sticking in the throat has poor localizing value, as it may be seen in cases of esophageal as well as pharyngeal dysphagia. The sensation of food sticking in the chest, on the other hand, is generally associated with esophageal problems.

Dysphagia Screening

Given the high prevalence of dysphagia and its complications, a swallowing screening examination should be completed as part of every stroke patient's initial assessment.

Elements commonly evaluated on bedside screening are described in Table 11-2. Dysphagia screening is part of the practice guidelines for adult stroke rehabilitation care (86). The goals of swallowing screening examination are to identify possible signs of dysphagia and aspiration and identify patients in need of further evaluation. The water swallow test is commonly used as a screening tool. The patient continuously drinks a predetermined amount of water, usually three or four ounces, and clinicians observe for signs of aspiration or dysphagia (87–89). Other screening tests include items from history as well (90). This screening is usually performed by trained medical personnel. Results of this screening must be interpreted with caution as they have limited predictive ability, cannot detect silent aspiration, determine safety with other forms of food/liquids, or provide information regarding the mechanism of dysphagia. It is essential to have a high index of suspicion to improve sensitivity of screening.

Physical Examination

A physical examination of the upper aerodigestive tract, including cranial nerve testing, should be performed to assess structure and function. Symmetry, strength, and range of motion of the facial and oral muscles are examined in isolated and purposeful movements. Sensation to facial, lingual, labial, and palatal stimulation is assessed. Drooling and secretion management should be noted as they are associated with the ability to manage food and liquid boluses. Hearing and vision skills should be screened as well. Symmetry and strength of movement of the velopharynx is demonstrated through vocalization and by eliciting a gag reflex. The presence or absence of a gag reflex must not be used as a predictor of swallow safety. Some normal individuals have an absent gag

---

TABLE 11-2
Elements Commonly Evaluated on Bedside Screening

General Assessment
1. History of dysphagia or enteral feeding
2. Conciousness level: Altered alertness or arousal
3. Postural control
4. Difficulty managing oral secretions
5. Weak voluntary cough

Swallow challenge (One teaspoon of water followed by three ounces of water)
1. No laryngeal elevation
2. Coughing
3. Choking
4. Wet or "gurgly" vocal quality

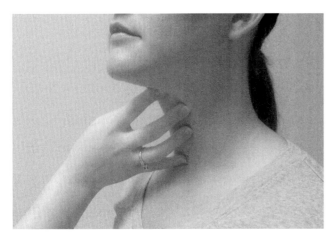

FIGURE 11-5

Palpation of the larynx. Each finger is used to palpate a different structure: middle finger, hyoid bone; fourth finger, top of thyroid cartilage; fifth finger, cricothyroid notch.

reflex; individuals with severe dysphagia can have intact gag reflexes (91).

The larynx is manually palpated for abnormalities at rest and during a volitional swallow of saliva (Figure 11-5). Laryngeal function is further assessed by eliciting a volitional cough and assessing vocal quality. Respiratory control is observed at rest, during speech, and through sustained phonation. Cognition and communication skills, including orientation, attention, memory, and insight, should be examined, as impairments in cognition can negatively impact outcomes (92, 93).

Clinical Swallow Evaluation

If the presence of dysphagia is suggested by the screening examination or the patient complains of symptoms associated with swallowing dysfunction, that individual should be referred for a complete clinical swallow evaluation. The clinical (or bedside) swallow evaluation (CSE) examines an individual's potential risk for dysphagia and aspiration with various food and liquid consistencies and is usually performed by a speech language pathologist. Findings are used to guide decision-making on further instrumental examinations, safe means of alimentation, and an appropriate treatment plan. During a CSE, clinicians complete a thorough oral, pharyngeal, and laryngeal motor and sensory assessment. Liquids and solid foods are presented. Oral function is observed for ability to manage substances with adequate lip, tongue, plus jaw control and movement. This includes adequate mastication and maneuvering of liquid and solid boluses and ability to propel boluses into the pharynx without oral residual. The timing and strength of the pharyngeal swallow is assessed through palpation of the tongue base, hyoid,

and larynx. Clinicians look for signs of overt aspiration before, during, or after the swallow occurs. While silent aspiration cannot be reliably detected during a bedside examination, several clinical signs are associated with risk of aspiration. These include dysphonia, dysarthria, weak cough, abnormal laryngeal elevation, impaired control of secretions, cough after swallow, and voice change after swallow (94–97).

Clinical tools provide additional information and assist in making judgments during the CSE. Using cervical auscultation with a stethoscope, clinicians may listen to the sounds of swallowing for coordination, timing, and pre- and post-swallow breath sounds. Clear classification of the sounds heard and their physiological implications have yet to be described (98, 99). Decline in pulse oximetry during swallowing has been explored as a tool to predict aspiration; however, evidence has been contradictory (100, 101).

Checklists have been suggested as tools to help guide assessment. One formal CSE tool is the Mann Assessment of Swallowing Ability (MASA), a standardized swallowing test that uses a checklist to place individuals in categories that describe their risk of dysphagia and aspiration (102).

The CSE relies on indirect information to make judgments regarding swallow abnormalities. While clinician judgments regarding the presence of abnormal oral and pharyngeal function have reasonable reliability, they are not perfect, and they may fail to identify some patients with dysphagia and aspiration. In addition, the presence or absence of aspiration, the timing and cause of aspiration, and the effectiveness of compensatory maneuvers cannot be reliably determined with a CSE (28, 88, 100). Instrumental examination of swallowing is essential to the comprehensive assessment of patients with clinical signs of dysphagia or at high risk of silent aspiration.

Instrumental Assessment Tools

Videofluoroscopic Swallowing Studies.   The Videofluoroscopic swallowing study (VFSS) is the gold standard in swallowing assessment. This procedure is typically performed by a speech language pathologist along with a radiologist or physiatrist. During a VFSS, the patient ingests liquids and solids with barium or other radiopaque contrast while motion radiographic images are produced and recorded. The purpose of this test is to identify the structural or functional abnormalities related to swallowing and to identify circumstances for safe swallowing (103). Clinicians make observations of structure and function that cannot be made during a CSE. These include oral bolus control and propulsion, pharyngeal transport, timing and coordination of the swallow, presence and depth of laryngeal penetration or aspiration, and possible causes for aspiration or laryngeal penetration. In this context,

TABLE 11-3
Penetration-Aspiration Scale

Aspiration Risk	Score	Classification	Description
No risk	1	Normal	No airway invasion
	2	Mild	Bolus enters into airway, remains above the vocal folds with clearing
Risk of aspiration	3	Moderate	Bolus enters into airway, remains above the vocal folds without clearing
	4	Moderate	Bolus contacts vocal folds with airway clearing
	5	Moderate	Bolus contacts vocal folds without airway clearing
Positive aspiration	6	Severe	Bolus enters trachea; clears into the larynx or out of the airway
	7	Severe	Bolus enters trachea; not cleared despite attempts
	8	Severe	Bolus enters trachea; no attempt is made to clear

From Ref. 104.

laryngeal penetration is defined as contrast entering the larynx but not passing through the vocal folds. Aspiration is defined as contrast passing through the larynx and vocal folds. The penetration-aspiration scale (104) is a semi-quantitative tool for describing the degree or severity of laryngeal penetration and aspiration (Table 11-3). However, it is not typically used in clinical practice.

Use of standardized VFSS procedure improves its reliability and clinical utility (Table 11-4) (105). Images of the swallow should be obtained in both the lateral and anteroposterior views to determine laterality of swallow dysfunction. Observations are made regarding motions of the tongue, jaw, soft palate, epiglottis, hyoid bone, larynx, pharyngeal walls, and UES. Additional observations are made regarding timing and extent of bolus flow, including timing of swallow, retention of contrast after swallowing, and the presence of penetration or aspiration. Performing and interpreting a VFSS requires analysis of the mechanism of swallowing dysfunction. This analysis will suggest opportunities for treatment. The VFSS also provides opportunity to test compensatory maneuvers such as modifications of posture or bolus characteristics that may improve the safety and efficiency of swallowing.

TABLE 11-4
Videofluorographic Swallow Study Protocol

Lateral projection, patient sitting upright in usual position of comfort
Speech sample ("candy, candy") to visualize velar motion
Command swallow: 5 ml of thin liquid from a spoon
Drink thin liquid from a cup (patient controls rate and volume)
Command swallow: 5 ml nectar-thick liquid from a spoon
Drink nectar-thick liquid from a cup (patient controls rate and volume)
Eat 1 tsp pudding from spoon
Eat 1 tsp soft food (e.g., chicken salad sandwich spread) from a spoon
Eat shortbread cookie (e.g., ½ of a Lorna Doone)
Compensatory techniques as appropriate
Other food consistencies as indicated
Anteroposterior (AP) projection, sitting upright (neck slightly extended if safe)
Phonation of "e" (as in "he") several times in succession to visualize vocal fold and arytenoids motion
Command swallow: thin or nectar-thick liquid, 5 or 10 ml
Compensatory techniques or other foods as appropriate
Additional swallows as needed for imaging the esophagus

From Ref. 105.

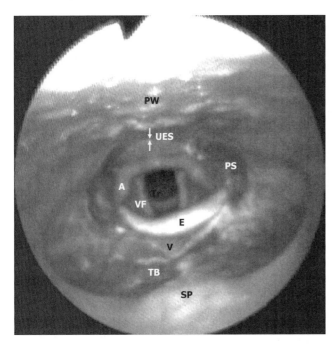

FIGURE 11-6

Fiberoptic endoscopic image of the pharynx. A, Arytenoid; E, Epiglottis; PS, Pyriform sinus; PW, posterior pharyngeal wall; SP, Soft palate; TB, Tongue base; Tr, Trachea; UES, Upper esophageal sphincter; V, Valleculae; VF, Vocal folds (Modified from Physical Medicine and Rehabilitation, Third edition, Randall L. Braddom Ed., Rehabilitation of Patients with Swallowing Disorders, Page 608, © 2007, with permission from Elsevier)

Radiation exposure limits the duration of the VFSS, so the VFSS is brief and provides only a window into the swallow function. However, the radiation dose and relative risk of radiation related complications are low (106).

Fiberoptic Endoscopic Evaluation of Swallowing. The fiberoptic endoscopic evaluation of swallowing (FEES) is a bedside procedure in which a nasally inserted flexible endoscope is used to directly view the nasopharynx and larynx during swallowing (Figure 11-6). During this procedure, individuals swallow various consistencies of food and liquids dyed for visualization.

The FEES is a useful procedure for evaluating the laryngeal and pharyngeal anatomy and assessing vocal cord function (107, 108), and it is highly sensitive for detecting silent aspiration (109). However, the pharynx is not directly visible during a swallow because its closure produces a white-out effect on the image. The FEES is ideal for cases where radiation exposure is a concern. Its portability makes it a valuable tool for critical care patients or patients who are unable to tolerate transportation to a radiology suite. Disadvantages of the FEES procedure include the inability to:

- Directly observe a swallow
- Observe critical pharyngeal swallow events
- Observe the oral and esophageal stages of swallowing

The inability to evaluate tongue base retraction, pharyngeal constriction, epiglottic tilt, and UES opening limit the utility of FEES for analyzing swallow mechanics and pathophysiology.

Other Tools. Other instrumental tools can be useful in further assessing swallowing. Esophagoscopy is useful in assessing anatomical abnormalities of the esophagus. Functional or physiological disorders are better assessed with radiologic studies. Manometry measures pressures in the pharynx and esophagus during swallowing. It is primarily used to analyze motor disorders of the esophagus. Electromyography (EMG) is useful in diagnosing dysphagia in motor unit disorders and as a biofeedback tool in dysphagia therapy. It provides little information regarding the mechanism of swallowing, so it cannot be a guide for rehabilitation. Ultrasound may be used in diagnosis of oral dysfunction, but it does not provide information on pharyngeal or esophageal function.

Treatment of Dysphagia after Stroke

The primary treatment principles in dysphagia management are amelioration of the underlying disease process, prevention of complications, compensation for an unsafe swallow, improvement of swallowing via therapy, and use of environmental modifications. A basic tenet of dysphagia rehabilitation is that the best exercise for swallowing is swallowing. This means it is important to determine the circumstances for safe swallowing before initiating a swallowing therapy program. Successful management of dysphagia requires adherence to these principles. As with evaluation, therapeutic management of the dysphagic stroke patient requires an interdisciplinary approach.

Prior to initiation of dysphagia therapy, the stroke patient must be stabilized medically. This includes providing recurrent stroke prevention, minimizing or preventing complications, and ensuring proper management of general health functions (110). Depending on the clinical presentation, a period where the patient receives no oral feeding might be indicated. Recent studies have demonstrated no difference in outcomes when comparing early tube feedings and avoidance of it (111, 112). In addition to inability to safely take oral nutrition due to dysphagia, nutritional intake may be reduced by poor appetite caused by depression and medication effects, lack of dentures, cognitive levels, or impaired arm function. Nutritional status should be closely monitored by following body weight and blood chemistries (113). Intravenous fluids may be needed to improve fluid intake. Some individuals may be able to tolerate supplemental water and ice chips despite dysphagia.

TABLE 11-5
National Dysphagia Diet

NDD Solids	Description
Level 1	Dysphagia-Pureed (homogenous, very cohesive, pudding-like, requiring very little chewing ability)
Level 2	Dysphagia-Mechanical Altered (cohesive, moist, semi-solid foods, requiring some chewing)
Level 3	Dysphagia-Advanced (soft foods that require more chewing ability)
Regular	(all foods allowed)
NDD liquids	**Description in centipoise (cP)**
Thin	1–50 cP (liquid viscosity similar to water*)
Nectar	51–350 cP (liquid viscosity similar to cream soup)
Honey-like	351–1, 1,750 cP (liquid viscosity similar to honey or molasses)
Spoon-thick	Greater than 1,750 cP (liquid viscosity similar to ketchup)

*Water has a viscosity of 1 centipoise at 20°C (68°F).

From Ref. 116.

Allowing water intake as part of the therapeutic diet may increase compliance with dietary recommendations and overall satisfaction (114), but it may lead to aspiration. Dysphagia management teams need to carefully consider an individual's risk of developing pneumonia, taking into account CSE and instrumental assessment results prior to allowing water in patients who aspirate.

Swallowing therapy is associated with successful outcomes, including return to oral feeding (115). Therapeutic programs must be individualized to the physiological and behavioral needs of the individual. A number of therapy techniques can be utilized to compensate for oral and pharyngeal control deficits and reduce the occurrence of penetration and aspiration. Environmental modifications should be employed, including reduction of distractions, proper seating and positioning, modifying bolus volume and rate, use of straws, and use of adaptive equipment.

Direct Swallowing Therapy Techniques

Direct swallowing therapy focuses on diet modification and behavioral compensations to improve swallowing efficiency and safety while allowing for oral nutrition. The therapy plan is individualized and based on the mechanism of swallowing dysfunction in the particular individual with dysphagia. A VFSS is necessary to determine the circumstances for safe swallowing for a dysphagic stroke patient and should be performed prior to initiating direct swallowing therapy.

Regular solid foods may be too difficult to effectively masticate and manipulate. Solid foods can be mechanically altered to make them softer, reduce particle size, or simplify consistencies to assist in mastication and food transport. Liquid viscosities can be altered to compensate for specific deficits. Thin liquids are generally the most difficult liquid consistency to tolerate for most dysphagic

stroke patients because they are difficult to control and may be aspirated before or during the swallow. Use of various levels of thickened liquids provides better oral and pharyngeal control and timing and may prevent aspiration. For other individuals, thin liquids are better tolerated because the major issue is lack of propulsive force or poor opening of the UES. Patients with these deficits may retain liquids in the pharynx and aspirate after swallowing. The National Dysphagia Diet, published by the American Dietetic Association, provides labels and descriptions of frequently used levels of food and liquid consistencies (Table 11-5) (116). Given the variety in pathophysiology of swallowing, these descriptions are not comprehensive, and clinicians must individualize diets based on specific findings in clinical and instrumental exams.

Altered bolus presentations—liquids by teaspoon, elimination of straws, decreased volume—can reduce aspiration risk and improve bolus transport in some patients. These strategies must be tested during the VFSS to determine their effectiveness and safety before their use in therapeutic diets. In addition to diet modifications, postural maneuvers are frequently utilized to facilitate safe and efficient swallowing. These postures are not effective for all dysphagic individuals and can be dangerous if utilized inappropriately. Careful clinical examination and testing during instrumental assessment ensure their appropriate use.

The chin tuck maneuver reduces laryngeal penetration and aspiration by improving laryngeal closure and preventing posterior loss of control of the bolus (28, 117, 118). This is accomplished by reducing the laryngohyoid distance and the hyoid-mandibular distance. The chin tuck maneuver also weakens pharyngeal contractions and can cause aspiration in patients with weakened pharyngeal muscles and tongue base retraction (37, 119).

Rotation of the head to the affected (weak) side is useful in individuals with unilateral pharyngeal weakness and impaired UES opening. This maneuver alters the bolus pathway and propels the bolus through the pharynx on the unaffected side. Head rotation also aids in UES dynamics and pharyngeal clearance (120). Tilting the head away from the weak side can also divert the bolus through the stronger side of the pharynx.

Use of neck extension posture can be beneficial for individuals with impaired anteroposterior oral propulsion. Extending the neck provides gravity assist for the bolus to move through the oral cavity. Caution should be used when attempting this technique if pharyngeal control is impaired, as it may cause aspiration. A reclining position can be useful in individuals who retain food in the pharynx after the swallow and experience overflow aspiration. The reclining posture elevates the laryngeal aditus (entry) relative to the hypopharynx, inhibiting overflow aspiration.

Two related behavioral techniques can be used to reduce aspiration. The supraglottic swallow technique involves holding the breath before and during swallowing and coughing after swallow. This produces closure of the larynx prior to swallowing to prevent aspiration. In the super-supraglottic swallow, the breath holding is combined with valsalva maneuver, which closes the laryngeal vestibule in addition to adducting the vocal folds (121).

Several compensatory techniques can improve pharyngeal clearance. The effortful swallow technique is used to compensate for impaired pharyngeal constriction. Individuals are instructed to swallow hard. This technique assists pharyngeal clearance by increasing tongue base retraction (122). When food is retained in the pharynx after a swallow, a subsequent liquid swallow can be used to clear residue. If residue occurs consistently, it may be useful to alternate solids and liquids. The double-swallow technique uses a volitional swallow to assist in clearing pharyngeal residue. In the case of severe retention after swallowing, individuals often require three or more volitional swallows. The Mendelsohn maneuver increases the extent and duration of UES opening by voluntarily prolonging contraction of the suprahyoid muscles (123). This can improve pharyngeal clearance.

Intraoral prostheses can be beneficial in selected individuals with decreased lingual and palatal strength and range of motion (124). Palatal augmentation assists individuals with oral stage transfer deficits. A device is fit to improve contact of the tongue with the hard palate. A palatal lift prosthesis elevates the palate to compensate for velopharyngeal insufficiency. Use of a one-way speaking valve for individuals with tracheostomy restores expiratory airflow after the swallow, allowing for coughing and clearing the airway.

Oral sensory stimulation involves use of altered temperature and taste to improve timing of the pharyngeal swallow. This technique is based on the premise that oral afferent information assists in swallowing initiation. Presentation of a sour bolus improves onset of oral swallow, reduces pharyngeal delay time, and improves swallow efficiency (125). Presentation of larger bolus volumes acts similarly by increasing swallow response time. Stimulation of the faucial arches with a chilled laryngeal mirror improves the swallow initiation when provided immediately before the swallow (126).

Neuromuscular electrical stimulation (NMES) is a relatively new treatment for oropharyngeal dysphagia. Tetanic stimulation is delivered via surface electrodes overlying the submental and anterior neck muscles, and individuals are asked to swallow (127). It is suggested that NMES contracts the muscles used for swallowing and improves swallow function (128). Although this technique is increasing in popularity among clinicians, its effects on swallow biomechanics are not well understood. Initial evidence indicates that NMES can stimulate only superficial muscles and not the pharyngeal muscles, and it can actually inhibit laryngeal elevation (129–131). Surface electrical stimulation may instead be useful as a resistance exercise in individuals with reduced laryngeal elevation (130, 132). Further research into the actual effects of NMES needs to be completed before surface electrical stimulation can be recommended as treatment for dysphagia.

Indirect Swallowing Therapy Techniques

Indirect therapy involves use of exercise to improve flexibility, strength, and coordination of oral, pharyngeal, and respiratory muscles for swallowing. Common indirect therapy techniques are summarized in Table 11-6.

Oral exercises are designed to target motions used in the oral stages of swallowing. Oral control exercises include rapid lingual lateralization, rotary lingual movements, suck-and-swallow movements to assist in posterior bolus propulsion, simulated chewing via lateralization of gauze or sponges to improve bolus manipulation, and simulated labial seal to reduce labial leakage.

Oral muscles can be strengthened with resistance exercise. Lingual muscles are strengthened by pushing the tongue against a tongue blade, pushing the tongue into a cheek, and pulling the tongue posteriorly while being held anteriorly. Labial muscles are strengthened by maintaining closure on a moving tongue blade and squeezing lips closed to resistance. Mandibular strengthening is achieved by opening and closing the jaw to resistance. Oral flexibility is improved through lateral, anterior, and rotary stretching of the tongue; protrusion and retraction of the lips; and mandibular opening and closure.

Pharyngeal exercises are designed to improve range of motion and strength of the tongue base, pharyngeal muscles, and laryngeal muscles. Lingual protrusion and retraction improves tongue base contact with the pharyngeal wall. The Masako tongue-holding maneuver

TABLE 11-6
Common Indirect Therapy Techniques with Brief Descriptions

THERAPY TECHNIQUES	BRIEF DESCRIPTION
Oral cavity	
Oral motor control exercises (jaw, tongue, lip)	Jaw opening and closing
	Tongue rotation, lateralization, protrusion, retraction
	Lip protrusion, lateralization, opening/closing
	Stretching and increasing range of motion
Relaxation and ROM* (jaw, tongue, lip)	Opening/closing the jaw against resistance
Resistance exercise (jaw, tongue, lip)	Pushing the tongue against resistance
Pharynx	
Laryngeal elevation exercise	Volitional laryngeal elevation by saying a high-pitched "ee"
Vocal cord adduction exercise	Pushing wall or table, uttering "ah" simultaneously
Masako maneuver	Swallowing with the tongue tip held anteriorly outside the mouth
Sensory stimulation	Tactile stimulation of the faucial arches with cold or sour stimuli
UES opening	
Shaker exercise	Active head raising (neck flexion) in the supine position
UES dilatation	Expansion of a balloon catheter in the UES

ROM*, range of motion

increases strength and duration of tongue base contact with the pharyngeal wall. In this technique, the tongue tip is held anteriorly outside of the mouth while swallowing (133). Shaker exercises strengthen the anterior submental muscles, improving UES opening during the swallow and thereby reducing food retention in the pharynx (134, 135). In this exercise, the patient lies supine and lifts the head against resistance of gravity, flexing the neck, and looking at the toes (Figure 11-7). The patient lifts the head three times for one minute each and then performs 30 consecutive head lifts without holding.

Laryngeal muscles are stimulated through sustained elevation exercises. Maintaining a high-pitch sound (for example, "ee"), performing effortful swallows, and using the Mendelsohn maneuver can improve laryngeal elevation during swallowing. Hard glottal attacks (forceful volitional closure of the vocal cords) and pushing-pulling exercises (phonation while pulling or pushing an object like a chair) improve vocal cord adduction to strengthen the cough response and vocal cord closure during swallowing.

Electromyography (EMG) biofeedback is an adjunct therapy that allows individuals to visualize force of muscle contraction. By increasing awareness of muscle activity, individuals are often able to effect greater control of those muscles (136). EMG can be used to record submental and infrahyoid activity during swallowing therapy, assisting the patient in contracting those muscles. EMG may be beneficial in training effortful swallows, sustained

pharyngeal contraction, lip closure, and tongue mobility (137). Laryngoscopy can provide visual feedback when teaching a patient to perform laryngeal exercises. It provides direct visualization of the vocal cords and larynx, and it can be useful in completing vocal cord adduction exercises and learning breath control techniques, for example, the supraglottic swallow.

Pharyngeal Bypass

When safe alimentation is not possible, pharyngeal bypass measures may be employed, eliminating the need for oropharyngeal swallowing and providing nutrition and hydration. Short-term feeding—that is, less than 30 days—can be accomplished via nasogastric (NG) tubes. NG tubes have risks, and they can result in numerous complications, including reflux aspiration, improper positioning, dislodgement, and ulceration of pharyngeal and esophageal tissue. Long-term feeding options include percutaneous gastrostomy (PEG) tubes and percutaneous jejunostomy (PEJ) tubes. While use of a PEG tube does not prevent aspiration pneumonia in acute stroke (138, 139), there is a reduction in the number of aspiration cases when compared to continued oral feeding (140). Aspiration and pneumonia from PEG tubes can be minimized through measures such as head elevation, good hygiene with bag and line handling, continuous drip feeding (as opposed to bolus feeding), and consistent monitoring for gastric residue (141). PEJ tubes are indicated for individuals with chronic aspiration of tube feedings or impaired

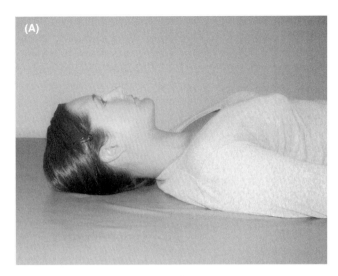

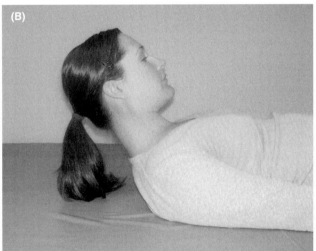

FIGURE 11-7

Shaker exercises. (A) The patient is instructed to lay flat on his or her back on the floor or bed. (B) Patient holds the head off the floor or bed, looking at his or her feet for one minute without raising the shoulders from the floor or bed. The second part of the exercise involves the same movement (without sustaining the head lift) for 30 repetitions.

gastric motility (142). PEG tubes can provide uninterrupted feeding, which is not possible with NG feeding, resulting in improved nutrition (143). Many individuals who will return to oral nutrition after stroke benefit from PEG use in order to allow exercise and therapeutic oral feeding to continue (144). As with any surgery, infection is a risk with performance of PEG or PEJ tubes.

Surgical and Pharmacological Management

Surgical options for dysphagia are rarely used in the United States. One exception to this is dilatation of the esophagus or UES, which are performed in the case of stricture, web, or setonosis. Cricopharyngeal myotomy is a surgical procedure

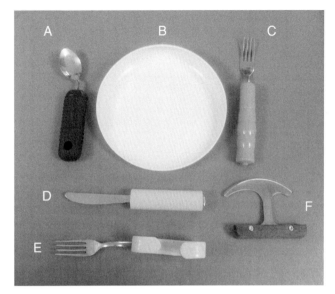

FIGURE 11-8

Assistive devices used for feeding. (A) Wide grip, weighted utensils. These utensils have soft-ribbed handles and bendable shafts. They are weighted to help keep hands steady. The extra handle weight provides help for individuals with limited hand control. The shaft can be bent for either right or left handed use. (B) Tapered front scoop dish. Nonskid feet keep the plate from sliding. Curved edge simplifies scooping food. Specially suited for individuals who have limited flexibility, motor coordination, or feed using one hand, for example, one who had a hemiparetic stroke. (C) Universal grip aid. These aids can be used with conventional flatware. Provide better grip by increasing friction and handle size. (D) Foam grip aid. Increases handle size, providing a large, more comfortable grip and better control of the utensil. (E) Universal feeding cuff. For individuals with little to no grip. Securely attaches the utensil to the hand for feeding. (F) Rocking "T" knife. For individuals with a weak grasp. Cuts food with a rocking motion. Wooden handle fits the hand and safety edge reduces risk of injury.

that disrupts the cricopharyngeus muscle to reduce UES pressure and improve bolus flow from the pharynx to the esophagus. Laryngeal diversion procedures are performed in cases of severe intractable aspiration caused by dysphagia (145, 146). The larynx is separated from the upper airway, and a permanent tracheostomy is performed (147). While laryngeal diversion eliminates aspiration, significant consequences include loss or reduction of upper airway functions like phonation, cough, or smell as well as potential for persistent pharyngeal dysphagia.

There are no specific pharmacological treatments for oral or pharyngeal dysphagia, but some symptoms may be managed with medication. Anticholinergic medications can reduce salivary flow in individuals with sialorrhea and chronic aspiration of oral secretions (148). Botulin toxin injections have been used in cases of oromandibular

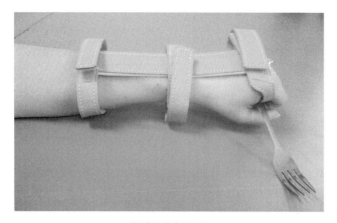

FIGURE 11-9

Wrist support with universal cuff. Allows self-feeding for individuals with weak grip and weak wrist or wrist drop.

or lingual dystonia, trismus, cricopharyngeal dysfunction, and sialorrhea.

Additional Considerations

Oral care is an often overlooked, but critical, concept in dysphagia management. Proper oral care before and

after meals reduces the bacterial load in the mouth, thereby reducing the risk of developing aspiration pneumonia (19). Proper positioning is important in dysphagia management (149). Individuals should be seated upright during and after meals to maximize effectiveness of rehabilitation techniques and reduce the risk of gastroesophageal reflux with subsequent aspiration. Adaptive equipment is used by individuals with motor disabilities in order to improve self-feeding. Some examples of adaptive equipment are pictured in Figures 11-8 and 11-9.

CONCLUSION

Although dysphagia after stroke has been associated with increased incidence of complications, morbidity, and mortality, early identification of feeding difficulties can impact long-term outcomes and improve quality of life. Early assessment and treatment are vital to preventing complications during the acute phase to allow for normal recovery of swallowing function. For those individuals whose swallowing function does not recover spontaneously, sophisticated therapeutic options that can be tailored to address individual needs are available.

References

1. Miller RM, Chang MW. Advances in the management of dysphagia caused by stroke. *Phys Med Rehabil Clin N Am* 1999; 10:x, 925–941.
2. Groher ME, Bukatman R. The prevalence of swallow disorders in two teaching hospitals. *Dysphagia* 1986; 1:3–6.
3. Martino R, Foley N, Bhogal S, et al. Dysphagia after stroke: Incidence, diagnosis, and pulmonary complications. *Stroke* 2005; 36:2756–2763.
4. Paciaroni M, Mazzotta G, Corea F, et al. Dysphagia following stroke. *Eur Neurol* 2004; 51:162–167.
5. Axelsson K, Asplund K, Norberg A, Eriksson S. Eating problems and nutritional status during hospital stay of patients with severe stroke. *J Am Diet Assoc* 1989; 89: 1092–1096.
6. Gordon C, Hewer RL, Wade DT. Dysphagia in acute stroke. *Br Med J (Clin Res Ed)* 1987; 295:411–414.
7. Kidd D, Lawson J, Nesbitt R, MacMahon J. The natural history and clinical consequences of aspiration in acute stroke. *QJM* 1995; 88:409–413.
8. Wade DT, Hewer RL. Motor loss and swallowing difficulty after stroke: Frequency, recovery, and prognosis. *Acta Neurol Scand* 1987; 76:50–54.
9. Horner J, Massey EW, Brazer SR. Aspiration in bilateral stroke patients. *Neurology* 1990; 40:1686–1688.
10. Teasell R, Foley N, Fisher J, Finestone H. The incidence, management, and complications of dysphagia in patients with medullary strokes admitted to a rehabilitation unit. *Dysphagia* 2002; 17:115–120.
11. Teasell RW, McRae M, Marchuk Y, Finestone HM. Pneumonia associated with aspiration following stroke. *Arch Phys Med Rehabil* 1996; 77:707–709.
12. Daniels SK, Brailey K, Priestly DH, et al. Aspiration in patients with acute stroke. *Arch Phys Med Rehabil* 1998; 79:14–19.
13. Holas MA, DePippo KL, Reding MJ. Aspiration and relative risk of medical complications following stroke. *Arch Neurol* 1994; 51:1051–1053.
14. Chokshi SK, Asper RF, Khandheria BK. Aspiration pneumonia: A review. *Am Fam Physician* 1986; 33:195–202.
15. Petroianni A, Ceccarelli D, Conti V, Terzano C. Aspiration pneumonia—pathophysiological aspects, prevention, and management: A review. *Panminerva Med* 2006; 48:231–239.
16. Pepe PE, Potkin RT, Reus DH, et al. Clinical predictors of the adult respiratory distress syndrome. *Am J Surg* 1982; 144:124–130.
17. Spilker CA, Hinthorn DR, Pingleton SK. Intermittent enteral feeding in mechanically ventilated patients: The effect on gastric pH and gastric cultures. *Chest* 1996; 110: 243–248.
18. Bartlett JG, Gorbach SL, Finegold SM. The bacteriology of aspiration pneumonia. *Am J Med* 1974; 56:202–207.
19. Yoneyama T, Yoshida M, Ohrui T, et al. Oral care reduces pneumonia in older patients in nursing homes. *J Am Geriatr Soc* 2002; 50:430–433.
20. Choi-Kwon S, Yang YH, Kim EK, et al. Nutritional status in acute stroke: Undernutrition versus overnutrition in different stroke subtypes. *Acta Neurol Scand* 1998; 98:187–192.
21. Unosson M, Ek AC, Bjurulf P, et al. Feeding dependence and nutritional status after acute stroke. *Stroke* 1994; 25:366–371.
22. Martineau J, Bauer JD, Isenring E, Cohen S. Malnutrition determined by the patient-generated subjective global assessment is associated with poor outcomes in acute stroke patients. *Clin Nutr* 2005; 24:1073–1077.
23. Mann G, Hankey GJ, Cameron D. Swallowing function after stroke: Prognosis and prognostic factors at six months. *Stroke* 1999; 30:744–748.
24. Smithard DG, O'Neill PA, England RE, et al. The natural history of dysphagia following a stroke. *Dysphagia* 1997; 12:188–193.
25. Ickenstein GW, Stein J, Ambrosi D, et al. Predictors of survival after severe dysphagic stroke. *J Neurol* 2005; 252:1510–1516.
26. Wilkinson TJ, Thomas K, MacGregor S, et al. Tolerance of early diet textures as indicators of recovery from dysphagia after stroke. *Dysphagia* 2002; 17:227–232.
27. Parker C, Power M, Hamdy S, et al. Awareness of dysphagia by patients following stroke predicts swallowing performance. *Dysphagia* 2004; 19:28–35.
28. Logemann JA. *Evaluation and Treatment of Swallowing Disorders.* 2nd ed. Austin, TX: Pro-Ed, 1998.
29. Daniels SK, Foundas AL. Swallowing physiology of sequential straw drinking. *Dysphagia* 2001; 16:176–182.
30. Dua KS, Ren J, Bardan E, et al. Coordination of deglutitive glottal function and pharyngeal bolus transit during normal eating. *Gastroenterology* 1997; 112:73–83.
31. Palmer JB, Rudin NJ, Lara G, Crompton AW. Coordination of mastication and swallowing. *Dysphagia* 1992; 7:187–200.
32. Hiiemae KM, Palmer JB. Food transport and bolus formation during complete feeding sequences on foods of different initial consistency. *Dysphagia* 1999; 14:31–42.
33. Casas MJ, Kenny DJ, Macmillan RE. Buccal and lingual activity during mastication and swallowing in typical adults. *J Oral Rehabil* 2003; 30:9–16.
34. Matsuo K, Saitoh E, Takeda S, et al. Effects of gravity and chewing on bolus position at swallow onset [Japanese]. *Jpn J Dysphagia Rehabil* 2002; 6:179–186.
35. Mioche L, Hiiemae KM, Palmer JB. A postero-anterior videofluorographic study of the intra-oral management of food in man. *Arch Oral Biol* 2002; 47:267–280.

36. Palmer JB, Hiiemae KM, Liu J. Tongue-jaw linkages in human feeding: A preliminary videofluorographic study. *Arch Oral Biol* 1997; 42:429–441.

37. Bulow M, Olsson R, Ekberg O. Videomanometric analysis of supraglottic swallow, effortful swallow, and chin tuck in healthy volunteers. *Dysphagia* 1999; 14:67–72.

38. Saitoh E, Shibata S, Matsuo K, et al. Chewing and food consistency: Effects on bolus transport and swallow initiation. *Dysphagia* 2007; 22:100–107.

39. Kendall KA, McKenzie S, Leonard RJ, et al. Timing of events in normal swallowing: A videofluoroscopic study. *Dysphagia* 2000; 15:74–83.

40. Martin-Harris B, Brodsky MB, Michel Y, et al. Breathing and swallowing dynamics across the adult lifespan. *Arch Otolaryngol Head Neck Surg* 2005; 131:762–770.

41. Perlman AL, Palmer PM, McCulloch TM, Vandaele DJ. Electromyographic activity from human laryngeal, pharyngeal, and submental muscles during swallowing. *J Appl Physiol* 1999; 86:1663–1669.

42. Thexton AJ, Crompton AW, German RZ. Electromyographic activity during the reflex pharyngeal swallow in the pig: Doty and Bosma (1956) revisited. *J Appl Physiol* 2006.

43. Kahrilas PJ, Logemann JA, Lin S, Ergun GA. Pharyngeal clearance during swallowing: A combined manometric and videofluoroscopic study. *Gastroenterology* 1992; 103:128–136.

44. Palmer JB, Tanaka E, Ensrud E. Motions of the posterior pharyngeal wall in human swallowing: A quantitative videofluorographic study. *Arch Phys Med Rehabil* 2000; 81:1520–1526.

45. Cook IJ, Dodds WJ, Dantas RO, et al. Opening mechanisms of the human upper esophageal sphincter. *Am J Physiol* 1989; 257:G748–59.

46. Ohmae Y, Logemann JA, Kaiser P, et al. Timing of glottic closure during normal swallow. *Head Neck* 1995; 17:394–402.

47. Palmer JB, Hiiemae KM. Eating and breathing: Interactions between respiration and feeding on solid food. *Dysphagia* 2003; 18:169–178.

48. Shaker R, Dodds WJ, Dantas RO, et al. Coordination of deglutitive glottic closure with oropharyngeal swallowing. *Gastroenterology* 1990; 98:1478–1484.

49. Logemann JA, Kahrilas PJ, Cheng J, et al. Closure mechanisms of laryngeal vestibule during swallow. *Am J Physiol* 1992; 262:G338–344.

50. Hiss SG, Treole K, Stuart A. Effects of age, gender, bolus volume, and trial on swallowing apnea duration and swallow/respiratory phase relationships of normal adults. *Dysphagia* 2001; 16:128–135.

51. Martin BJ, Logemann JA, Shaker R, Dodds WJ. Coordination between respiration and swallowing: Respiratory phase relationships and temporal integration. *J Appl Physiol* 1994; 76:714–723.

52. Ertekin C, Aydogdu I. Electromyography of human cricopharyngeal muscle of the upper esophageal sphincter. *Muscle Nerve* 2002; 26:729–739.

53. Shaw DW, Cook IJ, Gabb M, et al. Influence of normal aging on oral-pharyngeal and upper esophageal sphincter function during swallowing. *Am J Physiol* 1995; 268:G389–396.

54. Jones B, ed. *Normal and Abnormal Swallowing: Imaging in Diagnosis and Therapy.* 2nd ed. New York: Springer-Verlag, 2003.

55. Broussard DL, Altschuler SM. Brain stem viscerotopic organization of afferents and efferents involved in the control of swallowing. *Am J Med* 2000; 108:Suppl 4a:79S–86S.

56. Jean A. Brain stem control of swallowing: Neuronal network and cellular mechanisms. *Physiol Rev* 2001; 81:929–969.

57. Aydogdu I, Ertekin C, Tarlaci S, et al. Dysphagia in lateral medullary infarction (wallenberg's syndrome): An acute disconnection syndrome in premotor neurons related to swallowing activity. *Stroke* 2001; 32:2081–2087.

58. Ertekin C, Kiylioglu N, Tarlaci S, et al. Voluntary and reflex influences on the initiation of swallowing reflex in man. *Dysphagia* 2001; 16:40–47.

59. Miller AJ. Deglutition. *Physiol Rev* 1982; 62:129–184.

60. Miller AJ. Characteristics of the swallowing reflex induced by peripheral nerve and brain stem stimulation. *Exp Neurol* 1972; 34:210–222.

61. Shaker R, Ren J, Bardan E, et al. Pharyngoglottal closure reflex: Characterization in healthy young, elderly, and dysphagic patients with predeglutitive aspiration. *Gerontology* 2003; 49:12–20.

62. German RZ, Palmer JB. Anatomy and development of oral cavity and pharynx. *GI Motility Online* 2006:doi:10.1038/gimo5.

63. Shaker R, Ren J, Podvrsan B, et al. Effect of aging and bolus variables on pharyngeal and upper esophageal sphincter motor function. *Am J Physiol* 1993; 264:G427–432.

64. Kim H, Chung CS, Lee KH, Robbins J. Aspiration subsequent to a pure medullary infarction: Lesion sites, clinical variables, and outcome. *Arch Neurol* 2000; 57:478–483.

65. Hamdy S, Rothwell JC, Aziz Q, Thompson DG. Organization and reorganization of human swallowing motor cortex: Implications for recovery after stroke. *Clin Sci (Lond)* 2000; 99:151–157.

66. Martin RE, Sessle BJ. The role of the cerebral cortex in swallowing. *Dysphagia* 1993; 8:195–202.

67. Miller AJ. *The Neuroscientific Principles of Swallowing and Dysphagia.* vol 1. 1st ed. San Diego: Singular Publishing Group Inc., 1999.

68. Hamdy S, Rothwell JC, Brooks DJ, et al. Identification of the cerebral loci processing human swallowing with H2(15)O PET activation. *J Neurophysiol* 1999; 81:1917–1926.

69. Hamdy S, Aziz Q, Rothwell JC, et al. The cortical topography of human swallowing musculature in health and disease. *Nat Med* 1996; 2:1217–1224.

70. Hamdy S, Aziz Q, Rothwell JC, et al. Explaining oropharyngeal dysphagia after unilateral hemispheric stroke. *Lancet* 1997; 350:686–692.

71. Hamdy S, Aziz Q, Rothwell JC, et al. Recovery of swallowing after dysphagic stroke relates to functional reorganization in the intact motor cortex. *Gastroenterology* 1998; 115:1104–1112.

72. Hamdy S. The organisation and reorganisation of human swallowing motor cortex. *Suppl Clin Neurophysiol* 2003; 56:204–210.

73. Ertekin C, Aydogdu I, Tarlaci S, et al. Mechanisms of dysphagia in suprabulbar palsy with lacunar infarct. *Stroke* 2000; 31:1370–1376.

74. Hatch JP, Shinkai RS, Sakai S, et al. Determinants of masticatory performance in dentate adults. *Arch Oral Biol* 2001; 46:641–648.

75. Bourdiol P, Mioche L, Monier S. Effect of age on salivary flow obtained under feeding and nonfeeding conditions. *J Oral Rehabil* 2004; 31:445–452.

76. Ship JA, Pillemer SR, Baum BJ. Xerostomia and the geriatric patient. *J Am Geriatr Soc* 2002; 50:535–543.

77. Daniels SK, Corey DM, Hadskey LD, et al. Mechanism of sequential swallowing during straw drinking in healthy young and older adults. *J Speech Lang Hear Res* 2004; 47:33–45.

78. Robbins J, Hamilton JW, Lof GL, Kempster GB. Oropharyngeal swallowing in normal adults of different ages. *Gastroenterology* 1992; 103:823–829.

79. Tracy JF, Logemann JA, Kahrilas PJ, et al. Preliminary observations on the effects of age on oropharyngeal deglutition. *Dysphagia* 1989; 4:90–94.

80. Bardan E, Xie P, Brasseur J, et al. Effect of ageing on the upper and lower oesophageal sphincters. *Eur J Gastroenterol Hepatol* 2000; 12:1221–1225.

81. Leslie P, Drinnan MJ, Ford GA, Wilson JA. Swallow respiratory patterns and aging: Presbyphagia or dysphagia? *J Gerontol A Biol Sci Med Sci* 2005; 60:391–395.

82. Selley WG, Flack FC, Ellis RE, Brooks WA. Respiratory patterns associated with swallowing: Part 1. The normal adult pattern and changes with age. *Age Ageing* 1989; 18:168–172.

83. Hinchey JA, Shephard T, Furie K, et al. Formal dysphagia screening protocols prevent pneumonia. *Stroke* 2005; 36:1972–1976.

84. Neumann S, Bartolome G, Buchholz D, Prosiegel M. Swallowing therapy of neurologic patients: Correlation of outcome with pretreatment variables and therapeutic methods. *Dysphagia* 1995; 10:1–5.

85. Smithard DG, O'Neill PA, Parks C, Morris J. Complications and outcome after acute stroke: Does dysphagia matter? *Stroke* 1996; 27:1200–1204.

86. Bates B, Choi JY, Duncan PW, et al. Veterans Affairs/Department of defense clinical practice guideline for the management of adult stroke rehabilitation care: Executive summary. *Stroke* 2005; 36:2049–2056.

87. DePippo KL, Holas MA, Reding MJ. Validation of the three-oz water swallow test for aspiration following stroke. *Arch Neurol* 1992; 49:1259–1261.

88. Tohara H, Saitoh E, Mays KA, et al. Three tests for predicting aspiration without videofluorography. *Dysphagia* 2003; 18:126–134.

89. Wu MC, Chang YC, Wang TG, Lin LC. Evaluating swallowing dysfunction using a 100-ml water swallowing test. *Dysphagia* 2004; 19:43–47.

90. Logemann JA, Veis S, Colangelo L. A screening procedure for oropharyngeal dysphagia. *Dysphagia* 1999; 14:44–51.

91. Leder SB. Gag reflex and dysphagia. *Head Neck* 1996; 18:138–141.

92. Martin BJ, Corlew MM. The incidence of communication disorders in dysphagic patients. *J Speech Hear Disord* 1990; 55:28–32.

93. Palmer JB, DuChane AS. In: Felsenthal G, Garrison SJ,Steinberg FU, ed. *Rehabilitation of the Aging and Elderly Patient.* Rehabilitation of swallowing disorders in the elderly 275–287. Baltimore: Williams & Wilkins; 1994.

94. Daniels SK, McAdam CP, Brailey K, Foundas AL. Clinical assessment of swallowing and prediction of dysphagia severity. *Am J Speech Lang Pathol* 1997; 6:17–24.

95. Linden P, Kuhlemeier KV, Patterson C. The probability of correctly predicting subglottic penetration from clinical observations. *Dysphagia* 1993; 8:170–179.

96. McCullough GH, Wertz RT, Rosenbek JC. Sensitivity and specificity of clinical/bedside examination signs for detecting aspiration in adults subsequent to stroke. *J Commun Disord* 2001; 34:55–72.

97. Ramsey DJ, Smithard DG, Kalra L. Early assessments of dysphagia and aspiration risk in acute stroke patients. *Stroke* 2003; 34:1252–1257.

98. Leslie P, Drinnan MJ, Finn P, Ford GA, Wilson JA. Reliability and validity of cervical auscultation: A controlled comparison using videofluoroscopy. *Dysphagia* 2004; 19:231–240.

99. Stroud AE, Lawrie BW, Wiles CM. Inter- and intra-rater reliability of cervical auscultation to detect aspiration in patients with dysphagia. *Clin Rehabil* 2002; 16:640–645.

100. Leder SB. Use of arterial oxygen saturation, heart rate, and blood pressure as indirect objective physiologic markers to predict aspiration. *Dysphagia* 2000; 15:201–205.

101. Smith HA, Lee SH, O'Neill PA, Connolly MJ. The combination of bedside swallowing assessment and oxygen saturation monitoring of swallowing in acute stroke: A safe and humane screening tool. *Age Ageing* 2000; 29:495–499.

102. Mann G. *MASA: The Mann Assessment of Swallowing Ability.* 1st ed. New York: Singular, 2002.

103. Palmer JB, Monahan DM, Matsuo K. In: Braddom RL, Buschbacher RM, Chan L, et al, eds. *Physical Medicine and Rehabilitation.* 3rd ed. Rehabilitation of patients with swallowing disorders 597. Philadelphia: Elsevier, Inc., 2007.

104. Rosenbek JC, Robbins JA, Roecker EB, et al. A penetration-aspiration scale. *Dysphagia* 1996; 11:93–98.

105. Palmer JB, Kuhlemeier KV, Tippett DC, Lynch C. A protocol for the videofluorographic swallowing study. *Dysphagia* 1993; 8:209–214.

106. Zammit-Maempel I, Chapple CL, Leslie P. Radiation dose in videofluoroscopic swallow studies. *Dysphagia* 2006.

107. Kidder TM, Langmore SE, Martin BJ. Indications and techniques of endoscopy in evaluation of cervical dysphagia: Comparison with radiographic techniques. *Dysphagia* 1994; 9:256–261.

108. Langmore SE. *Endoscopic Evaluation and Treatment of Swallowing Disorders.* New York: Thieme Medical Publishers, 2001.

109. Leder SB, Sasaki CT, Burrell MI. Fiberoptic endoscopic evaluation of dysphagia to identify silent aspiration. *Dysphagia* 1998; 13:19–21.

110. Duncan PW, Zorowitz R, Bates B, et al. Management of adult stroke rehabilitation care: A clinical practice guideline. *Stroke* 2005; 36:e100–143.

111. Dennis MS, Lewis SC, Warlow C, FOOD Trial Collaboration. Routine oral nutritional supplementation for stroke patients in hospital (FOOD): A multicentre randomised controlled trial. *Lancet* 2005; 365:755–763.

112. Dennis MS, Lewis SC, Warlow C, FOOD Trial Collaboration. Effect of timing and method of enteral tube feeding for dysphagic stroke patients (FOOD): A multicentre randomised controlled trial. *Lancet* 2005; 365:764–772.

113. Ganger D, Craig RM. Swallowing disorders and nutritional support. *Dysphagia* 1990; 4:213–219.

114. Garon BR, Engle M, Ormiston C. A randomized study to determine the effects of unlimited intake of water in patients with identified aspiration. *J Neuro Rehab* 1997; 11:139–148.

115. Neumann S. Swallowing therapy with neurologic patients: Results of direct and indirect therapy methods in 66 patients suffering from neurological disorders. *Dysphagia* 1993; 8:150–153.

116. McCallum SL. The national dysphagia diet: Implementation at a regional rehabilitation center and hospital system. *J Am Diet Assoc* 2003; 103:381–384.

117. Ayuse T, Ayuse T, Ishitobi S, et al. Effect of reclining and chin-tuck position on the coordination between respiration and swallowing. *J Oral Rehabil* 2006; 33:402–408.

118. Welch MV, Logemann JA, Rademaker AW, Kahrilas PJ. Changes in pharyngeal dimensions affected by chin tuck. *Arch Phys Med Rehabil* 1993; 74:178–181.

119. Bulow M, Olsson R, Ekberg O. Videomanometric analysis of supraglottic swallow, effortful swallow, and chin tuck in patients with pharyngeal dysfunction. *Dysphagia* 2001; 16:190–195.

120. Ohmae Y, Ogura M, Kitahara S, et al. Effects of head rotation on pharyngeal function during normal swallow. *Ann Otol Rhinol Laryngol* 1998; 107:344–348.

121. Ohmae Y, Logemann JA, Kaiser P, et al. Effects of two breath-holding maneuvers on oropharyngeal swallow. *Ann Otol Rhinol Laryngol* 1996; 105:123–131.

122. Hind JA, Nicosia MA, Roecker EB, et al. Comparison of effortful and noneffortful swallows in healthy middle-aged and older adults. *Arch Phys Med Rehabil* 2001; 82:1661–1665.

123. Ding R, Larson CR, Logemann JA, Rademaker AW. Surface electromyographic and electroglottographic studies in normal subjects under two swallow conditions: Normal and during the Mendelsohn manuever. *Dysphagia* 2002; 17:1–12.

124. Light J. Review of oral and oropharyngeal prostheses to facilitate speech and swallowing. *American Journal of Speech Language Pathology* 1995; 4:15.

125. Logemann JA, Pauloski BR, Colangelo L, et al. Effects of a sour bolus on oropharyngeal swallowing measures in patients with neurogenic dysphagia. *J Speech Hear Res* 1995; 38:556–563.

126. Rosenbek JC, Roecker EB, Wood JL, Robbins J. Thermal application reduces the duration of stage transition in dysphagia after stroke. *Dysphagia* 1996; 11:225–233.

127. Freed ML, Freed L, Chatburn RL, Christian M. Electrical stimulation for swallowing disorders caused by stroke. *Respir Care* 2001; 46:466–474.

128. Blumenfeld L, Hahn Y, Lepage A, et al. Transcutaneous electrical stimulation versus traditional dysphagia therapy: A nonconcurrent cohort study. *Otolaryngol Head Neck Surg* 2006; 135:754–757.

129. Humbert IA, Poletto CJ, Saxon KG, et al. The effect of surface electrical stimulation on hyolaryngeal movement in normal individuals at rest and during swallowing. *J Appl Physiol* 2006; 101:1657–1663.

130. Ludlow CL, Humbert I, Saxon K, et al. Effects of surface electrical stimulation both at rest and during swallowing in chronic pharyngeal dysphagia. *Dysphagia* 2006.

131. Suiter DM, Leder SB, Ruark JL. Effects of neuromuscular electrical stimulation on submental muscle activity. *Dysphagia* 2006; 21:56–60.

132. Leelamanit V, Limsakul C, Geater A. Synchronized electrical stimulation in treating pharyngeal dysphagia. *Laryngoscope* 2002; 112:2204–2210.

133. Fujiu M, Logeman JA. Effect of tongue holding maneuver on posterior pharyngeal wall movement during deglutition. *Am J Speech Lang Pathol* 1996; 5:25–47.

134. Shaker R, Easterling C, Kern M, et al. Rehabilitation of swallowing by exercise in tube-fed patients with pharyngeal dysphagia secondary to abnormal UES opening. *Gastroenterology* 2002; 122:1314–1321.

135. Shaker R, Kern M, Bardan E, et al. Augmentation of deglutitive upper esophageal sphincter opening in the elderly by exercise. *Am J Physiol* 1997; 272:G1518–1522.

136. Crary MA, Carnaby Mann GD, Groher ME, Helseth E. Functional benefits of dysphagia therapy using adjunctive sEMG biofeedback. *Dysphagia* 2004; 19:160–164.

137. Crary MA, Groher ME. Basic concepts of surface electromyographic biofeedback in the treatment of dysphagia. *American Journal of Speech Language Pathology* 2000:116.

138. Dziewas R, Ritter M, Schilling M, et al. Pneumonia in acute stroke patients fed by nasogastric tube. *J Neurol Neurosurg Psychiatry* 2004; 75:852–856.

139. Kadakia SC, Sullivan HO, Starnes E. Percutaneous endoscopic gastrostomy or jejunostomy and the incidence of aspiration in 79 patients. *Am J Surg* 1992; 164:114–118.

140. Nakajoh K, Nakagawa T, Sekizawa K, et al. Relation between incidence of pneumonia and protective reflexes in post-stroke patients with oral or tube feeding. *J Intern Med* 2000; 247:39–42.

141. Davis AE, Arrington K, Fields-Ryan S, Pruitt JO. Preventing feeding-associated aspiration. *Medsurg Nurs* 1995; 4:111–119.

142. Kirby DF, Delegge MH, Fleming CR. American gastroenterological association medical position statement: Guidelines for the use of enteral nutrition. American Gastroenterological Association, 1995.

143. Norton B, McLean KA, Holmes GK. Outcome in patients who require a gastrostomy after stroke. *Age Ageing* 1996; 25:493.

144. James A, Kapur K, Hawthorne AB. Long-term outcome of percutaneous endoscopic gastrostomy feeding in patients with dysphagic stroke. *Age Ageing* 1998; 27:671–676.

145. Snyderman CH, Johnson JT. Laryngotracheal separation for intractable aspiration. *Ann Otol Rhinol Laryngol* 1988; 97:466–470.

146. Takano Y, Suga M, Sakamoto O, et al. Satisfaction of patients treated surgically for intractable aspiration. *Chest* 1999; 116:1251–1256.

147. Tomita T, Tanaka K, Shinden S, Ogawa K. Tracheoesophageal diversion versus total laryngectomy for intractable aspiration. *J Laryngol Otol* 2004; 118:15–18.

148. Hockstein NG, Samadi DS, Gendron K, Handler SD. Sialorrhea: A management challenge. *Am Fam Physician* 2004; 69:2628–2634.

149. Larnert G, Ekberg O. Positioning improves the oral and pharyngeal swallowing function in children with cerebral palsy. *Acta Paediatr* 1995; 84:689–692.

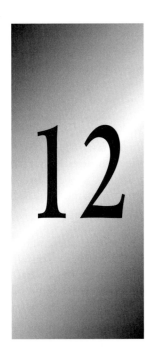

12 Right Hemispheric Neurobehavioral Syndromes

Kenneth M. Heilman

This chapter will provide an over-view of some of the major neuro-behavioral syndromes associated with right hemisphere strokes. Perhaps the three most common and disabling disorders associated with isolated right hemisphere injury are the neglect syndrome; emotional disorders, including disorders of emotional communication and emotional experience; and visuospatial disorders. Each of these major syndromes has several components, and the most common components of these neurobehavioral disorders will be discussed. Unfortunately, a detailed discussion of all the neurobehavioral disorders associated with right hemisphere injury would require writing a text rather than a chapter; thus, some of the less common neurobehavioral disorders that can be associated with right hemisphere disease—including some forms of amusia, identity disorders such as prosopagnosia, delusional misidentifications such as Capgras and reduplicative para-amnesia, and disorder of automatic speech and auditory agnosia for familiar voices—have not been included. There is another chapter in this text that discusses visuospatial disorders, so this domain is only briefly reviewed.

NEGLECT AND RELATED DISORDERS

Definitions

Neglect is the failure to report, respond, or orient to meaningful or novel stimuli presented in a portion of space when this failure cannot be accounted for by either an elemental sensory or motor defect (1).

Neglect is a common and severely disabling neurobehavioral disorder that is most commonly induced by discrete lesions such as cerebral infarctions and hemorrhages of the right hemisphere. However, neglect can also be induced by tumors, trauma, and degenerative diseases that primarily involve the right hemisphere. Of all the behavioral disorders caused by focal hemispheric brain damage, neglect diagnosed at time of the acute injury has the poorest prognosis for independent living. Studies have shown that patients with neglect are less likely to be able to live independently than even patients with global aphasia and a right hemiparesis.

There are many forms of neglect that are distinguished by several different factors, including:

1. Input or output demands (inattention or sensory neglect versus intentional or motor neglect)

2. Modality of input and type of output
3. Means of eliciting, including unilateral versus bilateral stimuli or movements or extinction
4. Domains of neglect, including spatial, personal, and representational
5. Spatial distribution of neglect, including the frame of reference (viewer-centered, environmentally centered, and object-centered); location of neglect in the three spatial planes, including horizontal at the intersection of the coronal and transverse planes (right versus left or contralesional versus ipsilesional), vertical at the intersection of the sagittal and coronal planes (up versus down), and radial at the intersection of the transverse and sagittal planes (proximal versus distal)

In this chapter, we will discuss the signs and symptoms associated with the different forms of this disorder, the means by which patients may be assessed for neglect and related disorders, as well as the management and treatment of these disorders. Because of length restrictions, we will not be able to discuss the pathophysiology of all these disorders. For further reading about pathophysiology, we suggest Heilman et al. (1).

CLINICAL SYNDROMES, SIGNS, AND TESTING

Sensory Inattention

Unawareness.   Sensory inattention is a form of selective unawareness that can be defined by its modality (tactile, visual, or auditory) and its distribution (hemispatial or personal). Sensory inattention may also be associated with an ipsilesional attentional bias and an inability to disengage from stimuli in ipsilesional space.

To clinically test for inattention, the patient is presented with stimuli (visual, tactile, and auditory) or no stimuli to either the ipsilesional or contralesional sides of the body in random order. Each time a stimulus or nonstimulus is presented, the examiner says, "Now!" The patient is then instructed to tell the examiner if the stimulus was on the right, left, or not present (none). If the patient makes more errors on one than the other side (for example, more contralesional than ipsilesional errors), he or she has evidence of unilateral sensory inattention.

When a patient consistently fails to detect contralesional stimuli, it is possible that he or she has a primary sensory defect rather than inattention. Inattention is sometimes confused with sensory defects and vice versa. There are, however, several means by which inattention might be dissociated from a primary sensory defect caused by deafferentation. In the tactile

modality, hemi-anesthesia (for example, from thalamic lesions) can be differentiated from inattention by the use of cold water caloric stimulation. Thus, if a patient has left-sided inattention, cold water caloric stimulation of the left ear will allow this person to feel the tactile stimulus (2). In the auditory modality, hemispheric lesions do not cause contralesional hemispatial deafness. Hence, if a patient fails to detect auditory stimuli (for example, snapping fingers or speech) presented on one side of space, he or she has inattention. In the visual modality, inattention may be viewer-centered hemispatial whereas a true hemianopia will be hemiretinal. Thus, the patients with visual inattention who cannot detect visual stimuli (for example, the examiner's moving fingers) in contralesional hemispace might be able to detect these stimuli if their eyes are deviated to the ipsilesional side (such that the contralesional retinal field now falls in ipsilesional hemispace) (3). However, if they have a true hemianopia (for example, to the left), the defect will be retinotopic, and they will still be unable to see stimuli presented to the contralesional visual field (for example, to the left) even when their eyes are deviated to ipsilesional (for example, to the right) hemispace. Psychophysiologic techniques such as evoked potentials or galvanic skin responses may also help demonstrate that a defect is inattention rather than deafferentation, and structural imaging might demonstrate that the lesion either does or does not injure afferent pathways.

Sensory Extinction to Simultaneous Stimulation (Extinction).   Many patients who are first unaware of stimuli may recover and be able to detect isolated stimuli, but, when they are presented with two or more simultaneous stimuli that are intermixed with unilateral stimuli to either the right or left side of the body and no stimuli, they may demonstrate unawareness of the contralesional stimulus (extinction). Many patients never demonstrate inattention to unilateral stimuli, but they still might demonstrate sensory extinction. Extinction can be found in the visual, tactile, and auditory modalities. Although most often the simultaneous stimuli are presented to the right and left sides of the body and the patient fails to recognize the contralesional stimuli, when two stimuli are given on one side of the body, extinction to the stimulus in the contralesional position can also go undetected.

Action-Intentional or Motor Neglect

There are several forms of motor or intentional neglect. These are distinguished by the means of testing and the behavior demonstrated by the patient.

Motor neglect, or limb akinesia, can appear to be a hemiplegia, but, when patients who have motor neglect of a limb are studied using brain imaging and transcranial magnetic stimulation, these studies reveal that their corticospinal motor system is intact. Unlike patients with true hemiplegia who will attempt to move their weak limbs, these patients often do not appear like they are attempting to move. There are some patients who have this limb akinesia only when the limb is on the contralesional side of the body, but, when the limb is brought over to the ipsilesional side, they might be able to use it. This disorder has been termed hemispatial akinesia. There are other patients who have difficulty moving their heads, eyes (for example, gaze paresis), or even arms in a contralesional direction, and this disorder is called a directional akinesia. Some patients are able to move their eyes, heads, or arms in both directions, but, at rest, they will have their eyes, arms, or heads deviated to one (ipsilesional) side. When this occurs with the eyes, it is called gaze palsy, but this is a misnomer because there really is no paralysis or weakness. These should be called intentional directional biases.

Hypokinesia is a milder form of intentional neglect where a patient is able to move a limb or his or her head and eyes, but there is a delay in initiating these movements. One of the best means for testing for hypokinesia is by performing reaction times. Hypokinesia can be found in tests of the limbs (limb hypokinesia), as a function of hemispace (hemispatial akinesia) and in a direction (directional hypokinesia). Directional akinesia and hemispatial hypokinesia can also be observed during eye and head movements.

Motor impersistence is the inability to sustain a movement or posture. When testing for motor impersistence, the examiner asks the patient to maintain a posture for a given period of time. Motor impersistence may also be seen in the limbs, eyes, or head. It may also be hemispatial or directional.

Hypometria is when a patient makes abnormally small movements. Hypometria can also be induced by impersistence, such that the reduction of movement amplitude is caused by the movement being prematurely discontinued. Hypometria can be seen with the limbs, head, and eye movements. However, hypometria can also be induced by other factors such as perceptual disorders, inattention, and abnormal spatial representations.

Motor Extinction. Some patients who can move the contralesional limb alone have difficulty initiating movement of this limb at the same time as they are starting to move the ipsilesional limb. To test for motor extinction, the patients should be able to move each forelimb independently. Then the patient is asked to close his or her eyes, put his or her hands on his or her lap, and lift the hand(s) that are touched by the examiner. The examiner randomly touches the right, left, or both hands. To distinguish sensory extinction from motor extinction, the patient should also be tested for sensory extinction by

asking the patient to tell the examiner which hand(s) have been touched.

Spatial Neglect

Contralesional Spatial Neglect. Spatial neglect can occur in all three dimensions of space: horizontal (right/left), vertical (up/down) and radial (near/far) as well as in a combination of these dimensions. Spatial neglect can also occur in near (peripersonal) or far (extrapersonal) space. Therefore, tests that assess spatial neglect should test all these dimensions. However, in this discussion, we will primarily focus on horizontal neglect. There are three bedside tests that are commonly used to assess patients for the presence of spatial neglect: line bisection, target cancellation, and drawing. Each of these tests may assess different functions.

In the line bisection task, the patient is presented with a line and asked to place a mark with a pen or pencil at the middle of the line. Longer lines are more likely to detect neglect than shorter lines are. Typically, when patients with contralesional (for example, left) spatial neglect attempt to bisect long lines, they deviate their bisection mark toward the injured (for example, right) hemisphere. However, with very short lines, they might error by placing their attempted bisection mark on the portion of the line that is in contralesional hemispace (for example, on the left side). This phenomenon is called the "crossover effect." Placing the entire line in the portion of space that is on the side opposite the injured hemisphere is more likely to detect neglect than placing the line in ipsilateral hemispace.

When performing the cancellation test, a sheet of paper with many targets, such as randomly placed, small, linear segments, is placed before the patient, and the patient is asked to mark out or cancel all the targets. Patients with neglect will often fail to cancel the targets that are positioned in the contralesional (for example, left) hemispace. To increase the sensitivity of this task, the number of targets can be increased, or the patient can be asked to selectively cancel target stimuli that are placed among foils. The use of foils that are difficult to discriminate from the targets, (for example, target Ts in a background of Ls) can also be used to increase the sensitivity of the task.

Drawing should be tested by having a patient copy some simple objects, such as a house with an evergreen (pine) tree to one side and a bush on the other side.

In addition to occurring in the three dimensions of space, spatial neglect can have three different reference frames: viewer-centered, object-centered, and environmentally centered. If a patient with neglect fails to draw the object on the contralesional side of the paper, the patient most likely has viewer-centered neglect. However, if the patient attempts to draw all three objects but only draws one side of these objects, then the patient has object-centered neglect. To determine if a patient has environmentally centered neglect, the patient performs line bisection tasks while upright and lying flat on his or her side. While lying flat, if he or she is presented with a line that is parallel to the long axis of his or her body—that is, vertical in relation to the body, but horizontal in respect to the environment—and the patient deviates his or her attempted bisection in the same direction he or she deviated when upright, and also does not deviate when performing the line bisection task with lines that are in his or her transverse plane, he or she has environmentally centered neglect.

In addition to demonstrating contralesional spatial neglect with the line bisection, cancellation, and drawing tasks, patients with neglect might also be impaired when reading and writing such that they might fail to read or write a part of a sentence or a part of a word.

Ipsilesional Neglect.   When performing a task such as line bisection, patients with neglect will most often deviate to the side (for example, to the right) of hemispheric injury (contralesional neglect). Some patients, however, will deviate in the opposite direction, and this is called ipsilesional neglect. Unlike the cross-over effect mentioned above, ipsilesional neglect can be observed even when using long lines.

Attentional vs. Intentional Spatial Neglect.   A series of studies have revealed that the reason patients fail to correctly perform tasks such as the line bisection or cancellation is because they have an attentional disturbance. This attentional disturbance might alter performance on these tasks by several means. Normally, attention is related to awareness. When we are inattentive to something, either that item does not reach awareness, or awareness is not maintained. If we are not aware of an item or part of an item, we do not interact with it. Thus, patients with spatial neglect might be unaware of a segment of a line (for example, the left side), only bisect the portion of which they are aware, and thus deviate to one side. Similarly, they might be unaware of cancellation targets on one side of a paper and thus fail to cancel these targets.

People can vary the degree of attention they allocate to an object or part of an object, and objects or parts of objects that are strongly attended appear to have a greater magnitude than objects that receive less attention. For example, when we first drive down a new road, we pay more attention than when returning, and this causes the road to appear longer when going than returning. Thus, when patients with spatial neglect view a line, the segment of the line (for example, contralesional) to which they are inattentive might appear shorter than its actual size, and the segment to which they are strongly attending will appear longer. This attentional asymmetry will induce a misperception, and

patients will have a deviation of their attempted bisection toward the segment that appears longer. In order to determine the size of something like a line or to find all the targets, a person has to be able to move their attention. If a person has a strong attentional bias toward an object or a part of space, he or she might have difficulty disengaging his or her attention and moving his or her attention to other parts of space. Patients with neglect often have problems with disengaging their attention from a portion of space (for example, ipsilesional) and thus neglect the opposite portion of space (for example, contralesional).

In addition to the correct allocation of attention, in order to correctly bisect a line, cancel targets, or copy a picture, a person has to move his or her eyes and arms to different parts of space. Some patients, as mentioned above, might have types of motor neglect where they fail to explore with their eyes or move their arms into a part of space (for example, the contralesional left space).

To dissociate attentional from intentional hemispatial neglect, the clinician can use a variety of techniques including video cameras with an image reversal system and a monitor, strings and pulleys, and mirrors. All of these techniques can dissociate the direction of action (for example, leftward) from the direction of sensory feedback (for example, rightward). Thus, if reversed, feedback causes a patient to change the side of his or her bias—for example, from a right-sided bias on the line bisection in the direct condition to a leftward bias on the reversed feedback condition—then this patient has primarily an attentional neglect. However, if the bias does not change in the reverse condition, the patient has a primarily intentional spatial neglect.

Asomatognosia and Personal Neglect

Patients with personal neglect may fail to groom or even dress one side of their bodies. Patients with asomatognosia do not recognize that parts of their body belong to them. To test for asomatognosia, the examiner can take a portion of the body (for example, the left arm and hand) contralateral to the hemispheric injury and bring it into ipsilateral (for example, the right) hemispace and visual field. To make certain the patient sees this part of his or her body, the examiner can write a number on it. The examiner then asks the patient to read the number on this body part (for example, his or her hand). If the patient can recognize this number, the examiner can then ask the patient whether this body part belongs to him or her or to the examiner. If the patient denies that this body part belongs to him or her, he or she has asomatognosia. To more formally test for personal neglect, the examiner can perform a type of cancellation task where the examiner puts little pieces of sticky paper on a different portion of the patient's body and asks the patient to remove all the pieces of paper. The examiner can also perform a type of line bisection task where a large horizontal line is placed before the subject who is asked to show, by pointing, the position on the line that is directly across from the middle of his or her chest, right shoulder, and left shoulder. Patients with personal neglect will often shift their midline and contralesional shoulder to the ipsilesional side. Patients with asomatognosia and personal neglect might also have lost or degraded their representations of their body. (See the next section.) Some of these patients will also demonstrate allesthesia and allokinesia. When touched on the contralesional (for example, left) side of their body and asked where they were touched, they might claim that they were touched on the right. When asked to move the contralesional side of their body, they might move the ipsilesional side.

Representational-Imagery Neglect

Representational-imagery neglect may be spatial or personal. When patients with retrograde imagery neglect are asked to recall details of a scene with which they were familiar before the onset of their illness, they might only report those details that are ipsilateral to their lesion. This disorder can be also be anterograde, such that after a patient has a stroke and is showed a scene in which he or she is able to recognize all the objects, and then several minutes to an hour later is asked to recall what he or she saw earlier, this patient might only report those parts of the scene that were presented ipsilateral to the hemispheric injury.

When performing a task where patients are required to imagine a contralesional part of their body, they also may fail (4).

Anosognosia and Anosodiaphoria

Patients with neglect can be unaware of their illness and/or disability. For example, many patients with neglect also have weakness of their contralesional arm. But, when asked about weakness, the patients may explicitly deny their hemiparesis. They might also deny a sensory loss and hemianopia. Anosognosia is most often seen during the acute phase of illness. After being repeatedly told that they have a disability, most patients with anosognosia will usually acknowledge their illness, but they appear unconcerned or even joke about their disabilities, which is called anosodiaphoria.

Pathophysiology of Neglect

Attention. Since the work of Morrizzi and Magoun (5), it has been known that the reticular activating system (RAS) is important in mediating arousal. When an organism is presented with a novel or significant stimulus, it becomes behaviorally and electrophysiologically aroused. An organism that cannot become aroused cannot normally attend. Therefore, arousal is a critical element in the systems that mediate attention, and the portions of the brain that appear to be important in mediating arousal are the mesencephalic reticular formation and portions of the thalamus. Unilateral injury to either of these structures produces neglect.

Attention must also be selective, and Sokolov (6) posited that the cortex selects which stimuli to attend. In humans, attentional neglect is most commonly associated with lesions that involve the posterior superior temporal lobe and the adjacent inferior parietal lobe of the right hemisphere. This temporoparietal region receives afferent (input) information from the cortical visual, auditory, and tactile association areas and sends projections to the RAS. There are, however, other areas where lesions in humans have been reported to induce neglect, for example, the lateral frontal lobe and the medial frontal lobe, which includes the cingulate gyrus. The frontal lobes are critical for mediating long-term, prospective, goal-oriented behaviors, and the cingulate gyrus is highly connected with other portions of the limbic system that are important in mediating behaviors induced by biological needs and emotions. The human brain can only process a limited number of stimuli and sensory input into the brain often exceeds its processing capacity. In order to decide what and where to attend, the regions of the brain that makes these computations must get information about long-term goals, emotions, and needs. Because each parietal lobe is a convergence area that receives input from the lateral frontal lobe and the cingulate gyrus as well as information from sensory processing systems that indicate the type of stimulus (what) and its spatial position (where), the temporoparietal cortex is able to compute where and to what stimuli a person's attention should be directed.

Imagery. The posterior superior temporal and inferior parietal cortices also have strong reciprocal relations with the hippocampus. Damasio (7) has posited that the hippocampus is important for the retroactivation of sensory association areas. Therefore, lesions of the posterior temporal-inferior parietal region might interfere with retroactivation and induce the imagery and representational defects described by Bisiach and Luzzatti (8).

Action-Intention

As mentioned above, attention is the process by which the brain triages incoming stimuli according to its importance to a person's long-term goals as well as his or her immediate needs and drives. In addition to the limited input processing capacity, the brain also has a limited ability to prepare and control motor actions directed to the environment. "Selective intention" is the term used to denote the process by which the brain triages environmentally directed actions. As mentioned above, a complete failure of this action-intentional system induces a total inability to initiate movements termed akinesia. Milder defects in the action-intentional systems may induce a delay in the initiation of movement called hypokinesia. In some cases, movements must be sustained. A failure to sustain movements is called impersistence, and impersistence might produce hypometria. All these action-intentional deficits can involve different body parts and can be directional or hemispatial.

Whereas the reticular activating system is important for the cortical arousal required for attentional processing, in a parallel fashion, the basal ganglia-dopaminergic system appears to be important in the action-intentional system. Thus, unilateral injury to the basal ganglia or dopaminergic system will produce forms of unilateral or asymmetrical action-intentional neglect. The basal ganglia receive glutaminergic projections from the premotor cortices of the lateral and medial frontal lobes. Deciding whether to act and where to act requires

- Knowledge of long-term goals (mediated by the prefrontal lobes)
- Knowledge of drives-needs and emotions (mediated by the limbic system)
- Cognitive knowledge of how to act (mediated by the temporal parietal regions)

Thus, damage to any of these regions can also induce action-intentional neglect. Although both sensory attentional and action-intentional neglect can be induced by damage to either the temporal-parietal or frontal lobes (both lateral and medial), in general, injury to the frontal lobes is more likely to induce primarily action-intentional neglect and injury to the parietal lobes, that is, sensory-attentional neglect. However, in order for a person to successfully interact with the environment, the intentional and attentional systems have to be interactive, and the frontal and parietal lobes are strongly connected.

Right-Left Asymmetries of Attention and Intention Neglect

Whereas neglect can be seen with either right or left hemisphere lesions, in humans, neglect is more common and severe with right than left hemisphere lesions. These asymmetries of neglect appear to be related to asymmetrical attentional and intentional representations of the body and space. Electrophysiological and functional imaging studies suggest that, whereas the left hemisphere attends primarily to the right side or in a rightward direction, the right hemisphere can attend to both sides or in both directions (9). Similarly, whereas the left hemisphere can

prepare for right-sided or rightward actions, the right hemisphere can help prepare for actions on both sides or in both directions.

Treatment of Neglect

Underlying Diseases. Whereas stroke (infarction and hemorrhage) is the most common cause of elements of the neglect syndrome, neglect can be induced by any disease that injures or destroys the networks that are important in mediating attention and intention. Therefore, clinicians always need to evaluate patients to learn the cause and, when possible, treat the underlying disease and attempt to prevent additional brain injury.

Pharmacological Treatments. As shown in experimental animals, neglect can be induced by unilaterally injuring (MPTP) (10) or interrupting (hydroxydopamine) (11) the dopaminergic system. Corwin et al. (12) demonstrated in rats that dopamine agonists reduce neglect. Fleet et al. (13) reported two patients who improved on tests of neglect when treated with a dopamine agonist, and there have been several other reports supporting the efficacy of this treatment. There are, however, no double-blinded controlled studies using this treatment. There have been other reports of patients treated with dopaminergic agents, but these did not show an improvement in neglect or their neglect became worse with this treatment (14).

This patient, however, had a lesion that involved subcortical structures that included the basal ganglia in one hemisphere. It is possible that the dopamine agonist could not induce a change in the injured hemisphere, but it could mediate up-regulation in the uninjured hemisphere, increasing the ipsilesional bias. Based on this report, it is recommended that, before patients are treated with dopaminergic medications, they be carefully assessed before and after the initiation of treatment to make certain there is improvement. In addition, because many patients improve with time, it is important to perform periodic medication withdrawal with testing before and after the withdrawal.

Behavioral Treatments

Environmental Shifts. When assessing neglect, the clinician often finds that moving objects into ipsilesional hemispace improves detection. Prisms may move visual images, and Frensel prisms have been used to treat neglect (15). This prism treatment appears to even be more effective when the patients with neglect are trained to find their midsagittal space while wearing these prisms. Although prism treatments appear to improve laboratory test performance, they do not dramatically influence activities of daily living.

In addition to using prisms, there are other means of shifting the environment that seem to help neglect. Cold caloric stimulation of the left ear (16), optokinetic nystagmus (17), and vibration of the neck muscles (18) can also improve neglect, but there is little evidence that these effects last for many minutes after the stimulation has terminated.

Training. The use of operant training techniques has been used to train patients with neglect to explore and scan contralesional hemispace (19). This system uses self-cueing (for example, "look left"). Unfortunately, this training often fails to generalize to other tasks, activities of daily living, and instrumental activities (20, 21).

Cueing. One means of getting the spatially inattentive patient to attend to contralesional hemispace is to provide them with attentional cues. Novel stimuli are powerful, that is, "bottom-up" cues that can be presented in contralesional hemispace. Novel visual (22), auditory (23), and tactile cues have been used to help patients with neglect direct their attention to the contralesional hemispace.

Self-initiated motor cues might also be helpful. Halligan and Marshall (24) demonstrated that, when patients with neglect from a right hemisphere lesion perform with their left hand, their performance is more normal than when they perform with their right hand. Although many patients with neglect have hemiplegia, Robertson and North (25) showed that any attempted movement of the left arm improves performance. Finger movements of the left hand, even when this hand or arm cannot be viewed by the patient, might improve performance.

Monocular Eye Patching. Monocular eye patching is based on the work of Sprague (26), who produced neglect (asymmetrical exploration and orienting) in animals by ablating a posterior portion of the neocortex. He subsequently reduced this orienting asymmetry by ablating the superior colliculus on the opposite side of the animals' brains. In mammals, the retina (both temporal and nasal) in each eye projects more strongly to the contralateral than ipsilateral colliculus. Posner and Rafal (27) suggest that perhaps unilateral spatial neglect in patients can be reduced by decreasing the visual input into the colliculus of the nonlesioned hemisphere. Patching the eye that is ipsilateral to the lesioned hemisphere might reduce the activation of the contralateral colliculus, and this decrease in activation might be similar to the ablation of the colliculus. The reason why a reduction of collicular activation would improve neglect is not known, but the colliculus might influence posterior neocortical activation, and a reduction of cortical activation of the intact hemisphere might reduce the ipsilesional attentional bias. Butter and Kirsch (28) tested this means of treatment and did demonstrate a reduction of left-sided neglect with a right eye patch. Barrett et al. (29), however, reported a patient with left-sided neglect who was made worse by patching the right eye, but the reason for this response is not known.

Forced Use. Some individuals with milder upper extremity hemiparesis following stroke have been treated with a procedure called constrained induced-forced use therapy, where the therapist places the less affected hand in a mitt and intensively trains the paretic upper extremity using an array of tasks that are behaviorally reinforced (30). Recent randomized clinical trials now provide evidence that this approach produces significant and functionally relevant gains in upper extremity function (see chapter 17) for some stroke survivors. Patients with right hemisphere lesions and neglect often have a limb akinesia (limb motor neglect) that can either mimic a hemiparesis or enhance the disability associated with a hemiparesis. As mentioned above, motor neglect can be dissociated from a hemiparesis, by lesion location, and TMS (31). Although there are no controlled studies assessing constraint-induced movement therapy for the treatment of limb akinesia or motor neglect, the methods theoretically might prove successful.

Patients with neglect often demonstrate a directional akinesia of their eyes, such that they fail to move their eyes in a contralesional direction and fail to explore contralesional visual hemispace. Having patients wears glasses where the ipsilesional half of each lens is covered with an opaque material might force patients with neglect and who want to see to learn to move their eyes in a contralesional direction. Most recently there have been studies in which the use of prisms appeared to successfully treat patients with spatial neglect (32).

Management of the Environment and Safety Considerations. The sensory-attentional and action-intentional disorders associated with neglect dramatically reduce a person's capacity to successfully interact with his or her environment. In order to reduce disability and make the environment safer for both the patient and others, patients with these disorders must have their environment altered to reduce the risk of injury and to increase the possibility for successful interaction with environmental stimuli. Patients with even the mildest forms of neglect should not drive vehicles or use machinery that has the potential to injure themselves or others. Neglect is often in reference to the patients' body rather than to the objects in the environment. Therefore, patients could be positioned and the environment arranged such that environmental stimuli take place on the ipsilesional (for example, the right side) of the patient's body.

President Wilson had a large hemisphere stroke. Senators were concerned that this stroke would make him incapable of governing the country, so they went to visit him. However, before they came, Wilson's wife, who was doing much of the governing, placed him so that his left side was against a wall and his right side was facing the senators. After their visit, the senate delegation claimed that Wilson was fit to govern.

One of the problems with rearranging a patient's environment is that, if that person is never required to attend or act in contralesional hemispace, it is possible that this will curtail or retard recovery.

Because patients with neglect have a reduced attentional capacity and have difficulty dealing with more than one stimulus, there should be a reduction of competing or distracting stimuli. In addition, because patients with neglect also have a reduction of sustained attention and vigilance, the most important stimuli or actions should take place first.

EMOTIONAL DISORDERS ASSOCIATED WITH RIGHT HEMISPHERE DYSFUNCTION

Communicative Disorders

In this section, we will discuss changes in emotional communication that can be caused by injury to the right hemisphere. These communicative disorders are organized by modality (visual-facial and verbal auditory prosody) as well as into afferent (receptive) and efferent (expressive) subtypes.

Receptive Disorders

Emotional Faces.   The development of an appropriate emotional state, as well as the ability to successfully communicate with others, often depends upon perceiving and comprehending visual stimuli, such as facial expressions, gestures, and scenes.

When patients with right versus left hemisphere lesions were asked to name the emotion being expressed by faces, as well as to discriminate whether two faces were displaying the same or different emotional expressions, right hemisphere-damaged individuals were impaired (33), and this impairment could not be explained by facial discrimination or visuospatial disorders. Investigators from other laboratories have also reported that right hemisphere-damaged stroke patients are more impaired than their left hemisphere counterparts in recognizing or categorizing facial emotions (34, 35, 36). In general, these defects in identifying facial affect by right hemisphere-damaged patients are not valence dependent, such that patients have trouble recognizing both positive (happy) and negative (sad or angry) emotional expressions.

Based on stimulation studies of epileptic patients, Fried et al. (37) found that the posterior portion of the superior temporal gyrus was the area critical for the comprehension and discrimination of emotional faces. The finding that patients with damage to this area not only fail to correctly name emotional faces but also cannot discriminate between the same and different emotional expressions suggests that these patients might have an iconic representational deficit. In addition, Blonder et al. (38) gave patients with these face comprehension deficits sentences that either describe emotional expressions or emotion-invoking stories. The patients with right hemisphere damage, when compared to control subjects, were impaired in comprehending the emotions associated with expressions but not stories, suggesting that these patients had degradation of emotional expressive representations. In addition, Bowers et al. (39) demonstrated that the patients with right hemisphere damage had deficits of facial emotional imagery, but not object imagery, providing evidence that these representations are, at least in part, iconic. There are studies, however, that also suggest that the discrimination of emotional faces might depend on motor-imitation or movement mirroring (40).

Affective Prosody.   When people with a meaningful relationship have a disagreement, one of the partners frequently says to the other, "It's not what you said, but how you said it." This expression indicates that speech might carry more than one message. In addition to communicating a propositional message, which requires lexical, syntactic, and phonemic encoding and decoding, speech may simultaneously communicate a message by the use of prosody. Although prosody, which is expressed by making changes in pitch, tempo, amplitude, and rhythm, may also convey linguistic content (for example, declarative versus interrogative sentences), prosody is frequently used to convey an emotional message.

Since Paul Broca's reports of right-handed patients who were aphasic because they suffered with left hemisphere strokes, it has been repeatedly demonstrated that, in greater than 95% of right-handed people, it is the left hemisphere that mediates propositional language. Hughlings-Jackson (41), however, noted that a patient with a nonfluent aphasia remained capable of expressing emotional speech prosody and posited that it might be the uninjured right hemisphere that was mediating this skill. However, no systematic studies of emotional prosody were reported until Heilman et al. (42) and Tucker et al. (43) indicated that, when compared to left hemisphere-injured aphasic patients, those with right hemisphere injury were frequently impaired at comprehending and expressing emotional speech prosody. Although similar findings were reported by Ross (44), not all investigators found differences between right and left hemisphere-damaged patients. Further evidence for the dominant role of the right hemisphere in comprehending affective intonations comes from studies that demonstrate preserved abilities in patients with left hemisphere lesions. We have examined patients with global aphasia (45) who have destroyed their entire left peri-Sylvian speech cortex and have pure word deafness (normal speech output and reading, but impaired speech comprehension and repletion) induced by injury to the left auditory cortex (46), who comprehended speech very poorly but had no difficulty recognizing emotional intonations of speech.

The defect underlying the impaired comprehension of emotional prosody is not entirely known, but Tucker et al. (47) attempted to determine whether patients with right hemisphere disease could discriminate between affective intonations of speech without having to verbally classify or denote these intonations and found that patients with right hemisphere disease performed more poorly on this task than patients with left hemisphere disease did. We suspect that the right hemisphere contains the auditory representations of the prototypical emotional prosodies, and degradation of these representations or an inability to access them could impair both comprehension and discrimination of emotional prosody.

In normal conversation and experimental tasks, emotional prosody is often superimposed on propositional speech, and the poor performance of right hemisphere-damaged patients on emotional prosody tasks might, in part, be related to distraction. Thus, after right hemisphere damage, the intact left hemisphere might be able to comprehend emotional prosody, but it is distracted by the propositional semantic message. To learn if distraction plays a role in the impaired comprehension of emotional prosody associated with right hemisphere damage, we presented right and left hemisphere-damaged subjects an emotional prosody task that varied in the degree of conflict between the emotional message conveyed by the prosody and that conveyed by the propositional content (48) and found that the right hemisphere-damaged group was more disrupted when the propositional and prosodic emotional messages were highly conflicting than when they were less conflicting. However, in a subsequent study when the verbal semantic message was deleted by filtering the speech, the patients with right hemisphere damage were still more impaired than those with left, suggesting that, while the left hemisphere is capable of some processing of emotional prosodic information, the right is dominant (48).

Visual and Auditory Verbal Processes. The comprehension of spoken and written words by aphasic left hemisphere-damaged patients is improved when emotional words or phrases are used (49). These observed improvements suggest that the right hemisphere has a lexical-semantic system that can process emotional words better than non-emotional words. It is also possible that the increased arousal, which typically accompanies emotional stimuli, is the critical factor.

Support for the former lexical postulate comes from the work of Borod and coworkers (50), who tested right and left hemisphere-injured patients with emotional and non-emotional sentence and word discrimination tests. They found that the patients with right hemisphere damage were more impaired than those subjects with left hemisphere damage on the emotional discrimination tests. Other studies, however, suggest that lesions of the right hemisphere do not specifically disrupt lexical semantic knowledge about emotions or emotional situations (51). Patients with right hemisphere lesions appear to have intact conceptual knowledge about emotions that are communicated verbally, as long as this communication does not involve verbal descriptions of nonverbal affect signals (38).

Expressive Defects

Speech and Writing. We demonstrated that many patients with right hemisphere disease cannot express affective speech prosody (expressive affective aprosodia) (43). Typically, these patients speak in a flat monotone and often verbally denoted the target affect. Similar findings have been reported by Ross and Mesulam (52), who described two patients who could not express affectively intoned speech but who could comprehend affective speech prosody. Ross (44) postulated that right hemisphere lesions may disrupt the comprehension, repetition, or production of affective speech in the same manner that left hemisphere lesions disrupt propositional speech.

There is little or no evidence to suggest that patients with right hemisphere dysfunction are impaired at expressing emotions using propositional speech or writing, but Bloom et al. (53) reported that right hemisphere-damaged patients used fewer words when denoting emotions in their spontaneous speech. However, this might be related to other factors such as the decreased arousal associated with right hemisphere injury.

Facial Expressions. Buck and Duffy (54) reported that right hemisphere-damaged patients were less facially expressive than left hemisphere-damaged patients, and these findings have been repeatedly replicated and similar deficits have also been observed in more naturalistic settings outside the laboratory (38). In contrast to these studies, when using the facial action scoring system (55), other investigators have reported no differences in facial emotion expressiveness between right and left hemisphere-damaged patients (56). The reason for this discrepancy remains unclear; however, the observation that normal people express emotions more intensely on the left side of the face (57) supports the postulate of right hemisphere dominance.

Treatments

Communication Disorders. Rosenbek and associates (58) have demonstrated that both imitative treatment and cognitive-linguistic treatments might help patients with expressive aprosodia. However, there have been no well-controlled studies of either the treatment of comprehension disorders of aprosodia or of disorders of facial emotional communication.

VISUOSPATIAL FUNCTIONS

Angle and Face Matching

Based on observations of patients with discrete lesions and corpus callosum disconnection, neuropsychologists have proposed functional hemispheric asymmetries; for example, the left hemisphere is dominant for mediating speech and language, and the right hemisphere is dominant for visuospatial functions. In regard to intrahemispheric localization, it has been thought that injury to the posterior portions of the right hemisphere's cerebral cortex, including the parietal lobes, induces visuospatial dysfunction (59). However, Trojano et al. (60) tested patients with right and left hemisphere damage using many tests of visuospatial ability, including judgment of line orientation, angle, and mental rotation as well as the copying portions of the Rey Complex Figure Test, and found that there were no significant differences between those with right and left hemisphere injuries. Although many studies suggest that injury to the language-dominant left hemisphere might also induce visuospatial deficits, there are only two well known visuospatial tests that left hemisphere-damaged patients often perform normally and that right hemisphere-damaged patients often appear to perform poorly. One of these tests is the judgment of line orientation (61). Patients see a series of pages where there are two line segments that are drawn at different angles from each other and the side of the page on which they are presented. The patients subsequently perform a recognition test, selecting the angle on a protractor like display. The second test is a face matching test (61), where patients attempt to match photographs of faces of people who are unknown to the subjects. These photographs are taken from different perspectives so that subjects cannot correctly perform this task by simply making same-different decisions.

Constructional Apraxia

An impaired ability to copy and make drawings is called constructional apraxia. Patients with both left and right hemisphere injury might demonstrate constructional apraxia. Several investigators, however, have suggested that the patients with left hemisphere disease often demonstrate different forms of errors than those with right hemisphere injuries. The patients with left hemisphere lesions appear to have problems with planning and organizing their drawing; therefore, their productions tend to be simplified and impoverished. For example,

when attempting to draw a three-dimensional cube, the patients with left hemisphere damage might draw several attached rectangles. In contrast, the patients with right hemisphere lesions have problems correctly producing the spatial relationships between the components of the drawing. When attempting to draw a cube, patients with right hemisphere disease will have problems displaying the correct angles between the lines that form the cube. Patients with right hemisphere damage also frequently demonstrate elements of spatial neglect and thus might fail to copy-draw the left side of objects.

Topographic Disorientation and Image Rotation

Patients can have topographic disorientation for several reasons. They might have impaired spatial orientation and an inability to recall the spatial relationships of landmarks or a failure to recognize landmarks. These disorders, however, are most often seen with bilateral hemispheric dysfunction, but a defect in the acquisition of topographic relationships has been reported to be associated with right medial temporal lobe dysfunction (62).

There are many defects of imagery (see 63 for a review). However, several studies have suggested that lesions of the right parietal lobe are most likely to induce this deficit (64).

Dressing Apraxia

The visuospatial deficit that might cause the greatest disability is dressing apraxia. This deficit is most commonly associated with degenerative diseases such as corticobasal degeneration, but focal right hemisphere lesions might also induce dressing apraxia. However, many patients with right hemisphere lesions such as stroke have neglect and related disorders. Thus, these patients might be inattentive or unaware of the left side of space and/or the left side of their body. This inattention-unawareness induces a failure to dress the left side of the body, but there are some patients without neglect who also have trouble with dressing. To test for dressing apraxia, patients are often given a jacket that is inside out and asked to put on this jacket.

Unfortunately, there are no systematic studies of treating this disorder or the other visuospatial disorders mentioned above.

CONCLUSIONS

For many years, physicians and surgeons believed that except for the motor and sensory systems, the right hemisphere was "silent" and did not play a critical role in controlling higher-order cognitive functions. Therefore, if the surgeon had to take a brain biopsy or insert a tube through the cortex into the ventricles, they would operate on the right hemisphere. Over the last several decades, however, it has become apparent that the right hemisphere mediates many of human beings' most important cognitive functions, such attending to relevant stimuli, as well as deciding when to initiate an action, when to persist at an action, when to complete an action, and even when not to act. Emotions play a critical role in our lives, and the right hemisphere appears to be dominant for verbal-prosodic and facial emotional communications. In addition, spatial operation, such as drawing and dressing, appears to be mediated by the right hemisphere.

Overall, most of the more recent studies of disability have demonstrated that damage to the right, as opposed to the left hemisphere, is more likely to induce severe disabilities that reduce independence. Thus, rather than being the "non-dominant" hemisphere, the right hemisphere in many respects appears to be the "governing" hemisphere. Health providers who deal with patients that have suffered with hemispheric injuries or degeneration must understand the right hemisphere's functions—and hopefully this chapter will aid this understanding.

References

1. Heilman KM, Watson RT, Valenstein E. Neglect and related disorders. In: Heilman KM, Valenstein E, eds. *Clinical Neuropsychology*. 4th ed. New York: Oxford University Press, 2003:296–346.
2. Vallar G, Sterzi R, Bottini G, et al. Temporary remission of left hemianesthesia after vestibular stimulation: A sensory neglect phenomenon. *Cortex* 1990; 26:123–131.
3. Nadeau SE, Heilman KM. Gaze-dependent hemianopia without hemispatial neglect. *Neurology* 1991; 41(8):1244–1250.
4. Coslett HB. Evidence for a disturbance of the body schema in neglect. *Brain Cogn* 1998; 37(3):527–544.
5. Moruzzi G, Magoun HW. Brainstem reticular formation and the activation of the EEG. *Electroencephalogr. Clin Neurophysiol* 1949; 1:455–473.
6. Sokolov YN. *Perception and the Conditioned Reflex*. Oxford: Pergmon Press, 1963.
7. Damasio AR. Locked multiregional retroactivation: A systems-level proposal for the neural substrates of recall and recognition. *Cognition* 1989; 33(1–2):25–62.
8. Bisiach E, Luzzatti C. Unilateral neglect of representational space. *Cortex* 1978; 14:29–133.
9. Heilman KM, Van Den Abell T. Right hemisphere dominance for attention: The mechanisms underlying hemispheric asymmetries of inattention (neglect). *Neurology* 1980; 30:327–330.
10. Schneider JS, McLaughlin WW, Roeltgen DP. Motor and nonmotor behavioral deficits in monkeys made hemiparkinsonian by intracarotid MPTP infusion. *Neurology* 1992; 42(8):1565–1572.
11. Ungerstedt U. Brain dopamine neurons and behavior. In: Schmidt FO, Woren FG, eds. *Neurosciences*. Vol. 3. Cambridge, MA: MIT Press, 1974:695–703.
12. Corwin JV, Kanter S, Watson RT, et al. Apomorphine has a therapeutic effect on neglect produced by unilateral dorsomedial prefrontal cortex lesions in rats. *Exp Neurol* 1986; 36:683–698.
13. Fleet WS, Valenstein E, Watson RT, Heilman KM. Dopamine agonist therapy for neglect in humans. *Neurology* 1987; 37:1765–1771.
14. Barrett AM, Crucian GP, Schwartz RL, Heilman KM. Adverse effect of dopamine agonist therapy in a patient with motor-intentional neglect. *Arch Phys Med rehabil* 1999; 80(5):600–603.
15. Rossi PW, Kheyfets S, Reding MJ. Fresnel prisms improve visual perception in stroke patients with homonymous hemianopia or unilateral visual neglect. *Neurology* 1990; 40(10):1597–1599.
16. Rubens AB. Caloric stimulation and unilateral visual neglect. *Neurology* 1985; 35:1019–1024.
17. Pizzamiglio L, Frasca R, Guariglia C, et al. Effect of optokinetic stimulation in patients with visual neglect. *Cortex.* 1990 Dec; 26(4):535–540.
18. Karnath HO. Subjective body orientation in neglect and the interactive contribution of neck muscle proprioception and vestibular stimulation. *Brain* 1994; 117(5):1001–1012.
19. Diller L, Weinberg J. Hemi-inattention in rehabilitation: The evolution of a rational remediation program. In: Weinstein EA, Friedland RR, eds. *Advances in Neurology*. Vol. 18. New York: Raven Press, 1977.
20. Gouvier WD, Cubic B. Behavioral assessment and treatment of acquired visuoperceptual disorders. *Neuropsychol Rev* 1991; 2(1):3–28.
21. Gouvier WD. Assessment and treatment of cognitive deficits in brain-damaged individuals. *Behav Modif.* Jul 1987; 11(3):312–328.
22. Butter CM, Kirsh NL, Reeves GC. The effect of lateralized stimuli on unilateral spatial neglect following right hemisphere lesions. *Restorative Neurology & Neuroscience* 1990; 2:39–46.
23. Maguire A. Reducing neglect by introducing ipsilesional global cues. *Brain Cogn* 2000; 43(1–3):328–332.
24. Halligan PW, Marshall JC. Laterality of motor response in visuo-spatial neglect: A case study. *Neuropsychologia* 1989; 27:1301–1307.
25. Robertson IH, North N. Spatio-motor cueing in unilateral left neglect: The role of hemispace, hand and motor activation. *Neuropsychologia* 1992; 30(6):553–563.
26. Sprague JM, Meikle TH. The role of the superior colliculus in visually guided behavior. *Exp. Neurol.* 1965; 11:115–146.
27. Posner MI, Rafal RD. Cognitive theories of attention and rehabilitation of attentional deficits. In: Mier MJ, Benton AL, Diller L, eds. *Neuropsychological Rehabilitation*. New York: Guilford, 1987.
28. Butter CM, Kirsch N. Combined and separate effects of eye patching and visual stimulation on unilateral neglect following stroke. *Arch Phys Med Rehabil* 1992; 73(12):1133–1139.
29. Barrett AM, Crucian GP, Beversdorf DQ, Heilman KM. Paradoxical effect of monocular eye patching in attentional neglect. Presented at the American Society of Rehabilitation meeting, April 1998. (Abstract in *Journal of Neurologic Rehabilitation* 1998; 12:42–43.)
30. Taub E, Uswatt G. Constraint-induced movement therapy: Answers and questions after two decades of research. *NeuroRehabilitation* 2006; 21(2):93–95.
31. Triggs WJ, Gold M, Gerstle G, et al. Motor neglect associated with a discreet parietal lesion. *Neurology* 1994; 44:1164–1166.
32. Michel C, Pisella L, Prablanc C, Rode G, Rossetti Y. Enhancing visuomotor adaptation by reducing error signals: Single-step (aware) versus multiple-step (unaware) exposure to wedge prisms. *J Cogn Neurosci* 2007; 19(2):341–350.
33. DeKosky S, Heilman KM, Bowers D, Valenstein E. Recognition and discrimination of emotional faces and pictures. *Brain Lang* 1980; 9:206–214.
34. Cicone M, Waper W, Gardner H. Sensitivity to emotional expressions and situation in organic patients. *Cortex* 1980; 16:145–158.
35. Etcoff N. Perceptual and conceptual organization of facial emotions. *Brain Cognition* 1984; 3:385–412.
36. Borod J, Koff E, Perlman-Lorch J, Nicholas M. The expression and perception of facial emotions in brain damaged patients. *Neuropsychologia* 1986; 24:169–180.
37. Fried I, Mateer C, Ojemann G, et al. Organization of visuospatial functions in human cortex. Evidence from electrical stimulation. *Brain* 1982; 105(Pt 2):349–371.
38. Blonder LX, Bowers D, Heilman KM. The role of the right hemisphere in emotional communication. *Brain* 1991; 114(pt 3):1115–1127.
39. Bowers D, Blonder LX, Feinberg T, Heilman KM. Differential impact of right and left hemisphere lesions on facial emotion and object imagery. *Brain* 1991; 114 (Pt 6):2593–2609.
40. Jacobs DH, Shuren J, Bowers D, Heilman KM. Emotional facial imagery, perception, and expression in Parkinson's disease. *Neurology* 1995; 45(9):1696–1702.
41. Hughlings Jackson J. *Selected Writings of John Hughlings Jackson*. Taylor J, ed. London: Hodder and Stoughton, 1932.
42. Heilman KM, Scholes R, Watson RT. Auditory affective agnosia: Disturbed comprehension of affective speech. *J Neurol Neurosurg Psychiatry* 1975; 38:69–72.
43. Tucker DM, Watson RT, Heilman KM. Affective discrimination and evocation in patients with right parietal disease. *Neurology* 1977; 17:947–950.
44. Ross, ED. The aprosodias: Functional-anatomic organization of the affective components of language in the right hemisphere. *Ann Neurol* 1981; 38:561–589.
45. Barrett AM, Crucian GP, Raymer AM, Heilman KM. Spared comprehension of emotional prosody in a patient with global aphasia. *Neuropsychiatry Neuropsychol Behav Neurol* 1999B; 12(2):117–120.
46. Kanter SL, Day AL, Heilman KM, Gonzalez-Rothi LJ. Pure word deafness: A possible explanation of transient deteriorations after extracranial-intracranial bypass grafting. *Neurosurgery* 1986; 18(2):186–189.
47. Tucker, DM, Watson RT, Heilman KM. Affective discrimination and evocation in patients with right parietal disease. *Neurology* 1977; 17:947–950.
48. Bowers D, Coslett HB, Bauer RM, et al. Comprehension of emotional prosody following unilateral hemispheric lesions: Processing defect versus distraction defect. *Neuropsychologia* 1987; 25(2):317–328.
49. Reuterskiöld C. The effects of emotionality on auditory comprehension in aphasia. *Cortex* 1991; 27(4):595–604.
50. Borod JC, Andelman F, Obler LK, et al. Right hemisphere specialization for the identification of emotional words and sentences: evidence from stroke patients. *Neuropsychologia* 1992; 30(9):827–844.
51. Blonder LX, Burns A, Bowers D, et al. Right hemisphere facial expressivity during natural conversation. *Brain and Cognition* 1993; 21(1): 44–56.

52. Ross ED, Mesulam MM. Dominant language functions of the right hemisphere? Prosody and emotional gesturing. *Arch Neurol* 1979; 36:144–148.

53. Bloom R, Borod JC, Obler L, Gerstman L. Impact of emotional content on discourse production in patients with unilateral brain damage. *Brain and Language* 1992; 42:153–164.

54. Buck R, Duffy RJ. Nonverbal communication of affect in brain damaged patients. *Cortex* 1980; 16:351–362.

55. Ekman P, Friesen WV. *Facial Action Coding System*. Palo Alto, CA: Consulting Psychologists Press, 1978.

56. Mammucari A, Caltagirone C, Ekman P, et al. Spontaneous facial expression of emotions in brain damaged patients. *Cortex* 24; 1988:521–533.

57. Sackeim H, Gur R, Saucy M. Emotions are expressed more intensely on the left side of the face. *Science* 1978; 202:434–436.

58. Rosenbek JC, Rodriguez AD, Hieber B, et al. Effects of two treatments for aprosodia secondary to acquired brain injury. *J Rehabil Res Dev* 2006; 43(3):379–390.

59. Ratcliff G. Spatial thought, mental rotation and the right cerebral hemisphere. *Neuropsychologia*. 1979; 17(1):49–54.

60. et al. Relationships between constructional and visuospatial abilities in normal subjects and in focal brain-damaged patients. *J Clin Exp Neuropsychol* 2004; 26(8):1103–1112.

61. Benton AL, Sivan AB, Hamsher K. *Contributions to Neuropsychological Assessment: A Clinical Manual*. 2nd ed. New York: Oxford University Press, 1994.

62. Habib M, Sirigu A. Pure topographical disorientation: A definition and anatomical basis. *Cortex* 1987; 23(1):73–85.

63. Farah MJ. Disorders of Visual-Spatial Perception and Cognition. In Heilman KM, Valenstein E, eds. *Clinical Neuropsychology*. New York: Oxford University Press, 2003.

64. Corballis MC. Mental rotation and the right hemisphere. *Brain Lang* 1997; 57(1):100–121.

13 Memory, Executive Function, and Dementia

Steven M. Greenberg

POST-STROKE COGNITIVE DYSFUNCTION: THE SCOPE OF THE PROBLEM

Cognitive impairment following symptomatic stroke, one of the most important aspects of stroke recovery, has historically also been one of the least appreciated. Despite the self-evident importance of cognitive function to quality of life, widely used scales of stroke-related disability, such as the Barthel index (1), have typically focused on motor-dependent skills, such as ambulation, transfers, bathing, toileting, and feeding, without reference to cognition. One contributor to this tendency to exclude cognition from the stroke recovery field may have been the belief that dementia is caused primarily by Alzheimer's disease (AD) and is largely unrelated to cerebrovascular disease. With increased understanding of the key role played by vascular injury in cognitive dysfunction (2) and of possible overlaps and synergies between vascular processes and AD (3), however, has come greater appreciation of the cognitive dysfunction that follows stroke.

Stroke is a potent risk factor for cognitive impairment and dementia. Studies of hospitalized stroke patients using prospective follow-up (4) or analysis of Medicare Part A inpatient claims (5) estimated an approximately 10-fold increased risk for dementia and a prevalence of 20 to 25% (6). Prospective population-based studies (7–9) have yielded smaller—but still quite substantial

(approximately twofold)—increases in risk for dementia following stroke. As not all cognitive impairment meets criteria for "dementia" (10, 11) and not all cerebrovascular disease is diagnosed as "stroke," these figures likely underestimate the full contribution of vascular disease to cognitive dysfunction.

Once present, post-stroke dementia is a major risk for mortality, independent of age, Barthel index, and comorbid medical disease (12), underlining the importance of this complication from the stroke rehabilitation perspective. Post-stroke dementia also causes attrition from research follow-up(13), another factor likely to lead to underestimates of its true prevalence.

Post-stroke cognitive dysfunction, like post-stroke dysfunction of any type, occurs only in subjects who survive their stroke. Improvements in stroke survival would therefore be predicted to increase the prevalence of post-stroke cognitive dysfunction, a trend that indeed appears to be underway. In an analysis of Medicare Part A inpatient claims from approximately 42,000 subjects age 65 and older participating in the National Long-Term Care Survey (5), a comparison of the time periods 1984–1990 and 1991–2000 demonstrated a 53% increase in the age-adjusted rate of all dementia types, with the greatest increase (87%) occurring in those subjects with symptomatic stroke. These secular trends occurred in the setting of increased one-year stroke survival from 53% to 65% over the same time interval, suggesting that gains in stroke survival may indeed be contributing to the increasing burden posed by post-stroke cognitive dysfunction. Further, both cerebrovascular and AD pathology is markedly age dependent, suggesting that the prevalence of each will rise with the aging of the population. The net effect of improved stroke survival, an aging population, and steady age-specific stroke rates is thus predicted to be a major increase in the population of patients affected by post-stroke cognitive dysfunction.

THE SPECTRUM OF POST-STROKE COGNITIVE DYSFUNCTION

Two issues have stood as barriers to a full appreciation of the role of vascular factors in cognitive impairment. One is the heterogeneity of the vascular contribution to cognitive dysfunction. The vascular role can range from relatively pure instances of cognitive devastation caused by one or a few discrete infarctions with no apparent contribution from other neurologic disorders, to the more common situation where diffuse vascular injury combines with neurodegenerative processes like AD to produce a mixed impairment. The second complicating issue has been the types of cognitive impairments that can result from vascular injury. These also span a spectrum from frank dementia (defined as deficits of multiple cognitive domains, including memory, that interfere with functional activities (14)) to cognitive impairments not meeting these criteria but nonetheless causing substantial functional limitation.

Vladimir Hachinski, the first to disseminate the term "multi-infarct dementia," (15) has since argued eloquently that the field should essentially bypass these questions by considering vascular cognitive impairment as a spectrum of disorders with varying types of vascular contributors and varying types of cognitive deficits (16). The following discussion of post-stroke cognitive impairment will emulate this approach by considering first the range of factors (related to both the stroke and the patient in whom it occurs) that determine the likelihood of subsequent cognitive impairment and then the array of cognitive deficits that can occur following stroke.

Determinants of Impairment

Stroke Factors.   The effect of strokes on cognition likely represents the cumulative effects of location, number, and volume. In a subset of syndromes defined as "strategic" infarctions (17, 18), location is the overriding factor allowing single discrete infarctions to cause multi-domain cognitive impairment. Among these strategic locations are

1. The paramedian thalamus, typically supplied by branches from the distal basilar or proximal posterior cerebral arteries. Infarctions in this territory can give rise to widespread disturbances in memory, spatial processing, and personality as well as language (if the dominant side is included) (19).
2. The inferomedial temporal cortex, fed by the posterior cerebral arteries. If the dominant side is affected, this leads to verbal memory and verbal-visual impairments, such as alexia and color anomia (20).
3. The dominant angular gyrus, fed by branches of the middle cerebral artery. This leads to impairments of memory, language, and affect (21,22).
4. The parieto-temporal association cortex in the territory of the middle cerebral arteries, leading to inattention and behavioral abnormalities.
5. The frontal lobe, fed by the anterior cerebral artery. This produces deficits in memory and initiative.

Neuropathological studies have also pointed to lacunar infarctions in regions such as the basal ganglia, thalamus, and hippocampus or the medial temporal lobe as mimicking strategic stroke syndromes (23). In practice, the preponderance of single strategic infarcts causing vascular cognitive impairment appear to occur in the posterior circulation (24).

The remainder of the spectrum of strokes causing cognitive dysfunction is comprised of multiple infarctions, clinically symptomatic or asymptomatic, that collectively impair cognition. In multivariable analyses controlling for other potential contributors to dementia (see below), studies have implicated the total volume of infarcts in left and right vascular territories (25–27)—or more specifically, the volume of infarction in limbic and multimodal association cortex (28)—as predictors of stroke-related dementia. Efforts to identify specific radiographic features distinguishing patients with and without post-stroke dementia, however, have proven difficult. In a study of 125 subjects with stroke, none of the radiographic characteristics proposed as supporting a diagnosis of vascular dementia (17) (such as involvement of the bilateral thalami, medial temporal lobes, or basal ganglia) were overrepresented among those with dementia (29). These data suggest that the risk of post-stroke dementia may depend substantially on factors other than the stroke itself, in particular the pre-existing state of the brain in which it occurs.

Patient Factors.   Among demographic factors, age, low education level, and possibly male sex and non-white race have been demonstrated as risks for post-stroke dementia (8, 25, 27, 30, 31). The extent of pre-existing cerebrovascular disease also appears to contribute to the likelihood that a subsequent stroke will impair cognition, as suggested by positive associations with history of prior stroke, the extent of white-matter lesions on neuroimaging, and vascular risk factors, such as diabetes mellitus, cigarette use, or elevated low-density lipoprotein (25, 27, 30–32). The latter findings are consistent with broader studies of the general population, linking vascular risk factors of all types (including midlife hypertension, midlife cholesterol, diabetes/hyperinsulinemia, plasma homocysteine, tobacco use, metabolic syndrome, and a composite score of atherosclerosis) with impairments of cognition (33–48).

Presence of pre-existing AD pathology may be another key determinant of the effects of stroke on cognition, in keeping with the increasingly accepted concept that cerebrovascular disease and AD act synergistically in generating cognitive impairment (49, 50). Supporting an important role for underlying AD is the observation that atrophy of the medial temporal lobe is a strong predictor of post-stroke dementia (27, 29). Similarly, pre-stroke cognitive impairment has been identified to predict post-stroke impairment (51). Some studies (52) (though not all (53)) have also identified the AD-associated apolipoprotein E (APOE) ε4 allele as a genetic risk for post-stroke dementia. Interpretation of this finding is potentially confounded by the fact that APOE ε4 also has associations with ischemic stroke (54) and cerebral amyloid angiopathy (55). With the development of noninvasive markers for senile plaques (56), assessing the interaction of stroke with AD pathology in determining post-stroke cognition will be increasingly feasible.

In summary, the situation where widespread cognitive impairment can be attributed to individual strategic strokes appears to be the exception rather than the rule. Post-stroke cognitive impairment instead generally represents the cumulative effects of location, number, and size of strokes (both incident and remote) and white matter lesions—"a matter of strokes large and small" in Fisher's widely quoted formulation (57)—and pre-existing brain pathologies, in particular, AD.

Characteristics of Impairment

Although stroke-related cognitive impairment might be expected to manifest immediately following the triggering stroke, studies have emphasized the ongoing incidence of newly diagnosed dementia months or even years post-stroke. This phenomenon might be partly related to difficulties in diagnosing dementia during the medically active early post-stroke period, but very likely also reflects an increased vulnerability of stroke patients to ongoing vascular and neurodegenerative events. Among 154 stroke survivors initially free of dementia, the incidence of new dementia remained substantially greater than in elderly controls, with cumulative incidence of approximately 10% at one year post-stroke, 15% at two years, and 22% at three years (58). Approximately two-thirds of the incident dementias in this study could be attributed to recurrent stroke, intercurrent medical illnesses potentially causative of brain hypoxia (such as seizure, heart failure, or pneumonia), or borderline post-stroke cognitive test scores that left the patient close to meeting dementia criteria during follow-up. The remaining one-third had no clinically evident cause or event. Similarly high rates of incident cognitive impairment during the years following stroke have been identified in other prospective studies (59, 60), with recurrent stroke or borderline post-stroke cognitive status again acting as risk factors (8, 59, 61).

Studies comparing the cognitive profile of AD and vascular dementia have often emphasized the relatively greater impairments of episodic memory in AD and increased impairments on tasks requiring executive function and working memory, such as picture arrangement or object assembly, in vascular disease (62, 63). Deficits in *short-term episodic memory* are nonetheless a common feature of post-stroke cognitive impairment, even in those not meeting criteria for dementia (64, 65). Memory impairment following stroke can be due to infarction of medial temporal lobe structures directly involved in memory storage (23). Another possible mechanism is damage to white matter structures involved in memory retrieval through connections with the medial temporal lobe. In a functional MRI study of older, cognitively normal subjects, T2-hyperintensities in the dorsal prefrontal cortical white matter correlated with decreased activation of the medial temporal lobe and worse performance on an episodic memory task (66). These experiments raise the intriguing possibility that vascular lesions may contribute to memory impairment through a kind of disconnection mechanism even without direct damage to the medial temporal brain regions.

Executive function is the other prominent cognitive domain commonly affected following stroke. Executive function is a somewhat ill-defined, but nonetheless central, component of the cognitive abilities required for day-to-day functioning. It represents a constellation of higher-order skills used to manipulate available information to plan and execute complex activities. Among the elemental skills felt to comprise executive function are allocation of attention, mental flexibility, processing speed, set maintenance, set shifting, working memory, and error correction. Its importance to real-life functioning is demonstrated by strikingly high correlations in the elderly with institutionalized versus non-institutionalized level of care (67) and with formal scales of activities of daily living (ADLs) (68, 69). In a study of 337 testable stroke survivors (mean age 70.2 ± 7.6), executive dysfunction (performance at least 1.5 standard deviations below the mean for elderly control subjects on eight tests) was present in 40.6% of subjects and was associated with more than a doubling of deficits on measurements of basic ADLs (69).

A useful methodological advance for studying executive function following stroke has been the introduction of the diagnostic category "vascular cognitive impairment, no dementia" (CIND) (70) to reflect subjects with substantial cognitive deficits without sufficient memory loss, functional impairment, or other multi-domain deficits to meet criteria for dementia (14). Cognitive features typical of CIND include deficits related to executive function in areas such as sequencing, attention, working memory, and cognitive processing speed (71). Analysis of 92 hospital-based subjects diagnosed with CIND found less memory impairment but essentially the same extent of executive dysfunction as 33 similarly aged subjects diagnosed with vascular dementia (65). Another notable finding from this study was that even those stroke survivors that were considered to have *no* significant cognitive impairment demonstrated worse executive function than stroke-free controls (with no difference in memory scores), indicating that executive function may indeed be the most sensitive cognitive domain to the effects of stroke.

Other cognitive domains have been less extensively studied following stroke. A population-based study found no stroke-associated decline in *visuospatial* or *language* performance (64), whereas the above-noted study of hospitalized stroke patients without significant cognitive impairment demonstrated subtle deficits in these areas (65). Increasing attention has focused on post-stroke *depression* and *anxiety* as other possible manifestations of vascular dementia (72), with psychomotor retardation as perhaps the most prominent neuropsychiatric feature to be seen in specific association with cognitive impairment (73).

MANAGEMENT OF POST-STROKE COGNITIVE DYSFUNCTION

The high prevalence of cognitive impairment following stroke (even in subjects felt clinically to have no significant cognitive impairment (65)) argues that cognitive screening and follow-up should be a fundamental component of the stroke rehabilitation process. No cognitive test battery has emerged as a standard protocol for this purpose, however. Widely used instruments, such as the Mini-Mental State Examination (MMSE) (74) and the full or abbreviated Cambridge Cognitive Examination (CAMCOG) (75, 76) for example, offer little testing of executive function and are therefore not ideal for the post-stroke setting. The National Institute of Neurological Disorders and Stroke–Canadian Stroke Network's (NINDS-CSN) vascular cognitive impairment working group (77) recently addressed the issue of cognitive testing by proposing three protocols requiring approximately 60, 30, or five minutes

for administration (Table 13-1). Tests in the full 60-minute protocol address four primary cognitive domains: executive/activation, language, visuospatial, and memory, as well as items such as the Neuropsychiatric Inventory Questionnaire (NPI-Q) to capture neurobehavioral change and mood. Items addressing the executive/activation domain in the 60- and 30-minute protocols are tests of semantic and phonemic fluency, digit-symbol coding, and trailmaking (the latter being an optional supplemental task in the 30-minute battery). The five-minute protocol, designed for ease of use as well as potential administration by telephone, tests phonemic fluency, orientation, and immediate and delayed recall; the NINDS-CSN authors note that instructions and norms in English and French for this short battery are publicly available for noncommercial use (www.mocatest.org). Although the NINDS-CSN cognitive stroke batteries were not designed (and have not been validated) for the specific purposes of identifying and tracking post-stroke impairment, they represent logical, well-established instruments that appear promising as potential standards for future clinical use.

Once the presence of cognitive impairment is established, the question turns to potential non-pharmacologic and pharmacologic approaches to treatment. Cognitive rehabilitation is a widely used non-pharmacologic treatment for post-stroke impairment (78) but has had little experimental testing. A Cochrane Review, published in 2000, of cognitive therapy for post-stroke memory impairment found only a single study of 12 subjects meeting criteria (79), underlining the importance of further work in this area.

Pharmacologic approaches to post-stroke cognitive impairment can be divided into disease-modifying treatments to prevent future declines and symptomatic treatments aimed at improving the current level of functioning. Among disease-modifying treatments, secondary stroke prevention is of paramount importance, as longitudinal studies of patients with symptomatic (8, 58, 61) or clinically silent (9) stroke demonstrate recurrent stroke as a major contributor to subsequent cognitive decline. Current guidelines for secondary stroke prevention (80, 81) include 1) antihypertensive treatment, with the strongest evidence favoring angiotensin-converting enzyme inhibitors and diuretics; 2) glucose control to near-normoglycemic levels; 3) aggressive treatment of dyslipidemia, with recent evidence favoring use of high-dose atorvastatin through a wide range of baseline cholesterol levels (82); 4) antiplatelet, anticoagulant, or vascular reperfusion therapy as dictated by stroke evaluation (81); and 5) lifestyle modifications, such as smoking cessation, reduction of heavy alcohol use, increased physical activity, and weight loss if overweight. The most relevant data for prevention of post-stroke cognitive decline came from the randomized controlled PROGRESS study, in which perindopril plus optional indapamide significantly reduced the risk of both

TABLE 13-1
NINDS-CSN (77) Cognitive Test Battery for Vascular Cognitive Impairment

60-MINUTE PROTOCOL	30-MINUTE PROTOCOL	5-MINUTE PROTOCOL
Animal Naming	Animal Naming	Five-Word Memory Task (registration, recall, recognition)
Controlled Oral Word Association Test	Controlled Oral Word Association Test	Six-Item Orientation
WAIS-III Digit Symbol-Coding	WAIS-III Digit Symbol-Coding	One-Letter Phonemic Fluency
Trailmaking Test	Hopkins Verbal Learning Test—Revised	*Supplemental Tests* Remainder of Montreal Cognitive Assessment (www.mocatest.org)
Boston Naming Test (2nd Edition, Short Form)	Center for Epidemiologic Studies-Depression Scale	Animal Naming
Rey-Osterrieth Complex Figure Copy	NPI-Q	Trailmaking Test
Hopkins Verbal Learning Test—Revised (with List Learning Strategies)	*Supplemental Tests*	MMSE
NPI-Q	MMSE	
Center for Epidemiological Studies-Depression Scale Informant Questionnaire for	Trailmaking Test	
Informant Questionnaire for Cognitive Decline in the Elderly (short form)		
MMSE		
Supplemental/Alternate Tests Rey-Osterrieth Complex Figure Memory		
Boston Naming Recognition		
Digit Symbol-Coding Incidental Learning		
California Verbal Learning Test – 2		

cognitive decline (MMSE drop of ≥3 points in 9.1% of treated versus 11% of placebo, representing a 19% risk reduction) and progression of white matter lesions (mean increase in white matter hyperintensity volume of 0.4 mm^3 versus 2.0 mm^3) (83, 84). These data suggest that this or similar drug combinations may be useful through a wide range of baseline blood pressures for prevention of post-stroke cognitive decline.

The association between markers of AD, such as medial temporal atrophy and apolipoprotein E ε4, and post-stroke cognitive decline suggest that AD pathology also contributes to this process. Slowing of AD progression is therefore a rational approach for stroke patients with cognitive impairment but has not yet been demonstrated for any available agent. Rapidly growing understanding of the pathogenesis of AD provides grounds for optimism

that disease-modifying agents will soon emerge (85), however, and serve as promising candidates for prevention of cognitive decline following stroke.

Trials of symptomatic treatments for post-stroke cognitive impairment have focused largely on medications already demonstrated to provide symptomatic benefit in AD (Table 13-2) (86). A pooled analysis (87) of two 24-week randomized, controlled trials (88, 89) of the acetylcholinesterase inhibitor (AChEI) donepezil in patients diagnosed with vascular dementia found improvement of approximately two points on the Alzheimer's Disease Assessment Scale—cognitive subscale (ADAS-cog) and a significant increase in the proportion of subjects with global improvement (37% and 30% on 5 and 10 mg of donepezil versus 27% on placebo). These modest improvements appear slightly smaller than those achieved using the same agent for

TABLE 13-2
Medications with Demonstrated Efficacy for Vascular Cognitive Impairment

Agent (Trade Name)	Initial Dose	Titration Schedule/ Effective Dose	Most Common Adverse Effects
Donepezil (87–89) (Aricept)	5 mg/day, single dose	Increase 5 mg/day after 4 to 6 weeks 5 to 10 mg/day	Nausea, diarrhea, vomiting, sleep disturbances
Galantamine (90) (Razadyne or Razadyne ER, previously Reminyl)	8 mg/day, single dose (extended release formulation) or two divided doses	Increase 8 mg/day every 4 to 6 weeks 16 to 24 mg/day	Nausea, diarrhea, vomiting, anorexia
Memantine(91, 92) (Namenda)	5 mg/day, single dose	Increase 5 mg/day every week 20 mg/day, two divided doses	Dizziness, confusion, fatigue

AD (86), possibly reflecting the lesser tendency of vascular dementia subjects in the placebo arm to decline during the study period, compared to placebo-treated AD subjects. Slightly larger effects on cognitive testing and global functioning were noted in a 6-month randomized, controlled trial of the AChEI galantamine in subjects diagnosed with vascular dementia or AD plus cerebrovascular disease (90). Finally, two 28-week randomized, controlled trials of the uncompetitive NMDA antagonist memantine in subjects diagnosed with vascular dementia reported improvements relative to placebo of approximately two points on ADAS-cog, with statistically insignificant improvements in global functioning (91, 92).

Practical steps that merit strong consideration in patients with cognitive impairment following stroke are screening for and treating post-stroke depression (93) and reduction or withdrawal of medications contributing to cognitive slowing, such as psychotropic or anticholinergic agents. Studies in animal models of brain injury have highlighted the possibility that common classes of drugs

may slow the post-stroke recovery process (94), although the relevance of these data to human stroke recovery remains largely unknown. Other potential symptomatic approaches to post-stroke cognitive impairment have not been tested by large, randomized trials and remain of unclear effectiveness. These include stimulants, such as methylphenidate or modafinil (95), and antidepressants (in the absence of diagnosed depression) (96).

In summary, the treatment approach to post-stroke cognitive impairment is based on aggressive secondary stroke prevention and symptomatic treatment. Although the US Food and Drug Administration has not approved agents for the specific indication of vascular dementia, the AChEIs donepezil and galantamine appear to be rational choices, with the possibility of further efficacy from added memantine, as has been demonstrated in moderate to severe AD (97). Among the highest priorities for future studies will be to identify vasculoprotective or anti-AD agents with specific effects on preventing further cognitive decline in stroke patients.

References

1. Mahoney FI, Barthel DW. Functional evaluation: The Barthel Index. *Md State Med J* 1965; 14:61–65.
2. O'Brien JT, Erkinjuntti T, Reisberg B, et al. Vascular cognitive impairment. *Lancet Neurol* 2003; 2(2):89–98.
3. Iadecola C, Gorelick PB. Converging pathogenic mechanisms in vascular and neurodegenerative dementia. *Stroke* 2003; 34(2):335–337.
4. Tatemichi TK, Desmond DW, Mayeux R, et al. Dementia after stroke: Baseline frequency, risks, and clinical features in a hospitalized cohort. *Neurology* 1992; 42(6):1185–1193.
5. Ukraintseva S, Sloan F, Arbeev K, Yashin A. Increasing rates of dementia at time of declining mortality from stroke. *Stroke* 2006; 37(5):1155–1159.
6. van Kooten F, Koudstaal PJ. Epidemiology of post-stroke dementia. *Haemostasis* 1998; 28(3–4):124–133.
7. Ivan CS, Seshadri S, Beiser A, et al. Dementia after stroke: The Framingham Study. *Stroke* 2004; 35(6):1264–1268.
8. Kokmen E, Whisnant JP, O'Fallon WM, et al. Dementia after ischemic stroke: A population-based study in Rochester, Minnesota (1960–1984). *Neurology* 1996; 46(1):154–159.
9. Vermeer SE, Prins ND, den Heijer T, et al. Silent brain infarcts and the risk of dementia and cognitive decline. *N Engl J Med* 2003; 348(13):1215–1222.
10. Erkinjuntti T, Ostbye T, Steenhuis R, Hachinski V. The effect of different diagnostic criteria on the prevalence of dementia. *N Engl J Med* 1997; 337(23):1667–1674.
11. Pohjasvaara T, Mantyla R, Ylikoski R, et al. Comparison of different clinical criteria (DSM-III, ADDTC, ICD-10, NINDS-AIREN, DSM-IV) for the diagnosis of vascular dementia. *Stroke* 2000; 31(12):2952–2957.
12. Tatemichi TK, Paik M, Bagiella E, et al. Dementia after stroke is a predictor of long-term survival. *Stroke* 1994; 25(10):1915–1919.
13. Desmond DW, Bagiella E, Moroney JT, Stern Y. The effect of patient attrition on estimates of the frequency of dementia following stroke. *Arch Neurol* 1998; 55(3):390–394.
14. *Diagnostic and Statistical Manual of Mental Disorders, 4th Edition: DSM-IV.* Washington, DC: American Psychiatric Association, 1994.
15. Hachinski VC, Lassen NA, Marshall J. Multi-infarct dementia: A cause of mental deterioration in the elderly. *Lancet* 1974; 2(7874):207–210.
16. Hachinski V. Vascular dementia: A radical redefinition. *Dementia* 1994; 5(3–4):130–132.

17. Roman GC, Tatemichi TK, Erkinjuntti T, et al. Vascular dementia: Diagnostic criteria for research studies. Report of the NINDS-AIREN International Workshop. *Neurology* 1993; 43(2):250–260.

18. Tatemichi TK. How acute brain failure becomes chronic: A view of the mechanisms of dementia related to stroke. *Neurology* 1990; 40(11):1652–1659.

19. Graff-Radford NR, Eslinger PJ, Damasio AR, Yamada T. Nonhemorrhagic infarction of the thalamus: Behavioral, anatomic, and physiologic correlates. *Neurology* 1984; 34(1):14–23.

20. De Renzi E, Zambolin A, Crisi G. The pattern of neuropsychological impairment associated with left posterior cerebral artery infarcts. *Brain* 1987; 110 (Pt 5):1099–1116.

21. Benson DF, Cummings JL. Angular gyrus syndrome simulating Alzheimer's disease. *Arch Neurol* 1982; 39(10):616–620.

22. Nagaratnam N, Phan TA, Barnett C, Ibrahim N. Angular gyrus syndrome mimicking depressive pseudodementia. *J Psychiatry Neurosci* 2002; 27(5):364–368.

23. Vinters HV, Ellis WG, Zarow C, et al. Neuropathologic substrates of ischemic vascular dementia. *J Neuropathol Exp Neurol* 2000; 59(11):931–945.

24. Auchus AP, Chen CP, Sodagar SN, et al. Single stroke dementia: Insights from 12 cases in Singapore. *J Neurol Sci* 15 2002; 203–204:85–89.

25. Desmond DW, Moroney JT, Paik MC, et al. Frequency and clinical determinants of dementia after ischemic stroke. *Neurology* 14 2000; 54(5):1124–1131.

26. Pohjasvaara T, Mantyla R, Salonen O, et al. How complex interactions of ischemic brain infarcts, white matter lesions, and atrophy relate to poststroke dementia. *Arch Neurol* 2000; 57(9):1295–1300.

27. Pohjasvaara T, Mantyla R, Salonen O, et al. MRI correlates of dementia after first clinical ischemic stroke. *J Neurol Sci* 2000; 181(1–2):111–117.

28. Zekry D, Duyckaerts C, Belmin J, et al. The vascular lesions in vascular and mixed dementia: The weight of functional neuroanatomy. *Neurobiol Aging* 2003; 24(2):213–219.

29. Ballard CG, Burton EJ, Barber R, et al. NINDS AIREN neuroimaging criteria do not distinguish stroke patients with and without dementia. *Neurology* 28 2004; 63(6):983–988.

30. Gorelick PB, Brody J, Cohen D, et al. Risk factors for dementia associated with multiple cerebral infarcts: A case-control analysis in predominantly African-American hospital-based patients. *Arch Neurol* 1993; 50(7):714–720.

31. van Kooten F, Bots ML, Breteler MM, et al. The Dutch Vascular Factors in Dementia Study: Rationale and design. *J Neurol* 1998; 245(1):32–39.

32. Moroney JT, Tang MX, Berglund L, et al. Low-density lipoprotein cholesterol and the risk of dementia with stroke. *JAMA* 1999; 282(3):254–260.

33. Breteler MM. Vascular risk factors for Alzheimer's disease: An epidemiologic perspective. *Neurobiol Aging* 2000; 21(2):153–160.

34. de Leeuw FE, de Groot JC, Oudkerk M, et al. Hypertension and cerebral white matter lesions in a prospective cohort study. *Brain*. 2002; 125(Pt 4):765–772.

35. Elias MF, Wolf PA, D'Agostino RB, et al. Untreated blood pressure level is inversely related to cognitive functioning: The Framingham Study. *Am J Epidemiol* 1993; 138(6):353–364.

36. Hofman A, Ott A, Breteler MM, et al. Atherosclerosis, apolipoprotein E, and prevalence of dementia and Alzheimer's disease in the Rotterdam Study. *Lancet* 1997; 349(9046):151–154.

37. Juan D, Zhou DH, Li J, et al. A 2-year follow-up study of cigarette smoking and risk of dementia. *Eur J Neurol* 2004; 11(4):277–282.

38. Kivipelto M, Helkala EL, Laakso MP, et al. Apolipoprotein E epsilon4 allele, elevated midlife total cholesterol level, and high midlife systolic blood pressure are independent risk factors for late-life Alzheimer disease. *Ann Intern Med* 2002; 137(3):149–155.

39. Launer LJ, Masaki K, Petrovitch H, et al. The association between midlife blood pressure levels and late-life cognitive function: The Honolulu-Asia Aging Study. *JAMA* 1995; 274(23):1846–1851.

40. Luchsinger JA, Mayeux R. Cardiovascular risk factors and Alzheimer's disease. *Curr Atheroscler Rep* 2004; 6(4):261–266.

41. Luchsinger JA, Tang MX, Shea S, Mayeux R. Hyperinsulinemia and risk of Alzheimer disease. *Neurology* 2004; 63(7):1187–1192.

42. Ott A, Slooter AJ, Hofman A, et al. Smoking and risk of dementia and Alzheimer's disease in a population-based cohort study: The Rotterdam Study. *Lancet* 1998; 351(9119):1840–1843.

43. Ott A, Stolk RP, van Harskamp F, et al. Diabetes mellitus and the risk of dementia: The Rotterdam Study. *Neurology* 1999; 53(9):1937–1942.

44. Razay G, Vreugdenhil A, Wilcock G. The metabolic syndrome and Alzheimer disease. *Arch Neurol* 2007; 64(1):93–96.

45. Reitz C, Luchsinger J, Tang MX, Mayeux R. Effect of smoking and time on cognitive function in the elderly without dementia. *Neurology* 2005; 65(6):870–875.

46. Seshadri S, Beiser A, Selhub J, et al. Plasma homocysteine as a risk factor for dementia and Alzheimer's disease. *N Engl J Med* 2002; 346(7):476–483.

47. Skoog I, Lernfelt B, Landahl S, et al. 15-year longitudinal study of blood pressure and dementia. *Lancet* 1996; 347(9009):1141–1145.

48. Vanhanen M, Koivisto K, Moilanen L, et al. Association of metabolic syndrome with Alzheimer disease: A population-based study. *Neurology* 2006; 67(5):843–847.

49. Esiri MM, Nagy Z, Smith MZ, et al. Cerebrovascular disease and threshold for dementia in the early stages of Alzheimer's disease. *Lancet* 1999; 354(9182):919–920.

50. Snowdon DA, Greiner LH, Mortimer JA, et al. Brain infarction and the clinical expression of Alzheimer disease: The Nun Study. *JAMA* 1997; 277(10):813–817.

51. Barba R, Martinez-Espinosa S, Rodriguez-Garcia E, et al. Poststroke dementia: Clinical features and risk factors. *Stroke* 2000; 31(7):1494–1501.

52. Slooter AJ, Tang MX, van DC, et al. Apolipoprotein E epsilon4 and the risk of dementia with stroke: A population-based investigation. *JAMA* 1997; 277(10):818–821.

53. Arpa A, del Ser T, Goda G, et al. Apolipoprotein E, angiotensin-converting enzyme and alpha-1-antichymotrypsin genotypes are not associated with post-stroke dementia. *J Neurol Sci* 2003; 210(1–2):77–82.

54. McCarron MO, Delong D, Alberts MJ. APOE genotype as a risk factor for ischemic cerebrovascular disease: A meta-analysis. *Neurology* 1999; 53(6):1308–1311.

55. Greenberg SM, Rebeck GW, Vonsattel JPV, et al. Apolipoprotein E e4 and cerebral hemorrhage associated with amyloid angiopathy. *Ann Neurol* 1995; 38:254–259.

56. Klunk WE, Engler H, Nordberg A, et al. Imaging brain amyloid in Alzheimer's disease with Pittsburgh Compound-B. *Ann Neurol* 2004; 55(3):306–319.

57. Fisher CM. Dementia in cerebral vascular disease. In: JF Toole, RG Siekert, JP Whisnant, eds. *Cerebral Vascular Diseases, Sixth Conference*. New York: Grune & Stratton, 1968:232–236.

58. Tatemichi TK, Paik M, Bagiella E, et al. Risk of dementia after stroke in a hospitalized cohort: Results of a longitudinal study. *Neurology* 1994; 44(10):1885–1891.

59. Serrano S, Domingo J, Rodriguez-Garcia E, et al. Frequency of cognitive impairment without dementia in patients with stroke: A two-year follow-up study. *Stroke* 2006. 2007; 38(1):105–110.

60. Treves TA, Aronovich BD, Bornstein NM, Korczyn AD. Risk of dementia after a first-ever stroke: A 3-year longitudinal study. *Cerebrovasc Dis* 1997; 7:48–52.

61. Srikanth VK, Quinn SJ, Donnan GA, et al. Long-term cognitive transitions, rates of cognitive change, and predictors of incident dementia in a population-based first-ever stroke cohort. *Stroke* 2006; 37(10):2479–2483.

62. Kertesz A, Clydesdale S. Neuropsychological deficits in vascular dementia vs. Alzheimer's disease: Frontal lobe deficits prominent in vascular dementia. *Arch Neurol* 1994; 51(12):1226–1231.

63. Looi JC, Sachdev PS. Differentiation of vascular dementia from AD on neuropsychological tests. *Neurology* 1999; 53(4):670–678.

64. Reitz C, Luchsinger JA, Tang MX, et al. Stroke and memory performance in elderly persons without dementia. *Arch Neurol* 2006; 63(4):571–576.

65. Stephens S, Kenny RA, Rowan E, et al. Neuropsychological characteristics of mild vascular cognitive impairment and dementia after stroke. *Int J Geriatr Psychiatry* 2004; 19(11):1053–1057.

66. Nordahl CW, Ranganath C, Yonelinas AP, et al. White matter changes compromise prefrontal cortex function in healthy elderly individuals. *J Cogn Neurosci* 2006; 18(3):418–429.

67. Royall DR, Cabello M, Polk MJ. Executive dyscontrol: An important factor affecting the level of care received by older retirees. *J Am Geriatr Soc* 1998; 46(12):1519–1524.

68. Bell-McGinty S, Podell K, Franzen M, et al. Standard measures of executive function in predicting instrumental activities of daily living in older adults. *Int J Geriatr Psychiatry* 2002; 17(9):828–834.

69. Pohjasvaara T, Leskela M, Vataja R, et al. Post-stroke depression, executive dysfunction and functional outcome. *Eur J Neurol* 2002; 9(3):269–275.

70. Rockwood K, Wentzel C, Hachinski V, et al. Prevalence and outcomes of vascular cognitive impairment: Vascular Cognitive Impairment Investigators of the Canadian Study of Health and Aging. *Neurology* 2000; 54(2):447–451.

71. Desmond DW. The neuropsychology of vascular cognitive impairment: Is there a specific cognitive deficit? *J Neurol Sci* 2004; 226(1–2):3–7.

72. Ballard C, Neill D, O'Brien J, et al. Anxiety, depression and psychosis in vascular dementia: Prevalence and associations. *J Affect Disord* 2000; 59(2):97–106.

73. Naarding P, de Koning I, dan Kooten F, et al. Depression in vascular dementia. *Int J Geriatr Psychiatry* 2003; 18(4):325–330.

74. Folstein MF, Folstein SE, McHugh PR. Mini-mental state: A practical method for grading the cognitive state of patients for the clinician. *J Psychiatr Res* 1975; 12(3):189–198.

75. de Koning I, Dippel DW, van Kooten F, Koudstaal PJ. A short screening instrument for poststroke dementia: The R-CAMCOG. *Stroke* 2000; 31(7):1502–1508.

76. de Koning I, van Kooten F, Dippel DW, et al. The CAMCOG: A useful screening instrument for dementia in stroke patients. *Stroke* 1998; 29(10):2080–2086.

77. Hachinski V, Iadecola C, Petersen RC, et al. National Institute of Neurological Disorders and Stroke–Canadian Stroke Network vascular cognitive impairment harmonization standards. *Stroke* 2006; 37(9):2220–2241.

78. Cuesta GM. Cognitive rehabilitation of memory following stroke: Theory, practice, and outcome. *Adv Neurol* 2003; 92:415–421.

79. Majid MJ, Lincoln NB, Weyman N. Cognitive rehabilitation for memory deficits following stroke. *Cochrane Database Syst Rev* 2000(3):CD002293.

80. National clinical guidelines for stroke: A concise update. *Clin Med* 2002; 2(3):231–233.

81. Sacco RL, Adams R, Albers G, et al. Guidelines for prevention of stroke in patients with ischemic stroke or transient ischemic attack: A statement for healthcare professionals from the American Heart Association/American Stroke Association Council on Stroke: Co-sponsored by the Council on Cardiovascular Radiology and Intervention: The American Academy of Neurology affirms the value of this guideline. *Stroke* 2006; 37(2):577–617.

82. Amarenco P, Bogousslavsky J, Callahan AIII, et al. High-dose atorvastatin after stroke or transient ischemic attack. *N Engl J Med* 2006; 355(6):549–559.

83. Dufouil C, Chalmers J, Coskun O, et al. Effects of blood pressure lowering on cerebral white matter hyperintensities in patients with stroke: The PROGRESS (Perindopril Protection Against Recurrent Stroke Study) Magnetic Resonance Imaging Substudy. *Circulation* 2005; 112(11):1644–1650.

84. Tzourio C, Anderson C, Chapman N, et al. Effects of blood pressure lowering with perindopril and indapamide therapy on dementia and cognitive decline in patients with cerebrovascular disease. *Arch Intern Med* 2003; 163(9):1069–1075.

85. Citron M. Strategies for disease modification in Alzheimer's disease. *Nat Rev Neurosci* 2004; 5(9):677–685.

86. Lleo A, Greenberg SM, Growdon JH. Current pharmacotherapy for Alzheimer's disease. *Annu Rev Med* 2006; 57:513–533.

87. Roman GC, Wilkinson DG, Doody RS, et al. Donepezil in vascular dementia: Combined analysis of two large-scale clinical trials. *Dement Geriatr Cogn Disord* 2005; 20(6):338–344.

88. Black S, Roman GC, Geldmacher DS, et al. Efficacy and tolerability of donepezil in vascular dementia: Positive results of a 24-week, multicenter, international, randomized, placebo-controlled clinical trial. *Stroke* 2003; 34(10):2323–2330.

89. Wilkinson D, Doody R, Helme R, et al. Donepezil in vascular dementia: A randomized, placebo-controlled study. *Neurology* 2003; 61(4):479–486.

90. Erkinjuntti T, Kurz A, Gauthier S, et al. Efficacy of galantamine in probable vascular dementia and Zleheimer's disease combined with cerebrovascular disease: A randomised trial. *Lancet* 2002; 359(9314):1283–1290.

91. Orgogozo JM, Rigaud AS, Stoffler A, et al. Efficacy and safety of memantine in patients with mild to moderate vascular dementia: A randomized, placebo-controlled trial (MMM 300). *Stroke* 2002; 33(7):1834–1839.

92. Wilcock G, Mobius HJ, Stoffler A. A double-blind, placebo-controlled multicentre study of memantine in mild to moderate vascular dementia (MMM500). *Int Clin Psychopharmacol* 2002; 17(6):297–305.

93. Chen Y, Guo JJ, Zhan S, Patel NC. Treatment effects of antidepressants in patients with post-stroke depression: A meta-analysis. *Ann Pharmacother* 2006; 40(12):2115–2122.

94. Goldstein LB. Potential effects of common drugs on stroke recovery. *Arch Neurol* 1998; 55(4):454–456.

95. Zorowitz RD, Smout RJ, Gassaway JA, Horn SD. Neurostimulant medication usage during stroke rehabilitation: The Post-Stroke Rehabilitation Outcomes Project (PSROP). *Top Stroke Rehabil* 2005; 12(4):28–36.

96. Turner-Stokes L, Hassan N. Depression after stroke: A review of the evidence base to inform the development of an integrated care pathway. 2. Treatment alternatives. *Clin Rehabil* 2002; 16(3):248–260.

97. Tariot PN, Farlow MR, Grossberg GT, et al. Memantine treatment in patients with moderate to severe Alzheimer disease already receiving donepezil: A randomized controlled trial. *JAMA* 2004; 291(3):317–324.

14 Central Post-Stroke Pain

Fatemeh Milani

P ain is a common symptom among stroke survivors, and may result from several potential causes. These include central nervous system pathology, dysfunction of affected extremities (e.g. peripheral neurogenic or nociceptive pains), or psychogenic pain. The perception of pain itself is also multifaceted, and dependent on the organic as well as affective state of each patient.

Because of the multiple potential causes of pain in stroke survivors, it is imperative that a thorough differential diagnosis be considered, and that the pain is not automatically attributed to central pain syndrome after stroke. Patients with stroke are predisposed to certain primary and secondary conditions that affect their limbs, and that may present with pain after stroke. Some of the more common conditions are listed in Table 14-1. Similarly, one must always consider the possibility that a patient may have more than one reason for his or her pain. In other words, there may be more than one pain-inducing pathology in a single patient.

Central post-stroke pain (CPSP) is defined as pain associated with vascular lesions of the central nervous system. CPSP can cause marked discomfort and distress that may interfere with a patient's full participation in a rehabilitation program, thus impeding functional recovery. As symptoms are often vague and difficult to characterize, the proper diagnosis may be delayed, thereby prolonging patient suffering and further impeding recovery.

HISTORY

Two French neurologists, Dejerine and Roussy, first described post-stroke pain in 1906, naming the condition "thalamic syndrome." Their definition of the syndrome included the following characteristic findings:

1. Mild hemiplegia that improves rapidly
2. Persistent superficial hemi-anesthesia, sometimes replaced by cutaneous hyperesthesia, and always accompanied by marked and persistent impaired deep sensation
3. Mild hemiataxia and more or less complete astereognosis
4. Severe, often intolerable persistent paroxysmal pain affecting the hemiparetic side that does not respond to analgesic treatments and that interferes with sleep
5. Choreoathetoid movements of the involved limbs (1).

In 1969, Cassinari and Pagni suggested that the syndrome could occur following lesions occurring anywhere along the

---

TABLE 14-1

Primary and Secondary Conditions Commonly Causing Pain in the Limbs of Stroke Patients

---

Complex regional pain syndrome (reflex sympathetic dystrophy/shoulder-hand syndrome, as previously known in earlier literature)
Deep venous thrombosis
Arthropathy
Fractures secondary to falls or other trauma
Shoulder impingement syndrome
Shoulder malalignment related to muscle weakness and spasticity
Adhesive capsulitis of the shoulder
Spasticity
Brachial plexus and axillary nerve injuries due to shoulder subluxation or improper handling of involved upper extremity
Heterotopic ossification, especially at the elbow
Compression neuropathy secondary to poor positioning
Decubitus ulcers

---

course of spinothalamic pathways (2). Case reports of post-stroke pain occurring with the lesions of the brain stem, thalamus, subcortical white matter, and even possibly of the cerebral cortex have appeared in the medical literature since the initial description of "thalamic syndrome" (2–8). The term "Central Post-Stroke Pain" (CPSP) is now preferred, given the variety of locations within the brain that may be involved in this syndrome (7, 9).

EPIDEMIOLOGY

Nearly 700,000 Americans suffer from a stroke each year. It is estimated that approximately 8% of stroke patients develop CPSP, with different studies estimating the incidence to be between 2% and 11%. Incidence of CPSP may increase with age, with one report that approximately 11% of stroke patients over the age of 80 develop CPSP (10).

ETIOLOGY

In the thalamus, lesions of the ventral posteromedial (VPM) and ventral posterolateral (VPL) nuclei are commonly associated with central pain (11). These lesions are commonly of vascular origin, but in some cases are neoplastic. Bogousslavsky et al. found that only 3 of 18 patients with thalamic infarcts affecting the ventral posterior nucleus developed CPSP (12). However, in the case of vascular lesions, since multiple sites can cause central pain, the terms "thalamic syndrome" and "pseudo-thalamic pain" are no longer utilized, and are rather placed under the umbrella of central post-stroke pain.

CPSP may occur following lesions at any level in the spino-thalamo-cortical pathway (mainly lateral medulla oblongata, thalamus, posterior limb of internal capsule, cortical and subcortical zones in the post central gyrus and insular region). Either hemorrhagic or ischemic strokes in the spinothalamic cortical pathway may cause CPSP. However, due to the fact that ischemic infarcts are more common than cerebral hemorrhages (85% vs. 15%), most cases of CPSP are seen in patients with infarcts (2, 8, 13).

PATHOPHYSIOLOGY

The exact pathophysiologic mechanism of CPSP is not known, but several potential mechanisms have been proposed. Dejerine & Roussy hypothesized that an irritable focus causes this pain syndrome (1). Boivie proposed that CPSP originates from hyperirritability in surviving cells in a lesion along the pain pathway (spinothalamic, thalamocortical pathways) (13).

CLINICAL PRESENTATION

The onset of pain is immediately after the stroke in about 20% of patients, and develops within the first month post-stroke in an additional 50% of patients. The remaining 30% of patients develop CPSP between one month and three years following the stroke (7).

The affected area varies, ranging from the entirety of the involved side of the body, to a small anatomic area such as the face or hand, or even a small portion of an anatomic location such as a particular portion of the hand, depending on the location of the lesion. Large ventroposterior thalamic or posterior limb of internal capsule lesions can cause hemibody pain. Central pain involving small areas in patients with superficial cortical and subcortical lesions were reported by Mitchel et al (3). The area with sensory loss is almost invariably more extensive than the area with pain. In fact, in some cases with extensive sensory deficits, only a small portion of this area is associated with concomitant pain.

In brainstem lesions, impairments in facial sensation are generally ipsilateral to the lesion, whereas extremity involvement is contralateral, and the distribution of central pain may follow the same pattern.

The pain in CPSP has been described in many different ways, including burning, aching, stabbing, shooting, pricking, lancinating, constricting, crushing, cramping, pins and needles, stings, or pruritus. Pain is experienced as either deep, superficial, or both. Burning sensation is probably the most common type of pain (60%), and is considered a "classic" presentation for this syndrome. However, burning pain is rare in patients with cortical/subcortical lesions (3, 14).

Pain may be continuous or intermittent, with continuous pain being more common. The pain intensity may vary spontaneously, or vary depending on external, internal, or psychological stimuli. There is also variation in the intensity of different forms of central pain in patients experiencing more than one type of pain symptom (13).

An abnormal response to external stimuli, or dysesthesia, is the most common abnormal sensation in patients with CPSP. Central dysesthesia is associated with a delayed onset of symptoms after application of a stimulus, in contrast to dysesthesia due to peripheral nerve pathology, which is immediately perceived. Central dysesthesia most often results in a burning sensation (15, 16).

Bizarre pains and sensations in a stroke patient should alert the clinician to the possibility of CPSP. Hyperalgesia, an exaggerated perception of painful stimuli, is another feature of CPSP, as is hyperesthesia, an exaggerated response to noxious stimuli. A hallmark of CPSP, present in over 50% of patients, is allodynia, the perception of non-painful stimuli as painful. Allodynia may be induced by thermal, tactile stimuli, or by movement in a portion of the overall area affected by pain. In movement allodynia, pain occurs with both active and passive movement of the joints, putting patients at high risk for the development of contractures. Moreover, pain during walking can interfere with ambulation. Muscle pains such as constriction (the sensation of very tight clothing), cramping, and crushing can be very distressing to patients. Visceral pain such as burning pain with urination, rectal pain, and chest pain in the absence of local visceral pathology is very rare (13, 15, 16).

Hypoesthesia, a weaker-than-normal sensory reaction to stimuli, is also common in CPSP. It is reported that about 95% of patients with CPSP have impaired pain and temperature sensations. In a study by Bovie et al. in 1989, it was found that every patient had hypoesthesia to temperature, but that only 50% had hypoesthesia to touch, vibration, and kinesthesia (15).

Autonomic instability is also seen in CPSP. However, it is not clear if it is a manifestation of CPSP, or superimposed reflex sympathetic dystrophy (complex regional pain syndrome type 1). Motor involvement, when present, is mostly mild. Pain is mild in about one-third of affected patients, and moderate to severe in the other two-thirds.

Most patients with CPSP develop two to four different types of painful symptoms, either at the same location or at different parts of an involved area. Apparently, similar lesions in the same area of the central nervous system may cause different pain symptoms in different patients (7). As such, no specific area can be definitively correlated with a particular type of pain. Moreover, there is no algorithm currently available to accurately predict the incidence of CPSP or the type of pain a patient will suffer.

TREATMENT

Treatment of CPSP remains a challenge. Most reported treatments for CPSP are based on individual case reports and small case series. It is often necessary to try several different empiric treatments in order to maximize clinical results in each individual patient. Among the best measures of pain intensity is the Visual Analogue Scale, although some stroke patients are not able to use the scale because of language or cognitive deficits. Response to treatment is shown by decrease in pain intensity, or shorter duration of high intensity pain in patients with fluctuating pain intensity. In some cases, improvement can be demonstrated by a reduction in the size of the painful area (17).

Pharmacologic Therapy

The pharmacologic treatment of CPSP is similar to the treatment of peripheral neuropathic pain, with antidepressants and antiepileptics serving as first-line agents.

Antidepressants. Tricyclic antidepressants (TCAs) inhibit neuronal reuptake of serotonin and noradrenalin. Their mechanism of action is most likely augmentation of endogenous pain inhibitory mechanisms through their noradrenergic effects. The analgesic effects of TCAs start in the second week of administration. The degree of response to each TCA is highly idiosyncratic, but in general the most effective is amitriptyline, followed by nortriptyline, desipramine, maprotiline, and doxepin in order of decreasing efficacy.

In a double-blind, four-week crossover study, 10 of 15 patients with CPSP, with a mean age of 66 years, showed a response to amitriptyline given at a starting dose of 25 mg, increased to a final dose of 75 mg. There was no difference in response to medication between patients with thalamic lesions (5 patients) and those with nonthalamic lesions. A correlation was noted between pain relief and the plasma concentration of amitriptyline, with a level greater than 300 nmol/l associated with a clinical effect. However, they found little correlation between oral dose and plasma level (18).

TCAs have a long half-life, and the entire daily dose can be taken at bedtime to prevent daytime sedation. For amitriptyline, starting doses of 10–25 mg are generally recommended, with 10 mg being preferred in the elderly. The dose should be increased weekly as tolerated, to a target dose of 50–75 mg. Patients should be informed that the effects of TCAs on pain appear to be unrelated to their antidepressant effects. One must also consider that all TCAs have anticholinergic effects that can cause side effects in stroke patients, particularly the more elderly patients. It is the recommendation of the

American Geriatric Society that TCAs be used with caution in patients older than 65 years of age.

Antiepileptics. Antiepileptic drugs (AEDs) decrease pathological neuronal activity by blocking ion channels. These medications have been used frequently in CPSP, even though early studies were not promising. Carbamazepine has continued to be used for CPSP, even though a placebo controlled study of 15 patients showed that, when given in doses up to 800 mg per day, carbamazepine did not provide a statistically significant improvement in pain (18).

Second generation AEDs may be more effective for the treatment of CPSP. Gabapentin, a second generation AED, has been widely utilized for CPSP, but no placebo controlled study has been performed to evaluate its efficacy. Clinical experience suggests that dosages as high as 1000 mg three times daily may be needed to control the pain. Even in high doses, Gabapentin is generally well-tolerated, although patients may experience transient fatigue or lethargy for a day or two following a dosage increase. Higher dosages should be tapered rather than abruptly discontinued.

Lamotrigine, another second generation AED, suppresses the release of glutamate and blocks sodium channels. It has been shown to be effective for CPSP in a randomized placebo-controlled trial of 30 patients treated over an 18-week period. The minimal effective dose was found to be 200 mg per day (19).

Topiramate, which is yet another second generation AED, was studied in seven patients with CPSP refractory to other medications (amitriptyline, lamotrigine, gabapentine, mexiletine), but was found not to be effective (20). However, there are no published studies of the effects of topiramate on CPSP in patients who are not refractory to other medications.

Pregabaline is chemically and structurally similar to gabapentin, though more potent than gabapentin in reducing neuronal calcium currents. Although it has been used for treatment of CPSP, there are no published studies regarding its efficacy.

Local Anesthetics and Antiarrhythmic Medications. Local anesthetic and antiarrhythmic medications have structural similarities to antiepileptic drugs, leading to attempts to use them for CPSP and other neuropathic pain syndromes. Because of their effect on cardiac conduction, these medications are contraindicated in patients with second or third degree atrioventricular (AV) block. In a double-blind, placebo-controlled study, lidocaine was administered intravenously to six patients with chronic CPSP and 10 patients with spinal cold injury with chronic central pain. Moderate or complete pain relief was reported by 69% of patients when receiving lidocaine, as opposed to 38% of patients when receiving placebo. Effects lasted up to 45 minutes (21). However, since lidocaine was administered intravenously, this therapy is not practical for routine clinical use. A subsequent study was performed in which 12 patients were treated with oral mexiletine, based on its structural similarity to lidocaine. Mexiletine was administered for 4 to 12 weeks starting at 200 mg per day, with a maximum dose of 800 mg per day, but no significant beneficial effects on pain were seen (16, 21).

Analgesics. Conventional analgesics, including opioids, are generally ineffective for the treatment of CPSP. Studies by Arner and Meyerson found minimal clinical response to opioids (22). In a double-blind, placebo-controlled study of 15 patients, Attal et al found that intravenous morphine provided decreased pain for up to 120 minutes, but did not provide a significant improvement in evoked pain over placebo, except for brush allodynia (23). In a subsequent study with oral morphine, a high rate of drop-out was noted due to lack of efficacy, and only three patients remained on the medication after one year. As such, it appears that only a small fraction of patients with CPSP demonstrate a significant clinical response to narcotic analgesics. Therefore, other agents should be used as initial therapy, and any trials of narcotic analgesics should be closely monitored for effectiveness, and continued only if clinical efficacy is clearly obtained.

Other Medications. The alpha-2 adrenergic agonist clonidine has not been studied in CPSP, but propranolol, a beta-2 adrenergic receptor antagonist, was found to potentiate the effects of doxepin in an open-label trial of CPSP (24).

A controlled study found that that the opioid antagonist naloxone, given as a 10 mg per day injection, was not superior to placebo (25). Similarly, calcium channel blockers are not effective for pain relief, but may decrease sensations of coldness. Neuroleptics have been tried without benefit, and are best avoided in view of their potential for serious side effects, such as tardive dyskinesia. Regional sympathetic blockade has not shown to provide any long-term benefit in patients with CPSP (13, 17, 26).

Nonpharmacologic Interventions

Rehabilitative Techniques. *Transcutaneous nerve stimulation.* Transcutaneous nerve stimulation (TENS) is used in one of two modes—high frequency (70 to 100 Hz) or low frequency (1 to 4 Hz). In a trial of 15 patients with CPSP, Leijon and Boivie showed significant pain relief in 4 of 15 patients after a trial of high and low frequency TENS (27). Three subjects benefited from ipsilateral high frequency (70 Hz) and low frequency (2 Hz) TENS, and two patients also obtained pain relief with contralateral stimulation. Ipsilateral stimulation provided clinically significant and long-lasting results in 20% of patients, and decreased pain in 40% of patients. However, 30% of patients reported transient increased pain. Considering the mild adverse effects of TENS, a trial is worth considering for patients with CPSP, and treatment should be continued in patients who respond. Note that this treatment should be avoided in patients with a cardiac pacemaker or defibrillator.

Desensitization techniques. Rubbing affected areas with materials of different textures, starting from soft and advancing to rough, for desensitization can be helpful. In addition, the use of contrast baths may be effective for hand desensitization.

Joint contractures prevention. Stroke patients with weakness and spasticity are commonly known to be prone to developing contractures. In addition, CPSP patients with movement allodynia are at high risk for developing joint contractures. In order to prevent increased pain, therapists should grasp affected extremities gently; once the extremity is grasped, the therapist should not change his or her hand location, and should use steady movements without sudden stops and starts. In addition, appropriate splints and orthotics should be utilized to prevent contractures and facilitate appropriate positioning.

Psychological interventions. Patients must be reassured that CPSP is a misperception, and that pain is related to cerebral pathology and not to other diseases or local pathology in other organs. Patients may be trained to use relaxation techniques and self-hypnosis. Biofeedback may also decrease muscle tension and increase limb temperature, improving patient comfort (17, 28).

Surgical Interventions. Surgery is generally not considered until all forms of medical, rehabilitative, and psychological treatment have failed.

Thalamotomy of the ventrobasal complex, post central gyrus cortectomy, and cingulotomy are irrevocable procedures with low probabilities of long-term success. Moreover, such procedures are frequently complicated by unacceptable morbidity such as new dysesthesias, hemiparesis, cognitive deficits, and even death. In the present era, destructive neurosurgery may be excluded as an option.

Deep brain stimulation has been found to be effective in some patients with thalamic pain syndromes. It should be considered in selected patients with severe, treatment-resistant pain.

Spinal cord stimulation increases the level of gamma aminobutyric acid (GABA), which is an inhibitory neurotransmitter. It can be considered in patients in whom pain is localized to a single limb. However, Tasker, based on patients' responses and review of the literature, reached the conclusion that spinal cord stimulation was not beneficial enough to be routinely recommended for central pain (8).

Chronic sub-threshold stimulation of the motor cortex in seven patients resulted in excellent or good pain control in all patients (29). Stimulation is directed to the area of the motor cortex that controls function in the involved limb(s). The observation that clinically effective stimulation does not produce muscle contraction suggests that the mechanism involves activation of cortical interneurons rather than pyramidal tract neurons.

Duration of Therapy

The duration of therapy should be tailored to each individual patient. In general, if a treatment results in resolution or significant improvement in pain, the treatment regimen should be maintained for at least a six-month period. Thereafter, gradual tapering of medications should be attempted. If pain recurs, the previous regimen should be immediately resumed. When devising long-term treatments, one must consider the fact that many patients will require life-long treatment (17).

CONCLUSION

CPSP develops in between 2% and 11% of patients suffering stroke. The condition can be extremely distressing and debilitating, and may interfere with rehabilitation and recovery following a stroke. Recognition of this condition, and differentiation from other causes of pain in a stroke patient, are crucial for a physician managing patients during the post-stroke period. Appropriate medical and rehabilitative care can minimize the symptoms and impact of this condition on patients with CPSP. Future studies may better define the etiology and pathogenesis of this condition. Pharmacologic and other medical advances may improve therapeutic outcomes, while reducing the morbidity and adverse effects of current treatments.

References

1. Dejerne J., Roussy G. Le Syndrome Thalamique. *Revue Neurologique* 1906; 14:521–523.
2. Cassinari V, Pagni CA. *Central Pain. A Neurological Survey*, Cambridge, MS: Harvard University Press, 1969.
3. Mitchel D, Courent B, Conver SP, et.al. Douleurs corticales: Etude clinique, electrophysiologique et topographiede 12 Case. *Revue Neurologique* 1990; 146:405–411.
4. Bowsher D, Leijon G, Thomas KA. Central post stroke pain: Correlation of MRI with clinical pain characteristics and sensory abnormalities. *Neurology* 1998; 51:1352–1358.
5. Davidson C, Schick W. Spontaneous pain and other subjective sensory disturbances: Clinical pathological study. *Neurology* 1935; 34:1204–1237.
6. Schmahmann JD, Leifer D. Parietal pseudothalamic pain syndrome: Clinical features and anatomic correlates. *Archives of Neurology* 1992; 49:1032–1037.
7. Leijon G, Boivie J, Johansson I. Central post stroke pain: Neurological symptoms and pain characteristics. *Pain* 1989; 36:13–25,27–36.
8. Tasker R. Pain resulting from nervous system pathology (central pain). In Bonica JJ, ed. *The Management of Pain*. Philadelphia, PA: Lee A Febiger, 1990. 264–280.

9. Jensen TS, Lenz FA. Central post stroke pain: A challenge for the scientist and the clinician. *Pain* 1995; 61:161–164.

10. Bowsher D. Some population data about Central Post Stroke Pain. *Proc. 9th World Congress Pain* 1999:435. Abstract.

11. Hassler R. Diezentrale systeme des schmerzes. *Acta Neurochirugical* 1960; 8:353–423.

12. Bogousslavsky J, Regli F, Uske A. Thalamic infarcts: Clinical syndromes, etiology and prognosis. *Neurology* 1988; 38:837–848.

13. Boivie J. Central pain. In: Wall PD, Melzack R, eds. *Text Book of Pain*. 3rd ed. London: Churchill Livingstone, 1994. 871–902.

14. Kimyai-Asadi A, Nousari HC, Kimyai-Asadi T, Milani F. Post stroke prutitus. *Stroke* 1999; 30:692.

15. Boivie J, Leijon G, Johansson I. Central post-stroke pain. A study of the mechanisms through analysis of the sensory abnormalities. *Pain* 1989; 37:173–185.

16. Nicholson BD. Evaluation and treatment of central pain syndrome. *Neurology* 2004; 62(Suppl 2):530–536.

17. Bowsher, David. The mangement of central post stroke pain. *Post Grad Med Journal*, 1995; 71:598–604.

18. Leijon G, Boivie, J. Central post stroke pain. A controlled trial of amitriptyline and carbamazepine. *Pain* 1989; 36:27–36.

19. Vestergaard K, Andersen G, Gottrup H, Kristensen BT. Lamotrigine for the post stroke pain: A randomized controlled trial. *Neurology* 2001; 56:184–190.

20. Canavero S, Bonicalzi V, Paolotti, R. Lack of effect of topiramate for central pain. *Neurology* 2002; 58:831–832.

21. Attal N, Gaude V, Barasseur L, et al.Intravenous lidocaine in central pain: A double blind, placebo-controlled, psychophysical study. *Neurology* 2000:54:564–74.

22. Arner S, Meyerson BA. Genuine resistance to opioids—Fact or fiction? *Pain* 1991; 47:116–118.

23. Attal N, Guirimand F, Brasseur L, et al. Effects of IV morphine in central pain: A randomized placebo-controlled study. *Neurology* 2002; 58:554–563.

24. Tourian AY. Narcotic responsive "thalmic" pain treatment with proprarolol and tricyclic antidepressants. *Pain* 1987, suppl. 4:s411.

25. Bainton T, Fox M, Bowsher D, Wells C. A double blind trial of naloxone in central post stroke pain. *Pain* 1992:48.

26. Loh L, Nathan PW, Schott, GD. Pain due to lesion of central nervous system removed by sympathetic block. *British Medical Journal* 1981; 282:1026–1028.

27. Leijon G, Boivie J. Central post stroke pain: The effects of high and low frequency TENS. *Pain* 1989; 38:187–191.

28. Mohr JP, Choi DW, Grotta JG, et al. Pathophysiology, diagnosis and management. In *Text Book of Stroke*, 4th edition. London: Churchill Livingstone, 2004. 1093.

29. Tsubokawa T, Katayama T, Hirayama T, Koyama S. Treatment of thalamic pain by chronic motor cortex stimulation. *Pacing Clin Electrophysiology* 1991; 14(1):131–134.

15 Visual, Ocular Motor, and Vestibular Deficits

David Solomon
Judith E. Goldstein

S trokes commonly impact the ocular, visual, and vestibular systems. The variability and breadth in visual effects alone are remarkable. They include reduced vision, visual field defects, diplopia, pupil abnormalities, eye movement disorders, and cortical blindness. It can be the impact on the visual system alone that causes loss of independence in a given individual. It also may be that a carefully tailored rehabilitative plan of therapy that can be responsible for regaining an active, independent life (1, 2). Despite the potential functional effects from vision loss secondary to stroke, historically, there has not been a systematic treatment approach as is present in language, speech, and motor rehabilitation.

Like most other aspects of the neurologic system, the location and method of the cerebral insult will determine the type and magnitude of the deficits. For the purposes of visual and functional impact, we will restrict this discussion to postchiasmal loss. Approximately 30% of stroke admissions are found to have homonymous hemianopsia or hemineglect (3, 4), and 70% of all hemianopias result from stroke. Hemianopsia is likely the most debilitating and common visual complication of stroke that must be addressed during rehabilitation.

Homonymous hemianopsia can cause significant problems with mobility, driving, navigation, visual exploration, and reading. The impact on the combination of these disabilities make visual recovery and rehabilitation critical for independent living and vocational concerns (5). Without recovery, visual field disorders and visuospatial deficits are associated with an adverse prognosis in outcome studies according to life table analysis (6–8).

Although therapies for speech, language, motor disorders, and cognitive dysfunction are universally accepted and implemented as part of stroke rehabilitation, vision-sensory and oculomotor disorders are still widely neglected. The most likely reason is that rehabilitation strategies in vision have shown limited success (9). They require lengthy therapy of a typically unmotivated cohort and, when successful, often entail a specialized clinical skill set that is not readily accessible in most rehabilitation facilities.

RECOVERY FROM VISUAL SEQUELE

The traditional idea that a lesion to the striate cortex results in total and permanent blindness in corresponding visual field has been challenged. Rather, individuals with occipital lesions may in fact retain certain visual function through subcortical mechanisms (10). The most recent school of thought regarding neurogenesis and neuroplasticity (2) may offer new ground on which to base rehabilitation strategies. Even prior to rehabilitation, however, some individuals with homonymous hemianopsia experience spontaneous visual recovery of vision depending on the underlying pathology (11–12). In less than 10% of cases, individuals with homonymous hemianopsia caused by ischemia fully recover their visual field (13–15). This recovery is largely complete within the first 10 days from the time of stoke. Recovery of a partial defect occurs within the first 48 hours and is typically complete within 10–12 weeks (13–15). The extent of visual recovery negatively correlates with age and other comorbidities. The documented course of recovery shows that vision returns to the affected field in definite stages, starting with perception of light, motion, form, color, and, lastly, stereognosis (16–17). In addition to spontaneous visual improvement, we see improvement from natural compensatory strategies that occur within the visual system; these are likely associated with some degree of cortical reorganization and individual adaptation. This is evident in hemianopic patients where it is thought that cognitive influences alter eye movement patterns. For example, the fixation point in a hemianope may be directed into the blind field, with the theory that this positioning provides more visual information available to the unaffected field. We also see compensatory alterations in saccadic patterns and activity.

KEY AREAS OF VISUAL IMPACT

Visual Acuity (VA)

After stroke, the ultimate, best-corrected acuity, or clarity, will impact an individuals reading and mobility ability, including risk for falls (18). These are important considerations in the rehabilitation plan and prognosis. In one series, 14% of patients had visual impairment that benefited from refractive correction alone (19). After bilateral postchiasmatic lesions, visual acuity often declines with great variability (20). Generally, the more posterior the lesion, the more symmetrical the acuity and visual field loss. With that said, many patients retain good visual acuity after stroke.

Measuring visual acuity (VA) in a stroke patient can be the most challenging of tasks. Because of aphasia and cognitive impairment, it is frequently necessary to deviate from Snellen acuity. Portable charts with numbers can work well, as there are fewer optotypes and verbalization of numbers in aphasic patients often provides better success than letters. Matching characters and tracing can be an effective testing method when detailed explanation can be repeated and reinforced. With severe aphasia, alternatives such as tumbling E, Landolt C, and the Cardiff visual acuity test are helpful in obtaining measurable responses, although correlation to Snellen visual acuities can be poor (21). Line and letter isolation can also help to assist patient focus and limit confusion. It is important to take the necessary time to measure visual acuity and provide a careful trial frame refraction. Improved spectacle correction, whenever possible, can assist with training of visual processing skills, speech and language therapy, and improved safety in activities of daily living. In cases where visual field cuts are also present, it is necessary to distinguish for the patient and family members that spectacles do not eliminate field loss; therefore, many of the problems with mobility and reading will exist even with new glasses.

Homonymous Visual Field Disorders (HVFD)

Although homonymous visual field disorders (HVFD) are not solely vascular in origin, 70% of all occurrences are a result of arterial infarctions (22). The remaining nonstroke causes include head trauma, brain tumor, neurosurgical procedures, and multiple sclerosis (23). Approximately 70% of all HVFD cases are thought to have visual field sparing of five degrees or less (Figure 15-1) (9). This is known as macular or foveal sparing. Significant controversy exists as to whether macular sparing is real, the relevance of it, and whether it represents perimetric artifact. It does not help predict the location of the lesion within the retrochiasmal visual pathway (24–26).

HVFD represents one of the most debilitating causes of impairment after stroke. Effects on mobility and navigation are shown early on. Individuals frequently bump into people, trip over unseen objects, spill when pouring, and may miss half the food on their plate. Visual-motor skills are often impaired because of visual exploratory deficits in the blind and intact hemifield caused by small amplitude saccades and disorganized visual search patterns (6, 27–28).

Reading is the other primary functional complaint frequently reported by patients with HVFD. Parafoveal visual field or, more appropriately, preview area, along with visual acuity have been correlated with impaired reading. For efficient reading, it is necessary to scan ahead using the preview area to assist with planning for rightward reading saccades (29–30). During reading from left to right, the necessary window for fluent reading seems to extend three to four characters to the left of fixation and seven to eleven letter spaces to the right of it. (This can also be translated to five degrees to the right of fixation.) (31). Right-sided loss will typically cause greater reading impairment than left-sided loss, as the former forces reading into the scotoma or blind area and eliminates the possibility of anticipatory scanning. This will limit reading speed (9). This deficit is also known as hemianopic alexia (32). This disorder is evident through

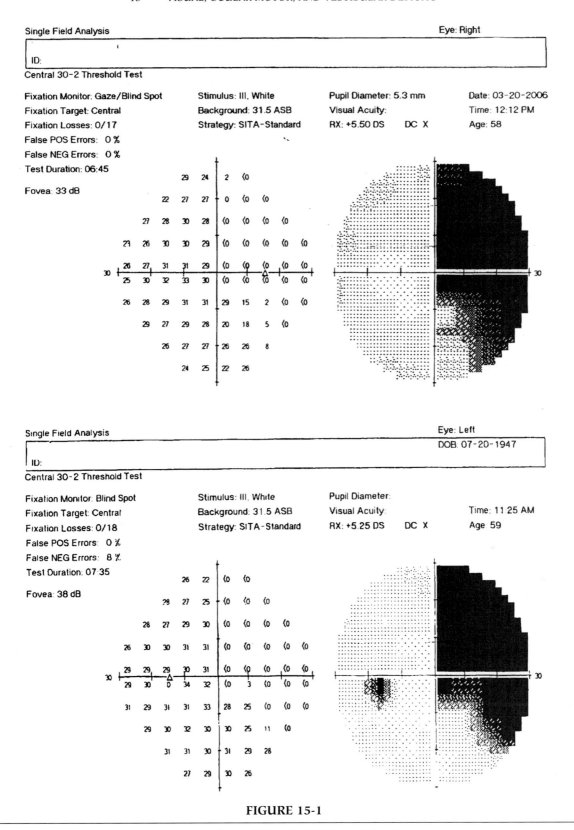

FIGURE 15-1

Incomplete right homonymous hemianopsia in right eye (above) and left eye (below).

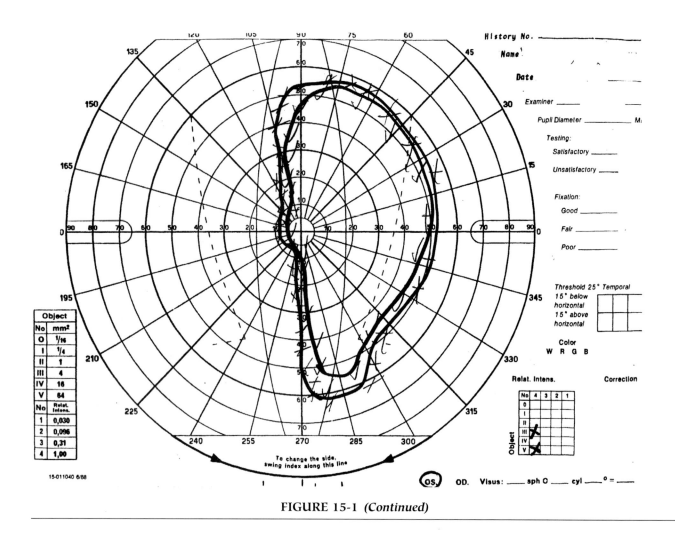

FIGURE 15-1 *(Continued)*

disrupted eye movement scanpaths, prolonged fixations, inappropriate small amplitude saccades to the right, and saccadic regressions (29). Left-sided loss primarily accounts for deficits in omissions in the first letter or word on a line and is often responsible for difficulty with return eye movements to the beginning of a new line of text.

VISUOSPATIAL PERCEPTION DEFICITS

Disorders of perception may be a poor prognostic factor for rehabilitation of stroke outcomes (33–34). One of the most common perceptual deficits is unilateral inattention or visuospatial neglect (VSN). VSN is defined as neglect of relevant visual stimuli when doing activities on the contralesional side (35). It occurs more frequently with right hemispheric lesions, and spontaneous recovery can occur within the first three months, with maximal recovery in the first month (33, 36). It is clear that

deficits in visual space perception create difficulties with orientation, mobility, and visual search. These patients often bump into objects on their left side and can get lost in familiar environments. VSN can be present with and without a HVFD. Presence of both likely points to greater neurologic damage from the stroke and therefore represents an even poorer prognostic indicator for recovery and rehabilitation.

EYE MOVEMENT DISORDERS

Ocular misalignment was found in 28% of cortical stroke patients; however, most of these did not experience double vision (37). Diplopia was reported in 38% of consecutive patients with posterior circulation stroke admitted to a rehabilitation service (38). Although up to 15% of stroke rehabilitation patients have had brain stem involvement, there is a relative lack of research in rehabilitating these cases (39). More

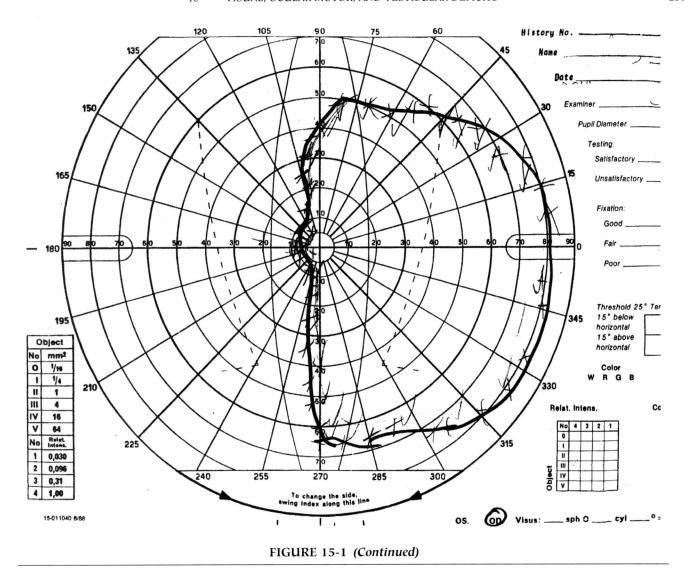

FIGURE 15-1 *(Continued)*

detailed descriptions of posterior circulation oculomotor deficits are provided in Chapter 6. When internuclear ophthalmoplegia is the predominant or only manifestation of a dorsal brain stem stroke, the prognosis is very good (40). Patching of the unaffected eye or placing semi-opaque tape over one of the lenses if the patient uses spectacles can provide symptomatic relief from double vision.

REHABILITATION STRATEGIES

Visual rehabilitative strategies can be divided into compensatory training and restoration therapy. Within these strategies, there exist different technical treatment approaches. As each case is unique, it is necessary to tailor therapy precisely for the individual because of the complexity and variety of effects from stroke. To be successful, these therapies should be implemented in a

task-oriented approach—for example, reading, writing, navigation, and so forth—and hopefully in coordination with other therapies, with the ultimate objective of improving functional outcomes at the goal level, that is, independent living, socialization, transportation, and so forth.

Decreased Visual Acuity and Optical Approaches

Decreased VA may exacerbate the impact of other impairments on overall disability (41). Initially, every effort should be made by the inpatient team to ensure that stroke patients have and wear their glasses. Objective and subjective, when possible, refractions through a trial frame should be performed to ensure best-lens correction is obtained. Although refraction will not address postchiasmal HVFD loss, it is not uncommon to find that these patients were not maximally optically refracted in their distance or near correction prior to the stroke.

To assist with clarity at near, a stronger, added power in the bifocal along with a directed, well-placed light source and appropriate material positioning may suffice. Consideration, however, must be given to the effect of bifocal use when navigation is already impaired from visual field and gait effects. Separate spectacles for mobility and reading may be the most advantageous regarding safety, although cognition and memory loss may limit possibilities. The use of low vision aids incorporating magnification can be of some assistance, depending on the severity of loss and the presence or absence of HVFD. Moderate-powered reading lenses and magnifiers may be of use for spot reading purposes, for example, mail, bills, and medicine bottles, understanding that, if a HVFD is present, tracking and fixation may complicate continuous reading. Video magnifiers, or closed-circuit television (CCTV) provides magnification and enhanced contrast of print material such as black writing on a white background. Additionally, as compared to spectacles and magnifiers, a greater field of view and viewing distance can be obtained. Video magnification is also now manufactured in a portable fashion, providing greater flexibility for affected individuals, especially those returning to work. These devices also have the ability to adjust color and contrast of print. Some of the devices also can provide moving or scrolling text, which can be of benefit in improving reading speed (42).

Technology has advanced to the degree that visual and auditory support through screen reading can enable restoration of function. Specialized software applications, such as Zoom Text Kurzweil 1000, now provide magnification of computer screen information, including both icons and text. The speech output component can read documents at varying speeds, like e-mail and Web pages. Handheld, portable speech output systems, such as Kurzweil NFB Reader, provide total auditory output of scanned text with the advantage of portability. These approaches can be most effective in cases where the functional reserve from vision is limited and auditory processing should be the primarily learning modality. In a vocational environment, this can reduce fatigue and increase work efficiency in a visually impaired individual.

Focused lighting and proper illumination is another treatment strategy that is often overlooked in the performance of activities of daily living, especially reading. Several types of lighting are now available, including full-spectrum, high-intensity, and halogen. Careful selection of appropriate lighting can be useful in the overall improvement of daily functioning, including reading, while being mindful of the negative effect of glare.

Optical Treatments in Homonymous Hemianopia

Optical approaches have shown mixed results in their treatment effects. The optical approach is either to relocate the field of view of the visual image or to expand field of view (43). The goal in the former is to take visual information present in the affected portion of the field and transfer it for processing in the functioning area of the field. The limitation in this approach is that a previous visible portion of the field is now unseen. Essentially, the relocation simply shifts the visual space, trading one scotoma (area of field loss) for another. This may be effective in training certain tasks, such as neglect and awareness, but field expansion is certainly the preferable option of the two. Both approaches are aimed at improving mobility, navigation, and awareness rather than reading.

Optical Field Relocation. Prisms and mirrors work by displacing the image from the nonseeing area to the seeing. A small dental mirror can be soldered to a padded tie clip and mounted nasally onto the spectacle plane in right or left orientation. This provides a larger angle compensation for the HVFD, as the patient can see the reflection of objects from the affected field (44). Significant limitations to this approach include dealing with the reversed image, exaggerated image movement, and cosmesis. Partially reflecting mirrors (beam splitters) and dichroic mirrors provide some improvement; however, many of the disadvantages continue to make them a less than satisfactory and uncommon treatment approach (45).

Full-diameter binocular prisms, or yoked prisms, have been used to shift the visual space and can be useful for both distance and near tasks such as mobility and reading. Typically, a prism of approximately 10–20 dioptors with the base toward the defect can be placed in training goggles or ground into spectacles, causing shifting of the image by five to ten degrees respectively into the seeing field. Different amounts of prism may be required for different tasks. This technique assumes that patients do not neutralize the effect by making compensatory eye movements of five to ten degrees. The effect of prism on individuals with normal vision and hemineglect suggest that some compensation and perhaps adaptation does take place (46–47). By using the prisms binocularly, diplopia is avoided; however, the beneficial effect on activities of daily living from yoked prisms is uncertain and not sustainable.

Binocular sector prisms work similarly to yoked prisms in that they shift the field of view. This approach reduces the amplitude of the scanning eye movements into the area of visual loss, as opposed to increasing awareness of the visual field (44). Rather than full-diameter placement, the prism is only placed on the hemianopic half of the spectacle consistent with the affected HVFD. Fresnel press-on prisms (12–18 dioptors) are typically used, as they are inexpensive and fairly easy to modify based on the patient responses. Prism placement should be as close to the visual axis as possible without impairing central acuity. As the patient scans into the area of field loss/ prism, everything is shifted into the seeing field, thereby lessening the need for large-amplitude saccades into the affected field. Once the object of interest is viewed through the prism, head movement is initiated to return sight of the object through the seeing field. Therefore, the intention of the prism is to spot objects in the blind field, reorient head positioning, and then view through the unaffected field. The limitations in this treatment strategy is that it requires intentional, self-directed scanning into the affected field/prism, which can be difficult in patients with neglect and cognitive impairment, and the scotoma induced by the prism jump at the transition of lens into prism, causing the jack-in-the-box phenomenon, which can be disconcerting to the patient (1). In one clinical trial using fresnel binocularly in stroke patients with HVFD or unilateral visual neglect, improvement of visual perceptual test scores were evident; however, they did not generalize to improvement in activities of daily living (4).

Optical Expansion of Field. Monocular sector prisms expand the field of view as scanning occurs into the blind field. The fresnel prisms are placed in a very similar fashion to the binocular prisms, except that only one lens is fitted and typically higher amounts of prism are used, 30 dioptors and greater (48–49). When gaze enters the affected field and prism, intentional confusion and diplopia result such that the patient appreciates the presence of an object that typically would not be visible because of the HVFD. Although diplopia can be lessened to be just off the visual axis, the confusion can still be bothersome. It is both the confusion and diplopia that make this treatment strategy less than desirable and should be avoided in cognitively impaired individuals.

A more promising approach to field expansion is through monocular sector prisms that are restricted to the peripheral field (superior, inferior, or both) of the lens and avoid central diplopia (43). A fairly new optical approach of field expansion incorporates the concept of vision multiplexing (50). Vision multiplexing refers to the transmission of two or more signals simultaneously in ways that permit these functionalities to be both separable and practical to the user. The peripheral prism of 40 dioptors is placed monocularly with base in the direction of the HVFD across the vertical midline of the spectacle lens above and below the visual axis so it can be effective in all lateral positions of gaze (Figure 15-2). The prism expands the field approximately 20 degrees by inducing peripheral diplopia by optically creating a peripheral exotropia. Central visual alignment is unaffected. This

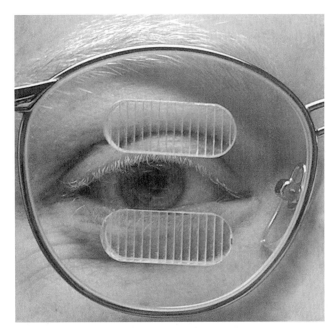

FIGURE 15-2

Prism correction for a right hemianopia. The prisms are worn only over the right eye. This depicts permanent prism placement, however temporary. Fresnel prisms are used during the extensive diagnostic and training period.

is typically less disturbing compared to other optical treatment modalities, as peripheral physiological diplopia occurs in normal vision and is rarely bothersome because of lack of attention to peripheral objects (51).

Field of view expansion with these prisms has been measured on binocular perimetric testing and shown improvement (43). Essentially, objects are detected through the peripheral prism, and vertical head movement is then initiated to sight the object through the carrier lens of the spectacle for clarity and accuracy of spatial positioning. Practically, the prisms enable individuals increased detection of obstacles above and below the line of sight, such as open cabinets or a trash can on the floor. Additionally, with improved mobility in unfamiliar situations, we would anticipate improvement in activities of daily living, increased confidence, and greater independence. Like all optical relocation and expansion strategies, vision multiplexing also requires good cognition as well as patient motivation and training.

Orientation and Mobility Training in Homonymous Hemianopia

When mobility is severely affected by field loss, cane use and sighted guide techniques can be considered effective rehabilitation strategies. In many cases over time, the mobility domain improves. Individuals who were once bumping into things subjectively report improvement with time. How much is related to the development of scanning strategies accommodating the change in visual input or the increased dependency on familiar environments reducing the chance of an incident is unknown. In most instances, hemianopia leads to a cessation in driving; therefore, individuals are typically accompanied on trips outside the home (See Chapter 43). Along with scanning and saccadic training, wall-trailing techniques, holding a partner's elbow or hand, cane-tapping, receiving verbal cues, and so forth can be effective in reducing the incidence of mishaps and falls caused by the visual impairment.

Restorative Approaches in Homonymous Hemianopia

HVFD restoration is rare beyond spontaneous improvement within the first one to three months. Factors predictive of visual field recovery are incomplete lesions, a shallow gradient in the profile of light sensitivity in perimetry and amblyopic transition zones, residual metabolism in the lesioned striate cortex, or activations on functional (f)MRI (52–55). fMRI studies also indicate that function in the blind fields may be mediated by extrageniculostriate pathways projecting to subcortical structures, including the superior colliculus and the pulvinar and ultimately to the ipsilesional extrastriate cortex via tecto-tectal pathways (56–57). Other recent fMRI studies have shown—via forced choice discrimination of facial expressions projected into the blind field—that unconscious emotional expression via the amygdala was expressed (58). The theory of residual visual function when the geniculostriate pathway has been damaged is termed as blindsight (10). In the future, fMRI or some similar tool may be the basis in determining on who best to initiate therapy and what type of therapy would be most beneficial.

Without fMRI yet in practical therapeutic use, different rehabilitative approaches have, at best, achieved visual field enlargement on average of five degrees through visual field training. There have been individual cases with remarkable recovery, but this is not the norm effect from training. It has been suggested that the factors predictive for recovery as mentioned above are likely responsible for the cases of recovery beyond the average. There are primarily two strategies clinically used for restorative field expansion: systematic practice of saccadic eye movements to improve visual scanning capabilities as well as light stimulation of the visual field border.

Saccadic Training Treatment for Visual Exploration. Patients with HVFD show disordered and slowed visual search in their blind hemifield. Their oculomotor behavior reveals less regular and accurate saccades directed

toward the affected side and an increase in the number of fixations (59). Various fixation and saccade parameters seem to correlate with increasing lesion age, but not its location or size. This may reflect the evolution of a compensatory eye movement strategy (60–61). 40% of hemianopic patients show dysfunction in saccadic activity, number of fixations, and, ultimately, scanpaths found in both the blind field and unaffected field, leading to longer search times (59). Scanpaths are series of saccades and fixations undertaken when viewing a structured scene. Functionally, this translates to both difficulties with navigation and visual exploration tasks, such as driving, crossing the street, bumping into objects, and finding objects on a table.

Systematic training of saccadic eye movement strategies does seem to provide valuable compensatory techniques, which transfers to improvement in ADLs (28). Treatment often includes a series of steps to improve the oculomotor function:

1. Training first with quick, large amplitude (30–40 degree) saccades into the scotoma
2. Systematic training on visual search tasks (that is, row by row or column by column)
3. Transfer of strategies into natural situations

Magnitude of improvement in visual search gain as evidence by decreases in search time, number of fixations, and lengths of scanpaths in both the intact and affected field cannot be justified completely by expansion of visual field that typically averages 6.7 degrees in 30–50% of patients (28). Of interest, head movements during eye movement training appear to not be of any benefit and perhaps delays rehabilitative progress (61–62). No differences in visual search effects have been found between the deliveries of early or late visual training, as has been shown for aphasia rehabilitation (28).

Positive treatment factors are pure occipital lesions without parietal or thalamic involvement and a good awareness of the scotoma and its effects on ADLs. Patients with VSN and cognitive impairment will likely have a more difficult rehabilitation course.

Saccadic Training Treatment for Reading. Reading difficulty in hemianopes is proportional to the extent of visual field loss and seems to correlate with the side of loss. In left-to-right reading, right homonymous hemianopes typically require more therapy than left, as these individuals are reading into their scotoma or blind area and do not have the anticipatory scanning-ahead capability necessary for efficient reading (63). This preview ability of seeing the shape and location of ensuing words allows for planning of reading saccades. Self-reported complaints are sometimes vague, including "I can't read like I used to" or frequent loss of place during reading.

During examination, patients will often be able to read a few lines of text without difficulty, thereby confusing the examiner as the findings do not appear consistent with the patient complaints. In many cases, it appears that the functional reserve is not adequate for prolonged reading, and fatigue ensues early on. Because of limitations in field recovery, we are reliant on rehabilitation strategies for reading.

Once maximal correction, low-vision aids, and lighting have been addressed, treatment involves compensatory training of eye movements with the objective of improving saccadic activity and decreasing reading errors:

- Reading of short, high-frequency words requiring few fixations
- Reading of increased word length and complexity
- Reading of numbers
- Transfer to reading material of importance to individual (books, magazines, computer, and so forth)

A clinical trial incorporating optokinetic therapy using moving text (right to left) in patients with hemianopic alexia is another training strategy to improve saccadic activity and reading speed (42).

Other effective strategies include using an L-shaped ruler in left-sided hemianopes to maintain place during reading and assist with appropriately returning eye movements to the next line of text. This can be also be accomplished by using finger placement on the left and right side of a column to limit omissions and loss of place. Typoscopes (a black card with a cutout for a line of text) can also facilitate tracking when glare or contrast is a complicating factor. Turning a book or document 45 to 90 degrees can be remarkably effective in moving the print into the unaffected field. In these cases, patients may read up or down, avoiding the scotoma. Therapy can improve reading speed and accuracy by enhancing oculomotor and compensatory strategies, which can generate small amounts of visual field recovery (64). Patients with homonymous hemianopia frequently do not return to their prehemianopic reading ability.

Visual Restoration Treatment (VRT). Since the advent of blindsight theory, the concept of visual restoration therapy (VRT) became more plausible; however, how much visual field restoration can actually be obtained after hemianopia is still uncertain. Some studies that repeatedly presented light stimuli at the visual field border did not exceed more than five degrees of visual field expansion in most cases (52, 65). It has been suggested that a minimum number of surviving neurons, of the order of 10%, may provide a sufficient substrate for visual recovery (66–67). However, intense controversy still exists over whether any training can be effectively used to provide visual field expansion.

A computerized software company, Nova Vision, offers VRT for treatment of visual field defects caused by optic nerve diseases and postchiasmal brain lesions. This technique operates through the stimulation of transition zone, or residual vision, evidenced by relative visual field defects (66). Once patients are determined appropriate for therapy through diagnostic testing, as evidenced by visual field deficits, that is, hemianopia and quandrantanopia, in-home computer therapy can be initiated. Patients undergo computerized stimulation perimetry in the home six days per week for an hour a day for six months. According to NovaVision, in postchiasmal disorders, the VRT sites improved perimetric performance in 30% of patients and scotoma border shift of 4.9 degrees. The appeal of the VRT is its ease of access as patients can perform the treatment at home, likely making compliance of therapy greater as compared to other treatment modalities.

VRT has significant limitations in its reliability data of fixation controls, false positives, and false negatives. VRT uses high-resolution perimetry to measure improvement changes in visual field. During an independent study using scanning laser ophthalmoscopy combined with microperimetry, no improvement in the absolute visual field border could be detected after VRT (68). It is still unclear whether frequent saccades toward the blind field or a raised level of attention is accounting for the reported expansion in visual field by Nova Vision studies (69). Despite the minimal evidence in significant visual field expansion with VRT, the subjective self-reported improvements in visual function were on the order of 72%, compared to 17% in the placebo group. Whether the subjective improvements are caused by the compensatory exploratory saccadic movements, increased attention, or something unique to VRT, this remains unknown. What is clear, however, is that both visual field expansion and patient-reported outcome measures should be considered when evaluating any rehabilitative therapy.

VESTIBULAR REHABILITATION AFTER STROKE

It is not possible to cover the field of vestibular rehabilitation in this chapter. Excellent textbooks have been written on the subject and deserve careful study. Rather, in this chapter, we will highlight the principles underlying recovery from vestibular injury and the impact that changes in vestibular function have on patients. First, we describe the types of symptoms and deficits that occur with lesions of the vestibular apparatus and central connections. Mechanisms of central compensation are discussed, including changes in neuronal firing that rebalances activity in the vestibular nuclei and mechanisms that restore dynamic vestibular function. Syndromes of neglect, while not caused by vestibular injury, may be transiently reversed by vestibular stimulation. Damage to pathways carrying graviceptive vestibular information can cause postural imbalance and visual misperception. Finally, discussion of diagnosis and treatment of benign paroxysmal positional vertigo is included because of the prevalence of this condition in the relevant stroke population.

It is important to emphasize that vestibular function is not synonymous with activity in the peripheral labyrinth of the inner ear. The perception of motion is unique among the senses in that it is multimodal. That is, visual stimuli can cause a feeling of movement indistinguishable from actual head acceleration, for example, feeling one's automobile is moving in reverse when a nearby bus begins moving forward. Auditory and somatosensory signals can similarly induce a sense of motion (vection).

Damage to peripheral and central vestibular structures can result in vertigo, postural imbalance, gait unsteadiness, oscillopsia (perceived movement of the visual scene), or disorientation. Oscillopsia that only occurs with head movement is usually caused by bilateral vestibular loss (70). When oscillopsia is present without head movement, it is generally caused by nystagmus or ocular oscillations.

Although the term *stroke* is generally reserved for infarction of central nervous system structures, identical mechanisms and blood vessels are involved when ischemia occurs in the vestibular labyrinth (71). The entire blood supply to the inner ear comes from the labyrinthine artery, a branch of the anterior inferior cerebellar artery (AICA). The syndrome of AICA stroke includes hearing loss, unilateral peripheral vestibular loss, facial numbness, as well as ipsilateral cerebellar ataxia (72). Vertigo and hearing loss can be the sole manifestation of AICA stroke, and ischemic lesions of the lateral pons at the root entry zone can mimic peripheral lesions (73). Rarely, vertigo can arise from stroke in the anterior circulation as well (74). Hemispheric stroke can affect the vestibular-ocular reflex, and the degree of involvement correlates with disequilibrium (75).

Vertigo is best understood as arising from an asymmetry in vestibular function. Unilateral vestibular loss (UVL), caused by a VIII nerve or labyrinthine lesion, can account for a range of acute symptoms and signs, including nystagmus, nausea and vomiting, vertigo, and imbalance. Central nervous system compensatory mechanisms must operate to balance and recalibrate the system after unilateral injury. A lesion that results in an imbalance between vestibular information from each side presents unique challenges to the central nervous system. In some ways, this may be analogous to the idea that hemineglect syndromes may arise because of a competition in directing attention to one or the other side. In order for postural balance to be restored, a neuronal balance must

be achieved within the vestibular nuclei. Very early after a unilateral lesion, transcription events occur, leading to a restoration of spontaneous firing on the damaged side. In rodent models, evidence of immediate early gene expression (Fos-like immunoreactivity) peaks as early as two hours after a lesion and is differentially expressed predominantly in the ipsilateral vestibular nuclei and contralateral inferior olive (76–77). Symmetric activity is increased in locus coeruleus, autonomic nuclei, and other reticular-related nuclei (78). Some pontine and medullary nuclei also show a second peak in Fos expression between one and seven days postlesion. These two phases of transcription in animal models correspond temporally with the early restoration of static balance and later adaptive mechanisms underlying dynamic recovery, respectively. This mechanism is remarkable. The central nervous system automatically adjusts for the presence of an acute lesion in order to restore function. Whereas recovery of paretic limb motor function involves recruitment of alternative pathways, in the vestibular system, there is evidence of repair occurring within hours of the lesion, which does not require any external inputs or stimuli (79).

The cerebellum is very important in modulation of vestibular function, and, when the cerebellum is affected by the stroke, vestibular rehabilitation is less effective (80). For patients who do not recover normal walking trajectory after appropriate physical therapy intervention, wearing a shoe with a built-in wedge under the lateral aspect of the ipsilesional foot can improve the ability to walk in a straight path (81).

Recovery Symptoms

A unique aspect of vestibular injury is that symptoms occur even during the recovery of function. Unlike recovery from a hemiparesis, patients who have some return of vestibular function often become symptomatic. A recovery in limb strength is always a good thing, while any change in peripheral vestibular function presents an additional challenge to the central nervous system, which needs to adapt to a moving baseline. The reason for this difference is that the vestibular system operates by comparing information from both sides in making a determination of how the head is oriented or moving through space. This push-pull arrangement has certain advantages. If labyrinthine function is completely lost on one side, the intact ear is still able to signal rotation in both directions because each side is capable of both in addition and excitation.

Acutely, a loss of function on one side is interpreted by the brain as rotation toward the intact side, accounting for the symptoms of vertigo and vestibulospinal manifestations of falling and veering toward the lesioned side. Early on, mechanisms are brought into play, which even out the activity in the brain stem vestibular nuclei so that the nystagmus and vertigo are decreased. The first response is to inhibit the function of the intact side so that the asymmetry is decreased. This is also the action of many of the medications used appropriately during the acute phase of the illness. Vestibular suppressant therapy, however, should be limited because, ultimately, the goal would be to maximize utilization of the remaining function rather than inhibiting it.

Once the nervous system has responded to the initial loss of peripheral function, a second phase of compensation requires an error signal to recalibrate the system under the new postinjury conditions. Two aspects of this compensation process are worth discussing. The first is adaptation, in which an overall decreased sensory signal can be used to drive a normal motor response. A common example of this process occurs when one is prescribed a new spectacle correction; there is a brief period of disorientation before the vestibular ocular reflex can be appropriately recalibrated for the new degree of lens-induced magnification or reduction of the size of visual field. The second aspect of compensation is habituation. By this, we mean the reduction of symptoms that result from a mismatch between the expected to sensory input from a given movement and the postinjury absent, or reduced, response.

Vestibular Effects on Cortical Processes

The vestibular system is important in navigation and spatial memory, domains that also have been localized to the hippocampus. The link between vestibular information and cognitive mechanisms underlying spatial memory and processing has been demonstrated using quantitative volumetric MRI imaging. Patients who have chronic bilateral peripheral vestibular loss were found to have a significant 16.9% decrease in hippocampal volume compared to controls. In addition to this selective atrophy of the hippocampus, these individuals also showed a deficit in performing a virtual navigation and spatial memory task, though general memory function was unaffected. A remarkable aspect of this study was that an intact vestibular system was required for performing a virtual task that did not involve any actual head or body motion (82).

Caloric stimulation of the labyrinth has also been demonstrated to transiently ameliorate left-sided visual neglect after right hemispheric stroke (83–84). A patient with left brain damage, however, also showed a transient remission in right-sided hemianesthesia after caloric stimulation (85).

VESTIBULAR REHABILITATION THERAPY

An individualized therapy program has been found to be most effective when treating patients in need of vestibular rehabilitation. In most cases, there is no one-size-fits-all approach. Each patient may have a predisposition toward relying upon one or another sensory modality (vision or somatosensation), or he or she may adapt a different motor strategy (walking slower, widening the base of support, and so forth). Early strategies used to cope with aberrant vestibular information can result in sensorimotor reorganization that is maladaptive in the chronic phase of the illness. Fear of instability leads to a slowing of gait and an overreliance on visual and somatosensory cues. Moreover, poor self-efficacy for falls that may follow stroke with vestibular symptomatology can be associated with dramatically reduced free living ambulatory activity and can discourage participation in rehabilitation. (See Chapter 28.) Hence, attention to vestibular symptoms and awareness of their impact on basic mobility function is critical for rehabilitation planning. Individuals with asymmetric vestibular stimulation will deviate from their intended path more when walking slowly than when running (86).

Standard vestibular therapy consists of a customized treatment program designed on the clinical examination and has demonstrated efficacy in improving balance and reducing dizziness (87). In addition to the usual methods to address strengthening and flexibility, activities emphasize the use of visual and somatosensory pathways to compensate for the vestibular deficit. Rehabilitation strategies tend to be customized to individual patients but devised according to rational principles. Habituation exercises are used to facilitate central nervous system tolerance of conflicting or novel sensory stimuli resulting from head motion (88). Postural control exercises are used to retrain the balance system, and general conditioning activities are included when appropriate (89). To avoid conflicting sensory information, patients frequently restrict their head movements. When there is a vestibular asymmetry, adaptation exercises are added to calibrate the relationship between labyrinthine signals as well as vestibular ocular and vestibulospinal motor commands. When there is bilateral vestibular loss, substitution exercises are indicated to promote the use of alternative strategies for gaze and posture control, utilizing visual and somatosensory information.

Although the signs and symptoms that occur without movement (spontaneous nystagmus and vegetative symptoms) resolve independently without intervention, the dynamic instability and head movement-provoked symptoms often require specific, but accessible, treatment (90). In a single-blind, randomized, controlled trial of primary care-delivered treatment, 170 patients with chronic dizziness were randomized to vestibular rehabilitation; the other received usual medical care. The treatment group received just one 30- to 40-minute appointment with a primary care nurse, who instructed the patient in a home exercise program that was reinforced with a treatment booklet and log (available online as an appendix to the article). At three months, there were significantly fewer spontaneous and provoked symptoms of dizziness as well as improved dizziness-related quality of life. Postural stability with eyes open and eyes closed was objectively improved. Benefits were maintained at six months. Clinically significant improvement occurred in 67% of treated patients, while only 38% of the control patients improved (91). For such a program to succeed, however, patients need to be motivated to carry out the exercises, even though they exacerbate the very symptoms targeted by the treatment. Patients must be reassured that they are not causing additional damage. Too often, patients abandon their exercises because, after several weeks of performing them, they still have the same symptoms of dizziness. What they often fail to realize is that they are doing much more activity before experiencing these same symptoms and are thus actually progressing in the therapy.

Patients with central vestibular dysfunction caused by stroke had a significant benefit from a customized treatment program that included balance and gait training, general strengthening and flexibility exercises, utilization of visual and somatosensory information, in addition to adaptation and substitution exercises, depending upon the results of the examination (80). In particular, stroke patients' scores on the Dynamic Gait Index improved by an average of 4.7 points, with a 4.0 point or more change considered clinically significant.

Chronic postural deficits were studied in 40 patients with hemiplegia after a single hemisphere stroke, who were at least 12 months post-stroke, using computerized dynamic posturography (EquiTest) in order to assess their ability to use sensory inputs separately and to effectively suppress inaccurate inputs in case of sensory conflict (92). Hemiplegic patients exhibited excessive sway when visual and somatosensory information were unavailable (eyes closed, sway-referenced support surface, and so forth), and over two-thirds had obvious difficulty when vision conflicted with vestibular information (sway-referenced vision and support surface) (93). Overreliance on visual input in hemiplegic patients was also demonstrated in a task that involved aligning a rod to the vertical when a frame is tilted to the right or left. Hemiplegic patients were twice as likely to be biased by the orientation of the frame when compared to controls (94). Chronic hemiplegic patients demonstrated significant improvement in postural control after they underwent a rehabilitation program, regardless of whether they performed their exercises with or without visual input; however, the vision-deprived group achieved greater improvement, suggesting the possibility that traditional treatment may have reinforced visual overreliance and limited potential benefit from treatment (95). The efficacy of vestibular rehabilitation in patients with abnormal sensory organization was demonstrated in a prospective study in which over half of the patients showed objective improvement in balance function (96). Spectacles used when walking should have lenses with a single-focal length, as use of bifocals or progressive lenses increases the risk of falls (97).

Why Some Patients Do Not Improve Following Vestibular Damage

Several factors that may delay or prevent recovery after vestibular loss include age, activity, medications, mood, fluctuating symptoms, or maladaptive strategies. Patients with vestibular deficits do not like to move their heads. In the case of dynamic symptoms, however, the brain only solves problems with which it is confronted. Several studies point to the importance of early intervention in treating a unilateral vestibular loss. Primates given a peripheral vestibular lesion regained postural and locomotor control much sooner if they were allowed to perform early active motor exploration (90). Cats subjected to motor restriction had a delayed recovery. If a seven-day interval of sensorimotor restriction was applied within the first three weeks of a unilateral vestibular loss, there was a delayed and limited recovery. Complete restoration of postural abilities was never achieved (98).

When patients have only peripheral lesions, vestibular suppressants are recommended only acutely to treat the vegetative symptoms of nausea and vomiting. Patients with vertigo caused by central lesions may benefit from more prolonged pharmacological treatment in combination with vestibular rehabilitation (99).

Graviceptive Pathways

The otolith organs in the vestibular labyrinth detect linear head acceleration. If the head is not moving, these inner ear structures are stimulated only by gravity and therefore provide information about how the head is oriented relative to the earth vertical (tilt) (100). The calcium carbonate crystals embedded in the otoconial membrane serve as the mass upon which gravity acts, resulting in deflection of hair cells and change in firing of primary afferents in the VIII nerve. (These crystals are the culprits in benign paroxysmal positional vertigo, described below.) Damage to the otoliths or their central projections results in components of the ocular tilt reaction, including skew deviation (vertical misalignment of the eyes not caused by muscle palsy), head tilt, and ocular torsion (rotation of the eyes about the line of sight) (101). When the body or head is tilted toward one side, the ipsilateral vestibular labyrinth is excited. Vestibulospinal pathways originating in the lateral vestibular nucleus facilitate ipsilateral extensor motor neurons, constituting the righting reflex. Following a unilateral loss, asymmetry in spinal reflexes results in decreased ipsilesional recruitment and relatively increased extensor activity on the opposite side (102). This contributes to patients' tendency to fall or lean toward the damaged side.

Brain stem strokes can cause lateropulsion of the body toward the side of a lateral medullary stroke or away from the side of a paramedian pontine infarction (103–105). In hemispheric stroke involving the posterolateral thalamus, a different phenomenon termed contraversive pushing may occur (106). This is the tendency for patients to use their nonparetic limbs to force their body away from the side of the stroke toward the paretic side. It was found acutely in up to 10% of acute strokes, without a predilection for right- or left-sided lesions, and its presence was associated with a longer period of time required to functional recovery (107).

Patients with acute unilateral peripheral vestibular lesions misperceive the visual vertical, tending to align a target line toward the side of the labyrinthine loss. When asked to align their bodies with the true upright, however, they performed as well as control subjects (108). By contrast, patients with contraversive pushing considered themselves upright when they were actually tilted 18 degrees toward their unaffected (ipsilesional) side, while their perception of the subjective visual vertical and head orientation were normal (109–110). Other studies, however, do show changes in subjective visual vertical following hemispheric stroke and suggest that its presence may influence balance recovery after stroke (111–112).

Benign Paroxysmal Positional Vertigo (BPPV) (113)

Although ischemia can predispose patients to the development of benign paroxysmal positional vertigo (BPPV), the occurrence of this common condition in the subacute or chronic stroke patient is probably more likely caused by the age of the population and their prolonged immobility. Acute management of stroke often includes maintenance of the head-down position, which could also promote the development of BPPV. It is important to recognize this condition so it is not confused with a recurrence of the patient's cerebrovascular disease. Often, BPPV symptoms are initially attributed to vertebral basilar insufficiency, although a careful history and brief examination is sufficient to distinguish these conditions, sparing the patient further evaluation or transfer from a rehabilitation facility back to an acute care setting. Imbalance and vertigo from BPPV may also interfere with the progress of rehabilitation in the post-stroke population.

Symptoms of BPPV are always brought about by changes in head position with respect to gravity. Rotation of the head, as if the patient is saying "no," when upright is generally the only head movement that does not provoke symptoms. Rolling over or getting in or out of bed and reaching to a high shelf when standing is also

provocative maneuvers. The diagnosis and localization can readily be made using the Dix-Hallpike maneuvers. This begins with the patient seated in the bed with the legs extended. The head is turned 45 degrees to one side, and then the patient is brought into the supine position. Observe the eye movements and query the patient about his or her typical symptoms of vertigo. Maintaining the head turn, the patient is then brought back into the sitting position. The head is turned 45 degrees to the other side, and the procedure is repeated. Generally, symptoms will only develop in the right- or left ear-down position, although bilateral cases do occur. Nystagmus that accompanies the symptoms of vertigo is a mixed-up beating and torsional nystagmus. This can best be observed by watching a scleral blood vessel in either eye. The nystagmus develops several seconds after the head is moved (latency) and usually lasts less than 30 seconds (duration). Although the vertical complement may be suppressed by visual fixation, the torsional nystagmus can be visualized without the use of any specialized equipment. The eyes rotate about the line of sight, and, when BPPV is responsible, the upper poles of the eyes beat toward the ground.

The diagnosis of BPPV is certain if four criteria are met:

- There is a several second latency before the onset of the nystagmus.
- The duration of the nystagmus is less than one minute.
- The nystagmus is elicited only in the appropriate head orientation.
- The direction of nystagmus matches the head position (114).

Treatment is extremely effective and can be performed readily at the bedside using the canalith repositioning procedure (CRP, or Epley maneuver) (115–116). Below is an illustration and instructions for treatment of left posterior semicircular canal benign paroxysmal positional vertigo. For right-sided BPPV, the same procedure would be performed, except the procedure would begin with the head turned to the right and follows in mirrored fashion.

Begin with patient sitting upright with legs extended (Figure 15-3). Turn the head 45 degrees toward the affected ear. This was determined by a positive response (upbeat and torsional nystagmus lasting less than 30 seconds), elicited by placing the patient in the left Dix-Hallpike position (A). Deliberately move the patient into the supine position, maintaining the head turn. Extend the neck just enough so that the downward ear is below the shoulder. Observe for the typical BPPV nystagmus. This is equivalent to a left Dix-Hallpike maneuver (B). Maintain each position for the duration of the nystagmus and symptoms, usually about 30 seconds.

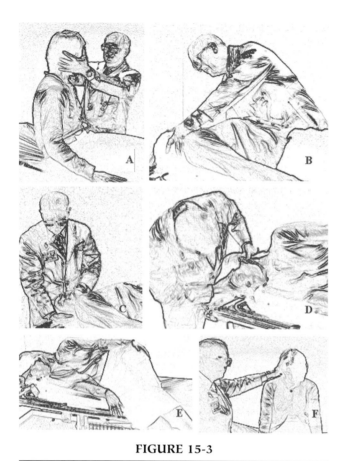

FIGURE 15-3

Canalith repositioning procedure for treatment of left posterior semicircular canal benign paroxysmal positional vertigo.

Unlike Dix-Hallpike testing, during which the patient would be brought back into a seated position, the CRP proceeds with the patient supine. Keeping the neck extended, rotate the head 90 degrees so that the unaffected (right) ear is now pointed 45 degrees downward (C). Rotate the patient's head another 90 degree so the nose is now pointed 45 degrees toward the ground (D). The patient rolls herself or himself into the right lateral decubitus position. Again observe for nystagmus, which should still be upbeat, with the torsional component (upper poles of the eyes) beating toward the affected (left) ear. The presence of nystagmus with a downbeat component indicates an ineffective procedure.

The patient is instructed to bring the knees up toward the chest and drop the legs over the edge of the table while the head is kept in the nose-down position (E). The patient is brought up into the sitting position, keeping the head rotated 45 degrees on the body to the right with the chin down (F). In the upright position, keeping the chin tucked down, the head is rotated straight ahead, and then the patient may assume a normal head position. Hold on to the patient when he or she is brought upright, as vertigo and imbalance may occur. The entire procedure may be repeated as often as necessary until no further nystagmus or symptoms are present. Instruct the patient to keep the head upright (no more than 45 degrees from the vertical) for the remainder of the day in order to inadvertently avoid reintroducing the debris into the semicircular canal. It is not necessary to have the patient sleep sitting up after the procedure.

CONCLUSION

Because of the limited objective evidence of strategic and effective approaches, the decision to treat and type of treatment for patients with visual, ocular motor, and vestibular impairments secondary to stroke needs to be individualized. The associated deficits, level of functional impairment, as well as desired tasks and goals identified by the patient and family must enter into the tailored rehabilitative plan. Recovery of dynamic control of balance and gait after vestibular damage requires exercises that often provoke symptoms of dizziness and should be performed as soon as possible after the stroke. Encouraging normal head movement (like the forced use of the paretic limb) decreases symptoms (habituation) and improves function (adaptation). Visual, vestibular, and somatosensory information can substitute for one another in a variety of tasks, but overreliance on one modality can be maladaptive and should be addressed explicitly in a customized rehabilitation program.

References

1. Nelles G, Esser J, Eckstein A, et al. Compensatory visual field training for patients with hemianopia after stroke. *Neurosci Lett* 2001; 306(3):189–192.
2. Buonomano DV, Merzenich MM. Cortical plasticity: From synapses to maps. *Annu Rev Neurosci* 1998; 21:149–186.
3. Pambakian AL, Kennard C. Can visual function be restored in patients with homonymous hemianopia? *Br J Ophthalmol* 1997; 81(4):324–328.
4. Rossi PW, Kheyfets S, Reding MJ. Fresnel prisms improve visual perception in stroke patients with homonymous hemianopia or unilateral visual neglect. *Neurology* 1990; 40(10):1597–1599.
5. Gianutsos R. In: Gentile M, ed. *A Therapists Guide to Evaluation and Treatment Options.* Vision rehabilitation following acsquired brain injury 267–294. Bethesda, MD: American Occupational Therapist Organization, 1997.
6. Kerkhoff G. Neurovisual rehabilitation: Recent developments and future directions. *J Neurol Neurosurg Psychiatry* 2000; 68(6):691–706.
7. Dombovy ML, Sandok BA, Basford JR. Rehabilitation for stroke: A review. *Stroke* 1986; 17(3):363–369.
8. World Health Organization (WHO). Cerebrovascular diseases: Prevention, treatment, and rehabilitation. *World Health Organization Tech Rep Ser No. 469* 1971:1–57.
9. Kerkhoff G. Restorative and compensatory therapy approaches in cerebral blindness: A review. *Restor Neurol Neurosci* 1999; 15(2–3):255–271.
10. Stoerig P, Cowey A. Blindsight in man and monkey. *Brain* 1997; 120 (Pt 3): 535–559.
11. Riddoch G. Dissociation of visual perceptions due to occipital injuries, with special reference to appreciation of movement. *Brain* 1917; 40:15–57.

12. Hine M. The recovery of fields of vision in concussion injuries of the occipital cortex. *Br J Ophthalmol* 1918; 2:12–25.

13. Gray CS, French JM, Bates D, et al. Recovery of visual fields in acute stroke: Homonymous hemianopia associated with adverse prognosis. *Age Ageing* 1989; 18(6):419–421.

14. Zihl J. Blindsight: Improvement of visually guided eye movements by systematic practice in patients with cerebral blindness. *Neuropsychologia* 1980; 18(1):71–77.

15. Pambakian A, Currie J, Kennard C. Rehabilitation strategies for patients with homonymous visual field defects. *J Neuroophthalmol* 2005; 25(2):136–142.

16. Kolmel HW, Tiel K. Homonymous hemianopsia due to posterior ischemia as a model for quantification of neurologic deficit. *Stroke* 1989; 20(4):559.

17. Kaul S, Du Boulay G, Kendall B, Russel R. Relationship between visual field defect and arterial occlusion in the posterior cerebral circulation. *J Neurol Neurosurg Psychiatry* 1974; 37:1022–1030.

18. Harwood RH. Visual problems and falls. *Age Ageing* 2001; 30 (Suppl 4):13–18.

19. Lotery AJ, Wiggam MI, Jackson AJ, et al. Correctable visual impairment in stroke rehabilitation patients. *Age Ageing* 2000; 29(3):221–222.

20. Frisen L. The neurology of visual acuity. *Brain* 1980; 103(3):639–670.

21. Johansen A, White S, Waraisch P. Screening for visual impairment in older people: Validation of the Cardiff Acuity Test. *Arch Gerontol Geriatr* 2003; 36(3):289–293.

22. Trobe JD, Lorber ML, Schlezinger NS. Isolated homonymous hemianopia: A review of 104 cases. *Arch Ophthalmol* 1973; 89(5):377–381.

23. Zhang X, Kedar S, Lynn MJ, et al. Homonymous hemianopias: Clinical-anatomic correlations in 904 cases. *Neurology* 28 2006; 66(6):906–910.

24. Sugishita M, Hemmi I, Sakuma I, et al. The problem of macular sparing after unilateral occipital lesions. *J Neurol* 1993; 241(1):1–9.

25. Bischoff P, Lang J, Huber A. Macular sparing as a perimetric artifact. *Am J Ophthalmol* 1995; 119(1):72–80.

26. Zhang X, Kedar S, Lynn MJ, et al. Homonymous hemianopia in stroke. *J Neuroophthalmol* 2006; 26(3):180–183.

27. Meienberg O, Zangemeister WH, Rosenberg M, et al. Saccadic eye movement strategies in patients with homonymous hemianopia. *Ann Neurol* 1981; 9(6):537–544.

28. Kerkhoff G, Munssinger U, Meier EK. Neurovisual rehabilitation in cerebral blindness. *Arch Neurol* 1994; 51(5):474–481.

29. Leff AP, Scott SK, Crewes H, et al. Impaired reading in patients with right hemianopia. *Ann Neurol* 2000; 47(2):171–178.

30. Zihl J. Eye movement patterns in hemianopic dyslexia. *Brain* 1995; 118 (4):891–912.

31. Rayner K, McConkie GW, Zola D. Integrating information across eye movements. *Cognit Psychol* 1980; 12(2):206–226.

32. Leff AP, Spitsyna G, Plant GT, Wise RJ. Structural anatomy of pure and hemianopic alexia. *J Neurol Neurosurg Psychiatry* 2006; 77(9):1004–1007.

33. Cassidy TP, Bruce DW, Lewis S, Gray CS. The association of visual field deficits and visuospatial neglect in acute right hemisphere stroke patients. *Age Ageing* 1999; 28(3):257–260.

34. Adams GF. Clinical outlook for stroke patients. *Gerontol Clin (Basel)* 1971; 13(4):181–188.

35. Heilman KM, Watson RT, Valenstein E. In: E HKaV, ed. *Clinical Neuropsychology*. Neglect and related disorders 279–336. Oxford: Oxford University Press, 1993.

36. Meerwaldt JD, van Harskamp F. Spatial disorientation in right hemisphere infarction. *J Neurol Neurosurg Psychiatry* 1982; 45(7):586–590.

37. Fowler MS, Wade DT, Richardson AJ, Stein JF. Squints and diplopia seen after brain damage. *J Neurol* 1996; 243(1):86–90.

38. Teasell R, Foley N, Doherty T, Finestone H. Clinical characteristics of patients with brain stem strokes admitted to a rehabilitation unit. *Arch Phys Med Rehabil* 2002; 83(7):1013–1016.

39. Kruger E, Teasell R, Salter K, et al. The rehabilitation of patients recovering from brain stem strokes: Case studies and clinical considerations. *Top Stroke Rehabil* 2007; 14(5):56–64.

40. Kim JS. Internuclear ophthalmoplegia as an isolated or predominant symptom of brain stem infarction. *Neurology* 2004; 62(9):1491–1496.

41. Kempen GI, Verbrugge LM, Merrill SS, Ormel J. The impact of multiple impairments on disability in community-dwelling older people. *Age Ageing* 1998; 27(5):595–604.

42. Spitzyna GA, Wise RJ, McDonald SA, et al. Optokinetic therapy improves text reading in patients with hemianopic alexia: A controlled trial. *Neurology* 2007; 68(22):1922–1930.

43. Peli E. Field expansion for homonymous hemianopia by optically induced peripheral exotropia. *Optom Vis Sci* 2000; 77(9):453–464.

44. Cohen JM. An overview of enhancement techniques for peripheral field loss. *J Am Optom Assoc* 1993; 64(1):60–70.

45. Duszynski LR. Hemianopsia dichroic mirror device. *Am J Ophthalmol* 1955; 39(6):876–878.

46. Welch RB, Bridgeman B, Anand S, Browman KE. Alternating prism exposure causes dual adaptation and generalization to a novel displacement. *Percept Psychophys* 1993; 54(2):195–204.

47. Rossetti Y, Rode G, Pisella L, et al. Prism adaptation to a rightward optical deviation rehabilitates left hemispatial neglect. *Nature* 1998; 395(6698):166–169.

48. Jose R, Smith A. Increasing peripheral field awareness with Fresnel prisms. *Optical J Rev Optom* 1976; 3:3–37.

49. Gottlieb D, inventor. Method of using a prism in lens for the treatment of visual field loss. US patent Patent [4,779,972], 1988.

50. Peli E. Treating with spectacle lenses: A novel idea!? *Optom Vis Sci* 2002; 79(9):569–580.

51. Bishop P. In: Moses R, ed. *Adler's Physiology of the Eye: Clinical Application*. Binocular vision 575–649. St. Louis: C.V. Mosby, 1981.

52. Zihl J, von Cramon D. Visual field recovery from scotoma in patients with postgeniculate damage: A review of 55 cases. *Brain* 1985; 108 (2):335–365.

53. Bosley TM, Rosenquist AC, Kushner M, et al. Ischemic lesions of the occipital cortex and optic radiations: Positron emission tomography. *Neurology* 1985; 35(4):470–484.

54. Kiyosawa M, Bosley TM, Kushner M, et al. Middle cerebral artery strokes causing homonymous hemianopia: Positron emission tomography. *Ann Neurol* 1990; 28(2):180–183.

55. Miki A, Nakajima T, Fujita M, et al. Functional magnetic resonance imaging in homonymous hemianopsia. *Am J Ophthalmol* 1996; 121(3):258–266.

56. Ptito A, Fortin A, Ptito M. Seeing in the blind hemifield following hemispherectomy. *Prog Brain Res* 2001; 134:367–378.

57. Barbur JL, Watson JD, Frackowiak RS, Zeki S. Conscious visual perception without V1. *Brain* 1993; 116 (6):1293–1302.

58. Morris JS, DeGelder B, Weiskrantz L, Dolan RJ. Differential extrageniculostriate and amygdala responses to presentation of emotional faces in a cortically blind field. *Brain* 2001; 124(6):1241–1252.

59. Zihl J. Visual scanning behavior in patients with homonymous hemianopia. *Neuropsychologia* 1995; 33(3):287–303.

60. Pambakian AL, Wooding DS, Patel N, et al. Scanning the visual world: A study of patients with homonymous hemianopia. *J Neurol Neurosurg Psychiatry* 2000; 69(6):751–759.

61. Kerkhoff G, Mumbinger U, Haaf E. Rehabilitation of homonymous scotomata in patients with postgeniculate damage of the visual system: Saccadic compensation training. *Restorative Neurology and Neuroscience* 1992; 4:245–254.

62. Zangemeister WH, Meienberg O, Stark L, Hoyt WF. Eye-head coordination in homonymous hemianopia. *J Neurol* 1982; 226(4):243–254.

63. Zihl J. Treatment of patients with homonymous visual field disorders. *Z Neuorpsychol* 1990; 2:95–101.

64. Kerkhoff G, MunBinger U, Eberle-Strauss G, Stogerer E. Rehabilitation of hemianopic alexia in patients with postgeniculate visual field disorders. *Neuropsychol Rehabil* 1992; 2:21–42.

65. Zihl J, von Cramon D. Restitution of visual function in patients with cerebral blindness. *J Neurol Neurosurg Psychiatry* 1979; 42(4):312–322.

66. Kasten E, Wust S, Behrens-Baumann W, Sabel BA. Computer-based training for the treatment of partial blindness. *Nat Med* 1998; 4(9):1083–1087.

67. Sabel B, Kasten E, Kreutz M. In: Freund JH SB, Witte OW, ed. *Brain Plasticity*. Recovery of vision after partial visual system injury as a model of postlesion neuroplasticity 251–276. Philadelphia: Lippincott-Raven, 1997.

68. Reinhard J, Schreiber A, Schiefer U, et al. Does visual restitution training change absolute homonymous visual field defects? A fundus controlled study. *Br J Ophthalmol* 2005; 89(1):30–35.

69. Sabel BA, Trauzettel-Klosinksi S. Improving vision in a patient with homonymous hemianopia. *J Neuroophthalmol* 2005; 25(2):143–149.

70. Herdman SJ. In: Herdman SJ, ed. *Vestibular Rehabilitation*. Assessment and management of bilateral vestibular loss 316–330. Philadelphia: F.A. Davis, 1994.

71. Solomon D. Distinguishing and treating causes of central vertigo. *Otolaryngol Clin North Am* 2000; 33(3):579–601.

72. Oas JG, Baloh RW. Vertigo and the anterior inferior cerebellar artery syndrome. *Neurology* 1992; 42(12):2274–2279.

73. Lee H, Ahn BH, Baloh RW. Sudden deafness with vertigo as a sole manifestation of anterior inferior cerebellar artery infarction. *J Neurol Sci* 2004; 222(1–2):105–107.

74. Brandt T, Botzel K, Yousry T, et al. Rotational vertigo in embolic stroke of the vestibular and auditory cortices. *Neurology* 1995; 45(1):42–44.

75. Catz A, Ron S, Solzi P, Korczyn AD. The vestibulo-ocular reflex and dysequilibrium after hemispheric stroke. *Am J Phys Med Rehabil* 1994; 73(1):36–39.

76. Kaufman GD, Shinder ME, Perachio AA. Correlation of fos expression and circling asymmetry during gerbil vestibular compensation. *Brain Res* 1999; 817(1–2):246–255.

77. Darlington CL, Lawlor P, Smith PF, Dragunow M. Temporal relationship between the expression of fos, jun, and krox-24 in the guinea pig vestibular nuclei during the development of vestibular compensation for unilateral vestibular deafferentation. *Brain Res* 1996; 735(1):173–176.

78. Gustave Dit Duflo S, Gestreau C, Tighilet B, Lacour M. Fos expression in the cat brain stem after unilateral vestibular neurectomy. *Brain Res* 3 1999; 824(1):1–17.

79. Darlington CL, Dutia MB, Smith PF. The contribution of the intrinsic excitability of vestibular nucleus neurons to recovery from vestibular damage. *Eur J Neurosci* 2002; 15(11):1719–1727.

80. Brown KE, Whitney SL, Marchetti GF, et al. Physical therapy for central vestibular dysfunction. *Arch Phys Med Rehabil* 2006; 87(1):76–81.

81. Ushio M, Murofushi T, Okita W, et al. The effectiveness of wedge shoes in patients with insufficient vestibular compensation. *Auris Nasus Larynx* 2007; 34(2):155–158.

82. Brandt T, Schautzer F, Hamilton DA, et al. Vestibular loss causes hippocampal atrophy and impaired spatial memory in humans. *Brain* 2005; 128(11):2732–2741.

83. Rubens AB. Caloric stimulation and unilateral visual neglect. *Neurology* 1985; 35(7):1019–1024.

84. Cappa S, Sterzi R, Vallar G, Bisiach E. Remission of hemineglect and anosognosia during vestibular stimulation. *Neuropsychologia* 1987; 25(5):775–782.

85. Bottini G, Paulesu E, Gandola M, et al. Left caloric vestibular stimulation ameliorates right hemianesthesia. *Neurology* 2005; 65(8):1278–1283.

86. Jahn K, Strupp M, Schneider E, et al. Differential effects of vestibular stimulation on walking and running. *Neuroreport* 5 2000; 11(8):1745–1748.

87. Horak FB, Jones-Rycewicz C, Black FO, Shumway-Cook A. Effects of vestibular rehabilitation on dizziness and imbalance. *Otolaryngology - Head & Neck Surgery* 1992; 106:175–180.

88. Telian SA, Shepard NT, Smith-Wheelock M, Kemink JL. Habituation therapy for chronic vestibular dysfunction: Preliminary results. *Otolaryngol Head Neck Surg* 1990; 103(1):89–95.

89. Shepard NT, Telian SA. Programmatic vestibular rehabilitation. *Otolaryngol Head Neck Surg* 1995; 112(1):173–182.

90. Lacour M. Restoration of vestibular function: Basic aspects and practical advances for rehabilitation. *Curr Med Res Opin* 2006; 22(9):1651–1659.

91. Yardley L, Donovan-Hall M, Smith HE, et al. Effectiveness of primary care-based vestibular rehabilitation for chronic dizziness. *Ann Intern Med* 2004; 141(8):598–605.

92. Nashner LM, Black FO, Wall C. Adaptation to altered support and visual conditions during stance: Patients with vestibular deficits. *J Neurosci* 1982; 2(5):536–544.

93. Bonan IV, Colle FM, Guichard JP, et al. Reliance on visual information after stroke. Part I: Balance on dynamic posturography. *Arch Phys Med Rehabil* 2004; 85(2):268–273.

94. Bonan I, Derighetti F, Gellez-Leman MC, et al. Visual dependence after recent stroke. *Ann Readapt Med Phys* 2006; 49(4):166–171.

95. Bonan IV, Yelnik AP, Colle FM, et al. Reliance on visual information after stroke. Part II: Effectiveness of a balance rehabilitation program with visual cue deprivation after stroke: A randomized controlled trial. *Arch Phys Med Rehabil* 2004; 85(2):274–278.

96. Cass SP, Borello-France D, Furman JM. Functional outcome of vestibular rehabilitation in patients with abnormal sensory-organization testing. *Am J Otol* 1996; 17(4):581–594.

97. Lord SR, Dayhew J, Howland A. Multifocal glasses impair edge-contrast sensitivity and depth perception and increase the risk of falls in older people. *J Am Geriatr Soc* 2002; 50(11):1760–1766.

98. Xerri C, Lacour M. Compensation deficits in posture and kinetics following unilateral vestibular neurectomy in cats: The role of sensorimotor activity. *Acta Otolaryngol* 1980; 90(5–6):414–424.

99. Hain TC, Uddin M. Pharmacological treatment of vertigo. *CNS Drugs* 2003; 17(2):85–100.

100. Kalb R, Solomon D. Space exploration, Mars, and the nervous system. *Arch Neurol* 2007; 64(4):485–490.

101. Brandt T, Dieterich M. Pathological eye-head coordination in roll: Tonic ocular tilt reaction in mesencephalic and medullary lesions. *Brain* 1987; 110 (3):649–666.

102. Lacour M, Roll JP, Appaix M. Modifications and development of spinal reflexes in the alert baboon (Papio papio) following a unilateral vestibular neurotomy. *Brain Res* 1976; 113(2):255–269.

103. Bjerver K, Silfverskiold BP. Lateropulsion and imbalance in Wallenberg's syndrome. *Acta Neurol Scand* 1968; 44(1):91–100.

104. Yi HA, Kim HA, Lee H, Baloh RW. Body lateropulsion as an isolated or predominant symptom of a pontine infarction. *J Neurol Neurosurg Psychiatry* 2006.

105. Nowak DA, Topka HR. The clinical variability of Wallenberg's syndrome: The anatomical correlate of ipsilateral axial lateropulsion. *J Neurol* 2006; 253(4):507–511.

106. Karnath HO, Ferber S, Dichgans J. The neural representation of postural control in humans. *Proc Natl Acad Sci U S A* 2000; 97(25):13931–13936.

107. Pedersen PM, Wandel A, Jorgensen HS, et al. Ipsilateral pushing in stroke: incidence, relation to neuropsychological symptoms, and impact on rehabilitation. The Copenhagen Stroke Study. *Arch Phys Med Rehabil* 1996; 77(1):25–28.

108. Anastasopoulos D, Haslwanter T, Bronstein A, et al. Dissociation between the perception of body verticality and the visual vertical in acute peripheral vestibular disorder in humans. *Neurosci Lett* 1997; 233(2–3):151–153.

109. Karnath HO, Ferber S, Dichgans J. The origin of contraversive pushing: Evidence for a second graviceptive system in humans. *Neurology* 14 2000; 55(9):1298–1304.

110. Perennou DA, Amblard B, Laassel el M, et al. Understanding the pusher behavior of some stroke patients with spatial deficits: A pilot study. *Arch Phys Med Rehabil* 2002; 83(4):570–575.

111. Bonan IV, Hubeaux K, Gellez-Leman MC, et al. Influence of subjective visual vertical misperception on balance recovery after stroke. *J Neurol Neurosurg Psychiatry* 2007; 78(1):49–55.

112. Yelnik AP, Lebreton FO, Bonan IV, et al. Perception of verticality after recent cerebral hemispheric stroke. *Stroke* 2002; 33(9):2247–2253.

113. Solomon D. Benign paroxysmal positional vertigo. *Curr Treat Options Neurol* 2000; 2(5):417–428.

114. Buttner U, Helmchen C, Brandt T. Diagnostic criteria for central versus peripheral positioning nystagmus and vertigo: A review. *Acta Otolaryngol* 1999; 119(1):1–5.

115. Epley JM. The canalith repositioning procedure: for treatment of benign paroxysmal positional vertigo. *Otolaryngology - Head & Neck Surgery* 1992; 107(3):399–404.

116. Furman JM, Cass SP. Benign paroxysmal positional vertigo. [Review] [48 refs]. *New England Journal of Medicine* 18 1999; 341(21):1590–1596.

IV

SENSORIMOTOR IMPAIRMENTS AND THEIR TREATMENT

16 Patterns of Locomotor Recovery after Stroke

Carol L. Richards
Francine Malouin
Francine Dumas

T he objective of this chapter is to examine different ways of evaluating the patterns of locomotor recovery after sustaining a cerebral stroke. It will

1. Review recovery trajectories after stroke obtained from longitudinal studies using categorical clinical measures of function and underlying mechanisms associated with recovery.
2. Argue for the use of walking speed as a marker of recovery.
3. Present data describing the recovery, from stroke onset to two years post-stroke, of walking speed and its relation to movements and muscle activations of the lower extremity in a cohort of subjects with a middle cerebral artery ischemic stroke who participated in a clinical trial (1).
4. Use data from a second clinical trial (2) to address three questions: Does the gait speed at baseline predict gait speed after therapy? Is locomotor recovery comparable in patients with right- or left-sided hemiparesis? Is the magnitude of locomotor recovery affected by the delay of rehabilitation therapy initiation in patients with subacute stroke?
5. Briefly review the kinetic patterns related to propulsion and generation of walking speed in healthy subjects.

6. Describe compensatory kinetic strategies chosen by persons with stroke to walk.
7. Summarize the concepts introduced and their clinical implications.

RECOVERY AFTER STROKE AS MEASURED BY LONGITUDINAL STUDIES USING CATEGORICAL CLINICAL MEASURES OF FUNCTION

Traditionally, studies have described patterns of recovery on the basis of repeated assessments of functional recovery by means of clinical measures that rate function on the basis of observations made by trained evaluators or clinical benchmarks. Thus, it is generally accepted that the recovery curve of function post-stroke rises rapidly in the first six weeks after stroke, when rehabilitation interventions supplement natural recovery, and that it reaches a plateau at about three months post-stroke, with little further recovery after six months (3–5) although there are reports of recovery much later post–stroke (6). Duncan et al. (5), on the basis of serial Fugl-Meyer (7) assessments over time, further demonstrated that the severity of motor impairment and the patterns of motor recovery were similar for the upper and lower extremities and that the most rapid recovery occurred within 30 days post-stroke. These results were confirmed and extended by the results of the Copenhagen Stroke Study (8–10) conducted in a cohort of 1,197 persons treated in the stroke unit of a hospital in Denmark. If the capacity to return home after rehabilitation is taken as a measure of recovery, 64% were discharged to their own home, while 15% were discharged to a nursing home, and 21% died during the hospital stay (8). Stroke severity, as determined by the Scandinavian Stroke Scale, was initially very severe in 19%, severe in 14%, moderate in 26%, and mild in 41% of the patients. After rehabilitation, 11% of survivors still had severe or very severe neurologic deficits, 11% had moderate deficits, and 78% had no or only mild deficits.

One might ask how stroke severity relates to return of function. In the Copenhagen Stroke Study, the time course of functional recovery (9) was described by weekly assessments with the Barthel Index (11). As expected, the time course of recovery was strongly related to stroke severity. Nevertheless, functional recovery was completed within 12.5 weeks from stroke onset in 95% of the patients, with best recovery attained by 8.5 weeks in those with initially mild stroke and within 20 weeks in those with very severe stroke. Furthermore, best functional recovery was reached by 80% of the patients with initial mild strokes within three weeks and by those with initial moderate strokes within seven weeks.

The time course of recovery of walking function and lower extremity paresis were also assessed by the Barthel Index and the Scandinavian Stroke Scale at weekly intervals in a subgroup of 804 patients in the Copenhagen Stroke Study (10). Initially, 51% had no walking function, 12% could walk with assistance, and 37% could walk independently. At the end of rehabilitation, 21% had died, 18% had no walking function, 11% could walk with assistance, and 50% were independent walkers. They also reported that a plateau in the Barthel Index score was attained in 95% of the patients within the first 11 weeks post-stroke and that, as expected, the rate and magnitude of recovery was related to both the level of initial impairment of walking function and the severity of lower extremity paresis. Thus, when using the Barthel Index as a measure of walking function, Jorgensen et al. (10) state that a valid prognosis of walking function in patients with mild or moderate leg paresis can be made in three weeks and that further recovery should not be expected after nine weeks.

The above-mentioned longitudinal studies indicate that patients with stroke can be expected to have at least some predictable degree of functional recovery in the first six months post-stroke and that the largest gains occur in the first month post-stroke. This non-linear pattern of recovery as a function of time is, however, not well understood. Several mechanisms have been evoked in an attempt to explain the "natural" recovery that occurs in the first weeks, including recovery of tissue in the restitution of penumbral tissue surrounding the lesion, resolution of the diaschisis, and recovery of neurotransmission in spared tissue near and remote from the infarct (12). This recovery process, which is presumed to underlie the recovery pattern early post-stroke, has been referred to as "spontaneous neurologic recovery" (13), and its contribution to the patterns of stroke recovery has been largely overlooked (14, 15). Kwakkel et al. (15) have proposed the use of progress of time as a surrogate, independent covariate to reflect spontaneous recovery and have shown by means of a regression model that it explains 16–42% of the observed improvements in body functions and activities in the first six to ten weeks after stroke onset.

NEURAL PLASTICITY AND BEHAVIORAL COMPENSATIONS

Rehabilitation is believed to modulate recovery by interacting in some way with natural recovery processes. It is very difficult, however, to tease out therapy effects when it is not possible, for obvious ethical reasons, to have a control group receiving no therapy and relegated to a natural recovery. Prediction models that are adjusted for the effects of time after stroke suggest that outcome is largely defined within the first weeks post-stroke, although functional improvement has been found to extend beyond six months post-stroke (15–17). The ground-breaking work of Nudo and colleagues (18, 19), who examined neural plasticity in an animal model of stroke using cortical lesions in primates, demonstrated the potential of task-specific training to modulate brain plasticity and heralded a new era in the field of neurorehabilitation post-stroke that is still evolving. In the past ten years there has been a dramatic change in the type and intensity of therapy provided to persons recovering from a stroke, as new information has emerged from animal and human studies of brain plasticity. These presumably more effective therapeutic approaches will likely alter the pattern of recovery.

Given the technical difficulties associated with recording from the brain as the persons walk, it is not surprising that studies describing the neural correlates of locomotor-related therapy are few. Miyai et al. (20), using an optical imaging system, found that body weight-supported treadmill training (BWSTT) led to a lower activation in the sensorimotor cortex (SMC) as assessed by task-related changes of oxygenated hemoglobin levels. Importantly, changes in the SMC activation correlated with changes in the cadence, and improvement in the asymmetry of SMC activation also correlated with improvement in gait asymmetry. In a second study, again with optical imaging, Miyai et al. (21) measured cortical activity in persons with sub-acute stroke before and after two months of inpatient rehabilitation. They concluded that locomotor recovery after stroke may be associated with improvement of asymmetry in SMC activation and enhanced premotor cortex activation in the affected hemisphere (21, 22).

Yen et al. (23) have recently reported a study using focal transcranial magnetic stimulation to document the relationship between motor improvement and corticomotor excitability change after gait training in persons with chronic stroke. They compared the effects of four weeks of general physical therapy in a control group (n = 7) to general physical therapy with the addition of BWSTT in an experimental group (n = 7). They found that, after general therapy, the patients improved their walking speed and cadence but had no significant changes in corticomotor excitability. The addition of BWSTT led to changes in corticomotor excitability. These changes in corticomotor excitability with BWSTT were correlated with improvements in balance and gait performance.

To date, fMRI studies attempting to document the neural correlates of recovery in locomotor function after stroke or cerebral palsy have used ankle dorsiflexion movements and tibialis anterior activation as a surrogate to assay motor control for walking during rehabilitation (24). Sullivan et al. (25) documented activity-dependent cortical reorganization using fMRI mapping of the brains of persons with stroke who practiced walking on a treadmill. The fMRI changes were correlated with faster over-ground walking speeds and more precise voluntary control of the tibialis anterior muscle. Recently, Philips et al. (26) demonstrated the feasibility of using fMRI to document changes in cortical activation during voluntary ankle movements before and after intensive BWSTT as a physiological marker of brain plasticity with training in children with cerebral palsy.

Also, one can question whether more effective, task-specific therapy, provided early and with sufficient intensity, will limit the development of disturbed motor control processes associated with spasticity, excessive coactivation, and paresis during walking (27). Furthermore, kinematic and kinetic studies have demonstrated that functional improvements in balance and gait or lower extremity function can occur without the restoration of "normal" motor control, indicating that behavioral compensation strategies for impaired motor control are an important part of the "recovery" of function after stroke (28–39). One can ask whether these behavioral compensations that reflect learned skills designed to overcome motor control impairments are part of the recovery process that is triggered when restoration of "normal" function is not possible.

WALKING SPEED AS A MARKER OF RECOVERY AFTER STROKE

Walking speed has been shown to be a robust indicator of walking capacity (40). Supporting the validity of walking speed as a measure of locomotor recovery is its positive correlation with motor recovery (39, 41, 42), static muscle strength of the lower extremity (43, 44), and the size of the "push-off" plantarflexor moment (35), with balance (45)

and the use of walking aids (46), and its negative correlation to spasticity of the plantarflexors (33). Faster walking speeds are also indicative of the quality of the lower extremity movements (38, 47). Moreover, the reliability of the clinical measurement of walking speed has been established for test-retest and between observer measurements (46–48), whereas repeated measurements of the simple, timed walking test over five and ten meters have been shown to be a responsive measure of walking performance in acute stroke (49). Gait speed, however, is not always the outcome of choice throughout the range of recovery. When subjects walk very slowly or need support from a person clinical outcomes, such as the Barthel (11) ambulation subscale or the Fugl-Meyer (7) leg subscore, may be more sensitive than walking speed (38). On the other hand, chronicling the full extent of walking recovery may require measures more demanding than gait speed alone (50).

Importantly, Perry et al. (51) related the level of walking speed attained by persons post-stroke to their capacity to participate in the community. Thus, to be able to be independent in the community the stroke survivor must be able to walk at about 80 cm/s, but this speed is too slow to cross wide streets in large cities (52). At the end of their rehabilitation phase, relatively few persons with stroke walk at this speed. For example, after two months of rehabilitation that included a task-specific locomotor physical therapy approach, only 15 of 62 persons had a walking speed of 80 cm/s or faster (2). Other studies have reported mean comfortable walking speeds of less than 80 cm/s at the end of intervention studies (1, 17, 48, 53). In a recent study, Schmid et al. (54) stratified gait speed after stroke into the following clinically meaningful ambulation classes based on the Perry et al. (51) study: household ambulation (<40 cm/s), limited community ambulation (40–80 cm/s), and full community ambulation (>80 cm/s). In sub-acute stroke survivors with mild or moderate deficits who participated in a randomized, clinical trial of stroke rehabilitation they (54) found that a gait speed gain leading to a transition to a higher class of ambulation results in better function and quality of life, especially for household ambulators, suggesting that an outcome assessment based on transitions between gait speed classifications yields potentially meaningful indicators of clinical benefit. Desrosiers et al. (55) also found disability measures of the lower extremity, including gait speed, to be highly correlated to handicap situations as measured by the Life-H outcome measure in persons after suffering a stroke, thus emphasizing the importance of mobility to promote social participation.

As mentioned above, the patterns of recovery—and in particular, walking recovery—post-stroke has essentially been defined by serial assessments made with categorical clinical measures up to six months post-stroke when these measures fail to show further improvement. When using walking speed as a marker of functional recovery, however, Richards et al. (39) found that walking speed continued to increase up to 12–18 months post-stroke and that the increase in speed was related to increases in both cadence and stride length, thus re-defining the time course of recovery. The recovery of gait speed, however, remained limited when compared to the gait speed of healthy, elderly persons asked to walk slowly (56), with the mean level of gait speed recovery attaining about 50% of the slow speed of the healthy subjects at 12 to 18 months post-stroke (39). The latter study documented recovery in a cohort of patients with an ischemic stroke due to a middle cerebral artery infarct who participated in a randomized, controlled trial comparing three physical therapy interventions (1, 57).

Kollen et al. (48) documented the recovery of walking speed in a prospective cohort longitudinal study of 101 persons with acute stroke who participated in a clinical trial designed to study the effects of augmented therapy (53). None of the participants were able to walk unassisted in the first week post-stroke. The mean interval between stroke onset and the first unassisted walk was 4.8 ± 2.9 weeks. They followed the subjects for 52 weeks, and because not all of the subjects progressed to unassisted walking, comfortable walking speed was measured in 85, and fast walking speed in 81, participants. The mean comfortable walking speed progressively increased from 3.7 cm/s to 63.5 cm/s at one year post-stroke, whereas the mean maximum speed increased from 7.1 cm/s to 85.1 cm/s, thus confirming the progressive increase in gait speed up to one year post-stroke. Moreover, they found a systematic difference between comfortable and fast walking speeds. Regression analyses applied cross-sectionally and longitudinally demonstrated that the relation between comfortable and maximum walking speed does not change over time after stroke. Maximum speed was estimated to be 1.32 times that of comfortable walking speed (48). This is an important finding because it makes it possible to estimate the maximum speed a subject can attain, without actually measuring it, to predict, for instance, the capacity to cross a wide street.

The works of Richards et al. (38) and Kollen et al. (48) have clearly shown that gait speed continues to increase beyond six months after stroke when clinical measures may fail to show further functional recovery. The following section reports the extension of the Richards et al (39) study of recovery in gait movements and muscle activations accompanying changes in gait speed in the 11 subjects that remained in the study at two years post-stroke (58).

RECOVERY, FROM STROKE ONSET TO TWO YEARS POST-STROKE, OF WALKING SPEED AND ITS RELATION TO MOVEMENTS AND MUSCLE ACTIVATIONS OF THE LOWER EXTREMITY

Table 16-1 gives selected subject characteristics for 11 patients with complete data followed from baseline to two years post-stroke. At six weeks post-stroke 23 of the

TABLE 16-1

Selected Characteristics of the Subjects Evaluated at Baseline One Week Post-Stroke and Two Years Post-Stroke. These Subjects Participated in a Randomized Controlled Trial That Evaluated the Effects of an Intensive Task-Oriented Gait Training Program (1, 57)

PATIENT NUMBER	AGE (YEARS)	GENDER/ AFFECTED SIDE	FUGL-MEYER LEG MOTOR SUBSCORE (MAXIMUM SCORE = 34)			BALANCE SCALE (MAXIMUM SCORE = 56)	
			B	6 WEEKS	2 YEARS	6 WEEKS	2 YEARS
206	82	W/L	30	23	NA	22	NA
207	69	M/L	22	25	32	43	51
113	66	M/L	14	30	31	52	54
211	65	W/L	19	28	31	52	NA
201	60	M/R	21	31	33	55	56
104	63	W/R	9	30	29	54	55
204	77	M/R	19	26	29	39	52
101	61	W/L	5	24	28	23	51
208	63	W/L	16	16	26	14	48
109	56	M/R	6	20	NA	40	NA
107	48	M/R	4	10	12	42	51
Mean ± 1 SD (n=11)	64.6 ± 9.3	W:5/R:5	15 ± 8.3	23.9 ± 6.5	27.9 ± 6.3	39.6 ± 14.2	52.3 ± 2.6

B: baseline; M: men; W: women; L: left; R: right; NA: not available

27 patients recruited into the study remained, and of these, 18 were able to walk, 15 with one-arm support for balance or independently, while three required maximal bilateral arm support to walk 4 m (38). Of the five patients who did not walk at six weeks post-stroke, one refused to be evaluated and four others were unable to walk, even with maximal bilateral support. At two years post-stroke, all of the patients remaining in the study could walk independently.

Figure 16-1 illustrates the recovery of gait speed over time in comparison to values obtained in healthy subjects walking slowly. At six weeks post-stroke, the gait speed of two patients (cases 113 and 211) fell within the confidence limits of the healthy controls, and a third (case 206) was close. The mean gait speed was 31.8 ± 19.9 cm/s (mean, ± 1SD, n = 11). At two years post-stroke, all the patients walked faster and six attained normal confidence limits. The mean speed almost doubled, rising to 62.8 ± 19.1 cm/s (n = 11), a speed that is still much below the 104.3 ± 19.3 cm/s free speed of healthy subjects walking under similar laboratory conditions (56).

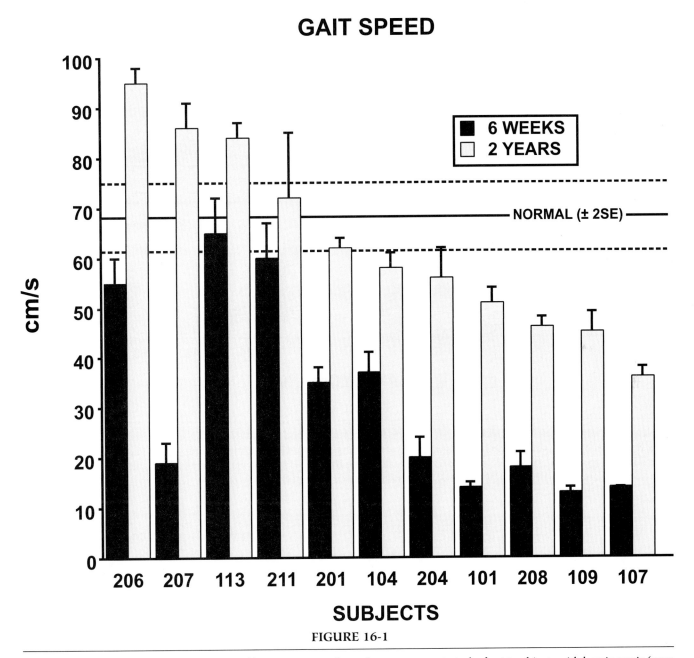

FIGURE 16-1

Bar graph representing changes in gait speed between six weeks and two years post-stroke for 11 subjects with hemiparesis (case numbers given on x-axis). Horizontal lines indicate mean and confidence limits of gait speed obtained in a group (n = 10) of healthy subjects (aged 58 ± 5.6 yrs) walking at 75% of their usual cadence (mean speed 68.3 ± 6.7 cm/s; ±2 SE, n = 8).

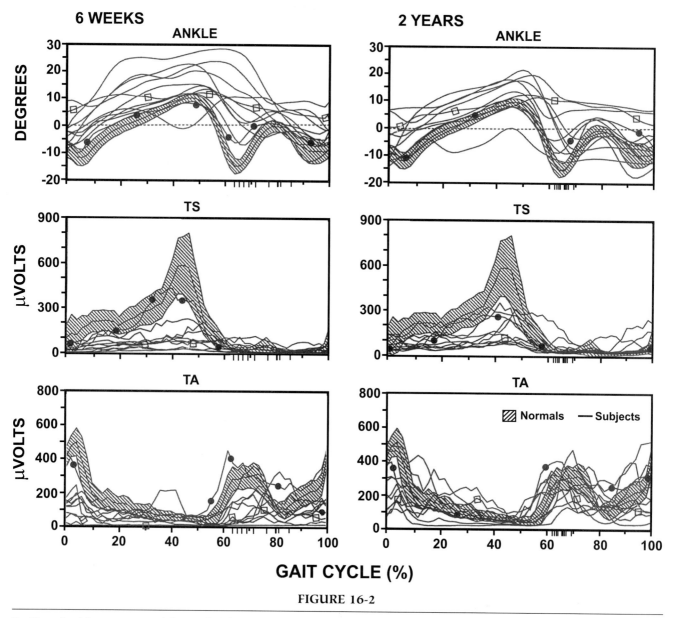

FIGURE 16-2

Profiles of ankle movements (obtained with a TRIAX electrogoniometer) and activations (surface EMG; rectified and time averaged; time constant = 20 ms) of the triceps surae (TS) and tibialis anterior (TA) muscles during gait of 11 subjects at six weeks and two years post-stroke in comparison with normal values (mean ± 2 SE, n = 8). The patients who walked slowest (case 109: open squares) and fastest (case 113: filled circles) at six weeks are indicated.

Recovery, as defined by comparison to healthy values, in the ankle movements and muscle activations that accompanied these changes in gait speed are shown in Figure 16-2.

In most cases the movement and activation profiles differ markedly from normal values at six weeks post-stroke and are closer to normal at two years post-stroke. Interestingly, the movement profiles (top row) appear to show better recovery than the muscle activation profiles, particularly the TS (middle row). As previously mentioned, the mean speed approximately doubles during this time frame, and

this increase in speed is related to both an increase in stride length (59–88 cm) and faster cadence (61–85 steps/min).

To examine more closely the relationship between gait speed and the patterns of movements and muscle activations with recovery, the 11 patients at two years post-stroke were divided into two groups: a slow-walking group (n = 5) and a fast-walking group (n = 6). The walking speed of patients in the fast group attained or surpassed the confidence limits of the healthy controls walking slowly.

As shown in Figure 16-3, the movement and muscle activation profiles during gait of the fast group (H-N) are

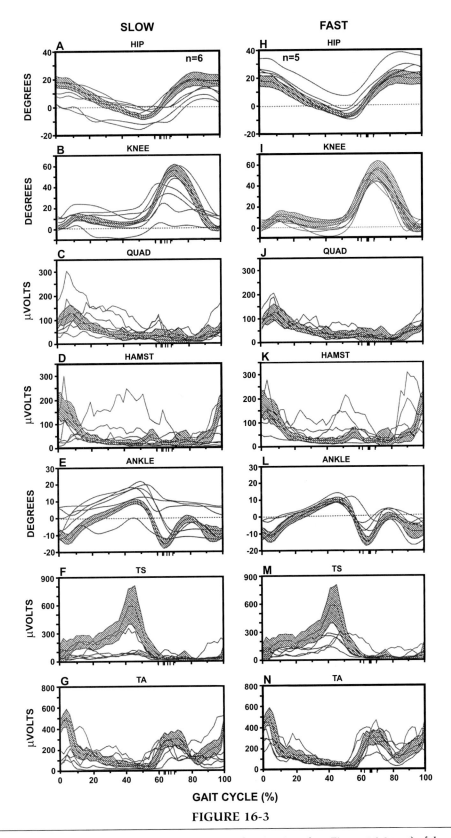

FIGURE 16-3

Comparison of the profiles of hip, knee, and ankle movements and activations (see Figure 16-2 text) of the quadriceps (QUAD), hamstrings (HAMST), triceps surae (TS), and tibialis anterior (TA) muscles during the gait cycle of a group of slow-walking (A–G) and a group of faster-walking (H–N) subjects at two years post-stroke with normal values. Thin lines represent the profiles of individual subjects. Shaded area gives mean and confidence limits for healthy controls (n = 8). Additional vertical lines on x-axis indicate end-of-stance phase, which ranged from 62 to 69% and from 60 to 67% of the gait cycle for the slow and fast groups, respectively.

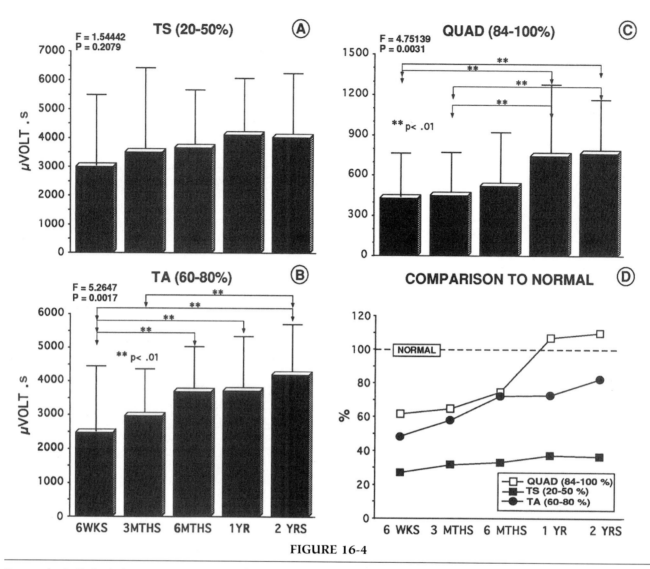

FIGURE 16-4

Bar graphs A–C, depicting recovery over time of selected muscle activation bursts of the triceps surae (TS), tibialis anterior (TA), and quadriceps (QUAD) muscles of 11 patients whose muscle activation profile were depicted in Figure 16-3. Values in A–C give mean + 1 SD. The area under specific activation bursts was used in comparisons. Three activation bursts were defined for the TA (0–16%, 60–80%, and 84–100%). These bursts are related to footfall control after foot contact, toe lift at swing phase initiation, and foot lift preparatory to foot contact at the end of the cycle. Activation bursts related to functional events in the gait cycle were also defined for the other muscles: TS (20–50%) and QUAD (84–100%). An analysis of variance for repeated measures and the Scheffe post-hoc test were used to compare changes over time (x-axis). Line graph in D compares recovery of the activation bursts (in % of values obtained in healthy subjects) in the three muscles. Statistical differences are indicated by asterisks (**: $p < 0.01$) and horizontal lines above bars in A–C.

generally (except for the HAMST activations which remain perturbed) closer to normal values. The TS "push-off" activation burst is larger for most of the patients in the fast group, but the recovery, or return to more normal values, is less than expected given the role of this activation burst in the generation of power needed to increase gait speed (36, 37, 59).

To further examine the recovery (recovery is used in the general sense and refers to return in the capacity to activate the muscle) in the muscle activation profiles over

time, the areas under functionally important activation bursts were compared (Figure 16-4).

As expected from the profiles shown in Figures 16-2 and 16-3, the "push-off" activation burst in the TS does not change over time in this group of patients. In contrast, the TA activation burst that is related to foot lift at swing phase initiation (60–80% of the gait cycle) shows recovery up to two years post-stroke. The recovery in this burst is representative of recovery in the two other TA activation bursts (0–16% and 84–100% of the gait cycle)

TABLE 16-2

*Pearson Correlation Coefficients (r) Between Recovery (Change from Baseline to Two Years Post-Stroke)
in Gait Speed and Muscle Activation Burst That are Functionally Important During the Gait Cycle
in Persons with Chronic Stroke (n = 11)*

	GAIT SPEED	TS (20–50%)	TA (0–16%)	TA (60–80%)	TA (84–100%)	QUAD (84–100%)
Gait Speed	1	0.27	0.53	0.60**	0.20	0.22
TS (20–50%)		1	0.74**	0.59	0.64*	0.77**
TA (0–16%)			1	0.89**	0.79**	0.49
TA (60–80%)				1	0.86**	0.43
TA (84–100%)					1	0.41
QUAD (84–100%)						1

**: $p < 0.01$; *: $p < 0.05$; TS: triceps surae; TA: tibialis anterior; QUAD: quadriceps

which were correlated with the 60–80% gait cycle activation burst (r = 0.89 and 0.86, respectively, $p < 0.01$). The QUAD also improves over time but it shows its improvement later than that for the TA, the largest change occurring between six months and one year post-stroke in the late swing activation burst (84–100% of the gait cycle) that corresponds to knee extension preparatory to weight acceptance. Comparison of the magnitude of the activation bursts (TA, TS, and QUAD) in the patients with healthy values (Figure 16-4D) emphasizes the poor recovery of the TS at two years post-stroke.

Pearson correlation coefficients (Table 16-2) were calculated to further probe the interaction among the muscle activation bursts and gait speed during recovery, which was defined as the magnitude of change from baseline to two years post-stroke. Recovery in the TA bursts (0–16 and 84–100) was significantly associated (r = 0.74 and 0.64, respectively) with change in the TS (20–50%). Recovery in the QUAD, mainly a knee extensor, was most highly correlated (r = 0.77, $p < 0.01$) with recovery in the ankle extensors (TS). Recovery of gait speed, on the other hand, had a closer association with recovery in the TA (60–80%: r = 0.60, $p < 0.01$) than with the two extensor muscle groups.

In summary, these data describe the longitudinal recovery of gait in a cohort of patients with a middle cerebral artery ischemic stroke (1). One week post-stroke their Fugl-Meyer leg subscores (7) varied from 4 to 30, indicating a wide range of impairment, and this was later reflected in the variable locomotor recovery. Although the mean gait speed at six weeks post-stroke of about 30 cm/s doubled to a near normal slow gait speed at two years post-stroke, some patients attained a relatively good walking pattern, while others were left with a very perturbed pattern. These results also show a clear relationship between gait speed and the quality of gait movements and muscle activations at two years post-stroke, confirming

the findings of our earlier study (38) and in agreement with Wade et al. (47).

Recovery of activation profiles was not uniform among the muscles. The TA recovers consistently over time, whereas the QUAD recovers little until about one year post-stroke, and the TS was particularly resistant to change. The apparent resistance of the TS to recovery is a surprising and important result because of the importance of this muscle as a generator of propulsive force for walking and the emphasis put on the re-learning of "push-off" in locomotor rehabilitation approaches (36, 60, 61). One can ask whether the TS is more resistant to change for physiological reasons or, alternatively, if rehabilitation strategies are inadequate to provide the appropriate input to evoke recovery in this muscle. In this context, Colborne et al. (62) demonstrated that computer-assisted biofeedback (ankle position or EMG biofeedback) was more effective than conventional therapy to induce improved force impulses of the plantarflexors at "push-off". Furthermore, in a subgroup of 25 subjects participating in an RCT, Richards et al. (2) found that an improved "push-off" plantarflexor A2 power burst (see Figures 16-3 and 16-6 for illustrations of the muscle activations and power bursts) in late stance explained about 25% of the variance in the change in gait speed post-therapy. The close association between gait speed and recovery in the TA at two years post-stroke confirms and extends earlier findings (39) and suggests that the TA may be an important muscle to target in therapy given its recovery potential and association with gait speed recovery. Could it be that the TA is more easily controlled by voluntary drive (63) post-stroke, whereas the TS is under control of the subcortical postural system and less accessible to voluntary drive after a lesion of the corticospinal tract? Clearly, these questions provide ample motivation for continued research in this area.

THREE QUESTIONS ABOUT THE POTENTIAL FOR LOCOMOTOR RECOVERY, WITH WALKING SPEED AS A MARKER OF RECOVERY

To address these questions, data was reviewed from 62 persons with subacute stroke who participated in an RCT that compared the efficacy of two task-oriented PT programs to promote gait recovery (2). Since the therapeutic effects of both approaches were found to be similar, the subjects were pooled for these analyses. They received a total of about 38 hours of task-oriented physical therapy over two months.

What is the Relationship Between Gait Speed at Baseline (When Therapy was Initiated) and the Speed Attained Post Therapy?

Figure 16-5A illustrates the relationship between walking speed at baseline and walking speed after therapy. The relationship is significant ($p < 0.0001$) with an r of 0.62 and an R^2 of 0.40, indicating that about 40% of the change in gait speed from baseline can be explained by the initial gait speed. If subjects who walk at speeds less than 30 cm/s are considered to have a severe stroke then the clustering of the points in the lower left of the figure illustrates the tendency for smaller gains in this group of subjects.

Is the Magnitude of Locomotor Recovery Affected by the Time Post-Stroke of Therapy Initiation?

It is generally assumed that early initiation of therapy post-stroke promotes optimal results, and as discussed in section one, most of the functional recovery occurs in the first month post-stroke. Figure 16-5B examines the relationship between change in gait speed with therapy and time of therapy initiation in the rehabilitation center. These subjects likely had therapy in the acute setting prior to referral to the rehabilitation center. Also, later referrals tended to indicate more severe strokes. The relationship ($r = 0.38$) between change in gait speed with therapy and time post-stroke of therapy initiation is significant ($p < 0.003$) and indicates that about 14% of the change in gait speed can be attributed to the time of therapy initiation in the rehabilitation setting.

Is Locomotor Recovery Comparable in Patients with Right- or Left-Sided Hemiparesis?

Figure 16-5C that compares the change in gait speed with therapy in persons with left- or right-sided hemiparesis illustrates that recovery is similar ($p > 0.05$) in this group of subjects. This finding needs to be confirmed in other

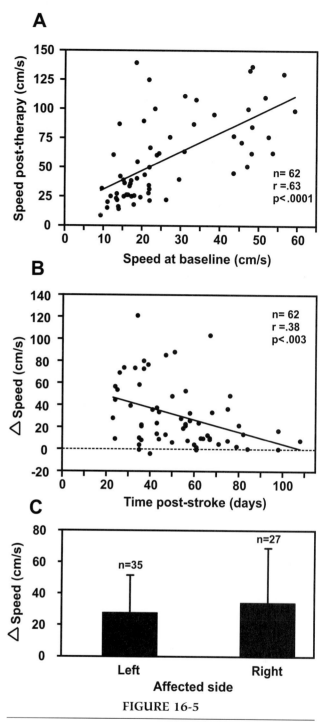

FIGURE 16-5

The association (Pearson Correlation Coefficients (r)) between walking speed at baseline and walking speed after therapy (A), change in gait speed with time post-stroke (B), and change in walking speed with therapy in persons with left- and right-sided hemiparesis (C) is illustrated in a cohort of 62 persons with sub-acute stroke who participated in a clinical trial (2).

groups of subjects with stroke of different severities and receiving other types of task-oriented training.

MUSCLE GROUPS CONTRIBUTING TO THE GENERATION OF ENERGY FOR FORWARD PROPULSION, THEIR RELATIVE CONTRIBUTIONS TO WALKING SPEED, AND STRATEGIES USED BY PERSONS WITH HEMIPARESIS

Kinetic analyses such as moment of force and power profiles over the gait cycle help to understand *why* a subject has a given movement pattern and gait speed. The reader is referred to Winter (59) and Olney et al. (35) for details of the equipment, data, and formulae required to calculate joint moments (a *moment* is defined as the turning effect of a force about any point) and power (the *power* generated by a moment is the product of the moment acting at an axis and the angular velocity of the rigid body about that axis). The method of calculation of muscle power is such that power generation (above zero on the y-axis) indicates that the power burst is achieved by a concentric contraction (at least for muscles crossing a single joint), thus further helping understand the force deficit. *Work* is the integral of power, with concentric and eccentric contractions producing positive and negative work, respectively. Since the seminal work of Winter (59) the contributions of the major muscle groups of the lower extremity contributing to the work of walking have become well known. The three major bursts of energy generation and the propulsive force for forward progression come from the hip extensors in early stance (H1 in Figure 16-6), the plantarflexors at "push-off" (A2 in Figure 16-6), and the hip flexors at "pull-off" (H3 in Figure 16-6) in late stance and early swing. The knee extensors in early stance (K2) produce a small amount of positive work. Most of the absorption is provided by the ankle plantarflexors (A1), the hip flexors (H2), the knee extensors (K1 and K3), and the knee flexors (K4).

Winter (59) further showed in healthy subjects that faster walking speeds were related to larger power generation bursts, particularly of the ankle plantarflexors at push-off (A2), that contributed most (about 75%) of the propulsive force, with the H3 hip flexor burst and the H1 hip extensor burst contributing most of the remainder. The contribution of the knee to the propulsive force was considered to be minimal. Many studies have since confirmed the influence of speed on energy generation (64–66). A recent study (66) that examined the effects of three metronome-induced cadences (60, 80, and 120 steps/min) on energy generation and absorption in healthy subjects found that the mean relative contribution of the ankle to mechanical energy generation was about 60% at the slowest cadence and fell to about 44% at the fastest cadence. On the other hand, the 24% contribution of the hip at the slowest

cadence rose to about 38% at the fastest cadence, while that of the knee increased from 16% to 19%. These findings indicate a large contribution from the hip muscles to the modulation of walking speed, while the ankle muscles are relatively insensitive to changes in speed—findings that are in agreement with previous studies (64, 65, 67). The variability, however, suggested that individual subjects likely used different strategies.

Do Persons with Stroke Employ the Same Kinetic Strategies to Produce Gait Speed as Healthy Subjects?

A stroke results in a walking disability because locomotor control is impaired. Although the impairment may be associated with different types of disturbed motor control (27, 32–34, 68), the net result is a diminished capacity of the lower extremity muscles to act on the skeletal levers to produce rotational force at the hip, knee, and ankle. The impaired force output, in turn, results in altered power generation and absorption and can result in intra-limb and inter-limb compensatory gait patterns in which stronger muscle groups attempt to counter deficiencies by generating more than their normal work (35, 36, 61). In the first study examining the capacity for power generation in persons with chronic stroke, Olney et al. (35) divided a group of 30 subjects into slow (25 cm/s, SD 5 cm/s, n = 10), intermediate (41 cm/s, SD 8 cm/s, n = 10), and fast walkers (63 cm/s, SD 8 cm/s, n = 10). Each subgroup comprised ten subjects, for a total of thirty. They reported that in all three groups the mean A2 power burst was smaller than that of healthy controls and, furthermore, that its magnitude was related to walking speed. The H3 power burst, on the other hand, tended to be larger than in healthy controls, suggesting that persons with stroke compensate for a poor "push-off" burst by pulling off more at the hip. Not unexpected, given that walking is a bipedal task, they also reported that even if the power-generating capacity of the less-affected lower extremity differed from healthy values, the less-affected side performed a greater proportion of the positive work than the affected side at all speeds, approximately in a 60:40 ratio. From simulations, Higginson et al. (69) have shown that the contributions of individual muscles to the support moment in mid-stance of a person with stroke differ from those of neurologically healthy older subjects. The slower walking speed of persons with stroke, although no doubt a factor, cannot explain these differences in kinetic strategies because persons with stroke walking at similar speeds may use quite different power combinations (30, 70).

Data obtained from subgroups of the same cohort of patients that participated in the RCT (2) described in the previous section are used to illustrate the concepts relating to power generation and the production of gait speed. Figure 16-6 gives a comparison of the mean moment and

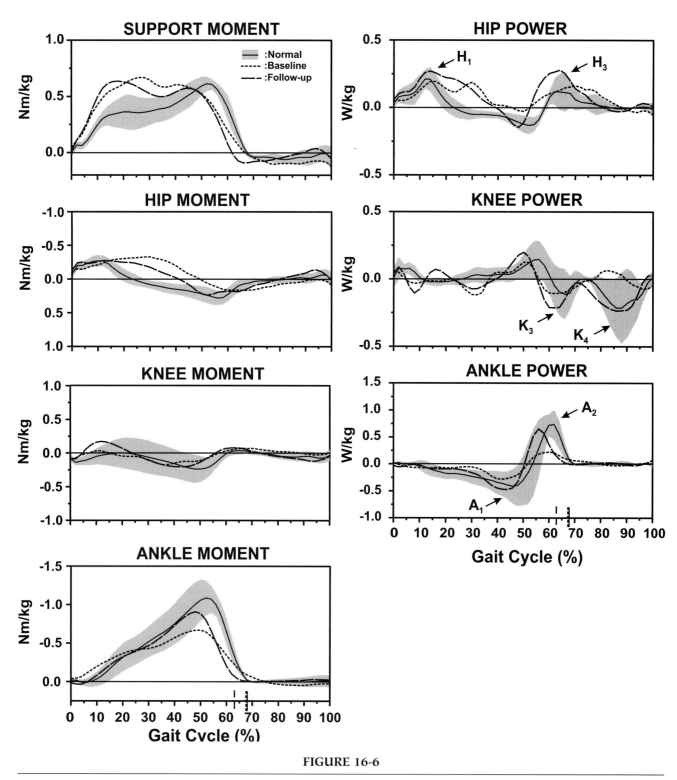

FIGURE 16-6

Comparison of the mean moment and power profiles for 19 subjects with sub-acute stroke who participated in the Richards et al. trial (2) before and after two months of task-oriented therapy with values obtained in healthy elderly controls walking slowly (59 ± 7 cm/s, n = 5). Profile of moments and power (y-axis) are given in relation to the gait cycle in percent (x-axis). Mean baseline values for the subjects (dotted line) are compared to mean post-therapy values (interrupted line). Profiles in healthy controls represent mean ± 2 SD. The mean gait speed in the persons with stroke rose from 42 cm/s to 68 cm/s post-therapy. Hip (H1 and H3) and ankle (A2) power generation and knee (K3 and K4) and ankle (A1) power absorption bursts are indicated.

TABLE 16-3

Selected Subject Characteristics of the Slow and Fast Walkers. Subjects Walking ≥70 cm/s Post-Therapy were Considered to be Fast Walkers, While those Walking <70 cm/s were Slow Walkers. These Subjects Participated in a Randomized, Controlled Trial Evaluating the Effects of Task-Oriented Gait Training (2). Measures of Strength were Obtained with a Hand-Held Dynamometer

	SLOW WALKERS (N = 13)	FAST WALKERS (N = 8)
Age (years)	67 ± 12	56 ± 11
Ashworth scale	2.4 ± 1.4	1.1 ± 1.1
Fugl-Meyer leg motor subscore	21.3 ± 6.1*	26.8 ± 3.5
Barthel ambulation subscore	20 ± 9.6	18 ± 8.5
Isometric hip flexor strength (Nm)	34 ± 23	48 ± 30
Isometric ankle plantarflexor strength (Nm)	16 ± 6	19 ± 6
Gait speed (cm/s)	28 ± 13*	52 ± 19
Change in gait speed with therapy (cm/s)	12 ± 12*	34 ± 20

*: $p < 0.05$

power profiles produced by the affected side of 19 persons with stroke before (1.4 ± 0.5 months post-stroke onset) and about two months after task-oriented locomotor training with values obtained in 5 healthy elderly persons walking at about 60% of their free gait speed (59 ± 7 cm/s). When comparisons are made with power profiles obtained from healthy subjects walking at free speed, the magnitude of the differences between the subjects with hemiparesis and the healthy subjects are much larger. As illustrated by the hip and ankle power profiles, the A2 ankle "push-off" power burst and the H1 hip extensor burst in early stance and the H3 hip "pull-off" burst in late stance and early swing phase increased after therapy. This increased power generation at the hip and ankle was associated with a mean increase in gait speed of 26 cm/s (42 to 68 cm/s). In this group of patients (n = 19), Richards et al. (37) found the peak of the A2 and H3 power bursts to be significantly correlated to gait speed (r = 0.62, p < 0.01, r = 0.85, p < 0.01, respectively) post-therapy. At the end of the RCT (n = 63), Richards et al. (2) reported a near-doubling of gait speed after therapy and reported that in 25 of these subjects with pre- and post-kinetic gait analyses the increased gait speed was associated (r = 0.52, p = 0.003, n = 25) with an increase in the A2 ankle power generation burst of the affected leg.

To further explore the choice of kinetic strategies used by persons with hemiparesis, bilateral kinetic analyses were made in a subgroup of 21 patients who participated in the RCT (Table 16-3) before and after task-oriented therapy for two months (see Richards et al. (2) for details).

The Relationship of Bilateral Ankle and Hip Power Bursts to Gait Speed

Because we were particularly interested in the trade-off between a "push-off" (A2) or a "pull-off" (H3) strategy to create gait speed (dependent variable) the following variables (A2 peak power and H3 peak power on both the *affected* and *less affected* sides) were entered in the step-wise regression analyses, one on the baseline and the second on the post-therapy values (Table 16-4).

The regression analysis on the *baseline* values revealed that the peak A2 and H3 power bursts on the *affected* side explained as much as 84% (R^2) of the variance in gait speed in these sub-acute subjects who had an average gait speed of 40 cm/s. The results of the second stepwise regression analysis using the same bilateral kinetic variables *post-therapy* (Table 16-4), however, show that the contribution of the *less-affected side* becomes important with the H3 on the *non-affected* side replacing the *affected* H3 peak obtained in the baseline analysis. The A2 peak on the *affected* side and the H3 peak on the *less-affected* side thus explain about 82% of the variance in gait speed post-therapy that had improved to an average of 58 cm/s. These results confirm the importance of the ankle A2 power burst both before and after therapy and demonstrate an interlimb strategy to gain speed post-therapy. Because the trade-off between hip and ankle power generators during walking is highly dependent on walking speed (30, 66, 70), comparisons of results in patients with different walking speeds are difficult. For example, in a group of subjects with chronic stroke who followed an 8- to 10-week training program Parvataneni et al. (70) found that the mean gait speed increased from a mean of 69 ±31 cm/s to 83 ± 33 cm/s (n = 28). When the change in gait speed was regressed on the chosen predictor variables of change in positive work, the first variable selected was the affected H1, which alone accounted for 66% of the variation in change of gait speed. A2 was the second variable selected, which, together with the affected H1, accounted for 75% of the variation in gait speed. A second model, which included only the affected and

TABLE 16-4

Step-Wise Regression Analyses of the Relationship Between Peak A2 and H3 Power Bursts on the Affected and Less-Affected Sides of 21 Persons with Stroke While Walking at Comfortable Speed, with Gait Speed Before Therapy (Baseline) in the First Model and with Gait Speed after Therapy in the Second Model.

	R	R SQUARE	ADJ R SQUARE	STD ERROR
Model at baseline				
1. A2, affected side	0.812	0.660	0.637	11.65
2. A2, affected side	0.917	0.841	0.818	8.26
H3, affected side				
Model after therapy				
1. A2, affected side	0.846	0.716	0.697	14.61
2. A2, affected side	0.907	0.822	0.797	11.97
H3, less-affected side				

less-affected H1, accounted for 74.3% of the variation in gait speed. These models resulting from the regression analyses confirm that subjects with hemiparesis increase their gait speed with a combination of H1, H3, and A2 work on the affected side and H1 and H3 on the less-affected side (70). Clinically, this suggests that the gait speed of subjects with similar characteristics could be increased with appropriate changes in a combination of these positive work variables during gait.

Changes in Hip and Ankle Power with Recovery

To further examine the relationship of changes in the A2 and H3 peak power bursts bilaterally with gait speed, the 21 subjects were divided into fast (≥70 cm/s post therapy) and slow (≤69 cm/s post therapy) walkers (Table 16-3). Figure 16-7 illustrates the relationship between changes (post- minus pre-therapy values) in the H3 and A2 peak power bursts bilaterally in the two groups.

In the group of fast walkers, the points cluster mainly in the upper right quadrants for both the affected and less-affected sides, indicating an increase in both the H3 and A2 power bursts. In one subject, the hip power decreased post-therapy, while in another the ankle power decreased. Among the slow walkers, the points tend to cluster more near the intersection point of the quadrants, indicating that the changes are smaller. On the affected side, two subjects had concomitant decreases in the A2 and H3 bursts, while five had little change in the A2 burst. Only three had concomitant increases in both the hip and ankle powers. This graphical representation emphasizes the very small, lack of, or even negative changes in the power-producing capacity of the ankle plantarflexors and hip flexors on the affected side despite two months of task-oriented gait training. The magnitude of the correlations between change in the ankle plantarflexors and the hip flexors

once again demonstrates the variability in the choice of kinetic strategy used by the subjects during walking. The similar correlations for both the affected and less-affected sides in the slow and fast walkers may be related to a matching of the sense of effort (71).

One can also question whether persons after stroke are capable of tapping into their full dynamic strength potential during walking. Milot et al. (71, 72) have used a muscular utilization ratio (MUR) that relates the net moment produced during gait to the muscle's maximal capacity to quantify the level of effort in key muscle groups used by healthy persons and persons with chronic stroke during walking. When compared to a group of healthy individuals (72) they found the MUR values to be higher in the persons with hemiparesis, that the weakest paretic muscle groups had the highest level of effort during gait, and that persons with chronic stroke walking at self-selected and maximal speeds increase their MURs with gait speed. Thus, in a group of persons with stroke walking at a relatively fast mean self-selected speed (73 ± 27 cm/s, n = 17) the peak MURs on the affected side were 64%, 46%, and 33%, respectively, for the plantarflexors, hip flexors, and hip extensors. These values rose to 77%, 72%, and 58% at the maximal speed (126 ± 39 cm/s). Thus, the plantarflexors were the most used muscle group at self-selected speed, while at maximal speed, although the MUR value of all three muscle groups increased, that of the hip muscles increased more than the ankle. Thus, the analysis of the MURs concur with that of the positive work generated at different speeds (66) during walking, with both showing the contribution of the plantarflexors to remain relatively constant at self-selected and maximal speeds, while the use of the hip muscles is increased at maximal speed.

In a subsequent study, Milot et al. (73) examined the effects of increased plantarflexor and hip flexor muscle strength following an isokinetic strengthening program on the levels of effort (MURs) during gait of

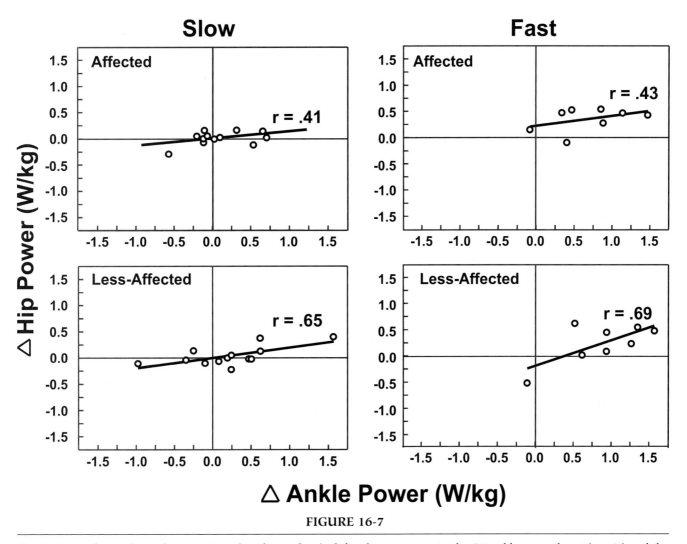

FIGURE 16-7

Concomitant change (post-therapy minus baseline values), defined as recovery, in the A2 ankle power burst (x-axis) and the H3 hip power burst on the affected and less-affected sides of the group of slow (n = 13) and fast walkers (n = 8) described in Table 16-3. Correlations obtained with Pearson Correlation Coefficients.

a group of 24 persons with chronic stroke walking at both self-selected and maximal speeds. They observed a reduction in MUR ratios of 12–17% in the affected plantarflexors and hip flexors and strength gains that were associated with a significant but small increase in gait speeds post-training. Thus, as the subjects became stronger, they apparently favored a reduction in the levels of effort during walking instead of substantially increasing their gait speed. A logical extension of this work would be to test whether the decreased level of effort leads to better functional endurance during walking.

Interestingly, both healthy individuals and persons with stroke have similar MUR values for the muscle groups between sides at both self-selected and maximal speeds (72). This observation of similar levels of effort on the affected and less-affected sides despite a more pronounced weakness of the affected distal muscles led to the interpretation that the asymmetrical gait pattern

of persons with hemiparesis could represent a means of preserving a similar, perceived sense of effort between the affected and less-affected sides. Simon and Ferris (74), building on work that has suggested that healthy individuals use a sense of effort more than proprioceptive feedback to gauge force production in the upper limbs, recently demonstrated a similar mechanism in the control of asymmetrical force in the lower limbs in healthy subjects, providing evidence that the limb force asymmetry was related to neural factors rather that differences in mechanical capabilities between the limbs.

SUMMARY

This chapter has examined recovery after stroke as determined by different methods of evaluation. The use of clinical measures or the attainment of benchmarks, such as discharge from rehabilitation or the ability to walk with help or unassisted, provide an assessment of recovery of function that can be used to evaluate change related to therapy and in the planning of care programs. Such measures, however, do not assess change in biomechanical or neural variables related to locomotor control in relation to normal values. When an increase in gait speed is used as a surrogate for recovery the poor recovery of the majority of stroke survivors, even after two months of therapy, becomes very obvious. Only the minority attain gait speeds that allow them to ambulate freely in the community (51, 54), and it is those who walk at speeds less than 40 cm/s that benefit most from a change in category (54). Nevertheless, few are able to cross busy streets in large cities (17, 52). It is also important to realize that gait speed can continue to increase up to two years post-stroke without formal therapy after discharge from rehabilitation, and that persons with chronic stroke can increase their gait speed with task-oriented circuit training (16, 17).

These results also showed that gait speed at therapy initiation—at least in the subacute state when therapy in the rehabilitation center was started—predicts 40% of the variance in gait speed after two months of task-oriented therapy. As expected, the change in the slowest walkers, which were likely the most severely affected, was small. The time of therapy initiation was also related to the recovery of gait speed, even though therapy was delayed because of constraints related to transfer from an acute hospital. Although the axiom "the earlier, the better" is used to describe the optimal time of therapy initiation, little is known about the optimal time, and further studies are indicated to guide therapy. In this group of stroke survivors the recovery in gait speed was similar in persons with right and left hemiparesis. Again, these findings need to be confirmed in groups of persons with different severities, times of therapy initiation, and types of therapy.

Although the movement profiles of hip, knee, and ankle during the gait cycle tend to improve with increasing gait speed, they will only rarely return to "normal." Moreover, these abnormal gait movements are associated with patterns of muscle activations that differ in both the timing and amplitude from normal values. Comparison of functionally important activation bursts in the TS, TA, and QUAD muscles over time, with normal values, revealed that the TA showed the most recovery and the TS the least. The late change in the QUAD also suggested that muscles may have different temporal patterns of recovery. Although these findings were obtained in a small number of subjects and need to be confirmed in other longitudinal studies of recovery, they are intriguing and worthy of further study. The lack of recovery in the TS is particularly worrisome because of its role in propulsion and the emphasis placed on it in locomotor

therapy. On the other hand, these findings suggest that the TA has an untapped and poorly understood potential in locomotor recovery.

Comparisons of the power and work profiles during gait in persons after stroke, with normal values, have revealed that persons after stroke tend to compensate for a poor power generation at the ankle by increasing the generation of power at the hip, and that with therapy they may choose to produce gait speed by adopting a strategy that depends on the hip of the less-affected leg. Although variable, these compensatory, power-generating strategies again point to the poor recovery in the ankle "push-off" power-generating burst and the use of compensatory strategies involving the hip power generators to increase walking speed.

RESEARCH FRONTIERS

Defining Recovery

The term "recovery" has been used almost indiscriminately to describe changes in locomotor behavior after stroke. These changes, however, may be due to true recovery of biomechanical and motor control mechanisms, to compensatory mechanisms, or a combination of both. More precise definitions of "recovery" and "compensations" would be very helpful in advancing our understanding of the types of changes that occur over time or with therapy after stroke. A better understanding of true recovery, as opposed to compensations, would be helpful in guiding therapeutic choices.

Recovery in Persons with Severe Stroke

We also need to better understand how recovery occurs in the more severely affected persons and how best to promote their recovery, because most of our present information comes from persons with mild and moderate strokes. In this view, a recent fMRI study (75) shed new light on possible mechanisms involved in brain reorganization in pure motor stroke, associated with severe motor deficits. They showed increased activation in a contralesional network following proprioceptive passive training over a four-week period. Although the addition of passive training did not yield better motor outcomes than Bobath therapy, their findings suggest the existence of neural correlates of proprioceptive integration in the contralesional hemisphere. These are preliminary results (75), and further studies need to confirm the possible link between proprioceptive priming and return of function. They are, nevertheless, intriguing and lead to the question of the possibility of transfer of these findings to persons with severe locomotor impairments.

Clinical Correlates to Guide Recovery

Another approach could be to determine from a quantitative gait analysis the levels of power generation at the hip and ankle and from these measures determine the prognosis for true recovery of dynamic force and the choice of therapy. Evaluations of the power-generating and absorption capacity of lower extremity muscles should ideally be task specific because changes in the motor control mechanisms of persons after stroke may lead to a loss of the capacity to activate muscles during walking but not during voluntary contractions in the sitting position (76). Correlation studies, however, have demonstrated that high correlations can be expected between the force measured with a myometer during isometric contractions and walking speed (37, 43, 44). A better understanding of the relation of such clinical measures of force with the recovery of biomechanical parameters during gait would also be of benefit in predicting recovery and possibly more targeted therapy approaches.

Dose-Response Characteristics of Interventions

Despite much work in the last 20 years that has demonstrated the value of task-specific locomotor training (1, 2, 16, 17, 57, 77–79) , we know surprising little about the optimal dose-response characteristics of the intervention, such as the optimal time to start therapy post-stroke once the person is medically stable, the ideal intensity per day, if therapy should be provided on alternate days, if types of therapeutic approaches should be combined, or how many weeks or months therapy should be provided. Physical therapy approaches can be seen as a black box filled with different components, with the specific effects of each component unknown but the total package shown to improve function. The recent STEPS randomized clinical trial (78) is an example of a trial that attempted to determine the effects of task-specific or lower-extremity strength training (or their combination) to improve walking ability in persons with chronic stroke. They were able to show that task-specific BWSTT was more effective in improving walking speed and maintaining these gains after six months than resisted leg cycling alone. More importantly, they showed that combining BWSTT with lower-extremity strength training (limb-load resistive leg cycling or muscle-specific resistive exercise) on alternate days did not enhance walking outcomes. The authors interpreted the lack of added benefit from strength training as overtraining. The superior efficacy of the BWSTT to promote improved gait outcomes over muscle strengthening, on the other hand, is most likely related to the specificity of the training concept. This study (78) emphasized the need to better understand the type of muscle strengthening exercises (isometric, isotonic, isokinetic, strengthening while performing locomotor tasks) that result in increased strength and can best be transferred to improved gait outcomes (42). It also showed the importance of optimal scheduling of training sessions when programs that incorporate moderate- to high-intensity endurance and resistive training are combined.

Sense of Effort and Force-Scaling

The finding that as persons with chronic stroke became stronger they apparently favor a reduction in the levels of effort during walking instead of substantially increasing their gait speed (71) opens a new area of inquiry into the mechanisms controlling the symmetry of effort at self-selected walking speeds. These investigators (72) have also shown that normalizing joint moments during gait to the maximum joint moment capabilities led to similar effort levels in the affected and less-affected limb of persons with chronic stroke during walking. Thus, it seems that sense of effort is an important factor in determining lower-limb muscle activations in persons with hemiparesis. Force matching studies (74, 80) thus suggest that, in addition to strengthening the affected lower extremity muscles, rehabilitation approaches should also address the impaired force scaling ability. Simon et al. (81) advocate that symmetry-based resistance has the potential to improve both force scaling ability and limb strength because subjects can learn to scale muscle activations more appropriately to achieve a desired force outcome. This would enable persons with stroke to better match paretic limb forces to task requirements during activities of daily living.

Neural Correlates of Therapeutic Gains

Another avenue in understanding the specific effects of therapy is to examine the neural correlates of therapeutic gains. In this context, Dobkin (82) has recommended the use of serial fMRIs as a physiological indicator for "dose-response" interactions during a rehabilitative intervention. An example of such a study is that of Dong et al. (83) who questioned whether the brain activation midway through two weeks of constraint-induced arm therapy (84) might capture adaptations induced by the initial week of training that could be used to predict post-therapeutic changes in hand function. They found a relationship between brain activation during treatment and functional gains and concluded that there was a use for serial fMRIs in predicting the success and optimal duration for a focused therapeutic intervention.

Functional Cognition and Walking Competency

Even though up to 65% of stroke survivors have new onset or worsening of cognitive deficits after stroke (85–88) that interfere with functional recovery and the potential benefits of rehabilitation (86, 88, 89) and lead to falls (90), the rehabilitation of cognitive deficits, and in particular the impact of cognitive deficits on walking competency, have been largely ignored. Members of the rehabilitation theme of the Canadian Stroke Network have identified cognitive deficits as a priority area for research (91), and recognizing the need, the National Institute of Neurological Disorders and Stroke (NINDS) and the Canadian Stroke Network have joined together to establish criteria for systematic study of cognitive deficits associated with stroke (92). In a recent paper devoted to conceptualizing functional cognition in stroke, Donavan et al. (86) have defined functional cognition "as the ability to accomplish everyday activities that rely heavily on cognitive abilities." Walking competency (17) implies that, in addition to the physical capacity to walk fast enough to cross streets and far enough to be able to walk about in the community, a person also has the planning abilities to navigate among others and to find his/her way, as well as to make locomotor adjustments to meet the demands of the changing environment.

There is a growing body of literature from both the aging and clinical populations that examines the role of cognition in locomotion. The main approach to study the interaction between cognitive processing and motor behavior is the dual task paradigm. Thus, Plumer-D'Amato et al. (93) have shown that, in persons with stroke living in the community, speech produced more gait interference than memory and visuospatial tasks and that, even though the participants were mobility impaired, they prioritized the cognitive tasks. Future research is needed to determine if dual task training can help reduce gait decrements in dual task situations. The use of virtual reality paradigms, on the other hand, provide the opportunity to combine physical locomotor training on the treadmill with cognitive training that is goal directed and motivating for persons with chronic stroke. Our research team has developed a walking simulator that mimics changes in the terrain as subjects walk on a self-paced treadmill into increasingly challenging virtual environments (94) that require the subjects to meet time constraints while dealing with terrain changes and avoiding collisions with obstacles that cross their path. Preliminary findings show that persons with stroke, in addition to improving their walking capacity, also gain a sense of self-efficacy in dealing with the changing environment from this type of practice, which is transferred to their everyday life (95) Moreover, adaptations of the trunk and hip movements prior to terrain changes suggest that subjects learn to make anticipatory adjustments (96). A randomized, controlled pilot trial is currently underway to evaluate the efficacy of a VR-based locomotor training program in comparison to training on the same treadmill with perturbations

similar to those experienced by the VR-group as they move through the virtual environments but instead view a series of slides. A case study of one person with chronic stroke who followed both the control and the VR-training programs found the VR-training to be more motivational and to lead to improved planning and decision-making and a sense of self-efficacy that carried over into real life (97). These preliminary findings warrant further study, first to confirm the findings and then to determine the characteristics of the subjects most likely to benefit from such an approach.

Further studies are also needed to better understand the importance of self-efficacy, defined as a judgment of one's ability to organize and execute given types of performances (98), in the success of locomotor training programs. For example, Salbach et al. (99, 100) found that enhancing balance self-efficacy in addition to functional walking capacity, when compared to enhancing functional walking capacity alone, may lead to greater improvement, not only in perceived health status, but also in physical function, Much work is needed to better elucidate the interaction between cognitive function and walking competency as well as the development of adequate rehabilitation programs to target impaired cognitive function in persons with stroke.

Another alternative for locomotor retraining in patients with severe motor impairment is the use of mental practice through motor imagery (101). Using transcranial magnetic stimulation Pascual-Leone and colleagues (102) reported that mental practice produced representational changes in the brain comparable to those yielded by physical practice. Moreover, they found that subjects who had mentally practiced a one-handed piano exercise for five sessions and then added only one physical session reached the same level of performance as those who practiced physically for five sessions. The latter findings suggest that part of the behavioral improvement seen in the mental practice may be latent, waiting to be expressed after minimal physical practice. Mental practice in subjects who cannot walk or with limited walking capacity could thus have a preparatory effect on the task, hence increasing the efficiency of subsequent physical training (102). The priming effects of mental practice have been extended to movements of the lower limbs in a Positron Emitted Tomography study (103). Indeed, after five days of intense mental practice of a foot movement sequence, subjects were able to complete the sequences of foot movement faster, both mentally and physically. In addition, similar dynamic changes during both modalities (imagination and execution) were observed, hence demonstrating that learning a sequential motor task through motor imagery practice produces cerebral changes similar to those observed after physical practice of the same task (103). Combining physical and mental practice has also been found to promote the learning of a foot movement sequence after stroke (104). To date, positive effects of mental practice on gait speed and step length have been reported after stroke in series of patients with chronic stroke (105, 106). The potential of motor imagery could also be explored for training cognitive (planning, anticipation) and motor skills required to navigate safely in various indoor or outdoor environments, for negotiating stairs and inclines, or for avoiding fixed or moving obstacles.

For patients who have difficulty or are unable to engage in motor imagery, action observation remains an interesting alternative for developing their walking capacity (107, 108). This suggestion is based on findings that, like the imagination, the execution and the observation of a movement are controlled by more or less the same brain areas (109–111). Indeed, mirror neurons in the premotor cortex and the inferior parietal cortex not only discharge during the performance of a goal-directed movement but also while observing the movements performed by another person. Thus, when a person sees an action performed by someone else, neurons that represent that action are activated in the observer's premotor cortex so that, automatically, motor representations involved in the execution of that action are activated. Hence, observing an action directly activates the motor commands needed for performing that action.

ACKNOWLEDGEMENTS

This work over the years has been supported by grants from the National Health Research and Development Program of Canada, the Canadian Stroke Network, the Canadian Institutes of Health Research, the Canadian Foundation for Innovation, and the "Fonds de la recherche en santé du Québec." C. L. Richards is the holder of a Tier I Canada Research Chair in Rehabilitation and the Laval University Research Chair in Cerebral Palsy. The authors thank D. Tardif and F. Comeau for technical assistance.

References

1. Richards CL, Malouin F, Wood-Dauphinee S, et al. Task-specific physical therapy for optimization of gait recovery in acute stroke patients. *Arch Phys Med Rehabil* 1993; 74:612–620.
2. Richards CL, Malouin F, Bravo G, et al. The role of technology in task-oriented training in persons with subacute stroke: A randomized controlled trial. *Neurorehabil Neural Repair* 2004; 18(4):199–211.
3. Twitchell TE. The restoration of motor function following hemiplegia in man. *Brain* 1951; 74(4):443–480.
4. Skilbeck CE, Wade DT, Hewer RL, Wood VA. Recovery after stroke. *J Neurol Neurosurg Psychiatry* 1983; 46:5–8.
5. Duncan PW, Goldstein LB, Horner RD, et al. Similar motor recovery of upper and lower extremities after stroke. *Stroke* 1994; 25:1181–1188.
6. Bach-y-Rita P, ed. *Recovery of Function: Theoretical Considerations for Brain Iinjury Rehabilitation.* Baltimore: University Park Press, 1980.
7. Fugl-Meyer AR, Jaaskp L, Leyman I, et al. The post-stroke hemiplegia patient. I. A method for evaluation of physical performance. *Scand J Rehabil Med* 1975; 7:13–31.
8. Jorgensen HS, Nakayama H, Raaschou HO, et al. Outcome and time course of recovery in stroke. I. Outcome: The Copenhagen Stroke Study. *Arch Phys Med Rehabil* 1995; 76:399–405.
9. Jorgensen, HS, Nakayama H, Raaschou HO, et al. Outcome and time course of recovery in stroke. II. Time course of recovery: The Copenhagen Stroke Study. *Arch Phys Med Rehabil* 1995; 76:406–412.
10. Jorgensen HS, Nakayama H, Raaschou HO, Olsen TS. Recovery of walking function in stroke patients. The Copenhagen Stroke Study. *Arch Phys Med Rehabil* 1995; 76:27–32.
11. Mahoney FD, Barthel DW. Rehabilitation of the hemiplegic patient: A clinical evaluation. *Arch Phys Med Rehabil* 1954; 35:359–362.
12. Kwakkel G, Kollen B, Lindeman E. Understanding the pattern of functional recovery after stroke: Facts and theories. *Restor Neurol Neurosci* 2004; 22:281–299.
13. Newman M. The process of recovery after hemiplegia. *Stroke* 1972; 3:702–710.
14. Gresham GE. Stroke outcome research. *Stroke* 1986; 17(3):358–360.
15. Kwakkel G, Kollen B, Twisk J. Impact of time on improvement of outcome after stroke. *Stroke* 2006; 37:2348–2353.
16. Dean CM, Richards CL, Malouin F. Task-related training improves performance of locomotor tasks in chronic stroke: A randomized, controlled pilot study. *Arch Phys Med Rehabil* 2000; 81:409–417.
17. Salbach NM, Mayo NE, Wood-Dauphinee S, et al. A task-orientated intervention enhances walking distance and speed in the first year post stroke: A randomized controlled trial. *Clin Rehabil* 2004; 8(5):509–519.
18. Nudo RJ, Plautz EJ, Frost SB. Role of adaptive plasticity in recovery of function after damage to motor cortex. *Muscle Nerve* 2001; 24:1000–1019.
19. Nudo RJ, Plautz EJ, Milliken GW. Adaptive plasticity in primate motor cortex as a consequence of behavioral experience and neuronal injury. *Semin Neurosci* 1997; 9:13–23.
20. Miyai I, Suzuki M, Hatakenaka M, Kubota K. Effect of body weight support on cortical activation during gait in patients with stroke. *Exp Brain Res* 2006; 169:85–91.
21. Miyai I, Yagura H, Hatakenaka M, et al. Longitudinal optical imaging study for locomotor recovery after stroke. *Stroke* 2003; 34:2866–2870.
22. Miyai I, Yagura H, Oda I, et al. Premotor cortex is involved in restoration of gait in stroke. *Ann Neurol* 2002; 52:188–194.
23. Yen CL, Wang RY, Liao KK, et al. Gait training induced change in corticomotor excitability in patients with chronic stroke. *Neurorehabil Neural Repair* 2008; 22:22–30.
24. Dobkin BH, Firestine A, West M, et al. Ankle dorsiflexion as an fMRI paradigm to assay motor control for walking during rehabilitation. *Neuroimage* 2004; 23:370–381.
25. Sullivan KJ, Dobkin BH, Tavakol M, et al. Post-stroke cortical plasticity induced by step training. *Proc Soc Neurosci* 2001; 27; Program No. 624.14.
26. Phillips JP, Sullivan KJ, Burtner PA, et al. Ankle dorsiflexion fMRI in children with cerebral palsy undergoing intensive body-weight supported treadmill training: A pilot study. *Dev Med Child Neurol* 2007; 49:39–44.
27. Knutsson E, Richards CL. Different types of disturbed motor control in gait of hemiparetic patients. *Brain* 1979; 102:405–430.
28. Cirstea MC, Ptito A, Levin MF. Arm reaching improvements with short-term practice depend on the severity of the motor deficit in stroke. *Exp Brain Res* 2003; 152:476–488.
29. Garland SJ, Willems DA, Ivanova TD, Miller KJ. Recovery of standing balance and functional mobility after stroke. *Arch Phys Med Rehabil* 2003; 84:1753–1759.
30. Kim CM, Eng JJ. Magnitude and pattern of 3D kinematic and kinetic gait profiles in persons with stroke: Relationship to walking speed. *Gait & Posture* 2004; 20:140–146.
31. Kollen B, van de Port I, Lindeman E, et al. Predicting improvement in gait after stroke: A longitudinal study. *Stroke* 2005; 36:2676–2680.
32. Lamontagne A, Malouin F, Richards CL. Contribution of passive stiffness to ankle plantarflexor moment during gait after stroke. *Arch Phys Med Rehabil* 2000; 81:351–358.
33. Lamontagne A, Malouin F, Richards CL. Locomotor-specific measure of spasticity of plantarflexor muscles after stroke. *Arch Phys Med Rehabil* 2001; 82:1696–1704.
34. Lamontagne A, Malouin F, Richards, CL, Dumas F. Mechanisms of disturbed motor control in ankle weakness during gait after stroke. *Gait & Posture* 2002; 15:244–255.
35. Olney SJ, Griffin MP, Monga TN, McBride ID. Work and power in gait of stroke patients. *Arch Phys Med Rehabil* 1991; 72:309–314.
36. Olney SJ, Richards CL. Hemiplegic gait following stroke. I. Characteristics. *Gait & Posture* 1996; 4:136–148.
37. Richards CL, Malouin F, Dumas F, Lamontagne A. Recovery of ankle and hip power during walking after stroke. *Can J Rehabil* 1998; 11:271–273.
38. Richards CL, Malouin F, Dumas F, Tardif D. Gait velocity as an outcome measure of locomotor recovery after stroke. In: Craik RL, Oatis CA, eds. *Gait Analysis: Theory and Application.* St Louis, MO: Mosby, 1995; 25:355–364.

39. Richards CL, Malouin F, Dumas F, Wood-Dauphinee S. The relationship of gait speed to clinical measures of function and muscle activations during recovery post-stroke. In: *Proceedings of the Second North American Congress of Biomechanics*, 1992:299–302.

40. Wade DT. *Measurement in Neurological Rehabilitation*. Oxford, UK: Oxford University Press, 1992.

41. Brandstater ME, de Bruin H, Gowland C, Clark BM. Hemiplegic gait: Analysis of temporal variables. *Arch Phys Med Rehabil* 1983; 64:583–587.

42. Richards CL, Olney SJ. Hemiparetic gait following stroke. 2. Recovery and physical therapy. *Gait & Posture*1996; 4:149–162.

43. Bohannon RW, Andrews AW. Correlation of knee extensor muscle torque and spasticity with gait speed in patients with stroke. *Arch Phys Med Rehabil* 1990; 71:330–333.

44. Bohannon RW. Strength of lower limb related to gait velocity and cadence in stroke patients. *Physiother Can* 1986; 38:204–206.

45. Bohannon RW. Selected determinants of ambulatory capacity in patients with hemiplegia. *Clin Rehabil* 1989; 3:47–53.

46. Holden MK, Gill KM, Magliozzi MR, et al. Clinical gait assessment in the neurologically impaired: Reliability and meaningfulness. *Phys Ther* 1984; 64:35–40.

47. Wade DT, Hewer RL. Functional abilities after stroke: Measurement, natural history and prognosis. *J Neurol Neurosurg Psychiatry* 1987; 50.177–182.

48. Kollen B, Kwakkel G, Lindeman E. Hemiplegic gait after stroke: Is measurement of maximum speed required? *Arch Phys Med Rehabil* 2006; 87:358–363.

49. Salbach NM, Mayo NE, Higgins J, et al. Responsiveness and predictability of gait speed and other disability measures in acute stroke. *Arch Phys Med Rehabil* 2001; 88:1204–1212.

50. Richards CL, Malouin F, Dean C. Gait in stroke: Assessment and rehabilitation. In: Duncan PW, ed. *Clin Geriatr Med* 1999; 15(4):833–855.

51. Perry J, Garrett M, Gronley JK, Mulroy SJ. Classification of walking handicap in the stroke population. *Stroke* 1995; 26: 982–989.

52. Robinett CS, Vondran MA. Functional ambulation velocity and distance requirements in rural and urban communities: A clinical report. *Phys Ther* 1988; 68(9):1371–1373.

53. Kwakkel G, Wagenaar RC, Twisk JW, et al. Intensity of leg and arm training after primary middle cerebral-artery stroke: A randomised trial. *Lancet* 1999; 354:191–196.

54. Schmid A, Duncan PW, Studenski S, et al. Improvements in speed-based gait classifications are meaningful. *Stroke* 2007; 38(7):2096–2100

55. Desrosiers J, Noreau L, Robichaud L, et al. Validity of the assessment of life habits in older adults. *J Rehabil Med* 2004; 36(4):177–182.

56. Richards CL, Cioni M, Malouin F, et al. Changes in gait of patients with Parkinson's Disease induced by sensory cues and L-Dopa. *Proceedings of the 6th Biennial Conference of the Canadian Society for Biomechanics* Quebec City, Canada. 1990:199–202.

57. Malouin F, Potvin M, Prevost J, et al. Use of an intensive task-oriented gait training program in a series of patients with acute cerebrovascular accidents. *Phys Ther* 1992; 72:781–789; discussion 789–793.

58. Richards CL, Malouin F, Dumas,F, Wood-Dauphinee S. Longitudinal study of locomotor recovery up to two years after stroke. XVIIth Conference on Postural and Gait Research. *Gait & Posture* 2005; 21(suppl 1):S110.

59. Winter DA. *The Biomechanics and Motor Control of Human Gait: Normal, Elderly and Pathological*. Waterloo: University of Waterloo Press, 1991.

60. Olney SJ. Training gait after stroke: A biomechanical perspective. In: *Science-Based Rehabilitation. Theories into Practice*. Refshauge K, Ada L, Ellis E, eds. Sydney: Butterworth Heinemann, 2005; 8:159–184.

61. Olney SJ, Griffin MP, McBride ID. Multivariate examination of data from gait analysis of persons with stroke. *Phys Ther* 1998; 8:814–828.

62. Colborne GR, Olney SJ, Griffin MP. Feedback of ankle joint angle and soleus electromyography in the rehabilitation of hemiplegic gait. *Arch Phys Med Rehabil* 1993; 74(10):1100–1106.

63. Capaday C, Lavoie BA, Barbeau H, et al. Studies on the corticospinal control of human walking. 1. Responses to focal transcranial magnetic stimulation of the motor cortex. *J Neurophysiol* 1999; 81(1):129–139.

64. Chen IH, Kuo KN, Andriacchi TP. The influence of walking speed on mechanical joint power during gait. *Gait & Posture* 1997; 6:171–176.

65. Graf A, Judge JO, Ounpuu S, Thelen DG. The effect of walking speed on lower-extremity joint powers among elderly adults who exhibit low physical performance. *Arch Phys Med Rehabil* 2005; 86(11):2177–2183.

66. Teixeira-Salmela LF, Nadeau S, Milot MH, et al. Effects of cadence on energy generation and absorption at lower extremity joints during gait. *Clin Biomech* 2008, doi:10.1016/j.clinbiomech.2008.02.007.

67. Andriacchi TP, Ogle JA, Galante JO. Walking speed as a basis for normal and abnormal gait measurements. *J. Biomech.* 1977; 10:261.

68. Shiavi R, Bugle HJ, Limbird T. Electromyographic gait assessment. 2. Preliminary assessment of hemiparetic synergy patterns. *J Rehabil Res Dev* 1987; 24:24–30.

69. Higginson JS, Zajac FE, Neptune RR, et al. Muscle contributions to support during gait in an individual with post-stroke hemiparesis. *J Biomech*. 2006; 39:1769–1777.

70. Parvataneni K, Olney SJ, Brouwer B. Changes in muscle group work associated with changes in gait speed of persons with stroke. *Clin Biomech* 2007; 22(7):813–820.

71. Milot MH, Nadeau S, Gravel D. Muscular utilization of the plantarflexors, hip flexors and extensors in persons with hemiparesis walking at self-selected and maximal speeds. *J Electromyogr Kinesiol* 2007; 17(2):184–193.

72. Milot MH, Nadeau S, Gravel D, Requião LF. Bilateral level of effort of the plantar flexors, hip flexors, and extensors during gait in hemiparetic and healthy individuals. *Stroke* 2006; 37(8):2070–2075.

73. Milot MH, Nadeau S, Gravel D, Bourbonnais D. Effect of increases in plantarflexor and hip flexor muscle strength on the levels of effort during gait in individuals with hemiparesis. *Clin Biomech* 2008; 23(4):415–423.

74. Simon AM, Ferris DP. Lower limb force production and bilateral force asymmetries are based on sense of effort. *Exp Brain Res* 2008; 187(1):129–138.

75. Dechaumont-Palacin S, Marque P, De Boissezon X, et al. Neural correlates of proprioceptive integration in the contralesional hemisphere of very impaired patients shortly after a subcortical stroke: An fMRI study. *Neurorehabil Neural Repair* 2008; 22:154–165.

76. Crenna P. Spasticity and "spastic" gait in children with cerebral palsy. *Neurosci Biobehav Rev* 1998; 22(4):571–578

77. Ada L, Dean CM, Hall JM, et al. A treadmill and overground walking program improves walking in persons residing in the community after stroke: A placebo-controlled, randomized trial. *Arch Phys Med Rehabil* 2003; 84:1486–1491.

78. Sullivan KJ, Brown DA, Klassen T, et al. Effects of task-specific locomotor and strength training in adults who were ambulatory after stroke: Results of STEPS randomized clinical trial. *Phys Ther* 2007; 87:1–23.

79. Van de Port IG, Wood-Dauphinee S, Lindeman E, Kwakkel G. Effects of exercise training programs on walking competency after stroke: A systematic review. *Am J Phys Med Rehabil* 2007; 86:935–951.

80. Mercier C, Bertrand AM, Bourbonnais D. Differences in the magnitude and direction of forces during a submaximal matching task in hemiparetic subjects. *Exp Brain Res* 2004; 157(1):32–42.

81. Simon AM, Gillespie B, Ferris DP. Symmetry-based resistance as a novel means of lower limb rehabilitation. *J Biomech* 2007; 40:1286–1292.

82. Dobkin BH. Rehabilitation and functional neuroimaging dose-response trajectories for clinical trials. *Neurorehabil Neural Repair* 2005; 19(4):276–282.

83. Dong Y, Dobkin BH, Cen SY, et al. Motor cortex activation during treatment may predict therapeutic gains in paretic hand function after stroke. *Stroke* 2006; 37:1552–1555.

84. Winstein CJ, Miller JP, Blanton S, et al. Methods for a multisite randomized trial to investigate the effect of constraint-induced movement therapy in improving upper extremity function among adults recovering from a cerebrovascular stroke. *Neurorehabil Neural Repair* 2003; 17:137–152.

85. Ballard C, Stephens S, McLaren A, et al. Mild cognitive impairment and vascular cognitive impairment in stroke patients. *Int Psychogeriatr* 2003; 15(1):123–126.

86. Donavan NJ, Kendall DL, Heaton SC, et al. Conceptualizing functional cognition in stroke. *Neurorehabil Neural Repair* 2008; 22(2):122–135.

87. Tatemichi TK, Desmond DW, Stern Y, et al. Cognitive impairment after stroke: Frequency, patterns, and relationship to functional activities. *J Neuol Neurosurg Psychiatry* 1994; 57:202–207.

88. Zinn S, Dudley TK, Bosworth HB, et al. The effect of poststroke cognitive impairment on rehabilitation process and functional outcome. *Arch Phys Med Rehabil* 2004; 85:1084–1090.

89. Paolucci S, Antonucci G, Gialloreti LE, et al. Predicting stroke inpatient rehabilitation outcome : The prominent role of neuropsychological disorders. *Eur Neurol* 1996; 36:385–390.

90. Liu-Ambrose T, Pang MYC, Eng JJ. Executive function is independently associated with performances of balance and mobility in community-dwelling older adults with mild stroke: Implications for falls prevention. *Cerebrovasc Dis* 2007; 23:203–210.

91. Bayley M, Hurdowar A, Teasell R, et al. Priorities for stroke rehabilitation research and knowledge translation: Results of a 2003 Canadian Stroke Network Consensus Conference. *Arch Phys Med Rehabil* 2007; 88(4):526–528.

92. Hachinski V, Iadecola C, Petersen RC, et al. National Institute of Neurological Disorders and Stroke Canadian Stroke Network Vascular Cognitive Impairment Harmonization Standards. *Stroke* 2006; 37:2220–2241.

93. Plummer-D'Amato P, Altman LJP, Saracino D, et al. Interactions between cognitive tasks and gait after stroke: A dual task study. *Gait & Posture* 2008; 27(4):683–688.

94. Fung J, Richards, CL, Malouin F, et al. A treadmill and motion coupled virtual reality system for gait training post-stroke. *Cyberpsychol Behav* 2006; 9(2):157–162.

95. Richards CL, Malouin F, McFadyen BJ, et al. A virtual reality-based locomotor training program to promote walking competency after stroke. World Confederation for Physical Therapy Congress, Vancouver. *Physiotherapy* 2007; 93(Suppl 1):S104.

96. Richards CL, McFadyen BJ, Malouin F, et al. Virtual reality (VR) training to promote anticipatory gait control post stroke. 2nd International Congress on Gait & Mental Function, Amsterdam, Feb 1–3, 2008. *Parkinsonism & Related Disorders* 2008; 14(Suppl 1): S66 (P2.089).

97. Richards CL, Malouin F, McFadyen BJ, et al. Training in virtual reality improves locomotor self-efficacy after stroke: A single subject design study. FICCDAT Conferences, Toronto, June 17–19, 2007, 369–370.

98. Bandura A. *Self-Efficacy: The Exercise of Control*. New York: WH Freeman, 1997.

99. Salbach NM, Mayo NE, Robichaud-Ekstrand S, et al. The effect of a task-oriented walking intervention on improving balance self-efficacy poststroke: A randomized controlled trial. [Published erratum in: *J Am Geriatr Soc* 2005; 53:1450]. *J Am Geriatr Soc* 2005; 53:576–582.

100. Salbach NM, Mayo NE, Robichaud-Ekstrand S, et al. Balance self-efficacy and its relevance to physical function and perceived health status after stroke. *Arch Phys Med Rehabil* 2006; 87:364–70.

101. Jackson PL, Lafleur MF, Malouin F, et al. Potential role of mental practice using motor imagery in neurologic rehabilitation. *Arch Phys Med Rehabil* 2001; 82:1133–1141.

102. Pascual-Leone A, Nguyet D, Cohen LG, et al. Modulation of muscle responses evoked by transcranial magnetic stimulation during the acquisition of new fine motor skills. *J Neurophysiol* 1995; 74:1037–1045.

103. Jackson PL, Lafleur MF, Malouin F, et al. Functional cerebral reorganization following motor sequence learning through mental practice with motor imagery. *Neuroimage* 2003; 20:1171–1180.

104. Jackson PL, Doyon J, Richards CL, Malouin F. The efficacy of combined physical and mental practice in the learning of a foot-sequence task after stroke: A case report. *Neurorehabil Neural Repair* 2004; 18:106–111.

105. Dickstein R, Dunsky A, Marcovitz E. Motor imagery for gait rehabilitation in post-stroke hemiparesis. *Phys Ther* 2004; 84:1167–1177.

106. Dunsky A, Dickstein R, Ariav C, et al. Motor imagery practice in gait rehabilitation of chronic post-stroke hemiparesis: Four cases. *Int J Rehabil Res* 2006; 29: 351–356.

107. Buccino G, Solodkin A, Small SL. Functions of the mirror neuron system: Implications for neurorehabilitation. *Cogn Behav Neurol* 2006; 19:55–63.

108. Pomeroy VM, Clark CA, Miller JS, et al. The potential for utilizing the "mirror neurone system" to enhance recovery of the severely affected upper limb early after stroke: A review and hypothesis. *Neurorehabil Neural Repair* 2005; 19:4–13.

109. Decety, J., Grèzes, J. Neural mechanisms subserving the perception of human actions. *Trends Cogn Sci* 1999; 3:172–178.

110. Gallese V, Fadiga L, Fogassi L, Rizzolatti G.. Action recognition in the premotor cortex. *Brain* 1996; 119:593–609.

111. Iseki K, Hanakawa T, Shinozaki J, et al. Neural mechanisms involved in mental imagery and observation of gait. *Neuro Image* 2008; doi:10.1016/j.

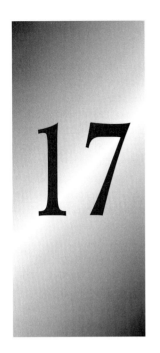

17 Task-Oriented Training to Promote Upper Extremity Recovery

Carolee J. Winstein
Steven L. Wolf

ask-oriented training has emerged as the dominant approach to motor restoration for stroke-induced motor impairments. This chapter provides the background and context for the emergence of a task-oriented approach to promote functional recovery after stroke (Section II). To move beyond a simplistic interpretation of "task-oriented" training, we elaborate on what the multi-disciplinary scientific community would term the "active ingredients" and propose three criteria for effective training programs to promote functional recovery (Section III). In the next section, we use the criterion-based definition and make the case that constraint-induced movement therapy is a special class of task-oriented training (Section IV). In Section V, we draw from the extensive foundations in the behavioral sciences of motor control and learning to consider the "pharmacokinetics" of training, including practice schedules, practice time and intensity of training, the organization of training, and the contents of training. In Section VI, we review each of the 10 principles of experience-dependent neural plasticity in the context of task-oriented training. Section VII gives two examples of emerging innovative task-oriented training approaches to upper limb rehabilitation, one a multi-modal combination intervention, and the other, a fully-defined evidence-based hybrid combination of constraint-induced movement therapy and skill-based/impairment-mitigating

motor skill training with embedded motivational enhancements. Finally, Section VIII provides a brief overview of four related research frontiers in neurorehabilitation.

I. EMERGENCE OF TASK-ORIENTED TRAINING FOR NEUROREHABILITATION

The 2006 National Institutes of Health, National Institute for Neurological Disorders and Stroke (NINDS) Stroke Progress Review Group summarized what it considered to be the most significant scientific accomplishments since its last published guidelines in 2001. The Recovery and Rehabilitation workgroup remarked that there had been a substantial increase in the understanding of how training parameters and subject characteristics change response to motor rehabilitation. In particular, the workgroup concluded that *task-oriented training* had emerged as the dominant approach to motor restoration. Other findings from the motor learning field including the delivery schedule of training, motivation, and contextual factors are now under active study. In addition, characteristics of treatment participants, including severity of motor deficits and co-existing sensory or cognitive impairments, are also under investigation. Further, the panel identified that clinical trials in this area have proven more challenging than previously anticipated, with variables in dosing, timing, and duration adding to their inherent complexity. This area encompasses unmet needs, the resolution of which could yield large potential benefits. Most importantly, one of the key unresolved scientific questions revolves around establishing the "pharmacokinetics" of training: Dosing, timing of administration, half-life, and resolving the question of whether the training paradigm matters (1).

What Is Task-Oriented Training?

As this approach is emergent within the field of neurorehabilitation, yet lacking clear criteria, there is considerable variability in the literature as to what constitutes a task-oriented training (TOT) program. From a disablement/enablement perspective such as the World Health Organization's International Classification of Disability and Functioning (2), task-oriented training is best described as a top-down approach to rehabilitation (see Top-Down Model) (3). This approach is one that addresses activity limitations, rather than the specific and isolated remediation of impairments (4–7) or specific movement kinematics (i.e., body functions/structures). In more recent literature, this top-down approach has variously been referred to as a "motor learning" or "movement science" approach to rehabilitation (8), "task-specific training" (4), "task-related training" (9–12), "functional task practice" (13) or "goal-directed training" (7, 14, 15). Task-oriented training is based on more recent integrated models of motor control, motor learning, and behavioral neuroscience, where active participation and skill acquisition are critical components of recovery. Consistent with this patient-centered perspective of motor control, the manner in which voluntary movement is elicited after a paralyzing stroke represents the best efforts to achieve "functional task goals" given the constraints imposed by the stroke-induced impairments, the personal attributes, the environment, and the demands of the task (16–18). With these assumptions, and considering this conceptual framework, the patient is viewed as an *active problem-solver*, and *rehabilitation is focused on acquisition of skills* for performance of meaningful and relevant tasks. In addition, these tasks should be challenging to achieve, involve real objects and activities, and be goal-directed in nature. These activities are therefore distinct from rote or exercise-based movements that can be abstract and without a preconceived and task-based functional goal (5, 19–21).

Therefore, the desired outcome of a task-oriented training program is **skill**. In turn, skill can be defined as the ability to achieve a goal (the task) with consistency, flexibility, and efficiency. This definition of "skill" provides a useful framework for measuring how well the outcome has been achieved (22). The identification of skill as the critical outcome of TOT differentiates it from mere practice of activities of daily living (ADL) or compensatory training. In spite of the fact that there is little evidence to

support the efficacy of repeated task-practice, simplistic and imprecise discussions of TOT often include practice of ADL as an example. In this context, it is unfortunate that the Ottawa Panel evidence-based clinical practice guidelines (EBCPG) for post-stroke rehabilitation defined interventions related to "task-oriented training" as treatments that involved dividing activities of daily living into component parts (23). Individual components of the larger task were then practiced until the patient was able to complete the component adequately. Component parts were then combined, and the overall task was practiced with repetition. Any intervention that divided required tasks into individual components was included in the Ottawa Panel EBCPG under the general classification of "task-oriented training," including tasks such as seated reaching, adapted games, and repetitive elbow joint movements. This classification of TOT is not consistent with the supporting evidence, and misses the essential and critical outcome of TOT that is skill-based.

It should be obvious from this discussion that a precise and evidence-based definition of task-oriented training is essential to stimulate further advances in neurorehabilitation. There is, however, a clear distinction between TOT approaches and the more traditional bottom-up neuromuscular re-education approaches that dominated neurorehabilitation well into the 1980s.

How Is TOT Different From Neuromuscular Re-Education?

When one reviews a magnificent compendium of work that characterized rehabilitative efforts to improve movement among patients with central nervous system deficits that is housed within the landmark Northwestern University Special Therapeutic Exercise Project (NUSTEP) volume (24), one is struck by the outstanding efforts set forth among a dedicated group of clinicians, whose collective treatment formulations were derived from elements of fundamental neurophysiology. The emergence of such "approaches" as advocated, for example, by Brunnstrom, Bobath, Rood, Knott, and Doman-Delgado were sincere efforts to guide clinical practice by encouraging clinicians to treat patient impairments using specific directives. These efforts at "neuromuscular reeducation" were appreciated by physical and occupational therapists because they provided some of the initial foundations and translation of the science for implementation of clinical practice. Many of these techniques are still in use; however, even with their births and subsequent evolution, their collective value has been hampered by a series of concerns, the significance of which become more meaningful with the development of more sophisticated assessment tools, and with advances in scientific exploration. Among these concerns are the fact that the bases for most "neuromuscular reeducation techniques" were never externally validated; that is, the relevance and verification of observations extracted from animal preparations had not been confirmed in a convincing fashion among human patients before the formulation of specific techniques were disseminated. Second, very few outcome measures existed, and those that did lacked confirmatory validation until subjected to study and refinement that did not begin until the mid-1980s. Moreover, many procedures permitted use of compensatory behaviors rather than optimizing function within the context of maximal utilization of the impaired anatomy. Last, much of the emphasis of neuromuscular re-education was focused on the impairment level of disablement (i.e., "body functions/structures" in the ICF framework) without considering adequately the implications or relevance to voluntary participatory behaviors (i.e., "activity" in the ICF framework) or the importance of changes in life roles or health related quality of life (i.e., "participation" in the ICF framework).

II. CRITERION-BASED TOT: WHAT ARE THE ACTIVE INGREDIENTS?

In this section, we summarize relevant evidence from neuroscience, neurology, and the motor control and learning literatures to develop a short list of strong candidates for consideration as "active" ingredients for the prospective design of an effective task-oriented training program to promote post-stroke upper extremity recovery.

Evidence is emerging from animal and human studies to suggest that *behavioral demands* and *motor skill training* may be critical drivers to cortical reorganization associated with positive functional outcomes following a stroke or stroke-like lesion in animals (25–28). In non-disabled adults, the kinematics of arm and hand movements have been shown to be uniquely constrained by the behavioral goals of the movement and the characteristics of the to-be-grasped object, such as spatial location and object shape and size (29–32). After stroke, there is evidence to suggest that the emergent movement kinematics are organized differently for real objects compared with simulated or artificial objects. Upper limb movement kinematics were more efficient when the goal-directed activity included reaching for a ringing telephone, compared to simulated contexts such as reaching for a stick (15) or no object (32, 33). Thus, the fidelity of the task in the natural context seems to be a critical ingredient of effective task-oriented training programs. (This observation and its relationship to the recently discovered mirror-neuron system is touched upon in the section on Research Frontiers at the end of this chapter). In addition, greater transfer of training to life activities might be anticipated from such task-oriented training, particularly given the focus on familiar everyday tasks, and transfer to unpracticed tasks might be possible given the focus on the development of problem-solving

strategies. It is well known that training programs which are designed to enforce the *practice of problem-solving* are usually more effective for learning than those which are drill-like and enforce mere repetition of the previous solution to the movement problem (34, 35).

Taken together, and compiled from perspectives including brain, cognitive, and the social sciences, we propose a minimum of three active ingredients thought to be critical for an effective task-oriented training program. The program must be:

1) **Challenging** enough to require new learning, and engagement with attention to solve the motor problem (28).
2) **Progressive and optimally adapted** such that over practice, the task-demand is optimally adapted to the patient's capability and the environmental context; not too simple or repetitive to not challenge, and not too difficult to cause a failure of motor learning or a low sense of competence (36, 37). Extending the environmental context outside the laboratory or clinic is an important aspect of an optimally adapted patient-centered program. This reinforces the "real-life" benefits through a virtuous cycle that becomes self-sustaining.
3) Interesting enough to invoke **active participation** to engage a "particular type of repetition" that Bernstein referred to as "problem-solving." There is considerable evidence that voluntary movement elicits motor learning more than passively induced movement (38). This criterion is inextricably tied to the residual voluntary motor control capacity (i.e., residual corticospinal tract), as well as the meaningfulness and functionality of the task.

It should be noted that these three criteria (i.e., challenge, progressive and optimally adapted, active participation) may not be independent, but rather complimentary in nature and thought to be important for the most effective task-oriented training programs. We return to these criteria later (see "Considerations from the Neuroscience Perspective," below). It is perhaps no coincidence in the context of this discussion that the recent Ontario Stroke Rehabilitation Consensus Panel (39) defined stroke rehabilitation as a: 1) progressive, 2) dynamic, 3) goal-oriented process aimed at enabling a person with an impairment to reach his or her optimal physical, cognitive, emotional, communicative, and/or social functional level.

III. CONSTRAINT-INDUCED MOVEMENT THERAPY: A SPECIAL CLASS OF TOT?

In this section, we review the evidence from a family of forced-use and constraint-induced movement therapies. Using our criterion-based definition of task-oriented training, we suggest that forced-use/CIMT therapies constitute a special class of task-oriented training.

During the last decade, a class of intervention studies that has addressed the suboptimal recovery of upper extremity function, and for which there is mounting evidence, is the family of forced-use and constraint-induced movement therapy protocols (40–50). Along with the recently published phase III multi-site EXCITE trial results (51, 52), there have been several small (46, 53) and one larger-scale study (48) showing efficacious results for constraint-induced movement therapy in restoring motor function in patients with upper extremity motor impairments. A modified protocol was shown to be effective in outpatient (41, 42), clinic (44), and home settings (43), and even feasible in the acute in-patient setting (40).

Constraint-induced movement therapy protocols combine the use of a constraint (restraint mitt worn on the less-affected limb) and training of the affected arm and hand. The restraint device can be thought to exert an indirect effect on paretic limb use by preventing compensatory use of the less-affected limb for some tasks, while the task-specific training with the paretic limb can be thought to exert a direct effect on paretic limb use. Several studies of constraint-induced movement therapy used a training duration of 14 days (two weeks), in which 10 of those days included six hours per day of supervised in-laboratory training with the participant's less-affected upper extremity placed in a protective safety mitt for a goal of 90% of their waking hours (46, 48, 49, 54). One study compared the effectiveness of a six hour per day training protocol to one half as long (three hours per day) and found that while the shorter training period produced significant and functionally relevant treatment effects, the longer training protocol produced even greater efficacy in young adolescent participants (55). Because the two groups had equivalent restraint use times, Sterr and colleagues suggest that the major factor contributing to the gains in upper extremity function comes from the massed practice, which occurs during training (54). In essence, task-oriented training may exert a greater influence on recovery than the restraint when overcoming the effects of learned-nonuse, but this hypothesis is controversial with other findings using a modified protocol showing that reduced levels of training relative to mitt use are also effective (41, 42, 56). We will return to this point later in our discussion of practice time (see "Practice Time or Intensity of Training," below).

In addition to mitt use, two distinct training procedures were employed with these participants as they practiced functional task activities: shaping or adaptive task practice (ATP) and standard task practice (TP). The former is a training method based on the principles of behavioral training (49, 57–59) that can also be described in terms of motor learning derived from adaptive or part-task practice (60–65). In this approach, a motor or behavioral objective (task goal) is approached in small steps, by successive approximation (i.e., parts of the task), or the task is made more difficult in accordance with a participant's motor capabilities, or the speed of performance is progressively increased. Each functional activity is practiced for a set of 10 trials, and explicit feedback is provided regarding the participant's performance with each trial. Standard task practice is less structured (for example, the tasks are not set up to be carried out as individual trials of discrete movements); they involve functionally-based activities performed continuously for a period of 15 to 20 minutes (e.g., wrapping a present, writing a letter). In successive periods of task practice, the spatial requirements of the activity or other parameters (such as duration) can be changed to require more demanding control of limb segments for task completion. Global feedback about overall performance is provided at the end of the 15- to 20-minute period. For the majority of signature protocol CIMT studies, the training tasks are selected for each participant using the following criteria: 1) specific joint movements that exhibit the most pronounced deficits, 2) the joint movements that trainers believe have the greatest potential for improvement, and 3) participant preference among tasks that have similar potential for producing specific improvements.

For the EXCITE trial, a large bank of tasks was created for each type of training procedure. Additional tasks could be submitted and added to the bank of approved tasks only after receiving approval from the EXCITE Training Core. The task bank consisted of 71 ATP activities (e.g., ring toss, nuts and bolts, pouring from mug) and 42 TP activities (e.g., setting table, dusting, eating with chopsticks). All practice items were considered "task-oriented" and were items from a broad range of everyday activities including: food preparation, dining, cleaning, home maintenance, laundry, office, recreational, and instrumental activities of daily living.

Based on published CIMT protocol descriptions, including shaping procedures to progress task difficulty, the provision of optimal challenge, and multi-faceted approaches to encourage active participation (e.g., behavioral contract, constraint mitt), we suggest that CIMT be considered a special class of task-oriented training. The most important difference, and one we will return to later in the section on emerging approaches (see "Emerging Innovative Approaches to Upper Limb Rehabilitation," below), is that forced-use/CIMT protocols tend to negate other approaches for training, such as bimanual task practice (66), and arm use is promoted more than skill acquisition. While disentangling the individual contributions to arm and hand improvements of the constraint (i.e., mitt use) and the task-oriented training component embedded in CIMT protocols is not possible, there is emerging support for the effectiveness of task-oriented upper limb training in the subacute phase following stroke, particularly in those individuals who had suffered their first-ever stroke incident resulting in mild to moderate unilateral upper limb paresis.

In all clinical trials during the subacute phase, and one case study, participants who received task-oriented training, without using a constraint, demonstrated significant improvements in upper limb motor impairment and in activity limitations immediately post-intervention (11, 13, 66, 67); however, significant between-group differences in favor of task-oriented training were most apparent when long term upper limb outcomes were evaluated many months following the intervention (13). One interpretation of these findings is that in the subacute phase, there has been less opportunity (less time) for robust learned-non use strategies to dominate, and patients in this phase are less likely to benefit from an approach that emphasizes the reversal of learned-non-use compared to one that emphasizes motor re-learning through skill acquisition, problem-solving, and self-management.

IV. MOTOR CONTROL AND LEARNING CONSIDERATIONS

There is a significant body of work from movement and psychological science that deals with the behavioral aspects of motor control and learning in non-disabled populations. Such knowledge can provide important direction to the implementation of task-oriented training to promote upper extremity recovery (69, 70). Earlier, we highlighted the importance of establishing the so-called "pharmacokinetics" of task-oriented training including: dosing, timing of administration, half-life, and the nature of the training paradigm. In this section, we draw from the motor learning and control literature to guide an analysis of these important parameters of training.

Massed Versus Distributed Practice Schedules

In the motor learning literature, the term "massed" practice is defined as a set of practice trials in which the performance-rest ratio is high and the proportion of rest between practice attempts is relatively shorter than the amount of time spent practicing. In contrast, "distributed" practice refers to a set of practice trials in which the performance-rest ratio is low and the rest time between trials is longer than the amount of time spent practicing (64). Although there are no direct comparisons (massed vs. distributed) in the neurorehabilitation literature, there is a long history of this debate in the motor learning literature (71).

The effectiveness for motor learning of various task performance and rest schedules seems to depend on the nature of the tasks that are practiced. For discrete tasks, such as tossing a ball or fastening a button, reducing the rest time (i.e., massed practice) has little or no influence on learning, and in some cases less rest may even be beneficial. However, for continuous tasks, such as handwriting, fatigue-like states are more apt to build up within a performance bout, suggesting that massed practice would be undesirable. The majority of the laboratory findings in non-disabled populations would support this notion—less rest between performance epochs degrades performance and has a detrimental effect on learning (72).

In the clinical literature, especially that used to describe the signature CIMT protocol, the term "massed practice" has been used to mean high intensity training conducted, for example, daily using a schedule of six hours per day in the laboratory one-on-one with a "trainer." While there is no doubt that the saying, "practice makes perfect" bears some truth and there is ample evidence to support the notion that "practice" is the most important variable for motor learning, conventional wisdom suggests that the design of that practice (schedule, duration), and the contents of practice (task-specificity) are equally important factors to consider when attempting to optimize the effectiveness of task-oriented training.

A concentrated "massed practice" schedule may be impractical to implement in today's health care environment. On the other hand, a more distributed schedule, while a departure from the signature CIMT massed schedule, is closer to that prescribed in more recent reports that have used a modified CIMT protocol (42, 56, 73–75). Finally, such a distributed schedule is attractive from a practical perspective, both to the patient and clinic; clinics consider a therapy visit to be approximately 45 minutes to an hour, and customary out-patient therapy for stroke ranges from two to three times per week for up to 10 weeks. Together, there is considerable practical and empirical support for implementing a task-specific practice program using these more distributed training schedules for upper extremity neurorehabilitation (23, 66).

Practice Time or Intensity of Training

Practice time, or the amount of time engaged with specific tasks, appears to be a major factor contributing to the effectiveness of constraint-induced movement therapy. However, in general clinical practice and even for published protocols, a precise quantification of task-specific practice is usually no more explicit than the length of stay or the total minutes or hours of each particular therapy delivered (76, 77). The considerable outcomes and effectiveness research surrounding constraint-induced movement therapy have seldom focused on an explicit characterization of the intervention itself, including the very nature of the repetitions inherent to task-practice. The signature CIMT protocol calls for a minimum of six hours per day of supervised training; however, from a task-oriented training perspective, the metric that is of interest is the amount of actual time practicing and time on task with the more impaired limb. Recently, we undertook such an analysis on one of the seven sites from the EXCITE RCT (78).

This retrospective analysis of a two-week (range 11 to 16 days) administration of the signature CIT protocol revealed that on average, participants tolerated approximately four hours of daily task-specific practice, or 62% of in-laboratory time. Further, we showed that there was 100% compliance with the specified six-hour minimum supervised in-laboratory time averaged across the 10 days. The significant correlation between Mean Daily Practice Time (time on task) and in-laboratory time in the context of the large between-subject ranges for Practice Time prompts the question concerning the impact of training time and outcomes. For example, do participants who have longer training times benefit more from constraint-induced movement therapy than those with shorter training times? While outside the scope of our single-site "time-on-task" project, a subsequent analysis was recently performed on the entire EXCITE database to address this.

In fact, when all participants enrolled into the EXCITE Trial and who underwent 10 days of CIMT ($N = 169$) were examined for change scores on a primary outcome measure, the Wolf Motor Function Test (79, 80), there was no apparent relationship between intensity of training and outcome until the nature of the training was included in the analysis (81). Apparently spending an excessive amount of training time in adaptive task practice training, which, arguably implements a "problem solving" approach, yielded greater improvements with less overall practice time among those participants classified in the higher functional level, compared to other EXCITE participants. The lack of an overall intensity-to-outcome relationship along with the more detailed subgroup analysis suggests that total time spent practicing is less important than the nature of what is practiced. As such, task-specificity may be more important than intensity of training (34, 82). We return to this topic later in the chapter (see "Task-specificity and contents of training," below).

From our single-site analysis, there was considerable variability (2.83 to 5.04 hours per day) across participants in Mean Daily Practice Time, and the proportion of Task Practice and Adaptive Task Practice that constituted practice time, however this variability did not appear to depend on functional level. In fact, two of the three in the low functional group were among the lowest for the entire group in Practice Time (22 and 23% below the mean), while the other had the third highest overall practice time at 20% above the mean. Instead, independent of functional level, it appears that those who engaged in more total practice time also engaged in more time on Adaptive Task Practice/Shaping. However, this

was not the case between total practice time and Task Practice Time. Therefore, other factors besides motor capability were more important in determining the time on task practice and the relative proportion of Adaptive Task Practice and Task Practice engaged in by any given participant. Individual subject motor capability, motivational and behavioral factors likely influenced important training parameters, such as task progression, training intensity, and choice of ATP/TP components. An understanding of these factors which are beyond training intensity, but relevant to the implementation of individualized patient-centered therapy programs, will be important for future developments in clinical practice (83).

Both the full-study and single-site EXCITE (78, 81) analyses were limited to the temporal components of task-specific training, and the two classifications of tasks, ATP and TP, that represent only one of the active ingredients for efficacy of CIMT. The motor learning literature would suggest that there may be other critical elements of task-specific training that are important for the design of effective programs. We describe a few of these macro-level elements in the next sections.

Practice Schedules and Organization of Tasks

Random vs. Blocked Task Order Practice. The motor learning literature describes the contextual interference effect as an important and compelling variable for consideration in motor learning. For non-disabled learners, a practice schedule that promotes *interference* has been shown to be beneficial for skill learning (84–87). One way to manipulate interference during practice of multiple tasks is to change the order in which tasks are practiced. For example, a random practice order in which tasks are practiced in a quasi-random order (i.e., C-A-B, A-B-C, B-C-A, where each letter represents a different task) is thought to introduce more interference than a blocked practice order in which each task is practiced repeatedly prior to switching to the next task (i.e., A-A-A, B-B-B, C-C-C).

Results from studies investigating the effects of practice order on motor learning typically show that a random practice order enhances motor learning compared with a blocked practice order and total number of trials is held constant across the two conditions. This phenomenon is known as the Contextual Interference (CI) effect (88–91). The CI effect elicited under random practice (i.e., high-interference) conditions has been explained in part by the additional planning and parameter specification which is required when different tasks are being practiced within the same session. For random order practice, every trial necessitates parameter specification and action planning; both processes now are thought to implement a stronger memory representation of the practiced tasks (92–96). This enhanced processing related to the CI effect may in part take the form of increased cortical motor activity.

Transcranial magnetic stimulation (TMS) is a technique that can introduce a transient perturbation to modulate cortical motor activity by means of noninvasive stimulation of the human brain (97). Recently we used single-pulse TMS in healthy non-disabled participants as an identical external perturbation during both blocked and random practice (98). The TMS perturbation centered over primary motor cortex during practice selectively disrupted motor learning under random, but not the blocked practice condition, suggesting that TMS may have interfered with those essential brain processes evoked distinctly by random practice. Increased cortical activity during random practice can be hypothesized as necessary neural processing in order to repeatedly specify, with every practice trial, kinematic parameters, such as the amplitude or timing of the movement. Several neuroimaging studies support this hypothesis by demonstrating broad activation in primary and secondary cortical motor regions, such as primary motor (M1) and sensory (S1) cortex, dorsal and ventral premotor cortex (PMd and PMv), supplementary motor area (SMA), and posterior parietal cortices when subjects attempt to perform tasks requiring skillful action, or when subjects are trained in high-interference practice conditions (99–109).

These studies, together with the recent TMS perturbation results, provide compelling support for the hypothesis that variable or random order task practice conditions evoke extensive task-related activity in cortical motor regions. This observation suggests that task-specific practice order, such as that used to invoke the contextual interference effect, might offer an important "active" ingredient to the design of effective task-oriented training programs for stroke neurorehabilitation.

Task-Specificity and the Contents of Training. There is no doubt that behavioral experience can enhance function after brain injury. Studies of the effects of enriched environments show that rats exposed to complex housing environments pre- and/or post-injury typically have improved functional outcomes compared to animals in standard housing (110, 111). Further, general exercise, such as wheel running, which influences neuronal circuitry of brain and spinal cord when initiated pre- and post-injury is associated with activity-dependent plasticity. A landmark study conducted more than a decade ago showed that physical exercise has a direct, positive impact on enriching the blood supply (i.e., angiogenesis) to a brain region that is engaged by the exercise (112), but physical exercise by itself generated no changes in the elaboration of brain connections. In models of injury, exercise is beneficial for restoring plasticity-related proteins after spinal cord injury (113, 114) increasing axonal regeneration in sensory neurons (115), and protecting

from damage caused by cerebral ischemia (116). However, there is no evidence that the running rat or hamster has better memories, faster or more competent thinking, or stronger, more refined and more flexible control of its actions, because it spent all day on the running wheel. It seems that for the latter benefits to occur, for fundamental processes including remembering, reasoning, and fine motor control, *new experiences and learning* are a necessary and critical driver.

In support of this idea, recent work using animal models of stroke suggest that functional brain remodeling may be critically contingent upon the behavioral demands of the training and the acquisition of motor skills associated with learning a novel task (25, 28). Animals trained in skilled upper limb tasks show differential changes in the functional reorganization of the motor cortex compared either to animals that had the unaffected limb restrained but received no additional training (117), or to animals that received an identical intensity of training in unskilled upper limb movement tasks that demanded less movement precision (28, 118). The adult animals that were exposed to motor skill training demonstrated enlargement of the motor cortex representation of the wrist and digits, while comparable changes in functional reorganization of the cortical maps were not found in the animals that undertook repetitive unskilled upper limb activities. Thus, although exercise can be beneficial in some ways, learning motor skills results in neuronal structural and functional plasticity in the motor cortex and cerebellum that is not found with simple exercise or repetition of previously learned skills (25, 117–121)

Recently, Maldonado and colleagues used a unilateral ischemic lesion model and asked if exercise could be used as a positive modulator of motor skill "re-learning" in young and older rats. Motor skill training consisted of daily practice of the impaired forelimb in a tray-reaching task (task-specific training). Exercised rats had free access to running wheels for six hours per day. In the young adult rats (task-specific training group), motor skill training significantly enhanced skilled reaching recovery compared to controls (no activity or exercise groups). However, exercise did not significantly enhance performance when administered alone or in combination with task-specific training. Further, there was no major benefit of exercise in older rats, and no effects of exercise in a measure of coordinated forelimb placement or in immunocytochemical measures of several plasticity-related proteins (BDNF, NMDAR-1, spinophilin, MAP-2) in the motor cortex. Thus the Maldonado et al.'s results support the importance of task-specific training over general exercise, either alone or combined, for improving skilled reaching after unilateral ischemic lesions of the sensorimotor cortex in rats (26).

Studies in humans regarding the relative effects of the content of training on cortical plasticity and associated functional recovery of the upper limb are less conclusive. In contrast, a recent phase II RCT, Strength Training Effectiveness Post Stroke (STEPS), was designed to determine the effects of combined task-specific and strength training interventions to improve walking ability in individuals post-stroke (four months to five years post-stroke). In brief, the trial randomized eligible participants into one of four interventions four days per week for six weeks (24 sessions): 1) a locomotor-specific training group using body-weight supported treadmill training (BWST) two times a week, and an upper extremity sham exercise on alternate days of the four-day training; 2) a loaded cycling training group using a specially-designed limb-loaded cycling (CYCLE) program two times a week, combined on alternate days with the same upper extremity sham exercise; 3) BWST combined with CYCLE on the alternate two days of the four-day program; and 4) BWST combined with lower extremity strengthening exercises on the two alternate days. Sullivan and colleague (2007) reported that the BWST training resulted in improvements in walking speed and endurance, and the CYCLE training resulted in similar gains in endurance but not walking speed, thus highlighting the importance of task-specific training. In addition, the BWST combined with either the loaded CYCLE or lower extremity strengthening did not improve outcomes over BWST alone (see Chapter 20, Walking Recovery and Rehabilitation after Stroke). In the end, the BWST training resulted in a clinically meaningful change in walking speed that persisted at the six months post follow-up test, and regardless of whether or not it was combined with a strengthening program (122). We return to the idea of combined approaches (e.g., strength training and task-oriented training) in a later section (see "Emerging Innovative Approaches," below).

In non-injured humans, learning-associated activation of the primary motor cortex was found to be greater than the activation associated with simple repetitive motor use (123, 124). Investigations of CIMT showed both increased use of the affected upper limb and changes in cortical activation post-training (125–133). However, the specific contribution of task-oriented training compared with the "forced-use" associated with the constraint of the non-paretic limb cannot be determined without a control group (134).

Nelles and colleagues conducted a small RCT and compared the effects of upper limb TOT and a similar intensity of passive movements and muscle stretching activities in 10 subacute stroke participants (27). The TOT group showed a trend toward diminished motor impairments (UL Fugl-Meyer) and significantly increased activation in several sensori-motor regions of the brain (bilateral parietal, premotor, contralateral precentral, and postcentral areas). In contrast, the control participants did not exhibit comparable changes in the fMRI BOLD signal response. Similar results were obtained in a study that used computer-aided training of finger tracking in 10 chronic stroke participants. Here the researchers found a significant shift in activation from the unaffected to the affected hemisphere in the primary sensory and motor areas and premotor cortices after training and associated improvements in manual dexterity, compared to pre-training (135). Recently, this same group compared the effects of two weeks of computer-aided training of finger tracking to repetitive simple finger movements in 20 mildly impaired chronic stroke participants (136). Surprisingly, they found no differences between the two training groups in performance of clinical tests, including the Box and Block and Jebsen-Taylor hand function test; however, both groups showed improvements on these tests compared with pre-training levels. Similar findings prevailed for the fMRI activation results, with no consistent patterns or trends.

Compared to the animal studies, those in humans are less conclusive about the relative effects of the contents of training on cortical plasticity and associated upper limb functional recovery after stroke; however, there are several additional variables that deserve consideration. Some of these variables were identified earlier (see "Emergence of Task-Oriented Training for Neurorehabilitation," above) as dosing, timing of administration (acute, subacute, chronic), half-life, and consideration of whether the training paradigm matters. In addition, participant characteristics, especially the *severity* of motor deficits are considered in the next sections.

Severity of Motor Deficits. Two studies in particular highlight the importance of matching the task-specific training program to the participant characteristics, especially the severity of motor deficits. Salbach and colleagues reported on the efficacy of a task-oriented intervention in enhancing competence in walking in people after stroke (137). This was a two-center observer-blinded, stratified, block-randomized controlled trial with 91 patients (44 experimental, 47 control) who exhibited a residual walking deficit within one year of first or recurrent stroke. Forty-four participants were randomized into a task-oriented training program administered during three 90-minute sessions per week for six weeks. The TOT consisted of functional tasks designed to strengthen the lower extremities and enhance walking balance, speed, and distance. Forty-seven participants were randomized into the control intervention that consisted of task-oriented upper limb practice of functional, unilateral, and bilateral tasks chosen to improve gross and fine manual dexterity. Baseline six-minute walk test was not different between groups (Experimental 209 m, Control 204 m), but the change was significant with task-specific training group showing a 40 (+/− 72) m improvement compared to the control (UL task-specific group) showing a 5 (+/1 66) m improvement. More importantly, people with mild, moderate, or severe walking deficits at baseline improved on average of 36 (+/1 96), 55 (+/− 56) and 18 (+/− 23) m, respectively. For this study, the best responders to the task-oriented training program for walking were those who presented with a moderate walking deficit at baseline. The other important point is that all patients could walk at baseline, though some much slower than others.

Two years later, this same group published the results of the task-oriented intervention on arm function in people with stroke using the control group ($n = 47$) data from the same RCT described above (138). They reported that the 27 hours of upper extremity task-oriented training distributed over six weeks did not improve voluntary movement or manual dexterity of the affected arm. However, a closer look at the baseline upper limb motor deficit of the "control" group provided a reasonable explanation for these negative findings. Indeed, these results were not surprising when considering the heterogeneous sample that was selected based on walking impairment, rather than arm impairment. Sixteen percent of the patients had no distal (wrist/fingers) movement capability. It is well known that if no hand dexterity is apparent by six weeks after stroke, the likelihood of achieving hand function at six months is poor (139). For this RCT, the primary outcome for arm function was the Box and Block test, with secondary outcomes including the Nine-hole peg test, maximum grip strength, and the TEMPA, focused primarily on distal movement capability. This study underscores the need for well-designed investigations with inclusion criteria that are appropriately matched to the specific task-oriented training intervention, in this case one that necessitated active participation that was clearly beyond the capability of at least 16% of the participant group. It is not surprising therefore that the task-oriented training program was not beneficial in this group of stroke survivors who effectively could not actively participate to the degree that would lead to a meaningful improvement in upper extremity function (see 140 for more discussion).

Timing of Task-Oriented Training. Evidence from animal studies suggest that timing of training may play a critical role in its effectiveness in restoring or improving performance, enhancing the survival and neural reorganization of the surviving peri-lesional tissue, and establishing effective neural reorganization of the contralesional hemisphere (55, 141, 142). While intensive training commenced too early post-lesion has been shown to have deleterious effects in animals (143–145), a modified CIMT protocol commenced within the first two weeks following stroke in humans was shown to be safe (40). In animal models, a delay in training results in poorer behavioral recovery and poorer preservation of penumbral areas representing the distal forelimbs (55, 146). In humans, the

optimal therapeutic window after stroke for rehabilitation of the upper limb remains to be established (147). Regardless of severity, there is preliminary evidence to suggest that earlier, more aggressive therapy results in better upper limb outcomes (148, 149). It is likely that the therapeutic window for rehabilitation might depend upon the severity of the stroke, as well as the presence of other co-morbidities (150). Imaging studies provide evidence of ongoing cortical reorganization of motor systems for several months after stroke (151). Improvements in function have been observed from clinical measures in the first three to six months post-stroke, after which relatively less change may be seen if no further intervention is undertaken (152). As mentioned earlier, changes in cortical activation and improvements in affected upper limb function have been reported with training in chronic stroke participants (130–132); however, there are several compelling arguments for introducing a task-oriented approach earlier post-stroke, during the immediate outpatient interval, especially for those who exhibit a mild to moderate upper limb impairment.

Although the exact proportion of stroke survivors who are mildly to moderately impaired is not known, conservative estimates range between 5% and 30%. These are individuals who return to the community but with significant disablement (153). The paucity of dose-equivalent designs in the stroke upper extremity clinical trial literature, and including the recent EXCITE trial (52), highlights an important need in this area (154, 155). Unlike EXCITE, a task-oriented intervention that targets the immediate post-acute period provides several advantages for the patient with a mild to moderate motor deficit. This timing is considered optimal for several reasons:

1) It enables a supportive interaction between processes associated with experience-dependent and injury-induced cortical reorganization that are known to influence functional recovery (156, 157)
2) It is possible that earlier intervention may allow for more optimal cortical re-organization and potentially less use of behavioral compensatory strategies (55, 158)
3) It may attenuate the detrimental effects of maladaptive compensatory strategies (e.g., learned non-use) currently promoted during inpatient rehabilitation (159), that may with time be reinforced and become more difficult for the patient and clinician to reverse (6)
4) It is not so early as to be overly aggressive during a more vulnerable period both physiologically and psychologically (156, 160)
5) The outpatient environment is a more practical setting for a distributed, relatively high dose of upper extremity task-specific training, especially given the already dwindling acute inpatient length of stay (155, 1598). Indeed, recently, Lang and colleagues

showed that affected upper extremity use is minimal during the inpatient rehabilitation stay in patients with mild to moderate acute hemiparesis (161).

Dosing of Task-Oriented Training.   The recent ASA/AHS endorsed Clinical Practice Guidelines (162) review the evidence for therapy intensity and duration. While the heterogeneity of the studies combined with borderline results in many trials limits the specificity and strength of any conclusions overall, the trials support the general concept that rehabilitation can improve functional outcomes, particularly in patients with lesser degrees of impairment. There is weak evidence for a dose-response relationship between intensity of the rehabilitation intervention and functional outcomes. For example, Sterr and colleagues demonstrated that while both groups improved, six hours of CIMT led to greater improvements at one month on the WMFT and MAL than three hours delivered daily, over a two-week period in 15 adults with chronic hemiparesis (53). Despite limitations of these individual studies, the conclusions among several systematic reviews are fairly consistent: Two meta-analyses both concluded that greater intensity produces slightly better outcomes (163, 164). Kwakkel (164) reported a small but statistically significant intensity effect relationship in the rehabilitation of stroke patients. The literature specific to upper extremity treatment is mixed. Other than EXCITE, there are no multi-center trials in the literature.

The recently completed Very Early Constraint Induced Movement Therapy (VECTORS) phase II trial (Dromerick, PI) begins within 14 days of stroke onset. VECTORS was a single center pilot randomized controlled clinical trial of the early application of CIMT. Participants were assigned using adaptive randomization into the control group (two hours traditional Occupational Therapy), a dose-matched CIMT group (two hours shaping, six hours per day constraint), or the high dose CIMT group (three hours shaping, 90% waking hours constraint) at inpatient rehabilitation admission. Inclusion criteria included ischemic or hemorrhagic stroke within 28 days of onset; no prior stroke-related neurologic impairment; need for inpatient rehabilitation; NIH Stroke Scale (NIHSS) aphasia, command, consciousness, and sensory items < 1; NIHSS neglect = 0; and persistently hemiparetic upper extremity with some residual voluntary movement. Blinded raters evaluated subjects at randomization, end of treatment (14 days), and the primary endpoint (90 days). The pre-specified primary dependent measure was the total Action Research Arm Test (ARAT) at 90 days after randomization. A subsample ($n = 9$) underwent MRI imaging (apparent diffusion coefficient [ADC] mapping) at study baseline and Day 7–9 to determine if new neuronal injury occurred during study treatment. Fifty-two participants (mean age 63.9 +/− 14 yrs) were randomized 9.6 (+/− 4.5) days after onset. Mean NIHSS was 5.3 (+/− 1.8); mean ARAT score was 22.5 (+/− 15.6); 77% had ischemic stroke. Groups were equivalent at baseline on all randomization variables. As expected, all groups improved with time on the total ARAT score. Of particular importance, the high-dose CIMT group had significantly worse scores at Day 90 compared to the other two groups. No significant differences were found between the dose-matched CIMT and control groups at Day 90. A similar time by group interactions was observed using the Wolf Motor Function Test Functional Ability score. No clinical safety issues were encountered; ADC maps revealed no evidence of new neuronal damage. The VECTORS study did not support the hypothesis that CIMT therapy is superior to equal doses of conventional therapy in the acute inpatient rehabilitation setting. A dose response relationship was observed, where a *higher dose* of CIMT was associated with *less motor recovery*. These results highlight the need for clinical trial designs that directly and empirically determine the efficacy of specific treatments at specific delivery schedules during each phase of stroke care.

For our recent NIH funded phase III stroke rehabilitation trial, Interdisciplinary Comprehensive Arm Rehabilitation Evaluation (I-CARE), we chose a distributed dose of 30 hours of training for scientific and pragmatic reasons. We included a comparison control group, an observation only, usual and customary (UCC) outpatient therapy. We expect considerable variation in the UCC dose both by site and across the five-year monitoring period. These observation data will be important in the end from a policy standpoint, and should be useful to estimate the cost if more prescriptive practice guidelines were to be implemented, especially if a higher dose can be shown to produce better outcomes. Pilot data from a multi-site outpatient survey suggests that 30 hours distributed over 10 weeks would be on the higher side of what is commonly prescribed, but still practical in that it would allow patients to participate in other concurrent therapy services (e.g., physical therapy and speech therapy). Thirty hours is 33% more than what we used in our single site phase II trial that commenced during inpatient rehabilitation and extending to outpatient (20 hours distributed over 4–6 weeks) (13); it is 50% of that used for EXCITE (60 hours over 2 weeks) during the 3–9 month post-outpatient period (49); twice that used by Page and colleagues (56) (15 hours over 10 weeks, 30-minute sessions, 3 times per week) in a recent phase I acute trial of mCIT, and 55% of that prescribed in the recent home-based RCT of a multifaceted therapeutic exercise program (54 hours over 12 weeks) in subacute stroke (165). Therefore the 30-hour dose is well within the range of previous intervention trials shown to be effective, and it is practical for the outpatient environment, yet it is likely higher than the usual average dose that is prescribed for this patient group.

CONSIDERATIONS FROM THE NEUROSCIENCE PERSPECTIVE

Recently Kleim and Jones (166) reviewed a growing body of neuroscience research that used a variety of models of learning, neurologic disease, and trauma from the perspective of basic neuroscientists, but in a manner intended to be useful for the development of more effective clinical rehabilitation interventions. Because neural plasticity is believed to be the basis for both motor learning in the intact brain and relearning in the damaged brain that occurs through physical rehabilitation, the recent advances in understanding experience-dependent neural plasticity can inform the application of task-oriented training interventions. Kleim and Jones argue that the "qualities and constraints of experience-dependent neural plasticity are likely to be of major relevance to rehabilitation efforts in humans with brain damage. However, some research topics need much more attention in order to enhance the translation of this area of neuroscience to clinical research and practice" (166) (p. S225).

In this section, each of the 10 Kleim/Jones principles of experience-dependent neural plasticity are reviewed in the context of task-oriented training. For each principle, we consider a literal translation as it pertains to the promotion of upper extremity recovery and, where appropriate, include current behavioral perspectives from available motor control and learning research.

Principle 1: Use It or Lose It

Failure to drive specific brain functions can lead to functional degradation. Principle 1 suggests that any intervention that encourages or promotes "use" of the paretic limb would be appropriate. Task-oriented training, CIMT, Bilateral arm training, and functional task practice are just a few programs from the clinical evidence-based literature that would qualify for application of Principle 1. (See "What is Task-Oriented Training," above, and "Emerging Innovative Approaches," below, for details).

Principle 2: Use It and Improve It

Training that drives a specific brain function can lead to an enhancement of that function. Principle 2 implies that the "use" promoting intervention must be progressed so that neural adaptation is driven at the same time that the motor control and skill improves. This concept maps back nicely to the second active ingredient of task-oriented training—*progressive and optimally adapted* (see "Criterion-Based TOT: What Are the Active Ingredients?" above). An implicit message contained within Principle 2 is that to "improve" at something, you need to start by practicing what you cannot already do. The challenge for the clinician and patient is to develop enough drive or motivation to continue practicing something that at the present time is difficult. Lee and Wishart offer some possible solutions to what they describe as motor learning conundrums (36). Basically, the patient will need to understand that investing in "difficult" practice now will pay off mightily in the future.

Principle 3: Specificity

The nature of the training experience dictates the nature of the plasticity. Principle 3 implies that *specificity* of training is important. Indeed, *specificity* effects are one of the oldest and most common findings in learning and memory research (e.g., 167). Later in the twentieth century, work in the transfer of skills again supported a specificity effect, with the general finding that transfer of training was small unless the skills were essentially identical to one another (168). Similarly, a specificity effect was found in experiments in which participants learned a task during practice and then performed it under similar or changed conditions in a transfer test (e.g., 169). As predicted by the specificity effect, performance was usually most effective when the transfer conditions matched those conditions that were available during the practice session. Therefore, there is considerable evidence suggesting that motor skills are represented in memory in a highly specialized way (170). This idea of "specificity" overlaps considerably with what we refer to earlier as the "contents" of training. The evidence for the importance of "specificity" is detailed earlier (see "Task-Specificity and Contents of Training," above). Although general exercise and strengthening programs are thought to be effective when combined with task-oriented training programs, the benefits are usually expressed at the system level (i.e., physiology, musculoskeletal) and not at the level of the specific task or skill that is being trained.

Principle 4: Repetition Matters

Induction of plasticity requires sufficient repetition. Principle 4 suggests that repeated attempts to solve the motor problem benefits plasticity and learning. There is considerable evidence for this idea that comes from the motor learning literature and is reviewed earlier (see "Motor Control and Learning Considerations," above). What is less understood is how the organization of those repetitions (e.g., massed vs. distributed) should be structured for the best outcomes. What is clear from the evidence to date is that mere repetition of simple tasks that are well within the capability of the performer will most certainly not induce neural plasticity or learning (28).

Principle 5: Intensity Matters

Induction of plasticity requires sufficient training intensity. Principle 5 implies that the dose, frequency, and duration of training are important parameters in the design of any effective task-oriented training program. Intensity is usually defined as an exceptionally great concentration, power, or force. In the field of physics, it is the amount or degree of strength of electricity, light, heat, or sound per unit area or volume. In earlier sections (see "Practice Time or Intensity of Training," and "Practice Schedules and Organization of Tasks"), we reviewed the studies that have manipulated the "intensity" of training by varying parameters of dose, frequency, and duration. There is considerable evidence to support this idea, however, explicit guidelines for what constitutes a "sufficient" level of intensity is sorely lacking. The so-called "pharmacokinetics" includes "dosing of training" and has been identified as both a challenge and an important unmet need in the design of clinical trials in rehabilitation (see "Research Frontiers," below, for more discussion). The importance of "therapy dose" in neurorehabilitation is reflected in a recent trend for clinical trials of complex interventions to include at least one dose-equivalent control group in the design (171, 172).

Principle 6: Time Matters

Different forms of plasticity occur at different times during training. Principle 6 implies that timing of an intense, task-oriented training program is an important factor. Most of the clinical research up until recently has been conducted in the chronic phase of stroke recovery. The reason for this choice is complicated and multifaceted (e.g., confounded by spontaneous recovery; safety concerns related to glutamatergic toxicity from the animal studies), but also an unfortunate one, especially in light of the more recent studies suggesting that an earlier time frame would likely have a greater impact on important outcomes (55, 141, 146). We review the evidence related to "timing" earlier (see "Timing of Task-Oriented Training," above).

Principle 7: Salience Matters

The training experience must be sufficiently salient to induce plasticity. Principle 7 implies that the training must have the quality or state of being "salient." It must be prominent or stand out conspicuously or be noticeable. There has been considerable discussion in the literature about the nature of the recovery process from the patient's perspective (e.g., 173, 174). Barker and colleagues (2007) (174) reported that the single most important factor that contributed to upper limb recovery, from the perspective of the stroke survivor and through self-report, was "use

of the arm in everyday tasks." From this, we suggest that a task-oriented training program that includes everyday tasks will likely be viewed as most salient in the context of the recovery process.

Principle 8: Age Matters

Training-induced plasticity occurs more readily in younger brains. Principle 8 implies that the more successful task-oriented training programs will be those that target the younger stroke survivors. We are not aware of any evidence that directly supports this idea. However, because age is often a covariate with other important factors that do modify responsiveness to intense rehabilitation programs, and recovery processes such as advanced cardio-vascular disease, diminished cognition, endurance, and motivation, we cannot rule it out as an important consideration.

Principle 9: Transference

Plasticity in response to one training experience can enhance the acquisition of similar behaviors. Principle 9 suggests the notion of transfer of training that has long been a topic of debate in the motor learning literature, and seems to contrast sharply with that of Principle 3, dealing with specificity. However, there is considerable evidence that motor control is highly flexible and non-specific. This notion of generalization comes from a long history of work showing that well-learned tasks, such as handwriting, are quite independent of the effector system that is typically used to execute them (175–178). It was Bernstein (34, 178) who suggested that such a flexible organization of the system's many degrees of freedom represents the hallmark of skilled motor behavior. Schema theory (179, 180) suggested that motor skills were represented by two structures stored in memory—the generalized motor program (GMP) and a separate structure, called the recall schema, was responsible for specifying the parameters that were needed to scale the GMP's output to the specific environmental demands and conditions. With practice, the schema comes to represent the relationship between the parameters of the GMP and the outcome associated with each movement attempt. The schema is therefore a rule that expresses the relationship among variables (parameters and outcome) rather than a set of specific memories for each movement attempt. One important prediction from schema is that practice within a class of actions that is conducted using a variable practice (e.g., reach and grasp of different sized objects) schedule will develop a stronger schema for the action than one that is conducted using a constant practice (e.g., reach and grasp to the same sized object) schedule. The prediction is that the stronger schema is better for transference. There is considerable support for this prediction in the motor learning literature, especially for novice or young learners (92). However, to our knowledge, no one has as yet examined it in the design of task-oriented training programs to promote upper extremity recovery. Our analysis of the task-training records from the EXCITE trial suggests that there is considerable variability in the order that tasks are practiced in a session, which would likely promote the development of a stronger schema and a higher probability for transference (78); however a more systematic examination of these data is needed to advance our understanding in this area.

Principle 10: Interference

Plasticity in response to one experience can interfere with the acquisition of other behaviors. Principle 10 suggests that the effects of experience-dependent plasticity might impede the induction of new, or the expression of existing, plasticity within the same circuitry. This interference ultimately can impair learning or re-learning. While there are several aspects to Principle 10, the most salient one for consideration here is the idea that some behavioral experience may drive plasticity within residual brain areas in a direction that could impede or interfere with optimal behavioral recovery. For example, the development of "bad habits" or compensatory strategies early after stroke may be more difficult to re-direct than if an optimal strategy were promoted from the earliest opportunity (181). Recently, the notion of "learned baduse" was introduced with evidence from a rat model of motor cortex stroke. These researchers found that after the acute post-stroke period, the lesioned rats made few gestures, but thereafter gesture number escalated with recovery time and eventually exceeded preoperative levels (182). At the same time, there is incomplete recovery of skilled reaching behaviors and an excessive frequency of these inappropriate gestures, supporting the notion that this "learned baduse" might compete or interfere with successful reaching behaviors. The implications of this for rehabilitation and task-oriented training are to avoid training repetitive behaviors (blocked order practice) that can lead to a decline rather than an improvement in performance (183). Some evidence for this is described earlier (see "Random vs. Blocked Practice," above).

Together, these ten principles of experience-dependent neural plasticity were used to provide a consistent structure for a back-translation to the design of effective task-oriented training programs to promote upper extremity recovery after stroke. In some cases, the translation was clear, direct, and intuitive (e.g., use it or lose it), but in others (e.g., interference), the translation was not so obvious, and clearly there was not enough clinical research to provide the necessary guidance for a meaningful translation. In those cases, we drew from the existing body of work in the behavioral movement sciences to propose a direction and stimulate impetus for more research to begin filling in these important research gaps. Several lines of research that will be important for advancing knowledge in this area are described later (see "Research Frontiers," below).

EMERGING INNOVATIVE APPROACHES TO UPPER LIMB REHABILITATION

In the Clinical Trials section of the 2006 Stroke Progress Review Group report, "multi-modality combination interventions" were identified as an emergent research area. Specifically, the report stated that, "In the past five years, clinical trials for the treatment, prevention, and rehabilitation of stroke have moved from evaluation of a single or multiple drug treatments to trials that involve combinations of drugs and devices, devices that release drugs, and devices and programs of physical therapy. For example, ongoing acute intervention trials of ischemic stroke include the use of thrombolytic drugs plus clot-removal devices (e.g. concentric retriever), thrombolytic drugs and ultrasound therapy, and combination of devices. The use of drug-eluting stents, currently used in the coronary circulation, may be considered for occlusive disease in the cerebrovasculature. Finally, several ongoing trials of stroke recovery are evaluating the use of devices, drugs, and cell therapies added to standard or modified physical therapy." (1)

The recently completed industry-sponsored (Northstar Neuroscience, Inc.) pivotal trial of targeted sub-threshold epidural cortical stimulation delivered concurrently with intensive rehabilitation therapy is an example of just such a multi-modality combination intervention (184). We describe the intervention briefly here as an example of a task-oriented training program that was effectively combined with the cortical stimulation device in patients with chronic hemiparetic stroke. Details of the pre-clinical animal and preliminary safety and efficacy trial are described in the phase I/II trial reports and case report published previously (185–187).

Multi-Modal Combination Intervention: The Everest Clinical Trial

Both investigational and control patients began rehabilitation treatment approximately two to four weeks following randomization into the Everest Clinical Trial (Northstar Neuroscience, Inc.). The rehabilitation protocol was administered in a standardized fashion over six weeks, providing a total of approximately 2.5 hours of treatment on each therapy day divided into two daily sessions. Therapy was delivered five days a week for the first four weeks, and then three days a week for the later two weeks. Thus a total of 26 therapy days were provided, amounting to 65 treatment hours. Investigational patients receive cortical stimulation (CS) during rehabilitation, while control patients receive rehabilitation alone and using the same dosing and duration.

All treating therapists were required to undergo an initial certification and receive a passing score allowing them to deliver a standardized rehabilitation protocol, and had to re-certify their competence in the protocol techniques every six months for the duration of the trial. The protocol was based on the contemporary task-oriented approach (also known as systems model of motor control) as described by Bass-Haugen and colleagues (188). This approach applies the principles of motor control research to occupational therapy, emphasizing the role of the environment and its interaction with the person performing the task. The model explains motor behavior as the interplay between the individual's motor abilities, the task requirement, and the environment. The focus of the therapy is targeted to the hemiplegic upper limb, but does not exclude bimanual activities. For practical application of task-oriented therapy, the therapist was required to have an adequate understanding of the movement patterns needed for a particular task, as well as the individual's motor patterns that may interfere with successful task performance. In collaboration with the patient, the therapist helps solve the motor problem by manipulating the structure of the task to be performed, by remediation of the patient's impairment (e.g., improve scapular alignment and stability, or improve functional reach), or by changing environmental variables, as by using equipment such as a built-up grip.

Because functional upper limb movement requires coordination of shoulder, elbow, and distal joints, a sequence of pre-functional and functional activities that address components of upper limb movement and use were presented to the patient. The focus of these therapeutic activities was primarily on distal movements, because cortical electrode placement was targeted over cortex that was active during hand and wrist motion. If, however, the patient had challenges with proximal arm stability impacting distal hand function, some portion of the therapy sessions was used to address proximal motor control. Functional movements such as grasp, release, and reach were emphasized. In addition, activities of daily living were practiced, including self-care and other tasks that are meaningful to the patient and require the affected upper limb. Upon completion of the six-week protocol, patients were provided with exercises to continue at home, at the discretion of the patient and therapist.

Although patients were expected to participate in all 26 sessions, a missed therapy session did not influence subsequent study participation. Study investigators instructed patients not to participate in additional physical or occupational therapy during the six-week rehabilitation protocol or during the four-week follow-up period.

To our knowledge, this is the first example in the field of neurorehabilitation that has combined the use of a behavioral training program (i.e., task-oriented training) with that of an investigational device in a multi-modal combination intervention designed to promote upper extremity recovery for stroke hemiparesis. We expect there will be more innovative and combination rehabilitation therapies tested in the near future, that embody a similar chemotherapy-cocktail approach for the treatment of various forms of cancer. For stroke rehabilitation, task-oriented training is but one of the most effective ingredients of a full spectrum, multi-dimensional approach to restoration and recovery.

Proposing an Integrated Model: Accelerated Skill Acquisition Program (ASAP)

In this section, we propose an integrated model of task-oriented training that is evidence-based and theoretically defensible. As discussed earlier (see "Constraint-Induced Movement Therapy: A Special Class of TOT," above), the family of forced-use and constraint-induced movement therapy protocols have addressed the suboptimal recovery of upper extremity function; including the recently completed phase III EXCITE clinical trial. There is now considerable evidence for efficacy of this approach in the subacute and chronic phases of recovery (41, 43, 48, 52, 189–199). In contrast, recent findings from the VECTORS phase II acute trial suggest that this intensive approach, administered too early after stroke, is not as effective as a lower dose of CIMT or dose equivalent usual and customary therapy (200).

Another set of interventions for which there is RCT level evidence also features focused task-oriented training, and is based in large part on motor control and learning principles, including motivational considerations (71, 201). This class of interventions subsumes more diverse approaches and modalities, including impairment-focused arm training (202–204), bilateral training (205, 206), and movement science/motor learning focused training (138, 207–209), but nonetheless with a common emphasis on systematic, progressed task-specific practice, and without constraint of the less impaired limb. In three recent systematic reviews, arm-focused interventions that contain targeted task-oriented training, including the family of CIMT interventions, emerge as the single most important element for overcoming the disabling consequences of stroke in mildly to moderately impaired participants (140, 210, 211). To this end, Van Peppen and colleagues recommend that training be applied intensively, early after onset and with at least 16 hours of additional therapy beyond current practice.

Our own review of clinical trials published within the last 10 years, pertaining to upper extremity stroke recovery, revealed a consistent pattern of findings. We grouped the studies into five functional categories broadly defined based on the nature of the intervention. These were: 1) **technology-based** (robotics, VR, computer games), 2) **functional electrical stimulation** (alone or combined with therapy or a device), 3) **adjunctive drug administration** (e.g., botox alone or combined with therapy), 4) **structured voluntary therapeutic exercise** (i.e., task-specific training, impairment-based, behavioral training, CIT, mCIT, bimanual training-BATRAC, functional training, movement science based, BASIS, AAT), and 5) **other** (mental practice, passive ROM, acupuncture). The studies with the highest level of evidence (design, control, number of subjects), the least expense to implement (i.e., no expensive equipment necessary), and most easily translatable into the current rehabilitation practice environment were in those grouped together into "structured voluntary therapeutic exercise." This grouping made up 41% of the 130 trials reviewed (54 out of 130). We examined this subgroup further by chronicity (acute, subacute, chronic), control group comparison (no control, dose-equivalent), and follow-up endpoint (immediate, short-term, longer term endpoint). Twenty-three percent (13 out of 54) had a comparison control group with some form of equivalent dose (e.g., attention control or conventional therapy). Of those, the majority (58%) as noted earlier, were conducted during the chronic phase of recovery and applied various forms of CIT (7 out of 13); one of these also included patients in the subacute stage (42). Only two studies were conducted in the subacute phase (44, 212), and three others in the acute phase (13, 40, 56). The two subacute studies varied widely in the dose of training from 1.3 hours over eight 10 minute sessions (212), to the application of forced-use (mitt use) for 6 hours per day for the duration of inpatient rehabilitation (44). Only one RCT of task-specific training administered in the outpatient setting in subacute stroke (88–117 days post-stroke) compared the effects of 18 2-hour sessions (6 week duration) to a dose-equivalent conventional therapy group (207). Not surprisingly, and consistent with a specificity effect, performance improved significantly more for the task-training group on the tasks that were practiced (balance, ADL, IADL) and tested over the six week time course. Unfortunately, the persistence of these findings was not examined longer-term (207).

Together, published meta-analyses (140), a focused clinical trial review, recent practice guidelines (23, 162), recommended strategies (66, 159, 213), and our collective research experience lead to the formulation of an approach toward an integrated, evidence-based intervention that embodies the elements that contribute to upper extremity task-oriented training **as a fundamental basis for skill reacquisition** among patients with hemiparetic upper extremities. Task-oriented training (skill) would be integrated with means to mitigate underlying mutable

impairments (capacity), and optimize internal motivation (motivation). We note that the literature on upper extremity recovery through task-oriented practice shows no sign of this convergence toward a single label that we call Accelerated Skill Acquisition Program (ASAP). This construct is intended to capture the best, scientifically-derived and evidence-based, investigational practice. ASAP is derived based on a logical and tightly connected conceptual framework from which it was developed.

Conceptual Framework and Foundations of ASAP. A pathway from impairment reduction, to functional capability, to more general use of restored limbs in real-world contexts, is often implicitly assumed but less frequently embedded into therapeutic practice protocols. We propose that **skill** (motor learning and self-management), **capacity** (impairment mitigation), and **motivation** (intrinsic drive) together form the foundation for effective incorporation of the paretic upper extremity into life activities (Figure 17-1). This conceptual model derives from the foundational and applied neuromotor and psychological sciences (64, 71, 139, 214–216). As noted above, the three elements that define ASAP include: 1) task-specific practice (skill); 2) impairment mitigation (capacity); and 3) motivational enhancements (motivation). As mentioned earlier (see "Constraint-Induced Movement Therapy," above), task-specific practice is considered to be the most important element of CIMT with some, including its originator (Edward Taub) claiming that it is more important than constraint of the less-affected limb (47). The scientific rationale and evidence for impairment mitigation (capacity) comes from a growing body of work showing the importance of fundamental impairments, including strength and control (6, 13, 165, 202–204, 213, 217, 218), for restoration of upper extremity function. In contrast, CIMT protocols do not recognize physical impairments such as weakness or incoordination as direct targets for

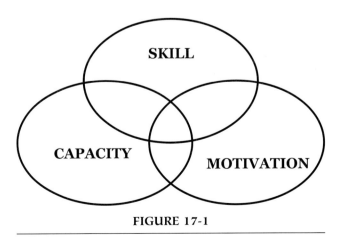

FIGURE 17-1

Conceptual model showing three active ingredients.

intervention (213, 219). Similarly, the scientific rationale and evidence for motivational enhancements, as well as the pursuit of meaningful goals for sustainable behavioral change, comes from a growing body of work showing the importance of self-regulation, self-management, and self-efficacy for behavioral change that supports beneficial outcomes (214, 215, 220–223). In most cases, the motivational enhancements strengthen self-confidence and support patient control or autonomy (intrinsic motivation). This provides support for the important conceptual linkage between the capacity for intrinsic motivation and the development of self-efficacy. Capacity increases, such as those induced by highly structured practice and the mitt in CIT, support self efficacy through performance progress, but provide extrinsic motivation for affected limb use. Thus, in the case of CIMT as a task oriented treatment, we might remind patients about the helpfulness of mitt use (especially in activities requiring unimanual use) and encourage its use to optimize functional change, thus supporting participants' autonomy and therefore adherence (221, 224, 225).

Further Elaboration of Asap: Key Elements.   Targeted task-oriented training (skill) emerges in three recent systematic reviews as the single most important attribute for the disabling consequences of stroke in mildly to moderately impaired participants (140, 210, 211) (see "Emergence of Task Oriented Training for Neurorehabilitation," above). Likewise, the fundamental problem that ASAP addresses is conceived as the learning or re-learning of motor skills to optimally affect neural reorganization (66, 226), as well as skills to self-direct post-training activities. Development of skill is facilitated by the amelioration of impairments (e.g., muscle weakness, low self-efficacy) to enhance capacity. Attention to motor learning, motor control (e.g., goal-directed whole tasks with natural synergies) (227), and exercise physiology (e.g., overload in terms of training load/intensity, speed) principles are relevant. Social-cognitive psychological theories of motivation have long been used in motor learning /performance and clinical contexts (e.g., 228–230), and are applied in this integrated model for immediate and particularly longer-term participant motivation. These theories assume that intrinsic sources of motivation, including perceptions of self-determination (choice, control, collaboration) and self-efficacy (confidence in one's capabilities), are key contributors of continued choice, effort, and persistence to use paretic limbs, which in turn leads to mitigation of disability and of self-imposed participation restrictions. These concepts are reminiscent of the successful strategies used in falls prevention programs that combine balance training with development of self-efficacy for tasks (e.g., stairs, bathtub, curbs) that were initially perceived as unachievable, in large part because of low self-efficacy.

Impairment focused mitigation (capacity): Given that there is a strong relationship between impairment level and motor recovery (139, 231–234), interventions designed to remediate impairments should impact functional capabilities as well (203, 204, 235–237). Subacute patients between three weeks and six months post-stroke who received impairment-focused arm ability training realized improved functional capability, immediately and at the one year follow-up, in timed motor performance tests (TEMPA) compared to control subjects (204). This enhanced capacity has also been correlated with a change in neural activation patterns (203, 231). We found that strength training alone without functional training induced short-term, but not persistent longer-term improvements in a group of mildly to moderately impaired subacute patients (13). On the other hand, functional task training alone induced both short-term and longer term improvements in both upper extremity use and isometric torque (13), suggesting that impairment mitigation combined with task-specific practice would be optimal for inducing longer-term changes (217). These results would lead us to believe that time in therapy directed at the mitigation of impairments would be well spent. Of note, and consistent with our findings with a functional task training protocol (13), the CIT protocol used in EXCITE did not directly target impairments, yet, between group differences emerged at one year for the two force items (grip strength, lift weight) on the WMFT. This finding suggests that there is some benefit to fundamental impairments (strength in this case) that is achieved through the "activity" domain manifest through increased "use" of the limb in daily life.

Task-specific training includes bimanual activities (skill): Many everyday activities involve the coordinated use of two hands (238) to accomplish separate movements in an inter-dependent manner, and some in which the two limbs move in parallel to achieve the goal. A series of studies from the University of Maryland (205, 206, 239) has examined the effects of a six-week bilateral arm training program on the neural correlates, fine motor coordination, and functional activity outcomes of individuals with chronic stroke hemiparesis. These preliminary studies suggest post-intervention improvements in paretic and non-paretic limb strength, range of motion, motor control, and functional abilities with bilateral training (206), accompanied by modest fMRI changes in cerebral and cerebellar activation patterns (205). In a separate study, we (240) found increases in aiming velocity for the paretic arm only when this activity was coupled with the non-paretic limb for a task analogous to catching a fast-moving mosquito. The ASAP approach requires that at least one of the participant-selected tasks be bimanual. Together, bilateral movements that invoke natural movement synergies and facilitate effects on motor coordination are seen as integral to real-world goal-directed skill acquisition, in which practice during and after training is important.

Motivational enhancements (motivation): Following self-efficacy theory, individuals' self-efficacy for functional performance, coping, or self-management element has prospectively predicted health-related behavior adherence, physical functioning and disability, and health outcomes in diverse medical conditions, including stroke (222, 241–250). Converging theory and empirical evidence, as well as quality initiatives in patient-centered care and evidence-based practice (251, 252), suggest that health care provided in a manner that supports individuals' self-determination, including autonomy, preferences, and active participation in medical decision making (222, 253–257), improves adherence to health providers' recommendations and enhances clinical outcomes mediated by intervening health-related behaviors. From a motor learning perspective, active involvement and a more distributed practice schedule facilitates deeper and more effective information processing for skill acquisition (35, 66, 258, 259). A number of structured interventions to affect patient participation in health decisions and health behaviors have been developed, including a 20-minute module to activate patient questioning of health care providers (253), motivational interviewing by health professionals (82, 260), and the use of instruments or interventions with goal-setting features (261, 262). For the I-CARE clinical trial, and specifically within ASAP, we embed a structural element to enhance active patient involvement in collaborative decision-making and problem-solving in motor skill and self-management skill learning, to enhance participants' self-directed behavior that includes collaboration about mitt use. The clinician could select a structured, simple, and straightforward representation of active patient-centered collaboration (in training task selection, scheduling, and mitt use) with problem-solving discussion (regarding injury prevention, movement skill development, exercise/training principles, performance, compensatory strategies, and with self-directed elaboration for participation) throughout the treatment plan. Table 17-1 translates the ASAP elements, including collaboration and problem-solving, into a 15-session dose of ASAP.

In summary, an evaluation of current task-oriented therapy practices and the state of phase II and III clinical trial evidence led to the proposed integrated model. The proposal represents a theoretically sound and evidence-based set of elements combined together into ASAP. In turn, ASAP represents a fully-defined, evidence-based, hybrid combination of constraint-induced movement therapy and skill-based/impairment-mitigating motor skill training with embedded motivational enhancements. A phase III multi-site clinical trial (I-CARE) is currently underway to test the effectiveness of ASAP administered to patients with mild to moderate impairments during the early post-acute outpatient interval, and to compare the effects of ASAP to that of an equivalent dose of usual and customary outpatient therapy on upper extremity functional recovery measured one year later.

RESEARCH FRONTIERS

In this section, we briefly highlight four important research frontiers that have relevance to task-oriented training to promote upper extremity recovery after stroke.

Predictive Models for the Proper Dosing of Therapy

This area is particularly challenging and identified by the NINDS Stroke Progress review group as one of the important unmet needs of the current strategic planning process. Recently, this problem was approached using a biologically plausible model of bilateral reaching movements to investigate the mechanisms and conditions leading to effective rehabilitation (263). This type of approach has promise, and may provide the needed stimulus for the design of hypothesis-driven clinical trials that incorporate patient-specific characteristics with predictive models for determining the proper therapy dose. Recently, several papers have used quantitative measures of anatomical and functional neural capacity (e.g., corticospinal tract) to determine functional potential in chronic stroke (264), or to determine the relationship between CST injury and peduncular asymmetry (265). Given that neural capacity largely determines potential for recovery and the choice of an appropriate rehabilitation strategy (140), patient-specific models that include neural resources would be particularly appealing to optimize healthcare services.

Multi-Modality Therapy Programs

A second research frontier includes the development of *multi-modality therapy programs* that combine several complimentary modalities, such as a drug with an intense program of task-oriented training, or a behavioral intervention with a socially-assisted robot (266). There has been very little work of this sort, in part because much of the foundational research is still needed (267), but we think it is only a matter of time before we begin to see more biologically motivated multi-modality therapy programs designed to promote restoration of function after stroke. Progress is being made in the development of training algorithms and testing, including selected TOT (and ASAP) principles in robotics assisted rehabilitation of the UE (e.g. progressing games simulating elements of functional reach with varying or progressive impedance control training algorithms) such as that used in ADAPT, a new robotic task-practice system, designed to deliver

TABLE 17-1

Example Case: Integration of ASAP Elements over Fifteen 2-hour Sessions

ELEMENT(S)	DESCRIPTION	COMMENTS
ORIENTATION SESSION		
MOTIVATION: Collaboration agreement	Participant oriented to ASAP purpose and principles, organization, action planning. Future sessions are scheduled.	
MOTIVATION: Task collaboration	Designate 4 specific tasks (including ones with bimanual, strength, dexterity requirements), including one as his priority task.	Priority task selected was use of his impaired arm and hand to eat, including management of utensils and mug. Other chosen tasks: card manipulation (shuffling, dealing, holding, placing), writing, handyman tool use (e.g., hammer).
TRAINING DAYS	Assess vitals signs	Within normal limits (all days)
MOTIVATION: Brief self-efficacy assessment for priority task	Patient asked how confident he was in performing specific chosen task. Then asked to problem-solve by providing thoughts on what could be done to increase confidence in next week (Day 1: "Exercise; what else is there?").	Brief self-efficacy assessments 4 times, including first and last sessions. Initial brief self-efficacy score = 4 for eating/management of utensils/mug. Later scores were 5 (middle session) and 7 (end of training).
MOTIVATION and SKILL: Action plans for self-management skills/extended practice	Set-up (end of sessions) and debriefing (beginning of sessions) of participant's action plans.	Participant reported on home tasks of writing and eating with impaired arm/hand (day 8), tasks of writing and lifting boxes in garage (day 15).
TRAINING DAYS		
SKILL: task-specific practice (priority task) and **IMPAIRMENT MITIGATION**: coordination, selective movement, precision; force modulation, and **MOTIVATION**: collaboration and challenge	Eating skills (use of knife for cutting, pouring liquid into varied size mugs/cups). Progressed from use of knife with built-up handle (Day 1); knife without build-up for cutting around targets in simulated food, drinking from mug filled with varied amounts of water in mug (Day 8); use of knife without built-up handle to cut muffin, break and peel an egg, placed various-sized beans into varied-size containers. Task practiced for 25–30 minutes in different participant-selected order each day.	Participant limited by decreased grip strength and fine motor control; reported difficulty with cutting and fork and spoon use (Day 1). Participant limited by decreased forearm pronation, shoulder abduction with internal rotation, selective use (coordination) of the arm and hand (Day 8). Participant directed practice session with ideas to increase the level of difficulty and challenge (Day 15).
SKILL: task-specific practice and **IMPAIRMENT MITIGATION**: speed, intersegmental coordination, selective finger movement, and **MOTIVATION**: collaboration and challenge	Card manipulation (shuffling, dealing, holding, placing). Participant challenged to speed up movements. Repetitions timed. Task practiced for 25–30 minutes in different order each day.	Day 1: Participant prompted to self-assess difficulty of task and begin problem-solving with therapist to increase challenge, implemented 5-point difficulty rating scale. Day 8: Participant dealt cards farther away from midline and body, able to deal and pick up card faster than previous day. Day 15: Participant chose to vary the type of hand technique to pick up cards, such as finger to thumb, to sliding card to edge of table; reports playing cards with friends.

TABLE 17-1
(Continued)

ELEMENT(S)	DESCRIPTION	COMMENTS
TRAINING DAYS		
SKILL: task-specific practice and **IMPAIRMENT MITIGATION**: precision; force modulation; coordination; selective movement, and **MOTIVATION**: collaboration and challenge	Writing (use of pencil for printing and cursive writing). Participant progressed from use of a pencil with built-up handle and pencil manipulation on table top (Day 1), to copying a paragraph, writing in large and small print and cursively (Day 8), to writing without built-up handle, writing on triplicate form, drawing a picture (Day 15). Task practiced for 25–30 minutes in different order each day.	Day 1: Participant required 80.04 seconds to pick up pencil and print name; reported 3 out of 5 difficulty. Participant chose order of writing tasks; stated on day 6 "...writing is a little better...I can read it." Participant reported being pleased with his writing; chose to draw a picture; able to write 3/4 of a page in 10 minutes (Day 15).
SKILL: task-specific practice and **IMPAIRMENT MITIGATION**: precision; force modulation; load/intensity; endurance work to fatigue; coordination; selective movement, and **MOTIVATION**: collaboration and challenge	"Handyman" activities (hammering, taking measurements at varied angles, heights, surfaces with ruler and making measurements with pencil; sanding wood; pulling duct tape off a roll and placing on wall at varied heights, plugging cords in/removing from socket). Grip strength targeted. Task practiced for 25–30 minutes in different order each day.	Day 1: missed nail on 10 of 25 attempts; Days 8 and 15: Participant offered suggestions for activity progression based on level of difficulty (e.g., reach farther from body when taking measurements).
MOTIVATION: Task collaboration	Tasks chosen by participant for next day Assess vital signs, pain, and fatigue	Order of tasks practice differed. Vitals: within normal limits (all days); pain absent; fatigue 6 and 5 out of 10 on Days 8 and 15.
	Exit interview (Day 15)	Participant reported that he resumed playing cards with friends and playing games with grandchildren such as building houses out of cards, coloring, jigsaw puzzles; preparing to get his driver's license and is glad to have practiced writing his signature; reported being pleased with the program and expressed appreciation "... you have changed my life and I thank you."

Case Analysis-Integration of ASAP Elements.

task-oriented training (268). Robotics technology is not a mutually exclusive approach, but rather elements of TOT can be (and are) built into or combined with it to maximize the benefit of training.

Mirror Neuron System

A third exciting research frontier involves the *mirror neuron system* (269). Evidence for a human mirror neuron system is mounting (270, 271). However, there still is considerable controversy and confusion about the homologue to the primate mirror neuron system in the human (272). A provocative review suggested that the mirror neuron system might provide a useful circuitry to enhance recovery of the severely affected upper limb early after stroke (273). Recently, another group provided empirical support for the use of observation with intent to imitate in stroke rehabilitation to augment physical therapy and promote motor function (274). This notion represents a very exciting and potentially important alternative circuit for driving recovery after stroke.

Attention and Motor Skill Learning

Finally, the area of *attention and motor skill learning* is an important one for motor retraining (275). There is considerable evidence that a simple manipulation of attentional focus can benefit motor learning (276–278). Instructional manipulations that focus attention on external cues are more effective for motor learning than those that direct attention on internal cues (i.e., the moving limb or pressure under the feet). Fasoli and colleagues tested this simple concept in an experiment dealing with functional reach actions in persons with and without cerebrovascular accident (279). One group was instructed to focus on the to-be-grasped object, and the other was instructed to focus on their arm movements. The results showed that both non-disabled and disabled groups performed the tasks more effectively (e.g., more effective movement kinematics) if given external rather than internal focus instructions. This finding suggests that participants with stroke and controls preplanned these functional actions to a greater extent and used more automatic control processes when they focused externally. The importance of this work for task-oriented training in rehabilitation is tremendous. It suggests that the nature of the instructions about attentional focus can impact the effectiveness of the training program, and could be as important as the specific training paradigm for determining the most effective dose of training. For example, a task-oriented training program administered using instructions for an external focus of attention might achieve a clinically meaningful outcome with greater efficiency (e.g., shorter time, smaller dose), than one using instructions for an internal focus of attention. This area is clearly important for future developments and in conjunction with determining the pharmacokinetics of task-oriented training.

CONCLUSION/SUMMARY

We find ourselves in a particularly exciting time for neurorehabilitation, repair, and recovery, with an exponential growth in understanding the basic social, cognitive, and neuroscience surrounding effective rehabilitation (280). In this chapter, we merely scratch the surface of what only recently emerged as the dominant approach to motor restoration, "a task-oriented approach." Contrary to current medical reimbursement models that support early acute and sub-acute stages of rehabilitation, substantial evidence supports the effectiveness of TOT in the post-sub-acute and chronic stages of recovery. More work is needed to determine the requisite and optimal TOT dosing in the early acute and sub-acute recovery stage (e.g., VECTORS trial). Further, more work is needed to study ways to optimize the clinical translation of TOT across different care settings to maximize outreach and dissemination. We are encouraged by how much is known, and at the same time, how little is known, for example about the "pharmacokinetics" of training. Building a strong theoretical foundation will be important for future advances in this exciting field of neurorehabilitation. We hope this chapter provides a beginning and impetus for these future advances in rehabilitation science.

References

1. NINDS Stroke Progress Review Group. http://www.ninds.nih.gov/find_people/groups/stroke_prg/09_2006_stroke_prg_report.htm.
2. World Health Organization. *International Classification of Functioning, Disability and Health*. Geneva: World Health Organization, 2001.
3. Gordon J. Assumptions underlying physical therapy interventions: Theoretical and historical perspectives. In: Car J, Shepard RD, eds. *Movement Science: Foundation for Physical Therapy in Rehabilitation*. 2nd ed. Gaithersburg, MD: Aspen, 2000:1–31.
4. Ada L, Canning CG, Carr J, Kilbreath SL, Shephed R. Task-specific training of reaching and manipulation. In: Bennett K, Castiello U, ed. *Insights into the Reach to Grasp Movement*. Vol 105. Amsterdam: Elsevier, 1994:239–265.
5. Carr J, Shepherd RB. *Stroke Rehabilitation: Guidelines for Exercise and Training to Optimize Motor Skill*. London: Butterworth-Heinemann, 2003.
6. Winstein CJ, Wing AM, Whitall J. Motor control and learning principles for rehabilitation of upper limb movements after brain injury. In: Boller F, Grafman J, eds. *Handbook of Neuropsychology*. Vol. 9. 2nd ed. Amsterdam: Elsevier Science B.V., 2003:77–137.
7. Mastos M, Miller K, Eliasson AC, Imms C. Goal-directed training: Linking theories of treatment to clinical practice for improved functional activities in daily life. *Clinical Rehabilitation* 2007; 21:47–55.
8. Carr J, Shepherd RB. A motor learning model for stroke rehabilitation. *Physiotherapy* 1989; 75:372–380.
9. Dean C, Shepherd RB. Task-related training improves the performance of seated reaching tasks after stroke. A randomised controlled trial. *Stroke* 1997; 28:722–728.
10. Richards C, Malouin F, Dean C. Gait in stroke: Assessment and rehabilitation. *Clinics in Geriatric Medicine* 1999; 15:833–855.
11. Blennerhassett J, Dite W. Additional task-related practice improves mobility and upper limb function early after stroke: A randomised controlled trial. *Australian Journal of Physiotherapy* 2004; 50(4):219–224.
12. Thielman GT, Dean CM, Gentile AM. Rehabilitation of reaching after stroke: Task-related training versus progressive resistive exercise. *Arch Phys Med Rehabil* 2004; 85(10):1613–1618.
13. Winstein CJ, Rose DK, Tan SM, Lewthwaite R, Chui HC, Azen SP. A randomized controlled comparison of upper-extremity rehabilitation strategies in acute stroke: A pilot study of immediate and long-term outcomes. *Arch Phys Med Rehabil* 2004; 85(4):620–628.
14. Trombly C. Occupation: Purposefulness and meaningfulness as therapeutic mechanisms. *American Journal of Occupational Therapy* 1995; 49:960–972.
15. Trombly C, Wu, C. Effect of rehabilitation tasks on organization of movement after stroke. *American Journal of Occupational Therapy* 1999; 53:333–347.
16. Bongaardt R, Meijer OG. Bernstein's theory of movement behavior: Historical development and contmeporary relevance. *Journal of Motor Behavior* 2000; 32:57–71.
17. Newell K. On task and theory specificity. *Journal of Motor Behavior* 1989; 21:91–96.
18. Shepherd R, Carr J. An emergent or dynamical systems view of movement dysfunction. *Australian J of Physiotherapy* 1991; 37:4–5, 17.
19. Newell K. Motor skill acquisition. *Annual Reviews in Psychology* 1991; 42:213–237.
20. Shumway-Cook A, Woollacott M. *Motor Control: Translating Research into Clinical Practice*. 3rd ed. Philadelphia, PA: Lippincott Williams & Wilkins, 2007.
21. Wu CY, Wong MK, Lin KC, Chen HC. Effects of task goal and personal preference on seated reaching kinematics after stroke. *Stroke* 2001; 32(1):70–76.
22. Quinn L, Gordon J. Documenting functional status: A skill-based model. In: . *Functional Outcomes Documentation for Rehabilitation*. St. Louis: J. Saunders, 2003:63–77.
23. Ottawa Panel, Khadilkar A, Phillips K, et al. Ottawa panel evidence-based clinical practice guidelines for post-stroke rehabilitation. *Topics in Stroke Rehabilitation* 2006; 13(2):1–269.
24. An Exploratory and Analytical Survey of Therapeutic Exercise: Northwestern University Special Therapeutic Exercise Project (STEP). *American Journal of Physical Medicine* 1967; 46(1): .

25. Adkins D, Boychuk J, Pemple MS, Kleim JA. Motor training induces experience-specific patterns of plasticity across motor cortex and spinal cord. *Journal of Applied Physiology* 2006; 10:1776–1782.

26. Maldonado M, Allred RP, Felthauser EL, Jones TA. Motor skill training, but not voluntary exercise, improves skilled reaching after unilateral ischemic lesions of the sensorimotor cortex in rats. *Neurorehabilitation and Neural Repair* 2008; 22(3):250–261.

27. Nelles G, Jentzen W, Jueptner M, Muller S, Diener HC. Arm training induced brain plasticity in stroke studied with serial positron emission tomography. *NeuroImage* 2001; 13(6 Pt 1):1146–1154.

28. Plautz EJ, Milliken GW, Nudo RJ. Effects of repetitive motor training on movement representations in adult squirrel monkeys: Role of use versus learning. *Neurobiol Learn Mem* 2000; 74(1):27–55.

29. Marteniuk R, Leavit JL, MacKenzie CL, Athenes S. Functional relationships between grasp and transport components in a prehension task. *Human Movement Science* 1990; 9:149–176.

30. van Vliet P. An investigation of the task specificity of reaching: Implications for retraining. *Physiotherapy Theory and Practice* 1993; 9:69–76.

31. Weir P, MacKenzie CL, Marteniuk RG, Cargoe SL. Is object texture a constraint on human–prehension—Kinematic evidence. *Journal of Motor Behavior* 1991; 23:205–210.

32. Wu C, Trombly CA, Lin K, Tickle-Degnen L. Effects of object affordances on reaching performance in persons with and without cerebrovascular accident. *American Journal of Occupational Therapy* 1998; 52:447–456.

33. van Vliet P, Sheridan M, Kerwin DG, Fentem P. The influence of functional goals on the kinematics of reaching following stroke. *Neurology Report* 1995; 19:11–16.

34. Bernstein N. *The Co-ordination and Regulation of Movements.* London: Oxford: Pergamon Press, 1967.

35. Lee TD, Swinnen SP, Serrien DJ. Cognitive effort and motor learning. *Quest* 1994; 46:328–344.

36. Lee TD, Wishart LR. Motor learning conundrums (and possible solutions). *Quest* 2005(57):67–78.

37. Sanger T. Failure of motor learning for large initial errors. *Neural Computation* 2004; 16(9):1873–1886.

38. Lotze M, Braun C, Birbaumer N, Anders S, Cohen LG. Motor learning elicited by voluntary drive. *Brain* 2003; 126(Pt 4):866–872.

39. The Consensus Panel on the Stroke Rehabilitation System: Time is Function. In: HSFO, ed. Ontario, Canada 2007.

40. Dromerick AW, Edwards DF, Hahn M. Does the application of constraint-induced movement therapy during acute rehabilitation reduce arm impairment after ischemic stroke? *Stroke* 2000; 31(12):2984–2988.

41. Page SJ, Sisto S, Levine P, McGrath RE. Efficacy of modified constraint-induced movement therapy in chronic stroke: A single-blinded randomized controlled trial. *Arch Phys Med Rehabil* 2004; 85(1):14–18.

42. Page SJ, Sisto SA, Levine P, Johnston MV, Hughes M. Modified constraint induced therapy: A randomized feasibility and efficacy study. *J Rehabil Res Dev* 2001; 38(5):583–590.

43. Pierce SR, Gallagher KG, Schaumburg SW, Gershkoff AM, Gaughan JP, Shutter L. Home forced use in an outpatient rehabilitation program for adults with hemiplegia: A pilot study. *Neurorehabil Neural Repair* 2003; 17(4):214–219.

44. Ploughman M, Corbett D. Can forced-use therapy be clinically applied after stroke? An exploratory randomized controlled trial. *Arch Phys Med Rehabil* 2004; 85(9):1417–1423.

45. Roberts PS, Vegher JA, Gilewski M, Bender A, Riggs RV. Client-centered occupational therapy using constraint-induced therapy. *Journal of Stroke and Cerebrovascular Diseases* 2005; 14(3):115.

46. Taub E, Miller NE, Novack TA, et al. Technique to improve chronic motor deficit after stroke. *Arch Phys Med Rehabil* 1993; 74(4):347–354.

47. Taub E, Uswatte G, Morris DM. Improved motor recovery after stroke and massive cortical reorganization following Constraint-Induced Movement Therapy. *Phys Med Rehabil Clin N Am* 2003; 14(1 Suppl):S77–91, ix.

48. van der Lee JH, Wagenaar RC, Lankhorst GJ, Vogelaar TW, Deville WL, Bouter LM. Forced use of the upper extremity in chronic stroke patients: Results from a single-blind randomized clinical trial. *Stroke* 1999; 30(11):2369–2375.

49. Winstein CJ, Miller JP, Blanton S, et al. Methods for a multisite randomized trial to investigate the effect of constraint-induced movement therapy in improving upper extremity function among adults recovering from a cerebrovascular stroke. *Neurorehabil Neural Repair* 2003; 17(3):137–152.

50. Wolf SL, Lecraw DE, Barton LA, Jann BB. Forced use of hemiplegic upper extremities to reverse the effect of learned nonuse among chronic stroke and head-injured patients. *Exp Neurol* 1989; 104(2):125–132.

51. Wolf S, Winstein CJ, Miller JP, Thompson PA, Taub E, Uswatte G, Morris D, Blanton S, Nichols-Larsen D, Clark PC. Retention of upper limb function in stroke survivors who have received constraint-induced movement therapy: The EXCITE randomized trial. *Lancet Neurology* 2008; 7(1):33–40.

52. Wolf SL, Winstein CJ, Miller JP, et al. Effect of constraint-induced movement therapy on upper extremity function 3 to 9 months after stroke: The EXCITE randomized clinical trial. *JAMA* 2006; 296(17):2095–2104.

53. Sterr A, Elbert T, Berthold I, Kolbel S, Rockstroh B, Taub E. Longer versus shorter daily constraint-induced movement therapy of chronic hemiparesis: An exploratory study. *Arch Phys Med Rehabil* 2002; 83(10):1374–1377.

54. Sterr A, Freivogel S, Schmalohr D. Neurobehavioral aspects of recovery: Assessment of the learned nonuse phenomenon in hemiparetic adolescents. *Arch Phys Med Rehabil* 2002; 83(12):1726–1731.

55. Barbay S, Front SB, Nudo RJ, Dancause N, Plautz EJ, Friel FM, Stowe AM. Behavioral and neurophysiological effects of delayed training following a small ischemic infarct in primary motor cortex of squirrel monkeys. *Experimental Brain Research* 2006; 169:106–116.

56. Page SJ, Levine P, Leonard AC. Modified constraint-induced therapy in acute stroke: A randomized controlled pilot study. *Neurorehabil Neural Repair* 2005; 19(1):27–32.

57. Morgan MG. The shaping game: A teaching technique. *Behav Ther* 1974; 5(2):271–272.

58. Panyan M. *How to Use Shaping.* Lawrence, Kansas: H&H Enterprises, 1980.

59. Skinner B. *The Technology of Teaching.* New York: Appleton-Century-Crofts, 1968.

60. Holding D. *Principles of Training.* New York: Pergamon, 1965.

61. Kelley C. What is adaptive training? *Human Factors* 1969; 11:547–556.

62. Lintern G, Gopher D. Adaptive training of perceptual motor skills: Issues results and future directions. *International Journal of Man-Machine Studies* 1978; 10:521–551.

63. Mane A, Adams JA, Donchin E. Adaptive and part-whole training in the acquisition of a complex perceptual-motor skill. *Acta Psychol (Amst)* 1989; 71:179–196.

64. Schmidt RA, Lee TD. *Motor Control and Learning: A Behavioral Emphasis.* 4th ed. Champaign, IL: Human Kinetics, 2005.

65. Winstein C. Designing practice for motor learning: Clinical impressions. In: Lister M, ed. *Contemporary Management of Motor Control Problems: Proceedings of the II Step Conference.* Alexandria, VA: Foundation for Physical Therapy, 1991:65–76.

66. Dobkin BH. Strategies for stroke rehabilitation. *Lancet Neurol* 2004; 3(9):528–536.

67. Desrosiers J, Bourbonnais D, Corriveau H, Gosselin S, Bravo G. Effectiveness of unilateral and symmetrical bilateral task training for arm during the subacute phase after stroke: A randomized controlled trial. *Clin Rehabil* 2005; 19(6):581–593.

68. Flinn N. A task-oriented approach to the treatment of a client with hemiplegia. *American Journal of Occupational Therapy* 1995; 49:560–569.

69. Rosenbaum DA. The Cinderella of psychology: The neglect of motor control in the science of mental life and behavior. *The American Psychologist$* 2005; 60(4):308–317.

70. Winstein C, Knecht HG. Movement science and its relevance to physical therapy. *Physical Therapy* 1990; 70:759–762.

71. Krakauer JW. Motor learning: Its relevance to stroke recovery and neurorehabilitation. *Curr Opin Neurol* 2006; 19(1):84–90.

72. Lee TD, Genovese ED. Distribution of practice in motor skill acquisition: Different effects for discrete and continuous tasks. *Res Q Exerc Sport* 1989; 60(1):59–65.

73. Levine P, Page SJ. Modified constraint-induced therapy: A promising restorative outpatient therapy. *Top Stroke Rehabil* 2004; 11(4):1–10.

74. Page SJ, Elovic E, Levine P, Sisto SA. Modified constraint-induced therapy and botulinum toxin A: A promising combination. *Am J Phys Med Rehabil* 2003; 82(1):76–80.

75. Page SJ, Sisto S, Johnston MV, Levine P, Hughes M. Modified constraint-induced therapy in subacute stroke: A case report. *Arch Phys Med Rehabil* 2002; 83(2):286–290.

76. DeJong G, Horn SD, Gassaway JA, Slavin MD, Dijkers MP. Toward a taxonomy of rehabilitation interventions: Using an inductive approach to examine the "black box" of rehabilitation. *Arch Phys Med Rehabil* 2004; 85(4):678–686.

77. Whyte J, Hart T. It's more than a black box; it's a Russian doll: Defining rehabilitation treatments. *Am J Phys Med Rehabil* 2003; 82(8):639–652.

78. Kaplon R, Prettyman M, Kushi C, Winstein C. Six hours in the laboratory: A quantification of practice time during constraint-induced therapy (CIT). *Clinical Rehabilitation* 2007; 21(10):950–958.

79. Morris DM, Uswatte G, Crago JE, Cook EW, 3rd, Taub E. The reliability of the Wolf Motor Function Test for assessing upper extremity function after stroke. *Arch Phys Med Rehabil* 2001; 82(6):750–755.

80. Wolf SL, Catlin PA, Ellis M, Archer AL, Morgan B, Piacentino A. Assessing Wolf Motor Function Test as outcome measure for research in patients after stroke. *Stroke* 2001; 32(7):1635–1639.

81. Wolf SL, Newton H, Maddy D, Blanton S, Zhang Q, Winstein CJ, Morris DM, Light K. The EXCITE trial: Relationship of intensity of constraint induced movement therapy to improvement in the wolf motor function test. *Restorative Neurology and Neuroscience* 2007; 25(5–6):549–562.

82. Bell KR, Temkin NR, Esselman PC, et al. The effect of a scheduled telephone intervention on outcome after moderate to severe traumatic brain injury: A randomized trial. *Arch Phys Med Rehabil* 2005; 86(5):851–856.

83. Sterr A, Szameitat A, Shen S, Freivogel S. Application of the CIT concept in the clinical environment: Hurdles, practicalities, and clinical benefits. *Cogn Behav Neurol* 2006; 19(1):48–54.

84. Battig WF. Transfer and verbal pretraining to motor performance as a function of motor task complexity. *Journal of Experimental Psychology* 1956; 51:371–378.

85. Battig WF. Facilitation and interference. In: Bilodeau EA, ed. *Acquisition of Skill.* New York: Academic Press, 1966.

86. Battig WF. The flexibility of human memory. In: Cermak LS, Craik, FIM, eds. *Levels of Processing in Human Memory.* Hillsdale, New Jersey: Earlbaum, 1979.

87. Guadagnoli MA, Lee TD. Challenge point: A framework for conceptualizing the effects of various practice conditions in motor learning. *J Mot Behav* 2004; 36(2):212–224.

88. Giuffrida CG, Shea JB, Fairbrother JT. Differential transfer benefits of increased practice for constant, blocked, and serial practice schedules. *J Mot Behav* 2002; 34(4):353–365.

89. Meira CM, Tani G. The contextual interference effect in acquisition of dart-throwing skill tested on a transfer test with extended trials. *Perceptual and Motor Skills* 2001; 92(1):910–918.

90. Perez CR, Meira CM, Tani G. Does the contextual interference effect last over extended transfer trials? *Perceptual and Motor Skills* 2005; 100(1):58–60.

91. Wright DL, Magnuson CE, Black CB. Programming and reprogramming sequence timing following high and low contextual interference practice. *Res Q. Exercise Sport* 2005; 76(3):258–266.

92. Hall KG, Magill RA. Variability of practice and contextual interference in motor skill learning. *Journal of Motor Behavior* 1995; 27(4):299–309.

93. Lee TD. Transfer-appropriate processing: A framework for conceptualizing practice effects in motor learning. In: O.G. Meijer KR, ed. *Complex Movement Behaviour: The Motor-Action Controversy.* North-Holland: Elsevier Science Publishers B.V., 1988:201–215.

94. Lee TD, Magill RA. The locus of contextual interference in motor-skill acquisition. *J. Exp Psychol: Human Learning and Memory* 1983; 9:730–746.

95. Lee TD, Magill RA. Can forgetting facilitate skill acquisition? In: Goodman D, Wilberg RB, Franks IM, eds. *Differing Perspectives in Motor Learning, Memory and Control.* North-Holland: Elsevier Science Publishers B.V., 1985:3–21.

96. Shea JB, Zimny ST. Contextual effects in memory and learning movement information. In: Magill RA, ed. *Memory and Control of Action.* Amsterdam: Elsevier, 1983:345–366.

97. Hallett M. Transcranial magnetic stimulation and the human brain. *Nature* 2000; 406(6792):147–150.

98. Lin C, Fisher BE, Winstein CJ, Wu AD, Gordon J. Contextual interference effect: Elaborative-processing or forgetting-reconstruction? A post-hoc analysis of TMS-induced effects on motor learning. *Journal of Motor Behavior* 2008; 40.

99. Aoki T, Tsuda H, Takasawa M, Osaki Y, Oku N, Hatazawa J, Kinoshita H. The effect of tapping finger and mode differences on cortical and subcortical activities: A PET study. *Exp Brain Res* 2005; 160(3):375–383.

100. Chung SC, Min BC, Kim CJ, Cho ZH. Total activation change of visual and motor area due to various disturbances. *J. Physiol Anthropol Appl Human Science* 2000; 19(2):93–100.

101. Demiralp T, Karamursel S, Karakullukcu YE, Gokhan N. Movement-related cortical potentials: Their relationship to the laterality, complexity and learning of a movement. *International Journal of Neuroscience* 1990; 51(1-2):153–162.

102. Gorbet DJ, Staines W.R., Sergio L.E. Brain mechanisms for preparing increasingly complex sensory to motor transformations. *Neuroimage* 2004; 23(3):1100–1111.

103. Hatfield BD, Haufler AJ, Hung TM, Spalding TW. Electroencephalographic studies of skilled psychomotor performance. *J. Clin Neurophysiology* 2004; 21(3):144–156.

104. Lewis PA, Wing AM, Pope PA, Praamstra P, Maill RC. Brain activity correlates differentially with increasing temporal complexity of rhythms during initialization, synchronisation, and continuation phases of paced finger tapping. *Neuropsychologia* 2004; 42(10):1301–1312.

105. Meister I, Krings T, Foltys H, Boroojerdi B, Muller M, Topper R, Thron A. Effects of long-term practice and task complexity in musicians and nonmusicians performing simple and complex motor tasks: Implications for cortical motor organization. *Human Brain Mapping* 2005; 25(3):345–352.

106. Schubotz RI, von Cramon DY. A blueprint for target motion: fMRI reveals perceived sequential complexity to modulate premotor cortex. *Neuroimage* 2002; 16(4):920–935.

107. Seidler RD, Noll DC, Thiers G. Feedforward and feedback processes in motor control. *Neuroimage* 2004; 22(4):1775–1783.

108. Sergio LE, Kalaska JF. Changes in the temporal pattern of primary motor cortex activity in a directional isometric force versus limb movement task. *J. Neurophysiology* 1998; 80(3):1577–1583.

109. Zhang J, Riehle A, Requin J. Analyzing neuronal processing locus in stimulus-response association tasks. *J. Math Psychol* 1997; 41(3):219–236.

110. Kolb B, Gibb R. Environmental enrichment and cortical injury: Behavioral and anatomical consequences of frontal cortex lesions. *Cerebral Cortex* 1991; 1(2):189–198.

111. Will B, Galani R, Kelche C, Rosenzweig MR. Recovery from brain injury in animals: Relative efficacy of environmental enrichment, physical exercise or formal training (1990–2002). *Progress in Neurobiology* 2004; 72(3):167–182.

112. Isaacs KR, Anderson BJ, Alcantara AA, Black JE, Greenough WT. Exercise and the brain: Angiogenesis in the adult rat cerebellum after vigorous physical activity and motor skill training. *J. Cerebral Blood Flow Metab* 1992; 12(1):110–119.

113. Hutchinson KJ, Gomez-Pinilla F, Crowe JJ, Ying Z, Basso DM. Three exercise paradigms differentially improve sensory recovery after spinal cord contusion in rats. *Brain* 2004; 127(6):1403–1414.

114. Ying Z, Roy RR, Edgerton VR, Gomez-Pinilla F. Exercise restores levels of neurotrophins and synaptic plasticity following spinal cord injury. *Exp Neurol* 2005; 193(2):411–419.

115. Molteni R, Zheng J-Q, Ying Z, Gomez-Pinilla F, Twiss JL. Voluntary exercise increases axonal regeneration from sensory neurons. *Proc Natl Acad Sci U.S.A.* 2004; 101(22):8473–8478.

116. Wang RY, Yang YR, Yu SM. Protective effects of treadmill training on infarction in rats. *Brain Research* 2001; 922(1):140–143.

117. Nudo RJ, Wise BM, SiFuentes F, Milliken GW. Neural substrates for the effects of rehabilitative training on motor recovery after ischemic infarct. *Science* 1996; 272(5269):1791–1794.

118. Kleim JA, Barbay S, Nudo RJ. Functional reorganization of the rat motor cortex following motor skill learning. *J Neurophysiol* 1998; 80(6):3321–3325.

119. Black JE, Isaacs KR, Anderson BJ, Alcantara AA, Greenough WT. Learning causes synaptogenesis, whereas motor activity causes angiogenesis, in cerebellar cortex of adult rats. *Proc Natl Acad Sci U.S.A.* 1990; 87(14):5568–5572.

120. Markham JA, Greenough WT. Experience-driven brain plasticity: Beyond the synapse. *Neuron Glia Biology* 2004; 1(4):351–363.

121. Monfils MH, Plautz EJ, Kleim JA. In search of the motor engram: Motor map plasticity as a mechanism for encoding motor experience. *Neuroscientist* 2005; 11(5):471–483.

122. Sullivan KJ, Brown DA, Klassen T, Mulroy S, Ge T, Azen SP, Winstein CJ, (PTClin-ResNet) PTCRN. Effects of task-specific locomotor and strength training in adults who were ambulatory after stroke: Results of the STEPS randomized clinical trial. *Physical Therapy* 2007; 87(12):1580–1602.

123. Karni A, Meyer G, Jezzard P, Adams MM, Turner R, Ungerleider LG. Functional MRI evidence for adult motor cortex plasticity during motor skill learning. *Nature* 1995; 377(6545):155–158.

124. Pascual-Leon A, Dang M, Cohen LG, Brasil-Neto P, Cammoroto A, Hallett M. Modulation of muscle responses evoked by transcranial magnetic stimulation during the acquisition of new fine motor skills. *J Neurophysiol* 1995; 74:1037–1045.

125. Liepert J, Uhde I, Graf S, Leidner O, Weiller C. Motor cortex plasticity during forced-use therapy in stroke patients: A preliminary study. *Journal of Neurology* 2001; 248(4):315–321.

126. Kopp B, Kunkel A, Muhlnickel W, Villringer K, Taub E, Flor H. Plasticity in the motor system related to therapy-induced improvement of movement after stroke. *Neuroreport* 1999; 10(4):807–810.

127. Liepert J, Bauder H, Wolfgang HR, Miltner WH, Taub E, Weiller C. Treatment-induced cortical reorganization after stroke in humans. *Stroke* 2000; 31(6):1210–1216.

128. Levy CE, Nichols DS, Schmalbrock PM, Keller P, Chakeres DW. Functional MRI evidence of cortical reorganization in upper-limb stroke hemiplegia treated with constraint-induced movement therapy. *Am J Phys Med Rehabil* 2001; 80(1):4–12.

129. Liepert J, Uhde I, Graf S, Leidner O, Weiller C. Motor cortex plasticity during forced-use therapy in stroke patients: A preliminary study. *Journal of Neurology* 2001; 248(4):315–321.

130. Johansen-Berg H, Dawes H, Guy C, Smith SM, Wade DT, Matthews PM. Correlation between motor improvements and altered fMRI activity after rehabilitative therapy. *Brain* 2002; 125(Pt 12):2731–2742.

131. Hamzei F, Liepert J, Dettmers C, Weiller C, Rijntjes M. Two different reorganization patterns after rehabilitative therapy: An exploratory study with fMRI and TMS. *Neuroimage* 2006; 31(2):710–720.

132. Liepert J. Motor cortex excitability in stroke before and after constraint-induced movement therapy. *Cogn Behav Neurol* 2006; 19(1):41–47.

133. Dong Y, Winstein CJ, Albistegui-Dubois R, Dobkin BH. Evolution of fMRI activation in perilesional primary motor cortex and cerebellum with rehabilitation training-related motor gains after stroke: A pilot study. *Neurorehabil Neural Repair* 2007; vol 21(5):412–428.

134. Dobkin BH. Interpreting the randomized clinical trial of constraint-induced movement therapy. *Arch Neurol* 2007; 64(3):336–338.

135. Carey JR, Kimberley TJ, Lewis SM, et al. Analysis of fMRI and finger tracking training in subjects with chronic stroke. *Brain* 2002; 125(Pt 4):773–788.

136. Carey JR, Durfee WK, Bhatt E, Nagpal A, Weinstein SA, Anderson KM, Lewis SM. Comparison of finger tracking versus simple movement training via telerehabilitation to alter hand function and cortical reorganization after stroke. *Neurorehabilitation and Neural Repair* 2007; 21:216–232.

137. Salbach NM, Mayo NE, Wood-Dauphinee S, Hanley JA, Richards CL, Cote R. A task-orientated intervention enhances walking distance and speed in the first year post stroke: A randomized controlled trial. *Clin Rehabil* 2004; 18(5):509–519.

138. Higgins J, Salbach NM, Wood-Dauphinee S, Richards CL, Cote R, Mayo NE. The effect of a task-oriented intervention on arm function in people with stroke: A randomized controlled trial. *Clin Rehabil* 2006; 20(4):296–310.

139. Kwakkel G, Kollen BJ, van der Grond J, Prevo AJ. Probability of regaining dexterity in the flaccid upper limb: Impact of severity of paresis and time since onset in acute stroke. *Stroke* 2003; 34(9):2181–2186.

140. Barreca S, Wolf SL, Fasoli S, Bohannon R. Treatment interventions for the paretic upper limb of stroke survivors: A critical review. *Neurorehabil Neural Repair* 2003; 17(4):220–226.

141. Biernaskie J, Chernenko G, Corbett D. Efficacy of rehabilitative experience declines with time after focal ischemic brain injury. *The Journal of Neuroscience* 2004; 24(5):1245–1254.

142. Nudo RJ. Mechanisms for recovery of motor function following cortical damage. *Current Opinion in Neurobiology* 2006; 16(6):638–644.

143. Risedal A, Zeng J, Johansson BB. Early training may exacerbate brain damage after focal brain ischemia in the rat. *J. Cerebral Blood Flow Metab* 1999; 19:997–1003.

144. Humm JL, Kozlowski DA, James DC, Gotts JE, Schallert T. Use-dependent exacerbation of brain damage occurs during an early post-lesion vulnerable period. *Brain Res* 1998; 783(2):286–292.

145. Kozlowski D, James DC, Schallert T. Use-dependent exaggeration of neuronal injury following unilateral sensorimotor cortex lesions. *J of Neuroscience* 1996; 16:4776–4786.

146. Hsu JE, Jones TA. Time-sensitive enhancement of motor learning with the less-affected forelimb after unilateral sensorimotor cortex lesions in rats. *European J of Neuroscience* 2005; 22:2069–2080.

147. Nelles G. Cortical reorganization-effects of intensive therapy. *Restorative Neurology and Neuroscience* 2004; 22:239–244.

148. Ottenbacher KJ, Jannell S. The results of clinical trials in stroke rehabilitation research. *Archives of Neurology* 1993; 50:37–44.

149. Horn SD, DeJong G, Smout RJ, Gassaway J, James R, Conroy B. Stroke rehabilitation patients, practice, and outcomes: Is earlier and more aggressive therapy better? *Arch Phys Med Rehabil* 2005; 86(12 Suppl 2):S10–S114.

150. Teasell R, Bitensky J, Salter K, Bayona NA. The role of timing and intensity of rehabilitation therapies. *Top Stroke Rehabil* 2005; 12(3):46–57.

151. Rossini PM, Dal Forno G. Neuronal post-stroke plasticity in the adult. *Restorative Neurology and Neuroscience* 2004; 22:193–206.

152. Duncan PW, Lai SM, Keighley J. Defining post-stroke recovery: Implications for design and interpretation of drug trials. *Neuropharmacology* 2000; 39(5):835–841.

153. Duncan PW, Wallace D, Studenski S, Lai SM, Johnson D. Conceptualization of a new stroke-specific outcome measure: The stroke impact scale. *Top Stroke Rehabil* 2001; 8(2):19–33.

154. van der Lee JH. Constraint-induced therapy for stroke: More of the same or something completely different? *Curr Opin Neurol* 2001; 14(6):741–744.

155. Weinrich M, Stuart M, Hoyer T. Rules for rehabilitation: An agenda for research. *Neurorehabil Neural Repair* 2005; 19(2):72–83.

156. Turton A, Pomeroy V. When should upper limb function be trained after stroke? Evidence for and against early intervention. *NeuroRehabilitation* 2002; 17(3):215–224.

157. Paolucci S, Antonucci G, Grasso MG, et al. Early versus delayed inpatient stroke rehabilitation: A matched comparison conducted in Italy. *Arch Phys Med Rehabil* 2000; 81(6):695–700.

158. Hodics T, Cohen LG, Cramer SC. Functional imaging of intervention effects in stroke motor rehabilitation. *Archives of Physical Medicine and Rehabilitation* 2006; 87: S36–S42.

159. Dobkin BH. Clinical practice. Rehabilitation after stroke. *N Engl J Med* 2005; 352(16):1677–1684.

160. Dromerick AW, Lang CE, Powers WJ, et al. Very Early Constraint Induced Movement Therapy (VECTORS): Phase II trial results. *International Stroke Conference*. San Francisco, CA: American Heart Association, 2007.

161. Lang CE, Wagner JM, Edwards DF, Dromerick AW. Upper extremity use in people with hemiparesis in the first few weeks after stroke. *J Neurol Phys Ther* 2007; 31(2):56–63.

162. Duncan PW, Zorowitz R, Bates B, et al. Management of adult stroke rehabilitation care: A clinical practice guideline. *Stroke* 2005; 36(9):e100–143.

163. Kwakkel G, Kollen BJ, Wagenaar RC. Long term effects of intensity of upper and lower limb training after stroke: A randomised trial. *J Neurol Neurosurg Psychiatry* 2002; 72(4):473–479.

164. Kwakkel G, Wagenaar RC, Twisk JW, Lankhorst GJ, Koetsier JC. Intensity of leg and arm training after primary middle-cerebral-artery stroke: A randomised trial. *Lancet* 1999; 354(9174):191–196.

165. Duncan P, Studenski S, Richards L, et al. Randomized clinical trial of therapeutic exercise in subacute stroke. *Stroke* 2003; 34(9):2173–2180.

166. Kleim JA, Jones TA. Principles of experience-dependent neural plasticity: Implications for rehabilitation after brain damage. *J Speech Lang Hear Res* 2008; 51(1): S225–239.

167. Thorndike EL. *Educational Psychology*. New York: Columbia University Press, 1913.

168. Schmidt R, Young DE. Transfer of movement control in motor skill learning. In: SM Cormier JH, ed. *Transfer of Learning*. Orlando, Fl: Academic Press, Inc, 1987:47–79.

169. Tremblay L, Proteau L. Specificity of practice: The case of powerlifting. *Res Q. Exercise Sport* 1998; 69:284–289.

170. Keetch KM, Schmidt RA, Lee TD, Young DE. Especial skills: Their emergence with massive amounts of practice. *J Exp Psychol* 2005; 31(5):970–978.

171. Luft AR, Hanley DF. Stroke recovery—Moving in an EXCITE-ing direction. *JAMA* 2006; 296(17):2141–2143.

172. Wolf SL, Winstein CJ, Miller JP, Blanton S, Clark PC, Nichols-Larsen D. Looking in the rear view mirror when conversing with back seat drivers: The EXCITE trial revisited. *Neurorehabilitation and Neural Repair* 2007; 21(5):379–387.

173. Barker RN, Brauer SG. Upper limb recovery after stroke: The stroke survivors' perspective. *Disabil Rehabil* 2005; 27(20):1213–1223.

174. Barker RN, Gill TJ, Brauer SG. Factors contributing to upper limb recovery after stroke: A survey of stroke survivors in Queensland Australia. *Disability and Rehabilitation* 2007; 29(13):981–989.

175. Lashley KS. The problem of cerebral organization in vision. In: Cattell J, ed. *Visual Mechanisms*. Biological Symposia, volume 7. Lancaster, PA: Jacques Catell Press, 1942.

176. Raibert MH. *Motor Control and Learning by the State-Space Model*. Cambridge: Massachusetts Institute of Technology, 1977.

177. Rijntjes M, Dettmers C, Buchel C, Kiebel S, Frackowiak RS, Weiller C. A blueprint for movement: Functional and anatomical representations in the human motor system. *J Neurosci* 1999; 19(18):8043–8048.

178. Bernstein NA. On dexterity and its development. In: Latash ML, Turvey MT, eds. *Dexterity and Its Development*. Mahwah, NJ: Erlbaum, 1996:3–244.

179. Schmidt RA. A schema theory of discrete motor skill learning. *Psychological Review*, 1975; 82(4):225–260.

180. Schmidt RA. Motor schema theory after 27 years: Reflections and implications for a new theory. *Res Q Exerc Sport* 2003; 74(4):366–375.

181. Allred RP, Maldonado MA, Hsu JE, Jones TA. Training the 'less-affected' forelimb after unilateral cortical infarcts interferes with functional recovery of the impaired forelimb in rats. *Restorative Neurology and Neuroscience* 2005; 23(5-6):297–302.

182. Alaverdashvili M, Foroud A, Lim DH, Whishaw IQ. "Learned baduse" limits recovery of skilled reaching for food after forelimb motor cortex stroke in rats: A new analysis of the effect of gestures on success. *Brain Research* 2008; 188:281–290.

183. Roby-Brami A, Feydy A, Combeaud M, Biryukova EV, Bussel B, Levin MF. Motor compensation and recovery for reaching in stroke patients. *Acta Neurol Scand* 2003; 107(5):369–381.

184. Harvey RL, Winstein CJ. A randomized trial of cortical stimulation, combined with rehabilitation, for arm function following stroke: The Everest clinical trial study design. *Neurorehabilitation and Neural Repair*, in press.

185. Brown JA, Lutsep H, Cramer SC, Weinand M. Motor cortex stimulation for enhancement of recovery after stroke: A case report. *Neurol Research* 2003; 25(8):815–818.

186. Brown JA, Lutsep HL, Weinand M, Cramer SC. Motor cortex stimulation for the enhancement of recovery from stroke: A prospective, multicenter safety study. *Neurosurgery* 2006; 58(3):464–473.

187. Levy R, Ruland S, Weinand M, Lowry D, Dafer R. Cortical stimulation for the rehabilitation of patients with hemiparetic stroke: A multicenter feasibility study of safety and efficacy. *J. Neurosurgery* 2008; 108(4):707–714.

188. Bass-Haugen J, Mathiowetz V, Flinn N. Optimizing motor behavior using the occupational therapy task oriented approach. In: Radomiski MV, Trombly, CA, Latham, CA, eds. *Occupational Therapy for Physical Dysfunction*. 6th ed. Baltimore: Lippincott Williams & Wilkins. 2008.

189. Blanton S, Wolf SL. An application of upper-extremity constraint-induced movement therapy in a patient with subacute stroke. *Phys Ther* 1999; 79(9):847–853.

190. Dettmers C, Teske U, Hamzei F, Uswatte G, Taub E, Weiller C. Distributed form of constraint-induced movement therapy improves functional outcome and quality of life after stroke. *Arch Phys Med Rehabil* 2005; 86(2):204–209.

191. Hakim RM, Kelly SJ, Grant-Beuttler M, Healy B, Krempasky J, Moore S. Case report: A modified constraint-induced therapy (mCIT) program for the upper extremity of a person with chronic stroke. *Physiother Theory Pract* 2005; 21(4):243–256.

192. Kunkel A, Kopp B, Muller G, et al. Constraint-induced movement therapy for motor recovery in chronic stroke patients. *Arch Phys Med Rehabil* 1999; 80(6):624–628.

193. Miltner WH, Bauder H, Sommer M, Dettmers C, Taub E. Effects of constraint-induced movement therapy on patients with chronic motor deficits after stroke: A replication. *Stroke* 1999; 30(3):586–592.

194. Page SJ, Sisto S, Johnston MV, Levine P. Modified constraint-induced therapy after subacute stroke: A preliminary study. *Neurorehabil Neural Repair* 2002; 16(3):290–295.

195. Page SJ, Sisto SA, Levine P. Modified constraint-induced therapy in chronic stroke. *Am J Phys Med Rehabil* 2002; 81(11):870–875.

196. Sabari JS, Kane L, Flanagan SR, Steinberg A. Constraint-induced motor relearning after stroke: A naturalistic case report. *Arch Phys Med Rehabil* 2001; 82(4):524–528.

197. Suputtitada A, Suwanwela NC, Tumvitee S. Effectiveness of constraint-induced movement therapy in chronic stroke patients. *J Med Assoc Thai* 2004; 87(12):1482–1490.

198. Tarkka IM, Pitkanen K, Sivenius J. Paretic hand rehabilitation with constraint-induced movement therapy after stroke. *Am J Phys Med Rehabil* 2005; 84(7):501–505.

199. Taub E, Uswatte G, King DK, Morris D, Crago JE, Chatterjee A. A placebo-controlled trial of constraint-induced movement therapy for upper extremity after stroke. *Stroke* 2006; 37(4):1045–1049.

200. Dromeick AW, Lang CE, Powers WJ, Wagner JM, Sahrmann SA, Videen TO, Birkenmeier R, Hahn MG, Wolf SL, Edwards DF. Very Early Constraint Induced Movement Therapy (VECTORS): Phase II trial results. *AHA International Stroke Meeting*. San Francisco, California, 2007.

201. Rosenbaum DA, Carlson RA, Gilmore RO. Acquisition of intellectual and perceptual-motor skills. *Annu Rev Psychol* 2001; 52:453–470.

202. Platz T. Impairment-oriented training (IOT)—Scientific concept and evidence-based treatment strategies. *Restor Neurol Neurosci* 2004; 22(3–5):301–315.

203. Platz T, van Kaick S, Moller L, Freund S, Winter T, Kim IH. Impairment-oriented training and adaptive motor cortex reorganisation after stroke: A fTMS study. *J Neurol* 2005; vol 82(7):961–968.

204. Platz T, Winter T, Muller N, Pinkowski C, Eickhof C, Mauritz KH. Arm ability training for stroke and traumatic brain injury patients with mild arm paresis: A single-blind, randomized, controlled trial. *Arch Phys Med Rehabil* 2001; 82(7):961–968.

205. Luft AR, McCombe-Waller S, Whitall J, et al. Repetitive bilateral arm training and motor cortex activation in chronic stroke: A randomized controlled trial. *JAMA* 2004; 292(15):1853–1861.

206. Whitall J, McCombe Waller S, Silver KH, Macko RF. Repetitive bilateral arm training with rhythmic auditory cueing improves motor function in chronic hemiparetic stroke. *Stroke* 2000; 31(10):2390–2395.

207. Chan DY, Chan CC, Au DK. Motor relearning programme for stroke patients: A randomized controlled trial. *Clin Rehabil* 2006; 20(3):191–200.

208. Langhammer B, Stanghelle JK. Bobath or motor relearning programme? A comparison of two different approaches of physiotherapy in stroke rehabilitation: A randomized controlled study. *Clin Rehabil* 2000; 14(4):361–369.

209. van Vliet PM, Lincoln NB, Foxall A. Comparison of Bobath based and movement science based treatment for stroke: A randomised controlled trial. *J Neurol Neurosurg Psychiatry* 2005; 76(4):503–508.

210. Kwakkel G, Kollen B, Lindeman E. Understanding the pattern of functional recovery after stroke: Facts and theories. *Restor Neurol Neurosci* 2004; 22(3–5):281–299.

211. Van Peppen RP, Kwakkel G, Wood-Dauphinee S, Hendriks HJ, Van der Wees PJ, Dekker J. The impact of physical therapy on functional outcomes after stroke: What's the evidence? *Clin Rehabil* 2004; 18(8):833–862.

212. Dickstein R, Heffes Y, Laufer Y, Abulaffio N, Shabtai EL. Repetitive practice of a single joint movement for enhancing elbow function in hemiparetic patients. *Percept Mot Skills* 1997; 85(3 Pt 1):771–785.

213. Sunderland A, Tuke A. Neuroplasticity, learning and recovery after stroke: A critical evaluation of constraint-induced therapy. *Neuropsychol Rehabil* 2005; 15(2):81–96.

214. Bandura A. Self-efficacy: Toward a unifying theory of behavioral change. *Psychol Rev* 1977; 84(2):191–215.

215. Bandura A. *Self-Efficacy: The Exercise of Control*. New York: Freeman, 1997.

216. Nudo RJ. Functional and structural plasticity in motor cortex: Implications for stroke recovery. *Phys Med Rehabil Clin N Am* 2003; 14(1 Suppl):S57–76.

217. Patten C, Dozono J, Schmidt SG, Jue ME, Lum PS. Combined functional task practice and dynamic high intensity resistance training promotes recovery of upper-extremity motor function in post-stroke hemiparesis: A case study. *J Neurol Phys Ther* 2006; 30(3):99–115.

218. Zackowski KM, Dromerick AW, Sahrmann SA, Thach WT, Bastian AJ. How do strength, sensation, spasticity and joint individuation relate to the reaching deficits of people with chronic hemiparesis? *Brain* 2004; 127(Pt 5):1035–1046.

219. Taub E, Uswatte G, Elbert T. New treatments in neurorehabilitation founded on basic research. *Nat Rev Neurosci* 2002; 3(3):228–236.

220. Jones F. Strategies to enhance chronic disease self-management: How can we apply this to stroke? *Disabil Rehabil* 2006; 28(13–14):841–847.

221. Kendall E, Catalano T, Kuipers P, Posner N, Buys N, Charker J. Recovery following stroke: The role of self-management education. *Soc Sci Med* 2007; 64(3):735–746.

222. Williams GC, McGregor HA, Sharp D, et al. Testing a self-determination theory intervention for motivating tobacco cessation: Supporting autonomy and competence in a clinical trial. *Health Psychology* 2006; 25(1):91–101.

223. Williams GC, McGregor HA, Zeldman A, Freedman ZR, Deci EL. Testing a self-determination theory process model for promoting glycemic control through diabetes self-management. *Health Psychol* 2004; 23(1):58–66.

224. Hart T, Evans J. Self-regulation and goal theories in brain injury rehabilitation. *J Head Trauma Rehabil* 2006; 21(2):142–155.

225. Siegert RJ, Taylor WJ. Theoretical aspects of goal-setting and motivation in rehabilitation. *Disabil Rehabil* 2004; 26(1):1–8.

226. Nudo RJ, Plautz EJ, Frost SB. Role of adaptive plasticity in recovery of function after damage to motor cortex. *Muscle Nerve* 2001; 24(8):1000–1019.

227. Wu C, Trombly CA, Lin K, Tickle-Degnen L. A kinematic study of contextual effects on reaching performance in persons with and without stroke: Influences of object availability. *Arch Phys Med Rehabil* 2000; 81(1):95–101.

228. Ewart CK, Stewart KJ, Gillilan RE, Kelemen MH. Self-efficacy mediates strength gains during circuit weight training in men with coronary artery disease. *Med Sci Sports Exerc* 1986; 18(5):531–540.

229. Sniehotta FF, Scholz U, Schwarzer R, Fuhrmann B, Kiwus U, Voller H. Long-term effects of two psychological interventions on physical exercise and self-regulation following coronary rehabilitation. *Int J Behav Med* 2005; 12(4):244–255.

230. Taylor CB, Bandura A, Ewart CK, Miller NH, DeBusk RF. Exercise testing to enhance wives' confidence in their husbands' cardiac capability soon after clinically uncomplicated acute myocardial infarction. *Am J Cardiol* 1985; 55(6):635–638.

231. Carey LM, Abbott DF, Egan GF, Bernhardt J, Donnan GA. Motor impairment and recovery in the upper limb after stroke: Behavioral and neuroanatomical correlates. *Stroke* 2005; 36(3):625–629.

232. Feys H, De Weerdt W, Nuyens G, van de Winckel A, Selz B, Kiekens C. Predicting motor recovery of the upper limb after stroke rehabilitation: Value of a clinical examination. *Physiother Res Int* 2000; 5(1):1–18.

233. Fritz SL, Chiu YP, Malcolm MP, Patterson TS, Light KE. Feasibility of electromyography-triggered neuromuscular stimulation as an adjunct to constraint-induced movement therapy. *Phys Ther* 2005; 85(5):428–442.

234. Shelton FD, Volpe BT, Reding M. Motor impairment as a predictor of functional recovery and guide to rehabilitation treatment after stroke. *Neurorehabil Neural Repair* 2001; 15(3):229–237.

235. Butefisch C, Hummelsheim H, Denzler P, Mauritz KH. Repetitive training of isolated movements improves the outcome of motor rehabilitation of the centrally paretic hand. *J Neurol Sci* 1995; 130(1):59–68.

236. Lum PS, Burgar CG, Shor PC, Majmundar M, Van der Loos M. Robot-assisted movement training compared with conventional therapy techniques for the rehabilitation of upper-limb motor function after stroke. *Arch Phys Med Rehabil* 2002; 83(7):952–959.

237. Platz T. [Evidence-based arm rehabilitation—A systematic review of the literature]. *Nervenarzt* 2003; 74(10):841–849.

238. Barreca S, Gowland CK, Stratford P, et al. Development of the Chedoke Arm and Hand Activity Inventory: Theoretical constructs, item generation, and selection. *Top Stroke Rehabil* 2004; 11(4):31–42.

239. McCombe Waller S, Whitall J. Fine motor control in adults with and without chronic hemiparesis: Baseline comparison to nondisabled adults and effects of bilateral arm training. *Arch Phys Med Rehabil* 2004; 85(7):1076–1083.

240. Rose DK, Winstein CJ. Bimanual training after stroke: Are two hands better than one? *Top Stroke Rehabil* 2004; 11(4):20–30.

241. Arnstein P. The mediation of disability by self efficacy in different samples of chronic pain patients. *Disabil Rehabil* 2000; 22(17):794–801.

242. Bandura A. Health promotion by social cognitive means. *Health Educ Behav* 2004; 31(2):143–164.

243. Bodenheimer T, Lorig K, Holman H, Grumbach K. Patient self-management of chronic disease in primary care. *JAMA* 2002; 288(19):2469–2475.

244. Brody BL, Roch-Levecq AC, Gamst AC, Maclean K, Kaplan RM, Brown SI. Self-management of age-related macular degeneration and quality of life: A randomized controlled trial. *Arch Ophthalmol* 2002; 120(11):1477–1483.

245. Garg S, Johnston-Brooks CH, Lewis MA. Self-efficacy impacts self-care and HbA1c in young adults with Type I diabetes. *Psychosom Med* 2002; 64:43–51.

246. Hellstrom K, Lindmark B, Wahlberg B, Fugl-Meyer AR. Self-efficacy in relation to impairments and activities of daily living disability in elderly patients with stroke: A prospective investigation. *J Rehabil Med* 2003; 35(5):202–207.

247. Kohler CL, Fish L, Greene PG. The relationship of perceived self-efficacy to quality of life in chronic obstructive pulmonary disease. *Health Psychol* 2002; 21(6):610–614.

248. Rejeski WJ, Miller ME, Foy C, Messier S, Rapp S. Self-efficacy and the progression of functional limitations and self-reported disability in older adults with knee pain. *J Gerontol B Psychol Sci Soc Sci* 2001; 56(5):S261–265.

249. Robinson-Smith G, Johnston MV, Allen J. Self-care self-efficacy, quality of life, and depression after stroke. *Arch Phys Med Rehabil* 2000; 81(4):460–464.

250. Sharma L, Cahue S, Song J, Hayes K, Pai YC, Dunlop D. Physical functioning over three years in knee osteoarthritis: Role of psychosocial, local mechanical, and neuromuscular factors. *Arthritis Rheum* 2003; 48(12):3359–3370.

251. Institute of Medicine. *Crossing the Quality Chasm: A New Health Care System for the 21st Century*. Washington, D.C.: National Academy Press, 2001.

252. Guadagnoli E, Ward P. Patient participation in decision-making. *Soc Sci Med* 1998; 47(3):329–339.

253. Greenfield S, Kaplan S, Ware JE, Jr. Expanding patient involvement in care. Effects on patient outcomes. *Ann Intern Med* 1985; 102(4):520–528.

254. Greenfield S, Kaplan S, Ware JE, Jr. Expanding patient involvement in care. Effects on patient outcomes. *Ann Intern Med* 1985; 102(4):520–528.

255. Norris SL, Engelgau MM, Narayan KM. Effectiveness of self-management training in type 2 diabetes: A systematic review of randomized controlled trials. *Diabetes Care* 2001; 24(3):561–587.

256. Thompson CE, Wankel LM. The effects of perceived activity choice upon frequency of exercise behavior. *J Appl Soc Psychol* 1980; 10(5):436–443.

257. Williams GC, McGregor H, Zeldman A, Freedman ZR, Deci EL, Elder D. Promoting glycemic control through diabetes self-management: Evaluating a patient activation intervention. *Patient Educ Couns* 2005; 56(1):28–34.

258. Ezekiel HJ, Lehto NK, Marley TL, Wishart LR, Lee TD. Application of motor learning principles: The physiotherapy client as a problem-solver. III: Augmented feedback. *Physiother Can* 2001; 53(1):33–39.

259. Wulf G. Self-controlled practice enhances motor learning: Implications for physical therapy. *Physiotherapy* 2007; 93:96–101.

260. Miller WR, Rollnick S. *Motivational Interviewing: Preparing People for Change*. 2nd ed. New York: Guilford Press, 2002.

261. Carswell A, McColl MA, Baptiste S, Law M, Polatajko H, Pollock N. The Canadian Occupational Performance Measure: A research and clinical literature review. *Can J Occup Ther* 2004; 71(4):210–222.

262. Stuifbergen AK, Becker H, Timmerman GM, Kullberg V. The use of individualized goal setting to facilitate behavior change in women with multiple sclerosis. *J Neurosci Nurs* 2003; 35(2):94–99, 106.

263. Han CE, Arbib MA, Schweighofer N. Stroke rehabilitation reaches a threshold. *PLOS Computational Biology*, in press.

264. Stinear CM, Barber A, Smale PR, Coxon JP, Fleming MK, Byblow WD. Functional potential in chronic stroke patients depends on corticospinal tract integrity. *Brain* 2007; 130:130–180.

265. Mark VW, Taub E, Perkins C, Gauthier LV, Uswatte G, Ogorek J. Poststroke cerebral peduncular atrophy correlates with a measure of corticospinal tract injury in the cerebral hemisphere. *Am J Neuroradiology* 2008; 29:354–358.

266. Mataric MJ, Eriksson J, Feil-Seifer DJ, Winstein CJ. Socially assistive robotics for post-stroke rehabilitation. *J. Neuroengineering and Rehabilitation* 2007; 19(4:5).

267. Nadeau SE, Wu SS. CIMT as a behavioral engine in research on physiological adjuvants to neurorehabilitation: The challenge of merging animal and human research. *Neuro-Rehabilitation* 2006; 21(2):107–130.

268. Choi YG, Gordon J, Schweighofer N. ADAPT—Adaptive automated robotic task practice system for stroke rehabilitation. *IEEE International Conference on Robotics and Automation (ICRA)*. Pasadena, CA, USA 2008.

269. Fadiga L, Fogassi L, Pavesi G, Rizzolatti G. Motor facilitation during action observation: A magnetic stimulation study. *J. Neurophysiology* 1995; 73(6):2608–2611.

270. Avenanti A, Bolognini N, Maravita A, Aglioti SM. Somatic and motor components of action simulation. *Curr Biol* 2007; 17(24):2129–3135.

271. Heiser M, Iacoboni M, Maeda F, Marcus J, Mazziotta JC. The essential role of Broca's area in imitation. *European J of Neuroscience* 2003; 17(5):1123–1128.

272. Dinstein I, Thomas C, Behrmann M, Heeger DJ. A mirror up to nature. . *Curr Biol* 2008; 18(1):R13–18.

273. Pomeroy VM, Clark CA, Miller JSG, Baron J-C, Markus HS, Tallis RC. The potential for utilizing the "mirror neuron system" to enhance recovery of the severely affected upper limb early after stroke: A review and hypothesis. *Neurorehabilitation Neural Repair* 2005; 19(1):4–13.

274. Ertelt D, Small S, Solodkin A, Dettmers C, McNamara A, Binkokski F, et al. Action observation has a positive impact on rehabilitation of motor deficits after stroke. *Neuroimage* 2007; 36(Suppl 2):T164–173.

275. Wulf G. Self-controlled practice enhances motor learning: Implications for physical therapy. *Physiotherapy* 2007; 93:96–101.

276. McNevin NH, Wulf G, Carlson C. Effects of attentional focus, self-control, and dyad training on motor learning: Implications for physical rehabilitation. *Phys Ther* 2000; 80(4):373–385.

277. Wulf G, Hob M, Prinz W. Instructions for motor learning: Differential effects of internal versus external focus of attention. *Journal of Motor Behavior* 1998; 30(2):169–179.

278. Wulf G, McNevin NH, Fuchs T, Ritter F, Toole T. Attentional focus in complex skill learning. *Res Q Exerc Sport* 2000; 71(3):229–239.

279. Fasoli SE, Trombly CA, Tickle-Degnen L, Verfaellie MH. Effect of instructions on functional reach in persons with and without cerebrovascular accident. *Am J Occup Ther* 2002; 56(4):380–390.

280. Ochsner KN. Current directions in social cognitive neuroscience. *Curr Opin Neurobiol* 2004; 14(2):254–258.

18 Neuromuscular Electrical Stimulation for Motor Restoration in Hemiplegia

John Chae
Lynne R. Sheffler

This chapter provides a comprehensive review of the clinical uses of neuromuscular electrical stimulation (NMES) in stroke rehabilitation. NMES refers to the electrical stimulation of an intact lower motor neuron (LMN) to cause contraction of paralyzed or paretic muscles. Clinical applications of NMES provide either therapeutic or functional benefit. In therapeutic applications, NMES may lead to a specific effect that enhances function, but it does not directly provide function. An example of therapeutic effect of NMES is motor relearning, defined as "the recovery of previously learned motor skills that have been lost following localized damage to the central nervous system" (1). Functional electrical stimulation (FES) refers to the use of NMES to directly accomplish functional tasks (2). Functional tasks may include standing, ambulation, or activities of daily living (ADL). Devices that provide FES are also referred to as neuroprostheses.

In order to provide a foundation for the various clinical applications, the neurophysiology of NMES and components of NMES systems are briefly reviewed. Specific therapeutic applications include post-stroke motor relearning and reduction of hemiplegic shoulder pain. Specific neuroprosthetic, or functional, applications include upper and lower limb motor movement for ADL and mobility, respectively. Perspectives on future developments and clinical applications of NMES are also presented.

NEUROPHYSIOLOGY OF NMES

NMES is initiated with the excitation of peripheral nervous tissue. The term stimulus threshold defines the lowest level of electrical charge that generates an action potential. The all-or-none phenomenon of the action potential produced by natural physiologic means is identical to the action potential induced by NMES. Nerve fiber recruitment and resultant force characteristics of muscle contraction are modulated by both stimulus pulse width (3) and stimulus frequency (4). Other variables include distance from the stimulating electrode and membrane capacitance. Direct muscle stimulation is possible, but it requires significantly greater current than nerve stimulation (5). Thus, clinical NMES systems stimulate either the nerve directly or the motor point of the nerve proximal to the neuromuscular junction.

The nerve fiber recruitment properties elicited by NMES differ from those elicited by normal physiologic means. An action potential produced by normal physiologic mechanisms initially recruits the smallest diameter neurons prior to recruitment of larger diameter fibers, such as alpha motor neurons. However, the nerve fiber recruitment pattern mediated by NMES follows the principle of reverse recruitment order, wherein the nerve stimulus threshold is inversely proportional to the diameter of the neuron. Thus, large diameter nerve fibers, which innervate larger motor units, are recruited preferentially. Recent work by Lertmanorat proposed the clinical applicability of a reshaping of the extracellular voltage, which may allow the reversal of the reverse recruitment order elicited by NMES (6).

NMES is delivered as a waveform of electrical current characterized by stimulus frequency, amplitude, and pulse width. The minimum stimulus frequency that generates a fused muscle response is approximately 12 Hz. Higher stimulus frequencies generate higher forces, but they also result in rapid fatigue. An optimal NMES system utilizes the minimal stimulus frequency, which produces a fused response. Ideal stimulation frequencies range from 12–16 Hz for upper limb applications and 18–25 Hz for lower limb applications. Greater muscle force generation is accomplished by either increasing the pulse duration or the stimulus amplitude to activate neurons at a greater distance from the activating electrode. Parameters for safe stimulation for implanted NMES systems have been experimentally established (5).

Skeletal muscle contains fast and slow muscle fibers, which are distinguished on the basis of contraction kinetics. Slow-twitch, oxidative Type I fibers generate lower forces, but they are fatigue-resistant. Fast-twitch, glycolytic Type II fibers generate higher forces, but they fatigue more rapidly (7). Disuse muscle atrophy common in an UMN injury is characterized by conversion of type I muscle fibers to type II fibers (8). An ideal application of NMES allows preferential stimulation of fatigue-resistant type I fibers. However, NMES systems preferentially recruit type II fibers because of lower stimulation thresholds. Chronic electrical stimulation at a frequency of 10–12 Hz facilitates reversal of fiber type conversion secondary to motor unit plasticity (9). This reversal of fiber type conversion may be related to the motor neuron firing patterns that control expression of contractile proteins and metabolic enzymes in muscle fibers during electrostimulation (10).

SYSTEM COMPONENTS

Most clinically available NMES systems fall into two broad categories: transcutaneous (surface) and implanted (percutaneous, epimysial, epineural, intraneural, and cuff) systems. NMES systems are either voltage- or current-regulated. Despite the variable motor response, voltage-regulated stimulation is more common with transcutaneous NMES systems. As impedance (resistance) increases because of electrode-skin interface issues, current is decreased (Ohm's law:

V (voltage) = I (current) × R (resistance)). Current density as opposed to absolute voltage determines the potential for tissue injury. Because of less variability in resistance and the need for muscle contraction consistency and repeatability, constant current applications are more common in implanted NMES systems.

The simplest electrode is the transcutaneous electrode, which is applied to the skin and stimulates directly over the peripheral nerve or motor point. The motor point is the muscle location that exhibits the most robust contraction at the lowest level of stimulation. Transcutaneous electrodes pose a risk of tissue injury, particularly in patients with concomitant sensory and/or cognitive deficits. Activation of cutaneous pain receptors, difficulties in positioning, poor selectivity, insecure fixation on moving limbs, skin irritation, and cosmesis are common limitations of transcutaneous electrodes. While a constant voltage transcutaneous NMES system minimizes the risk of high current densities associated with tissue-electrode interface fluctuations, variability in muscle stimulation and inconsistent functional response can result. Transcutaneous electrodes are more commonly used for therapeutic applications (11).

The minimally invasive percutaneous intramuscular electrode reduces the risk of tissue injury (12). However, it poses other safety concerns, including the risk of displacement or breakage associated with anchoring of the external lead, electrode-related infection, and granuloma formation secondary to retained electrode fragments (13). All percutaneous electrodes connect to lead wires that exit the skin and connect to the stimulator. The advantages of the percutaneous electrode are the elimination of skin resistance and cutaneous pain issues, greater muscle selectivity, and lower stimulation currents. Percutaneous electrodes are particularly usefully in activating small, deep muscle such as the intrinsic muscles of the hand. In general, they should be limited to short-term applications in the order of four to eight weeks.

Surgically implanted electrodes designed for long-term use include epimysial, epineural, intraneural, and helix (cuff) electrodes. These electrodes all require open surgical procedures, connection to implanted lead wires, and the implantation of a stimulator that receives power and command instructions through a radio-frequency (RF) telemetry link to an external control unit (ECU). Epimysial electrodes are sutured directly to the epimysium or fascia of the target muscle (14). Epineural electrodes are sutured to connective tissue directly surrounding the nerve (15). Intraneural electrodes that penetrate to the intrafascicular bundles are presently limited to research applications (16). Direct nerve stimulation is most commonly achieved via a nerve cuff electrode, which, by encompassing the nerve trunk, requires approximately one-tenth of the current necessary for intramuscular stimulation (17).

For neuroprostheses, there is the added requirement of volitional control to carry out specific functional tasks. FES control system design presents a significant challenge to correlate user intent to functional performance. Most clinical FES systems employ open-loop control with sensory feedback limited to residual visual and proprioceptive input. A closed-loop control system allows for continuous real-time modification of the stimulation pattern based on sensory feedback. Given the nonlinear and temporal variability of contractile muscle forces, a closed-loop system modulated by sensor-derived feedback signals offers clear advantage (18, 19). An optimal FES control system allows for consistent and predictable response to external perturbations, including changing muscle loads and internal time variations such as fatigue.

A special case of an electrode/stimulator system that does not fit well into the traditional classification scheme is the injectable microstimulator (20). The 2–3 cm long device functions as stimulator, electrode, and receiver. Each is individually addressable and injected into the target muscle or soft tissue contiguous to a specific nerve or a motor via a minimally invasive procedure. The first-generation device was glass-encased with an external tantalum capacitor electrode. A second-generation device may be more durable and less susceptible to mechanical and electrostatic trauma (21). The device receives power and digital command data via a single external RF. A battery-powered microstimulator is presently under development.

MOTOR RELEARNING

Basic Science and Theoretical Considerations

Following experimental and clinical brain injury, goal-oriented, active repetitive movement training of a paretic limb enhances motor relearning. Asanuma and Keller demonstrated that electrical stimulation of the somatosensory cortex—alone or in conjunction with thalamic stimulation in an animal model—induces long-term potentiations (LTP) in the motor cortex (22). They hypothesized that repetitive movement-associated, proprioceptive, and cutaneous afferent impulses induce LTP in the motor cortex, modify the excitability of specific motor neurons, and thereby facilitate motor relearning (23). Nonhuman primate research demonstrated findings consistent with this hypothesis. After local damage to the motor cortex, goal-oriented, active repetitive movement training of the paretic limb shaped subsequent functional reorganization in the adjacent, intact cortex, and the undamaged motor cortex played an important role in motor relearning. Specific types of behavioral experiences that induce long-term plasticity in motor maps were repetitive movements that entail the development of motor skills. That is, the

motor tasks were new and therefore required significant cognitive effort to learn and complete. Training to acquire new skills, such as retrieving food pellets from a small or rotating well, were associated with task-specific cortical reorganization. However, this was not the case with repetitive movement tasks that did not require new skill acquisition, that is, motor tasks are already mastered and are therefore easy to carry out and require minimal to no cognitive effort (24, 25).

If goal-oriented, repetitive movement therapy facilitates motor relearning, electrical stimulation-mediated, goal-oriented repetitive movement therapy may also facilitate motor relearning. There is evidence that electrical stimulation of the peripheral nerve is associated with concomitant physiologic changes in the brain. Electrical stimulation to a peripheral nerve was associated with activation of both sensory and motor structures in the brain as well as reduction of intracortical inhibition (26, 27). fMRI studies showed activation of the contralateral somatosensory cortex and bilateral supplementary motor areas in response to NMES-mediated wrist extension activity (28). Another fMRI study showed a dose-response relationship between fMRI images and NMES of the lower limb muscles (29). These data suggest that repetitive movement therapy mediated by NMES has the potential to facilitate motor relearning via cortical mechanisms.

NMES can be used by stroke survivors with hemiparesis who do not have sufficient residual movement to take part in volitional, active repetitive movement therapy. Regardless of cortical or spinal mechanisms, the experimental and theoretical considerations suggest that the necessary prerequisites for NMES-mediated motor relearning include repetition, novelty of activity, concurrent volitional effort, and high functional content.

Three forms of NMES are available for motor relearning: cyclic NMES, EMG/biofeedback mediated NMES, and neuroprostheses. Cyclic NMES contracts paretic muscles at a set duty cycle for a preset time period without any input from the patient beyond turning the device on and off. The patient is a passive participant and does not require cognitive investment in the form of either initiation of muscle contraction, interpretation of afferent signals, or functionality of motor task. EMG- or biofeedback-mediated NMES couples afferent feedback to NMES-induced repetitive movement therapy. These techniques may be applied to patients who can partially activate a paretic muscle based on the presence of EMG activity or change in joint position, but they are unable to generate sufficient muscle contraction for adequate exercise or functional purposes. While the patients using cyclic NMES are passive participants, EMG- or biofeedback-mediated NMES requires greater cognitive investment, which may result in greater therapeutic benefit. The third type of NMES includes neuroprosthetic applications, which provide FES for completion of ADLs and mobility tasks. Because repetitive movement training is performed in the context of meaningful, functional behavioral tasks, neuroprostheses have a theoretical advantage over both cyclic and EMG/biofeedback-mediated NMES for motor relearning. Neuroprosthesis applications are discussed in greater detail in a later section.

Upper Limb Applications

Several randomized clinical trials evaluated the efficacy of cyclic NMES in enhancing upper limb motor relearning (30–34). In general, studies demonstrated improved outcomes in motor impairment at end of treatment with mild to moderately impaired subjects benefiting most. Enduring effects were seen among acute stroke survivors, but not for chronic stroke survivors (30, 31). All studies evaluated activity limitation, but only half demonstrated short-term positive effects (31, 34).

In the most methodologically sound study to date, Powell and associates reported significantly higher isometric wrist extension torques for the treatment group at the end of treatment and at 32 weeks relative to controls (31). The grasp and grip subscores of the Action Research Arm Test were significantly higher for the treatment group at the end of treatment, but not at 32 weeks. A post-hoc subset analysis indicated that the intervention is most effective for those with residual wrist extension torque at study entry.

The strengths of these studies rest on their randomized designs. However, numerous methodological limitations render the results difficult to interpret, including inadequate blinding, unequal treatment intensity, inconsistent follow-up beyond end of treatment, inadequate accounting of dropouts, and failure to use intent-to-treat analysis. Nevertheless, even with the methodological limitations, these randomized trials do suggest that cyclic NMES enhances the upper limb motor relearning of stroke survivors. The effect may be more clinically relevant for acute stroke survivors and for those with milder baseline impairments. However, the effect of cyclic NMES on activity limitations remains uncertain.

Several clinical trials evaluated EMG biofeedback, position, or EMG-triggered NMES for upper limb motor relearning (35–40). In general, these studies demonstrated improved outcomes in motor impairment at end of treatment. In the few studies that evaluated activity limitations, improved outcomes were noted (38, 39). There was also evidence of central mechanisms using neurophysiologic assays, such as reaction time and fMRI (36, 37, 39).

In the most recent of these studies, Kimberly and associates carried out a double-blinded, randomized clinical trial among 16 chronic stroke survivors (39).

Over a three-week period, the treatment group received 60 hours of NMES therapy applied to the extensor muscles of the hemiplegic forearm to facilitate hand opening. The control group received sham treatment, but participants were asked to extend the finger in a repetitive manner. The EMG-triggered NMES group demonstrated significant improvements in measures of grasp and release of objects (Box and Block Test and Jebsen Taylor Hand Function), isometric finger extension strength, and self-rated activity limitation (Motor Activity Log). In addition, using fMRI and a finger-tracking task, an index of cortical intensity in the ipsilateral somatosensory cortex (relative to hemiparetic limb) increased significantly from pretest to posttest following treatment. The participants receiving sham treatments failed to improve on any of the outcome measures except isometric finger extension strength.

As with the cyclic NMES studies, numerous methodological deficiencies limit the interpretation of results, including inadequate blinding, paucity of follow-up data, inability to assess equality between treatment groups, and small sample sizes. Nevertheless, data suggests that EMG- and biofeedback-mediated NMES reduces upper limb motor impairment and these changes, to at least some degree, translate into improvements in activity limitations.

Finally, hand neuroprostheses may facilitate motor relearning. Studies evaluating hand neuroprostheses for persons with hemiplegia are reviewed later in this chapter. In the two earliest studies of hand neuroprostheses for hemiplegia, the primary objective was to demonstrate improvement in ADL function, not motor relearning (41, 42). However, both studies parenthetically reported evidence of improved motor ability when the device was turned off after a period of use. More recent studies evaluated neuroprostheses to specifically demonstrate a motor relearning effect. Alon and associates evaluated a hybrid brace-NMES device that incorporates transcutaneous electrodes into a brace for hand grasp and release (Figure 18-1) (43). The device was originally developed for the spinal cord injury (SCI) tetraplegia population (44). The authors reported significant improvements in motor impairment and activity limitations relative to baseline after five weeks of training. A controlled trial using the same device corroborated these findings (45). In another controlled trial, Popovic and associates demonstrated that performing intensive exercises with the assistance of a neuroprosthesis results in significant improvement in upper limb motor function among acute stroke survivors (46).

Overall, the literature suggests that NMES is effective in reducing motor impairment. However, the effect on upper limb-related activities limitation remains unknown. This is consistent with the results of a systematic review of randomized clinical trials of

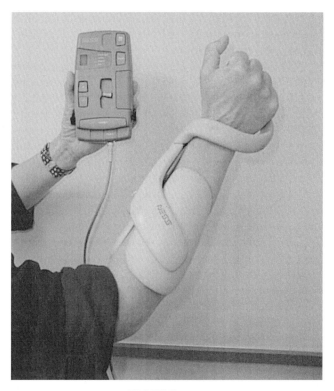

FIGURE 18-1

A hybrid brace-transcutaneous neuroprosthesis system that is worn on the hand and forearm. The exoskeleton positions the wrist in a functional position, and the five transcutaneous electrodes built into the exoskeleton stimulates specific muscles to provide coordinated hand opening and closing. (NESS H200, courtesy, Bioness Inc., Santa Clarita, CA.)

NMES interventions for motor relearning. The authors concluded that the literature:

> ...suggests a positive effect of electrical stimulation on motor control. [However] No conclusion can be drawn with regard to the effect on functional ability [activity]. (47)

The authors further concluded that the effect appears to be more significant for those with milder impairments.

Lower Limb Applications

Lieberson and associates described the first single-channel transcutaneous peroneal nerve stimulator to provide ankle dorsiflexion during the swing phase of gait for stroke survivors However, they also commented:

> On several occasions we observed, after training with the electrophysiologic brace [peroneal nerve stimulator]...patients acquire the ability of dorsiflexing the foot by themselves. (48)

Subsequent case series using implanted and transcutaneous systems described similar observations of improved ambulation function, more normal EMG muscle activation patterns, emergence of EMG signals in previously silent muscles, increased strength of EMG activity, and decreased co-contraction of antagonist muscles (49–55).

Controlled studies using single- or dual-channel transcutaneous cyclic NMES corroborated these findings. NMES combined with biofeedback was associated with improved knee and ankle joint angles, ambulation velocity, symmetry in stance, and knee extension torque (56, 57). Cyclical NMES alone also improved the strength of paretic ankle dorsiflexors (58, 59). In a recent double-blind, randomized clinical trial, Yan and associates reported that cyclic NMES reduces spasticity, strengthens ankle dorsiflexors, improves mobility, and increases home discharge rate after acute inpatient stroke rehabilitation (60).

Because gait deviation in hemiplegia is not limited to ankle dysfunction, several studies evaluated multichannel transcutaneous stimulation systems, such as a neuroprosthesis. Two case series demonstrated improvements in qualitative and quantitative measures of gait after training with a six-channel transcutaneous neuroprosthesis system (61, 62). The devices provided ankle dorsiflexion, knee flexion and extension, and hip extension. A follow-up controlled trial demonstrated significantly greater improvement in gait performance and motor function among participants treated with the neuroprosthesis, compared to those treated with conventional therapy (63).

As the number of electrodes increase, transcutaneous systems are difficult to implement and maintain clinically. The practicality of multichannel transcutaneous lower limb systems is further limited by reduced muscle selectivity, poor reliability of stimulation, and pain of sensory stimulation. Accordingly, Daly and associates developed and implemented a multichannel percutaneous system to facilitate lower limb motor relearning and mobility (64). A single-blinded, randomized clinical trial demonstrated that percutaneous NMES mediated ambulation training improves gait components and knee flexion coordination relative to controls (65).

As with upper limb applications, controlled studies of NMES for lower limb motor relearning exhibit significant methodological limitations. Specific limitations include inadequate blinding in most studies, small sample sizes, limited follow-up data, and outcomes limited to impairment measures only. Nevertheless, the preponderance of evidence suggests that NMES in the form of cyclic stimulation, neuroprostheses, or in combination with biofeedback is effective in facilitating lower limb motor relearning. A recent meta-analysis concluded that "FES is effective at improving gait speed in subjects post-stroke" (66). However, it was unclear whether NMES improved overall mobility function.

Summary, Clinical Considerations, and Future Directions

Despite the numerous methodological limitations of controlled trials to date, the weight of the scientific evidence suggests that NMES-mediated repetitive movement therapy reduces motor impairment in upper and lower limb hemiplegia. There is some evidence that the effect is more robust and enduring among acute stroke survivors relative to chronic stroke survivors. However, it remains uncertain whether the effect translates into clinically relevant improvements in ADLs and mobility for upper and lower limb applications, respectively. Although there are theoretical basis for expecting that EMG- or biofeedback-mediated NMES is more effective than cyclic NMES, to date, there are no direct comparison studies demonstrating the superiority of one over the other (67). At present, there are inadequate numbers of controlled trials to conclude that neuroprostheses facilitate motor relearning. However, because of its high functional content, neuroprostheses may ultimately prove to be the most effective NMES approach for facilitating motor relearning. Finally, the optimal dose and stimulation parameters remain to be elucidated.

A number of single- and dual-channel transcutaneous NMES devices are now commercially available for clinical implementation. However, in view of the methodological limitations of published controlled trials and the uncertain effect on ADLs and mobility, it is not possible to offer definitive clinical recommendations. Nevertheless, because the effect on motor impairment is consistent throughout the various studies and the NMES does not appear to be harmful, a select group of stroke survivors may benefit from NMES therapy. At this time, there are limited motor relearning options for those with severe upper limb motor impairments. Therefore, acute stroke survivors with no volitional finger extension may be offered cyclic NMES of the finger extensor (31, 68). If there is evidence of volitionally activated muscle contraction or EMG activation, EMG-triggered NMES should be considered (38, 69). For those with good proximal control but minimal distal movement, the hybrid orthosis- NMES system may be offered (43, 70). With the emergence of additional volitional movement, other motor relearning strategies, such as constraint-induced therapy, may be implemented (71). Similarly, acute stroke survivors with no volitional ankle dorsiflexion may benefit from cyclic peroneal nerve stimulation (59, 60). EMG-triggered NMES may be applied to those with evidence of volitional activation (72). If the stroke survivor has some ability to ambulate, gait training with a peroneal nerve stimulator may facilitate lower limb motor relearning (73, 74). Similar principles could be applied to proximal muscles and multiple muscles. However, at this time,

multichannel transcutaneous and percutaneous lower limb NMES systems are not as clinically accessible and are limited to research applications.

Optimal timing of treatment has not been determined. Nevertheless, because therapeutic benefit may be related to acuity, onset of treatment in the acute rehabilitation service should be considered. Patients and family should be trained by an experienced therapist, and treatment should be continued and completed in the home environment. Optimal dosing and duration have not been determined. However, based on studies reporting positive results, patients should be treated for at least one hour a day for a minimum of three weeks. Two hours of treatment per day for eight weeks is recommended.

Care must be taken to implement NMES in the context of the stroke survivors' clinical status. Many stroke survivors have concomitant cardiac conditions. Cardiac status should be clinically monitored during ambulation training with NMES. Many stroke survivors also have cardiac pacemakers. NMES should not be used with patients with demand-type pacemakers. The effects of NMES on fetal development and health are not known. Therefore, the application of NMES during pregnancy should also be avoided. At this time, there is no evidence that NMES causes seizures. Nevertheless, NMES should be used with caution with stroke survivors with poorly controlled seizures. Finally, the clinician should maintain surveillance for electrical burns, especially with stroke survivors with sensory and cognitive impairments. A more complete discussion of safety issues and contraindications can be found elsewhere (75).

Future investigations on NMES for motor relearning should address issues on two fronts. First, the effect of NMES on motor relearning and impact on clinical outcomes should be confirmed by addressing the methodological limitations of prior studies. Future studies should be large, multicenter, randomized clinical trials, which should be at least single-blinded. Future studies should carefully define the subject populations, identify potential confounds, and evaluate long-term outcomes using valid and reliable measures of motor impairment, energy consumption, activity limitations, and quality of life. These trials should directly compare the various types of NMES, such as EMG-triggered NMES, cyclic NMES, and neuroprostheses, to identify the most effective paradigm and the populations that will likely benefit from each approach. The second front for future investigations is refinement of stimulation technique to maximize patient compliance and clinical outcomes. Studies should determine the optimal dose and prescriptive parameters. Systems that increase cognitive investment by requiring initiation, maintenance, and termination of NMES, such as an EMG-controlled NMES system (76) should be considered. Future studies should also investigate more natural proxies for cognitive intent, such as cortical control (77). Neuroprostheses that provide clear, functional benefit to a broad range of stroke survivors should be developed in order to provide goal-oriented, repetitive movement therapy in the context of functional and meaningful tasks. Finally, basic studies should further investigate mechanisms in order to optimize the treatment paradigm.

POST-STROKE SHOULDER PAIN

Theoretical Considerations

Shoulder pain is a common complication following stroke (78). Postulated causes include adhesive capsulitis, impingement syndrome, complex regional pain syndrome, brachial plexopathy, spasticity, and subluxation (79). Figure 18-2 shows a theoretical framework describing the genesis and maintenance of post-stroke shoulder pain. The framework postulates that the initial spasticity and weakness lead to mechanical instability and immobility of the glenohumeral joint. These conditions cause pain directly or place the capsule and extracapsular soft tissue at risk for micro- and macrotrauma, subsequently leading to inflammation, immobility, and pain. In view of the importance of repetitive and functional use of the limb for motor recovery, as reviewed earlier, the immobility exacerbates the state of the already paretic muscles (heavy, dashed line in Figure 18-2). The cycle repeats with worsening of the condition. Numerous treatment approaches have been reported, but with limited success (80). However, transcutaneous and intramuscular NMES of the supraspinatus, trapezius, and deltoid muscles to reduce subluxation and improve biomechanical integrity may be an effective strategy for reducing post-stroke shoulder pain.

Transcutaneous Systems

To date, nine controlled clinical trials evaluated the effectiveness of transcutaneous NMES for the treatment of hemiplegic shoulder pain (81–89). Note that the two publications by Wang and associates included separate trials for acute and chronic stroke survivors and the two studies reported different outcomes from the same study (88, 89). The majority of these studies evaluated NMES as a treatment modality (81–83, 85, 86, 88, 89). One evaluated prevention, and another evaluated a combination of treatment and prevention (84, 87). Approximately half of the studies evaluated acute stroke survivors (82–84, 87–89). The other half evaluated combination of acute and chronic stroke survivors or chronic stroke survivors only (81, 85, 86, 88, 89).

Radiographic glenohumeral subluxation was the most consistently evaluated outcome measure. Seven of eight studies that evaluated radiographic inferior glenohumeral subluxation reported improvements (81–83, 87–89). However, the effect at end of treatment was significant only for acute stroke survivors (81–84, 87, 88). Among these, only two reported sustained effect beyond end of treatment (82, 84).

Six of nine studies evaluated pain-free passive lateral rotation range of motion (ROM) (82, 84, 86, 87, 89). One study reported significant and sustained improvements in the treatment group compared to controls (82). Two studies reported improvements based on within group analysis (84, 86). That is, the studies lacked sufficient power to demonstrate differences between groups. Three studies reported no significant effect.

Six of nine studies evaluated motor impairment (82–84, 87, 89). Two acute studies reported improvements at end of treatment and at follow-up (82, 89). One

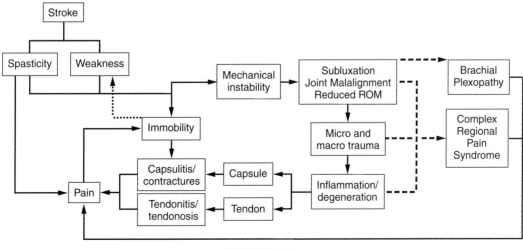

FIGURE 18-2

Theoretical framework describing the genesis and maintenance of hemiplegic shoulder pain.

acute study demonstrated improvement at end of treatment, but not at follow-up (84). Three studies (two acute and one chronic) reported no improvements in motor impairment (83, 87, 89).

As with NMES for motor relearning, numerous methodological limitations make these results difficult to interpret. Limitations include uncertain generalizability, small sample sizes (with concomitant limited power), inadequate or no blinding of outcomes, assessment, and limited, long-term follow-up.

The problem of small sample sizes and insufficient power may be addressed via meta-analyses. Two meta-analyses of the efficacy of NMES for the treatment of hemiplegic shoulder pain have been reported. A Cochrane review concluded that NMES improves pain-free passive ROM and reduces subluxation, but it does not improve motor impairment (90). Ada and Foongchomechey concluded that NMES reduces or prevents subluxation and improves motor impairment in the acute population, but not in the chronic population (91). The differences in the conclusion between the two meta-analyses are likely caused by the differences in inclusion criteria used to accept specific studies.

The individual clinical trials in conjunction with the results of the two meta-analyses suggest that transcutaneous NMES reduces glenohumeral subluxation, improves pain-free lateral rotation ROM, and reduces motor impairment. These effects may be more prominent among acute stroke survivors.

Intramuscular Systems

Despite the evidence for therapeutic benefit, the clinical use of transcutaneous NMES for post-stroke shoulder subluxation and pain is limited for several reasons. First, many stroke survivors are not able to tolerate the discomfort of cutaneous stimulation. Second, it is difficult to confirm stimulation of deeper muscles, such as the supraspinatus, without activating the overlying superficial muscle such as the trapezius. And third, clinical skill is required to place electrodes and adjust stimulation parameters to provide optimal, consistent, and tolerable treatment. Intramuscular NMES systems may be able to address these limitations. Intramuscular systems bypass the cutaneous nociceptors and are better tolerated than transcutaneous NMES. Because the electrodes are implanted into the motor points, the hassle factor associated with donning and doffing the device is reduced. Because the electrodes are implanted, repeatability and reliability of stimulation are enhanced, minimizing the need for skilled care. And, finally, because of the selectivity of intramuscular stimulation, the best muscles to stimulate can be identified, and current intensity on multiple channels can be titrated easily. Two intramuscular electrical stimulation systems are under investigation: an injectable system with an external antenna and a percutaneous system with an external stimulator.

The injectable microstimulator, which was previously described, is presently under investigation for the treatment of hemiplegic shoulder dysfunction. The device is injected into the motor point of specific muscles, that is, supraspinatus and deltoids, or contiguous to a target nerve, that is, suprascapular or axillary, via a minimally invasive procedure under local anesthesia. Preliminary results from a randomized clinical trial demonstrated reduction in shoulder subluxation and increase in the thickness of the stimulated muscles (92). The effect on shoulder pain remains under investigation. The devices are permanently implanted, and, if shoulder subluxation or pain recurs, additional treatments may be provided without an additional invasive procedure. However, the need for a large garment antenna may interfere with daily activities and compromise clinical acceptance.

The percutaneous system includes helical intramuscular electrodes, a pager-size stimulator, and a connector (Figure 18-3). Electrodes are placed in the upper trapezius, supraspinatus, middle deltoid, and posterior deltoid via a minimally invasive procedure under local anesthesia. The device may be worn on a belt while the patient goes about his or her daily business. Electrodes traverse the skin and remain across the skin for the duration of treatment. After completion of treatment, the electrodes are removed by gentle traction. A multicenter clinical trial among chronic stroke survivors demonstrated that the system reduces shoulder pain and improves pain-related quality of life

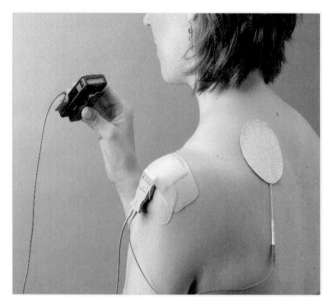

FIGURE 18-3

A percutaneous intramuscular electrical stimulation system for treatment of hemiplegic shoulder pain. The pager-size stimulator is connected to the implanted electrodes via a connector that can be disconnected when not in use. (RestoreStIM, courtesy, NeuroControl Corporation, North Ridgeville, OH.)

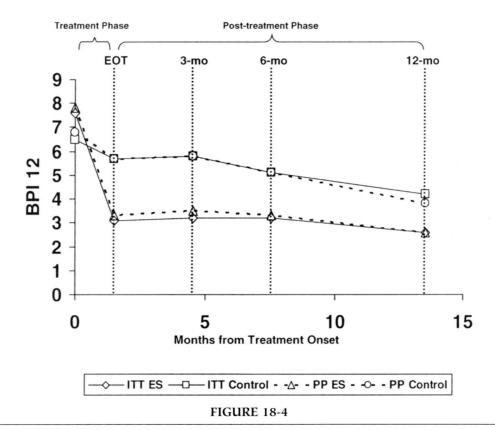

FIGURE 18-4

Results of a multicenter randomized clinical trial of percutaneous intramuscular electrical stimulation (ES) for the treatment of hemiplegic shoulder pain. Per-protocol (PP, dashed lines) and intent-to-treat (ITT, solid lines) approaches both showed that percutaneous intramuscular ES significantly reduces hemiplegic shoulder pain (Brief Pain Inventory Question 12) for up to 12 months after completion of treatment compared to controls who were treated with a cuffed hemisling. (Reproduced with permission, Chae et al., *Am J Phys Med Rehabil* 2005; 83:832–842, Lippincott Williams and Wilkins.)

for up to twelve months after completion of treatment (Figure 18-4) (93, 94). However, the system did not reduce glenohumeral subluxation or improve motor function. Although percutaneous NMES was effective in reducing post-stroke shoulder pain, the use of percutaneous wire electrodes poses the risk of electrode-related infections.

Summary, Clinical Considerations, and Future Directions

In spite of the methodological limitations, the preponderance of evidence suggest that transcutaneous NMES is effective in reducing post-stroke shoulder subluxation, increasing pain-free lateral rotation range of motion, and facilitating motor recovery. The therapeutic benefits appear to be more significant for those in the acute phase of stroke. Thus, a trial of transcutaneous NMES should be considered for those with flaccid hemiplegia—with or without subluxation—as a prophylactic measure to prevent the development of debilitating pain and facilitate motor recovery.

Transcutaneous NMES should also be considered as a treatment modality for those who already developed glenohumeral subluxation and pain. At present, it is unclear whether NMES renders any therapeutic benefit for those with post-stroke shoulder pain in the absence of glenohumeral subluxation.

Optimal timing of treatment onset has not been determined. However, as with motor relearning, stroke acuity and therapeutic benefit appear to be related. Thus, initiation of treatment during inpatient rehabilitation should be considered. Patients and family members should be trained by an experienced therapist to continue and complete the treatments at home. Although optimal dose and duration have not been determined, most studies with positive effects provided treatment for greater than four hours daily for a minimum of four weeks. Six hours of treatment daily for six weeks is recommended.

Additional studies are needed to address the previously noted methodological limitations in order to more definitively address the question of clinical efficacy. To date, only single-site studies of transcutaneous NMES for post-stroke shoulder dysfunction have been reported. A large, multicenter, single-blinded, randomized clinical trial is needed. As with any rigorous clinical trial, the study should carefully define the subject population, identify potential confounds, and evaluate long-term outcomes. The trial should be clinically relevant and focus on pain as the primary outcome with motor impairment, activity limitations, societal participation, and quality of life as secondary outcomes. Biomechanical and physiological measures may be included for elucidation of mechanisms. Finally, optimal timing, dose, and duration of treatment need to be determined.

Although transcutaneous NMES systems may ultimately prove effective for the treatment of post-stroke shoulder pain, clinical implementation may be difficult because of issues of pain of stimulation, compliance, reliability of stimulation, and need for skilled personnel. As noted previously, intramuscular systems may address these barriers to clinical implementation. However, intramuscular systems are investigational devices and are not clinically available. At present, the injectable and percutaneous systems are both undergoing clinical trials in support of FDA clearance for commercialization.

NEUROPROSTHESES

Introduction

A neuroprosthesis utilizes NMES to contract specific muscles in a specific sequence to allow the upper limb to perform ADLs or the lower limb to carry out mobility tasks. Motor relearning strategies, including therapeutic NMES, appear to be most effective for those with mild impairments (47). There are limited therapeutic options for those with more severe impairments. Although motor relearning may occur with regular use of a neuroprosthesis, the objective of a neuroprosthesis is the safe and efficient completion of functional tasks. Historically, neuroprostheses development focused on application to the SCI population. At present, neuroprostheses can provide grasp and release function for individuals with a complete cervical level SCI to facilitate performance of ADLs (95). Similarly, lower limb neuroprostheses can provide simple transfer function, navigation of architectural barriers, and limited ambulation for persons with complete paraplegia (96, 97).

All existing neuroprostheses consist of a stimulator that activates muscles, an input transducer, and a control unit. The control signal is derived from retained voluntary function. For example, a person with C5 complete tetraplegia usually has the ability to retract and protract the shoulder. A shoulder position transducer can detect this movement to generate a command signal for hand opening and closing. The user typically has control over electrically stimulated gross hand grasp opening and closing, but he or she does not have direct control over the activation of each muscle, thus simplifying the control task required by the user (98–100).

Upper Limb Applications

In view of the success of the hand neuroprosthesis in tetraplegia (95), it is reasonable to apply the technology to persons with hemiplegia. Four full-length publications in English language peer review journals evaluated the effectiveness of a hand neuroprosthesis for enhancing the upper limb function of stroke survivors (41, 42, 70, 101). All studies used limited sample sizes and open label designs with performance evaluated with and without the neuroprosthesis.

In 1973, Rebersek and Vodovnick published the first paper on the use of a hand neuroprosthesis in hemiplegia (42). Transcutaneous NMES opened the hand while closing was mediated by termination of the stimulation and subject's own volitional ability. The intensity of stimulation was proportionally controlled with a position transducer mounted on the contralateral, nonparalyzed shoulder. With training, subjects demonstrated progressive improvements in the number of hand positions they can maintain and the extent of hand opening using the device. A subset of subjects demonstrated progressive improvements in the number of plugs and baskets they could manipulate with the device. The authors noted that, without the stimulation, subjects performed less than 10% of the tasks. The feasibility of the device in enhancing upper extremity-related ADLs was not assessed.

In 1975, Merletti and associates evaluated a similar transcutaneous hand neuroprosthesis system (41). The device provided hand opening, but subjects again provided hand closure without the assist of the NMES. Subjects were trained to move a small plastic basket or bottle from one defined area to another and back again using the shoulder-mounted, position transducer-controlled stimulation. All subjects were able to perform the tasks with triceps and hand stimulation, although with varying degrees of success. None of the enrolled subjects could perform the assigned tasks without the stimulation or with hand stimulation only. The authors noted that the functional tasks required considerable amount of mental concentration. In several cases, voluntary effort to control the paretic limb produced tremors, spasticity, and erratic shoulder movement, which resulted in reduced performance.

Alon and associates tested the previously described hybrid NMES-orthosis neuroprosthesis (Figure 18-1) (70). Twenty-nine chronic stroke survivors participated in a home-based, three-week case series. Three ADL tasks were evaluated with and without the neuroprosthesis at baseline and at three weeks:

- Lifting a two-handled pot
- Holding a bag while standing with a cane
- Performing a subject-selected ADL task

The authors reported significant improvements in the percent of successful trials completing the ADL tasks.

Because of the limitations of transcutaneous NMES, Merletti and associates suggested that an implanted system would best meet the clinical needs of persons with hemiplegia (41). Accordingly, Chae and Hart evaluated four chronic stroke survivors implanted with percutaneous intramuscular electrodes to demonstrate adequacy of intramuscular NMES for hand opening and closing, identify control strategies that reliably open and close the hand under subject control, and demonstrate functional utility (101). The percutaneous hand neuroprosthesis was able to open a spastic hemiparetic hand as long as the limb was in a resting position, the wrist and proximal forearm were supported, subjects did not try to assist the stimulation, and an individual other than the participant modulated the stimulation. However, when subjects tried to assist the stimulation or complete a functional task, hand opening was significantly reduced because of increased finger flexor hypertonia, even with increased stimulation intensity. Similarly, electrically stimulated hand opening was significantly reduced following voluntary hand closure. Because of these limitations, a formal ADL evaluation was not pursued.

The benefits of the available hand neuroprosthesis systems are, at best, limited to a small number of selected simulated functional or grasp and release tasks. The clinical significance of these limited benefits is uncertain. In addition, two of the four studies reported that, when patients were asked to perform specific functional tasks, a significant degree of mental and physical effort was required, which was often associated with increased generalized hypertonia. In the face of increased hypertonia, the neuroprostheses could not open the hand effectively or reliably.

Lower Limb Applications

The initial application of neuroprostheses in hemiplegia focused on transcutaneous peroneal nerve stimulation to treat ankle dorsiflexion weakness. In a 1961 publication, Lieberson and associates described a stimulator that dorsiflexed the ankle during the swing phase of gait (48). The devices stimulated the common peroneal nerve near the head of the femur and activated both tibialis anterior and the peroneus longus and brevis muscles. In the only randomized study of transcutaneous peroneal stimulation, Burridge and associates demonstrated that stroke survivors treated with the device exhibit significantly greater increase in walking speed with the device relative to baseline without the device, while the control group did not (102). However, despite demonstrated effectiveness, transcutaneous peroneal nerve stimulation is not routinely prescribed in the United States for foot drop in hemiplegia. Likely reasons include difficulty with electrode placement, discomfort and inconsistent reliability of transcutaneous stimulation, insufficient medial-lateral

control during stance phase, lack of technical support, and the availability of custom-molded ankle-foot orthoses. However, recent FDA approval of three transcutaneous peroneal nerve stimulators (Figure 18-5) and demonstrated comparability of the peroneal nerve stimulator to an ankle-foot orthosis in improving hemiplegic gait may facilitate broader clinical prescription and usage of these devices (73, 103).

Nevertheless, transcutaneous systems have several inherent limitations, which might be addressable by implantable systems. An early study by Waters and associates reported significant increase in walking speed, stride length, and cadence with a single-channel implantable device relative to preimplantation performance (55). However, technical limitations included difficulty in balancing inversion and eversion, lack of an in-line connector, which necessitated removal of the entire implant in the event of component failure, and poor reliability of the heel switch and foot-floor contact transmitter. Kljajic and associates also reported significant benefits from a single-channel implantable stimulator relative to without stimulation (50). However, nearly half of all subjects required reimplantation because of electrode displacement or failure. At present, two multichannel implantable peroneal nerve stimulators are undergoing clinical investigations in Europe. A dual-channel device developed by the University of Twente and Roessingh Research and Development (The Netherlands) stimulates the deep and superficial peroneal nerves for better control of ankle dorsiflexion, eversion, and inversion (Figure 18-6) (104). A four-channel device, developed at Aalborg University (Denmark) utilizes a nerve cuff with four tripolar electrodes, oriented to activate different nerve fibers within the common peroneal nerve (105). Both devices have the CE mark in Europe. Finally, an injectable microstimulator, which is percutaneously placed via a minimally invasive procedure, is also under investigation for the correction of foot drop (106).

In order to address gait deviations caused by deficits proximal to the ankle, several studies evaluated multichannel transcutaneous systems (61–63). However, although these systems were clinically implemented as neuroprostheses, neuroprosthetic outcomes were not assessed. Instead, these studies focused on therapeutic or motor relearning effects and were therefore discussed in an earlier section.

Single-channel transcutaneous peroneal nerve stimulation appears effective in enhancing gait relative to no device and may be equivalent to an ankle-foot orthosis. A systematic review evaluated seven case series and one randomized clinical trial of transcutaneous peroneal nerve stimulation for hemiplegic gait. The pooled improvement in walking speed with the device relative to no device was 38% (107). The authors concluded that the "...review

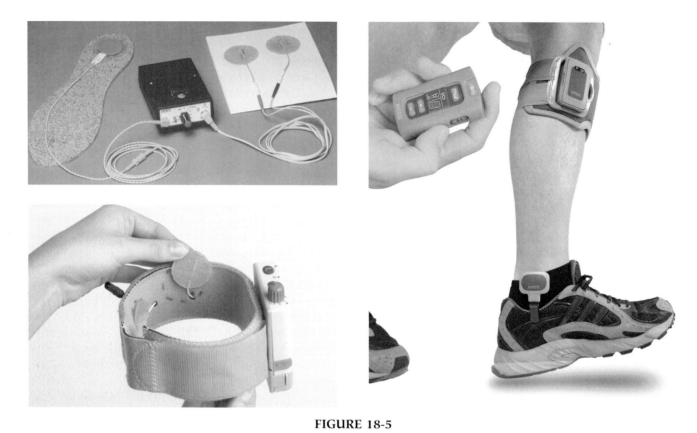

FIGURE 18-5

Three FDA approved transcutaneous peroneal nerve stimulators. The Odstock Dropped Foot Stimulator (Left-top, courtesy, Department of Medical Physics and Biomedical Engineering, Salisbury District Hospital, Salisbury, UK and NDI Medical, Cleveland, OH) and the wireless L300 (Left-bottom, courtesy, Bioness Inc., Santa Clarita, CA) both use a heel switch to trigger ankle dorsiflexion. The WalkAide (Right, courtesy, Hanger Orthopedic Group/Innovative Neurotronics, Bethesda, MD) uses a tilt sensor to trigger ankle dorsiflexion.

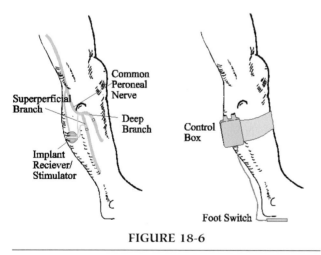

FIGURE 18-6

A two-channel implantable peroneal nerve stimulator (STIMuSTEP) allows individual stimulation of the deep and superficial branches of the common peroneal nerve for ankle dorsiflexion and eversion-inversion balance. (Courtesy, Department of Medical Physics and Biomedical Engineering, Salisbury District Hospital, Salisbury, UK.).

suggests a positive orthotic effect of functional electrical stimulation on walking speed."

Summary, Clinical Considerations, and Future Directions

At present, a hand neuroprosthesis may allow stroke survivors to complete a limited number of selected functional tasks. However, a clinically viable hand neuroprosthesis system that provides broad functional benefit is not yet available. The requirements for a clinically viable hand neuroprosthesis for person with hemiplegia are significant. Stroke survivors can perform most basic ADLs with the unaffected upper limb. Thus, in order to ensure added value, the system must allow stroke survivors to perform bilateral tasks or provide significant assistance to the unaffected upper limb in order to facilitate completion of additional tasks. Although distal function is usually more impaired than proximal function in hemiplegia, significant proximal deficits persist that impede the positioning of the hand. Therefore, in order to widen clinical indications, both distal and proximal control should be provided (108). Nearly all stroke survivors are ambulators. Thus, the system must have sufficient miniaturization to not interfere with mobility. The stroke survivor must be able to use the device with minimal effort to avoid triggering generalized hypertonia or associated reactions. The system must allow the user to perform functional tasks without impeding the function of the unaffected limb. Thus, control paradigms that produce effortless movement of the impaired upper limb without compromising the function of the intact limb should be incorporated into the system (109). Finally, the system must turn off overactive muscles to address the problems of spasticity, associated reactions, co-activations, co-contractions, and delay in termination of muscle contractions (101). Because motor relearning strategies appear to be limited to those with milder impairments, an upper limb neuroprosthesis is essential in improving the function and quality of life of those with more severe impairments. However, additional fundamental and clinical research is needed to develop a clinically viable upper limb neuroprosthesis for stroke survivors.

In contrast to upper limb neuroprostheses, lower limb neuroprostheses are closer to clinical viability. Specifically, transcutaneous peroneal nerve stimulators are now available for clinical implementation for stroke survivors with foot drop. Data suggests that these devices are superior to no device in improving overall mobility and may be equivalent to an ankle-foot orthosis (73, 102, 103). Patients should receive device and gait training from an experienced therapist. Eligibility criteria include:

1. Ankle dorsiflexion strength of ≤ 4/5 while standing
2. Presence of foot drop, resulting in gait instability or need for compensatory strategies such as circumduction, hip hiking, or vaulting
3. Passive ankle range of motion to neutral
4. Intact skin
5. Absence of edema
6. Berg balance score of at least 30/56 and tolerance to surface stimulation

Patients are not eligible if:

1. There is evidence of fixed plantarflexion contractures.
2. The ankle-foot orthosis is needed to prevent knee flexion collapse.
3. Genu recurvatum is not responsive to the peroneal nerve stimulator.
4. Patient is hypersensitive to electrode adhesives (103)

These criteria should be considered in the context of general warnings described in the Motor Relearning Section.

Implanted peroneal nerve stimulation devices are available in Europe and are likely to be equivalent to the transcutaneous devices with respect to function. They may be appropriate for those who experience significant improvement in mobility with the transcutaneous system, but have difficulty with electrode placement, skin irritation, painful sensation of stimulation, or donning and doffing of the device. However, in view of limited data, more definitive recommendations must await the emergence of additional clinical experience. At present, multichannel, multijoint systems are clinically less accessible and are limited to investigative purposes.

Although the development of lower limb neuroprostheses for hemiplegia is further along than upper limb systems, several issues remain to be further elucidated. First, transcutaneous systems can be limited by discomfort and difficulty with electrode placement for reliable muscle contraction. Percutaneous and implanted systems may address these issues, but potential benefits must be tempered with the risks and costs associated with an invasive procedure. Second, the indications for the level of complexity required for a specific individual remain undefined. Some individuals will require complex multichannel systems, while simple dorsiflexion assist devices will suffice for others. Third, it remains unclear as to when the motor relearning period ends and the indication for NMES for neuroprosthetic purposes begins. Nearly all studies with neuroprosthetic applications report some evidence of motor relearning, even among chronic stroke survivors. Finally, clinical relevance must be established by evaluating the effects of the intervention on mobility and quality of life and by comparing the neuroprosthetic system to a comparable standard of care such as the ankle-foot orthosis.

CONCLUSIONS

The principal goal of rehabilitation management of persons with hemiparesis is to maximize quality of life. NMES systems bypass the injured central circuitry to activate neural tissue and contract muscles to provide function to what is otherwise a nonfunctioning limb or structure. Recent advances in clinical medicine and biomedical engineering make the clinical implementation of NMES systems to enhance the ADL and mobility function of persons with hemiparesis more feasible.

NMES for motor relearning in hemiplegia is a promising application of goal-oriented, repetitive movement therapy. While rigorous, multicenter clinical trials to confirm effectiveness and fundamental studies to elucidate mechanisms are still needed, the approach is ready for clinical implementation in a limited scale for a select group of stroke survivors. Similarly, NMES for the treatment of shoulder subluxation and pain in hemiplegia has yielded encouraging results. While the community is ready for confirmatory, large-scale, multicenter clinical trials and more invasive approaches are being investigated, transcutaneous NMES may be clinically implemented in a select group of patients. The development of the hand neuroprosthesis for stroke survivors is in its infancy and must await further technical and scientific developments. Similarly, multichannel, multijoint lower limb neuroprostheses need further development. However, transcutaneous peroneal stimulators appear to be effective in improving hemiplegic gait and should be included in the clinical armamentarium.

Although this chapter focused on NMES, clinical practice is rarely limited to a single intervention. Thus, with the development of pharmacological interventions, neuronal regeneration and other innovations such as robotic therapy, mental imagery, virtual reality, and constraint-induced therapy, the future will likely embrace combination therapies to treat the myriad of motor dysfunction for persons with central nervous system paralysis (71, 110–116).

After decades of development, the clinical utility of NMES systems is becoming realized. By necessity, scientists and clinicians must continue to explore new ideas and improve upon the present systems. Components will be smaller, more durable, and more reliable. The issues of cosmesis and ease of donning and doffing will be a factor in the evolution of devices. Control issues will remain central, and the implementation of cortical control will dictate the nature of future generations of neuroprosthesis systems. Future developments will be directed by consumers. In the present health care environment where cost is an overwhelming factor in the development and implementation of new technology, the consumer will become one of technology's greatest advocates. Finally, the usual drive toward greater complexity will be tempered by the practical issues of clinical implementation where patient and clinician acceptances are often a function of a tenuous balance between the burden and cost associated with using a system and the system's impact on the user's quality of life.

References

1. Lee RG, van Donkelaar P. Mechanisms underlying functional recovery following stroke. *Can J Neurol Sci* 1995; 22:257–263.
2. Moe JH, Post HW. Functional electrical stimulation for ambulation in hemiplegia. *J Lancet* 1962; 82:285–288.
3. Szlavik RB, de Bruin H. The effect of stimulus current pulse width on nerve fiber size recruitment patterns. *Med Eng Phys* 1999; 21:507–515.
4. Adrian E. *The Physical Background of Perception.* Oxford: Clarendon Press, 1946.
5. Mortimer JT. In: Brookhart JM, Mountcastle VB, eds. *Handbook of Physiology: The Nervous System II.* Motor prostheses 155–187. Bethesda, MD: American Physiological Society, 1981.
6. Lertmanorat Z, Durand DM. Extracellular voltage profile for reversing the recruitment order of peripheral nerve stimulation: A simulation study. *J Neural Eng* 2004; 1:202–211.
7. Sieck GC, Prakash YS. Morphological adaptations of neuromuscular junctions depend on fiber type. *Can J Appl Physiol* 1997; 22:197–230.
8. Riley DA, Allin EF. The effects of inactivity, programmed stimulation, and denervation on the histochemistry of skeletal muscle fiber types. *Exp Neurol* 1973; 40:391–413.
9. Peckham PH, Mortimer JT, Marsolais EB. Alteration in the force and fatigability of skeletal muscle in quadriplegic humans following exercise induced by chronic electrical stimulation. *Clin Orthop Relat Res* 1976:326–333.
10. Kubis HP, Scheibe RJ, Meissner JD, et al. Fast-to-slow transformation and nuclear import/export kinetics of the transcription factor NFATc1 during electrostimulation of rabbit muscle cells in culture. *J Physiol* 2002; 541:835–847.
11. Benton LA, Baker LL, Bowman BR, Waters RL. *Functional Electrical Stimulation: A Practical Clinical Guide.* Downey, CA: Ranchos Los Amigos Medical Center, 1981.
12. Memberg W PP, Keith MH. A surgically implanted intramuscular electrode for an implantable neuromuscular stimulation system. *IEEE Trans Biomed Eng* 1994; 2:80–91.
13. Knutson JS, Naples GG, Peckham PH, Keith WM. Electrode fracture rate and occurrences of infection and granuloma associated with percutaneous intramuscular electrodes in upper limb functional electrical stimulation application. *J Rehabil Res Dev* 2003; 39:671–684.
14. Waters RL, Campbell JM, Nakai R. Therapeutic electrical stimulation of the lower limb by epimysial electrodes. *Clin Orthop* 1988:44–52.
15. Davis R, Houdayer T, Andrews B, et al. Paraplegia: Prolonged closed-loop standing with implanted nucleus FES-22 stimulator and Andrews' foot-ankle orthosis. *Stereotact Funct Neurosurg* 1997; 69:281–287.
16. Nannini N, Horch K. Muscle recruitment with intrafascicular electrodes. *IEEE Trans Biomed Eng* 1991; 38:769–776.
17. Sweeney JD, Mortimer JT. An asymmetric two-electrode cuff for generation of unidirectionally propagated action potentials. *IEEE Trans Biomed Eng* 1986; 33: 541–549.
18. Adamczyk MM, Crago PE. Input-output nonlinearities and time delays increase tracking errors in hand grasp neuroprostheses. *IEEE Trans Rehabil Eng* 1996; 4:271–279.
19. Lemay MA, Crago PE, Katorgi M, Chapman GJ. Automated tuning of a closed-loop hand grasp neuroprosthesis. *IEEE Trans Biomed Eng* 1993; 40:675–685.
20. Weber DJ, Stein RB, Chan KM, et al. BIONic WalkAide for correcting foot drop. *IEEE Trans Neural Syst Rehabil Eng* 2005; 13:242–246.
21. Arcos I, Davis R, Fey K, et al. Second-generation microstimulator. *Artif Organs* 2002; 26:228–231.
22. Asanuma H, Keller A. Neuronal mechanisms of motor learning in animals. *Neuroreport* 1991; 2:217–224.
23. Asanuma H, Keller A. Neurobiolgogical basis of motor relearning and memory. *Conc Neurosci* 1991; 2:1–30.
24. Nudo RJ, Plautz EJ, Frost SB. Role of adaptive plasticity in recovery of function after damage to motor cortex. *Muscle Nerve* 2001; 24:1000–1019.
25. Nudo RJ, Plautz EJ, Frost SB. Role of adaptive plasticity in recovery of function after damage to motor cortex. *Muscle Nerve* 2001; 24:1000–1019.
26. Ridding MC, Rothwell JC. Afferent input and cortical organisation: A study with magnetic stimulation. *Exp Brain Res* 1999; 126:536–544.
27. Spiegel J, Tintera J, Gawehn J, et al. Functional MRI of human primary somatosensory and motor cortex during median nerve stimulation. *Clin Neurophysiol* 1999; 110:47–52.
28. Han BS, Jang SH, Chang Y, et al. Functional magnetic resonance image finding of cortical activation by neuromuscular electrical stimulation on wrist extensor muscles. *Am J Phys Med Rehabil* 2003; 82:17–20.
29. Smith GV, Alon G, Roys SR, Gullapalli P. Functional MRI determination of a dose-response relationship to lower extremity neuromuscular electrical stimulation in healthy subjects. *Exp Brain Res* 2003; 150:33–39.
30. Chae J, Bethoux F, Bohinc T, et al. Neuromuscular stimulation for upper extremity motor and functional recovery in acute hemiplegia. *Stroke* 1998; 29:975–979.
31. Powell J, Pandyan AD, Granat M, et al. Electrical stimulation of wrist extensors in poststroke hemiplegia. *Stroke* 1999; 30:1384–1389.
32. Sonde L, Gip C, Ferneus S, et al. Stimulation with low frequency (1/7 Hz) transcutaneous electrical nerve stimulation (Low-TENS) increases motor function of post-stroke hemiparetic arm. *Scand J Rehabil Med* 1998; 30:95–99.
33. Sonde L, Kalimo H, Fernaeus SE, Viitanen M. Low TENS treatment on post-stroke paretic arm: A three-year follow-up. *Clin Rehabil* 2000; 14:14–19.
34. Wong AM, Su TY, Tang FT, et al. Clinical trial of electrical acupuncture on hemiplegic stroke patients. *Am J Phys Med Rehabil* 1999; 78:117–122.
35. Bowman BR, Baker L, Waters R. Positional feedback and electrical stimulation: An automated treatment for hemiplegic wrist. *Arch Phys Med Rehabil* 1979; 60:497–502.
36. Cauraugh J, Light K, Kim S, et al. Chronic motor dysfunction after stroke: Recovering wrist and finger extension by electromyography-triggered neuromuscular stimulation. *Stroke* 2000; 31:1360–1364.
37. Cauraugh JH, Kim S. Two coupled motor recovery protocols are better than one: Electroymogram-triggered neuromuscular electrical stimulation and bilateral movements. *Stroke* 2002; 33:1589–1594.
38. Francisco G, Chae J, Chawla H, et al. Electromyogram-triggered neuromuscular stimulation for improving the arm function of acute stroke survivors: A randomized pilot study. *Arch Phys Med Rehabil* 1998; 79:570–575.
39. Kimberley TJ, Lewis SM, Auerbach EJ, et al. Electrical stimulation driving functional improvements and cortical changes in subjects with stroke. *Exp Brain Res* 2004; 154:450–460.
40. Kraft GH, Fitts SS, Hammond MC. Techniques to improve function of the arm and hand in chronic hemiplegia. *Arch Phys Med Rehabil* 1992; 73:220–227.

41. Merletti R, Acimovic R, Grobelnik S, Cvilak G. Electrophysiological orthosis for the upper extremity in hemiplegia: Feasibility study. *Arch Phys Med Rehabil* 1975; 56:507–513.

42. Rebersek S, Vodovnik L. Proportionally controlled functional electrical stimulation of hand. *Arch Phys Med Rehabil* 1973; 54:378–382.

43. Alon G, Sunnerhagen KS, Geurts AC, Ohry A. A home-based, self-administered stimulation program to improve selected hand functions of chronic stroke. *NeuroRehabilitation* 2003; 18:215–225.

44. Nathan RH, Ohry A. Upper limb functions regained in quadriplegia: A hybrid computerized FNS system. *Arch Phys Med Rehabil* 1990; 71:415–421.

45. Alon G, Ring H. Gait and hand function enhancement following training with a multisegment hybrid orthosis stimulation system in stroke patients. *J Stroke Cerebrovasc Dis* 2003; 12:209–216.

46. Popovic DB, Popovic MB, Sinkjaer T, et al. Therapy of paretic arm in hemiplegic subjects augmented with a neural prosthesis: A cross-over study. *Can J Physiol Pharmacol* 2004; 82:749–756.

47. de Kroon JR, van der Lee JH, IJzerman MJ, Lankhorst GJ. Therapeutic electrical stimulation to improve motor control and functional abilities of the upper extremity after stroke: A systematic review. *Clin Rehabil* 2002; 16:350–360.

48. Lieberson W, Holmquest H, Scot D, Dow M. Functional electrotherapy: Stimulation of the peroneal nerve synchronized with the swing phase of the gait of hemiplegia patients. *Arch Phys Med Rehabil* 1961; 42:101–105.

49. Carnstam B, Larsson LE, Prevec TS. Improvement in gait following electrical stimulation. *Scand J Rehabil Med* 1977; 9:7–13.

50. Kljajic M, Malezic M, Acimovic R, et al. Gait evaluation in hemiparetic patients using subcutaneous peroneal electrical stimulation. *Scand J Rehabil Med* 1992; 24:121–126.

51. Stefancic M, Rebersek M, Merletti R. The therapeutic effects of the Ljubljana functional electrical brace. *Eur Medicophys* 1976; 12:1–9.

52. Takebe K, Basmajian J. Gait analysis in stroke patients to assess treatments of foot drop. *Arch Phys Med Rehabil* 1976; 10:75–92.

53. Takebe K, Kukulka C, Narayan M, et al. Peroneal nerve stimulator in rehabilitation of hemiplegic patients. *Arch Phys Med Rehabil* 1975; 56:237–240.

54. Taylor PN, Burridge JH, Dunkerley AL, et al. Clinical use of the Odstock dropped foot stimulator: Its effect on the speed and effort of walking. *Arch Phys Med Rehabil* 1999; 80:1577–1583.

55. Waters R, McNeal D, Perry J. Experimental correction of foot drop by electrical stimulation of the peroneal nerve. *J Bone Joint Surg* 1975; 57A:1047–1054.

56. Cozean CD, Pease WS, Hubbell SL. Biofeedback and functional electric stimulation in stroke rehabilitation. *Arch Phys Med Rehabil* 1988; 69:401–405.

57. Winchester P, Montgomery J, Bowman B, Hislop H. Effects of feedback stimulation training and cyclical electrical stimulation on knee extension in hemiparetic patients. *Phys Ther* 1983; 7:1096–1103.

58. Levin MF, Hui-Chan CW. Relief of hemiparetic spasticity by TENS is associated with improvement in reflex and voluntary motor functions. *Electroencephalogr Clin Neurophysiol* 1992; 85:131–142.

59. Merletti R, Zelaschi F, Latella D, et al. A control study of muscle force recovery in hemiparetic patients during treatment with functional electrical stimulation. *Scand J Rehabil Med* 1978; 10:147–154.

60. Yan T, Hui-Chan CW, Li LS. Functional electrical stimulation improves motor recovery of the lower extremity and walking ability of subjects with first acute stroke: A randomized placebo-controlled trial. *Stroke* 2005; 36:80–85.

61. Bogataj U, Gros N, Malezic M, et al. Restoration of gait during two to three weeks of therapy with multichannel electrical stimulation. *Phys Ther* 1989; 69:319–327.

62. Stanic U, Acimovic-Janezic R, Gros N, et al. Multichannel electrical stimulation for correction of hemiplegic gait: Methodology and preliminary results. *Scand J Rehabil Med* 1978; 10:75–92.

63. Bogataj U, Gros N, Kljajic M, et al. The rehabilitation of gait in patients with hemiplegia: A comparison between conventional therapy and multichannel functional electrical stimulation therapy. *Phys Ther* 1995; 75:490–502.

64. Daly JJ, Ruff RL, Haycook K, et al. Feasibility of gait training for acute stroke patients using FNS with implanted electrodes. *J Neurol Sci* 2000; 179:103–107.

65. Daly JJ, Roenigk K, Holcomb J, et al. A randomized controlled trial of functional neuromuscular stimulation in chronic stroke subjects. *Stroke* 2006; 37:172–178.

66. Robbins SM, Houghton PE, Woodbury MG, Brown JL. The therapeutic effect of functional and transcutaneous electric stimulation on improving gait speed in stroke patients: a meta-analysis. *Arch Phys Med Rehabil* 2006; 87:853–859.

67. de Kroon JR, Ijzerman MJ, Chae J, et al. Relation between stimulation characteristics and clinical outcome in studies using electrical stimulation to improve motor control of the upper extremity in stroke. *J Rehabil Med* 2005; 37:65–74.

68. Chae J, Bethoux F, Bohine T, et al. Neuromuscular stimulation for upper extremity motor and functional recovery in acute hemiplegia. *Stroke* 1998; 29:975–979.

69. Kimberley TJ, Lewis SM, Auerbach EJ, et al. Electrical stimulation driving functional improvements and cortical changes in subjects with stroke. *Exp Brain Res* 2004; 154:450–460.

70. Alon G, McBride K, Ring H. Improving selected hand functions using a noninvasive neuroprosthesis in persons with chronic stroke. *J Stroke Cerebrovasc Dis* 2002; 11:99–106.

71. Wolf SL, Winstein CJ, Miller JP, et al. Effect of constraint-induced movement therapy on upper extremity function three to nine months after stroke: The EXCITE randomized clinical trial. *JAMA* 2006; 296:2095–2104.

72. Fields RW. Electromyographically triggered electric muscle stimulation for chronic hemiplegia. *Arch Phys Med Rehabil* 1987; 68:407–414.

73. Stein RB, Chong S, Everaert DG, et al. A multicenter trial of a foot drop stimulator controlled by a tilt sensor. *Neurorehabil Neural Repair* 2006; 20:371–379.

74. Taylor P, Burridge J, Dunkerley A, et al. Clinical audit of five years provision of the Odstock dropped foot stimulator. *Artif Organs* 1999; 23:440–442.

75. DeVahl J. In: Wolf S, ed. *Electrotherapy in Rehabilitation.* Neuromuscular electrical stimulation (NMES) in rehabilitation 218–268. Philadelphia: F.A. Davis Company, 1992.

76. Chae J, Fang ZP, Walker M, Pourmehdi S. Intramuscular electromyographically controlled neuromuscular electrical stimulation for upper limb recovery in chronic hemiplegia. *Am J Phys Med Rehabil* 2001; 80:935–941.

77. Lauer RT, Peckham PH, Kilgore KL. EEG-based control of a hand grasp neuroprosthesis. *Neuroreport* 1999; 10:1767–1771.

78. Van Ouwenaller C, Laplace PM, Chantraine A. Painful shoulder in hemiplegia. *Arch Phys Med Rehabil* 1986; 67:23–26.

79. Bender L, McKenna K. Hemiplegic shoulder pain: Defining the problem and its management. *Disabil Rehabil* 2001; 23:698–705.

80. Snels IA, Dekker JH, van der Lee JH, et al. Treating patients with hemiplegic shoulder pain. *Am J Phys Med Rehabil* 2002; 81:150–160.

81. Baker LL, Parker K. Neuromuscular electrical stimulation of the muscles surrounding the shoulder. *Phys Ther* 1986; 66:1930–1937.

82. Chantraine A, Baribeault A, Uebelhart D, Gremion G. Shoulder pain and dysfunction in hemiplegia: Effects of functional electrical stimulation. *Arch Phys Med Rehabil* 1999; 80:328–331.

83. Chen CH, Chen TW, Weng MC, et al. The effect of electroacupuncture on shoulder subluxation for stroke patients. *Kaohsiung J Med Sci* 2000; 16:525–532.

84. Faghri PD, Rodgers MM, Glaser RM, et al. The effects of functional electrical stimulation on shoulder subluxation, arm function recovery, and shoulder pain in hemiplegic stroke patients. *Arch Phys Med Rehabil* 1994; 75:73–79.

85. Kobayashi H, Onishi H, Ihashi K, et al. Reduction in subluxation and improved muscle function of the hemiplegic shoulder joint after therapeutic electrical stimulation. *J Electromyogr Kinesiol* 1999; 9:327–336.

86. Leandri M, Parodi CI, Corrieri N, Rigardo S. Comparison of TENS treatments in hemiplegic shoulder pain. *Scand J Rehabil Med* 1990; 22:69–71.

87. Linn SL, Granat MH, Lees KR. Prevention of shoulder subluxation after stroke with electrical stimulation. *Stroke* 1999; 30:963–968.

88. Wang RY, Chan RC, Tsai MW. Functional electrical stimulation on chronic and acute hemiplegic shoulder subluxation. *Am J Phys Med Rehabil* 2000; 79:385–390; quiz 391–384.

89. Wang RY, Yang YR, Tsai MW, et al. Effects of functional electric stimulation on upper limb motor function and shoulder range of motion in hemiplegic patients. *Am J Phys Med Rehabil* 2002; 81:283–290.

90. Price CI, Pandyan AD. Electrical stimulation for preventing and treating post-stroke shoulder pain: A systematic Cochrane review. *Clin Rehabil* 2001; 15:5–19.

91. Ada L, Foongchomcheay A. Efficacy of electrical stimulation in preventing or reducing subluxation of the shoulder after stroke: A meta-analysis. *Aust J Physiother* 2002; 48:257–267.

92. Dupont A-C, Bagg SD, Creasey JL, et al. Clinical trials of BION Injectable neuromuscular stimulators. Sixth Annual Conference of the International Functional Electrical Stimulation Society, Cleveland, OH, June 16–20, 2001.

93. Chae J, Yu DT, Walker ME, et al. Intramuscular electrical stimulation for hemiplegic shoulder pain: A 12-month follow-up of a multiple-center, randomized clinical trial. *Am J Phys Med Rehabil* 2005; 84:832–842.

94. Yu DT, Chae J, Walker ME, et al. Intramuscular neuromuscular electrical stimulation for post-stroke shoulder pain: A multicenter randomized clinical trial. *Arch Phys Med Rehabil* 2004; 85:695–704.

95. Peckham PH, Keith MW, Kilgore KL, et al. Efficacy of an implanted neuroprosthesis for restoring hand grasp in tetraplegia: A multicenter study. *Arch Phys Med Rehabil* 2001; 82:1380–1388.

96. Davis JA, Jr., Triolo RJ, Uhlir J, et al. Preliminary performance of a surgically implanted neuroprosthesis for standing and transfers: Where do we stand? *J Rehabil Res Dev* 2001; 38:609–617.

97. Graupe D, Kohn KH. Functional neuromuscular stimulator for short-distance ambulation by certain thoracic-level spinal cord-injured paraplegics. *Surg Neurol* 1998; 50:202–207.

98. Hart RL, Kilgore KL, Peckham PH. A comparison between control methods for implanted FES hand-grasp systems. *IEEE Trans Rehabil Eng* 1998; 6:208–218.

99. Kilgore KL, Peckham PH. Grasp synthesis for upper extremity FNS. Part 1. Automated method for synthesising the stimulus map. *Med Biol Eng Comput* 1993; 31:607–614.

100. Kilgore KL, Peckham PH. Grasp synthesis for upper extremity FNS. Part 2. Evaluation of the influence of electrode recruitment properties. *Med Biol Eng Comput* 1993; 31:615–622.

101. Chae J, Hart R. Intramuscular hand neuroprosthesis for chronic stroke survivors. *Neurorehabil Neural Repair* 2003; 17:109–117.

102. Burridge JH, Taylor PN, Hagan SA, et al. The effects of common peroneal stimulation on the effort and speed of walking: A randomized controlled trial with chronic hemiplegic patients. *Clin Rehabil* 1997; 11:201–210.

103. Sheffler LR, Hennessey M, Naples GG, Chae J. Peroneal nerve stimulation versus an ankle-foot orthosis for correction of foot drop in stroke: Impact in functional ambulation. *Neurorehabil Neural Repair* 2006; 20:355–360.

104. Kenney L, Bultstra G, Buschman R, et al. An implantable, two-channel drop foot stimulator: Initial clinical results. *Artif Organs* 2002; 26:267–270.

105. Burridge J, Haugland M, Larsen B, et al. A Phase II study to evaluate the safety and effectiveness of the ActiGait implanted drop-foot stimulator in established hemiplegia. *J Rehabil Med* In-press.

106. Weber DJ, Stein RB, Chan KM, et al. Functional electrical stimulation using microstimulators to correct foot drop: A case study. *Can J Physiol Pharmacol* 2004; 82:784–792.

107. Kottink AI, Oostendorp LJ, Buurke JH, et al. The orthotic effect of functional electrical stimulation on the improvement of walking in stroke patients with a dropped foot: A systematic review. *Artif Organs* 2004; 28:577–586.

108. Kirsch RF, Acosta AM, van der Helm FC, et al. Model-based development of neuroprostheses for restoring proximal arm function. *J Rehabil Res Dev* 2001; 38:619–626.

109. Hoffer JA, Stein RB, Haugland MK, et al. Neural signals for command control and feedback in functional neuromuscular stimulation: A review. *J Rehabil Res Dev* 1996; 33:145–157.

110. Abbruzzese G, Assini A, Buccolieri A, et al. Changes of intracortical inhibition during motor imagery in human subjects. *Neurosci Lett* 1999; 263:113–116.

111. Bradbury EJ, McMahon SB. Spinal cord repair strategies: Why do they work? *Nat Rev Neurosci* 2006; 7:644–653.

112. Fasoli SE, Krebs HI, Hogan N. Robotic technology and stroke rehabilitation: Translating research into practice. *Top Stroke Rehabil* 2004; 11:11–19.

113. Goldstein LB. Neuropharmacology of TBI-induced plasticity. *Brain Inj* 2003; 17:685–694.

114. Krakauer JW. Motor learning: Its relevance to stroke recovery and neurorehabilitation. *Curr Opin Neurol* 2006; 19:84–90.

115. Krebs HI, Volpe BT, Aisen ML, Hogan N. Increasing productivity and quality of care: Robot-aided neurorehabilitation. *J Rehabil Res Dev* 2000; 37:639–652.

116. Rose FD, Brooks BM, Rizzo AA. Virtual reality in brain damage rehabilitation: Review. *Cyberpsychol Behav* 2005; 8:241–262;discussion 263–271.

19 Technological Aids for Motor Recovery[1]

Joel Stein
Richard Hughes
Susan E. Fasoli

Hermano Igo Krebs
Neville Hogan[2]

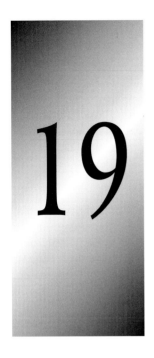

In contemporary society, the adoption of new technologies often is viewed as an inevitable component of progress. Stroke rehabilitation has been slower to adopt new technologically based therapeutic tools than many other areas of medicine and has largely remained a "hands-on" field. There are several arguments supporting the broader incorporation of technology into stroke rehabilitation. An economic case can be made that the field of stroke rehabilitation needs to take advantage of the potential labor-saving nature of these technologies. In an environment in which labor costs continue to rise and the costs of technology are falling, using technology to reduce the reliance on skilled human labor for stroke rehabilitation will undoubtedly be cost-effective in the long run. The need for more efficient delivery of exercise therapy is amplified by the growing evidence that more intensive exercise training is an important factor in enhancing motor recovery after stroke.

A second consideration in favor of increasing the adoption of technology in stroke rehabilitation is that technologically based therapies are able to provide treatments repetitively without risking therapist fatigue. This can be easily illustrated by analogy with the low-tech example of continuous passive motion (CPM) machines after total knee arthroplasty. These devices can provide many hours of slow, steady, passive range-of-motion exercises after surgery. While a human therapist is capable of performing similar exercises, he/she would not be able to sustain this effort for many hours.

Certain therapies and treatments can be provided only through the use of technology. For example, many virtual reality scenarios, such as an exercise used to control a flight simulator, would not be feasible for a disabled stroke survivor without the use of technology. The use of simulators often provides an opportunity to make a potentially tedious exercise much more interesting for the patient.

Similarly, robotic devices appear particularly well suited to facilitating motor learning. Evidence continues to accumulate that motor-learning principles, such as task repetition and progression, are critical elements of exercise programs to stimulate brain plasticity and recovery of motor function. Advances in robotic technology are increasingly capable of providing a flexible,

[1]Portions of this chapter are adapted from Stein J, Hughes R, Fasoli S, et al. Clinical applications of robots in rehabilitation. *Critical Reviews in Physical and Rehabilitation Medicine* 2005; 17(3):217–230, with permission from Begell House Publishing, Inc.

[2]Drs. H. I. Krebs and N. Hogan are co-inventors in the MIT-held patents for several of the robotic devices described in this chapter. They hold equity positions at Interactive Motion Technologies, Inc., the company that manufactures this type of technology under license to MIT.

programmable platform to engage stroke survivors in a growing array of interactive motor-learning activities.

Lastly, many stroke rehabilitation centers are seeking ways to distinguish themselves in a competitive marketplace. While this is not a strong argument for the adoption of new technologies, it is nonetheless likely a driving factor among some early adopters of new treatment technologies.

Robotic devices and virtual reality systems have been proposed as innovative technologies that may have particular application to stroke rehabilitation. This chapter describes the potential applications of these technologies as aids for rehabilitation and recovery in stroke survivors and discusses many of the specific systems currently in use and the evidence supporting their clinical efficacy.

WHAT ARE ROBOTS AND WHY USE THEM IN STROKE REHABILITATION?

The boundaries of robot technology overlap other emerging therapeutic technologies, such as electromechanical exercise devices and virtual reality therapy. Rehabilitation clinicians have employed electromechanical devices for decades. Continuous passive motion devices, treadmills, and isokinetic exercise machines perform automatic functions and can be programmed in advance. These relatively simple machines have primarily been used for orthopedic and sports medicine applications. Although some might consider these simple robots, we have used a somewhat stricter definition in this chapter.

The American Heritage Dictionary defines a robot as "(1) A mechanical device that sometimes resembles a human and is capable of performing a variety of often complex human tasks on command or by being programmed in advance. (2) A machine or device that operates automatically or by remote control" (2). In practice, general-purpose, anthropomorphic (human-appearing) robots have found little practical application in medicine, although they continue to captivate the popular imagination. The robots developed for rehabilitation have been specialized devices that bear little or no resemblance to humans and are of varying sizes, shapes, and complexity (see Figure 19-1). They share an increasing level of sophistication, with increasing capabilities and programmability.

USES OF ROBOTS IN STROKE REHABILITATION

Although the potential uses of robots in stroke rehabilitation are broad, we divide potential applications into two major categories: exercise training and as aids for activities of daily life (ADL). This chapter provides an overview of the arguments for and against the incorporation of these technologies into stroke rehabilitation in

these different roles and the various clinical circumstances in which they might prove useful. The development of robots for each of these potential applications is at different stages, ranging from limited clinical use (robot arms as ADL tools) to research only (powered orthoses). Clinical research results are reviewed, where applicable.

Robot-aided Exercise

Exercise is one of the key therapeutic modalities in stroke rehabilitation. Exercise treatments are most commonly provided under the direct personal supervision of physical therapists, occupational therapists, exercise physiologists, athletic trainers, or other practitioners. In many cases, this direct supervision is gradually withdrawn in favor of intermittent supervision as the patient progresses, and the patient is encouraged to engage in an independent exercise program at home or in a gym. This model of care requires extensive personnel time and, yet, is often unsuccessful in its ultimate goal of having patients independently performing exercises without direct supervision. Achieving long-term compliance with exercise programs remains a challenge in this traditional model of care because many patients discontinue exercises because of motivational factors.

The use of robots and virtual reality systems to assist in stroke rehabilitation has been proposed as a labor-saving approach for the provision of exercise therapy. Technology-guided exercise can, in principle, be substituted for exercise provided under the direct guidance of a therapist. Models for incorporating these devices into an exercise program include (1) having a single therapist provide supervision to several patients working with training systems simultaneously, (2) having a patient work at home with a robot or virtual reality system with remote supervision from a therapist, or (3) having a patient work independently with a technology-based training system, with periodic review and adjustment of their exercise program by a therapist.

The use of robots and virtual reality systems might enhance functional outcomes for certain conditions when compared with traditional exercise therapies. These systems offer a number of potential advantages over existing methods for the provision of therapeutic exercise. These potential advantages fall into two broad categories: economic savings through the use of automation and improved therapeutic outcomes.

The programmable nature of computer-based training devices allows the health care provider to design and institute an exercise program that is specific and well controlled. These devices can also be interactive and alter the therapy provided based on the patient's immediate reaction or response to treatment over time. The parameters of exercise that can be controlled through the use of robots include the nature of the exercise activity, the

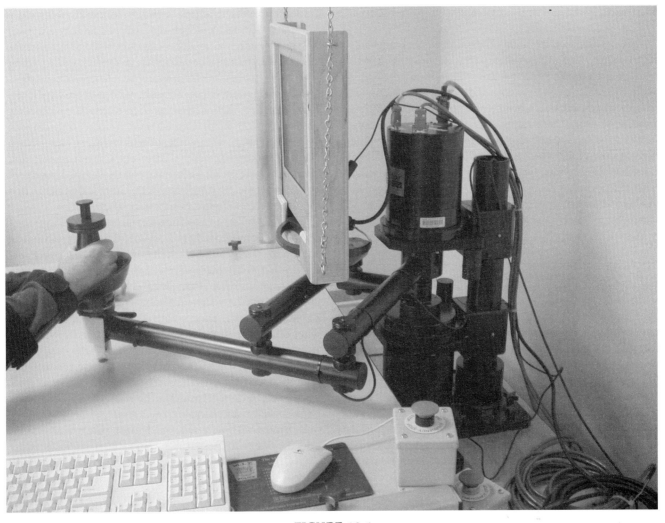

FIGURE 19-1

InMotion2 robot (Interactive Motion Technologies, Inc.), based on the MIT-Manus design, provides planar exercises for the upper limb involving shoulder and elbow movements.

movement pattern, the number of repetitions, the forces exerted by the robot on the patient, and others. Thus, there is the potential to deliver exercise in a more consistent fashion with robot aids and perhaps to improve the ultimate results of treatment.

For individuals with weakness, robots can provide physical assistance for task completion. Thus, for a stroke patient with some active movement at the shoulder and elbow, but unable to achieve antigravity strength, a robot might assist with a reaching movement. This capability is similar to that provided by a human therapist who provides individual treatment by facilitating/supporting movements in a weak patient but can be sustained for longer duration and more repetitions.

Resistance training has been studied as a therapy for post-stroke weakness (3, 4) and can be incorporated into robotic exercise (5, 6). While the possible therapeutic advantages of resistance training for hemiparetic stroke survivors continues to be studied, the availability of this mode of training in robotic exercise devices is an important capability and might be expected to be beneficial in certain clinical circumstances.

Robots can be designed and programmed to make repetitive exercise more interesting and enjoyable for a patient. Computer-based "video games" can be integrated with the robot training to provide a more stimulating therapy environment for the patient. Even relatively simple computer games, such as a "Pong"-type game, can relieve the boredom many patients associate with repetitive exercises. This ability to provide an interesting and structured environment for the performance of an exercise program holds promise as a means of improving compliance with exercise prescriptions in the future. More elaborate virtual reality visual displays are being developed, and some degree of convergence between the two approaches is likely.

Robots can collect data on exercise compliance and performance and allow the supervising practitioner to provide appropriate feedback to the patient regarding his/her exercise activities even when the practitioner is not physically present during the exercise session. This data can be stored electronically and reviewed at the convenience of the supervising therapist rather than at the time of the actual exercise. Compliance with prescribed exercise training can be directly measured rather than estimated from patient self-reports. From a research perspective, data obtained through robot devices have provided insights into the mechanisms of recovery of motor control after stroke (7–9).

Stationary Exercise Robots

Upper-limb robotic exercise training: Robotic devices for therapeutic exercise have been clinically tested for patients with neurologic diagnoses, including stroke, traumatic brain injury (TBI), multiple sclerosis, and spinal cord injury (SCI). Neurologic rehabilitation has been a particularly fertile field for robotic applications. For persons with stroke, it has been demonstrated that highly repetitive, task-specific exercise training can facilitate neuroplastic changes in the brain, with concomitant improved motor abilities and enhanced functional activity performance (10, 11). Robotic devices can provide such augmented exercise therapies in accurate and reproducible dosage; furthermore, they hold promise to become an economical complement to traditional, labor- and time-intensive neurologic rehabilitation.

Several research groups have tested the treatment effects of robotic therapy for poststroke, upper-limb motor recovery. The robots reported on in these clinical studies range in complexity from unimanual, single-joint devices to bimanual devices with multiple degrees of freedom. As with any emerging technology, devices are under development that have not yet been tested in clinical populations. This chapter focuses primarily on devices for which there are published reports in patient populations.

The MIT-Manus robot (InMotion2 robot, Interactive Motion Technologies, Inc., Cambridge, MA; see Figure 19-1) is a *two-degrees of freedom* robot that provides shoulder and elbow exercises in the horizontal plane. The patient's forearm and hand are supported and attached to the robot manipulandum with a splint. The MIT-Manus robot can administer active-assistive or resistive exercises or be programmed into a "passive" mode in which it provides neither resistance nor assistance. The design of the robot allows patients with a broad range of motor impairment to use this device. Even patients with severe weakness who are incapable of completing constraint-induced movement therapy can successfully

undergo exercise training with this robot. Training algorithms continue to be refined, and an adaptive active-assistive exercise mode has been developed that alters the amount of guidance or assistance provided to the patient based on his/her performance. An electromyographic-(EMG) triggered mode has been piloted in which the user's surface EMG activity is used to trigger the robotic assistance (12). In all exercise modes, subjects attempt to move the robotic arm while guided by target images on a computer monitor. Several different screen displays and accompanying motor tasks have been developed, although the best-studied "game" involves radial movements of a cursor in each of eight evenly spaced directions.

The MIT-Manus robot has been studied in a randomized controlled trial (13–15) of 76 patients within one month of stroke. Subjects in the treatment group received one hour of active-assistive exercises with the robot for the paretic arm five times per week for four weeks, and control subjects received sham exercise (i.e., with the robot in "passive" mode) with the robot once each week. The robotic therapy consisted of active-assistive reaching practice in the horizontal plane toward eight targets. All subjects received conventional rehabilitation therapy, per standard clinical practice, in addition to robotic therapy. At the end of treatment, the robot therapy subjects experienced significantly greater improvement in motor impairment on two scales (the Motor Status Scale [MSS] and the Medical Research Council Motor Power Scale [MRC]) for shoulder and elbow motor function. These improvements were maintained at the time of a three-year follow-up study (16).

The MIT-Manus robot has also been tested in four trials for persons with chronic hemiparesis after stroke. In one study (17), 42 subjects received either active-assistive or progressive-resistive reaching training for one-hour sessions, three times per week for six weeks. Subjects performed up to 18,000 point-to-point movements over the course of the trial. Subjects in the resistive and active-assistive treatment groups demonstrated significant impairment-level gains using several scales (Fugl-Meyer, MSS, MRC) that remained improved over baseline scores when measured at four-month follow-up evaluations. No differences in outcomes were detected between the resistance training and active-assistive training groups (5). The other studies of patients with chronic hemiparesis found similar improvements in motor function (18–21). Seventy-two subjects received active-assistive training using an adaptive training algorithm to adjust the amount of assistance to the person's movement ability using the MIT-Manus robot.

The benefits of robot-assisted upper-limb exercise therapy in these studies of MIT-Manus were seen primarily in shoulder and elbow movements, rather than in the wrist or hand. This is consistent with a specificity of training effect because the robot provides exercise only to these portions of the upper limb and keeps the wrist and hand immobilized in a splint. The magnitude of the changes in motor impairment has been clinically significant but modest, which would be expected given the limited nature of the robotic exercise. The training effects appear to persist over time (22). A related robot for wrist exercise has been developed, but the results of clinical trials of this device are not yet available. Devices to provide similar exercise to the hand are under development as well. Studies are underway to clarify if utilizing robotic modules serially for different limb segments (e.g., performing wrist exercises, followed by shoulder/elbow exercises) is more or less efficient than combining modules in multisegment configurations (e.g., wrist and shoulder/elbow exercises simultaneously) in achieving improved motor control. However, it is reasonable to speculate that the combined effects of training with multiple devices for different upper-limb segments will provide a larger benefit of overall motor function in the upper limb (23).

The mirror image movement enabler (MIME) robot is another device developed for upper-limb motor therapy after stroke (see Figure 19-2) (6). The MIME robot

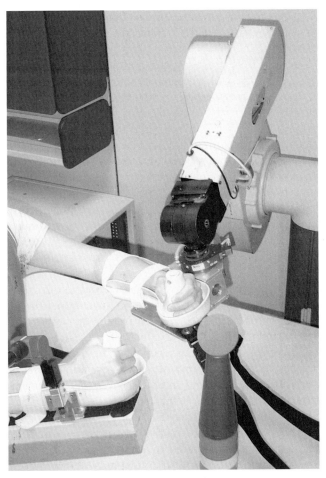

FIGURE 19-2

Mime robot, an upper limb robot with six degrees of freedom, designed to assist with reaching movements.

is a *six-degrees of freedom* robot that can administer four distinct modes of upper-limb reaching exercise in three dimensions. Similar to the MIT-Manus robot, the patient's forearm and hand are supported and attached to the robot with a splint. Unimanual exercises include passive, active-assistive, and active-constrained movements. During active-constrained exercise, the MIME robot resists reaching movements toward a target with a viscous field and provides a spring-like assist to movements in all other directions. Bimanual exercise is performed while subjects attempt to move both arms in simultaneous reaching movements; the robot assists the paretic limb's movements, as necessary, to mirror the less-impaired limb.

MIME robotic therapy has been compared to conventional neurodevelopmental technique-based therapy (NDT) in a study of 27 subjects with chronic hemiparesis after stroke in a randomized control trial (6). All subjects received 24 one-hour sessions over the course of two months. Subjects in the robotic treatment group practiced 12 reaching movements in four directions and three vertical levels. They received identical proportions of robot-guided passive and bimanual exercise and variable amounts of active-assisted and active-constrained exercise graded by individual motor ability. The NDT control group received exercises designed to facilitate a progression from mass upper-limb movement patterns to more isolated control, in the context of functional task performance. Immediate post-treatment results revealed that subjects in the robotic therapy group improved more than the control subjects for Fugl-Meyer Assessment scores (proximal section only), upper-limb strength measures, and free-reach distance. At six-month follow-up evaluations, the control group Fugl-Meyer scores improved relative to the treatment group such that the groups no longer differed significantly.

Reinkensmeyer and colleagues have developed the Assisted Rehabilitation and Measurement (ARM) Guide, a robot designed to administer active-assistive reaching practice in three dimensions (24). Although this robot provides only a single active degree of freedom, the linear track can be manually repositioned into different spatial orientations during the course of an exercise therapy session to allow a variety of movements. The patient's forearm and hand rest in a splint that attaches to a motorized, linear track, and the robot supports the arm against gravity and assists the patient to reach along the track. Visual feedback is provided through a computer monitor. Kahn and colleagues (25) tested the effects of the ARM Guide on reaching performance for patients with chronic hemiparetic stroke. Seven subjects received 24 one-hour robotic therapy sessions over the course of eight weeks, while another seven subjects received an equivalent dose of unassisted, goal-oriented reaching exercise. All subjects practiced repetitive reaching in multiple directions and vertical levels. After the trial, results of impairment-level measures were mixed. Neither group demonstrated improvements in free-reaching distance, all subjects showed improved straightness of reaching paths, and only the robotic therapy group showed improved movement smoothness. A timed measure of functional activities, the Functional Test for the Hemiparetic Upper Extremity, revealed significantly decreased performance times for the free-reach group and a trend toward improved performance for subjects who received robotic therapy. A one-degree of freedom robot with an adjustable track is available (26) (InMotion1 Linear Robot, Interactive Motion Technologies, Inc., 37 Spinelli Place, Cambridge, MA 02138, www.interactive-motion.com).

Hesse and colleagues tested a bimanual robotic therapy for its effects on distal motor impairment and function in a single-group exploratory study (27). This robotic arm trainer administered bimanual practice of wrist flexion/extension and forearm pronation/supination using active, passive, and resistive exercise. The robotic therapy was administered as an adjunct to a daily 45-minute comprehensive motor rehabilitation program. Twelve persons with chronic, hemiparetic stroke trained with the robot for fifteen 15-minute sessions over the course of three weeks. At the end of the robotic intervention, subjects showed reductions in wrist and finger spasticity as measured by the Modified Ashworth test, but there was no significant improvement in performance of functional motor activities according to Rivermead Motor Assessment scores. Participants reported favorable impressions of the robotic therapy.

A second study by Hesse and colleagues (28) compared this bimanual robotic training device to EMG initiated electrical stimulation of the paretic upper limb in hemiparetic individuals shortly after stroke (four to eight weeks post-stroke). Individuals receiving robot-aided exercise showed significantly larger improvements in Fugl-Meyer motor scores. The authors note that the robotic training group received a ten-fold increase in the number of repetitions than the EMG-triggered electrical stimulation, which they speculate was the reason for the different outcomes in the two groups.

Overall, published research on the use of robot-aided exercise for the upper limb after stroke is encouraging but not yet definitive. Differences in robot design and training algorithms make it difficult to compare studies and likely account for the variable results. Training-specific effects on motor function are evident and may be dose, device, and training-algorithm dependent. Further research needs to focus on expanding the scope of robot-aided exercise training to incorporate the entire upper limb and on continuing the exploration of the best training regimens and algorithms. Although stroke survivors are an appropriate population for study, consideration should be given to examining the effects of this type of training on other populations, such as individuals with spinal cord injury, traumatic brain injury, cerebral palsy, and others.

Lower extremity robotic exercise training: Robots for lower-limb use in neurologic rehabilitation have primarily been developed as devices for administering partial *body-weight–supported* treadmill gait training (BWST). BWST consists of partially unloading the weight of a neurologically impaired person suspended above a treadmill, while therapists manually assist the patient to step, shift weight, and maintain appropriate kinematic gait patterns during gait training. Several studies have reported improved gait performance after intensive BWST for persons with stroke (29), Parkinson's disease (30), and cerebral palsy (31), with inconclusive results after SCI (32, 33). BWST has not achieved wide translation into clinical practice, in no small part because it requires up to three therapists to perform physically demanding labor in often uncomfortable positions. One comparative study of BWST versus overground walking reported that therapists preferred to administer conventional gait training because of the physical demands imposed by the BWST (34).

Hesse and colleagues have developed a robotic device to automate BWST, called the electromechanical gait trainer (EGT) (35). Resembling an elliptical exercise trainer, the EGT uses footplates that move alternately to simulate stance and swing phases of a physiological gait pattern. A harness suspends patients above the footplates to provide for variable unweighting during gait training and reportedly serves to maintain the center of mass in a phase-dependent manner. Werner and colleagues (36) tested the EGT against conventional BWST in a randomized control trial involving 30 hemiparetic subjects who were four to twelve weeks after a stroke. All subjects required at least some physical assistance (Functional Ambulation Category [FAC] ≤ 2) for overground ambulation at baseline. Subjects were assigned to either an A-B-A or B-A-B crossover group. "A" consisted of two weeks of EGT therapy, and "B" consisted of two weeks of BWST therapy. They received experimental gait training 15–20 minutes daily in addition to conventional therapies for six weeks. At the end of treatment, both treatment groups demonstrated gains in FAC, gait velocity, and Rivermead Motor Assessment scores. The authors report that EMG measures of muscle activation patterns were similar for patients on both devices. The treatment group that received 2/3 epochs of EGT therapy had comparatively higher FAC scores, with more subjects able to ambulate independently; this advantage was no longer evident six months after treatment. Differences were reported in the amount of therapist assistance required for each treatment. At baseline, most patients using the EGT required one therapist, but they required two therapists for assistance using BWST. By the end of treatment, most patients could use the EGT without therapist assistance, whereas most patients needed assistance from one therapist while receiving BWST. The majority of subjects (23/30) reported that they preferred gait training with the EGT over the BWST.

A larger, multicenter study recently compared gait training with a combination of EGT plus conventional physical therapy with a group receiving conventional physical therapy alone in 155 subacute (average four to five weeks post-stroke) subjects (37). The EGT group showed a greater improvement in gait and ADL measures, both clinically and statistically, than the control group over the course of the four-week treatment protocol. Improved gait ability was maintained at six-month follow-up, though the difference in ADL ability was no longer evident.

Colombo and colleagues (38) have developed a lower-limb robot (driven gait orthosis [DGO]) for automated, intensive gait training. The DGO automates BWST by suspending two exoskeletal leg braces from a frame over a treadmill. Hip and knee motors in the exoskeletal braces are controlled by a computer to generate physiologically correct gait patterns for the patients who wear them. Ankle dorsiflexion is passively provided by elastic straps. The DGO requires a therapist operator but no direct human physical assistance while persons use the device for gait training. Studies examining the muscle activation patterns of subjects using the DGO compared with treadmill walking (39) and with manually assisted BWST (38, 40, 41) have shown conflicting results, and there is some evidence that users may reduce their effort during DGO assisted ambulation (41). A case series employing a DGO robot (Lokomat) (Hocoma AG, Industriestr 4b, CH-8604 Volkestwil, Switzerland; see Figure 19-3) found gait improvement in patients with chronic incomplete spinal cord injury (32). A randomized controlled pilot study

compared training with the Lokomat with conventional physical therapy in 30 acute stroke survivors (42), but it did not find any difference between the two groups with regard to functional measures of walking ability.

A clinical trial comparing gait training in stroke survivors with and without the Lokomat found that the magnitude of the gains seen with Lokomat training were smaller than those seen with non-robotic training (Hidler, personal communication).

A *two active* degree-of-freedom backdrivable robot for the ankle, the Anklebot, has been developed at MIT (Interactive Motion Technologies, Cambridge, MA; see Figure 19-4). No clinical studies have yet been reported with this device, however (23).

Potential Disadvantages and Limitations of Robot-aided Exercise. There are many characteristics of the present technology and robot design that limit the overall application of this type of therapeutic exercise. Generally speaking, existing robots are designed for very specific types of training and are limited in their degrees of freedom of motion. For example, the MIT-Manus robot provides

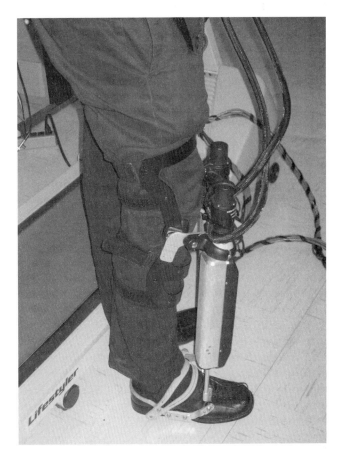

FIGURE 19-4

Anklebot (Interactive Motion Technologies, Inc.) is designed to assist and train ankle movements during gait.

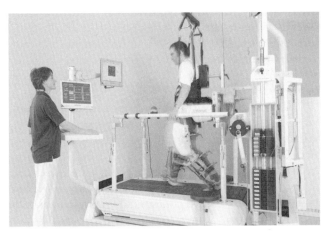

FIGURE 19-3

Lokomat robot (Hocoma, Inc.) provides partial body-weight support during assisted treadmill training.

only two degrees of freedom and is designed to provide reaching-type exercises for the shoulder and elbow (13). The MIME robot (6), although providing a larger number of degrees of freedom at the shoulder and elbow, does not include any robotic training for the wrist or hand. Solutions to this problem are being developed, including robots that provide multiple degrees of freedom at multiple joints at once as well as "robotic gyms," which provide several exercise robot tools analogous to "circuit training" in a gym (43).

Many existing upper-limb robots transmit force to the upper limb through a single point of contact, rather than exerting force at multiple limb segments. The rationale for this design is consistent with the paradigm shift introduced in early 1990s by two of the co-authors, H. I. Krebs and N. Hogan, that stimulated the growth of the area of therapeutic robotics: to assist the clinician delivering therapy and increase professional productivity (44). They designed their robots assuming that exercises requiring a small range of motion might suffice for these patients. Although it has the advantages of simplicity and perhaps safety, whether this limitation proves clinically relevant remains to be determined. At the moment, the best-studied robots (the MIT-Manus and MIME robots) are of this design, and robots that transmit force to multiple limb segments are exoskeletal in design.

Safety considerations have been addressed by robots for human exercise training, using a variety of approaches. The MIT-Manus robot uses an impedance controlled, "back-drivable" system for generating force that provides a highly compliant machine-user interface that allows the user's limb to deviate from the intended movement path while providing a progressive amount of corrective force to help the user achieve the desired position. This approach limits the corrective force and may reduce the risk of injury. Other robots, such as the MIME robot, have used more conventional machine-user interfaces with padding and safety cut-offs. These devices are not generally "back-drivable" and have a less compliant interaction with the user. Although not yet broadly used clinically, the robots being used to provide therapeutic exercise appear to have an excellent safety record. Whether such a record can be maintained outside of a carefully controlled research setting remains to be confirmed.

The development of training algorithms for robot-aided exercise remains in its early stages. Because of their programmable nature, there is no limit to the number of ways in which robot-assisted exercise can be designed. Questions remain regarding breaking down exercise tasks into simpler components versus performing more complex exercises, the importance of incorporating virtual environments, the most effective duration and frequency of training, the benefits of resistance training, and many other issues (45, 46). Fortunately, the availability of robotic exercise devices provides the scientific tools to answer these questions in the coming years.

Wearable Exoskeletal Robots/Robotic Orthoses

In contrast to the stationary exercise robots discussed above, robots are also being developed that are "wearable," known as wearable exoskeletal robots or powered orthoses. Such robots may be useful to provide therapeutic exercise (similar to stationary exercise robots) and/or as devices to help compensate for chronic weakness. (Note that robotic technology is being incorporated into prostheses as well [e.g., the "C-Leg"; Otto Bock USA, 2 Carlson Parkway, Suite 100, Minneapolis, MN 55447], but these are outside the scope of this chapter.) Wearable exoskeletal robots are in an earlier phase of development than stationary robots, and the benefits and risks of this approach are largely unknown. Potential advantages include the ability to move the location of therapy into a more "real-world" environment, rather than limiting treatment to a designated location in a health care facility.

Wearable exoskeletal robots may be deployed for two distinct but overlapping uses: as exercise devices and as compensatory aids (powered braces). Their use as exercise aids is similar in principle to the use of stationary robots—repetitive exercises facilitated (or even resisted) by the robot are used to improve motor control and/or strengthen muscles.

The use of wearable exoskeletal robots as compensatory aids has been proposed as a means of providing a "power assist" to chronically weak muscles. Such a robot might allow individuals to perform ADLs or ambulate independently despite severe weakness. Control and feedback mechanisms for this type of robot need further study and may vary with the nature and severity of weakness. A small pilot study of a powered elbow brace using surface EMG signals to control the level of torque provided found hemiparetic stroke survivors capable of using this device for exercise training (47). Improvements in motor control were seen, but larger studies are needed to further evaluate this technology (Myomo, Inc., 529 Main Street Suite 205; Boston, MA 02129, www.myomo.com).

Wearable exoskeletal robots may be capable of providing a substantial number of clinically relevant degrees of freedom, although practical considerations, including the bulk and weight of the exoskeletal robot, may limit the actual number of degrees of freedom achievable. The ability to apply forces at multiple limb segments, rather than at a single point of contact, adds both complexity and sophistication. Wearable exoskeletal robots have not yet achieved the same readiness for clinical application as stationary robots.

Potential disadvantages and limitations of wearable exoskeletal robots: Wearable exoskeletal robots need to function in a much more varied and less well-controlled environment than stationary robots. Accordingly, they may expose the user to unanticipated risks because situations arise that are beyond the intended activities of the robot. For ambulatory patients, issues such as falls while using a wearable exoskeletal robot need to be considered as a potential risk to both the user and the robotic device. The possibilities of striking oneself or being forced into an anatomically dangerous position are less easily prevented in a wearable exoskeletal robot design. Another design concern is the possibility of a mismatch between the machine kinematics and those of the limb(s) to which it is attached that could potentially generate forces large enough to cause injury. For certain movements, the bulkiness of the robot may directly reduce the usable range of motion. Issues of fit for individuals of varying size and shape need to be considered. Donning and doffing a wearable exoskeletal brace may also pose challenges and require the supervision of a skilled therapist.

Technical issues, such as a lightweight, portable power supply and actuators for wearable exoskeletal robots, remain a work in progress. Ideally, such robots would be lightweight, wearable devices that are as unobtrusive as possible. In reality, this goal has not yet been achieved. Power storage (i.e., batteries or their equivalent) is another limiting factor in wearable exoskeletal robotic design because existing power storage systems are suboptimal for this application. Actuators for wearable exoskeletal robots that are small, lightweight, durable, and generate sufficient force remain under development. Equally challenging is the need to develop effective and safe control systems for these devices. The use of surface or implantable EMG signals (48) or neural prostheses capable of capturing brain activity (49) are all under exploration and could potentially be applied to control powered orthoses.

Robots for ADL Assistance

Computer-based technologic aids have become an important component of assistive technology for individuals with severe disabilities. These devices have been used to aid in communication, to assist with powered mobility, and to assist in ADLs. Appropriately designed robotic devices may be useful to help with manipulating objects in the environment that the user is incapable of manipulating independently.

The Raptor® (Phybotics division of Applied Resources Corp., 1275 Bloomfield Avenue, Fairfield, NJ 07004; see Figure 19-5) and the ARM robot (Assistive Robotic Manipulator, also known as the Manus robot [not to be confused with the MIT-Manus robot]; Exact Dynamics, Edisonstraat 96, 6902 PK, Zevenaar, The Netherlands, www.exactdynamics.nl) are both robotic arms that mount on a power wheelchair. These robots are controlled by a joystick, keypad, or sip-and-puff interface

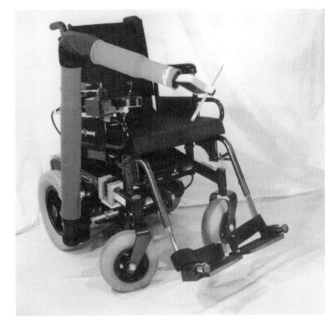

FIGURE 19-5

Raptor Robot (Phybotics, Inc.) is a wheelchair-mounted ADL robot arm that assists with reaching and grasping activities.

and can be used to pick up objects off the floor, open a refrigerator door and remove an item, etc. This type of robotic device is potentially useful for individuals with large brainstem strokes with bilateral weakness, as well as non-stroke conditions such as spinal cord injuries, limb deficiencies, and neuromuscular conditions.

This type of robot arm has a substantial number of degrees of freedom but may be slow and complex to master. The absence of proprioceptive feedback is compensated for by the use of visual monitoring of the robot's trajectory and target acquisition. The optimal terminal device (gripper) and force applied during robot grasp remain under study. Existing designs are capable of assisting in feeding, turning light switches on and off, and even opening doorknobs. There is little published research on the actual impact of these robots on independence in ADLs or number of hours of care needed. The psychological benefits of improved ability to manipulate one's own environment appear considerable, however, and are supported by case reports (50, 51) and small case series (52).

The Winsford Feeder (http://www.appliedresource. com/RTD/prod01.html) is a single-purpose feeding device that may be considered a simple robot. The user controls the device via a chin switch, rocker switch, or other switch. This simple robot reduces the amount of assistance needed by a disabled individual to self-feed. The device requires set up on the part of a caregiver but can provide meaningful improvements in independence. As with many sophisticated ADL aids, each prospective user needs to determine his or her own preferences for using a relatively complex device versus receiving assistance from a caregiver.

Potential Disadvantages and Limitations of ADL Robots. Technical issues include the absence of sensory feedback when using these devices, thus posing the risk of grasping an object too hard or not hard enough. These robot arm devices are slow and laborious to use and require patience, good perceptual abilities, and well-preserved cognitive abilities to master and use them appropriately. The risk of injury caused by misuse or errors appears small but has not been quantified.

The devices are designed for an intermediate degree of fine motor control. Tasks requiring very fine control, such as writing, or those that are bimanual in nature are not feasible with the current generation of devices.

Cost is a major consideration for ADL robots, as discussed below (see "Economic Considerations"). In contrast to exercise robots, which are typically used for a limited period of time in a therapeutic environment, ADL robots are intended for long-term use in a home setting. The Raptor robot costs approximately $14,000—a price that places this device outside the affordable range for most patients unless some funding source is identified.

Robotic Walkers

Robotic walkers have been proposed both as therapy aids during gait training and as functional aids during independent ambulation. The VA-PAMAID (Veterans Affairs Personal Adaptive Mobility Aid) is under development as a navigation aid for elderly individuals (53). Successful implementation of this type of robot will need to address issues of cost, weight, complexity, and stability.

Another type of robotic walker under development is designed to assist during gait training (KineAssist, ChicagoPT, LLC, Chicago, IL, www.chicagopt.com) (see Figure 19-6). This robot is designed to assist a physical therapist during gait training by providing external stabilization for the patient. The robot does not provide therapy per se, but rather facilitates conventional physical therapy training and reduces the need for additional staff members to provide physical assistance to the patient for safety. The robot is designed for a therapeutic environment rather than for use in the community, although it can be used outdoors on smooth surfaces. Limitations include a fairly large footprint, limiting use to relatively open areas. Clinical trials have not yet been conducted using this device.

VIRTUAL REALITY SYSTEMS

Virtual reality as been defined as "a realistic simulation of an environment, including three-dimensional graphics, by a computer system using interactive software and

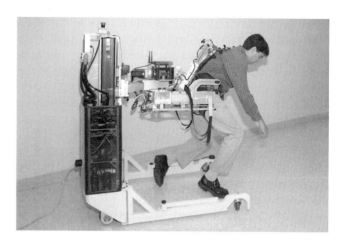

FIGURE 19-6

KineAssist (ChicagoPT, inc.) is a mobile robot to assist with gait training. The ability of the device to support a patient when losing balance is shown photo credit: Tom Probst, Movco Media Productions.

hardware" (54). Many computer/video games marketed for entertainment purposes utilize virtual reality to engage the user in highly complex environments, allowing the simulation of activities that would otherwise be impossible, impractical, or impermissible in real life.

Virtual reality (VR) shares some elements with robotic rehabilitation, with an emphasis on manipulating the sensory environment rather than the robotic approach of guiding movement. Sensory feedback in VR systems typically relies heavily on visual feedback, with auditory cues present in most systems as well. The incorporation of "haptic" (touch) feedback is present in some systems and provides another sensory modality that improves the simulation of the real world. An example of haptic feedback would be a handle held by the user that makes a brief shuddering movement when a simulated ball is hit with a simulated paddle.

Therapeutic use of virtual reality has been proposed for stroke survivors on several grounds. One potential advantage of virtual reality over conventional exercise is the ability to provide automated, continuous, real-time feedback regarding the accuracy of task performance. For example, a computer can provide an idealized trajectory for a reaching task and provide users with feedback regarding their success in adhering to this trajectory, including illustrating the movement needed to achieve the targeted trajectory.

Another proposed value of this technology over conventional exercise therapy is the ability to simulate activities that might otherwise pose excessive risk to the patient. For example, a virtual subway ride might provide the user with perturbations to standing balance comparable to those experienced during real subway ride, but do so in

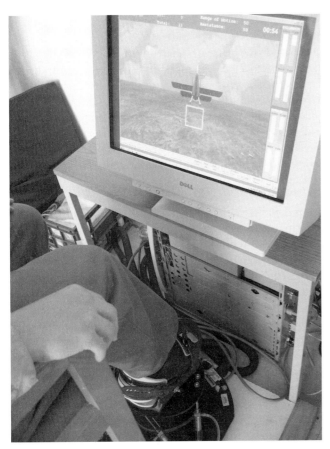

FIGURE 19-7

Rutgers Ankle platform and sample screen display showing flight simulator game.

an environment that provides safeguards (e.g., a harness) against falls and injury. Moreover, unlike a "real-world" activity, a virtual activity can be terminated at any time should the user become fatigued or at risk for injury.

Virtual reality is commonly implemented in the form of a "game," in which the user is provided with specific goals and some form of reward for success, such as an audible or visual signal or the accumulation of points. Games and virtual reality overlap in their implementations. Thus one could create a virtual environment in which a user perceives that he is walking through a virtual garden as he actually walks on a treadmill—an example of virtual reality without a game. Conversely, games may be created that are abstract and have little resemblance to a virtual environment, such as a "Pac-man" type game (in which a fantasy creature gobbles up "energy pills" in a two-dimensional maze). Practically speaking, however, most VR applications for rehabilitation do include some game elements to engage the user and direct their motor activity toward specific goals.

Perhaps the most cogent argument for incorporating virtual reality and other games into therapy for stroke

survivors is their ability to change tedious repetitive exercise tasks into engaging and challenging activities for the patient. The Rutgers ankle, for example, converts potentially tedious ankle dorsi/plantarflexion and inversion/eversion exercises into an engaging and even enjoyable flight simulator game (53) (see Figure 19-7). As with commercially available computer/video games used for entertainment, the motivation induced by the virtual games can be quite potent.

A number of upper-limb virtual reality training systems have been piloted, including some with telerehabilitation capabilities (56–58). Efforts to extend virtual reality training systems to the hand are ongoing. Virtual reality systems using a cyberglove and a haptic glove have been found feasible in pilot studies, with some evidence indicating improved motor performance in standard measures of upper-limb fine motor control, such as the Jebsen Test of Hand Function (58–61). While preliminary evidence of utility has been shown for several upper-limb virtual reality systems, definitive evidence of efficacy awaits larger, controlled clinical trials.

The T-WREX system consists of an exoskeletal orthosis that passively counterbalances the weight of the arm using elastic bands and provides a reduced-gravity virtual reality exercise program. Pilot studies suggest that use of this system by chronic hemiparetic stroke survivors is feasible and provide some preliminary evidence of efficacy (62). A commercial version of this device, the Armeo, is under development (see Figure 19-8) (Hocoma Inc., 100 Reservoir Park Dr., PO Box 553, Rockland, MA 02370).

Fewer lower-limb and mobility-oriented virtual reality systems have been developed. One system combining a

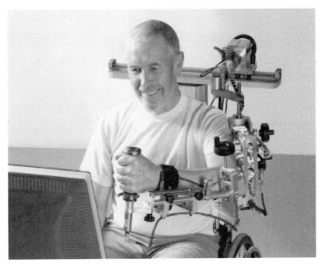

FIGURE 19-8

Armeo (Hocoma, Inc.) upper extremity virtual reality/exoskeletal training device.

virtual environment with a treadmill mounted on a six-degrees-of-freedom motion platform has been tested in a pilot study (63). The use of the system improved performance of the training tasks. A more recent study found that combining robotic therapy with virtual reality visual feedback was more effective in improving gait than a robotic system alone (Mirelman A, Bonato P, Deutsch JE. Effects of training with a robot–virtual reality system compared with a robot alone on the gait of individuals post stroke. *Stroke* [in press]). As with upper-limb training systems, larger and more definitive studies of efficacy are needed.

Virtual reality rehabilitation systems are becoming available for clinical use. The IREX is a virtual reality system intended for rehabilitation therapy that utilizes a motion capture system to integrate the user's movements with virtual games in a visual display (GestureTek Inc., 530 Lakeside Drive, Suite 270, Sunnyvale CA 94085). Pilot studies using this system for upper-limb retraining (64) and locomotor retraining (65) demonstrated improved motor function as well as concomitant changes in cortical activation patterns on fMRI (see Figure 19-9). Driving simulators are available from several vendors (e.g., DriveSafety, www.drivesafety.com) and have been shown to improve driving skills in stroke survivors (66).

Virtual reality therapy has been explored as a treatment for hemispatial neglect after stroke (67, 68). These and other computer-based training systems for treatment of neglect are discussed further in Chapter 12. Computer-based training has also been used for treatment of visual field defects after stroke, such as the Novavision VRT system (Novavision, Boca Raton, FL) and is discussed further in Chapter 15.

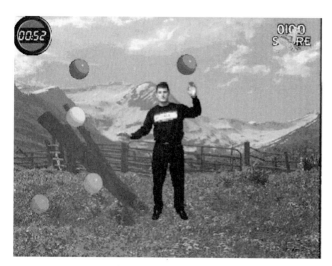

FIGURE 19-9

Sample screen display from the IREX system (Gesturetek, Inc).

Potential disadvantages and limitations of virtual reality systems: Highly immersive virtual reality systems, such as those utilizing head-mounted visual displays, have generally been avoided in patients with moderate or severe deficits after stroke because of concerns that the virtual environment may be overwhelming for these individuals. Some have argued that simplified games that do not seek to mimic reality are more appropriate for stroke survivors and have raised concerns that excessively realistic environments might interfere with successful motor retraining (69).

"Cybersickness," a form of motion sickness resulting from the mismatch between visual and vestibular sensory information, has been described in healthy individuals as well as those with disabilities undergoing rehabilitation. Delays between movements and their visual display appear to be a contributing factor. While clinicians treating patients with virtual reality systems need to be aware of this possible side effect, this issue has not been a major impediment in the development of virtual reality systems.

Virtual reality gait training studies have raised concerns regarding generalization to "real-world" environments with a distinct set of challenges (e.g. curbs, uneven or slippery surfaces) compared with the virtual training environment (63). Another study found that task performance in a virtual reality environment did not correlate strongly with "real-world" task performance of similar tasks (70). The errors seen in the virtual and the real-world environments differed as well. Despite efforts to match virtual reality simulations to real-world activities, discrepancies remain. Given the simulated nature of virtual reality, it is almost axiomatic that the training environment will fail to precisely duplicate all of the sensory stimuli present in the corresponding real-world task. These mismatches may be a limiting factor in this type of therapy.

ROBOTS AND VIRTUAL REALITY SYSTEMS FOR REMOTE PRESENCE AND TELEREHABILITATION

Many stroke survivors have difficulty leaving their home for rehabilitation and medical services. Traditional home care services are very labor intensive and inefficient, in large part because of the time required for travel between treatment locations. Telemedicine systems have been used as a component of home care, including some oversight of rehabilitation services (71).

Many robotic and virtual reality systems lend themselves to telerehabilitation and can be supervised remotely. Thus a stationary robotic device (particularly an upper-limb device) could be situated in a patient's home and remotely supervised by a therapist in a distant location. The feasibility of this approach has been demonstrated

(72, 73), but definitive trials of efficacy have not yet been performed.

In addition to these stationary telemedicine devices, mobile robotic devices have been proposed for use in the home that could "follow" the patient around his/her home and provide supervision of rehabilitation in different rooms and during varying activities. Robots have been proposed as a means of providing a mobile telerehabilitation link for homebound individuals. Mobile robots can provide visual and auditory links between a patient in a home environment and a medical provider in a remote location. As robots grow more sophisticated, autonomous interaction with the patient without the simultaneous involvement of a remote operator may be feasible to oversee medical care and safety in a home setting.

Issues of privacy could theoretically arise with these devices, although these seem easily addressed with appropriate protocols and devices. User acceptance, however, is less well established, and some individuals many nonetheless find such a device intrusive or undesirable. In particular, autonomous robots may be perceived as irritating or unwanted by the user.

Mobile telerehabilitation robots may encounter difficulties with obstacles in the home, such as stairs, rugs, furniture, etc. Robot vision systems remain in the early phase of development and are not yet capable of incorporation into home-based rehabilitation robots. Thus, environmental obstacles may limit their ability to successfully navigate and self-propel.

ECONOMIC CONSIDERATIONS

In more developed countries, such as the United States, Japan, and Western Europe, there has been a steady downward trend in the cost of technology-based devices, while at the same time, labor costs continue to rise. As a result, there has been an ongoing substitution of computer-based devices for workers, whenever feasible. Examples of this substitution abound and include the ubiquitous use of automated teller machines instead of bank tellers, the growing use of check-in kiosks in airports rather than airline representatives, and the continued growth of industrial robots in manufacturing to reduce the number of assembly line workers. Medicine is not immune to these trends, although it has been slower to adopt this approach than many other fields. One example of automation is the use of pharmacy dispensing systems that are now widespread in hospitals and help reduce the manual labor involved in managing medication inventories.

This trend of reducing the number of skilled workers required in favor of technological substitutes shows no sign of abating, and the economic forces that drive it are likely to persist or even accelerate. The aging of the population is now a major challenge in Japan, and the shortage of workers to assist older individuals is stimulating Japanese companies to explore devices to help bathe and care for the elderly. The United States population is also aging, and shortages of nurses and personal care attendants already plague health care systems in many areas of the United States.

The incorporation of newer technologies in rehabilitation depends in part on their cost and in part on reimbursement. In particular, assistive technology often is not adequately or not at all reimbursed by third-party payers because of annual caps on payment or definitions of "medically necessary devices." Although an ADL robot may provide substantial improvements in independence, it is not intended to directly treat the patient's medical condition, and thus may not be considered "medically necessary." Large randomized clinical trials comparing robotic and virtual reality systems with present rehabilitation techniques, and demonstrating "clinically meaningful improvement," need to be completed before third-party payers will reimburse their costs. Comparative costs for these systems also must fall substantially, or else the economics of incorporating these technologies into rehabilitation will remain unfavorable, unless research demonstrates added value in using these systems over present rehabilitation techniques.

Because of the novelty of therapeutic robots and virtual reality systems, these are still commonly used with direct supervision by a skilled caregiver (typically a physical or occupational therapist). Thus, little of the opportunity for these devices to be truly labor-saving has yet been realized. Over time, it is reasonable to expect that greater familiarity with these devices and simplified user interfaces will allow more autonomous use of technology aided exercise therapy. Therapy might be provided in a group setting in a "high-tech" gym with a therapy aide providing intermittent supervision or even in a home-based treatment program without the presence of a health care worker during treatment sessions.

The specialized design and limited range of activities that the current generation of devices provide, however, preclude using them as substitutes for human-provided therapy, even if they can be operated autonomously. As an example, an upper-limb exercise training robot cannot teach a stroke patient to dress herself or manage her hygiene, as an occupational therapist would. Thus, in the intermediate term, the likely role of robots and virtual reality systems are as adjuncts to skilled therapists—perhaps more of a rehabilitation "aide" than "therapist." Genuine cost savings appear at least several years in the future but seem inevitable as the efficiency of delivering these types of therapy improves. Ultimately, cost-effectiveness studies are needed to determine the appropriate utilization of these technologies.

RESEARCH FRONTIERS

Engineering advances in computer technology and in the implementation of clinical applications is proceeding at a rapid pace. Successful commercialization of one or more robotic and/or virtual reality devices is likely to enhance investment in industrial research and development, and further accelerate the rate of change.

As Yogi Berra is alleged to have said, "It's tough to make predictions, especially about the future." Many technological advances in stroke rehabilitation are impossible to foresee at this time.

One key question is the role of complexity in further technology development. Many new consumer technologies have become increasingly complex as new capabilities are added. While some consumers have avidly adopted these new technologies, others have found them confusing and distracting, as evidenced by the recent reemergence of simplified cell phones that lack built-in cameras, text messaging, and internet access in favor of simply functioning as a phone. Stroke survivors are often coping with perceptual and cognitive impairments, and concerns exist regarding their ability to effectively use highly complex systems. Cost concerns are also important, as more complex systems are generally more expensive than simpler systems. Ultimately, clinical trials will need to compare different approaches to determine the most effective strategy.

Larger randomized controlled trials of the efficacy of these treatment approaches are needed to validate preliminary evidence of efficacy seen in smaller studies. Research in the application of technologically based therapies will also need to clarify the relative efficacy and efficiency of strategies that seek to combine complex multiple limb segment training in a single activity versus training systems that use a more modular approach for training individual limb segments and movements. For example, it is not yet clear if it is better to perform upper-limb exercises incorporating the shoulder, elbow, wrist, and hand in a single movement versus individual exercises for these joints. Ultimately, randomized clinical trials will need to demonstrate "clinically meaningful improvement" in order to be accepted and reimbursed as effective therapies.

CONCLUSION

Stroke rehabilitation robots and virtual reality training systems are undergoing a phase of rapid development and testing and are likely to begin to appear in clinical settings on a regular basis within the next few years. Special purpose devices are likely to remain the mainstay of stroke rehabilitation technology for years to come, given the extraordinary complexity of attempting to create general purpose rehabilitation devices. Cost considerations and reimbursement issues are likely to grow in importance as the cost/benefit ratio of incorporating these technologies into stroke rehabilitation is debated.

References

1. Stein J, Hughes R, Fasoli S, et al. Clinical applications of robots in rehabilitation. *Critical Reviews in Physical and Rehabilitation Medicine* 2005; 17(3):217–230.
2. *The American Heritage® Dictionary of the English Language.* 4th ed. Boston: Houghton Mifflin Company, 2000.
3. Oullette, MM, LeBrasseur NK, Bean J, et al. High-intensity resistance training improves self-reported function and disability in long-term stroke survivors. *Stroke* 2004; 35:1404–1409.
4. Patten C, Lexell J, Brown HE. Weakness and strength training in persons with poststroke hemiplegia: rationale, method, and efficacy. *J Rehabil Res Dev.* 2004; 41(3A):293–312.
5. Stein J, Krebs HI, Frontera WR, et al. A comparison of two techniques of robot-aided upper limb exercise training after stroke. *Am J Phys Med Rehabil.* 2004; 83:720–728.
6. Lum PS, Burgar CG, Shor PC, et al. Robot-assisted movement training compared with conventional therapy techniques for the rehabilitation of upper-limb motor function after stroke. *Arch Phys Med Rehabil.* 2002; 83:952–959.
7. Krebs HI, Hogan N, Aisen ML, Volpe BT. Quantization of continuous arm movement in humans with brain injury. *Proc Natl Acad Sci U S A.* 1999; 96:4645–4649.
8. Rohrer B, Fasoli S, Krebs HI, et al. Movement smoothness changes during stroke recovery. *J Neurosci.* 2002; 22(18):8297–8304.
9. Rohrer B, Fasoli S, Krebs HI, et al. Submovements grow fewer, larger, and more blended during stroke recovery. *Motor Control.* 2004; 8(4):472–483.
10. Liepert J, Bauder H, Wolfgang HR, et al. Treatment-induced cortical reorganization after stroke in humans. *Stroke* 2000; 31:1210–1216.
11. Levy CE, Nichols DS, Schmalbrock PM, et al. Functional MRI evidence of cortical reorganization in upper-limb stroke hemiplegia treated with constraint-induced movement therapy. *Am J Phys Med Rehabil.* 2001; 80:4–12.
12. Dipietro L, Ferraro M, Palazzolo JJ, et al. Customized interactive robotic treatment for stroke: EMG-triggered therapy. *IEEE Transactions on Neural Systems & Rehabilitation Engineering* 2005; 13(3):325–334.
13. Aisen FL, Krebs HI, Hogan N, et al. The effect of robot-assisted therapy and rehabilitative training on motor recovery following stroke. *Arch Neurol.* 1997; 54:443–446.
14. Volpe BT, Krebs HI, Hogan N, et al. A novel approach to stroke rehabilitation: robot-aided sensorimotor stimulation. *Neurology.* 2000; 54(10):1938–1944.
15. Krebs HI, Volpe BT, Ferraro M, et al. Robot-aided neurorehabilitation: from evidence-based to science-based rehabilitation. *Top Stroke Rehabil.* 2002; 8:54–70.
16. Volpe BT, Krebs HI, Hogan N, et al. Robot training enhanced motor outcome in patients with stroke maintained over 3 years. *Neurology.* 1999; 53(8):1874–1876.
17. Fasoli SE, Krebs HI, Stein J, et al. Effects of robotic therapy on motor impairment and recovery in chronic stroke. *Arch Phys Med Rehabil.* 2003; 84:477–482.
18. Ferraro M, Palazzolo JJ, Krol J, et al. Robot-aided sensorimotor arm training improves outcome in patients with chronic stroke. *Neurology* 2003; 61:1604–1607.
19. Finley, MA, Fasoli, SE, Dipietro, L, et al. Short duration upper extremity robotic therapy in stroke patients with severe upper extremity motor impairment. *VA Journal Rehabilitation Research and Development* 2005; 42(5):683–692.
20. Daly, J, Hogan, N, Perepezko, E, et al. Response to upper limb robotics and functional neuromuscular stimulation following stroke. *VA Journal of Rehabilitation Research and Development* 2005; 42(6)723–736.
21. MacClellan, LR, Bradham, DD, Whitall, J, et al Robotic upper extremity neuro-rehabilitation in chronic stroke patients. *VA Journal of Rehabilitation Research and Development* 2005; 42(6)717–722.
22. Fasoli SE, Krebs HI, Stein J, et al. Robotic therapy for chronic motor impairments after stroke: follow-up results. *Arch Phys Med Rehabil.* 2004; 85:1106–1111.
23. Krebs, HI, Hogan, N, therapeutic robotics: a technology push. *Proceedings of IEEE* 2006; 94(9)1727–1738.
24. Reinkensmeyer DJ, Kahn LE, Averbuch M, et al. Understanding and treating arm movement impairment after chronic brain injury: progress with the ARM guide. *J Rehabil Res Dev.* 2000; 37(6):653–662.
25. Kahn LE, Zygman ML, Rymer WZ, Reinkensmeyer DJ. Effect of robot-assisted and unassisted exercise on functional reaching in chronic hemiparesis. *Conference Proceedings of the 23rd Annual International Conference of the IEEE Engineering in Medicine and Biology Society.* Istanbul 2001; 4(4132).
26. Krebs, HI, Ferraro, M, Buerger, SP, et al. rehabilitation robotics: pilot trial of a spatial extension for MIT-Manus. *Journal of NeuroEngineering and Rehabilitation, Biomedcentral* 2004; 1:5.

27. Hesse S, Schulte-Tigges G, Konrad M, et al. Robot-assisted arm trainer for the passive and active practice of bilateral forearm and wrist movements in hemiparetic subjects. *Arch Phys Med Rehabil* 2003; 84(6):915–920.

28. Hesse S, Werner C, Pohl M, et al. Computerized arm training improves the motor control of the severely affected arm after stroke: a single-blinded randomized trial in two centers. *Stroke* 2005; 36(9):1960–1966.

29. Sullivan KJ, Knowlton BJ, Dobkin BH. Step training with body weight support: effect of treadmill speed and practice paradigms on poststroke locomotor recovery. *Arch Phys Med Rehabil*. 2002; 83(5):683–691.

30. Miyai I, Fujimoto Y, Ueda Y, et al. Treadmill training with body weight support: its effect on Parkinson's disease. *Arch Phys Med Rehabil*. 2000; 81(7):849–852.

31. Schindl MR, Forstner C, Kern H, Hesse S. Treadmill training with partial body weight support in nonambulatory patients with cerebral palsy. *Arch Phys Med Rehabil* 2000; 81(3):301–306.

32. Wirz M, Zemon DH, Rupp R, et al. Effectiveness of automated locomotor training in patients with chronic incomplete spinal cord injury: a multicenter trial. *Arch Phys Med Rehabil*. 2005; 86(4):672–680.

33. Dobkin B, Apple D, Barbeau H, et al. Spinal cord injury locomotor trial group. weight-supported treadmill vs over-ground training for walking after acute incomplete SCI. *Neurology* 2006; 66(4):484–493,

34. Kosak MC, Reding MJ. Comparison of partial body weight-supported treadmill gait training versus aggressive bracing assisted walking post stroke. *Neurorehabil Neural Repair* 2000; 14(1):13–19.

35. Hesse S, Werner C, Uhlenbrock D, et al. An electromechanical gait trainer for restoration of gait in hemiparetic stroke patients: preliminary results. *Neurorehabil Neural Repair* 2001; 15:39–50.

36. Werner C, Von Frankenberg S, Treig T, et al. Treadmill training with partial body weight support and an electromechanical gait trainer for restoration of gait in subacute stroke patients: a randomized crossover study. *Stroke* 2002; 33(12):2895–2901.

37. Pohl M, Werner C, Holzgraefe M, et al. Repetitive locomotor training and physiotherapy improve walking and basic activities of daily living after stroke: a single-blind, randomized multicentre trial (DEutsche GAngtrainerStudie, DEGAS). *Clinical Rehabilitation* 2007; 21: 17–27.

38. Colombo G, Wirz M, Dietz V. Driven gait orthosis for improvement of locomotor training in paraplegic patients. *Spinal Cord* 2001; 39(5):252–255.

39. Hidler JM, Wall AE. Alterations in muscle activation patterns during robotic-assisted walking. *Clin Biomechanics* 2005; 20:184–193.

40. Dietz V, Muller R, Colombo G. Locomotor activity in spinal man: significance of afferent input from joint and load receptors. *Brain* 2002; 125(Pt 12):2626–2634.

41. Israel, JF, Campbell DD, Kahn JH, Hornby TG. Metabolic costs and muscle activity patterns during robotic- and therapist-assisted treadmill walking in individuals with incomplete spinal cord injury. *Phys Ther*. 2006; 86(11): 1466–1478.

42. Husemann B, Muller F, Krewer C, et al. Effects of locomotion training with assistance of a robot-driven gait orthosis in hemiparetic patients after stroke: a randomized controlled pilot study. *Stroke* 2007; 38(2):349–354.

43. Krebs HI, Volpe BT, Lynch D. Stroke rehabilitation: an argument in favor of a robotic gym [abstract]. Presented at the International Conference on Rehabilitation Robotics (ICORR), Chicago 2005. Digital Object Identifier 10.1109/ICORR.2005.1501089.

44. Krebs HI, Hogan N, Aisen ML, Volpe BT. Robot-aided neurorehabilitation. *IEEE Transactions on Rehabilitation Engineering* 1998; 6(1):75–87.

45. Fasoli, SE, Krebs. HI, Hogan, N. robotic technology and stroke rehabilitation: translating research into practice. *Topics in Stroke Rehabilitation* 2004; 11(4):11–19.

46. Fasoli, SE, Krebs, HI, Hughes, R, et al. Functionally-based rehabilitation robotics: A next step? *International Journal of Assistive Robotics and Mechatronics* 2006; 7(2), 26–30.

47. Stein J, Narendran K, McBean J, et al. EMG-controlled exoskeletal upper limb powered orthosis for exercise training post-stroke. *Am J Phys Med Rehabil*. 2007; 86:255–261.

48. Kuiken TA, Dumanian GA, Lipschutz RD, et al. The use of targeted muscle reinnervation for improved myoelectric prosthesis control in a bilateral shoulder disarticulation amputee. *Prosthet Orthot Int*. 2004; 28(3):245–253.

49. Friehs GM, Zerris VA, Ojakangas CL, et al. Brain-machine and brain-computer interfaces. *Stroke* 2004; 35(11 Suppl 1):2702–2705.

50. Bach JR, Zeelenberg AP, Winter C. Wheelchair-mounted robot manipulators. Long term use by patients with Duchenne muscular dystrophy. *Am J Phys Med Rehabil*. 1990; 69(2):55–59.

51. Hammel JM, Van der Loos HF, Perkash I. Evaluation of a vocational robot with a quadriplegic employee. *Arch Phys Med Rehabil*. 1992; 73(7):683–693.

52. Chaves E, Koontz AM, Garber S, et al. Clinical evaluation of a wheelchair mounted robotic arm. Presented at RESNA meeting, Atlanta, 2003. Accessed at http://www.resna.org/ProfResources/Publications/Proceedings/2003/Papers/sSPWinner/Chaves_SM.php on 12/27/06.

53. Rentschler AJ, Cooper RA, Blasch B, Boninger ML. Intelligent walkers for the elderly: performance and safety testing of VA-PAMAID robotic walker. *J Rehabil Res Dev*. 2003; 40(5):423–431.

54. Dictionary.com, Unabridged (v 1.1). Retrieved December 24, 2006, from Dictionary.com website: http://dictionary.reference.com/browse/virtual reality.

55. Deutsch JE, Latonio J, Burdea G, Boian R. Post–Stroke Rehabilitation with the Rutgers Ankle System—A case study. *Presence* 2001; 10:416–430.

56. Crosbie J, McDonough S, Lennon S, McNeill M. Development of a virtual reality system for the rehabilitation of the upper limb after stroke. *Studies in Health Technology & Informatics* 2005; 117:218–222.

57. Holden MK, Dettwiler A, Dyar T, et al. Retraining movement in patients with acquired brain injury using a virtual environment. *Stud Health Technol Inform* 2001; 81:192–198.

58. Kuttuva M. Boian R. Merians A. et al. The Rutgers Arm, a rehabilitation system in virtual reality: a pilot study. *Cyberpsychology & Behavior* 2006; 9(2):148–151.

59. Merians AS, Jack D, Boian R, et al. Virtual reality-augmented rehabilitation for patients following stroke. *Phys Ther*. 2002; 82:898–915.

60. Merians AS, Poizner H, Boian R, et al. Sensorimotor training in a virtual reality environment: does it improve functional recovery poststroke? *Neurorehabilitation & Neural Repair* 2006; 20(2):252–267.

61. Boian R, Sharma A, Han C, et al. Virtual reality-based post-stroke hand rehabilitation. *Studies in Health Technology & Informatics* 2002; 85:64–70.

62. Sanchez RJ, Liu J, Rao S, et al. Automating arm movement training following severe stroke: functional exercises with quantitative feedback in a gravity-reduced environment. *IEEE Transactions on Neural Systems & Rehabilitation Engineering* 2006; 14(3):378–389.

63. Fung J, Richards CL, Malouin F, et al. A treadmill and motion coupled virtual reality system for gait training post-stroke. *Cyberpsychology & Behavior* 2006; 9(2):157–162.

64. Jang SH, You SH, Hallett M, et al. Cortical reorganization and associated functional motor recovery after virtual reality in patients with chronic stroke: an experimenter-blind preliminary study. *Archives of Physical Medicine & Rehabilitation* 2005; 86(11):2218–2223.

65. You SH, Jang SH, Kim YH, et al. Virtual reality-induced cortical reorganization and associated locomotor recovery in chronic stroke: an experimenter-blind randomized study. *Stroke* 2005; 36(6):1166–1171.

66. Akinwuntan AE, De Weerdt W, Feys H, et al. Effect of simulator training on driving after stroke: a randomized controlled trial. *Neurology* 2005; 65(6):843–850.

67. Castiello U, Lusher D, Burton C, et al. Improving left hemispatial neglect using virtual reality. *Neurology* 2004; 62(11):1958–1962.

68. Katz N, Ring H, Naveh Y, et al. Interactive virtual environment training for safe street crossing of right hemisphere stroke patients with unilateral spatial neglect. *Disability & Rehabilitation* 2005; 27(20):1235–1243.

69. Krebs HI, Hogan N. Personal communication 2007.

70. Edmans JA, Gladman JR, Cobb S, et al. Validity of a virtual environment for stroke rehabilitation. *Stroke* 2006; 37(11):2770–2775.

71. Lewis JA, Boian RF, Burdea G, Deutsch JE. Remote console for virtual telerehabilitation. *Studies in Health Technology & Informatics* 2005; 111:294–300.

72. Piron L, Tonin P, Trivello E, et al. Motor tele-rehabilitation in post-stroke patients. *Medical Informatics & the Internet in Medicine* 2004; 29(2):119–125.

73. Carignan CR, Krebs HI. Telerehabilitation robotics: Bright lights, big future? *J Rehabil. Res. Dev.* 2006; 43(5): 695–710.

20 Walking Recovery and Rehabilitation after Stroke

Katherine J. Sullivan
Sara Mulroy
Steven A. Kautz

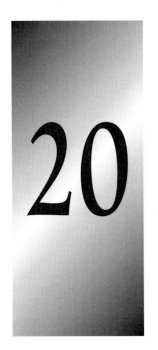otor control deficits are a common manifestation of and a major contributor to walking disability after stroke. As a result, limitations in mobility related to walking are evident in 75% of individuals who sustain a stroke each year (1). During the first six weeks post-stroke, the majority of stroke survivors will regain some ability to walk; however, 40% will have severe motor impairment that restricts functional walking to household ambulation. For those with mild to moderate motor impairment, independent walking ability is likely, but of those who achieve physical independence in walking, 60% will be limited in community ambulation (2). Furthermore, motor impairments that limit walking ability contribute to balance deficits after stroke. Individuals who have mild to moderate motor impairment and are functional ambulators after stroke have a 73% incidence of falls within the first six months post-stroke (3, 4). This culminates in a fourfold increase in falls risk after stroke and among those who fall, a tenfold increase in hip fracture.

The greatest predictor of community ambulation and participation in home and community mobility is walking speed (5). Perry et al. conducted a cross-sectional study of individuals with gait impairments after chronic stroke and classified them into one of six functional walking categories based on the degree of community ambulation and social interaction (5). The most significant difference between groups was preferred walking speed, with mean speeds ranging from slower than 0.4 meters per second (m/s) for household walkers, 0.4–0.8 m/s for limited community walkers, and faster than 0.8 m/s for unlimited community walkers. As expected, the higher the amount of community ambulation ability, the more likely one was to participate in social activities such as family outings, grocery shopping, going to church, etc. However, achieving the break point of faster than 0.8 m/s (1.8 mph) in walking speed only represents 60% of what is normal for most healthy adults (6). Thus, the functional impact of walking impairment after stroke is significant. Activity outcome measures of walking function such as the Barthel Index (BI) (7) or the Functional Independence Measure (FIM) (8) are poor indicators of community mobility and participation after stroke since the majority of stroke survivors can achieve high BI or FIM scores (i.e., independent walking 10 meters or less) without any consideration of walking speed.

The impact of motor control impairments and walking disability extends beyond the acute and subacute phases to the chronic phase post-stroke. Post-stroke, lower-extremity, motor control deficits contribute to specific lower-extremity primary and secondary motor impairments and activity restrictions that impact balance ability and walking skills and increases the risk of secondary complications related to impaired walking ability such as an increased risk of falls and hip fracture, and, ultimately, mobility limitations that restrict participation across the lifespan for an individual post-stroke. Walking recovery and rehabilitation after stroke includes therapeutic strategies that are designed to address the complicated and multivariate predictors of walking function. The overall purpose of this chapter is to describe all of the following:

1. Biomechanical features of post-stroke walking impairment
2. Primary and secondary motor impairments and recovery factors that contribute to activity restrictions in the acute and chronic phases post-stroke
3. Effects of stroke severity (i.e., severe compared to mild-moderate sensorimotor impairment) and secondary impairments on walking outcomes
4. Rehabilitation interventions for post-stroke walking recovery that are currently being used in practice to address the sensorimotor sequelae of stroke

BIOMECHANICS OF POST-STROKE GAIT

Stroke results in a constellation of sensorimotor impairments such as weakness, impaired selective motor control, spasticity, and proprioceptive deficits that interfere with the invariant features of normal adult gait. There is a wide range of walking ability after stroke that depends on the severity of these sensorimotor impairments. After stroke, there are obvious gait deviations that can be observed during observational gait analysis. Biomechanical gait characteristics such as spatiotemporal features (i.e., interlimb symmetry), kinematics (i.e., joint motion relationships within and between limbs), and kinetics (i.e., forces required for stance and forward progression) can be quantified in an appropriately instrumented gait lab. This section describes the biomechanical features of post-stroke gait since biomechanical analysis is an essential element for understanding the mechanisms of walking recovery and responsiveness to specific walking rehabilitation interventions.

Changes in Temporal Gait Characteristics

While asymmetry is a dominant characteristic of hemiparetic walking, the heterogeneity of the hemiparetic population has made it difficult to develop an integrative understanding of how spatiotemporal asymmetry is related to the underlying impairments. There are a multitude of variables that have been used to quantify spatiotemporal asymmetry, and inconsistent reporting of important variables has limited our understanding of the basis of asymmetry. For example, temporal asymmetry is often reported, while spatial asymmetry is not (or vice versa), with few studies reporting both variables

in detail. Additionally, the general speed dependence of spatiotemporal characteristics must also be considered when interpreting hemiparetic spatiotemporal data (9) because most persons with hemiparesis walk slowly with an altered stride length and/or cadence. Despite all of the complications that have limited a more detailed understanding of hemiparetic spatiotemporal asymmetry, some general relationships are beginning to emerge.

For example, walking speed is determined by a combination of cadence and stride length (distance between consecutive foot placements of the same foot in the direction of progression). While both are reduced in hemiparetic walking when compared to non-impaired persons walking at their self-selected speed (10), neither appears to be consistently different when compared to non-impaired persons walking at the same speed (9). This is likely explained by the mechanical constraints of walking and the required symmetry imposed by the definition of stride length and cadence. Hemiparetic subjects differ most dramatically from non-impaired individuals walking at the same speed in the spatiotemporal measures that indicate interlimb asymmetry.

There are two main temporal asymmetries in hemiparetic walking. First, it has been consistently reported that persons with hemiparesis spend significantly more time in stance phase on the non-paretic leg than on the paretic leg (10, 11). Note that this also requires that they spend significantly more time in swing phase on the paretic leg than on the non-paretic leg. Second, it has been somewhat less consistently reported that the double support phase preceding paretic leg foot-off (which we will define as paretic pre-swing) is longer in duration than is the initial paretic leg double support phase (which we will define as paretic weight acceptance). Olney et al. found an average increase in duration for 32 persons (25% vs. 20% of the gait cycle) (12). Similarly, de Quervain et al. also found that the paretic pre-swing phase was prolonged for 18 persons (13). However, Goldie et al. reported no significant differences in the duration of the two double support phases in a group of 42 persons (10).

The main spatial asymmetry of hemiparetic walking is characterized by differences in the paretic and non-paretic step length (i.e., paretic step length is the distance in the direction of progression that the paretic foot is placed in front of the non-paretic leg, and vice versa for non-paretic step length). While many studies have reported that on average the paretic step length is longer than the non-paretic step length, these studies typically find substantial variability and that some persons with hemiparesis exhibit substantial asymmetry in the opposite direction. Until recently there has been no mechanistic explanation advanced to explain this variability.

In a recent study, Balasubramanian et al. found that step length asymmetry was related to propulsive force generation during hemiparetic walking (14). Propulsive force generation was quantified from the forward directed component of the horizontal ground reaction forces (GRFs) by the time integral of the propulsive GRF (positive area under the GRF versus time curve), since it is that impulse that acts to accelerate the body forward. Paretic propulsion in particular is defined as the proportion of the total propulsive impulse produced by the paretic leg (i.e., impulse of paretic leg divided by sum of the impulses of the paretic and non-paretic legs). Paretic step ratio is used to quantify step-length asymmetry and is similarly defined as step length of the paretic leg divided by sum of the step lengths of the paretic and non-paretic legs. Specifically, these authors found that the subjects that generated the least paretic propulsion walked with relatively longer paretic steps, suggesting that increased propulsion by the non-paretic leg may be one mechanism contributing to production of a longer paretic step (Figure 20-1). Further, those with more severe hemiparesis (those dependent on abnormal flexor and extensor synergies) walk with the longest paretic steps relative to non-paretic (Figure 20-2). However, these results indicated that asymmetrical step lengths do not necessarily limit the self-selected walking speed (i.e., some subjects with longer paretic steps walk faster), likely because of other compensatory generation of propulsion by the non-paretic leg.

Changes in Kinematic Parameters

The kinematics of hemiparetic walking are altered in both legs relative to healthy walking, with the changes being necessarily consistent with the slower speed, slower

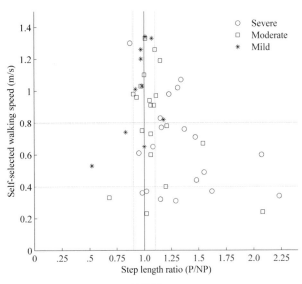

FIGURE 20-2

Relationship between step length asymmetry, walking speed, and hemiparetic severity. The solid vertical line indicates symmetric steps (SLR), vertical dashed lines indicate the SLR subdivisions at SLR = 0.9 and SLR = 1.1. Horizontal dashed lines indicate subdivisions of walking speeds (<0.4m/s, household walkers; 0.4–0.8m/s, limited community walkers; >0.8m/s, community walkers). Note that subjects with different SLR walk at all levels of walking speeds, yet the majority of those with severe hemiparesis walk asymmetrically at SLR greater than 1.1. From Balasubramanian et al. (14).

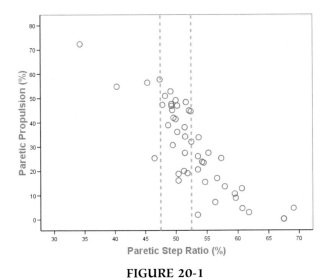

FIGURE 20-1

There is a strong relationship between step length asymmetry and paretic propulsion (r = −0.83, p = 0.001). Subjects with a longer paretic step generate less propulsion with their paretic leg. Modified from Balasubramanian et al. (14).

cadence, and greater asymmetry of hemiparetic walking. Paretic hip motion becomes more abnormal during pre-swing as self-selected walking speed declines (13). De Quervain et al. found that of 12 subjects studied post-stroke, seven with severe hemiparesis did not begin hip flexion until toe-off, five more did not begin hip flexion until the last third of pre-swing, and in the subjects with moderate hemiparesis, beginning hip flexion occurred at the midpoint of pre-swing (13). In contrast, the timing of non-paretic hip flexion was normal in even the slowest walkers. Ankle kinematics may also be important for the performance of paretic pre-swing since peak plantarflexion is less than in normal walking, even when the ankle is in a more plantarflexed (i.e., equinus) position throughout much of stance (11). Nine of twelve subjects with severe hemiparesis were found to have little or no plantarflexion in pre-swing (13).

Two studies performed detailed analyses in persons very early in the recovery phase (13, 15). Using the kinematic data, both studies classified subgroups of hemiparetic subjects with similar characteristics. Based on visual identification of common patterns of knee and ankle motion coupling, De Quervain et al. classified 18 subjects into four groups (13). Mulroy et al. used a nonhierarchical cluster analysis based on spatiotemporal characteristics and peak sagittal plane joint angles for each gait cycle phase and classified 47 subjects into four groups (15).

Subjects with slow walking speeds (i.e., severe hemiparesis) demonstrated more variable kinematics; however, similar kinematic patterns are described in the two studies. The "extension thrust" pattern described by De Quervain et al. was very similar to the "extended" pattern described by Mulroy et al. with increased ankle plantarflexion and knee hyperextension throughout stance, inadequate ankle dorsiflexion in pre-swing, and inadequate knee flexion in swing. Similarly, the "buckling-knee" pattern described by De Quervain et al. was similar to the "flexed" pattern described by Mulroy et al. with greatly increased ankle dorsiflexion and knee flexion throughout stance, decreased thigh extension in pre-swing, and decreased ankle dorsiflexion in swing. De Quervain et al. also described a "stiff-knee" pattern in which knee angle remained constant throughout stance at an angle of 20°–30° of flexion in combination with decreased ankle dorsiflexion. Mulroy et al. did not identify any subjects who exhibited a similar "stiff-knee" pattern in their study. Neither study identified a group of subjects with a fixed equinus deformity at this early stage of recovery, although others have reported it to be a major impairment during the later phases of recovery (16).

The kinematics of subjects who exhibit moderate to fast walking speeds (i.e., moderate to mild severity) tend to be more similar to those of nondisabled walkers, although some who are classified as the "extended" or "flexed" groups by Mulroy et al. are able to walk at these higher speeds. Mulroy et al. classified subjects into a "moderate" and "fast" group within this range, with the main difference being increased knee flexion in stance and decreased thigh extension and plantarflexion in pre-swing for the "moderate" group as compared to the "fast" group. De Quervain et al. appear to have combined these two groups into a single group, with intermediate characteristics.

The kinematics of the non-paretic leg differ from normal in a much more consistent fashion than did those of the paretic leg. Hip angles seem generally consistent with nondisabled walking at slower speeds with a shorter stride (13, 17). Those walking slowly tended to show the biggest differences at the ankle, where dorsiflexion in late stance is increased and the ankle plantarflexion in pre-swing is decreased or absent.

Changes in Kinetic Parameters

Generally, the ground reaction forces (GRFs) in hemiparetic walking are infrequently reported. Vertical forces have been investigated predominantly to determine symmetry of weight bearing. Three different patterns of vertical GRF are typically observed in the paretic leg: double-peaked with early and late peaks (similar to normal), one single peak in midstance, and a plateau with no discernable peak (18). Kim and Eng investigated 28 hemiparetic subjects of varying ambulatory ability and found that all but three had reduced vertical GRFs in the paretic leg and that symmetric weight distribution between the legs was related to increased temporal symmetry but not spatial symmetry during walking (19).

A recent study used the propulsion force as a performance measure to quantify the contribution of the paretic leg to hemiparetic walking (20). Lacking such a performance measure has been a significant barrier to understanding paretic leg motor performance during walking. Measures have typically focused on bilateral gait-related outcomes such as walking speed, over-ground ambulatory capacity, endurance, and balance. The biomechanical and mechanistic contributions of the paretic leg to such measures are not unique. For example, the same gait speed can be achieved with many levels of coordination of the paretic leg if the non-paretic leg provides different levels of compensatory output. Previously, estimates based on mechanical work calculations had suggested that the paretic leg does 30%–40% of the total mechanical work over the gait cycle, regardless of hemiparetic severity (17). However, these work estimates could be flawed because they may be dominated by the support of body weight and not a unique contribution of each leg to forward propulsion, this being a critical component of walking performance.

The purpose of the Bowden et al. study was to establish a quantifiable link between hemiparetic severity and paretic leg contribution to propulsion during walking using a measure based on the Anterior-Posterior (A-P) GRF. In particular, the measure defined the proportion of the summed propulsion from both legs generated by the paretic leg (PP). Total body forward propulsion by a leg is calculated by integrating over time (e.g., stance) the forward propulsion produced by that leg. PP is the ratio (in percent) of the total body forward propulsion produced by the paretic leg to the summed forward propulsion by both legs. Forty-seven participants with chronic hemiparesis walked at self-selected speeds. Spatiotemporal parameters and GRFs were collected. A-P GRF measures were correlated with both walking speed and hemiparetic severity (Figure 20-3). The percentage of propulsion generated by the paretic leg (PP) was found to be 16%, 36%, and 49% for those with severe, moderate, and mild hemiparesis (as assessed by Brunnstrom stages (21), respectively (Figure 20-4). Thus, PP provided a quantitative measure of the coordinated output of the paretic leg that indicates that the motor performance of the paretic leg can be assessed independently and corresponds to the severity of hemiparesis.

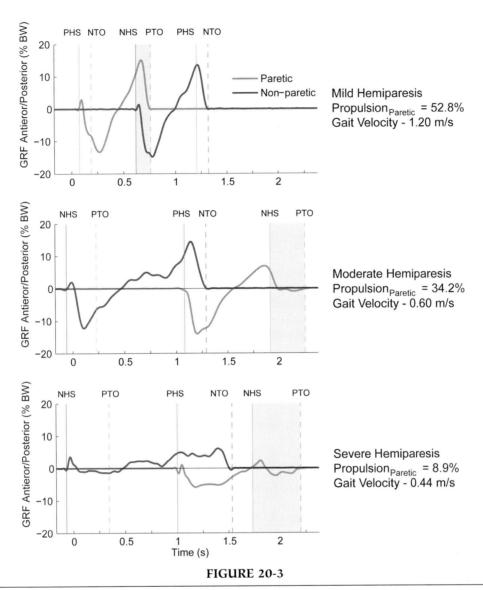

FIGURE 20-3

A-P GRFs for three subjects of differing hemiparetic severity. Positive values represent propulsion, and the positive area under the curve is the propulsive impulse. PHS indicates paretic heel strike; NTO, non-paretic toe off; NHS, non-paretic heel strike; PTO, paretic toe off. Increased hemiparetic severity was associated with decreased PP and decreases in self-selected walking speed. Modified from Bowden et al. (20).

Subsequently, additional studies used propulsion-based measures with success to explain step length asymmetry (14) and the consequences of abnormal electromyographic (EMG) timing (22) to assess the contribution of the paretic leg to hemiparetic walking. Forward body propulsion by a leg at any instant is defined as the force that acts on the body to accelerate it forward (represented by the red vector at hip in Figure 20-5a), which results from the anteriorly directed, forward ground reaction force (red vector parallel to ground in Figure 20-5a) acting on the leg at that instant.

PP is sensitive to differences in motor control not captured by multiconstruct measures such as gait speed, and therefore it may be an effective tool for distinguishing functional compensation by the non-paretic leg from physiological restitution of paretic leg performance. Quantifying forward propulsion provides great insight into overall paretic leg performance because it measures both the active generation of propulsive forces by muscles (e.g., plantarflexors) and the indirect contribution of other muscle activity (e.g., hip and knee flexors) through their influence on the walking mechanics. For example, in terminal stance, or pre-swing, of normal walking, the heel rises and the forefoot acts as a "rocker" that allows body forward progression (Figure 20-4a). An inverted pendulum representation of walking illustrates this contribution

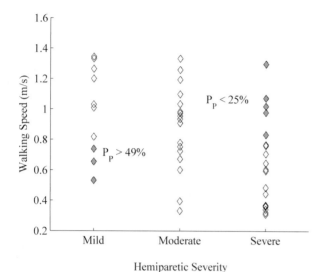

FIGURE 20-4

Individual walking speed data show that there is substantial variability in the weak relationship between walking speed and severity. Note, however, that PP helps explain much of this variation, as the five participants with severe hemiparesis who achieve faster walking speeds (>0.8 m/s) all demonstrate substantial decreases in PP, while the three participants with mild hemiparesis who walked >0.8 m/s have normal PP (>49%). From Bowden et al. (20).

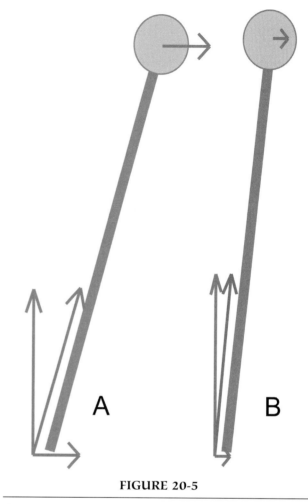

FIGURE 20-5

Illustration of the potential contribution of mechanics to the propulsive ground reaction force for two leg configurations in pre-swing. Reduced hip extension would result in decreased contribution to forward propulsion from walking mechanics.

to propulsion because the resultant ground reaction force acts along the axis of the leg (blue vector), which results in an anteriorly directed component (red vector parallel to ground) of a particular magnitude in direct relation to those walking mechanics. Thus, reduced propulsion will occur as a result of walking mechanics per se should early initiation of leg flexion prevent the foot from moving sufficiently posteriorly relative to the pelvis (i.e., should the hip not extend sufficiently; Figure 20-4b).

As would be expected during slow hemiparetic walking, joint moments and powers are greatly reduced when compared to non-disabled subjects walking at their self-selected speed. However, the differences are much reduced when compared with walking at a matched speed. In fact, it is remarkable the extent to which the paretic leg moment and power profiles are similar in pattern but reduced in amplitude in comparison to the non-paretic legs, which are mostly similar to those of matched speed control subjects (17). Thus, the main power generation bursts in hemiparetic walking are the same as that in non-disabled walking. There are the power generation burst associated with the ankle plantarflexor moment in pre-swing (commonly referred to as A2, as by Olney et al.) (17), the hip extension moment during initial double support (H1), and the hip flexion moment during pre-swing (H3). The A2 positive power burst associated with the ankle plantarflexor moment in pre-swing is usually greatly reduced

on the paretic side. H3 has also been found to be reduced in some subjects, especially those who walk most slowly, although it has been hypothesized for some subjects that H3 compensates for the absence of ankle plantarflexor power.

Ankle joint plantarflexor power (A2) was barely evident in the paretic leg in a group of 10 household walkers (17). In addition, when ankle moments during gait were compared with maximum isometric moments, it was suggested that the walking speed of 10 of 17 hemiparetic subjects was limited by plantarflexor weakness (although the four fastest walkers in that group appeared to compensate by increasing hip flexor moment) (23). Ankle moments are also substantially reduced in hemiparetic persons in comparison to slow walking controls, with household walkers having reduced moments compared to limited community walkers (17). In contrast to the paretic leg, the non-paretic leg A2 power generation is

equal to or greater than speed matched control subjects, as the A2 power bursts [...]
wo[...]
po[...]
pla[...]
spe[...]
an[...]
inc[...]
tro[...]
pre[...]
De[...]
and[...]
be a[...]
in tl[...]
be g[...]
non[...]
subs[...]
does[...]
tive[...]
doul[...]
ship[...]
posit[...]
bilit[...]
othe[...]
appe[...]
in slo[...]
burst[...]
a stud[...]
hemip[...]
Since[...]
Kim a[...]
for po[...]
This[...]
appro[...]
kinem[...]
to ach[...]
an aes[...]
T[...]
forces[...]
into tl[...]
Propul[...]
biome[...]
ground[...]
contrib[...]
potenti[...]
in the[...]
plantai[...]
pull off[...]

have been identified as the primary sources of power generation during normal and hemiparetic walking, with ankle plantarflexor power generation being particularly impaired in hemiparetic walking.

EARLY POST-STROKE PATTERNS OF RECOVERY

Immediately following stroke, the most common feature [of] motor impairment is either paresis or paralysis, par[tial] reduction or complete loss of the ability to generate [fo]rce in the muscles of the extremities contralateral to the [st]roke (26). At this time point post-stroke, the primary [co]ntributors to contralateral paresis are disruption of [th]e motor neural pathways leading to reduced motor [re]cruitment (27) and disuse atrophy (28). Consequently, [in] the early post-stroke phase the characteristic asym[m]etrical gait results primarily from inadequate muscle [fo]rce generation (29).

Abnormal Motor Unit Recruitment and Muscle Weakness

[Pa]resis in the lower extremity can impair both the ability [to] advance the limb for swing and to support body weight [du]ring stance (6, 11, 19). Support of body weight can [be] compromised by inadequate activation of the ankle [pla]ntar flexors, knee extensors, or hip extensors (30). [Pa]resis of the ankle dorsiflexors may result in poor foot [clea]rance in swing (29). If the hip flexors also are weak, [the a]bility to compensate by lifting the limb results in a toe [dra]g and limited step length.

Alterations in electromyographic (EMG) timing and [inten]sity during walking result from both reduced activa[tion] and from compensations for loss of force (15, 29). Few [studi]es have described muscle activity patterns in the early [post-]stroke phase (13, 15, 29, 31). The impact of reduced [musc]le activation and resultant weakness on the charac[teristi]c patterns of walking after stroke was identified in [in]dividuals at admission to acute rehabilitation and [again] at six months post-stroke (15). Four distinct gait pat[terns] were discerned. Those subjects in the two groups with [poore]r walking impairment walked at just 10% to 11% [of nor]mal velocity, and lower-extremity muscle strength [ranged] from 17% to 36% of normal with weakness most [marked] at the ankle. In both of the slower groups, marked [weakness] of the ankle plantar flexor muscles removed the [norma]l restraint of the tibia in stance. The pattern of walk[ing co]mpensation adopted initially was reflected in the [knee p]osition in mid-stance. The relative strength of the [proxima]l muscles in the paretic leg was the factor that [determ]ined which compensatory pattern was adopted. In [in]dividuals with greater strength in the knee exten[sors th]an in the hip extensors, the knee collapsed into [flexion] with the demand shifted to the quadriceps (Flexed [group).] In contrast, subjects with stronger hip extensors and weaker quadriceps thrust into hyperextension at the knee (Extended group) relying on passive stability at the knee and increased activation of the hip extensors for stance control and progression of body weight.

TABLE 20-1
*Mean EMG Intensity during Walking at Admission to Rehabilitation and
Six months after Stroke*

| | | EMG INTENSITY (% MAX MMT) | | | |
| | ABLE-BODIED | STROKE – ADMISSION | | STROKE – SIX MONTHS | |
		SLOW	*FAST*	*SLOW*	*FAST*
SMEMB	20	12 ± 11	18 ± 8	17 ± 10	21 ± 9
BF long	13	11 ± 9	13 ± 10	16 ± 14	17 ± 8
GMAX	18	17 ± 9	23 ± 9	21 ± 11	20 ± 8
VI	13	15 ± 9	29 ± 15	24 ± 16*	29 ± 17*
SOL	35	17 ± 13	30 ± 20	27 ± 19*†	36 ± 15*†
PB	20	5 ± 12	10 ± 8	7 ± 9*†	18 ± 17*†
ADL	14	9 ± 8	12 ± 7	15 ± 7*†	26 ± 11*†
RF	15	8 ± 7	12 ± 12	14 ± 10†	17 ± 11†
AT	25	10 ± 6	26 ± 18	20 ± 11*	28 ± 16*

SMEMB. Semimembranosus; BF long, long head of biceps femoris; GMAX, gluteus maximus; VI, vastus intermedius; SOL, soleus; PB, peroneus brevis; ADL, adductor longus; RF, rectus femoris; AT, anterior tibialis. * = significantly greater in Fast than in Slow; † = significantly greater at six months than at admission.

In the two faster groups (Fast and Moderate), walking velocity was 44% and 21% of normal, respectively. Ankle plantar flexion strength was less than normal (53% and 38% of normal), but not as markedly reduced as in the two slower groups (Flexed and Extended). This greater residual plantar flexion strength resulted in only mildly excessive knee flexion in stance for the Moderate group and normal extension in the group with the least walking impairment (Fast). Moreover, activation intensity was *greater than normal* at admission for the two faster groups in vastus intermedius and gluteus maximus, indicating increased proximal activity in stance as a substitution for reduced distal control (Table 20-1). The significant impact of reduced activation of the calf muscles on walking function in the acute post-stroke phase was confirmed by Lamontagne and colleagues, who documented that gastrocnemius EMG intensity during gait explained a full 52% of the variance in walking speed in the early post-stroke phase (29).

The swing-phase movement pattern in the acute phase was characterized by the amount of dorsiflexion achieved in mid-swing (15). The decreased activation of anterior tibialis in both of the two slower groups produced inadequate dorsiflexion in mid-swing (Table 20-1). While volitional ankle dorsiflexion strength also was less than normal in the two faster groups, the muscle response was adequate to achieve at least a neutral ankle in swing.

In addition to reduced EMG intensity, alterations in the timing of muscle activity have been identified during walking (13, 15, 31). In our study of walking recovery (15), at the early post-stroke assessment, onsets of muscle activity were delayed in the two groups with the slowest velocities for all hip and knee extensors that have a typical onset in mid- or terminal swing (gluteus maximus, gluteus medius, semimembranosus, biceps femoris, and vastus intermedius). This finding is indicative of a reduced need for limb deceleration in swing because of the subjects' very slow velocities. In contrast, EMG onsets for the faster subjects were premature in vastus intermedius and adductor longus, indicating that these subjects had the capacity to activate the muscles, but the decreased muscle force output required an early onset to achieve the desired swing-phase motions. Muscle activity was prolonged with cessations in mid-stance for the hamstrings and in terminal stance for gluteus maximus and vastus intermedius for subjects in all groups, indicating need for increased proximal stability in stance to substitute for the reduced plantar flexor activity distally. Rectus femoris activity was prolonged through swing for both fast and slow velocity groups, which may indicate either spasticity or the increased need for hip flexor force in swing. Because of its insertion below the knee, however, prolonged rectus femoris activity results in inhibition of the necessary knee flexion required for foot clearance and limb advancement. These results are consistent with those of den Otter and colleagues, who identified premature onset of gastrocnemius and prolonged activity through stance in biceps femoris and rectus femoris (31, 32). As they utilized surface electrodes to record EMG activity, the rectus femoris recording likely also reflects activity from the underlying vasti.

CHRONIC POST-STROKE PATTERNS OF RECOVERY

As time following stroke progresses, muscle strength, activation, and walking ability begin to improve (15, 33, 34). Incomplete recovery and development of additional impairments, however, can contribute to continued gait dysfunction (11, 13, 19, 35). Spasticity or contracture of the ankle plantar flexors can cause excessive plantar flexion and toe drag in swing and impede forward progression during stance (29, 35). Knee extensor or hamstring spasticity can inhibit limb advancement in swing (36). In the chronic post-stroke phase, disuse muscular atrophy compounds the initial neurologic injury, and consequently, muscle weakness remains prevalent despite the functional recovery during the acute phase (37). Decreases in activity level contribute to reduced cardiovascular fitness and endurance across the chronic phase post-stroke (see Chapter 23 for more information).

Abnormal Motor Unit Recruitment

In the study of walking recovery at six months post-stroke, consistent with improvement in walking speed, lower-extremity muscles, particularly distal ones, demonstrated increased activation intensity during walking compared to the early post stroke phase (15). Improved walking speed was associated most strongly with increased activation in soleus and adductor longus. Anterior tibialis intensity increased at the six-month assessment for subjects in the slow groups, while it remained unchanged for those in the faster groups at levels similar to those exhibited by able-bodied subjects. Subjects in the two faster groups exhibited a greater-than-normal intensity in both vastus intermedius and adductor longus in this later assessment. Those in the slow groups had greater than normal intensity only in vastus intermedius (Table 20-1).

Timing of muscle activity also improves with recovery but remains altered compared to normal phasing for most individuals (15, 31, 32, 38). The hip and knee extensors, which initially displayed a delayed onset late in terminal swing, began earlier in swing as recovery progressed at six months. Onsets were premature compared to normal timing for semimembranosus, vastus intermedius, and soleus. These premature onsets can interfere with the flexion necessary for limb advancement in swing. The swing-phase muscles—adductor longus, rectus femoris, and anterior tibialis—also displayed

earlier onsets at six months post stroke, resulting in premature activation.

The swing-phase movement pattern at six months was more influenced by the magnitude of knee flexion than ankle dorsiflexion, consistent with the improved anterior tibialis activity exhibited by subjects with slower initial walking speed (15). Those subjects who retained the extended pattern developed a stiff-legged gait with severely decreased knee flexion in swing. All four subject groups (e.g., fast, moderate; flexed, extended) demonstrated excessively prolonged activity of rectus femoris throughout swing, which would inhibit knee flexion. Only the intensity of adductor longus activity (a hip flexor in gait) differentiated those who displayed markedly reduced knee flexion in swing. It appears that individuals with sufficient activity in adductor longus were able to overcome the knee extension force from excessive activity of rectus femoris by generating a strong hip flexion force from adductor longus, resulting in thigh flexion and secondary knee flexion. Thus, restoration of walking function in the sub-acute post-stroke phase is accomplished both by restitution of distal muscle activation and greater than normal proximal muscle activity. (See Chapter 16 for similar discussion.)

Muscle Weakness

Although muscle strength improves from the acute to the chronic post-stroke phase (after six months), for most individuals, strength remains less than normal in the muscles of the lower-extremity contralateral to the side of the stroke (15, 33, 39). Ankle plantar flexion and dorsiflexion weakness still dominate in the slowest individuals. Neckel and colleagues documented greater than normal knee extension strength in a group of individuals who were at least one year post stroke (39). They postulated that knee extensor muscles may have been strengthened from increased activity during walking as part of a compensatory strategy. This is consistent with the finding of a greater-than-normal intensity of vastus intermedius activity (15).

Musculoskeletal models of walking have identified the function of muscle activity in normal walking and predicted the impact of paresis in individual muscles for subjects with pathology (40, 41). In walking at self-selected speed by able-bodied adults, a model of walking demonstrated that force production by plantar flexors in terminal stance and pre-swing is critical to trunk forward progression, swing initiation, and power generation (41). This is consistent with the robust finding of reduced ankle joint power that is strongly related to walking velocity after stroke (12, 42, 43).

Compensatory strategies to substitute for distal muscle weakness have been identified in the proximal musculature of the paretic leg as well as in muscles of the non-paretic limb (30, 40, 44, 45). Increased distal muscle co-activation in the non-paretic leg during the double-limb support phases was documented as a compensatory mechanism in subjects with more severe motor impairments (29, 45). Musculoskeletal modeling demonstrated that an individual with severe plantar flexion weakness and the flexed-knee post-stroke walking pattern would exhibit increased contributions from the paretic hip and knee extensor muscles in single-limb stance as an alternate source of stability confirming the experimental EMG evidence (30, 40). Later in stance phase, the model also identified that increased hip flexor activity can compensate for plantarflexor weakness and produce faster walking speeds (40). (See Chapter 16 for more information on the relationship between proximal and distal power strategies during walking.)

Abnormal Muscle Synergies

Clinical observations of volitional movement patterns in both the upper and lower extremities following stroke have been described as abnormal muscle synergies that are stereotypical combinations of secondary, unwanted motions that accompany the primary desired motion (21, 26, 39). During attempts of isolated, volitional joint movement, lower-extremity abnormal synergistic movement combinations have been described as massed extension of the entire limb with adduction and internal rotation and massed flexion with abduction and external rotation. Measurement of secondary torques during isolated, isometric contractions in subjects with stroke, however, did not confirm the patterns observed during attempted dynamic movements (39). Individuals who have impaired selective movement control can utilize these mass extension and flexion patterns of the lower extremity for stance and limb advancement during walking. The extent of

dependence on the abnormal synergy patterns and the strength of the patterns during walking vary greatly among individuals such that the subjects that depend on abnormal movement patterns for walking have greater functional impairment (46). The mass extension pattern does not have the normal graduated increases in muscle activation necessary for controlled knee flexion in initial double-limb support or ankle dorsiflexion in single-limb stance. The flexion pattern can limit stride length when knee extension in terminal swing is incomplete with continued hip and knee flexion. Excessive, premature ankle plantar flexion and hip extension in late swing often accompany attempted knee extension, which also impedes limb advancement and reduces stride length.

Spasticity

In his classic descriptive study of recovery after stroke, Twitchell described the timing and pattern of the onset of spasticity (26). He noted that spasticity began between 2 and 20 days post-stroke and was most common for the lower extremity in the ankle plantar flexors. Clinical measures of spasticity are related to both the intensity and duration of EMG activity elicited during passive stretching of the muscle (47).

In a study of walking recovery after stroke, the duration of EMG responses to a manual quick stretch was recorded as an indicator of spasticity at an average of 21 days post-stroke and again at six months post-stroke Table 20-2 (15). A normal EMG response to quick stretch lasts for less than 0.10 seconds. At both time periods adductor longus was the muscle that most frequently exhibited a prolonged response to quick stretch (greater than 3.0 seconds in over 80% of subjects). This excessive stretch sensitivity, however, was not related to increased functional deficits in walking. In fact, greater adductor longus activity

TABLE 20-2
Duration of EMG Activity Following Rapid Stretching at Admission to Rehabilitation and Six Months after Stroke

	ADMISSION					SIX MONTHS				
	% < 1 SEC	% 1–3 SEC	% > 3 SEC	MEAN SEC	MEDIAN SEC	% < 1 SEC	% 1–3 SEC	% > 3 SEC	MEAN SEC	MEDIAN SEC
Gluteus Maximus	90	6	4	0.44	0.12	90	8	2	0.33	0.10
Semimemb	45	15	40	2.03	1.14	32	19	49	2.49	2.96
Biceps Femoris	63	10	27	1.5	0.32	59	8	33	1.65	0.26
Adductor Longus	11	6	83	3.77	4.24	8	6	86	3.80	4.20
Rectus Femoris	65	14	21	1.25	0.36	53	10	37	1.94	0.84
Vastus Intermedius	76	10	14	0.98	0.24	74	13	13	0.97	0.38
Soleus	60	13	27	1.42	0.16	79	3	18	1.01	0.10
Anterior Tibialis	94	2	4	0.28	0.06	89	8	3	0.35	0.04

during gait was associated with greater (more normal) swing-phase knee flexion despite prolonged activation in rectus femoris. One-third to one-half of subjects exhibited prolonged responses to quick stretch in the hamstrings (semimembranosus and biceps femoris long head), rectus femoris, and soleus. Though less frequent, the impact of severe spasticity on walking in these muscles was greater than that of the adductor longus.

Spasticity of the hamstrings can limit knee extension in terminal swing and inhibit thigh flexion in initial swing with secondary decrease in peak swing knee flexion (36). Rectus femoris spasticity is a common contributor to reduced knee flexion in swing (36), and soleus spasticity can contribute to equinovarus, which can impair forward progression of body weight over the ankle in stance and impact foot clearance in swing (35). Both semimembranosus and rectus femoris demonstrated increased spasticity at the six-month test compared to the earlier evaluation, which corresponded with greater impairment in swing-phase knee flexion.

Although anterior tibialis does not often demonstrate increased response to passive stretch, excessive or continuous activity during walking is a common contributor to excessive subtalar joint varus (48). Although spasticity is not a strong determinant of walking function for the majority of individuals following stroke (49, 50), for those who do exhibit obstructive spasticity, both surgical interventions and anti-spasticity medication can produce increases in walking speed and reduce gait deviations at both the ankle and knee joints (35, 36, 51). (See Chapter 25 for more information.)

Joint Contractures

After stroke, longstanding weakness in a muscle group or spasticity in the antagonist group can result in increased passive stiffness and joint contractures (29, 47, 52). In the lower extremity the ankle plantar flexion contractures are the most common site for restrictions of joint motion, although inversion contractures are also common, and flexion contractures at the knee and hip joints develop occasionally, particularly in individuals with limited standing and walking function (35, 48, 53). Adequate passive joint mobility is necessary to obtain a stable passive alignment during the stance phase of gait.

Using a mechanical modeling simulation, Kagaya and colleagues (54) confirmed the clinical impression of the lower-extremity postures that produce maximal passive stability during stance, which comprised 5° of dorsiflexion at the ankle, 0° flexion at the knee, and 15° of extension at the hip (54, 55). The model predicted significant increases in muscle demand for postures at or greater than 6° of plantar flexion and 20° of flexion at the knee or hip joints. In a subsequent mechanical modeling simulation hip or knee flexion contractures of no greater than 15° or ankle plantar flexion contractures of less than 0° were required to maintain positive step length and forward movement of the center of gravity (54, 56). These theoretical models indicate that, while moderate to severe contractures are destabilizing, mild contractures may be accommodated, and in fact, mild ankle plantar flexion tightness (0°–5° of dorsiflexion) can augment support for weak calf muscles in stance (6, 45).

Proprioception

The influence of impaired joint position sense has proved to be more of a "yes/no" threshold rather than a scalar determinant of gait quality (5, 53). No significant difference in proprioceptive ability was identified between poor and good hemiparetic walkers (5, 19). Proprioception loss in the lower extremity tends to be more severe distally.

Absence or impaired proprioception in the ankle joint can be controlled with an ankle-foot orthosis that limits available motion at the ankle. If lack of proprioception extends to the knee joint, a knee-ankle-foot orthosis (KAFO) may be required to stabilize the knee in stance. If proprioception at the knee is impaired, but not absent, an unlocked KAFO may provide sufficient sensory input, but if joint position sense is absent at the knee, a locked KAFO is usually required for stability in stance. This is important for safety during walking since absent proprioception in the knee is related to the risk of frequent falls (57). The weight of the orthosis and increased energy cost of walking with an extended knee in swing typically result in KAFO use for household or exercise use only. If proprioception loss extends to the hip, potential for functional ambulation is typically limited. (See Chapter 31 for more detailed description of indicators for orthotic prescription.)

POST-STROKE WALKING REHABILITATION

Customary walking speed has been identified as the primary indicator of overall functional locomotor ability after stroke (5, 19). Moreover, improvements in walking speed categories following rehabilitation have been related to significant improvements in quality of life, confirming the impact that reduced walking speed has on functional mobility (58). Thus, the primary goals of walking rehabilitation programs are to develop walking ability at speeds and distances that are functionally significant for community ambulation. (See Chapter 16 for further discussion of walking speed as a global indicator of locomotor ability after stroke.)

In addition to gait training, walking rehabilitation programs address the various residual motor impairments identified as significant predictors of walking speed after stroke. Physical contributors to walking deficits post-stroke include selective motor control (i.e., synergy stage), muscle strength and balance (19, 49, 57, 60–65). It is beyond the scope of this chapter to address all physical rehabilitation intervention that may contribute to walking recovery. Rather, we focus on the main predictors of walking recovery and best-practice strategies based on current evidence as guides for the clinician in developing effective walking rehabilitation programs for their patients with stroke.

Predictors of Walking Recovery and Responsiveness to Rehabilitation Interventions

Improvement in walking after stroke is accomplished by a combination of natural recovery and rehabilitation intervention (66). Pre-morbid factors as well as stroke-related variables can impact an individual's ability to respond to intervention. Both older age and greater initial severity of stroke have been found to be predictors of poor outcome following rehabilitation (67, 68). This finding may give the erroneous impression that older individuals or those with severe stroke do not make significant or functionally useful gains in rehabilitation. In individuals with more severe involvement, functional improvement occurs more gradually and the magnitude of improvement is not as large as that seen in subjects with moderate or mild stroke (69). Moreover, the mechanisms underlying functional improvement may differ depending on initial impairment level.

Degree of Neurologic Damage and Multiple Comorbidities.   There are numerous covariates associated with motor recovery and responsiveness to therapy such as the pathophysiologic consequences and degree of neurologic damage directly related to the stroke as well as the personal and environmental factors associated with the individual. Cramer (70) discusses the impact that clinical variables such as stroke characteristics (e.g., location, volume, hemorrhagic or ischemic injury), time post-stroke, age, post-stroke depression, and other comorbidities have on recovery potential. With advances in imaging techniques such as functional magnetic resonance imaging and diffusion tensor imaging, the relationship between damage to neurologic structures, motor severity, and functional recovery potential are being elucidated (71).

In particular, the degree of pyramidal tract damage has been associated with both stroke severity and recovery potential for the upper extremity (72, 73). Case-series evidence for similar relationships in lower-extremity and walking recovery are emerging in adults and children with stroke at birth (55, 74). For both upper- and lower-extremity function, motor impairment severity measures such as the Fugl-Meyer motor assessment appear to be correlated with the degree of pyramidal tract damage. In other words, lower Fugl-Meyer motor scores indicate more synergistic movement patterns that are associated with a greater degree of pyramidal tract damage and less motor recovery potential. Thus, the clinical observations related to lower-extremity Fugl-Meyer (LEFM) scores and walking speed may be clinical predictors of both functional walking recovery and post-stroke brain damage. More importantly, therapeutic strategies for walking recovery most beneficial for individuals with mild to moderate stroke may differ compared to those with more severe stroke. (See Chapter 17 for more information on physiological and clinical predictors of recovery after stroke.)

Motor Severity.   Recovery of walking speed is most strongly linked to the magnitude of initial motor impairment, with less recovery in those individuals with the greatest initial severity (63). The strength of this relationship increases up to the first month post-stroke (21, 75). Prediction of further recovery after the first two to six months is less clear. The total score from the lower-extremity motor portion of the Fugl-Meyer test has been identified as a moderate predictor of both walking speed and stride length in patients after a stroke (63, 76). Walking speed was positively correlated with the Brunnstrom motor stage (measure of selective motor control) in the proximal limb, but not with the motor stages of the ankle or foot (64). The authors concluded that the ability to compensate for poor distal motor control determined the individual's walking speed.

Lower-extremity muscle strength in the paretic limb is strongly correlated with maximum walking speed post stroke (19, 49, 57, 60, 65, 77). Specific muscle groups that demonstrated the strongest relationship with walking velocity varied greatly between studies depending on the number of muscles investigated, the parameter used to quantify strength (hand dynamometer force, isometric or isokinetic torques), and the method of documenting gait velocity (comfortable or fast speeds, distance walked, with or without assistive devices and orthoses).

Studies that compared multiple muscle groups most frequently identified strength in the hip flexor (25, 61, 78) and ankle plantar flexor (19, 65) muscle groups as the strongest predictor of walking speed post stroke, although strength in the knee extensor (61, 62) hip extensor (60), and ankle dorsiflexors (57, 78) muscle groups were also identified as significantly related to gait speed. The dominance of ankle plantar flexion strength in the studies of multiple muscle groups is consistent with the relationship of calf strength and initial severity of the stroke (79). Moreover, the contribution of the hip flexors and ankle plantar flexors to maximizing walking speed has been related to their large bursts of power generation late in the terminal stance and pre-swing phases of the gait cycle (12, 17, 19, 23, 25).

Kosak and Reding investigated the effectiveness of gait training using a body-weight supported treadmill (BWST) in stroke subjects who required moderate assistance to ambulate prior to training (80). In a post-hoc analysis, they found locomotor outcomes varied based on the initial severity of neurologic impairments; training using the BWST was more effective for individuals who required moderate assistance to ambulate initially and presented with combined motor, sensory, and visual impairments. However, it should be noted that this study only investigated stroke patients with severe locomotor impairments and was not a study that compared different locomotor impairment severity levels.

In contrast, Sullivan and colleagues specifically investigated the effect of locomotor severity in chronic stroke (81). Neurologic motor impairment, functional locomotor ability, and locomotor severity were analyzed as potential factors that might contribute to treatment effectiveness. They demonstrated that initial walking speed was independently correlated to change in overground walking speed as a result of training with BWST. Lower-extremity motor impairment severity as measured by the LEFM score was correlated highly with the magnitude of walking speed improvement.

The mechanisms behind the functional recovery in walking stimulated by the gait training using a BWST after stroke are likely dependent on the individual's initial motor severity (82). The increase in free walking velocity after six weeks of training with BWST and strengthening exercises in 20 individuals who were six months to five years post stroke was related more strongly to initial LEFM score (r = 0.65) and isometric ankle plantar flexion torque (r = 0.57) than to initial walking velocity (r = 0.42). This finding indicates that those subjects with more preserved motor function in the paretic limb, particularly distally, have a better capacity for restoration of walking function, and it is also consistent with the finding that relatively fast walking speeds can be achieved after stroke with abnormal kinematic patterns through compensatory strategies (20, 83).

Subjects with higher initial LEFM scores (above 25) increased gait speed by improving the terminal stance mechanics of the paretic limb at both the ankle and hip. The increase in the plantar flexion power in terminal stance was associated with improved pre-swing hip flexion power, which contributes to increases in both cadence and stride length. In fact, soleus was the only muscle with a significant correlation between increased activation level and increased pre-swing *hip flexion power* (r = 0.54). The hip flexion power was likely augmented by the improved elastic recoil of the ankle plantar flexors assisting with swing initiation of the limb. Most of those individuals with higher LEFM scores also had stronger ankle plantar flexors (more preserved distal function) and responded to the intervention with

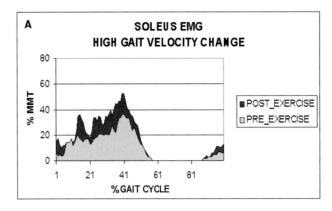

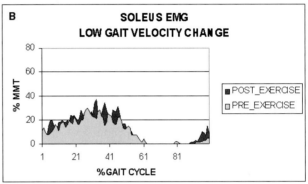

FIGURE 20-6

Change in soleus EMG during walking for subjects who demonstrated high gait velocity (top) and low walk gait velocity (bottom) increases with treadmill training with body-weight support.

increased activation intensity of the soleus to accomplish these improved mechanics (increased by 15% of maximum). This represents restitution of walking function (Figure 20-6).

In contrast, for those subjects with lower initial LEFM scores (and weaker plantarflexion strength), there was no correlation between change in ankle plantar flexion power and improved walking velocity (82, 84). Those subjects with low LEFM scores and a few individuals with higher LEFM scores but poor distal function improved paretic limb mechanics by other mechanisms (not related to increased soleus) including improved activity of proximal muscles (gluteus maximus, semimembranosus, and gluteus medius) leading to better knee and hip extension in stance, but no change in ankle plantar flexion power (85). Hip extension power absorption in terminal stance and hip flexion power generation in pre-swing, however, were related to improved velocity for those with low LEFM scores, indicating that these subjects relied on proximal muscle control of the paretic limb and increased swing-phase power of the non-paretic limb. This same proximal compensation pattern was documented in subjects without active ankle control from amputation at the ankle joint (Symes level) (86) and for those with reduced ankle power from high-heeled shoes (87).

The proximal muscles demonstrating increased activation in subjects with poor distal control are consistent with predictions of a simulation model developed by Jonkers and colleagues (44), who demonstrated that gluteus maximus, medial hamstrings, and gluteus medius would all contribute to hip extension and heel-off in single-limb stance. Thus, individuals with less severe initial motor involvement from the stroke demonstrated a greater capacity to restore distal control and walking function with intervention, and those with more severe distal motor impairment made more modest improvements by increased proximal and contralateral activity.

Standing Balance. Standing balance also has shown strong correlation with walking speed after stroke, particularly for individuals with more severe impairments (49, 84, 88). Patterson and colleagues (49) identified that the strongest predictor of both short- (30 feet) and long-distance (6 minute) walking speed in a cross-sectional analysis was the Berg Balance Score for subjects who walked at or below the median speed (49). In contrast, peak VO2 was the strongest predictor for the faster subjects. Standing balance and lower-extremity strength are strongly related after stroke, and this relationship is particularly strong for those with greater impairments (62).

Improvement in standing balance has been found to be correlated with increased walking speed after basic rehabilitation and muscle strengthening interventions, particularly for individuals with more severe impairments (62, 84). For subjects with less severe initial impairments, however, Pohl and colleagues documented that improvements in lower-extremity motor function and cardiovascular fitness were most strongly associated with increased walking speed (84). This suggests a hierarchy of functional substrates for walking with the ability to control balance during single-limb stance as a requisite skill for even slow walking and greater muscle strength, selective motor control, and fitness as determinants of faster walking speeds (49, 62).

Walking Rehabilitation Interventions

Determining the appropriate and most effective interventions to use for walking recovery is one of the primary roles of the physical therapist during the acute, subacute, and chronic phases post stroke. Evidence is building that innovations in post-stroke walking rehabilitation such as resisted lower-extremity strengthening, task-specific training, and aerobic training are more effective than conventional neurophysiologic approaches used by physical therapists (89–91). Recent innovations in therapeutic approaches to walking rehabilitation derive from understanding the biomechanical and neurologic

mechanisms that result in walking impairment after stroke.

As previously discussed in this chapter, post-stroke severity caused by primary motor impairments such as degree of lower-extremity weakness and selective motor control are significant predictors that contribute to the biomechanics of post-stroke gait and responsiveness to rehabilitation interventions. In addition, other secondary impairments such as balance dysfunction and deconditioning also contribute to post-stroke walking disability. Current evidence from rehabilitation research suggests that lower-extremity strength training, task-specific training such as body-weight supported treadmill training, and aerobic conditioning are interventions that contribute to gait recovery and increased community ambulation for individuals with walking disability after stroke (Figure 20-7).

Strength Training. Resisted strength training for the upper or lower limb after stroke has been questioned by therapists in the past because of the concern that resistance increases muscle spasticity and abnormal movement patterns. However, evidence is building that strength training leads to improvements in both lower-limb muscle strength and gait endurance post-stroke (91) without increasing spasticity (92, 93). The effectiveness of muscle strengthening to improve walking speed and endurance appears to relate to whether the strength training program is directed at single muscles or groups of muscles that are typically activated during the stance and swing phases of gait. For example, muscle strengthening for a single muscle group after stroke increases muscle strength but results in little or no improvement in walking speed or endurance (94). In contrast, strength training of multiple LE muscle groups is associated with modest functional changes in walking distance or improved balance and/or sit-to-stand ability but not increased walking speed (95–98). This finding is consistent with a recent study that used a resisted LE cycling task specifically designed to strengthen extensor and flexor groups with torque demands biased to emphasize the stance and swing phases of gait. The moderately high-intensity cycling program for 20–30 minutes of resisted cycling, two days a week for 6 six weeks, resulted in significant increases in post-intervention LE flexor torque production and walking endurance as measured by the distance walked in six minutes, but did not increase walking speed.

For individuals after stroke with moderate to mild walking impairment (i.e., baseline walking speeds approximately 0.30–0.80 m/s), strength programs that incorporate functional weight-bearing activities or dynamic high-intensity resistance training resulted in increases in strength of LE flexors and extensors that produced increases in walking speed, as well. Yang et al. used a program of progressive LE strengthening using functional

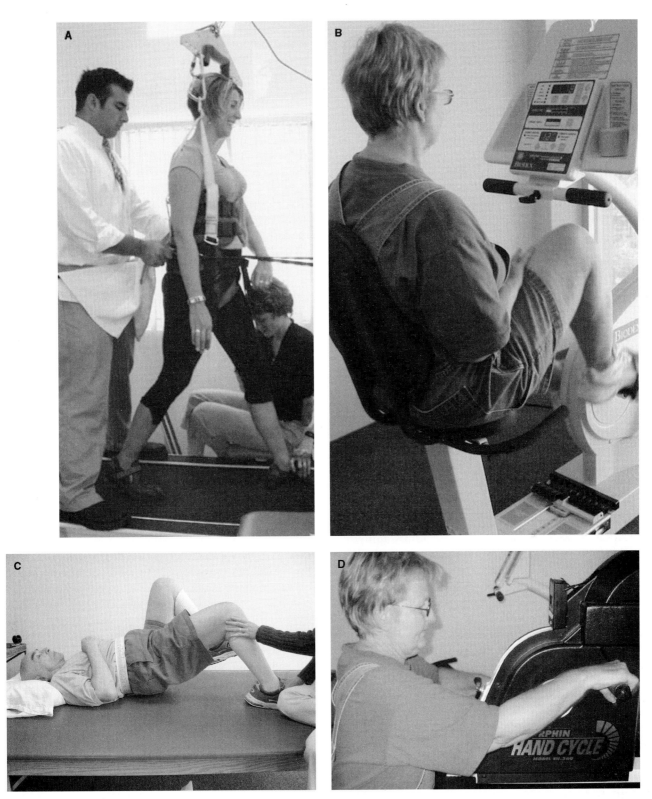

FIGURE 20-7

Rehabilitation interventions of treadmill training with body-weight support (top right), resisted lower-extremity cycling (top left), therapeutic progressive resistive exercise example (bottom left), and upper-extremity ergometry (bottom right).

weight bearing activities for exercise such as step climbing and single-limb heel raises to realize gains in LE strength and walking speed (99). Patten et al. found that a dynamic resistance training program of eccentric muscle strengthening using isokinetic exercises (15 sessions over five weeks) followed by clinic-based gait training (nine sessions over three weeks) resulted in increases in both gait speed and LE torque production (100). Increases in speed were not evident for the group that received concentric strength training with gait training. Together these findings suggest that functional task strengthening or strength training programs that emphasize the dynamic muscle control needed to support the kinematics, kinetics, and muscle activation of more normal gait are more effective strength training programs for walking recovery post stroke.

While it is evident that resisted LE strength training after stroke does not cause harm, there remains a relatively small body of literature that clearly elucidates the overall benefits or limitations of strength training. The recent Canadian Stroke Network (91) systematic review of LE strength training and mobility post stroke concludes that there is strong evidence that strength training improves distance walked after stroke but only moderate evidence that benefits extend to improved performance in other activities of daily living. Furthermore, our understanding of the appropriate dosing (i.e., intensity, frequency, duration) for significant strength gains in this group of patients with neurologic as well as peripheral mechanisms of weakness are not well understood. This lack of understanding is further complicated by lack of studies that have examined how principles of exercise that apply to healthy young and older adults apply to individuals with stroke. For example, a recent study that investigated the combined benefits of a rehabilitation program that alternated therapy days of LE strength training with high-intensity treadmill training with body weight support found evidence of overtraining (i.e., impaired strengthening) in the group that received successive days of LE muscle exercise with the group that received a program in which UE and LE exercise were provided on alternate days (101). Clearly, more investigation into maximizing the effects of resisted exercise post stroke is needed.

Task-Specific Training. Task-specific training is the repetitive practice of a task that is specific to the intended outcome. Treadmill training is a therapeutic modality that allows the individual with stroke to actively engage in repetitive stepping. Walking on a treadmill is an example of task-specific gait training that appears to be critical to the achievement of improved walking speed and endurance (95, 102–104). Treadmill training with body-weight support (TM-BWS) is an adaptation of treadmill walking that involves fitting the patient in a harness and

suspending them over a treadmill with a portion of the patient's body weight reduced so that a physical therapist, with help from another therapist or aide if needed, can assist the patient to step on the moving treadmill belt. Visintin et al. demonstrated that treadmill training with 40% body weight support (BWS) provided in early training that was progressively decreased over training sessions resulted in better walking outcomes for individuals in the acute and subacute phases post stroke than treadmill training without BWS (105).

In a control-comparison RCT of 80 individuals with chronic stroke who had severe to moderate walking impairment (average gait velocity: severe, 0.25 ± 0.12 m/s; moderate, 0.71 ± 0.12 m/s), Sullivan et al. demonstrated a statistically significant, and clinically meaningful, increase in both walking speed and distance that was maintained at a six-month follow-up for *any* of the exercise groups that received TM-BWS compared to the group that received resisted cycling (101). In this study, there were four exercise groups that received exercise four days per week for six weeks. Three of the groups received TM-BWS combined with another exercise such that the program included two days per week of TM-BWS alternated with two days per week of upper-extremity ergometry, progressive resistance LE exercise, or resisted cycling. The fourth group received two days per week of resisted cycling alternated with two days per week of upper-extremity ergometry. Each group was controlled for time in the exercise session (one hour per session) and intensity (moderately high). Moderate- to high-intensity TM-BWS sessions included 20 minutes of cumulative walking time on the treadmill at speeds that ranged from 1.8 to 2.3 mph. In addition to providing specific dose parameters and intervention protocol specifications for the exercise programs, this study demonstrated the overarching benefit of an exercise program that included TM-BWS for making long-term changes (six-month follow-up) in both walking speed and distance in individuals with chronic stroke.

Several recent systematic reviews have suggested that the collective findings on treadmill training or TM-BWS effectiveness compared to other gait interventions remain inconclusive (91, 106, 107). However, there is strong evidence that task-specific functional training performed at high intensity may be a critical factor that modulates gait training effectiveness (89, 108, 109). With task-specific gait therapies such as treadmill training or TM-BWS, responsiveness to this particular intervention is related to the training parameters used. Recent evidence consistently demonstrates that treadmill training at higher speeds (i.e., higher intensity), with or without body-weight support, is more effective for improving gait speed post stroke than training at slower speeds (81, 110, 111). These reports of differences in therapeutic effectiveness related to the type and dosing of the exercise program illustrate the importance of exercise prescription. Exercise prescription is a major contributor to therapy outcomes and most likely contributes to the inconclusive findings of systematic reviews that have not included trials in which training intensity is controlled.

Why are higher intensity, task-specific gait interventions more likely to achieve functionally significant changes in walking outcomes after stroke? We propose that walking rehabilitation that combines *specificity* of training intrinsic to walking with the *intensity* of walking at challenging speeds requires that the individual post stroke respond to and develop the gait dynamics and muscle activation patterns associated with more normal gait parameters. Thus, changes in walking recovery and response to appropriately selected and dosed walking interventions are related to the residual damage to the nervous system post stroke and the response of the nervous system to interventions that provide an appropriate dynamic stimulus to the nervous system to drive recovery. Long-term changes in performance are consistently achieved when the conditions of task practice are similar to the task and conditions in which long-term changes in performance are expected (112). For individuals post stroke, walking is a highly practiced functional task in which the learner has to reacquire the motor abilities associated with gait function; thus, improvements in walking outcomes post stroke appear to be more likely with task-specific interventions like treadmill walking with or without BWS. (See Chapter 17 for similar discussion.)

Aerobic Training. Deconditioning after stroke is a chronic health condition that is evident across the acute, subacute, and chronic phases post stroke (see Chapter 23 for more information). Aerobic training can be safely incorporated into rehabilitation exercise programs after stroke. Physical activity and exercise post stroke are highly recommended to address deconditioning and to reduce secondary risks for the post-stroke survivor (113). In addition, valuable evidence-based sources are now available for the rehabilitation specialist that provide heart rate and blood pressure guidelines to individually monitor the patient during moderately high exercise programs (for example, see: http://www.apta.org/AM/Template.cfm?Section=PFSP_Pocket_Guides&Template=/MembersOnly.cfm&ContentID=42129). While cardiovascular fitness is essential for good health after stroke, there is building evidence that specific types of aerobic programs are also associated with improved walking outcomes for the stroke survivor.

Pooled data from systematic reviews and well-designed RCTs reveal that walking outcomes such as walking speed and distance, functional tasks such as stair climbing, and increased community mobility and participation are positively impacted by aerobic training for patients with subacute and chronic stroke (91, 106, 114). Across these studies large-muscle activities such as walking, treadmill, stationary cycle, combined arm-leg ergometry, arm ergometry, and seated steppers were used. Exercise intensity among studies in which walking outcomes were improved ranged from 3 to 19 weeks, 20–40 minutes, three to five days per week at 50%–80% of heart rate reserve. Pooled data show that aerobic exercise had a small, statistically significant effect on walking speed 0.26 m/s (95% CI: 0.05–0.48, p = 0.008) and a moderate, statistically significant effect on walking distance 0.30 meters (95% CI: 0.06–0.55, p = 0.008).

Aerobic exercise training specifically designed to improve gait and gait-related activities is associated with greater clinically and statistically significant gains in walking outcomes (see systematic review by Van de port (115). Activities such as cycling, water-based exercise, and gait-oriented cardiovascular training resulted in greater post-intervention changes in walking speed 0.45 m/s (95% CI: 0.27–0.63) and distance 0.62 meters (95% CI: 0.30–0.95). Across the studies reviewed the most common exercise prescription (i.e., frequency, intensity, duration) averaged three times per week for 60 minutes across four weeks (ranges: 8–90 minutes; three to five time per week; 4–19 weeks). Exercise intensity in terms of percentage of heart rate maximum, heart rate reserve, or rate of perceived exertion was not reported.

The wide confidence intervals are most likely associated with the wide variety of exercise methods and prescriptions that ranged across the various trials. Once again, well-designed aerobic exercise rehabilitation clinical trials are needed to better understand the exercise method and aerobic training parameters that result in clinically significant walking recovery in individuals post stroke. However, efficacy for physical activity and aerobic training to improve walking outcomes after stroke is evident.

RESEARCH FRONTIERS

Future directions in walking rehabilitation therapies will most likely include the use of technology to enhance current walking rehabilitation interventions. Currently, technological advances in walking neurorehabilitation that are in either experimental (pre-clinical) or early phase I clinical trials are in the areas of lower-limb assisted robotics, implantable electrodes for neuromuscular function, and electrical stimulation.

Lower-limb assisted robotics are in development that will provide machine-assisted stepping since the physical demands during treadmill training are high for the therapist. Examples include both motorized (116) and gravity-balanced (117) exoskeletons that serve as gait-assisted orthotics during walking on a treadmill with a supportive harness and body-weight support. A recent clinical trial that examined walking outcomes in patients with chronic stroke demonstrated that therapist-assisted stepping was more effective than robotic-assisted stepping with a motorized exoskeleton (118). However, more study is needed to determine the optimal training paradigms that integrate the expertise of the therapy clinician with the most effective mechanical assistance.

Advances in technology and reduced device size have allowed neuromuscular electrical stimulation (NMES) to be used functionally as a neuroprosthesis. There is strong evidence that NMES, particularly peroneal nerve stimulation, in conjunction with gait training is an effective walking rehabilitation strategy (91). Surface electrode stimulation devices are readily available for clinical use; however, future research endeavors will most likely include the development of implantable electrode devices that will increase the effectiveness of NMES and increase ease of use and comfort for the patient (119). A recent study by Kottink et al. demonstrates initial evidence for the feasibility of NMES with implantable electrodes as an adjunct to walking rehabilitation therapy (120).

CONCLUSION

This chapter summarizes the temporal gait characteristics and kinematic and kinetic features associated with post-stroke gait dysfunction. Stroke severity affects the dynamic strategies used for walking after stroke. Stroke severity as measured by clinical assessments of LE motor impairment assessment (i.e., selective movement control, strength, spasticity) or functional walking ability (i.e., walking speed or distance) is also used as an indicator of stroke walking impairment severity and are associated with predictions of walking outcomes and disability after stroke. The capacity to recover movement control as indicated by changes in force production, increased movement selectivity, and appropriate motor unit activation and recruitment during walking appears to be related to the degree of corticospinal tract damage and the methods used during walking rehabilitation.

Walking recovery after stroke appears to be associated with rehabilitation strategies that incorporate strengthening of functional muscle groups with power and activation patterns that are more similar to those used in gait. Task-specific interventions such as treadmill walking with or without BWS are examples of effective rehabilitation strategies that incorporate the demands of gait into repetitive stepping and task-specific practice most similar to that of normal gait demands. Furthermore, aerobic training in gait-related activities or LE cycling tasks appear to be effective interventions to increase cardiovascular fitness associated with reduced activity levels after stroke. Collectively, these types of rehabilitation interventions improve walking outcomes and lead to enhanced participation and quality of life for individuals with stroke.

References

1. Duncan PW, Zorowitz R, Bates B, et al. Management of adult stroke rehabilitation care: a clinical practice guideline. Stroke 2005; 36(9):e100–143.
2. Jorgensen HS, Nakayama H, Raaschou HO, Olsen TS. Recovery of walking function in stroke patients: the Copenhagen Stroke Study. Arch Phys Med Rehabil. 1995; 76(1):27–32.
3. Forster A, Young J. Incidence and consequences of falls due to stroke: a systematic inquiry. BMJ. 1995; 311(6997):83–86.
4. Keenan MA, Perry J, Jordan C. Factors affecting balance and ambulation following stroke. Clin Orthop. 1984(182):165–171.
5. Perry J, Garrett M, Gronley JK, Mulroy SJ. Classification of walking handicap in the stroke population. Stroke Jun 1995; 26(6):982–989.
6. Perry J. Gait analysis: Normal and pathologic function. Thorofare, NJ: Slack, Inc., 1992.
7. Mahoney FI, Barthel DW. Functional evaluation: The Barthel Index. Md State Med J. 1965; 41:61–65.
8. Hamilton BB, Laughlin JA, Fiedler RC, Granger CV. Interrater reliability of the 7-level Functional Independence Measure (FIM). Scandinavian Journal of Rehabilitation Medicine 1994; 26(3):115–119.
9. Chen G, Patten C, Kothari DH, Zajac FE. Gait deviations associated with post-stroke hemiparesis: improvement during treadmill walking using weight support, speed, support stiffness, and handrail hold. Gait Posture 2005; 22(1):57–62.
10. Goldie PA, Matyas TA, Evans OM. Gait after stroke: initial deficit and changes in temporal patterns for each gait phase. Arch Phys Med Rehabil. 2001; 82(8):1057–1065.
11. Olney SR, CJ. Hemiparetic gain following stroke: Part I: Characteristics. Gait Posture. 1996; 4:136–148.
12. Olney SJ, Griffin MP, McBride ID. Temporal, kinematic, and kinetic variables related to gait speed in subjects with hemiplegia: a regression approach. Phys Ther. 1994; 74(9):872–885.
13. De Quervain IA, Simon SR, Leurgans S, et al. Gait pattern in the early recovery period after stroke. Journal of Bone & Joint Surgery - American Volume 1996; 78(10):1506–1514.
14. Balasubramanian CK, Bowden MG, Neptune RR, Kautz SA. Relationship between step length asymmetry and walking performance in subjects with chronic hemiparesis. Arch Phys Med Rehabil. 2007; 88(1):43–49.
15. Mulroy S, Gronley J, Weiss W, et al. Use of cluster analysis for gait pattern classification of patients in the early and late recovery phases following stroke. Gait & Posture 2003; 18(1):114–25.
16. Waters HJ, Perkin JM. Study of stroke patients in a single general practice. Br Med J (Clin Res Ed). 1982; 284(6318):791–793.
17. Olney SJ, Griffin MP, Monga TN, McBride ID. Work and power in gait of stroke patients. Arch Phys Med Rehabil. 1991; 72:309.
18. Wong AM, Pei YC, Hong WH, et al. Foot contact pattern analysis in hemiplegic stroke patients: an implication for neurologic status determination. Arch Phys Med Rehabil. 2004; 85(10):1625–1630.
19. Kim CM, Eng JJ. The relationship of lower-extremity muscle torque to locomotor performance in people with stroke. Physical Therapy 2003; 83(1):49–57.
20. Bowden MG, Balasubramanian CK, Neptune RR, Kautz SA. Anterior-posterior ground reaction forces as a measure of paretic leg contribution in hemiparetic walking. Stroke 2006; 37(3):872–876.
21. Brunnstrom S. Movement therapy in hemiplegia. New York: Harper & Row, 1970.
22. Turns LJ, Neptune RR, Kautz SA. Relationships between muscle activity and anteroposterior ground reaction forces in hemiparetic walking. Arch Phys Med Rehabil. 2007; 88(9):1127–1135.
23. Nadeau S, Gravel D, Arsenault AB, Bourbonnais D. Plantarflexor weakness as a limiting factor of gait speed in stroke subjects and the compensating role of hip flexors. Clin. Biomech. 1999; 14(2):125–135.
24. Parvataneni K, Olney SJ, Brouwer B. Changes in muscle group work associated with changes in gait speed of persons with stroke. Clin Biomech. 2007; 22(7):813–820.
25. Nadeau S, Arsenault AB, Gravel D, Bourbonnais D. Analysis of the clinical factors determining natural and maximal gait speeds in adults with a stroke. Am.J.Phys.Med.Rehabil. 1999; 78(2):123–130.
26. Twitchell TE. The restoration of motor function following hemiplegia in man. Brain 1951; 74:443–480.

27. Clark DJ, Condliffe EG, Patten C. Activation impairment alters muscle torque-velocity in the knee extensors of persons with post-stroke hemiparesis. *Clinical Neurophysiology* 2006; 117(10):2328–2337.

28. Andrews K, Brocklehurst JC, Richards B, Laycock PJ. The rate of recovery from stroke—and its measurement. *Int Rehabil Med.* 1981; 3(3):155–161.

29. Lamontagne A, Malouin F, Richards CL, Dumas F. Mechanisms of disturbed motor control in ankle weakness during gait after stroke. *Gait & Posture* 2002; 15:244.

30. Higginson JS, Zajac FE, Neptune RR, et al. Muscle contributions to support during gait in an individual with post-stroke hemiparesis. *Journal of Biomechanics* 2006; 39(10):1769.

31. Den Otter AR, Geurts ACH, Mulder TH, Dyusens J. Gait recovery is not associatted with changes in the temporal patterning of muscle activity during treadmill walking in patients with post-stroke hemiparesis. *Clinical Neurophysiology* 2006; 117:4.

32. Den Otter AR, Geurts AC, Mulder T, Duysens J. Abnormalities in the temporal patterning of lower-extremity muscle activity in hemiparetic gait. *Gait & Posture* 2007; 25(3):343.

33. Andrews AW, Bohannon RW. Short-term recovery of limb muscle strength after acute stroke. *Arch Phys Med Rehabil.* 2003; 84:125.

34. Jorgensen L, Jacobsen BK. Changes in muscle mass, fat mass, and bone mineral content in the legs after stroke: a 1 year prospective study. *Bone* 2001; 28 (6):655.

35. Pinzur MS, Sherman R, Dimonte-Levine P, et al. Adult-onset hemiplegia: changes in gait after muscle-balancing procedures to correct the equinus deformity. *Journal of Bone and Joint Surgery* 1986; 68A(8):1249.

36. Kerrigan DC, Gronley JK, Perry J. Stiff-legged gait in spastic paralysis: a study of quadriceps and hamstring activity. *American Journal of Physical Medicine* 1991; 70(6):294.

37. Hachisuka K, Umezu Y, Ogata H. Disuse muscle atrophy of lower limbs in hemiplegic patients. *Arch Phys Med Rehabil.* 1997; 78(1):13–18.

38. Kautz SA, Duncan PW, Perera S, et al. Coordination of hemiparetic locomotion after stroke rehabilitation. *Neurorehabilitation and Neural Repair.* 2005; 19(3):250.

39. Neckel N, Pelliccio M, Nichols D, Hidler J. Quantification of functional weakness and abnormal synery patterns in the lower limb of individuals with chronic stroke. *J Neuroengineering Rehabil.* 2006; 3(17):1.

40. Goldberg EJ, Neptune RR. Compensatory strategies during normal walking in response to muscle weakness and increased hip joint stiffness. *Gait & Posture* 2007; 25:360.

41. Zajac FE, Neptune RR, Kautz SA. Biomechanics and muscle coordination of human walking part II: Lessons from dynamical simulations and clinical implications. *Gait & Posture* 2003; 17:1.

42. Nadeau S, Gravel D, Arsenault AB, Bourbonnais D. Plantarflexor weakness as a limiting factor of gait speed in stroke subjects and the compensating role of hip flexors. *Clin Biomech.* 1999; 14(2):125–135.

43. Richards CL, Malouin F, Bravo G, et al. The role of technology in task-oriented training in persons with subacute stroke: a randomized controlled trial. *Neurorehabilitation & Neural Repair* 2004; 18(4):199–211.

44. Jonkers I, Stewart C, Spaepen A. The study of muscle action during single support and swing phase of gait: clinical relevance of forward simulation techniques. *Gait & Posture* 2003; 17:97.

45. Lamontagne A, Richards CL, Malouin F. Coactivation during gait as an adaptive behavior after stroke. *Journal of Electromyography and Kinesiology* 2000; 10:407.

46. Chen G, Patten C, Kothari DH, Zajac FE. Gait differences between individuals with post-stroke hemiparesis and non-disabled controls at matched speeds. *Gait & Posture* 2005; 22:51.

47. Cooper A, Musa IM, van Deursen R, Wiles CM. Electromyography characterization of stretch responses in hemiparetic stroke patients and their relationship with the Modified Ashworth scale. *Clin Rehabil.* 2005; 19(7):760.

48. Perry J, Waters RL, Perrin T. Electromyographic analysis of equinovarus following stroke. *Clinical Orthopaedics and Related Research* 1978; 131:47.

49. Patterson SL, Forrester LW, Rodgers MM, et al. Determinants of walking function after stroke: differences by deficit severity. *Arch Phys Med Rehabil.* 2007; 88(1):115–119.

50. Sommerfeld DK, Eek EU, Svensson A, et al. Spasticity after stroke: Its occurence and association with motor impairments and activity limitations. *Stroke* 2004; 35:134.

51. Francisco GE, Boake C. Improvement in walking speed in poststroke spastic hemiplegia after intrathecal baclofen therapy: a preliminary study. *Arch Phys Med Rehabil.* 2003; 84(8):1194.

52. Chung SG, van Rey E, Zhiqiang B, et al. Biomechanic changes in passive properties of hemiplegic ankles with spastic hypertonia. *Arch Phys Med Rehabil.* 2004; 85(1638):1646.

53. Keenan MA, Ure K, Smith CW, Jordan C. Hamstring release for knee flexion contracture in spastic adults. *Clinical Orthopaedics and Related Research* 1988; 236:221.

54. Kagaya H, Sharma M, Kobetic R, Marsolais EB. Ankle, knee, and hip moments during standing with and without joint contractures: simulation study for functional electrical stimulation. *Am J Phys Med Rehabil.* 1998; 77:49–54.

55. Dobkin BH, Firestine A, West M, et al. Ankle dorsiflexion as an fMRI paradigm to assay motor control for walking during rehabilitation. *Neuroimage* 2004; 23:370–381.

56. Kagaya H, Ito S, Iwani T, Obinata G, Shimada Y. A computer simulation of human walking in persons with joint contractures. *Tohoku Journal of Experimental Medicine* 2003; 200(1):31.

57. Soyuer F, Ozturk A. The effect of spasticity, sense, and waking aids in falls of people after chronic stroke. *Disability and Rehabilitation* 2007; 29(9):679.

58. Schmid A, Duncan PW, Studenski S, et al. Improvements in Speed-Based Gait Classifications Are Meaningful. *Stroke* 2007; 38(7):2096–2100.

59. Lin PY, Yang YR, Chen SJ, Wang RY. The relationship between ankle impairments and gait velocity and symmetry in people with stroke. *Arch Phys Med Rehabil.* 2006; 87(4):562.

60. Bohannon RW. Strength of lower limb related to gait velocity and cadence in stroke patients. *Physiother Can.* 1986; 38:204–206.

61. Hsu A, Tang P, Jan M. Analysis of impairments influencing gait velocity and asymmetry of hemiplegic patients after mild to moderate stroke. *Arch Phys Med Rehabil.* 2003; 84:1185.

62. Suzuki K, Imada G, Iwaya T, et al. Determinants and predictors of the maximum walking speed during computer-assisted gait training in hemiparetic stroke patients. *Arch Phys Med Rehabil.* 1999; 80:179.

63. Chae J, Johnston M, Hekyung K, Zorowitz R. Admission motor impairment as a predictor of physical disability after stroke rehabilitation. *Am J Phys Med Rehabil.* 1995; 74:218.

64. Chen CL, Chen HC, Tang SFT, et al. Gait performance with compensatory adaptations in stroke patients with different degrees of motor recovery. *Am J Phys Med Rehabil.* 2003; 82:925.

65. Bohannon RW. Selected determinants of ambulatory capacity in patients with hemiplegia. *Clinical Rehabilitation.* 1989; 3:47–53.

66. Richards CL, Olney S. Hemiparetic gait following stroke: Part II Recovery and physical therapy. *Gait and Posture* 1996; 4:149–162.

67. Kwakkel G, Kollen B, Lindeman E. Understanding the pattern of functional recovery after stroke: Facts and theories. *Restorative Neurology and Neuroscience* 2004; 22:281.

68. Lofgren B, Nyberg L, Gustafson Y. Rehabilitation of stroke patients who are older and severely affected: Short- and long term perspectives. *Top Stroke Rehab.* 2000; 6(4):20

69. Mayo NE. Epidemiology and recovery. *Physical Medicine and Rehabilitation; State of the Art Reviews* 1993; 7:1.

70. Cramer SCM. Functional Imaging in Stroke Recovery. *Stroke* 2004; 35(11): 2695–2698.

71. Stinear CM, Barber PA, Smale PR, et al. Functional potential in chronic stroke patients depends on corticospinal tract integrity. *Brain* 007; 130(Pt 1):170–180.

72. Binkofski F, Seitz RJ, Arnold S, et al. Thalamic metbolism and corticospinal tract integrity determine motor recovery in stroke. *Annals of Neurology* 1996; 39(4):460–470.

73. Feydy A, Carlier R, Roby-Brami A, et al. Longitudinal study of motor recovery after stroke: recruitment and focusing of brain activation. *Stroke* 2002; 33(6):1610–1617.

74. Phillips JP, Sullivan KJ, Burtner PA, et al. Ankle dorsiflexion fMRI in children with cerebral palsy undergoing intensive body-weight-supported treadmill training: a pilot study. *Developmental Medicine & Child Neurology* 2007; 49(1):39–44.

75. Duncan PW, Goldstein LB, Matchar D, et al. Measurement of motor recovery after stroke: Outcome assessment and sample size requirements. *Stroke* 1992; 23:1084.

76. Brandstater M, deBruin H, Gowland C, Clark BM. Hemiplegic gait: analysis of temporal variables. *Arch Phys Med Rehabil.* 1983; 64:583.

77. Bohannon RW. Relevance of muscle strength to gait performance in patients with neurologic disability. *J Neuro Rehab.* 1989; 3:97–100.

78. Lin SI. Motor function and joint position sense in relation to gait performance in chronic stroke patients. *Arch Phys Med Rehabil.* 2005; 86(2):197.

79. Hendricks HT, Pasman JW, van Limbeek J, Zwarts MJ. Motor evoked potential of the lower extremity in predicting motor recovery and ambulation after stroke: a cohort study. *Arch Phys Med Rehabil.* 2003; 84:1373.

80. Kosak MC, Reding MJ. Comparison of partial body weight-supported treadmill gait training versus aggressive bracing assisted walking post stroke. *Neurorehabilitation & Neural Repair.* 2000; 14(1):13–19.

81. Sullivan KJ, Knowlton BJ, Dobkin BH. Step training with body weight support: effect of treadmill speed and practice paradigms on poststroke locomotor recovery. *Arch Phys Med Rehabil.* 2002; 83(5):683–691.

82. Klassen TD, Mulroy SJ, Sullivan KJ. Gait parameters associated with responsiveness to a task-specific and/or strengthening program in individuals post-stroke. *J Neurol Phys Ther.* 2006; 29:4.

83. Kim CM, Eng JJ. Magnitude and pattern of 3D kinematic and kinetic gait profiles in persons with stroke: relationship to walking speed. *Gait & Posture* 2004; 20:140.

84. Pohl PS, Perera S, Duncan PW, et al. Gains in distance walking in a 3-month follow-up poststroke: What changes? *Neurorehabilitation and Neural Repair* 2004; 18:30.

85. Sullivan KJ, Klassen T, Mulroy S. Combined task-specific training and strengthening effects on locomotor recovery post-stroke: a case study. *Journal of Neurologic Physical Therapy* 2006; 30(3):130–141.

86. Dillon MP, Barker TM. Preservation of residual foot length in partial foot amputation: a biomechanical analysis. *Foot and Ankle International* 2006; 27 (2):110.

87. Esmail A, Walsh S, Walhein G, Gitter A. Kinetics of high-heeled gait. *J Am Podiatr Med Assoc.* 2003; 93:27.

88. Kollen B, van de Port I, Lindeman E, et al. Predicting improvement in gait after stroke: A longitudinal prospective study. *Stroke* 2005; 36:2676.

89. Kwakkel GP, van Peppen RMPT, Wagenaar RCP, et al. Effects of Augmented Exercise Therapy Time After Stroke: A Meta-Analysis. *Stroke* 2004; 35(11):2529–2536.

90. Van Peppen RPS, Kwakkel G, Wood-Dauphinee S, et al. The impact of physical therapy on functional outcomes after stroke: what's the evidence? *Clinical Rehabilitation* 2004; 18(8):833–862.

91. Foley NT, Bhogal, S. Mobility and the lower extremity. In: Teasell RFN, Salter K, Bhogal S, Jutai J, Speechley M., eds. *Evidence-Based Review of Stroke Rehabilitation.* Canadian Stroke Network; 2007:1–105.

92. Brown DA, Kautz SA. Increased workload enhances force output during pedaling exercise in persons with poststroke hemiplegia. *Stroke* 1998; 29(3):598–606.

93. Patten CL, J; Brown, HE. weakness and strength training in persons with poststroke hemiplegia: Rationale, method, and efficacy. *Journal of Rehabilitation Research & Development.* 2004; 41(3A):293–312.

94. Sharp SA, Brouwer BJ. Isokinetic strength training of the hemiparetic knee: effects on function and spasticity. *Arch Phys Med Rehabil.* 1997; 78(11):1231–1236.

95. Dean CMR, Malouin, F. Task-related circuit training improves performance of locomotor tasks in chronic stroke: a randomized, controlled pilot trial. *Arch Phys Med Rehabil.* 2000; 81(4):409–417.

96. Ouellette MM, LeBrasseur NK, Bean JF, et al. High-intensity resistance training improves muscle strength, self-reported function, and disability in long-term stroke survivors. *Stroke* 2004; 35(6):1404–1409.

97. Teixeira-Salmela LF, Olney SJ, Nadeau S, Brouwer B. Muscle strengthening and physical conditioning to reduce impairment and disability in chronic stroke survivors. *Arch.Phys. Med.Rehabil.* 1999; 80(10):1211–1218.

98. Weiss A, Suzuki T, Bean J, Fielding RA. High intensity strength training improves strength and functional performance after stroke. *American Journal of Physical Medicine & Rehabilitation* 79(4):369–376.

99. Yang Y-R, Wang R-Y, Lin K-H, et al. Task-oriented progressive resistance strength training improves muscle strength and functional performance in individuals with stroke. *Clinical Rehabilitation* 2006; 20(10):860–870.

100. Patten C, Dozono J, Jonkers I. Gait speed improves significantly following dynamic high-intensity resistance training in persons poststroke. *Stroke* 2007; 38(2):466–467.

101. Sullivan KJ, Brown DA, Klassen T, et al. Effects of task-specific locomotor and strength training in adults who were ambulatory after stroke: results of the STEPS randomized clinical trial. *Physical Therapy* 2007; 87(12):1580–1602; discussion 1603–1587.

102. Ada L, Dean CM, Hall JM, et al. A treadmill and overground walking program improves walking in persons residing in the community after stroke: a placebo-controlled, randomized trial. *Archives of Physical Medicine & Rehabilitation* 2003; 84(10):1486–1491.

103. Richards CL, Malouin F, Wood-Dauphinee S, et al. Task-specific physical therapy for optimization of gait recovery in acute stroke patients. *Arch Phys Med Rehabil.* 1993; 74(6):612–620.

104. Salbach NM, Mayo NE, Wood-Dauphinee S, et al. A task-orientated intervention enhances walking distance and speed in the first year post stroke: a randomized controlled trial. *Clinical Rehabilitation* 2004; 18(5):509–519.

105. Visintin M, Barbeau H, Korner-Bitensky N, Mayo NE. A new approach to retrain gait in stroke patients through body weight support and treadmill stimulation. *Stroke* 1998; 29(6):1122–1128.

106. Brosseau L WG, Hillel F, et al. Ottawa panel evidence-based clinical practice guidelines for post-stroke rehabilitation. *Topics in Stroke Rehabilitation* 2006; 13(2):1–26.

107. Moseley AM, Stark A, Cameron ID, Pollock A. Treadmill training and body weight support for walking after stroke. *Cochrane Database of Systematic Reviews* 2005 (4):CD002840.

108. Foley NT, Bhogal, Speechley, M. The efficacy of stroke rehabilitation. In: Teasell RFN, Salter K, Bhogal S, Jutai J, Speechley M., eds. *Evidence-Based Review of Stroke Rehabilitation.* Canadian Stroke Network; 2007:1–53.

109. Langhorne P, Wagenaar R, Partridge C. Physiotherapy after stroke: more is better? *Physiother Res Int.* 1996; 1(2):75–88.

110. Pohl MM. Speed-dependent treadmill training in ambulatory hemiparetic stroke patients: a randomized controlled trial. *Stroke* 2002; 33(2):553–558.

111. Lamontagne A, Fung J. Faster is better: implications for speed-intensive gait training after stroke. *Stroke* 2004; 35(11):2543–2548.

112. Schmidt RAL, *Motor Control and Motor Learning: A Behavioral Emphasis.* 4th ed. Champaign, IL: Human Kinetics, 2005.

113. Gordon NF, Gulanick M, Costa F, et al. Physical activity and exercise recommendations for stroke survivors: an American Heart Association scientific statement from the Council on Clinical Cardiology, Subcommittee on Exercise, Cardiac Rehabilitation, and Prevention; the Council on Cardiovascular Nursing; the Council on Nutrition, Physical Activity, and Metabolism; and the Stroke Council. Circulation 2004; 109(16):2031–2041.

114. Duncan P, Studenski S, Richards L, et al. Randomized Clinical Trial of Therapeutic Exercise in Subacute Stroke. *Stroke* 2003; 34(9):2173–2180.

115. Van de port 2007

116. Mayr A, Kofler M, Quirbach E, et al. Prospective, blinded, randomized crossover study of gait rehabilitation in stroke patients using the lokomat gait orthosis. *Neurorehabil Neural Repair.* 2007; 21(4):307–314.

117. Agrawal SK, Banala SK, Fattah A, et al. assessment of motion of a swing leg and gait rehabilitation with a gravity balancing exoskeleton. *Neural Systems and Rehabilitation Engineering, IEEE* 2007; 15(3):410–420.

118. Hornby TG, Campbell DD, Kahn JH, et al. Enhanced gait-related improvements after therapist- versus robotic-assisted locomotor training in subjects with chronic stroke: a randomized controlled study. *Stroke* 2008; 39(6):1786–1792.

119. Anke IR, Kottink AIR. The orthotic effect of functional electrical stimulation on the improvement of walking in stroke patients with a dropped foot: a systematic review. *Artificial Organs* 2004; 28(6):577–586.

120. Kottink AIR, Hermens HJ, Nene AV, et al. Therapeutic effect of an implantable peroneal nerve stimulator in subjects with chronic stroke and footdrop: a randomized controlled trial. *Phys Ther.* 2008; 88(4):437–448.

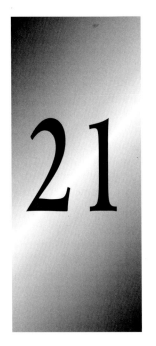

21

Recovery and Rehabilitation of Standing Balance after Stroke

Mark W. Rogers
Katherine M. Martinez

ifficulties with balance leading to disability are common occurrences after stroke. This chapter examines problems of standing balance accompanying stroke and its rehabilitation. The review will synthesize mostly recent information about these themes by:

1. Discussing the scope of the balance problem from the standpoint of interactive motor control factors that may normally contribute to sustaining standing balance
2. Identifying the functional balance limitations and changes in motor control factors that have been consistently identified after stroke and their relationship with falls
3. Examining the intervention approaches directed at improving balance
4. Introducing a protective stepping model of balance control for linking dynamic balance capacity, functional performance, and falls
5. Providing a glimpse of emerging new research frontiers in balance recovery after stroke

SCOPE OF THE BALANCE PROBLEM

Balance: A Multifaceted Control System

In mechanical terms, standing balance involves the maintenance of the relative position and motion of the body center of mass (COM) with respect to the base of support (BOS), usually represented by the feet in contact with the ground (1). Virtually limitless variations of body surface contact with the environment that provide support may reconfigure the BOS conditions that influence balance. Hence, the interplay between the COM position and motion (velocity or momentum) in relation to a stationary BOS (for example, feet-in-place and/or grasping a fixed rigid object) or moving BOS (for example, stepping and/or reaching to contact or grasp a secure surface) determines the moment-to-moment conditions of balance stability. The critical importance of the dynamic nature of these relationships is illustrated by observations showing that even healthy adults often naturally respond to balance challenges by rapidly changing their BOS through stepping or grabbing for support even when the COM is positioned well within the BOS boundaries (2). These responses have traditionally been considered to indicate falling in clinical assessments of balance, such the Rhomberg test (3). The complexity and multifaceted nature of the interactive factors that normally comprise the standing balance control system is represented in Figure 21-1 and discussed in this section.

Neural Factors

Concerning the neural control mechanisms by which standing balance may normally be achieved, much attention has been given to the role of spinal cord and brain stem-mediated postural reflexes involving visual, vestibular, and proprioceptive subsystems operating in a reactive mode of control (4–9). Anticipatory postural adjustments involving proactive control processes that may precede and accompany particularly voluntary goal-directed movements have been proposed to involve several higher-level brain centers, including motor cortical areas, basal ganglia, and the cerebellum (10). The interface between reactive and proactive neural control processes for standing balance is not well understood. This dichotomy appears to have somewhat limited current neuromotor approaches to balance rehabilitation after stroke by emphasizing either reactive responses to balance perturbations or practicing volitional balance tasks. (See Intervention Approaches.)

Although a commonly held view is that, in mammalian systems, including man, the balance regulatory system is phylogenetically old and operates relatively autonomously and automatically using polysynaptic relflex pathways involving the spinal cord and brain stem (6, 10), emerging perspectives suggest that standing balance may operate like any other form of movement by requiring planning, anticipation, and adaptive internal models (11, 12). For example, even during the quasi-static situation of stationary standing balance, sagittal plane sway regulation cannot be achieved by continuous muscle activation adjusted by reactive stretch reflexes at the ankles as generally believed (11). This is because the net series elastic component of the calf muscles is

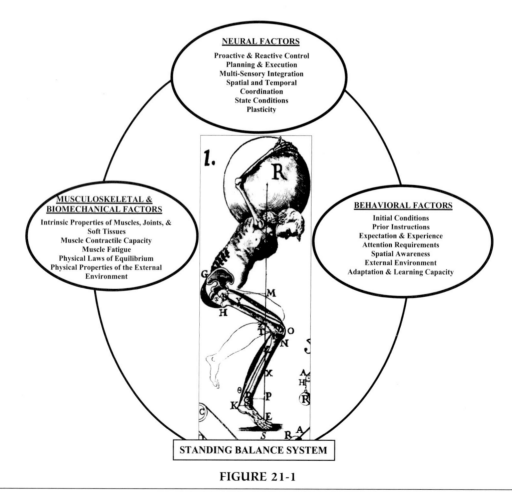

FIGURE 21-1

Conceptual scheme of the multifaceted interactive factors that normally comprise the human standing balance control system. Adapted from Borelli GA. De Motu Animalium, 1680.

disrupts the vestibular control of balance possibly by interrupting corticobulbar connections modulating brain stem balance areas. This perspective was supported by the results from the two subjects with discrete pyramidal tract lesions showing that the responses after a pontine stroke (that is, above the lower pons) were comparable to middle cerebral artery strokes, but those accompanying a medullary stroke (that is, below the vetibular nuclei) showed symmetrical GVS responses but asymmetrical TMS responses. Hence, these findings provide new insights pertaining to vestibular-mediated asymmetries of stance control that may contribute to the asymmetries of standing balance that have been consistently identified in most investigations of balance recovery after stroke.

Self-Produced Perturbations of Balance. Voluntary movements of the body segments and of the whole body exert challenges to sustaining standing balance because of their influences on the COM-BOS relationship as well as reactive forces acting on the body that must be counteracted to stabilize the segments and minimize their perturbation effects on balance. In many situations, voluntary movements are preceded and accompanied by anticipatory postural adjustments (APAs) that serve to minimize in advance the self-produced perturbations to balance induced by the goal-directed action or contribute to the evolving movement (10).

Predominantly cross-sectional studies of individuals with chronic stroke have generally found delayed and reduced APAs of the paretic lower limb muscles and increased activation of the nonparetic leg with reduced speed and amplitude of arm or leg movements that may be accompanied by difficulties with controlling balance (69, 84, 100, 106–112). A longitudinal prospective study (69) determined changes in EMG activation patterns of leg muscles (bilateral hamstrings and soleus) during rapid nonparetic limb arm flexion movements performed while standing in 27 subjects with chronic stroke (mean = 32.7 months post-stroke) undergoing a four-week rehabilitation program. Overall, after a month of rehabilitation treatment, arm acceleration was increased, and EMG-onset latencies in bilateral hamstring muscles occurred earlier relative to arm movement onset and were larger in magnitude, indicating improvements in APA responses. The changes in onset timing and probability of muscle recruitment at post-test approximated the muscle activation patterns of healthy subjects observed previously (110). Across the group, these changes were accompanied by clinically meaningful improvements in functional balance and mobility. However, when subjects were stratified into subgroups based on functional balance scores (Berg Balance Scale, Clinical Outcomes Variables Scale, 7-m comfortable gait speed), 12 subjects with low initial balance scores, which improved at post-test, did not have improvements in paretic muscle activation while

nonparetic-side APAs did improve. Another ten subjects showed an opposite trend whereby APA characteristics improved but functional measures did not. Respectively, these different patterns of recovery were consistent with the development of a compensatory strategy and true physiological recovery.

During natural speed voluntary leaning of the body as far as possible in different directions without moving the feet, hemiparetic subjects have difficulties in all directions and especially towards the paretic side (113). These problems with recovering weight-shifting ability have been examined in-depth longitudinally in 36 subjects who received inpatient rehabilitation beginning ten weeks after first-time stroke (intracerebral infarct or hematoma). Voluntary frontal plane weight-shifting guided by visual COP feedback was quantified by COP displacements under each foot when subjects could first stand unsupported for at least 30 seconds and after 2, 4, 8, and 12 weeks later. Weight-shifting speed increased by 33% over the first eight weeks and stabilized at a level that was slower than that of healthy control subjects. The imprecision of weight shifting continued to reduce by 25% over the 12 weeks of recovery and achieved normative values. Subjects retained a constant level of weight-transfer time asymmetry by being 23% slower toward the paretic leg compared with nonparetic-side transfers. Older age of greater than 65 years and the presence of visuospatial neglect were associated with a greater level of weight-shifting speed asymmetry but not with its recovery. Considering the coordinated inter-limb hip abductor-adductor muscle control that normally underlies lateral weight transfer and its impairment after stroke (100, 111, 112, 114), the persistence in weight-transfer time asymmetry may be indicative of difficulties with weight shifting to either side, as has been emphasized in other studies (109, 111, 115, 116).

Falls

Stroke is among the leading risk factors for falls in older adults (117). Between 23–73% of community-dwelling older adults with chronic stroke fall once or more within four to six months after discharge from hospital (117, 118). Community-based prospective studies have found that a history of stroke increases the risk of falling by two to sixfold (117, 119, 120). Compared with healthy adults, this population has more than seven times the risk of experiencing a fracture (121).

Despite the contributions of multiple risk factors to falls accompanying aging and the complicating effects of stroke (for example, environmental hazards, orthostatic hypotension, disorientation, and sedation), it is well-recognized that those who fall present greater impairments in balance and mobility functions, which have been consistently found to be among the most important risk factors for falls (123–126). In people with acute stroke (up to one month post-stroke) and subacute stroke (one to six months post-stroke), falls have been associated with balance and mobility impairments (78, 118, 127, 128) and cognitive deficits (78, 128–130). People with chronic stroke (more than six months post-stroke) who have fallen reported that they were usually either walking or dressing when falls occurred, and they have attributed their falls to loss of balance, misstepping, foot drag related to tripping, or a lack of concentration and poor judgment (131). However, among individuals with chronic stroke, the relationship between balance factors and falls is unclear (75).

For people with chronic stroke living in the community, studies of functional balance and mobility have either found a relationship with falls (131–134) or no relationship (75, 117, 135, 136). Part of the discrepancy in these findings appears to be related to whether or not fall prediction outcomes were focused on single fall events and/or multiple fall events (118, 131, 134–137). The level of stroke chronicity may also be an influential variable related to functional balance and falls (75, 135, 136). For example, a retrospective study of falls in 99 community-living subjects with chronic stroke (mean time post-stroke = 4 years, range = 1 to 24 years) found that clinical measures of balance (Berg Balance Scale), mobility (gait speed), and cognitive status (Mini-Mental Status Exam) did not discriminate between fallers and nonfallers (75). A major conclusion was that routine clinical tests of balance may not test those aspects required to prevent falling and that more sensitive measures of balance that include large components of reactive dynamic balance are needed. At least for the chronic stroke population, this report, together with the other inconsistencies in the literature, raises some caution when using functional tests of balance and mobility to determine fall risk outcomes.

Currently, relationships between changes in motor control factors affecting standing balance after stroke (impairments and compensations) and the risk of falls are largely unknown. One study (138) investigated acutely induced falls into a support harness following standing platform perturbations of balance in 44 subjects with single-episode chronic stroke (mean time post-stroke onset, about 3.5 years) involving variable lesion sites who were not currently receiving rehabilitation. EMG activity from leg muscles, GRFs, and kinematic recordings were used to characterize postural balance responses with subjects classified as either fallers (required harness support to prevent falling in one or more trials) or nonfallers (no support needed). One-fourth of the subjects fell during the forward displacement trials, leading to a backward balance disturbance with 7% of subject falling during posterior displacement trials. Comparison of balance responses for the anterior perturbations indicated slower paretic muscle activation timing

for the fallers in the tibialis anterior, rectus femoris, and biceps femoris muscles, with longer intramuscular onset timing intervals bilaterally. At perturbation onset, the nonparetic side ankle was more dorsiflexed, the paretic hip more flexed, and the trunk position more anterior for the nonfallers compared with the fallers. At the completion of perturbation, the trunk position was more posterior, and the backward velocity was greater for the faller group compared with the nonfaller group. The muscle activation timing differences and differences in kinematics between the groups were consistent with the possibility that they directly contributed to the large number of fall episodes among the faller group. However, the muscle onset timing delays of approximately 20–35 ms and intramuscular delays of less than 20 ms were relatively small, making their potential to directly cause loss of balance somewhat uncertain. Though, these changes might compound the overall balance stabilizing deficit. Furthermore, the initial postural conditions adopted by the nonfallers likely provided them with a compensatory mechanical advantage that somewhat offset the backward falling tendency produced by subsequent movement of the platform.

Behavioral factors influencing balance and mobility performance may also be an important determinant contributing to falls after stroke. Fall-related self-efficacy refers to the confidence an individual has in performing routine daily activities without falling or losing balance (139). An increasing number of studies in this area have reported significant relationships between fall-related self-efficacy (measured by the Falls Efficacy Scale or Activities-specific Balance Confidence Scale) and balance and mobility (140, 141) and falls (136, 141). It is striking that, while balance and mobility performance may not be a determinant of falls in some studies (75, 136, 141), fall-related self-efficacy is independently associated with balance, mobility, and falls in these reports. Therefore, increased attention should be given to assessing and treating behavioral factors underlying fall-related self-efficacy associated with falls and fractures after stroke.

Site of Brain Lesion

To date, there have been relatively few studies that have examined the relationship between the specific location of the brain lesion causing stroke and the recovery of standing balance. The majority of information has addressed balance outcomes relative to the side of hemispheric stroke. In general, these reports have indicated that acute and more chronic problems with balance recovery are more marked for right hemispheric lesions compared with left-sided insults (142–147). Other studies, however, have not been able to confirm this general finding (82, 103, 148). Right hemispheric lesion effects on balance have been linked with hemispatial neglect manifested by lack of awareness or acknowledgement of objects or people on the side of the body opposite of the lesion (149). Right hemisphere neural networks are thought to be important for both spatial attention and postural awareness of verticality (149). Brain imaging studies (150) in healthy human subjects have implicated a network of cortical neurons activated by vestibular activity (inferior parietal lobe, temperoporietal junction, posterior insula, and frontal eye fields) mainly in the right hemisphere of right hand-dominant individuals with neglect. This vestibular cortical network may also be involved with spatial orientation of the body relative to gravity (150). It may also play a more general role in representing the physical laws of motion by producing an internal model of gravity that estimates gravitational effects on the body and external objects (151). One such problem involves "the pusher syndrome," in which patients push toward the paretic side, especially while standing, and this may lead to falling (142). Vestibular cortical areas are frequently damaged after right middle cerebral artery stroke, resulting in neglect (103, 144, 145). Stroke lesions involving parietotemporal and parieto-insular vestibular cortical areas result in major difficulties with balance control (103, 144, 145). Thus, problems with multisensory integration of balance-related information and/or reduced spatial awareness of vertical orientation may be major contributors to deficits in standing balance following stroke.

INTERVENTION APPROACHES

Recent intervention studies for standing balance post-stroke are limited and can be categorized into five areas:

1. Exercise programs including group and individual activities
2. Biofeedback training
3. Sensory training
4. Cognitive strategies
5. External devices

Each area addresses a different aspect of the multifaceted motor control problem of standing balance. Some interventions emphasize a task-orientated approach to stroke rehabilitation, and others focus on the impairment level of the problem. This section addresses the outcomes of recent intervention studies on standing balance post-stroke.

Exercise Programs

Exercise programs can take many forms ranging from group, individual, functional training, or impairment-based approaches. Twelve of the exercise intervention programs included in Table 21-1 incorporate functional strengthening activities such as step-ups, sit-to-stand, and practice of balance tasks such as reaching and standing on unstable surfaces in the intervention training (76, 152–161). Each program was supervised by a therapist who provided individually tailored modifications to the prescribed tasks so as to progressively challenge the individual capability of each participant. Varied sensorimotor challenges modified the difficulty level, complexity, and dosage utilized. These challenges allowed each participant the opportunity to develop effective strategies to deal with the many changing environmental conditions that may arise during daily balance tasks. Eight of the exercise interventions showed improvement in balance as measured by the Berg Balance Scale (BBS) with one study showing faster reaction time stepping and fewer induced falls on platform perturbation testing in the experimental group who performed progressive dynamic balance tasks that emphasized agility and a multisensory approach (76).

There was only one study that specifically investigated strength training and balance performance measures (160). This study used a 1RM (repetition maximum) defined as the maximum weight that could be correctly lifted within 5% of full range of motion. The lower extremity exercises were performed unilaterally on both the affected and nonaffected sides utilizing stack weight and pneumatic training machines. Significant improvement was noted in strength of both affected and nonaffected lower extremities and in balance measured by the BBS. An increase in single-leg stance time was noted, but was not significantly different between pre- and post-intervention testing. Studies in older adults have shown strength of lower extremities to be related to balance and falls (123). This study suggests that lower extremity strengthening may be beneficial to balance performance in people post-stroke.

Constraint-induced movement therapy (CIMT) has been shown to improve upper limb function in certain populations of individuals with chronic stroke (162–165). One key element in CIMT is mass practice of functional tasks and limited use of the unaffected limb (see Chapter 17, Task-Oriented Training to Promote Upper Extremity Recovery). Limiting the use of the unaffected lower limb through constraint is difficult during standing balance training. Application of CIMT in the lower extremity has been reported but with less success than with upper limb (166).

Two recent studies have investigated the use of intense practice for improving balance with subjects at least 10 months post-stroke (159, 167). The training consisted of functional tasks, similar to those listed in the previous exercise studies. Training occurred for three to six hours per day for ten days. Both studies showed improvement in balance with some retention up to three months post-training. Each session was delivered in a one-on-one session. These studies support the feasibility

TABLE 21-1

Results of Recent Studies on Post-Stroke Balance Interventions

Citation	Population Acute < 7 Months Chronic > 12 Months	Type of Intervention	Description of Intervention	Duration of Treatment	Results	Conclusions/Comments
Macko RF, et al., 2008 (156)	N = 20 Chronic	Exercise	Group exercise that included 12 minutes of obstacle course walking, standing exercise in parallel bars, seated upper- and lower-extremity stretching. Home exercise included similar tasks, such as walking, stair-climbing, and stretching.	Group exercise: 60 minutes twice per week for 8 weeks Home exercise: three times per week	Improvements noted in Berg Balance Scale scores, 6-minute walk, Short Physical Performance Battery scores, and Barthel Index scores (p < 0.001). No change in the Lawton ADL scores was noted. Geriatric Depression Scale (p < 0.01) and Stroke Impact Scale (SIS), Mobility, Participation, and Recovery also improved with adaptive physical activity (p < 0.03).	Adaptive physical activity has the potential to improve gait, balance, and basic but not instrumental activities of daily living profiles in individuals with chronic stroke. Improved depression and SIS scores suggest APA improves stroke-specific outcomes related to QOL.
English CK, et al., 2007 (154)	N = 68 Acute	Exercise	Circuit Training Group included 5–6 participants. Activities included sit to stand; weight bearing LE strengthening; walking through obstacles, steps, ramps, stairs, outdoor surfaces; reach and grasp; unilateral and bilateral manipulation of everyday items. Individual Therapy: 1:1 therapist/patient ratio, with session tailored to patient needs.	Circuit Training Group: two 90-minute sessions, 5 days per week for 4 weeks Individual Sessions: 60 minutes, 5 days per week for 4 weeks	Both groups showed improvements at 4 weeks in 5MWT (0.07m/s change), 2minWT (1.8m change), Berg Balance Scale (3.9 point change) that were not significant between groups.	Subjects in both group showed similar degrees of improvement. However, circuit therapy was associated with greater walking independence at discharge. This study demonstrated the safety and feasibility of circuit class therapy as an alternative model for inpatient rehabilitation after stroke.

Study	Sample	Type	Intervention	Results	Conclusions
Yang YR, et al., 2006 (161)	N = 48 Chronic	Exercise	Six workstations: Standing reaching, sit-to-stand, stepping forward and back, stepping sideways, step-ups, heel raises. Control: no intervention	30 minutes 3 times per week	Strength significantly improved for the exercise group for both the paretic and non-paretic legs. The control group had a 6.7% gain to 11.2% decline in strength. The exercise group showed significant improvements in all functional performance measures except the step test (balance measure). Step test significantly declined (−20.3%) in the control group with no change in functional test. There was a significant difference between groups in all measures. Strength gains were significantly associated with gain in functional tests.	Task-orientated progressive resistive strength training program could improve lower-extremity muscle strength in individuals with chronic stroke and could carry over into improvement in functional abilities. Lack of improvement in the step test may indicate that there are other components, such as balance and coordination, determining ability at this task.
Sullivan KJ, et al., 2006 (158)	N = 1 Chronic	Exercise	Body weight supported treadmill training at 1.5–2.5 mph, from 40% to 0% unloading. Locomotor-based strength training: cycle with lower extremities on a modified Biodex semi-recumbent isokinetic ergometer that offers resistance during both flexion and extension phases of pedaling at 120 rpm for 10 sets of 15–20 cyclic repetitions between 10–100 lbs.	24 sessions (12 alternating sessions of each program), 1-hour sessions 4 times per week for 6 weeks	Post-treatment Fugl-Meyer LE motor score increased from 21/34 to 24/34, Berg Balance score decreased from 52/54 to 49/56, free walking speed increased by 18%, fast walking speed increased by 15%, 6-minute walk increased by 4%. At 6-month follow-up, the Fugl-Meyer LE did not change, but the Berg Balance score increased to 54/56.	For the person in this case, clinically meaningful changes in walking function were associated with a combined therapeutic program that included both task-specific and LE strength training. Possible mechanisms associated with response to therapy were related to improved motor unit activation associated with increased strength in key muscles used in gait.

TABLE 21-1
(Continued)

Citation	Population Acute < 7 months Chronic > 12 months	Type of Intervention	Description of Intervention	Duration of Treatment	Results	Conclusions/Comments
Mount J, et al., 2005 (157)	N = 4 Chronic	Exercise	Group Balance Class: 5 minutes sitting trunk mobility exercises. 10 minutes in step-stance position, moving upper body and arms slowly weight shifting. 10 minutes of sitting on therapeutic ball moving arms and legs, shifting weight, reactive and proactive perturbations. Ending with standing and walking activities of various challenges tailored to each participant. Explicit instructions about balance strategies were provided and practiced.	1-hour sessions 2 times per week for 8 weeks	Participants' responses to the questionnaire and pre-test/post-test differences in scores on BBS and POMA suggest trends towards improvement in balance. Change in BBS +1 to +6. Change in POMA 0 to +3.5. All subjects reported improvement in balance during ADLs.	Group balance skill class for individuals post-stroke >6 months appears feasible. Further research is needed, to determine the effectiveness of this class for improving functional balance and decreasing incidence of falls.
Marigold DS, et al., 2005 (76)	N = 62 Chronic	Exercise	Agility program: chal-lenged dynamic balance, emphasized agility and a multisensory approach. Stretching/Weight Shift program: focused on stretching and weight shifting exercises with slow, low-impact move-ments both standing and on mats on the floor. Each group also included 5 minutes of warm-up	1-hour sessions, 3 times a week for 10 weeks	Both groups showed improvements in all clinical outcome mea-sures, with the agility group demonstrating greater improvement in step reaction time and paretic rectus femoris postural reflex onset latency than the stretch-ing/weight-shifting group. In addition, the agility group experienced fewer	Group exercise programs that include agility or stretching/weight-shifting exercises improve postural reflexes, functional balance, and mobility, and may lead to a reduction of falls in older adults with stroke.

Study	Type	Intervention	Duration	Results	Conclusions
		with walking and light stretching, and 5 minutes of cool-down with light stretching.		induced falls on the platform.	
Hart J, et al., 2004 (155)	N = 18 Chronic	Exercise (Tai Chi)	Study group: Tai Chi exercises led by certified Tai Chi instructor. Control group: group exercise focusing on improvement of balance, led by physical therapist	1 hour, twice a week, for 12 weeks	The study group showed improvement in social and general functioning, whereas the control group showed improvement in balance and speed of walking.	It is concluded that there are potential and not adverse effects in Tai Chi practice in stroke subjects.
Eng J, et al., 2003 (153)	N = 25 Chronic	Exercise	Community-based exercise: Light aerobic warm-ups (e.g., marching in place, arm swings), stretching (e.g., calf, hamstring stretches), functional lower-extremity strengthening with and without weights (e.g., sit-to-stand, up on toes), balance and weight shifts, aerobic stepping, walking circuit, and cool-down designed to meet the capacities of each subject.	1-hour sessions, 3 times per week, for 8 weeks	Improvement from the exercise program was found for all physical measures including Berg Balance Test, and these measures were retained 1 month post-intervention. Those with the poorest balance showed the greatest improvement in the BBS.	Short-term community-based exercise program can improve and retain mobility, functional capacity, and balance. Community-based programs have potential for improving activity tolerance and reducing risk for secondary complications common to stroke.
Duncan P, et al., 2003 (152)	N = 92 Acute	Exercise	Intervention group received range of motion and stretching, strengthening, balance, upper-extremity functional use, and endurance, performed in the home, supervised by therapist. Control group received services as prescribed by their physician.	36 ninety-minute sessions over 12 to 14 weeks	Both groups showed improvements in strength, balance, motor control, upper limb function, and gait velocity. The intervention group showed greater gain in balance, endurance, peak aerobic capacity, and mobility.	This structured, progressive program of therapeutic exercise in persons who have completed acute rehabilitation services produced gains in endurance, balance, and mobility beyond those attributed to spontaneous recovery and usual care.

TABLE 21-1
(Continued)

Citation	Population Acute < 7 months Chronic > 12 months	Type of Intervention	Description of Intervention	Duration of Treatment	Results	Conclusions/Comments
Weiss A, et al., 2000 (160)	N = 7 Chronic	Exercise	3 sets of 8–10 repetitions at 70% of 1 RM on weight-training machine both standing (hip flexion, abduction, and extension) and sitting (knee extension and leg press), performed unilaterally on both affected and intact side. 1 RM = maximum weight lifted correctly within 5% of full ROM.	Two sessions per week for 12 weeks	Lower-limb strength improved 68% on affected side, 48% on intact side during training, with largest increase seen in hip extension (affected side 88%, $p < 0.01$; intact side 103%, $p < 0.001$). Repeated chair-stand time decreased 21% ($p < 0.02$). Motor Assessment Scale improved 9% ($p < 0.04$), and Berg Balance scale improved 12% ($p < 0.004$).	Progressive resistance training in individuals one year after stroke improved affected- and intact-side lower-limb strength, with associated gains in chair-stand time, balance, and motor performance.
Fritz SL, et al., 2007 (167)	N = 8 Chronic	Exercise (massed practice)	Intervention: focused on using affected lower extremity more, repeatedly performing activities such as gait with and without assistive device, sit-to-stand, stair climbing, balance (tandem, single-leg stance, reaching), stretching, proprioceptive and coordination tasks, range of motion exercises, stepping over and around obstacles, LE exercises in sitting and standing, and motor re-education.	3 hours per day for 2 weeks	The overall effect size of the intervention was 0.72, with changes in balance having much greater effects than changes in gait or mobility. The group demonstrated an average improvement, from pre- to post-tests, of 12 points on the Berg Balance Scale, where a change of 6 is considered a minimal detectable change.	This intense mobility training was a feasible intervention for this sample, and demonstrated large effect sizes for balance outcome measures. Future studies incorporating more participants, a standard control, and more emphasis on gait would provide insight into the effectiveness and clinical relevance of this intervention.

Study	Subjects	Intervention	Description	Dosage	Results	Conclusion
Vearrier LA, et al., 2005 (159)	N = 10 Chronic	Exercise (massed practice)	Intensive massed-practice intervention: 15% impairment training (closed-chain PRE, stretching, aerobic exercise); 70% functional training (weight shifts, gait training to decrease orthosis, assistive device, compensations, and improve ambulation outdoors and over elevations); 10% problem-solving community ambulation barriers; 5% rest.	6 hours of 1-on-1 training for 10 days	A reactive balance ability, as measured by the mean time to stabilize the CoP after a balance perturbation, decreased from baseline to intervention and was maintained up to 3 months post. Significantly improved pre to post, and post to follow-up, were noted in BBS and ABC.	Intensive massed practice of standard physical therapy produced significant results in balance retraining with patients post-stroke. Findings support the need to offer additional practice to maximize the efficacy of physical therapy sessions.
Flynn SL, et al., 2007 (183)	N = 1 Chronic	Visual feedback with virtual reality games	The Eyetoy: Play 2 with 23 different game experiences aimed at accurate target-based upper-extremity motion, motor planning, dynamic sitting and standing balance, and eye-hand coordination. Can be used with up to 4 players either sitting or standing. Independent home exercise with weekly contacts by research team.	Twenty 1-hour sessions for 4.5 weeks	Clinically relevant improvements were found on the Dynamic Gait Index and trends toward improvement on the Fugl-Meyer, Berg Balance, UE functional index, Motor Activity Lob, and Beck Depression Inventory. Device use was feasible. Subject reported that games were motivating and enjoyable to play.	A low-cost virtual reality system was easily used in the home. In the future it may be used to improve sensory/motor recovery following stroke, as an adjunct to standard care physical therapy.
Betker AL, et al., 2006 (182)	N = 3 Not stated	Visual feedback via video game	To investigate whether coupling foot center of pressure (COP)-controlled video games to standing balance exercises will improve dynamic balance control and to determine whether the motivational and challenging aspects of the video games would increase a subject's desire to perform the exercises and complete the rehabilitation process.	Eight 45-minute sessions over 3 weeks	Post-exercise, subjects exhibited a lower fall count, decreased COP excursion limits for some tasks, increased practice volume, and increased attention span during training.	The COP-controlled video game-based exercise regime motivated subjects to increase their practice volume and attention span during training. This in turn improved subjects' dynamic balance control.

TABLE 21-1
(Continued)

Citation	Population Acute < 7 months Chronic > 12 months	Type of Intervention	Description of Intervention	Duration of Treatment	Results	Conclusions/Comments
Cheng PT, et al., 2004 (175)	N = 52 Acute	Visual feedback	Training Group: Rhythmic weight shifts of 7 seconds in duration, to eight targets on visual screen, positioned at 45° angles in a circle at 75% of LOS. Center starting target represents subject's COG. A trained therapist directly supervised each training session. Control Group: Conventional stroke rehabilitation.	20 minutes 5 days per week for 3 weeks	Significant improvement in dynamic balance (as measured by matching moving cursor) was found in the training group and was maintained for 6 months. No significant change was noted in static standing balance. At six months, 17.8% of training group had fallen, versus 41.7% of control group (p = 0.059)	Visual feedback rhythmic weight-shift training significantly improves dynamic balance function for hemiplegic stroke patients. The effects were sustained over 6 months. The benefits of training might decrease fall occurrence for hemiplegic stroke patients.
Cheng PT, et al., 2001 (179)	N = 54 Acute	Visual feedback with functional task training	Control group received conventional stroke rehabilitation. Experimental group received conventional treatment plus 30 minutes of symmetrical standing and 20 minutes of repetitive sit-to-stand training with biofeedback trainer.	Conventional rehabilitation plus 50-minute session 5 days per week for 3 weeks	Significant improvement in symmetrical sit-to-stand and stand-to-sit from initial test to 6-month follow-up, with the incidence of falls significantly decreasing in the experimental group (16.7%) versus the control group (41.7%) in the 6-month follow-up period.	Symmetrical body-weight distribution training may improve sit-to-stand performance and, consequently, decrease the number of falls by stroke patients.
Geiger RA, et al., 2001 (177)	N = 13 Acute	Visual feedback	Both groups received PT techniques aimed at improving strength, range of motion, balance, and mobility.	50 minutes, 2–3 times a week	Following intervention, both groups scored higher on the Berg Balance Scale and required less time to perform the	Although both groups demonstrated improvement following 4 weeks of physical therapy interventions,

Study	N / Stage	Intervention	Intervention Details	Duration	Results	Conclusion
			The treatment group received 35 minutes of PT and 15 minutes of visual biofeedback balance training, at 50–75% of their limits of stability.		Timed "Up & Go" Test. These improvements corresponded to increased independence of balance and mobility in the study population. However, a comparison of mean changes revealed no differences between groups.	no additional effects were found in the group that received visual biofeedback/forceplate training combined with other physical therapy.
Walker C, et al., 2000 (178)	N = 46 Acute	Visual feedback	Control group received conventional PT/OT until discharge. Visual Feedback (VF) received visual feedback on their Center of Gravity work on symmetrical weight bearing and shifting their weight to visual targets. Conventional (CV) received verbal & tactile cues for weight shifts and symmetrical stance.	2 hours per day, 5 days a week, plus 30 minutes for the 2 experimental groups until discharge	All groups demonstrated marked improvement over time for all measures of balance ability, with the greatest improvements occurring in the period from baseline to discharge. No between-group differences were detected in any of the outcome measures.	Visual feedback or conventional balance training in addition to regular therapy affords no added benefit when offered in the early stages of rehabilitation following stroke.
Lynch EA, et al., 2007 (192)	N = 21 Acute	Sensory training	Sensory Retraining: Education on nature and extent of sensory loss; practice in detection and localization of touch, hardness, texture, and temperature discrimination in sitting and standing with vision obscured; proprioception training of the big toe. Control Group: Assisted to stand for the same time period as the treatment group, with eyes closed. The rest of the time was supine in relaxation exercises with eyes closed.	2 weeks, ten 30-minute sessions	Significant improvement over time ($p < 0.05$) in light touch at 3 points on affected foot, BBS, 10m walk, use of walking aid. No significant difference was noted between groups in any of the outcome variables, except for light touch at the first metatarsal. The study had poor power (13%) to detect group effects, due to the small sample size.	Results of this pilot study are unable to support or refute the routine use of sensory retraining of the lower limb for people during inpatient rehabilitation after stroke. Further research with a larger sample size is required.

TABLE 21-1
(Continued)

Citation	Population Acute < 7 months Chronic > 12 months	Type of Intervention	Description of Intervention	Duration of Treatment	Results	Conclusions/Comments
Hillier SA, et al., 2006 (191)	N = 3 Chronic	Sensory training	Intensive sensory appreci- ation training, involving a hierarchy of sensory education, experiences, and interpretation.	45-minute sessions 3 times per week for 2 weeks	Testing post-intervention demonstrated statistically significant changes in light-touch appreciation for two subjects and in some postural control parameters in the third subject. Clinically favorable trends were shown in other measures.	This initial study shows promising results for the incorporation of sensory training in the lower limb post-stroke, particularly if consideration is given to motivation, attention, and functional application.
van Nes IJ, et al., 2006 (199)	N = 53 Acute	Sensory stimulation vibration	All subjects received 90 minutes of PT and 30 minutes of OT/SP. The experimental group received whole-body vibration 4 × 45 second stimulation (30 Hz frontal plan oscillations of 3mm amplitude). The music group received the same amount of exercise therapy on music.	Four 45-second sessions per day for 6 weeks	At baseline, both groups were comparable in terms of prognostic factors and outcome measures. At both 6 and 12 weeks follow-up, no clinically relevant or statistical differences in outcome were observed between the groups. No side effects were reported.	Daily sessions of whole-body vibration during 6 weeks are not more effective in terms of recovery of balance and activities of daily living than the same amount of exercise therapy on music in the post-acute phase of stroke.
Worms G, et al., 2006 (190)	N = 1 Chronic	Electrical sensory stimulation	Subjects were perturbed in eight different directions, with and without sensory stimulation on four muscles of the impaired leg.	20 minutes daily for 2 weeks.	Vertical ground reaction forces on the impaired side increased after stimulation.	The subject improved his ability to balance throughout the training, with the largest improvements during the final period when electri- cal stimulation was used.

Bayouk JF, et al., 2006 (194)	N = 16 Chronic	Sensory (vision deprived)	Task-oriented exercises, Part 1: Stepping various directions, stepping over various blocks, standing up from chair and Swiss ball, walking forward and backward, turning. Part 2: double-leg stance 10 seconds, tandem stance 10 seconds, rise from chair without arms, tandem walking forward and backward, single-leg stance. Experimental group performed Part 2 exercises with eyes open and closed, on firm and soft surfaces.	1-hour sessions twice a week for 8 weeks	Significant improvements (P < 0.05) in COP displacement under sensory conditions (1) and (2) for the experimental group only, and limited changes for the sit-to-stand in both groups after training. Significant improvements (P < 0.05) were also found in both groups for the walking test.	It is concluded that a task-oriented exercise program, assisted by sensory manipulation, is more effective at improving the standing balance of stroke subjects than a conventional task-oriented program.
Bonan IV, et al., 2004 (103)	N = 20 Chronic	Sensory (vision deprived)	5 minutes of tone inhibition, 1 hour to improve balance. Week 1: 30 minutes of exercise in supine or prone position. Week 2: sitting. Week 3: all fours or kneeling. Week 4: in upright posture. Each session also included 20 minutes of balance training on treadmill and stationary bike, and ended with 10 minutes of walking on foam rubber track with obstacles. The experimental group had their eyes covered for each session. The control group did not have their eyes covered.	1 hour, 5 days per week, for 4 weeks	After completing the program, balance, gait velocity, and self-assessment of gait improved significantly in all patients. Balance improved more in the vision-deprived group than in the free-vision group, but only significantly in ST1 and ST4.	Balance improved more after rehabilitation with visual deprivation than with free vision. Visual overuse may be a compensatory strategy for coping with initial imbalance exacerbated by traditional rehabilitation.

TABLE 21-1
(Continued)

Citation	Population Acute < 7 months Chronic > 12 months	Type of Intervention	Description of Intervention	Duration of Treatment	Results	Conclusions/Comments
Morioka S, Yagi F, 2003 (193)	N = 28 Acute	Sensory training	Both groups participated in PT/OT rehabilitation program. Experimental group also participated in exercise to discriminate hardness of rubber sponge under sole of foot while standing and blindfolded.	10 days over 2 weeks	Hardness discrimination decreased over the 10 days, but no significant improvement in two-point discrimination. More postural sway measures improved pre-post in the experimental group than in the control.	Hardness discrimination by the plantar sole may be effective as a supplemental exercise for standing balance. Improvement in postural sway may also be related to increased standing time.
Pohl M, et al., 2006 (212)	N = 28 Acute	Ankle-foot orthosis	Individually fabricated quasi-double-stop semi-ridge AFO approximately 20 cm high, encasing the ankle. Does not encase the metatarsophalangeal joints.	Immediate post-fabrication	AFO significantly improved weight bearing on affected leg, and decreased postural sway in stance. Also, gait parameters of double stance duration, symmetry ratios, and deceleration forces improved.	An individually designed functional in-shoe AFO can improve stance and gait parameters, even in a single use, in patient with hemiparesis.
Wang RY, et al., 2005 (213)	N = 42 Acute N = 61 Chronic	Ankle-foot orthosis	Use of AFO over time	N/A	Significant improvements noted in acute post-stroke subjects in weight-bearing distribution during quiet stance, body sway on foam (eyes open and eyes closed), movement velocity during LOS, and maximal excursion toward affected side. Such effects were not observed in subjects with chronic stroke.	For subjects with hemiparesis of short duration, the AFO improves symmetry in quiet and dynamic standing balances. It also increases speed and cadence. However, its effectiveness is minimal for patients of long duration.

Study	Sample	Intervention	Description		Results
Laufer Y, 2003 (210)	N = 24 Acute N = 6 Chronic N = 20 healthy elderly	Assistive device (canes)	No cane, straight cane, and quad cane, with three different foot positions: (1) heels aligned, (2) affected foot forward, (3) unaffected foot forward.	N/A	Straight cane reduced postural sway only in the affected-forward position, whereas quad cane reduced sway in all three positions. Asymmetrical weight bearing did not change across positions, even with walking aids. Quad cane appears to be more effective than standard cane in decreasing postural sway during stance. The use of a cane does not appear to adversely affect asymmetrical weight-bearing pattern in stance, even when base of support is decreased.
Maeda A, et al., 2001 (211)	N = 41 Chronic N = 36 healthy elderly	Assistive device (cane)	Standard Romberg position, with and without straight cane	N/A	There was a significant reduction in postural sway with the cane in both control and stroke subjects, and a greater sway reduction with a straight cane for stroke survivors than for healthy controls. The effects of body support with a cane on postural sway of patients with stroke were greater than upon that of healthy independent elderly. Decrease in postural sway is more dramatic in stroke survivors than in healthy independent elderly.
Chaudhuri S, et al., 2000 (212a)	N = 10 Acute	Assistive device (shoe lifts)	Shoe lifts of three different heights (6 mm, 9 mm, 12 mm) under the non-affected leg	N/A	During platform translations using no lift, there were longer onset latencies for the affected compared to the stronger limb ($p < 0.01$); however, the latencies were only significant for the larger translations. Decreased latencies occurred in the paretic limb when using the smaller lifts under the nonaffected leg, but this did not reach significance. Weight symmetry improved with the smaller lifts but did not reach significance, due to high variability. Lifts applied to the shoe of the stronger limb induced a body weight shift toward the paretic limb and resulted in improved symmetry of stand and postural control of individuals with hemiparesis.

TABLE 21-1
(Continued)

Citation	Population Acute < 7 months Chronic > 12 months	Type of Intervention	Description of Intervention	Duration of Treatment	Results	Conclusions/Comments
Orrell AJ, et al., 2006 (209)	N = 20	Motor learning	To keep a stabilometer platform horizontal for 60 seconds. The discovery learning group was instructed to discover rules of how to perform the balancing task. In the errorless learning group, a braking resistance of 2.5 kg was applied, in order to restrict movement of the stabilometer platform, which was progressively decreased by 0.5kg every 4 trials so that no resistance was given in the final 4 trials.	Twenty-four 60-second trials with 2-minute minimum break between trials	The balance performance of the discovery (explicit) learners after stroke was impaired by the imposition of the concurrent cognitive task load. In contrast, the performance of the errorless (implicit) learners (stroke and control groups) and the discovery learning control group was not impaired.	This provision of explicit information during rehabilitation may be detrimental to the learning/relearning and execution of motor skills in some people with stroke. The application of implicit motor learning techniques in the rehabilitation setting may be beneficial.

of intense practice and the need to offer additional practice to maximize usefulness of treatment interventions.

Numerous studies have been done investigating the effectiveness of Tai Chi exercise on balance in various populations of older adults (168–172). The majority of the studies have reported improvements in balance with Tai Chi. Tai Chi movements are typically slow, graceful, continual flows around a centrally aligned head, shoulder, and pelvis. During the movements, or Tai Chi forms, the body weight is constantly shifting over a stable base of support (173). Tai Chi has also been reported to improve proprioception in the elderly (172, 174). To date, only one study has examined the effects of Tai Chi on stroke survivors (155). This study found that the Tai Chi group did not improve their balance or walking compared to the control group, and there were no side effects of the Tai Chi training. The small sample size, the amount of Tai Chi instruction, and/or pregroup differences may have impacted the results.

Visual Feedback

Weight transfer is a component of balance that occurs in situations such as reaching, shifting weight from one leg to the other, or postural transitions. Weight transfer training to improve balance has achieved mixed outcomes. Two studies utilizing weight-shifting exercises, one by means of goal-orientated activities and the other using visual biofeedback, reported no statistical difference between usual care and the experimental group who received additional weight-shifting training (175, 176).

Visual feedback to enhance balance training also has shown mixed results. Two studies compared conventional therapy to conventional therapy plus visual feedback training and found no added benefit in balance outcome measure between the groups (177, 178). Another study used visual feedback with the task-specific training during sit-to-stand (179). This study reported significant improvement in symmetrical weight bearing, speed, and rate of rise during sit-to-stand. These changes were accompanied by a decrease in the incidence of falls in the visual feedback groups compared to the usual care control group at the six-month follow-up. These improvements are in contrast to the lack of improvements found in other visual feedback studies (177, 178, 180, 181) and may be related to the additional task practice of sit-to-stand and the potential increase in lower extremity strength. These variables, however, were not measured in this study.

Technological developments in the form of virtual reality have been applied in studies of upper limb function and locomotion. Only two studies have used balance as an outcome measure. In a study by Betker et al. (182), subjects who trained on custom-designed computer games reported increased motivation and practice time when using the system. Post-exercise, the subjects reportedly exhibited a decrease in the number of falls and an increase in the center of pressure excursion during 12 different standing balance tasks (182). A commercially available system (Sony PlayStation 2 gaming system) was used by Flynn et al. (183) with an individual who was two years post-stroke. A trend toward improvement in balance after 20 one-hour training sessions was reported (183). The commercially available Wii computer gaming systems has also been anecdotally reported to be utilized in some rehabilitation facilities. Virtual reality and computer gaming open up another avenue of visual feedback training for improving balance control, but the potential effectiveness of such training remains to be demonstrated in randomized, control trials.

Sensory Training

Diminished or altered sensation is a frequent impairment post-stroke, and it has been related to reduced standing balance and mobility (81, 102, 137, 184, 185). Several studies have shown promising results using sensory retraining in the upper limb (186–189); however, there are relatively few studies that have investigated sensory training for standing balance. One study used sensory electrical stimulation of four lower extremity muscles of the paretic leg and reported an increased ability to bear weight on the paretic side during standing balance perturbation testing compared to no sensory stimulation (190). More systematic sensory retraining of pressure detection, hardness, and texture identification under the foot has been reported in three studies (191–193). These studies of sensory retraining in the lower extremity reported encouraging results on changes in sensory measures but little impact on balance. Two of the studies showed improvement of sensory and balance measures over time in subjects with post-acute stroke (191, 192). However, only one of the studies found a difference in balance measures between the sensory training and control group (193). The positive findings from this study may be attributed to the increased standing time the sensory training group received.

Alteration of visual input is easily accomplished in the clinic by having the patient close their eyes or occluding his or her vision. One study compared two balance training programs with and without visual cues (103). Compared to the vision-free group, fewer falls were observed in the vision-deprived group with improvement in static standing balance (103). The authors concluded that vision deprivation forces patients to increase their use of somatosensory and vestibular information and a reliance on visual information may be a natural compensatory strategy for dealing with impaired balance early on in the rehabilitation process.

Another simple way to manipulate sensory inputs in balance training is by using soft and firm surfaces. Bayouk et al. (194) used the same exercise program with two groups of chronic stroke survivors. One group performed the exercise with their eyes open; the second group performed the balance tasks with their eyes open and closed and on soft and firm surfaces. The group who performed the exercises with their eyes closed did better in the balance tasks and the ten-meter walk (194). Tilt boards, dimly lighted environments, and uneven or variously textured surfaces are other ways to manipulate sensory inputs in the clinic and challenge the patient to utilize or alternate their use of various sensory systems.

Whole body vibration (WBV) has recently emerged as an intervention that has positive effects on neuromuscular and sensorimotor systems by presumably activating muscles and stimulating sensory receptors (195–198). An investigation of the added benefit of WBV on balance control and ADLs found that, although the treatment was well-tolerated and appreciated by the participant, there was no difference in outcomes with the WBV (199).

Impact of Attention on Balance Training

Standing balance control requires the integration of multiple systems, the ability to adapt to changes in the task and environment, and some degree of attention (50, 200, 201). Cognitive deficits post-stroke can occur in the domains of language, orientation, attention, memory, information processing, executive function, and learning. Studies have shown that performance of dual-task impacts balance in person post-stroke (200, 202–204), suggest that, after stroke, people utilize increased attention to maintain balance.

Current rehabilitation therapies typically involve persons receiving many complex and explicit instructions from the clinician on how to perform tasks and evaluation procedures. Recent work suggests that this type of information is less helpful and may in fact hinder implicit motor skill learning after stroke (205–208). These studies have been done with upper extremity tasks. Orrell et al. (209) investigated implicit motor learning on a dynamic balance task with and without concurrent cognitive load. They found that all groups (healthy controls and persons post-stroke) improved in the balance task, regardless of the task instructions. However, balance performance in the explicit learning group post-stroke was impaired during secondary cognitive loading and not impaired in either the implicit learning post-stroke group or the control groups. This suggested that providing explicit information may be detrimental to learning and execution of a dynamic balance motor task in some people after stroke.

External Devices

Assistive devices and lower extremity orthosis are frequently prescribed for individuals post-stroke to help with ambulation. These devices have also been shown to increase postural stability (210, 211). Canes decrease postural sway with some studies reporting that the quad cane is more effective in reducing sway (210). However, straight canes and quad canes do not appear to improve symmetrical weight bearing (210). Ankle foot orthosis (AFO), on the other hand, do increase symmetrical weight bearing and decrease postural sway initially, but this effect does not appear to be maintained over the long term (212, 213) One study utilizing a small lift under the shoe of the stronger lower extremity reported an immediate improvement in symmetry of stance and postural control of individuals with hemiparesis (212a). Canes, ankle foot orthosis, and lifts appear to be beneficial for improving standing balance in some situations by providing external support of body load and by increasing the BOS area; however, this may interfere with protective responses of the lower or upper limb (214).

Summary

The recent studies of standing balance rehabilitation after stroke presented in this section utilized a variety of intervention approaches. The common theme has been one of task-orientated practice under various environmental, sensory, motor, and cognitive challenges. Dosages varied between the studies from intensely concentrated, one-on-one rehabilitation sessions to group activities held twice per week. Guidelines for effective standing balance training following stroke remain unclear. However, one might consider two simple, straightforward modifications to augment one's current balance training program:

1. Incorporate more training activities with vision occluded as a method to challenge an individual to increase his or her awareness and use of other sensory information.
2. Minimize the amount of explicit information that is given during a treatment session to allow the person post-stroke time to process and learn the balance strategies that work best for him or her.

PROTECTIVE STEPPING: A MODEL FOR LINKING DYNAMIC BALANCE CONTROL, FUNCTIONAL OUTCOMES, AND RISK OF FALLS

As discussed earlier in this chapter, falls and associated injuries related to problems with standing balance are common and frequently debilitating secondary complications accompanying chronic stroke. The relationship between changes in balance control factors, functional balance and mobility, and falls in chronic stroke is poorly understood. For example, a recent retrospective study (75) found that clinical measures of balance, gait mobility, and cognitive status were not associated with falls. A major conclusion was that routine clinical tests may not assess the aspects of balance required to prevent falls and that more sensitive measures of balance that include large components of reactive dynamic balance are needed (75). To a large extent, such current deficiencies in knowledge that limit the development of the most effective rehabilitation interventions to improve standing balance and prevent falls and related disabilities after stroke are likely caused by the lack of comprehensive approaches linking physiological measures of dynamic balance, functional performance, and falls.

As a starting point to addressing the foregoing issues, it has been pointed out that the lack of information concerning the active use of limb movements, such as stepping or reaching to contact a stable support surface as a standing balance recovery mechanism, has been a neglected aspect of standing balance recovery after stroke (96). This is striking because accumulating evidence has indicated the importance of stepping for dynamic balance recovery during ADLs (215). Moreover, healthy, community-living older adults at risk of falls have an increased reliance on stepping, rather than feet-in-place balance responses (2, 54, 124, 215–221).

From a biomechanical standpoint, stepping modifies the BOS in relation to the position and motion of the COM to maintain balance. Protective stepping may be initiated in anticipation of an impending loss of balance or fall or in reaction to sensorimotor events following external perturbations to balance. Contrary to traditional views, reactive stepping may be initiated well before the COM reaches the limits of the BOS (2). Additionally, protective stepping shares many of the requirements of ongoing gait and therefore is an attractive framework for identifying physiological changes underlying impaired balance and mobility and falls among people with chronic stroke. Remarkably, however, no published studies that have examined the potential link between protective stepping, functional performance, and prospective falls among chronic stroke survivors could be located.

Measures of Protective Stepping Predict Future Falls in Healthy Older Adults

From our ongoing studies of generally healthy, community-living older adults at risk for falls, we have identified two key performance markers of protective stepping that are predictive of prospectively identified falls, including the percentage of trials with multiple recovery steps and first-step global length combining the A-P and M-L directions (219). These measures reflect the effectiveness of stepping to arrest the motion of the COM at foot landing (221). We have previously demonstrated that the distance between the COM and the margin of the BOS, coupled with the

COM velocity, is importantly related to effective balance recovery through stepping (2, 222). These safety margins are smaller for older fallers than nonfallers (2, 222). Hence, step placement relative to body position and motion is a fundamental means by which balance is sustained. Because stepping is often impaired in chronic stroke (Richards, Malouin, et al.), we propose that multiple stepping behavior and impaired step length regulation (as well as other factors) will be importantly related to clinical assessments of impairments, functional performance, and falls.

Data from our previous studies of protective stepping using waist-pull perturbations of standing balance in 51 generally healthy, community-living older individuals (mean age = 73.3 years) included subjects' prospective fall history for a period of one year after testing (219). Logistic regression analyses determined potential predictors of falls. Fall status was included as the dependent variable after dichotomization. Independent variables included percent total trials with multiple steps (rather than a single-recovery step) and first-step global length following multidirectional waist-pull perturbations that always induced stepping. Because controlling sideways balance during multidirectional stepping may be particularly problematic for older people (223–225) and is largely dependent upon hip joint abduction-adduction torques (225, 226), we also evaluated clinical measures of isokinetic hip abduction (AB) torque (60 degrees through a range of motion of 0–30 degrees).

Overall, 74% (14 out of 19) of the fallers and 31% (10 out of 32) of the nonfallers used multiple steps in 100% of the trials (Chi Square: p = 0.003) in response to lateral perturbations. Figure 21-2 shows the percent total trials with multiple recovery steps used by the fallers and nonfallers (K-W: p = 0.018). The fallers also had a

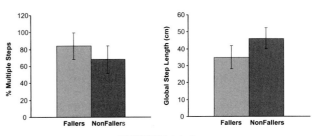

Protective Stepping Responses of Older Adults

FIGURE 21-2

Group means 1 SD for prospectively identified healthy older Fallers (n = 19) and NonFallers (n = 32) showing group differences between (left) first-step global length combining the A-P and M-L directions (Two-sample t-test: p < 0.003) and (right) between the percent of the total balance perturbation trials with multiple recovery steps in response to lateral waist-pulls K-W: (p < 0.018).

shorter (Two-sample t-test: p = 0.003) first-step global length (34 cm 13.9) than the nonfallers (46.1 cm 12.3). Differences in hip strength further discriminated between the groups, whereby fallers produced lower peak hip AB torque than nonfallers (t-test: p = 0.008).

The percent trials with multiple steps were first entered into the single-variable regression model. Then, global-step length was added using a forward stepwise method. The percent trials with multiple steps was the strongest predictive value for falls (odds ratio = 6.160, p = 0.005). Fallers who used multiple steps in 100% of the trials were 6.2 times more likely to fall than individuals who did not always use multiple steps. Single-variable analysis also showed that, for every decrease of 10 standardized units in step length, the odds of falling increased 2.0 times (odds ratio = 2.028, p = 0.006) and, for every decrease of 0.1 standardized units of peak isokinetic hip AB torque, the odds of falling increased 1.8 times.

The percent trials with multiple steps were combined with global-step length in the two variable models. This combination was not better in predicting fall status than the single-variable models. However, the percent multiple step-hip AB strength model was significantly (p < 0.016) improved over the percent multiple step model alone. Subjects who used multiple steps to recover their lateral balance 100% of the time and had lower peak isokinetic hip AB torque generation were 5.9 times more likely to fall.

We also determined the cutoff scores that provided the highest combination of sensitivity and specificity for predicting one or more falls. For example, in the protective stepping assessment, a cutoff score of 100% multiple steps resulted in 70.5% of the subjects being correctly identified as fallers or nonfallers, a sensitivity of 74%, and a specificity of 69%.

Protective Stepping Performance in Adults with Chronic Stroke Resembles Performance for Healthy, Older Fallers

The kinetic and kinematic characteristics of stepping following waist-pull perturbations of standing balance were evaluated in 10 independently ambulatory subjects with single-episode chronic stroke (mean age = 59.6 years). Three waist-pull trials at a single magnitude level (17.5 cm, 36 cm/s, 720 cm/s/s) were randomly applied in each of three directions:

- Straight forward (0 degrees)
- Diagonally forward at 30 degrees to the right (+ 30 degrees)
- To the left (− 30 degrees)

Subjects were placed in a safety harness and instructed to react naturally to prevent falling.

Overall, regardless of the direction of perturbation, subjects' first step was taken with their nonparetic leg in 66% of the trials. This indicated that they either selected to use and/or were limited to using their paretic leg more often for single-limb support rather than for relocating the BOS during the initial balance recovery step.

The data shown in Figure 21-3 further indicates that, regardless of perturbation direction, subjects used multiple recovery steps in a high percentage of the total

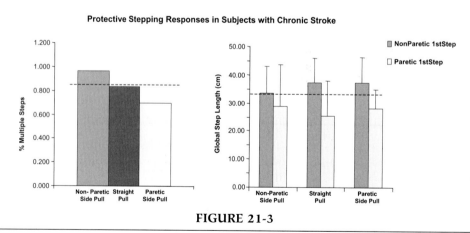

FIGURE 21-3

Means 1 SD for subjects with chronic stroke (n = 10) showing (left) the percent of the total trials with multiple recovery steps for each waist-pull direction and (right) the first-step global length (combined A-P and M-L displacement) for paretic and non-paretic limb steps for each direction of waist-pull perturbation. The broken horizontal lines indicate the levels of healthy elderly faller performance.

trials (pulls forward and toward paretic side = 70%, pulls straight forward = 83%, pulls forward and toward nonparetic side = 97%) that generally equaled and exceeded that of older fallers (83%) and occurred with a smaller magnitude of perturbation. Notably, steps taken in response to forward-diagonal waist-pulls toward the nonparetic side were almost always multiple recovery steps. This likely occurs because pulls to the nonparetic side cause passive loading of the nonparetic limb (and paretic limb unloading) that further complicates nonparetic limb stepping. In this case, subjects crossed over the midline of the body with a medially directed paretic limb step, which severely challenged their control of step landing.

In addition to the high incidence of multiple stepping responses, the initial global-step length (combined A-P and M-L directions; Figure 21-3) was shorter for paretic limb steps than for the step length identified for older fallers (Figure 21-2). These data from stroke subjects 13 years younger than the mean age of the older fallers suggest that they are at high risk of falling caused by impaired stepping performance.

To more fully determine the relationship between dynamic balance control and the functional impact of impairments in protective stepping and risk of falling, clinical assessments of balance and mobility (for example, Berg Balance Scale and 10-m timed walk) and prospective fall data are needed. Falls are tracked through monthly postcards mailed in at the end of each month for one year after testing. For each reported fall, a follow-up telephone call is made to ask about precipitating factors, and, if any injuries were sustained, the medical care sought. The use of monthly mail-in reporting and follow-up is among the most rigorous approaches (227).

Implications and Importance

Application of this or other models to people with chronic stroke will help to fill important deficiencies in knowledge, linking physiological measures of dynamic balance, functional performance, and falls. More elaborate applications of the framework would include assessing other potentially important factors such as changes in sensory systems, patterns of paresis, individuation of multijoint control, spasticity and joint mobility, response timing and multisegmental coordination, adaptive capacity, attention, and hemispatial neglect. Moreover, comprehensive approaches that attempt to link impairment level outcomes with functional and disability level outcomes, along with ecologically valid tests of dynamic balance recovery, will provide empirically grounded and evidence-based foundations for designing the most effective rehabilitation approaches to improving balance control, functional balance and mobility, and preventing falls.

RESEARCH FRONTIERS

This section provides a glimpse of selected research frontiers that have bearing on understanding the recovery of standing balance after stroke and on the development of the most effective rehabilitation interventions to enhance balance recovery and reduce related disabilities.

Cortical Control of Balance

A growing number of studies have begun to identify the involvement of cerebral cortical areas in the control of standing balance, a role that has been traditionally associated with spinal cord and brain stem systems. Using neural probes such as elecroencephalography, positron emission tomography, or transcranial magnetic stimulation, studies of healthy individuals have identified contributions of cortical mediated activity during standing (27), preceding or following external perturbation of stance (22–24, 26, 59, 228), and accompanying anticipatory postural adjustments during voluntary tasks (25, 29, 30, 33). Although understanding of the role of cortical areas in regulating standing balance is still quite limited, this area of investigation is of obvious potential significance to balance recovery after cerebral stroke. Thus, balance-related cortical involvement likely influences several important aspects of standing regulation that may be impaired after stroke, including:

1. Response preparation, planning, and selection
2. Adaptive control mechanisms
3. Attention and other cognitive resources

Information about the contributing roles of altered cortical mechanisms after stroke and their potential to be modified in the course of functional recovery by rehabilitation interventions such as those being applied to the upper limb (229–231) would be useful for developing the most effective balance intervention programs.

Changes in Skeletal Muscle

It is striking that there have been very few studies of fundamental physical and physiological properties of skeletal muscle after stroke, particularly as they relate to function and the recovery of balance and mobility. However, recent evidence from muscle biopsy (232) has indicated substantial structural and metabolic changes in muscle after stroke, including gross atrophy and shift to fast myosin heavy chain in paretic leg muscle that is associated with gait deficit severity. Evidence also suggests that inflammatory pathway activation and oxidative injury could lead to wasting, altered function, and impaired insulin action in skeletal muscle (232).

Other work (233) using computed tomography to examine changes in muscle composition in 60 subjects with chronic stroke demonstrated 20% lower muscle cross-sectional area and 25% higher intramuscular fat area in the paretic thigh compared to the nonparetic thigh. In older adults without stroke, this low-density lean tissue (fat infiltration) is associated with lower physical fitness levels (234, 235) and is implicated in muscle weakness (reduced contractile capacity) and reduced balance function (44, 55, 62, 103, 202, 234–237). Importantly, exercise training may modify or reverse skeletal muscle abnormalities in people with chronic stroke (238). Therefore, it would be important to determine the extent to which changes in skeletal muscle after stroke are contributing to balance problems. Further insights into this area could potentially shift or expand the focus of balance and mobility rehabilitation interventions by emphasizing the mitigating roles of muscle properties and mechanisms.

Balance Recovery: Physiological and Compensatory

As also discussed for locomotion in this volume (Richards et al.), difficulty with identifying and understanding balance recovery following stroke is further complicated by the presence of what are commonly thought to be compensatory mechanisms or behaviors that often develop together with improvements in motor control factors that normally contribute to sustaining balance, thought to represent true physiological recovery. In practical terms, it is likely that the two recovery states and their overlap represent a continuum of available solutions that the balance system uses to sustain the COM position and motion within the actual or projected stability limits defined by the BOS conditions.

An intriguing parallel situation to the recovery of balance exists for the recovery of upper limb function in chronic stroke, whereby an individual's potential for functional recovery of limb use can be predicted from neurophysiological (TMS) and imaging (fMRI) measures of neural capacity (239). A major finding of this work was that, in subjects without TMS motor-evoked potentials (MEPs) and a hemispheric cortical asymmetry level that exceeded a critical cutoff value, no functional gains in arm motor recovery were possible with practice training. In contrast, those individuals for whom MEPs could be elicited and who had lower cortical asymmetry were capable of arm motor improvements with training. Thus, corticospinal tract integrity predicted the clinical potential for functional arm recovery in people at about three years after the time of stroke onset. One suggestion

was that this approach can be used to help formulate goals for rehabilitation and identify patients for particular types of rehabilitation programs. The applicability of the findings with respect to true recovery and compensatory recovery processes is that those individuals identified to have residual neural capacity could be selected for programs emphasizing motor control factors while those with limited capacity might emphasize alternative compensatory solutions. If, as it appears, cortical areas are extensively involved in the control of standing balance (59, 60), then a similar, though possibly modified, algorithm could be developed to assess the balance recovery process.

To expand beyond the neural basis of recovery, it would also be informative to identify similar biological and physiological markers of skeletal muscle capacity and cognitive capacity after stroke to more fully capture the multifaceted nature of standing balance control problems. Overall, this line of investigation is an attractive and important research frontier for better understanding and optimizing the functional recovery and rehabilitation of balance and mobility after stroke.

SUMMARY

The rapid expansion of recent scientific and clinical knowledge has driven the field of rehabilitation to an unprecedented level of growth and understanding. At the forefront of these efforts has been the increasing development of interdisciplinary approaches blending clinical, experimental, and technological expertise. Inherently, the complex and multifaceted nature of the human standing balance system and the challenges to balance rehabilitation will continue to require such integrated approaches to identifying the different factors contributing to balance problems and the means by which they can be effectively treated. In this chapter, we have synthesized current information derived from many of these different approaches. In doing so, we have attempted to identify those areas in need of additional information, areas where information is lacking, and some promising newer areas of inquiry.

ACKNOWLEDGMENTS

The research presented in Section V, Protective Stepping: A Model for Linking Dynamic Balance Control, Functional Outcomes, and Risk of Falls, was supported by grants from the National Institutes of Health/National Institute on Aging (grant R01AG16780) to Mark W. Rogers and by the Foundation for Physical Therapy to Carolee J. Winstein.

References

1. Winter DA. *ABC: Anatomy, Biomechanics, and Control of Balance during Standing and Walking.* Waterloo, Ontario, Canada: Waterloo Biomechanics, 1995.

2. Pai YC, Rogers MW, Patton J, et al. Static versus dynamic predictions of protective stepping following waist-pull perturbations in young and older adults. *J Biomech* 1998; 31(12):1111–1118.

3. Krebs DE, Velyvis PH, Rogers MW. Vestibulopathy and the age effects on protective stepping during unperturbed standing. *Motor Control* 2000; 4(3):316–328.

4. Fitzpatrick R, Rogers DK, McCloskey DI. Stable human standing with lower-limb muscle afferents providing the only sensory input. *Journal of Physiology* 1994; 480(Pt 2): 395–403.

5. Gurfinkel VS, Ivanenko YuP, Levik YuS, Babakova IA. Kinesthetic reference for human orthograde posture. *Neuroscience* 1995; 68(1):229–243.

6. Horak FB, Macpherson JM. Postural orientation and equilibrium. In: Rowell LB, Shepherd JT, eds. *Handbook of Physiology, Section 12, Exercise: Regulation and Integration of Multiple Systems.* Oxford: Oxford University Press, 1996:255–292.

7. Jeka J, Kiemel T, Creath R, et al. Controlling human upright posture: Velocity information is more accurate than position or acceleration. *J Neurophysiol* 2004; 92(4):2368–2379.

8. Peterka RJ. Postural control model interpretation of stabilogram diffusion analysis. *Biol Cybern* 2000; 82(4):335–343.

9. Winter DA, Patla AE, Prince F, et al. Stiffness control of balance in quiet standing. *Journal of Neurophysiology* 1998; 80(3):1211–1221.

10. Massion J, Alexandrov A, Frolov A. Why and how are posture and movement coordinated? *Prog Brain Res* 2004; 143:13–27.

11. Loram ID, Maganaris CN, Lakie M. Human postural sway results from frequent, ballistic bias impulses by soleus and gastrocnemius. *J Physiol* 2005; 564(Pt 1):295–311.

12. Morasso PG, Baratto L, Capra R, Spada G. Internal models in the control of posture. *Neural Netw* 1999; 12(7–8):1173–1180.

13. Casadio M, Morasso PG, Sanguineti V. Direct measurement of ankle stiffness during quiet standing: Implications for control modeling and clinical application. *Gait Posture* 2005; 21(4):410–424.

14. Collins JJ, DeLuca CJ. Open-loop and closed-loop control of posture: A random-walk analysis of center-of-pressure trajectories. *Experimental Brain Research* 1993; 95:308–318.

15. Masani K, Popovic MR, Nakazawa K, et al. Importance of body sway velocity information in controlling ankle extensor activities during quiet stance. *J Neurophysiol* 2003; 90(6):3774–3782.

16. Allum JH, Bloem BR, Carpenter MG, et al. Proprioceptive control of posture: A review of new concepts. *Gait Posture* 1998;8(3):214–242.

17. Bloem BR, Allum JH, Carpenter MG, Honegger F. Is lower leg proprioception essential for triggering human automatic postural responses? *Exp Brain Res* 2000; 130(3):375–391.

18. Mergner T, Maurer C, Peterka RJ. A multisensory posture control model of human upright stance. *Prog Brain Res* 2003; 142:189–201.

19. Oie KS, Kiemel T, Jeka JJ. Human multisensory fusion of vision and touch: Detecting nonlinearity with small changes in the sensory environment. *Neurosci Lett* 2001; 315(3):113–116.

20. Peterka RJ. Sensorimotor integration in human postural control. *J Neurophysiol* 2002; 88(3):1097–1118.

21. Peterka RJ, Loughlin PJ. Dynamic regulation of sensorimotor integration in human postural control. *J Neurophysiol* 2004; 91(1):410–423.

22. Adkin AL, Quant S, Maki BE, McIlroy WE. Cortical responses associated with predictable and unpredictable compensatory balance reactions. *Exp Brain Res* 2006; 172(1):85–93.

23. Dietz V, Quintern J, Berger W, Schenck E. Cerebral potentials and leg EMG responses associated with stance perturbations. *Experimental Brain Research* 1985; 57:348–354.

24. Duckrow RB, Abu-Hasaballah K, Whipple R, Wolfson L. Stance perturbation: Evoked potentials in old people with poor gait and balance. *Clin Neurophysiol* 1999; 110(12):2026–2032.

25. MacKinnon CD, Bissig D, Chiusano J, et al. Preparation of anticipatory postural adjustments prior to stepping. *J Neurophysiol* 2007; 97(6):4368–4379.

26. Mochizuki G, Sibley KM, Esposito JG, et al. Cortical responses associated with the preparation and reaction to full-body perturbations to upright stability. *Clin Neurophysiol* 2008; 119(7):1626–1637.

27. Ouchi Y, Okada H, Yoshikawa E, et al. Brain activation during maintenance of standing postures in humans. *Brain* 1999; 122(Pt 2):329–338.

28. Quant S, Adkin AL, Staines WR, McIlroy WE. Cortical activation following a balance disturbance. *Exp Brain Res* 2004; 155(3):393–400.

29. Saitou K, Washimi Y, Koike Y, et al. Slow negative cortical potential preceding the onset of postural adjustment. *Electroencephalogr Clin Neurophysiol* 1996; 98(6):449–455.

30. Slobounov S, Hallett M, Stanhope S, Shibasaki H. Role of cerebral cortex in human postural control: An EEG study. *Clin Neurophysiol* 2005; 116(2):315–323.

31. Slobounov S, Wu T, Hallett M. Neural basis subserving the detection of postural instability: An FMRI study. *Motor Control* 2006; 10(1):69–89.

32. Staines WR, McIlroy WE, Brooke JD. Cortical representation of whole-body movement is modulated by proprioceptive discharge in humans. *Exp Brain Res* 2001; 138(2):235–242.

33. Yoshida S, Nakazawa K, Shimizu E, Shimoyama I. Anticipatory postural adjustments modify the movement-related potentials of upper extremity voluntary movement. *Gait Posture* 2008; 27(1):97–102.

34. Corbeil P, Blouin JS, Begin F, et al. Perturbation of the postural control system induced by muscular fatigue. *Gait Posture* 2003; 18(2):92–100.

35. Frontera WR, Hughes VA, Fielding RA, et al. Aging of skeletal muscle: A 12-yr longitudinal study. *J Appl Physiol* 2000; 88(4):1321–1326.

36. Yaggie JA, McGregor SJ. Effects of isokinetic ankle fatigue on the maintenance of balance and postural limits. *Arch Phys Med Rehabil* 2002; 83(2):224–228.

37. Nishikawa K, Biewener AA, Aerts P, et al. Neuromechanics: An integrative approach for understanding motor control *Integr Comp Biol* 2007; 47:16–54.

38. Loeb GE, Brown IE, Cheng EJ. A hierarchical foundation for models of sensorimotor control. *Exp Brain Res* 1999; 126(1):1–18.

39. Richardson AG, Slotine JJ, Bizzi E, Tresch MC. Intrinsic musculoskeletal properties stabilize wiping movements in the spinalized frog. *J Neurosci* 2005; 25(12): 3181–3191.

40. Rassier DE, Herzog W. Considerations on the history dependence of muscle contraction. *J Appl Physiol* 2004; 96(2):419–427.

41. Aoyagi Y, Stein RB, Mushahwar VK, Prochazka A. The role of neuromuscular properties in determining the end-point of a movement. *IEEE Trans Neural Syst Rehabil Eng* 2004; 12(1):12–23.

42. Spoor CW, van Leeuwen JL. Knee muscle moment arms from MRI and from tendon travel. *J Biomech* 1992; 25(2):201–206.

43. Narici MV, Maganaris CN. Plasticity of the muscle-tendon complex with disuse and aging. *Exerc Sport Sci Rev* 2007; 35(3):126–134.

44. Burleigh A, Horak FB. Influence of instruction, prediction, and afferent sensory information on the postural organization of step initiation. *J Neurophysiol* 1996; 75(4):1619–1628.

45. Rogers MW, Hedman LD, Johnson ME, et al. Triggering of protective stepping for the control of human balance: Age and contextual dependence. *Cogn Brain Res* 2003; 16(2):192–198.

46. Brauer SG, Woollacott M, Shumway-Cook A. The influence of a concurrent cognitive task on the compensatory stepping response to a perturbation in balance-impaired and healthy elders. *Gait Posture* 2002; 15(1):83–93.

47. Brown LA, Shumway-Cook A, Woollacott MH. Attentional demands and postural recovery: The effects of aging. *J Gerontol A Biol Sci Med Sci* 1999; 54(4):M165–M171.

48. Carpenter MG, Frank JS, Adkin AL, et al. Influence of postural anxiety on postural reactions to multidirectional surface rotations. *J Neurophysiol* 2004; 92(6):3255–3265.

49. Redfern MS, Muller ML, Jennings JR, Furman JM. Attentional dynamics in postural control during perturbations in young and older adults. *J Gerontol A Biol Sci Med Sci* 2002; 57(8):B298–303.

50. Woollacott M, Shumway-Cook A. Attention and the control of posture and gait: A review of an emerging area of research. *Gait Posture* 2002; 16(1):1–14.

51. Diener HC, Horak FB, Nashner LM. Influence of stimulus parameters on human postural responses. *J Neurophysiol* 1988; 59(6):1888–1905.

52. Horak FB, Diener HC, Nashner LM. Influence of central set on human postural responses. *J Neurophysiol* 1989; 62(4):841–853.

53. Maki BE, Whitelaw RS. Influence of expectation and arousal on center of pressure responses to transient postural perturbations. *Journal of Vestibular Research*. 1993; 3:25–39.

54. Mille ML, Rogers MW, Martinez K, et al. Thresholds for inducing protective stepping responses to external perturbations of human standing. *J Neurophysiol* 2003; 90(2):666–674.

55. Chong RKY, Horak FB, Woollacott MH. Time-dependent influence of sensorimotor set on automatic responses in perturbed stance. *Exp Brain Res* 1999; 124(4):513–519.

56. Henry SM, Fung J, Horak FB. Effect of stance width on multidirectional postural responses. *J Neurophysiol* 2001; 85(2):559–570.

57. McIlroy WE, Maki BE. Task constraints on foot movement and the incidence of compensatory stepping following perturbation of upright stance. *Brain Research* 1993; 616:30–38.

58. Zettel JL, McIlroy WE, Maki BE. Environmental constraints on foot trajectory reveal the capacity for modulation of anticipatory postural adjustments during rapid triggered stepping reactions. *Exp Brain Res* 2002; 146(1):38–47.

59. Jacobs JV, Horak FB. Cortical control of postural responses. *J Neural Transm* 2007; 114(10):1339–1348.

60. Maki BE, McIlroy WE. Cognitive demands and cortical control of human balance-recovery reactions. *J Neural Transm* 2007; 114(10):1279–1296.

61. Smith MT, Baer GD. Achievement of simple mobility milestones after stroke. *Arch Phys Med Rehabil* 1999; 80(4):442–447.

62. Berg K, Wood-Dauphinee S, Williams JI. The balance scale: Reliability assessment with elderly residents and patients with an acute stroke. *Scand J Rehabil Med* 1995; 27(1):27–36.

63. Jonsdottir J, Cattaneo D. Reliability and validity of the dynamic gait index in persons with chronic stroke. *Arch Phys Med Rehabil* 2007; 88(11):1410–1415.

64. Duncan PW, Weiner DK, Chandler J, Studenski S. Functional reach: A new clinical measure of balance. *J Gerontol* 1990; 45(6):M192–M197.

65. Kollen B, Kwakkel G, Lindeman E. Functional recovery after stroke: A review of current developments in stroke rehabilitation research. *Rev Recent Clin Trials* 2006; 1(1):75–80.

66. Benaim C, Perennou DA, Villy J, et al. Validation of a standardized assessment of postural control in stroke patients: The postural assessment scale for stroke patients (pass). *Stroke* 1999; 30(9):1862–1868.

67. Fugl-Meyer AR, Jaasko L, Leyman I, et al. The post-stroke hemiplegic patient. 1. A method for evaluation of physical performance. *Scandinavian Journal of Rehabilitation Medicine* 1975; 7(1):13–31.

68. Granger CV, Cotter AC, Hamilton BB, Fiedler RC. Functional assessment scales: A study of persons after stroke. *Arch Phys Med Rehabil* 1993; 74(2):133–138.

69. Garland SJ, Willems DA, Ivanova TD, Miller KJ. Recovery of standing balance and functional mobility after stroke. *Arch Phys Med Rehabil* 2003; 84(12):1753–1759.

70. Pyoria O, Era P, Talvitie U. Relationships between standing balance and symmetry measurements in patients following recent strokes (3 weeks or less) or older strokes (6 months or more). *Phys Ther* 2004; 84(2):128–136.

71. Tyson SF, DeSouza LH. Development of the Brunel Balance Assessment: A new measure of balance disability post-stroke. *Clin Rehabil* 2004; 18(7):801–810.

72. Collen FM, Wade DT, Robb GF, Bradshaw CM. The Rivermead mobility index: A further development of the Rivermead motor assessment. *Int Disabil Stud* 1991; 13(2):50–54.

73. Tyson SF, DeSouza LH. Reliability and validity of functional balance tests post-stroke. *Clin Rehabil* 2004; 18(8):916–923.

74. de Haart M, Geurts AC, Huidekoper SC, et al. Recovery of standing balance in post-acute stroke patients: A rehabilitation cohort study. *Arch Phys Med Rehabil* 2004; 85(6):886–895.

75. Harris JE, Eng JJ, Marigold DS, et al. Relationship of balance and mobility to fall incidence in people with chronic stroke. *Phys Ther* 2005; 85(2):150–158.

76. Marigold DS, Eng JJ, Dawson AS, et al. Exercise leads to faster postural reflexes, improved balance and mobility, and fewer falls in older persons with chronic stroke. *J Am Geriatr Soc* 2005; 53(3):416–423.

77. Pohl PS, Duncan PW, Perera S, et al. Influence of stroke-related impairments on performance in 6-minute walk test. *J Rehabil Res Dev* 2002; 39(4):439–444.

78. Teasell R, McRae M, Foley N, Bhardwaj A. The incidence and consequences of falls in stroke patients during inpatient rehabilitation: Factors associated with high risk. *Arch Phys Med Rehabil* 2002; 83(3):329–333.

79. Tyson SF, Hanley M, Chillala J, et al. Balance disability after stroke. *Phys Ther* 2006; 86(1):30–38.

80. Bohannon RW, Waters G, Cooper J. Perception of unilateral lower extremity weight bearing during bilateral upright stance. *Percept Mot Skills* 1989; 69(3 Pt 1):875–880.

81. Keenan MA, Perry J, Jordan C. Factors affecting balance and ambulation following stroke. *Clin Orthop Relat Res* 1984(182):165–171.

82. Niam S, Cheung W, Sullivan PE, et al. Balance and physical impairments after stroke. *Arch Phys Med Rehabil* 1999;80(10):1227–1233.

83. Engberg W, Lind A, Linder A, et al. Balance-related efficacy compared with balance function in patients with acute stroke. *Physiother Theory Pract* 2008;24(2):105–111.

84. Garland SJ, Ivanova TD, Mochizuki G. Recovery of standing balance and health-related quality of life after mild or moderately severe stroke. *Arch Phys Med Rehabil* 2007; 88(2):218–227.

85. Winter DA, Prince F, Frank JS, et al. Unified theory regarding a/p and m/l balance in quiet stance. *J Neurophysiol* 1996; 75(6):2334–2343.

86. Bohannon RW, Larkin PA. Lower extremity weight bearing under various standing conditions in independently ambulatory patients with hemiparesis. *Phys Ther* 1985; 65(9):1323–1325.

87. Corriveau H, Hebert R, Raiche M, Prince F. Evaluation of postural stability in the elderly with stroke. *Arch Phys Med Rehabil* 2004; 85(7):1095–1101.

88. Dickstein R, Abulaffio N. Postural sway of the affected and nonaffected pelvis and leg in stance of hemiparetic patients. *Arch Phys Med Rehabil* 2000; 81(3):364–367.

89. Dickstein R, Hocherman S, Dannenbaum E, Pillar T. Responses of ankle musculature of healthy subjects and hemiplegic patients to sinusoidal anterior-posterior movements of the base of support. *J Mot Behav* 1989; 21(2):99–112.

90. Dickstein R, Nissan M, Pillar T, Scheer D. Foot-ground pressure pattern of standing hemiplegic patients. Major characteristics and patterns of improvement. *Phys Ther* 1984; 64(1):19–23.

91. Eng JJ, Chu KS, Dawson AS, et al. Functional walk tests in individuals with stroke: Relation to perceived exertion and myocardial exertion. *Stroke* 2002; 33(3):756–761.

92. Genthon N, Rougier P, Gissot AS, et al. Contribution of each lower limb to upright standing in stroke patients. *Stroke* 2008; 39(6):1793–1799.

93. Mizrahi J, Solzi P, Ring H, Nisell R. Postural stability in stroke patients: Vectorial expression of asymmetry, sway activity and relative sequence of reactive forces. *Med Biol Eng Comput* 1989; 27(2):181–190.

94. Perennou D. Weight-bearing asymmetry in standing hemiparetic patients. *J Neurol Neurosurg Psychiatry* 2005; 76(5):621.

95. Sackley CM. Falls, sway, and symmetry of weight-bearing after stroke. *Int Disabil Stud* 1991; 13(1):1–4.

96. Geurts AC, de Haart M, van Nes IJ, Duysens J. A review of standing balance recovery from stroke. *Gait Posture* 2005; 22(3):267–281.

97. Hof AL. The equations of motion for a standing human reveal three mechanisms for balance. *J Biomech* 2007; 40(2):451–457.

98. Badke MB, Duncan PW. Patterns of rapid motor responses during postural adjustments when standing in healthy subjects and hemiplegic patients. *Phys Ther* 1983; 63(1):13–20.

99. Di Fabio RP, Badke MB, Duncan PW. Adapting human postural reflexes following localized cerebrovascular lesion: Analysis of bilateral long latency responses. *Brain Res* 1986; 363(2):257–264.

100. Kirker SG, Simpson DS, Jenner JR, Wing AM. Stepping before standing: Hip muscle function in stepping and standing balance after stroke. *J Neurol Neurosurg Psychiatry* 2000; 68(4):458–464.

101. Marigold DS, Eng JJ. The relationship of asymmetric weight-bearing with postural sway and visual reliance in stroke. *Gait Posture* 2006; 23(2):249–255.

102. Marigold DS, Eng JJ, Tokuno CD, Donnelly CA. Contribution of muscle strength and integration of afferent input to postural instability in persons with stroke. *Neurorehabil Neural Repair* 2004; 18(4):222–229.

103. Bonan IV, Yelnik AP, Colle FM, et al. Reliance on visual information after stroke. Part II: Effectiveness of a balance rehabilitation program with visual cue deprivation after stroke: A randomized controlled trial. *Arch Phys Med Rehabil* 2004; 85(2):274–278.

104. Di Fabio RP, Badke MB. Stance duration under sensory conflict conditions in patients with hemiplegia. *Arch Phys Med Rehabil* 1991; 72(5):292–295.

105. Marsden JF, Playford DE, Day BL. The vestibular control of balance after stroke. *J Neurol Neurosurg Psychiatry* 2005; 76(5):670–678.

106. Brunt D, Vander Linden DW, Behrman AL. The relation between limb loading and control parameters of gait initiation in persons with stroke. *Arch Phys Med Rehabil* 1995; 76(7):627–634.

107. Dickstein R, Dvir Z. Quantitative evaluation of stance balance performance in the clinic using a novel measurement device. *Physiother Can* 1993; 45(2):102–108.

108. Goldie PA, Matyas TA, Evans OM. Deficit and change in gait velocity during rehabilitation after stroke. *Arch Phys Med Rehabil* 1996; 77(10):1074–1082.

109. Goldie PA, Matyas TA, Evans OM, et al. Maximum voluntary weight-bearing by the affected and unaffected legs in standing following stroke. *Clin Biomech (Bristol, Avon)* 1996; 11(6):333–342.

110. Horak FB, Esselman P, Anderson ME, Lynch MK. The effects of movement velocity, mass displaced, and task certainty on associated postural adjustments made by normal and hemiplegic individuals. *J Neurol Neurosurg Psychiatry* 1984; 47(9):1020–1028.

111. Pai YC, Rogers MW, Hedman LD, Hanke TA. Alterations in weight-transfer capabilities in adults with hemiparesis. *Phys Ther* 1994; 74(7):647–657, discussion 657–659.

112. Rogers MW, Hedman LD, Pai YC. Kinetic analysis of dynamic transitions in stance support accompanying voluntary leg flexion movements in hemiparetic adults. *Arch Phys Med Rehabil* 1993; 74(1):19–25.

113. de Haart M, Geurts AC, Dault MC, et al. Restoration of weight-shifting capacity in patients with postacute stroke: A rehabilitation cohort study. *Arch Phys Med Rehabil* 2005; 86(4):755–762.

114. Hedman LD, Rogers MW, Pai YC, Hanke TA. Electromyographic analysis of postural responses during standing leg flexion in adults with hemiparesis. *Electroencephalogr Clin Neurophysiol* 1997; 105(2):149–155.

115. Laufer Y, Dickstein R, Resnik S, Marcovitz E. Weight-bearing shifts of hemiparetic and healthy adults upon stepping on stairs of various heights. *Clin Rehabil* 2000; 14(2):125–129.

116. Turnbull GI, Charteris J, Wall JC. Deficiencies in standing weight shifts by ambulant hemiplegic subjects. *Arch Phys Med Rehabil* 1996; 77(4):356–362.

117. Jorgensen L, Engstad T, Jacobsen BK. Higher incidence of falls in long-term stroke survivors than in population controls: Depressive symptoms predict falls after stroke. *Stroke* 2002; 33(2):542–547.

118. Forster A, Young J. Incidence and consequences of falls due to stroke: A systematic inquiry. *BMJ* 1995; 311(6997):83–86.

119. Herndon JG, Helmick CG, Sattin RW, et al. Chronic medical conditions and risk of fall injury events at home in older adults. *J Am Geriatr Soc* 1997; 45(6):739–743.

120. O'Loughlin JL, Robitaille Y, Boivin JF, Suissa S. Incidence of and risk factors for falls and injurious falls among the community-dwelling elderly. *Am J Epidemiol* 1993; 137(3):342–354.

121. Kanis J, Oden A, Johnell O. Acute and long-term increase in fracture risk after hospitalization for stroke. *Stroke* 2001; 32(3):702–706.

122. Guralnik JM, Branch LG, Cummings SR, Curb JD. Physical performance measures in aging research. *J Gerontol* 1989; 44(5):M141–M146.

123. Lord SR, Sherrington C, Menz HB, Close J. *Falls in older people: Risk factors and strategies for prevention.* 2nd ed. Cambridge: Cambridge University Press, 2007.

124. Luchies CW, Alexander NB, Schultz AB, Ashton-Miller J. Stepping responses of young and old adults to postural disturbances: Kinematics. *J Am Geriatr Soc* 1994; 42(5):506–512.

125. Nevitt MC, Cummings SR, Kidd S, Black D. Risk factors for recurrent nonsyncopal falls. A prospective study. *JAMA* 1989; 261(18):2663–2668.

126. Tinetti ME, Speechley M, Ginter SF. Risk factors for falls among elderly persons living in the community. *The New England Journal of Medicine* 1988;319(26):1701–1707.

127. Mayo NE, Korner-Bitensky N, Kaizer F. Relationship between response time and falls among stroke patients undergoing physical rehabilitation. *Int J Rehabil Res* 1990; 13(1):47–55.

128. Nyberg L, Gustafson Y. Patient falls in stroke rehabilitation. A challenge to rehabilitation strategies. *Stroke* 1995; 26(5):838–842.

129. Byers V, Arrington ME, Finstuen K. Predictive risk factors associated with stroke patient falls in acute care settings. *J Neurosci Nurs* 1990; 22(3):147–154.

130. Stapleton T, Ashburn A, Stack E. A pilot study of attention deficits, balance control, and falls in the subacute stage following stroke. *Clin Rehabil* 2001; 15(4):437–444.

131. Hyndman D, Ashburn A, Stack E. Fall events among people with stroke living in the community: Circumstances of falls and characteristics of fallers. *Arch Phys Med Rehabil* 2002; 83(2):165–170.

132. Hyndman D, Ashburn A. People with stroke living in the community: Attention deficits, balance, ADL ability, and falls. *Disabil Rehabil* 2003; 25(15):817–822.

133. Lamb SE, Ferrucci L, Volapto S, et al. Risk factors for falling in home-dwelling older women with stroke: The women's health and aging study. *Stroke* 2003; 34(2):494–501.

134. Mackintosh SF, Hill KD, Dodd KJ, et al. Balance score and a history of falls in hospital predict recurrent falls in the six months following stroke rehabilitation. *Arch Phys Med Rehabil* 2006; 87(12):1583–1589.

135. Ashburn A, Hyndman D, Pickering R, et al. Predicting people with stroke at risk of falls. *Age Ageing* 2008; 37(3):270–276.

136. Belgen B, Beninato M, Sullivan PE, Narielwalla K. The association of balance capacity and falls self-efficacy with history of falling in community-dwelling people with chronic stroke. *Arch Phys Med Rehabil* 2006; 87(4):554–561.

137. Yates JS, Lai SM, Duncan PW, Studenski S. Falls in community-dwelling stroke survivors: An accumulated impairments model. *J Rehabil Res Dev* 2002; 39(3):385–394.

138. Marigold DS, Eng JJ. Altered timing of postural reflexes contributes to falling in persons with chronic stroke. *Exp Brain Res* 2006; 171(4):459–468.

139. Powell LE, Myers AM. The activities-specific balance confidence (ABC) scale. *J Gerontol A Biol Sci Med Sci* 1995; 50(1):M28–M34.

140. Hellstrom K, Lindmark B, Wahlberg B, Fugl-Meyer AR. Self-efficacy in relation to impairments and activities of daily living disability in elderly patients with stroke: A prospective investigation. *J Rehabil Med* 2003; 35(5):202–207.

141. Pang MY, Eng JJ. Fall-related self-efficacy, not balance and mobility performance, is related to accidental falls in chronic stroke survivors with low bone mineral density. *Osteoporos Int* 2008; 19(7):919–927.

142. Karnath HO, Ferber S, Dichgans J. The origin of contraversive pushing: Evidence for a second graviceptive system in humans. *Neurology* 2000; 55(9):1298–1304.

143. Laufer Y, Sivan D, Schwarzmann R, Sprecher E. Standing balance and functional recovery of patients with right and left hemiparesis in the early stages of rehabilitation. *Neurorehabil Neural Repair* 2003; 17(4):207–213.

144. Miyai I, Mauricio RLR, Reding MJ. Parietal-insular strokes are associated with impaired standing balance as assessed by computerized dynamic posturography. *Neurorehabil and Neural Repair* 1997; 11(1):35–40.

145. Perennou DA, Leblond C, Amblard B, et al. The polymodal sensory cortex is crucial for controlling lateral postural stability: Evidence from stroke patients. *Brain Res Bull* 2000; 53(3):359–365.

146. Rode G, Tiliket C, Boisson D. Predominance of postural imbalance in left hemiparetic patients. *Scand J Rehabil Med* 1997; 29(1):11–16.

147. Spinazzola L, Cubelli R, Della Sala S. Impairments of trunk movements following left or right hemisphere lesions: Dissociation between apraxic errors and postural instability. *Brain* 2003; 126(Pt 12):2656–2666.

148. Sackley CM, Lincoln NB. Single-blind randomized controlled trial of visual feedback after stroke: Effects on stance symmetry and function. *Disabil Rehabil* 1997; 19(12):536–546.

149. Malhotra P, Coulthard E, Husain M. Hemispatial neglect, balance, and eye-movement control. *Curr Opin Neurol* 2006; 19(1):14–20.

150. Dieterich M, Bense S, Lutz S, et al. Dominance for vestibular cortical function in the nondominant hemisphere. *Cereb Cortex* 2003; 13(9):994–1007.

151. Indovina I, Maffei V, Bosco G, et al. Representation of visual gravitational motion in the human vestibular cortex. *Science* 2005; 308(5720):416–419.

152. Duncan P, Studenski S, Richards L, et al. Randomized clinical trial of therapeutic exercise in subacute stroke. *Stroke* 2003; 34(9):2173–2180.

153. Eng JJ, Chu KS, Kim CM, et al. A community-based group exercise program for persons with chronic stroke. *Med Sci Sports Exerc* 2003; 35(8):1271–1278.

154. English CK, Hillier SL, Stiller KR, Warden-Flood A. Circuit class therapy versus individual physiotherapy sessions during inpatient stroke rehabilitation: A controlled trial. *Arch Phys Med Rehabil* 2007; 88(8):955–963.

155. Hart J, Kanner H, Gilboa-Mayo R, et al. Tai chi chuan practice in community-dwelling persons after stroke. *Int J Rehabil Res* 2004; 27(4):303–304.

156. Macko RF, Benvenuti F, Stanhope S, et al. Adaptive physical activity improves mobility function and quality of life in chronic hemiparesis. *J Rehabil Res Dev* 2008; 45(2):323–328.

157. Mount J, Bolton M, Cesari M, et al. Group balance skills class for people with chronic stroke: A case series. *J Neurol Phys Ther* 2005; 29(1):24–33.

158. Sullivan K, Klassen T, Mulroy S. Combined task-specific training and strengthening effects on locomotor recovery post-stroke: A case study. *J Neurol Phys Ther* 2006; 30(3):130–141.

159. Vearrier LA, Langan J, Shumway-Cook A, Woollacott M. An intensive massed practice approach to retraining balance post-stroke. *Gait Posture* 2005; 22(2):154–163.

160. Weiss A, Suzuki T, Bean J, Fielding RA. High-intensity strength training improves strength and functional performance after stroke. *Am J Phys Med Rehabil* 2000; 79(4):369–376, quiz 391–394.

161. Yang YR, Wang RY, Lin KH, et al. Task-oriented progressive resistance strength training improves muscle strength and functional performance in individuals with stroke. *Clin Rehabil* 2006; 20(10):860–870.

162. Bowman MH, Taub E, Uswatte G, et al. A treatment for a chronic stroke patient with a plegic hand combining CI therapy with conventional rehabilitation procedures: Case report. *NeuroRehabilitation* 2006; 21(2):167–176.

163. Taub E, Uswatte G, Elbert T. New treatments in neurorehabilitation founded on basic research. *Nat Rev Neurosci* 2002; 3(3):228–236.

164. Taub E, Uswatte G, King DK, et al. A placebo-controlled trial of constraint-induced movement therapy for upper extremity after stroke. *Stroke* 2006; 37(4):1045–1049.

165. Wolf SL, Winstein CJ, Miller JP, et al. Retention of upper limb function in stroke survivors who have received constraint-induced movement therapy: The EXCITE randomised trial. *Lancet Neurol* 2008; 7(1):33–40.

166. Taub E, Uswatte G, Pidikiti R. Constraint-induced movement therapy: A new family of techniques with broad application to physical rehabilitation. A clinical review. [see comments]. *Journal of Rehabilitation Research & Development* 1999; 36(3):237–251.

167. Fritz SL, Pittman AL, Robinson AC, et al. An intense intervention for improving gait, balance, and mobility for individuals with chronic stroke: A pilot study. *J Neurol Phys Ther* 2007; 31(2):71–76.

168. Li F, Harmer P, Fisher KJ, et al. Tai chi and fall reductions in older adults: A randomized controlled trial. *J Gerontol A Biol Sci Med Sci* 2005; 60(2):187–194.

169. Qin L, Choy W, Leung K, et al. Beneficial effects of regular Tai Chi exercise on musculoskeletal system. *J Bone Miner Metab* 2005; 23(2):186–190.

170. Song R, Lee EO, Lam P, Bae SC. Effects of Tai Chi exercise on pain, balance, muscle strength, and perceived difficulties in physical functioning in older women with osteoarthritis: A randomized clinical trial. *J Rheumatol* 2003; 30(9):2039–2044.

171. Thornton EW, Sykes KS, Tang WK. Health benefits of Tai Chi exercise: Improved balance and blood pressure in middle-aged women. *Health Promot Int* 2004; 19(1):33–38.

172. Tsang WW, Hui-Chan CW. Effect of 4- and 8-wk intensive Tai Chi training on balance control in the elderly. *Med Sci Sports Exerc* 2004; 36(4):648–657.

173. Taylor-Piliae RE, Haskell WL. Tai Chi exercise and stroke rehabilitation. *Top Stroke Rehabil* 2007; 14(4):9–22.

174. Tsang WW, Hui-Chan CW. Effects of Tai Chi on joint proprioception and stability limits in elderly subjects. *Med Sci Sports Exerc* 2003; 35(12):1962–1971.

175. Cheng PT, Wang CM, Chung CY, Chen CL. Effects of visual feedback rhythmic weight-shift training on hemiplegic stroke patients. *Clin Rehabil* 2004; 18(7):747–753.

176. Howe TE, Taylor I, Finn P, Jones H. Lateral weight transference exercises following acute stroke: A preliminary study of clinical effectiveness. *Clin Rehabil* 2005; 19(1):45–53.

177. Geiger RA, Allen JB, O'Keefe J, Hicks RR. Balance and mobility following stroke: Effects of physical therapy interventions with and without biofeedback/forceplate training. *Phys Ther* 2001; 81(4):995–1005.

178. Walker C, Brouwer BJ, Culham EG. Use of visual feedback in retraining balance following acute stroke. *Phys Ther* 2000; 80(9):886–895.

179. Cheng PT, Wu SH, Liaw MY, et al. Symmetrical body weight distribution training in stroke patients and its effect on fall prevention. *Arch Phys Med Rehabil* 2001; 82(12):1650–1654.

180. Van Peppen RP, Kortsmit M, Lindeman E, Kwakkel G. Effects of visual feedback therapy on postural control in bilateral standing after stroke: A systematic review. *J Rehabil Med* 2006; 38(1):3–9.

181. Winstein CJ, Gardner ER, McNeal DR, et al. Standing balance training: Effect on balance and locomotion in hemiparetic adults. *Arch Phys Med Rehabil* 1989; 70(10):755–762.

182. Betker AL, Szturm T, Moussavi ZK, Nett C. Video game-based exercises for balance rehabilitation: A single-subject design. *Arch Phys Med Rehabil* 2006; 87(8):1141–1149.

183. Flynn S, Palma P, Bender A. Feasibility of using the Sony Playstation 2 gaming platform for an individual post-stroke: A case report. *J Neurol Phys Ther* 2007; 31(4):180–189.

184. Ryerson S, Byl NN, Brown DA, et al. Altered trunk position sense and its relation to balance functions in people post-stroke. *J Neurol Phys Ther* 2008; 32(1):14–20.

185. Smith DL, Akhtar AJ, Garraway WM. Proprioception and spatial neglect after stroke. *Age Ageing* 1983; 12(1):63–69.

186. Byl N, Roderick J, Mohamed O, et al. Effectiveness of sensory and motor rehabilitation of the upper limb following the principles of neuroplasticity: Patients stable post-stroke. *Neurorehabil Neural Repair* 2003; 17(3):176–191.

187. Carey LM, Matyas TA, Oke LE. Sensory loss in stroke patients: Effective training of tactile and proprioceptive discrimination. *Arch Phys Med Rehabil* 1993; 74(6):602–611.

188. Smania N, Montagnana B, Faccioli S, et al. Rehabilitation of somatic sensation and related deficit of motor control in patients with pure sensory stroke. *Arch Phys Med Rehabil* 2003; 84(11):1692–1702.

189. Yekutiel M, Guttman E. A controlled trial of the retraining of the sensory function of the hand in stroke patients. *J Neurol Neurosurg Psychiatry* 1993; 56(3):241–244.

190. Worms G, Matjacic Z, Gollee H, et al. Dynamic balance training with sensory electrical stimulation in chronic stroke patients. *Conf Proc IEEE Eng Med Biol Soc* 2006; 1:2150–2153.

191. Hillier S, Dunsford A. A pilot study of sensory retraining for the hemiparetic foot post-stroke. *Int J Rehabil Res* 2006; 29(3):237–242.

192. Lynch EA, Hillier SL, Stiller K, et al. Sensory retraining of the lower limb after acute stroke: A randomized, controlled pilot trial. *Arch Phys Med Rehabil* 2007; 88(9):1101–1107.

193. Morioka S, Yagi F. Effects of perceptual learning exercises on standing balance using a hardness discrimination task in hemiplegic patients following stroke: A randomized controlled pilot trial. *Clin Rehabil* 2003; 17(6):600–607.

194. Bayouk JF, Boucher JP, Leroux A. Balance training following stroke: Effects of task-oriented exercises with and without altered sensory input. *Int J Rehabil Res* 2006; 29(1):51–59.

195. Bruyere O, Wuidart MA, Di Palma E, et al. Controlled whole body vibration to decrease fall risk and improve health-related quality of life of nursing home residents. *Arch Phys Med Rehabil* 2005; 86(2):303–307.

196. Cardinale M, Bosco C. The use of vibration as an exercise intervention. *Exerc Sport Sci Rev* 2003; 31(1):3–7.

197. Cardinale M, Lim J. Electromyography activity of vastus lateralis muscle during whole-body vibrations of different frequencies. *J Strength Cond Res* 2003; 17(3):621–624.

198. Torvinen S, Kannus P, Sievanen H, et al. Effect of four-month vertical whole body vibration on performance and balance. *Med Sci Sports Exerc* 2002; 34(9):1523–1528.

199. van Nes IJ, Latour H, Schils F, et al. Long-term effects of 6-week whole-body vibration on balance recovery and activities of daily living in the post-acute phase of stroke: A randomized, controlled trial. *Stroke* 2006; 37(9):2331–2335.

200. Brown LA, Sleik RJ, Winder TR. Attentional demands for static postural control after stroke. *Arch Phys Med Rehabil* 2002; 83(12):1732–1735.

201. Shumway-Cook A, Woollacott M. Attentional demands and postural control: The effect of sensory context. *J Gerontol A Biol Sci Med Sci* 2000; 55(1):M10–M16.

202. Bensoussan L, Viton JM, Schieppati M, et al. Changes in postural control in hemiplegic patients after stroke performing a dual task. *Arch Phys Med Rehabil* 2007; 88(8):1009–1015.

203. Bowen A, Wenman R, Mickelborough J, et al. Dual-task effects of talking while walking on velocity and balance following a stroke. *Age Ageing* 2001; 30(4):319–323.

204. Marshall SC, Grinnell D, Heisel B, et al. Attentional deficits in stroke patients: A visual dual task experiment. *Arch Phys Med Rehabil* 1997; 78(1):7–12.

205. Boyd L, Winstein C. Explicit information interferes with implicit motor learning of both continuous and discrete movement tasks after stroke. *J Neurol Phys Ther* 2006; 30(2):46–57; discussion 58–59.

206. Boyd LA, Quaney BM, Pohl PS, Winstein CJ. Learning implicitly: Effects of task and severity after stroke. *Neurorehabil Neural Repair* 2007; 21(5):444–454.

207. Boyd LA, Winstein CJ. Impact of explicit information on implicit motor-sequence learning following middle cerebral artery stroke. *Phys Ther* 2003; 83(11):976–989.

208. Boyd LA, Winstein CJ. Providing explicit information disrupts implicit motor learning after basal ganglia stroke. *Learn Mem* 2004; 11(4):388–396.

209. Orrell AJ, Eves FF, Masters RS. Motor learning of a dynamic balancing task after stroke: Implicit implications for stroke rehabilitation. *Phys Ther* 2006; 86(3):369–380.

210. Laufer Y. The effect of walking aids on balance and weight-bearing patterns of patients with hemiparesis in various stance positions. *Phys Ther* 2003; 83(2):112–122.

211. Maeda A, Nakamura K, Higuchi S, et al. Postural sway during cane use by patients with stroke. *Am J Phys Med Rehabil* 2001; 80(12):903–908.

212a. Chaudhuri S, Aruin AS. The effects of shoe lifts on static and dynamic postural control in individuals with hemiparesis. *Arch Phys Med Rehabil* 2000; 81(11):1498–1503.

212. Pohl M, Mehrholz J. Immediate effects of an individually designed functional ankle-foot orthosis on stance and gait in hemiparetic patients. *Clin Rehabil* 2006; 20(4):324–330.

213. Wang RY, Yen L, Lee CC, et al. Effects of an ankle-foot orthosis on balance performance in patients with hemiparesis of different durations. *Clin Rehabil* 2005; 19(1):37–44.

214. Maki BE, Cheng KC, Mansfield A, et al. Preventing falls in older adults: New interventions to promote more effective change–in–support balance reactions. *J Electromyogr Kinesiol* 2008; 18(2):243–254.

215. Maki BE, McIlroy WE. Change-in-support balance reactions in older persons: An emerging research area of clinical importance. *Neurol Clin* 2005; 23(3):751–783, vi–vii.

216. Hsiao ET, Robinovitch SN. Biomechanical influences on balance recovery by stepping. *J Biomech* 1999; 32(10):1099–1106.

217. McIlroy WE, Maki BE. Age-related changes in compensatory stepping in response to unpredictable perturbations. *J Gerontol A Biol Sci Med Sci* 1996; 51(6):M289–M296.

218. Rogers MW, Hedman LD, Johnson ME, et al. Lateral stability during forward-induced stepping for dynamic balance recovery in young and older adults. *J Gerontol A Biol Sci Med Sci* 2001; 56(9):M589–M594.

219. Hilliard MJ, Martinez KM, Janssen I, et al. Lateral balance factors predict future falls in community-living older adults. *Arch Phys Med Rehabil* in press.

220. Hsiao ET, Robinovitch SN. Elderly subjects' ability to recover balance with a single backward step associates with body configuration at step contact. *J Gerontol A Biol Sci Med Sci* 2001; 56(1):M42–M47.

221. Schulz BW, Ashton-Miller JA, Alexander NB. Compensatory stepping in response to waist pulls in balance-impaired and unimpaired women. *Gait Posture* 2005; 22(3):198–209.

222. Patton JL, Hilliard MJ, Martinez K, et al. A simple model of stability limits applied to sidestepping in young, elderly, and elderly fallers. *Conf Proc IEEE Eng Med Biol Soc* 2006; 1:3305–3308.

223. Maki BE, Edmondstone MA, McIlroy WE. Age-related differences in laterally directed compensatory stepping behavior. *J Gerontol A Biol Sci Med Sci* 2000; 55(5):M270–M277.

224. Mille ML, Johnson ME, Martinez KM, Rogers MW. Age-dependent differences in lateral balance recovery through protective stepping. *Clin Biomech (Bristol, Avon)* 2005; 20(6):607–616.

225. Rogers MW, Mille ML. Lateral stability and falls in older people. *Exerc Sport Sci Rev* 2003; 31(4):182–187.

226. Johnson ME, Mille ML, Martinez KM, et al. Age-related changes in hip abductor and adductor joint torques. *Arch Phys Med Rehabil* 2004; 85(4):593–597.

227. Lord SR, Tiedemann A, Chapman K, et al. The effect of an individualized fall prevention program on fall risk and falls in older people: A randomized, controlled trial. *J Am Geriatr Soc* 2005; 53(8):1296–1304.

228. Taube W, Schubert M, Gruber M, et al. Direct corticospinal pathways contribute to neuromuscular control of perturbed stance. *J Appl Physiol* 2006; 101(2):420–429.

229. Harris-Love ML, Cohen LG. Noninvasive cortical stimulation in neurorehabilitation: A review. *Arch Phys Med Rehabil* 2006; 87(12 Suppl 2):S84–93.

230. Hummel FC, Cohen LG. Noninvasive brain stimulation: A new strategy to improve neurorehabilitation after stroke? *Lancet Neurol* 2006; 5(8):708–712.

231. Reis J, Swayne OB, Vandermeeren Y, et al. Contribution of transcranial magnetic stimulation to the understanding of cortical mechanisms involved in motor control. *J Physiol* 2008; 586(2):325–351.

232. Hafer-Macko CE, Ryan AS, Ivey FM, Macko RF. Skeletal muscle changes after hemiparetic stroke and potential beneficial effects of exercise intervention strategies. *J Rehabil Res Dev* 2008; 45(2):261–272.

233. Ryan AS, Dobrovolny CL, Smith GV, et al. Hemiparetic muscle atrophy and increased intramuscular fat in stroke patients. *Arch Phys Med Rehabil* 2002; 83(12):1703–1707.

234. Goodpaster BH, Carlson CL, Visser M, et al. Attenuation of skeletal muscle and strength in the elderly: The health ABC study. *J Appl Physiol* 2001; 90(6):2157–2165.

235. Hicks GE, Simonsick EM, Harris TB, et al. Trunk muscle composition as a predictor of reduced functional capacity in the health, aging, and body composition study: The moderating role of back pain. *J Gerontol A Biol Sci Med Sci* 2005; 60(11):1420–1424.

236. Goodpaster BH, Park SW, Harris TB, et al. The loss of skeletal muscle strength, mass, and quality in older adults: The health, aging and body composition study. *J Gerontol A Biol Sci Med Sci* 2006; 61(10):1059–1064.

237. Visser M, Kritchevsky SB, Goodpaster BH, et al. Leg muscle mass and composition in relation to lower extremity performance in men and women aged 70 to 79: The health, aging, and body composition study. *J Am Geriatr Soc* 2002; 50(5):897–904.

238. Ivey FM, Hafer-Macko CE, Macko RF. Task-oriented treadmill exercise training in chronic hemiparetic stroke. *J Rehabil Res Dev* 2008; 45(2):249–260.

239. Stinear CM, Barber PA, Smale PR, et al. Functional potential in chronic stroke patients depends on corticospinal tract integrity. *Brain* 2007; 130(Pt 1):170–180.

V

POST-STROKE
COMPLICATIONS AND
THEIR TREATMENT

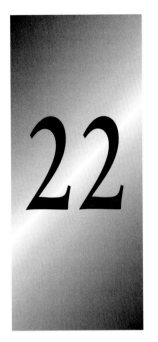

22 Secondary Prevention of Ischemic Stroke

Sandra M. Pinzon
Karen L. Furie

Survivors of a first-ever stroke or transient ischemic attack (TIA) are at high risk of a recurrent event, especially in the first year. Recurrent stroke, whether symptomatic or silent, increases the morbidity and mortality of cerebrovascular disease. Secondary prevention is of paramount significance in this at-risk population. The greatest risk reductions are seen with interventions (e.g., carotid revascularization) that target a specific stroke pathophysiologic mechanism. These interventions require rapid and accurate classification of the etiologic mechanism of infarction. It is critical to assess the cardiovascular risk profile and initiate aggressive management of vascular risk factors in all patients (1). Epidemiological studies have identified many of the determinants of recurrent stroke, and clinical trials have provided the data to generate evidence-based recommendations to reduce this risk.

The most current definition for an ischemic stroke requires either symptoms lasting more than 24 hours or imaging of an acute, clinically relevant ischemic lesion in patients with rapidly improving symptoms. In contrast, a TIA is a brief episode of neurologic dysfunction caused by a focal ischemia, with clinical symptoms lasting less than 1 hour and without radiographic evidence of infarction (2).

TIA and stroke share the same pathophysiological mechanisms. Adequate treatment and risk reduction depends on the accurate classification of the cause of ischemic symptoms, whether they are transient or permanent (Table 22-1) (3).

THERAPEUTIC APPROACH

Large Artery Atherosclerosis

Extracranial Carotid Disease. The benefit of carotid endarterectomy (CEA) was established by three prospective randomized trials: the North American Symptomatic Carotid Endarterectomy Trial (NASCET) (4), the European Carotid Surgery Trial (ECST) (5), and the Veterans Affairs Cooperative Study Program (6). These studies compared endarterectomy plus medical therapy with medical therapy alone. Among symptomatic patients with TIA or minor strokes and high-grade carotid stenosis (greater than 70%), each trial showed impressive relative and absolute risk reductions for those randomized to surgery. There was no significant benefit with surgery if the stenosis was less than 50%.

For patients with symptomatic carotid stenosis between 50% and 69% (moderate category), the results from NASCET and ECST demonstrated consistent benefit of lesser magnitude with CEA as compared to medical therapy. Patients over 75 years old, male, suffering from a recent stroke (rather than TIA), and with hemispheric

377

TABLE 22-1
*Ischemic Stroke Subtypes Rochester,
Minnesota Study*

Large vessel atherothrombotic disease: 16%
  -Extracranial carotid
  -Intracranial
Cerebral embolism from cardiac source: 20%
Small vessel lacunar disease (penetrating artery: 16%
Others (dissection, hypercoagulable states or sickle cell
  disease): 12%
Undetermined cause: 36%

---

symptoms are the populations deriving the greatest benefit from CEA. Intracranial stenosis, absence of leukoaraiosis, early surgery, and the presence of collaterals were also associated with better outcome (4, 5).

Stroke or TIA patients who undergo endarterectomy also need to be treated with maximal medical therapies to aggressively manage risk factors (antihypertensive, antithrombotic, and lipid-lowering therapies, lifestyle modification).

Other techniques: Extracranial-intracranial (EC-IC) bypass surgery was not found to provide benefit for patients with carotid occlusion distal to the carotid bifurcation. A more recent trial, the Carotid Occlusion Surgery Study, is examining the potential role of EC-IC bypass for carotid occlusion using positron emission tomography (PET) to identify the target population at highest risk and most likely to benefit from revascularization (7, 8).

The use of stents is under intense investigation in numerous trials and registries. To date, the data are limited by evolving stent technology and the proficiency of the operators. The Wallstent Trial randomized 219 symptomatic patients with 60%–90% stenosis to CEA or carotid artery angioplasty and stenting (CAS). The risk of perioperative stroke or death was 4.5% for CEA and 12.1% for CAS, and the risk of major stroke or death at 1 year was 0.9% for CEA and 3.7% for CAS (9).

The Stenting and Angioplasty with Protection in Patients at High Risk for Endarterectomy (SAPPHIRE) trial randomized 334 patients to endarterectomy or stenting with the use of an embolic protection device (10). Most of the benefit was detected in the lower risk of myocardial infarction (MI) for the stent compared with the high surgical risk endarterectomy cases.

Two randomized, multicenter trials (EVA3S and SPACE) compared complication rates and long-term complications between angioplasty stenting of the carotid artery and carotid endarterectomy in patients with a symptomatic carotid stenosis of at least 60%. EVA3S aimed to show superiority; unfortunately this study was stopped prematurely after the inclusion of

527 patients because of excessive risk in the carotid angioplasty-stenting cohort, despite the obligatory use of cerebral protection devices. The 30-day incidence of any stroke or death was 3.9% after endarterectomy and 9.6% after stenting; the relative risk of any stroke or death after stenting as compared with endarterectomy was 2.5 (95% CI, 1.2 to 5.1). At 6 months, the incidence of any stroke or death was 6.1% after endarterectomy and 11.7% after stenting (p=0.02) (11). In contrast, SPACE aimed to show non-inferiority between the two interventions and included 1,183 patients in the analysis. The rate of death or ipsilateral ischemic stroke from randomization to 30 days after the procedure was 6.84% with carotid artery stenting and 6.34% with carotid endarterectomy (absolute difference 0.51%, 90% CI–1.89% to 2.91%) (12). The upper CI is more than 2.5, which shows that non-inferiority was not achieved. However the difference was non-significant (13). There is still no available evidence to support the preferential use of carotid endarterectomy over carotid angioplasty and stenting or vice versa. Two further trials (the Carotid Revascularization Endarterectomy vs. Stenting Trial (CREST) and International Carotid Stenting Study (ICSS)) are ongoing.

At present, CAS is recommended in selected patients in whom the stenosis is difficult to access surgically and patients with high surgical risk, radiation induced stenosis, or restenosis after CEA. For patients with extracranial vertebrobasilar disease, medical treatment should be the first choice (antithrombotics, statins, and management of other risk factors). In exceptional circumstances, when patients continue to have symptoms despite maximal medical therapy, endovascular treatment may be considered. The efficacy of endovascular therapy is uncertain and is considered investigational in patients with hemodynamically significant intracranial stenosis who fail to medical therapy.

Cardiogenic Cerebral Embolism

Patients with cardiac conditions such as atrial fibrillation (AF), valvular heart disease, acute MI, cardiomyopathy, patent foramen ovale (PFO) with atrial septal aneurysm, left ventricular dysfunction, and other structural diseases have an increased risk of presenting a first-time ever and recurrent stroke and/or TIA because of the increased potential for the formation of intracardiac thrombi. These cardiac conditions are highly prevalent in the population at risk for stroke; therefore, it can be difficult to distinguish between a coincidental comorbidity and the true source of embolism. These patients often have multiple vascular risk factors in addition to the cardiac source of embolism. In some cases, this potential dissociation can make the selection of an antithrombotic agent or a decision regarding an intervention (e.g., PFO closure) complicated. It is always important to fully evaluate the patency of the large arteries before ascribing thromboembolism to a cardiac source (Table 22-2) (14).

Atrial Fibrillation. More than 75,000 cases of stroke per year are attributed to AF. Multiple clinical trials have demonstrated the superior therapeutic effect of warfarin compared with placebo in the prevention of thromboembolic events among patients with nonvalvular AF (15). The efficacy of warfarin has an overall RR (relative risk) reduction of 68% (95% CI, 50 to 79). Warfarin has also been shown to be relatively safe (16). A large case-control study and two RCTs (randomized controlled trial) suggest that the optimal INR (international normalized ratio) range for anticoagulation appears to be 2.0 to 3.0 (17).

TABLE 22-2

Recommendations for Patient with Cardioembolic Stroke Types

Risk Factor	Recommendation	Class/Level of Evidence
Atrial fibrillation	Anticoagulation with adjusted-dose warfarin (INR range 2.0–3.0) is recommended for patients with ischemic stroke or TIA with persistent or paroxysmal AF.	Class I, Level A
Valvular heart disease	Long-term warfarin therapy is rational with adjusted dose (INR 2.0–3.0) whether or not AF is present.	Class IIa, Level C
Rheumatic mitral Valve disease	Antiplatelet agents should not be added to warfarin to avoid additional bleeding risk.	Class III, Level C
	For patients who have a recurrent embolism while receiving warfarin, adding aspirin (81 mg/d) is suggested.	Class IIa, Level C
Mitral Valve Prolapse	Long-term antiplatelet therapy is reasonable.	Class IIa, Level C
Mitral Annular Calcification (MAC)	Antiplatelet therapy may be considered for patients with MAC not documented to be calcific.	Class IIb, Level C
	Patients with mitral regurgitation resulting from MAC without AF, antiplatelet therapy or warfarin may be considered.	Class IIb, Level C
Aortic Valve Disease	Antiplatelet therapy may be considered for patients who do not have AF.	Class IIa, Level C
Prosthetic Heart Valves	Oral anticoagulants are recommended for patients with modern mechanical valves (INR 2.5–3.5)	Class I, Level B
	For patients with mechanical valves who have an ischemic stroke or systemic embolism despite adequate therapy with anticoagulants, adding 75–100 mg/d of aspirin (INR 2.5–3.5) is rational.	Class IIa, Level B
	Anticoagulation with warfarin (INR 2.0–3.0) may be considered in patients who have bioprosthetic valves.	Class IIb, Level C
Acute MI and left ventricular thrombus	For patients with ischemic stroke caused by an acute MI in whom LV mural thrombus is identified by cardiac imaging, oral anticoagulation is reasonable (INR 2.0–3.0) for at least 3 months and up to 1 year.	Class IIa, Level B
	Aspirin should be used concurrently for the ischemic coronary artery disease patient during oral anticoagulant therapy in doses up 162 mg/d.	Class IIa, Level A
CARDIOMYOPATHIES	In this group of patients, either warfarin (INR 2.0–3.0) or antiplatelet therapy may be considered for prevention of recurrent strokes.	Class IIb, Level C
PATENT FORAMEN OVALE (PFO)	Antiplatelet therapy is reasonable to prevent a recurrent stroke.	Class IIa, Level B
	Warfarin should be used in patients with other indications for oral anticoagulation.	Class IIa, Level C
	PFO closure may be considered for patients with recurrent cryptogenic stroke despite medical therapy.	Class IIb, Level C

There is no evidence that combining anticoagulation with an antiplatelet agent further reduces the risk of stroke compared with anticoagulant therapy alone (18).

In general, the guidelines for prevention of stroke in patients with ischemic stroke or TIA recommend initiation of oral anticoagulation within 2 weeks of an ischemic stroke or TIA. In patients with large infarcts, hemorrhagic transformation of an ischemic stroke, or uncontrolled hypertension, additional delays may be appropriate.

Valvular Heart Disease. **Rheumatic mitral valve disease:** Recurrent embolism occurs in 30% to 65% of patients with rheumatic mitral valve disease who have a history of a previous embolic event (19, 20). Mitral valvuloplasty has not been shown to reduce the risk of thromboembolism. Multiple observational studies have reported that long-term anticoagulant therapy reduces the risk of systemic embolism in patients with rheumatic mitral valve disease (21, 22).

Mitral valve prolapse: Mitral valve prolapse (MVP) likely reflects a normal variant rather than a single disease process. Despite years of research, the symptomatology and significance of MVP remain controversial (23). No randomized trials have addressed the efficacy of selected antithrombotic therapies for this specific subgroup of stroke or TIA patients.

Mitral annular calcification: The incidence of systemic and cerebral embolism is not clear in patients with mitral annular calcification (MAC); however thrombus has been found in heavily calcified annular tissue at autopsy. Embolization of fibrocalcic material from the calcified mitral annulus may be an alternative mechanism of stroke in these patients (24, 25). Most uncomplicated stroke/TIA cases with MAC can be managed with antiplatelet therapy. For those patients who do not respond to medical management, valve replacement should be considered.

Aortic valve disease: No randomized trials have compared medical therapy in patients with stroke and aortic valve disease. Clinical features suggestive of cardioembolism, particularly recurrent embolism, may warrant long-term anticoagulation.

Patent foramen ovale (PFO): PFO is a congenital cardiac atrial defect that provides a conduit for peripheral venous clots to be shunted to the cerebral arterial circulation. The prevalence of PFO can be as high as 30% (26). Patients with PFO-associated strokes tend to be younger and are less likely to have traditional risk factors such as hypertension, hypercholesterolemia, or smoking (27, 28). PFO can be detected by transthoracic echocardiography using agitated saline injection. The current diagnosis of a hypercoagulable state or deep venous thrombosis in the lower extremities or pelvis in conjunction with the presence of PFO raises the suspicion of PFO as and etiology of embolic strokes (29). There has not been a definitive study to establish best medical therapy in the absence of

venous thrombus in the young. However the PICSS study showed no benefit to warfarin in a group of older, conventional stroke patients enrolled in the WARSS trial (30). The question of optimal management remains unresolved. Ongoing studies comparing PFO closure to best medical therapy may be informative in the future.

Non-cardioembolic Stroke or TIA

Recently published trials have contributed to the large body of evidence supporting the benefit of antiplatelet agents for stroke prevention in patients with history of non-cardioembolic ischemic stroke or TIA. In a meta-analysis of 21 randomized trials comparing antiplatelet therapy with placebo in 18,270 patients with prior stroke or TIA, antiplatelet therapy was associated with a 28% relative risk reduction in nonfatal strokes and a 16% reduction in fatal strokes (31).

Antiplatelets Agents

Aspirin. Two randomized controlled trials have demonstrated that aspirin, in doses ranging from 50 to 1300 milligrams per day (mg/d), prevented vascular events in patients with stroke or TIA, but that higher doses were associated with a greater risk of adverse effects such as gastrointestinal hemorrhage.

Clopidogrel. In the CAPRIE trial, which compared clopidogrel to aspirin, there was an approximately 8% reduction in stroke, MI, or vascular death in favor of clopidogrel (p=0.03) (32). The CAPRIE trial was not powered to detect treatment differences within patient subgroups, and there was significant patient heterogeneity with respect to the results for the various subgroups, with peripheral arterial disease (PAD) driving the main result. However when results for subgroups were compared, there was no significant difference between clopidogrel and ASA (aspirin) in patients with stroke or MI.

Overall, the safety of clopidogrel is comparable to that of aspirin, and it has clear advantages over ticlopidine, which is rarely used because of the risk of neutropenia. A few cases of thrombotic thrombocytopenic purpura have been described with clopidogrel.

Addition of Clopidogrel to Aspirin for Prevention of Vascular Events. The double-blind, randomized study Clopidogrel and Aspirin versus Aspirin Alone for the Prevention of Atherothrombotic Events (CHARISMA) randomized 15,603 subjects with cardiovascular disease or multiple risk factors to either 75 mg of clopidogrel plus a low dose of aspirin (75–162 mg) or a placebo plus aspirin (33). Thirty-five percent of subjects (n=4,320) qualified because of a history of cerebrovascular disease within 5 years of enrollment, significantly beyond the high-risk period for stroke recurrence. A third of these events were TIA. The median follow up was 28 months. There was no significant difference in rates of nonfatal ischemic stroke (1.9% vs. 2.4%, p=0.10). There was no difference in the rate of intracerebral hemorrhage (ICH) (0.3%). The combination therapy did not significantly increase the risk of severe or fatal bleeding, but there was a higher rate of moderate bleeding in the combination therapy arm. There was a reduction in a secondary endpoint, hospitalization for unstable angina, TIA, or revascularization (11.1% vs. 12.3%, p=0.02) in the combination therapy arm. In the subgroup of patients with a history of stroke, there was a trend toward a benefit from combination therapy, but it was nonsignificant.

Although clopidogrel plus aspirin is recommended over aspirin for acute coronary syndromes, recently published results of the Management of Atherothrombosis with Clopidogrel in High Risk Patients eith TIA or Stroke (MATCH) trial do not suggest a similar benefit ratio for stroke and TIA survivors. (34). Patients with a prior stroke or TIA plus additional risk factors (n=7,599) were allocated to 75 mg of clopidogrel or combination therapy with 75 mg of clopidogrel plus 75 mg of aspirin per day. There was no significant benefit of combination therapy compared with clopidogrel alone in reducing vascular events, death-related vascular events, or rehospitalization secondary to ischemic events. The risk of major hemorrhage was significantly increased in the combination group compared with clopidogrel alone, with a 1.3% absolute increase in life-threatening bleeding.

Aspirin and Dipyridamole. Several trials have evaluated the efficacy of aspirin in combination with dipyridamole. The European Stroke Prevention Study (ESPS-2) randomized 6,602 patients with prior stroke or TIA in three groups: (1) 50 mg/d of aspirin plus 400 mg/d of extended-release dipyridamole, (2) aspirin alone, (3) extended-release dipyridamole alone, and (4) a placebo. The risk of stroke was significantly reduced by 18% on aspirin alone, 16% with dipyridamole alone, and 37% with a combination of aspirin plus dipyridamole. The combination was superior to aspirin alone in reducing recurrence of stroke (23%) and 25% superior to dipyridamole alone (35). The most common side effect of dipyridamole was headache, which can represent an adherence issue during treatment. Bleeding was not significantly increased by dipyridamole.

Although a combination of aspirin and extended-release dipyridamole is suggested over aspirin alone, individual patient characteristics continue to play a role in selection of antiplatelet agents for recurrent stroke prevention. Aspirin, a combination of aspirin and extended-release dipyridamole, and clopidogrel all remain accepted options for initial therapy for patients with non-cardioembolic ischemic stroke and TIA; therefore the selection of an antiplatelet agent should be individualized on the basis of patient risk factors, tolerance, and other clinical characteristics.

OTHER CONDITIONS ASSOCIATED TO STROKE OR TIA

Hyperhomocysteinemia

Hyperhomocysteinemia is one of the causes that should be considered in a young patient with a history of stroke or TIA, but its causal relationship to stroke in the elderly remains controversial. In 1969 McCully observed premature atherosclerosis in young patients with homocystinuria because of the deficiency of methyltetrahydrofolate reductase (MTHFR). He hypothesized that elevated plasma homocysteine (Hcy) was atherogenic and could contribute to the risk of large and small vessel disease (36). Homocysteine has also been associated with hypercoagulability, suggesting that it could also affect the risk of cardioembolism. In recent years, several epidemiological studies have demonstrated an association between hyperhomocysteinemia and clinical vascular disease.

Homocysteine metabolism is regulated by genetic and nutritional factors. A family history of premature atherosclerotic disease and stroke should generate consideration of genetic screening for this disease. In addition it is important to consider vitamin B12, vitamin B6, and folate deficiencies as mechanisms for hyperhomocysteinemia. The VISP (Vitamins in Stroke Prevention) study compared the efficacy of high- (folic acid 2.5mg, B12 400µg, B6 25mg) and low-dose (folic acid 200µg, B12 6µg, B6 0.2mg) vitamins for secondary prevention of stroke or myocardial infarction in 3,600 subjects with recent stroke and failed to show a benefit of high-dose therapy despite a homocysteine-reducing effect (37). There is currently no evidence that reducing homocysteine levels with vitamin therapy leads to a reduction in rates of recurrent stroke. A large randomized clinical trial (VITATOPS) is still ongoing.

Hypercoagulable States

Inherited coagulation disorders such as antithrombin III, protein C or proteins S deficiency, prothrombin gene G20210A mutation, or Factor V Leiden (FVL) may contribute to strokes in pediatric or young populations. These abnormalities rarely contribute to stroke in adults and can be over-interpreted if only measured during acute stroke, when levels can be temporarily affected by the active thrombotic event (38). Several meta-analyses have studied the association between prothrombotic mutations and ischemic stroke, and this association appears to be very weak; however the mechanism of gene-environment interaction remains a major unanswered question (39).

Patients with ischemic stroke or TIA with an established, inherited thrombophilia should be evaluated for deep vein thrombosis, which is an indication for short- or long-term anticoagulant therapy. Adults with a history of recurrent thrombotic events may be considered for long-term anticoagulation, but this should be based on a careful assessment of the risks and benefits of therapy. Hypercoagulability may be a symptom of an underlying malignancy, and diagnostic studies should be performed to exclude this as a possible underlying cause.

The strongest link between a thrombophilic disorder and stroke is the association between antiphospholipid (APL) antibodies and stroke in young adults (less than 50 years of age) (40). The Antiphospholipid Antibodies in Stroke Aubstudy (WARSS/APASS) was the first study to compare randomly assigned warfarin (INR 1.4 to 2.8) with aspirin (325 mg) for the prevention of a second stroke in patients with APL antibodies. Patients with both lupus anticoagulant and anticardiolipin antibodies had a higher event rate (31.7%) than patients negative for both antibodies (24%), but this was not statistically significant. Antiplatelet agents appear reasonable as first-line therapy. For patients with stroke or TIA who meet the criteria for APL antibody syndrome, oral anticoagulation with a target INR of 2 to 3 is recommended.

Sickle Cell Disease

Sickle cell anemia is an autosomal recessive genetic disease that causes production of a defective form of hemoglobin, hemoglobin S (HbS). Central nervous system manifestations of vaso-occlusive crises include cerebral infarction (children), hemorrhage (adults), seizures, transient ischemic attacks, cranial nerve palsies, meningitis, sensory deficits, and acute coma. Ischemic strokes are common in children, and they tend to be recurrent. These patients are often maintained on transfusion programs to suppress HbS. A retrospective multicenter review of sickle cell disease (SCD) patients with stroke showed that a reduction of hemoglobin S to less than 30% was associated with a reduction in the rate of recurrence at 3 years from more than 50% to 10% (41). Some experts recommend transfusions only during the first 3 years after the stroke to avoid long-term complications such as iron overload. Transcranial Doppler can be used to monitor patients and identify those risk before they have a stroke (42). In addition, there appear to be genetic factors that identify a high-risk group (43). Two small

studies of secondary stroke prevention in children and young adults with stroke reported encouraging results using hydroxyurea to replace regular blood transfusion after 3 years of transfusion therapy (44). For cases of advanced occlusive disease, bypass surgery may be considered.

Cerebral Venous Sinus Thrombosis

Cerebral venous sinus thrombosis (CVST) results from occlusion of a venous sinus and/or cortical vein and usually is caused by a partial thrombus or an extrinsic compression. CVST can be caused by a multitude of factors including hypercoagulable state, extrinsic compression of the venous system, infection, dehydration, pregnancy, and oral contraceptives. CVST has highly variable clinical manifestations (alteration of consciousness, seizures, focal neurologic deficits, headache), making its diagnosis a challenge. Magnetic resonance (MR) venography or computed tomography (CT) venography is used to confirm the diagnosis.

Several trials and observational data have concluded that both unfractioned heparin (UFH) and low-molecular weight heparin (LMWH) are safe and effective in acute cerebral venous thrombosis followed by oral anticoagulation for 3 to 6 months. Anticoagulation is recommended, even in patients with hemorrhagic venous infarcts.

Arterial Dissections

Dissection, a tear in the subintimal layer of a large artery, is most common in the internal carotid artery as it enters the petrous bone and the vertebral arteries as they course through the foramen transversarium. Intracranial dissections are less common. Dissections lead to ischemic strokes through artery-to-artery embolism or by causing significant stenosis and occlusion of the proximal vessel (45). Dissections can also cause a pseudo-aneurysm, creating a source for thrombus formation. Intradural dissections can cause subarachnoid hemorrhage. Although the treatment is unproven unproven, patients are often treated with intravenous heparin followed by oral warfarin for 3 to 6 months. There has not been a trial comparing this approach to antiplatelet therapy. The duration of therapy is based on the period of anticipated high risk and the natural history of the vessel's repair. No studies have examined the safety and efficacy of therapy using different durations of anticoagulation. For patients with recurrent ischemic events, long-term anticoagulation may be considered. Endovascular therapy (stenting or occlusion) may be considered for patients who have definite recurrent ischemic events despite adequate antithrombotic therapy.

CONVENTIONAL MODIFIABLE STROKE RISK FACTORS

Hypertension

Hypertension is one of the most common global diseases. Because of the associated morbidity and mortality and the cost to society, hypertension is an important public health challenge. Hypertension is the single most important risk factor for stroke and also causes "silent" infarcts, which contribute to cognitive dysfunction (46, 47). There is a continuous association between both systolic and diastolic blood pressures (BPs) and the risk of ischemic stroke (48, 49). The Seventh Report of the Joint National Committee on Prevention, Detection, Evaluation and Treatment of High Blood Pressure (JNC-7) emphasized the importance of lifestyle modifications in the management of hypertension and makes the following recommendations:

- Lose weight if overweight
- Limit alcohol intake to no more than 1 oz (30 mL) of ethanol (i.e., 24 oz [720 mL] of beer, 10 oz [300 mL] of wine, 2 oz [60 mL] of 100 proof liquor) per day or 0.5 (15 mL) ethanol per day for women and people of lighter weight
- Increase aerobic activity (30–45 minutes most days of the week)
- Reduce sodium intake to no more than 100 millimoles per day (mmol/d; 2.4 g sodium or 6 g sodium chloride)
- Maintain adequate intake of dietary potassium (approximately 90 mmol/d)
- Maintain adequate intake of dietary calcium and magnesium for general health
- Stop smoking and reduce intake of dietary saturated fat and cholesterol for overall cardiovascular health

Initial therapy based on the JNC VII report recommendations is as follows (50):

- Prehypertension (systolic 120–139, diastolic 80–89): No antihypertensive drug is indicated.
- Stage 1 hypertension (systolic 140–159, diastolic 90–99): Thiazide-type diuretics are recommended for most. An ACE inhibitor, angiotensin II receptor blocker (ARB), beta-blocker, calcium channel blocker, or a combination of these may be considered.
- Stage 2 hypertension (systolic >160, diastolic < 100): Two-drug combination (usually thiazide-type diuretic and ACE inhibitor or ARB or beta-blocker or calcium channel blocker) is recommended for most.

- For the compelling indications, other antihypertensive drugs (e.g., diuretics, ACE inhibitor, ARB, beta-blocker, calcium channel blocker) may be considered as needed.

Seven published randomized controlled trials with a combined sample size of 15,527 participants with ischemic stroke, TIA, or ICH focused on the relationship between BP reduction and the secondary prevention of stroke and other vascular events (51). The patients were followed up for 2–5 years. Treatment with antihypertensive drugs was associated with significant reductions in all recurrent strokes, nonfatal recurrent stroke, MI, and all vascular events. The overall reductions in stroke and all vascular events were related to the degree of BP lowering achieved, but whether a particular class of antihypertensive drug offers a particular advantage for use in patients after ischemic stroke remains uncertain.

Blood pressure management is recommended for both prevention of recurrent stroke and prevention of other vascular events in persons who have had an ischemic stroke or TIA. Benefit has been seen with an average reduction of approximately 10/5 mmHg. The optimal drug regimen remains uncertain; however, the available data support the use of diuretics and the combination of diuretics and an ACEI (angiontensin converting enzyme inhibitor). The choice of specific drugs should be individualized and according to the JNC-7 Report. In patients with history of MI, a beta-blocker and ACE inhibitor are recommended. In patients with mild hypertension with increased cardiovascular risk, an ACE inhibitor or a calcium channel blocker were not found to be superior to low-dose thiazide diuretic therapy. However, the HOPE and EUROPA trials demonstrated that ACE inhibitors provided better outcomes than placebo.

Diabetes

Diabetes mellitus is a chronic disease that requires conscientious longitudinal medical attention. It is estimated that diabetes affects 8% of the adult population (52). Diabetes mellitus (DM) and age were the only significant independent predictors of recurrent stroke in a population-based study of stroke (53). In another community-based stroke study, the Oxfordshire Stroke Project, diabetes was an important factor that independently predicted stroke recurrence (hazard ratio [HR] 1.85; 95% CI 1.18 to 2.90; p<0.01), and it was estimated that 9.1% (95% CI 2.0– 20.2) of the recurrent strokes were attributable to diabetes. In the Stroke Data Bank, patients at the lowest risk of 2-year stroke recurrence were free of diabetes. Furthermore, diabetes has been shown to be a strong determinant for the presence of multiple lacunar infarcts in two different stroke cohorts (54).

Most of the available data on stroke prevention in patients with diabetes are on the primary rather than

TABLE 22-3
*LDL Cholesterol Goals and Cut Points for Therapeutic Lifestyle Changes (TLCs)
and Drug Therapy in Different Risk Categories*

RISK CATEGORY	LDL GOAL	LDL LEVEL AT WHICH TO INDICATE LIFESTYLE CHANGES	LDL LEVEL AT WHICH TO CONSIDER DRUG THERAPY
CHD or CHD risk equivalents	<100 mg/dl	>100 mg/dl	>130 mg/dl (100–129 mg/dl drug optional)
2+ risk factors	<130 mg/dl	>130 mg/dl	10 year risk 10%–20% >130 mg/dl 10 year risk <10% >160 mg/dl
0–1 risk factors	<160 mg/dl	>160 mg/dl	>190 mg/dl (160–189 mg/dl drug optional)

secondary prevention of stroke. Intensive treatments to control hyperglycemia, hypertension, dyslipidemia, and microalbuminuria have demonstrated reductions in the risk of cardiovascular events (55).

Thiazide diuretics, beta-blockers, ACEIs, and ARBs are beneficial in reducing cardiovascular events and stroke incidence in patients with diabetes (56). ACEIs and ARBs are preferred because they have been shown to reduce albuminuria and affect favorably the progression of diabetic nephropathy (52).

More meticulous control of lipids is now also recommended among diabetics with an LDL cholesterol (LDL-C) goal as low as 70 milligrams per deciliter (mg/dL) (57).

Glycemic control has been shown to reduce the occurrence of microvascular complications (nephropathy, retinopathy, and peripheral neuropathy) in several clinical trials and is recommended in multiple guidelines of both primary and secondary prevention of stroke and cardiovascular disease (58). Analysis of data from randomized trials suggests a continual reduction in vascular events with the progressive control of glucose to normal levels (59). Diet, exercise, oral hypoglycemic drugs, and insulin are recommended to reach glycemic control, targeting a goal of Hb A1C lower than 7%.

Dyslipidemia

The impact of lipid abnormalities on ischemic stroke has been somewhat controversial, although mounting evidence supports aggressive management for secondary prevention. The guidelines of the American Heart Association and the NCEP Adult Treatment Panel III (ATP III) define hypercholesterolemia as a blood cholesterol concentration of greater than or equal to 240 mg/dL. Desirable cholesterol concentrations are less than 200 mg/dL.

The 2006 American Heart Association/American Stroke Guidelines for prevention of recurrent stroke make the following recommends for lipid management in ischemic stroke and TIA patients:

1. Follow the national Cholesterol Educational Program III (NCEPIII) guidelines for patients with stroke or TIA who have elevated cholesterol (Table 22-3)
2. Administer statins and aim for a target cholesterol-lowering goal of low-density lipoprotein (LDL-C) lower than 100mg/dl for those with CHD (coronary heart disease) or symptomatic atherosclerotic disease, or LDL-C lower than 70mg/dl for very high-risk persons with multiple risk factors
3. Consider administration of statins for ischemic stroke or TIA patients with atherosclerotic stroke but no preexisting indications for statin therapy.

The Stroke Prevention by Aggressive Reduction in Cholesterol Levels (SPARCL) trial was a randomized, double-blind study designed to determine if 80 mg/d of atorvastatin or placebo would reduce the risk of fatal or nonfatal stroke in patients with no known CHD who had a stroke or TIA within the previous 6 months (60). The trial randomized 2,365 subjects to atorvastatin and 2,366 to placebo. There were no significant differences between the two treatment groups in the incidence of serious adverse events. However, there were 55 hemorrhagic strokes in the atorvastatin treatment group and 33 in the placebo group. Myalgia (5.5% vs. 6.0%), myopathy (0.3% vs. 0.3%), and rhabdomyolysis (0.1% vs. 0.1%) did not differ in the atorvastatin or placebo treatment groups (60).

The SPARCL results provide evidence that 80 mg/d of atorvastatin administered to patients with stroke or TIA and without known CHD reduces the risk of stroke and cardiovascular events, despite a small increase in the risk of hemorrhagic stroke. Additional clinical trial studies are needed to determine whether statins reduce the risk of recurrent ischemic stroke or TIA.

Other medications also used to treat dyslipidemia include niacin, fibrates, and cholesterol-absorption inhibitors. These agents can be used in stroke or TIA patients who cannot tolerate statins, but there is not sufficient data that support their efficacy.

Smoking

Smoking increases the risk of ischemic stroke in a dose-dependant fashion. In the Women's Health Initiative Study (WHI) of 39,783 patients, smoking fewer than 15 cigarettes a day had a relative risk of 1.93 for total hemorrhagic stroke. This risk increased to a risk ratio of 3.29 for women who smoke more than 15 cigarettes per day. The risk of intracerebral hemorrhage and subarachnoid hemorrhage were also increased in this population (RR2.67, 4.02, respectively). On average, smoking doubles the risk of stroke (61).

Patients should be approached during their acute hospitalization regarding the importance of a smoking cessation program. The use of nicotinic patch, alone or in combination with bupropion, may be considered. The potential risk for a reduction in seizure threshold associated with bupropion use may be a concern in patients with large cortical strokes.

Alcohol Intake

The role of alcohol is controversial. Studies are difficult to conduct because of multiple socioeconomic variables. Meta-analysis of multiple studies indicates that heavy alcohol consumption (>60 grams per day) increases the individual's risk for al stroke subtypes, especially intracerebral and subarachnoid hemorrhages, and also is correlated with increase in the incidence of hypertension (62). Therefore alcohol cessation is an important intervention for heavy drinkers.

MODIFIABLE RISK FACTORS EXCLUSIVE TO WOMEN

Oral contraceptive pills (OCPs) are a very common method of birth control globally, but the risk of stroke with OCPs—especially in conjunction with factors such as smoking, hypertension, genetic predisposition to thromboembolism, and migraine—has a major impact in secondary stroke prevention. Preparations with a high estrogen content (150 mcg) have been associated with both arterial and venous thromboembolism, and the third-generation OCP, containing gestodene or desogestrel and the same low dose of estrogen, has been associated with an increase in the risk of venous thromboembolic disease (63). In heavy smokers over the age of 35 and in women with previous thromboembolic events, OCPs are contraindicated.

Migraine with aura is an independent risk factor for stroke (64). The symptom of migraine with aura is associated with a 6–8 fold increase in risk of stroke for patients under the age of 45. There is a fear of stroke in migraine patients taking OCPs because the presence of two risk factors and their multiplicative effect on the overall risk of stroke. Therefore, the change in migraine symptoms and the development or change in aura should suggest discontinuation of OCPs. There is also evidence that the risk of stroke is high during the peripartum and postpartum period (65). In the Baltimore-Washington Cooperative Young Stroke Study, the relative risk of ischemic stroke during pregnancy increased from 0.7 to 8.7 six weeks postpartum. There is no definite guideline for the use of antiplatelet/antithrombotic therapy in stroke prevention for woman with a history pregnancy-related stroke. However, heparin is the preferred anticoagulant of choice during pregnancy, warfarin may be used between 13 and 36 weeks of gestation, and both heparin and warfarin may be used during breastfeeding (66).

SUMMARY

Stroke and TIA have great impact in the global public health, affecting millions of people of varied ethnicity, age, gender, and socioeconomic status and causing serious disabilities that affect the quality of life of these people. Therefore, stroke prevention is an important field of secondary prevention considering both conventional and population-specific risk factors. Modifiable risk factors such as hypertension, diabetes, smoking, obesity, and dyslipidemia should be aggressively managed. Workup for an etiology should be thorough, and more intensive measures maybe warranted.

References

1. Koennecke HC. Secondary prevention of stroke: a practical guide to drug Treatment. *CNS Drugs* 2004; 18(4):221–241.
2. Albers GW, Caplan LR, Easton JD, et a.l, for the TIA Working Group. Transient ischemic attack: proposal for a new definition. *N Engl J Med* 2002; 347:1713–1716.
3. Petty GW, et al., Ischemic stroke subtypes: a population-based study of incidence and risk factors. *Stroke* 1999; 30(12):1513–2516.
4. Barnett HJ, Taylor DW, Eliasziw M, et al. Benefit of carotid endarterectomy in patients with symptomatic moderate or severe stenosis: North American Symptomatic Carotid Endarterectomy Trial Collaborators. *N Engl J Med* 1998; 339: 1415–1425.
5. European Carotid Surgery Trialists' Collaborative Group. Randomised trial of endarterectomy for recently symptomatic carotid stenosis: final results of the MRC European Carotid Surgery Trial (ECST). *Lancet* 1998; May 9; 351(9113):1379–1387.
6. Carotid endarterectomy and prevention of cerebral ischemia in symptomatic carotid stenosis. Veterans Affairs Cooperative Studies Program 309 Trialist Group. *JAMA* 1991 Dec 18; 266(23):3289–3294.

7. Grubb RL Jr, et al., Importance of hemodynamic factors in the prognosis of symptomatic carotid occlusion. *JAMA* 1998; 280:1055–1060.

8. Schmiedek P, et al., Improvement of cerebrovascular reserve capacity by EC-IC arterial bypass surgery in patients with ICA occlusion and hemodynamic cerebral ischemia. *J Neurosurg* 1994; 81:236–244.

9. Alberts MJ, for the Publications Committee of the WALLSTENT. Results of a multicenter prospective randomized trial of carotid artery stenting vs. carotid endarterectomy. *Stroke* 2001; 32:325.

10. Yadav JS, et al., for the Stenting and Angioplasty with Protection in Patients at High Risk for Endarterectomy Investigators. Protected carotid stenting versus endartectomy in high-risk patients. *N Engl J Med* 2004; 351:1493–1501.

11. Jean-Louis Mas, et al., Endarterectomy versus stenting in patients with symptomatic severe carotid stenosis. *N Engl J Med* 2006; 355:1660–1671.

12. Ringleb PA, et al., SPACE collaborative group. 30 day results from the SPACE trial of stent-protected angioplasty versus carotid endarterectomy in symptomatic patients: a randomized non-inferiority trial. *Lancet* 2006; 368:1239–1247.

13. Ross Naylor, SPACE: not the final frontier. Comment. *Lancet* 2006; 368:1215–1216.

14. Sacco RL, et al., Guidelines for prevention of stroke in patients with ischemic stroke or transient ischemic attack. *A statement for Healthcare Professionals from the American Heart Association/American Stroke Association Council on Stroke* 2006; 37(2):577–617.

15. Risk factors for stroke and efficacy of antithrombotic therapy in atrial fibrillation: analysis of pooled data from five randomized controlled trials. *Arch Intern Med* 1994; 154:1449–1457.

16. Hylek EM, et al., An analysis of the lowest effective intensity of prophylactic anticoagulation for patients with nonrheumatic atrial fibrillation. *N Engl J Med* 1996; 335:540–546.

17. Secondary Prevention in non-rheumatic atrial fibrillation after transient ischaemic attack or minor stroke: EAFT (European Atrial Fibrillation Trial) Study Group. *Lancet* 1993; 342:1255–1262.

18. Adjusted-dose warfarin versus low intensity, fixed dose warfarin plus aspirin for high-risk patients with atrial fibrillation: stroke prevention in Atrial Fibrillation III randomized clinical trial. *Lancet* 1996; 348:633–638.

19. Carter AB. Prognosis of cerebral embolism. *Lancet* 1965; 2:514–519.

20. Friedberg CK. *Diseases of the Heart*. Philadelphia, Pa: WB Saunders, 1996.

21. Szekely P. Systemic embolization and anticoagulant prophylaxis in rheumatic heart disease. *BMJ* 1964; 1:209–212.

22. Roy D., et al., Usefulness of anticoagulant therapy in the prevention of embolic complications of atrial fibrillation. *Am Heart J* 1986; 112:1039–1043.

23. Avierinos JF, et al., Cerebral ischemic events after diagnosis of mitral valve prolapse: a community based study of incidence and predictive factors. *Stroke* 2003; 34(6):1339–1344.

24. Fulkenrson PK, et at., Calcification of the mitral annulus: etiology, clinical associations, complications and therapy. *Am J Med* 1979; 66:967–977.

25. Nestico PF, et al., Mitral annular calcification: clinical, pathophysiology, and echcardiographic review. *Am Heart J* 1984; 107(pt. 1):989–996.

26. Hagen PT, et al., Incidence and size of patent foramen ovale during the firs 10 decades of life: and autopsy study of 965 normal hearts. *Mayo Clin Proc* 1984; 59(1):17–20.

27. Lamy C, et al., Clinical and imaging findings in cryptogenic stroke patients with and without patent foramen Ovale: the PFO-ASA Study. Atrial Septal Aneurysm. *Stroke* 2002; 33(3):446–449.

28. Mas JL, et al., Recurrent cerebrovascular events associated with patent foramen ovale, atrial septal aneurysm or both. *N Engl J Med* 2001; 345(24):1740–1746.

29. Rodriguez CJ, et al., Hypercoagulable states in patients with patent foramen ovale. *Curr Hematol Rep* 2003; 2(5):435–441.

30. Homma S, et al., for the PFO in Cryptogenic Stroke Study (PICSS) Investigators. Effect of medical treatment in stroke patients with patent foramen ovale: Patent Foramen Ovale in Cryptogenic Stroke Study. *Circulation* 2002; 105:2625–2631.

31. Antithrombotic Trialists' Collaboration. Collaborative meta-analysis of randomized trials of antiplatelet therapy for prevention of death, myocardial infarction, and stroke in high risk patients. *BMJ* 2002; 324:71–86.

32. CAPRIE Steering Committee. A randomized, blinded, trial of Clopidogrel Versus Aspirin in Patients at Risk of Ischemic Events (CAPRIE): CAPRIE Steering Committee. *Lancet* 1996; 348:1329–1339.

33. Bhatt DL, Fox KA, Hacke W, et al., Clopidogrel and Aspirin versus aspirin alone for the prevention of atherothrombotic events. *N Engl J Med* 2006; 354(160):1706–1717.

34. Diener HC, et al., for the MATCH Investigators. Aspirin and clopidogrel compared with clopidogrel alone after recent ischaemic stroke or transient ischaemic attack in high-risk patients (MATCH): randomized, double blind, placebo-control trial. *Lancet* 2004; 364:331–337.

35. Diener HC, et al., European Stroke Prevention Stud, 2: dipyridamole and acetylsalicylic acid in the secondary prevention of stroke. *J Nurol Sci.* 1996; 143:1–13.

36. McCully KS. Vascuar pathology of homocysteinemia: implications for the pathogenesis of arteriosclerosis. *Am J Pathol* 1969; 56(1):111–128.

37. Toole, JF, Malinow MR, Chambless LE, et al. Lowering homocysteine in patients with ischemic stroke to prevent recurrent stroke, myocardial infarction, and death: the Vitamin Intervention for Stroke Prevention (VISP) randomized controlled trial. *JAMA* 2004; 291(5):565–575.

38. Hankey GJ, et al., Inherited thrombophilia in ischemic stroke and its pathogenic subtypes. *Stroke* 2001; 32:1793–1799.

39. Casas JP, Hingorani AD, et al., Meta-analysis of genetic studies in ischemic stroke: thirty-two genes involving approximately 18.000 cases and 58.000 controls. *Arch Neurol* 2004; 61:1652–1661.

40. Blohorn A, Guegan-Massardier E, Triquenot A, et al. Antiphospholipidantibodies in the acute case of cerebral ischaemia in young adults: a descriptive study of 139 patients. *Cerebrovas Dis* 2002; 13:156–162.

41. Pegelow GH, et al., Risk of recurrent stroke in patients with sickle cell disease treated with erythrocyte transfusions. *J Pediatr* 1995; 126:896–899.

42. Adams RJ, McKie VC, et al., Prevention of a first stroke by transfusions in children with sickle cell anemia and abnormal results on transcranial Doppler ultrasonography. *N Engl J Med* 1998; 339:5–11.

43. Sebastiani P, Ramoni MF, et al., Genetic dissection and prognostic modeling of overt stroke in sickle cell anemia. *Nat Genet* 2005; 37(4): 340–341.

44. The Stroke Prevention by Aggressive Reduction in Cholesterol Levels (SPARCL) investigators: High-dose atorvastatin after stroke or transients ischemic attack. *N Engl J Med* 2006; 355:549–559.

45. Lucas C, et al., Stroke patterns of internal carotid artery dissection in 40 patients. *Stroke* 1998; 29:2646–2648.

46. Kase CS, et al., Prevalence of silent stroke in patients presenting with initial stroke: the Framingham Study. *Stroke* 1989; 20(7):850–852.

47. Liao D, et al., Presence and severity of cerebral white matter lesions and hypertension, its treatment, and its control. THE ARIC Study. Atherosclerosis risk in Communities Study. *Stroke* 1996; 27(12); 2262–2270.

48. Rodgers A, et al., Blood pressure and risk of stroke in patients with cerebrovascular disease: the United Kingdom Transient Ischaemic Attack Collaborative Group. *BMJ* 1996; 313:147.

49. Wolf PA, et al., Cigarette smoking as a risk factor for stroke. The Framingham Study. *JAMA* 1998; 259(7):1025–1029.

50. Chobanian AV, Bakris GL, Black HR, et al. for the National Heart, Lung, and Blood Institute Joint National Committee on Prevention, Detection, Evaluation, and Treatment of High Blood Pressure; National High Blood Pressure Education Program Coordinating Committee. the seventh report of the joint national committee on prevention, detection, evaluation, and treatment of high blood pressure: the JNC 7 Report. *JAMA* 2003; 289:2560–2571.

51. Rashid P, Leonardi-Bee J, Bath P. Blood pressure reduction and secondary prevention of stroke and other vascular events: a systematic review. *Stroke* 2003; 34:2741–2748.

52. American Diabetes Association. ADA clinical practice recommendations. *Diabetes Care* 2004; 27:S1–S143.

53. Petty GW, Brown RD Jr., et al., Survival and recurrence after first cerebral infarction: a population based study in Rochester, Minnesota, 1975 through 1989. *Neurology* 1998; 50:208–216.

54. Mast H, et al., Hypertension and diabetes mellitus as determinants of multiple lacunar infarcts. *Stroke* 1995; 26:30–33.

55. Gaede P, et al., Multifactorial intervention and cardiovascular disease in patients with type 2 diabetes. *N Engl J Med* 2003; 348:383–393.

56. Hansson L, et al., Effects of intensive blood-pressure lowering and low dose aspirin in patients with hypertension: principal results of the Hypertension Optimal Treatment (HOT) randomized trial: HOT Study Group. *Lancet* 1998; 351:1755–1762.

57. Grundy SM, et al., for the National Heart, Lung, and Blood Institute; American College of Cardiology Foundation; and American Heart Association. Implications of recent clinical trials for the National Cholesterol Education Program Adult Treatment Panel III guidelines. *Circulation.* 2004; 110:227–239.

58. Grundy SM, et al., Prevention Conference VI: Diabetes and Cardiovascular Disease: executive summary: conference proceeding for healthcare professionals from a special writing group of the American Heart Association. *Circulation* 2002; 105:2231–2239.

59. American Diabetes Association. Standards of medical care for patients with diabetes mellitus. *Diabetes Care* 2003; 26(suppl 1):S33–S50.

60. The Stroke Prevention by Aggressive Reduction in Cholesterol Levels (SPARCL) investigators: high-dose atorvastatin after stroke or transients ischemic attack. *N Engl J Med* 2006; 355:549–559.

61. Wolf PA, et al., Cigarette smoking as a risk factor for stroke. The Framingham Study. *JAMA* 1998; 259(7):1025–1029.

62. Reynolds K, et al., Alcohol consumption and risk of stroke: a meta-analysis. *JAMA* 2003; 289(5):579–588.

63. Effect of different progestagens in low estrogen oral contraceptives on venous thromboembolic disease. World Heath Organization Collaborative Study of Cardiovascular Disease and Steroid Hormone Contraception. *Lancet* 1995; 346(8990): 1582–1588.

64. Lidegaard O. Oral Contraceptives, pregnancy and the risk of cerebral thromboembolism: the influence of diabetes, hypertension, migraine and previous thrombotic disease. *Br J Obstet Gynaecol* 1995; 102(2):153–159.

65. Kittner SJ, et al., Pregnancy and the risk of stroke. *N Engl J Med* 1996; 335(11):768–774.

66. Leys D, et al., Arterial ischemic strokes associate with pregnancy and puerperium. *Acta Neurol Belg* 1997; 97(1):5–16.

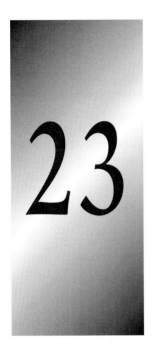

23 Prevention of Deconditioning after Stroke

Frederick M. Ivey
Richard F. Macko

Stroke leads to profound cardiovascular deconditioning that propagates neurologic disability and worsens cardiovascular disease risk factor profiles by promoting insulin resistance. Peak fitness levels for individuals with history of stroke are approximately half that found in age-matched sedentary controls, indicating significant functional aerobic impairment (1–3). Low fitness levels compromise the capacity of stroke patients to meet the elevated energy demands of hemiparetic gait (4–6). Further, this diminished physiological fitness reserve limits basic activities-of-daily-living (ADL) capacity, contributing to activity intolerance and subjective fatigue (7, 8).

The etiology of deconditioning after stroke is multifactorial; the product of physical inactivity, age-related declines, and hemiparetic body composition abnormalities that affect multiple physiological systems. Secondary biological abnormalities in hemiparetic body composition and tissue include gross muscular atrophy (9), increased intramuscular area fat (9), and a shift towards a fast twitch muscle fiber type (10–12). These unilateral tissue changes likely play a role in the poor fitness and high prevalence of insulin resistance seen after stroke. An emerging consensus is that poor fitness not only compromises a stroke survivor's functional abilities, but also increases atherothrombotic risk by contributing to the

Cardio-Metabolic Syndrome (13). Accelerated hemiparetic osteoporosis coupled with the heightened fall-risk also predispose to serious fractures (14). All of these stroke-related body composition and metabolic abnormalities are worsened by physical inactivity and advancing age. Section one of this chapter defines the profile of diminished physiological fitness reserve and details some of the underlying body composition and tissue-level abnormalities. We discuss the clinical implications of these findings in terms of functional impairment and risk factor profiles.

A number of studies now demonstrate that a variety of different exercise training modalities can be safely used to improve cardiovascular fitness following stroke (1, 3, 15–17). Increasing evidence from randomized studies further shows that structured exercise programs, particularly those employing task-repetitive locomotor training, can improve sensorimotor function even years after stroke (16, 18, 19). Hence, several exercise regimens are successful at both increasing fitness and improving gait patterning to reduce the energy costs of hemiparetic gait. This may ultimately improve mobility function and basic ADL capacity after stroke. Section two reviews the physiological and functional effects of exercise after stroke. While further research is needed to optimize exercise design, new evidence regarding dose-intensity and health benefits of exercise after stroke is presented. Current health care recommendations suggest exercise as an adjunct to best pharmacological treatment for optimal risk factor management of the Metabolic Syndrome (13).

Section three provides some general guidelines for implementing exercise programs after stroke. Goals should be oriented towards a multiple-physiological systems approach intended to improve fitness, sensorimotor function, and cardiovascular-metabolic health, and prevent or reduce deleterious body composition abnormalities that accompany disuse while aging with the chronic disability of stroke. The high prevalence of residual neurologic deficits and medical and cardiovascular comorbid conditions presents unique safety and feasibility issues related to implementation of exercise programs after stroke. Recommendations are provided for initial medical evaluation to optimize safety and overcome the barriers to exercise participation after stroke. We reference some evidence-based protocols and exercise progression formulas that have proven successful in research settings, and touch upon some future research directions that are likely to influence the practice of exercise to best promote health and wellness after stroke.

CARDIOVASCULAR HEALTH AND FITNESS AFTER STROKE

Cardiovascular health and fitness are integrally linked to exercise behaviors. In order to gain perspectives on the health impact of physical deconditioning following stroke, exercise behaviors must be considered across the phases of recovery. Conventional sub-acute stroke rehabilitation primarily focuses on optimizing basic activities of daily living skills, functional independence, and preventing complications during the crucial early sub-acute stroke period that can complicate recovery (20). It is not clear that conventional rehabilitation systematically provides an adequate exercise stimulus to reverse the profound physical deconditioning and associated hemiparetic muscular atrophy that worsen neurologic disability and cardiovascular health profiles in this sedentary population. In one study, cardiac monitoring of conventional physical therapy during the sub-acute stroke recovery period revealed that less than 3 minutes per session reached an aerobic intensity of 40% of measured heart rate reserve (HRR) (21). This level represents the lowest target for exercise in usual cardiac rehabilitation care. A large metropolitan catch-all area in the United States reported that after a stroke, a mean of 9 ± 5 outpatient physical therapy visits are attended by the typical patient. The same study went on to say that therapy has usually ended entirely between 30–180 days post stroke (15). Collectively, these findings suggest that conventional physical therapy during the sub-acute recovery phase provides an inadequate exercise stimulus to address the domains of physical and metabolic deconditioning.

Measuring Fitness Levels after Stroke

Several studies have measured cardiovascular fitness levels using open circuit spirometry after stroke (Table 23-1). Although exercise testing strategies have been diverse, the

---

TABLE 23-1
Studies on Peak Aerobic Fitness after Stroke

STUDY	SUBJECTS	TESTING DEVICE	MEAN VO₂ PEAK (MLS/KG/MIN)
Potempa et al. 1995 (3)	42 chronic stroke, 43–72 yrs.	Cycle Ergometer	15.9
Fujitani et al. 1999 (25)	2–49 mo. post-stroke (n=30), 53.6 yrs.	Cycle Ergometer	17.7
Rimmer et al. 2000 (17)	35 chronic stroke, 53 ± 8 yrs.	Cycle Ergometer	13.3
Mackay-Lyons 2002 (26)	29 sub-acute, 65 ± 14 yrs.	Treadmill 15% BWS	14.4
Duncan et al. 2003 (15)	92 sub-acute, 69 ± 10 yrs.	Cycle Ergometer	11.5
Kelly et al. 2003 (27)	17 sub-acute, 61 ± 16 yrs.	Semi-recumbent Cycle	15.0
Chu et al. 2004 (1)	12 chronic, 62 ± 9 yrs.	Cycle Ergometer	17.2
Ivey et al. 2005 (2)	131 chronic, 64 ± 7 yrs.	Treadmill Full BWS	13.6

BWS = Body weight support

general finding has been dramatically lower peak VO_2 levels in stroke survivors, contrasting with age-matched elderly who are physically inactive but otherwise healthy. Individuals in their sixties are expected to have peak oxygen levels ranging between 25 and 30 mL/kg/min depending on a number of factors (22, 23). Thus, the mean peak oxygen consumption level in stroke patients is roughly half that of age-matched individuals. This is partially a function of the extremely high energy cost of hemiparetic gait contributing to diminished physiological fitness reserve (5, 24).

Functional Consequences of Reduced Fitness after Stroke

The extremely low levels of peak oxygen consuming capacity found in stroke survivors can compromise functional mobility and are below the level required for some basic activities of daily living. The human body at rest consumes roughly 3.5 mLs/kg/min of oxygen, or 1 metabolic equivalent (MET) (28). The MET calculations associated with various forms of activity (29) reveal that light instrumental activities of daily living (IADLs) generally require approximately 3 METS of oxygen consumption, whereas more strenuous ADLs require approximately 5 METS or 17.5 mLs/kg/min. Notably, published MET values for different activities do not take into account neurologic disability, which may be associated with even higher energy requirements for gross motor activities due to biomechanical inefficiency (6).

The impact of low fitness on function after stroke is best illustrated when peak fitness values are considered in the context of the range of energy expenditure necessary to perform daily activities (Figure 23-1) (2).

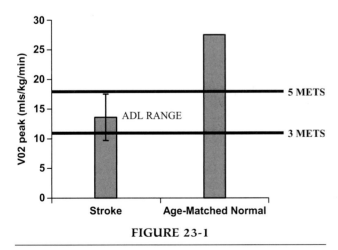

FIGURE 23-1

Peak aerobic fitness levels of N=131 chronic stroke patients relative to the energy requirements for activities of daily living. *Reproduced with permission from Topics in Stroke Rehabilitation.*

While peak values for age-matched healthy individuals far exceed the approximated ADL range, the exhaustion value falls in the middle of the zone for most stroke patients. (Figure 23-1) (2). Thus, many stroke patients must work to complete exhaustion to achieve the middle of the established ADL range, making mid- to upper- level ADLs either impossible or unsustainable.

Mechanisms Underlying Post-Stroke Deconditioning

Although consensus has emerged that stroke leads to extreme deconditioning, the underlying biological mechanisms have not been systematically investigated. The disability of stroke is widely attributed to brain injury alone, and the diminished fitness attributed to reduced "central" neural drive. However, there are a number of changes in skeletal muscle and surrounding tissues that propagate disability and contribute to low fitness levels, including gross muscular atrophy, muscle fiber type shift, tissue inflammation, and altered vasomotor function, as discussed in the following sections.

Role of Muscle Atrophy.   Reduced muscle mass plays a role in the ability to use oxygen in these patients. The level and quality of metabolically active tissue partially accounts for the amount of oxygen a person can utilize. Ryan et al. (30) confirm a strong relationship between thigh muscle mass by Dual Energy X-ray Absorbtiometry (DEXA) and peak VO_2. In this study, VO_2 was related to the lean muscle mass of both thighs, with lean mass predicting over 40% of the variance in peak aerobic fitness (30).

Stroke patients have reduced lean tissue mass that is related to the degree of neurologic disability. Bilateral mid-thigh CT scans are used to illustrate the severe atrophy caused by chronic hemiparesis (Figure 23-2) (9). There is extreme gross muscular atrophy in paretic leg mid-thigh CT scans, showing 20% lower muscle area compared to the non-paretic thigh. In addition, intramuscular area fat is 25% greater in the paretic thigh compared to the non-paretic thigh (9). Elevated intramuscular fat is linked to insulin resistance and its complications (11). These body composition abnormalities may impact whole-body metabolic health and function.

Unilateral Muscle Fiber-Type Changes.   Cellular changes in skeletal muscle may also contribute to poor fitness and worsening cardiovascular disease (CVD) risk after stroke. Prior studies of hemiparetic muscle reveal variable findings related to altered fiber type proportions, loss of type I muscle fibers, fiber atrophy, and reduced oxidative capacity (11, 12, 31–34). A slow-to-fast fiber type conversion has been reported (10, 11, 33). Skeletal muscles are composed of fibers that express different myosin heavy chain

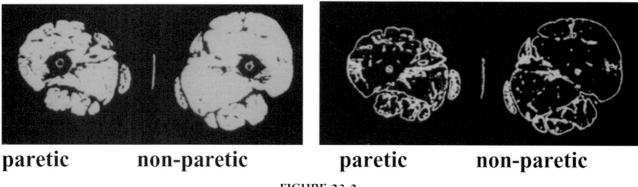

paretic   non-paretic   paretic   non-paretic

FIGURE 23-2

Bilateral CT scan illustrating muscle atrophy and elevated intramuscular area fat on the paretic side *Reproduced with permission from Topics in Stroke Rehabilitation.*

(MHC) isoforms. Slow (Type I) MHC isoform fibers have higher oxidative function, are more fatigue resistant, and are more sensitive to insulin-mediated glucose uptake. Fast (Type II) MHC fibers are recruited for more powerful movements, they fatigue rapidly and are less sensitive to the action of insulin (35). Routine ATPase staining of paretic leg muscle biopsies show elevated proportions of fast type II fibers in the paretic leg of stroke survivors (Figure 23-3) (2).

Similar findings are reported in the hemiparetic upper extremity (33). Further, densitometric analysis of MHC gel electrophoresis analyzing bilateral vastus lateralis biopsies shows significantly elevated proportion of fast MHC isoforms in the paretic vs. non-paretic leg (10). These findings contrast with the relatively equal proportions of slow and fast MHC fibers found in vastus lateralis of individuals without stroke (33). Interestingly, a shift to fast MHC composition in the paretic muscle is also seen in animals and humans after spinal cord injury (36). This suggests that neurologic alterations may be partially responsible for the shift of muscle phenotype. A switch to fast MHC can occur with muscle unloading or disuse. The relative

ATPase 4.6

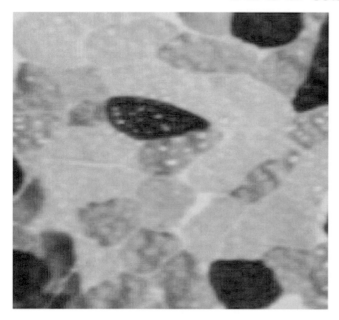
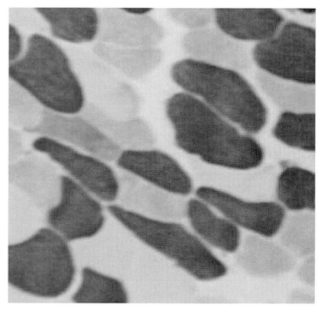

Paretic   Non-Paretic

FIGURE 23-3

Fiber-type shift on paretic side *Reproduced with permission from Topics in Stroke Rehabilitation.*

inactivity after stroke could also facilitate these changes. The shift to fast MHC is in contrast to the changes seen in normal aging, where fast MHC fibers are preferentially lost through denervation and slow MHC fiber density increases (37). Hence, this shift after stroke is an abnormal muscle molecular phenotype that would be expected to result in a more fatigable, insulin- resistant muscle.

Inflammatory Pathway Activation in Hemiparetic Muscle. The molecular mechanisms underlying muscular atrophy and insulin resistance after stroke are not fully understood. Bilateral biopsies from vastus lateralis muscle of chronic stroke patients reveal a nearly threefold increased tumor necrosis factor-alpha mRNA expression in hemiparetic leg muscle, compared to age-matched non-stroke controls (38). In addition, there is a significant 1.6-fold increased TNF-alpha mRNA expression in the non-paretic leg muscle of stroke patients compared to controls (38); evidence of a bilateral or systemic process conferring more widespread inflammatory effects. Immunohistochemical studies further show that TNF-alpha localizes to inter-fascicular space, as well as the muscle fascicle, suggesting that increased inflammatory cytokine production may arise from both muscle and surrounding adipocytes (2). The clinical significance is that TNF-alpha blocks insulin signaling and mediates muscle atrophy (39–42). Thus, inflammatory mechanisms may contribute to both muscular atrophy and insulin resistance after stroke.

Hemiparetic Osteoporosis. Hemiparetic osteoporosis is a clinically important body composition abnormality that is linked to duration of immobility, muscular atrophy, and poor cardiovascular fitness after stroke (43–45). Osteoporosis is more severe in the upper than lower extremity, but fracture risk is greater for the hip (43). Hip fracture risk is reported sevenfold elevated in the first year post-stroke, and 15% projected across five years (14), and is increased sevenfold for each 2 standard deviation decrease in femoral neck bone mineral density (46). Paretic leg femoral neck bone density declines up to 14% within a year after stroke (47); a period in which up to 73% experience a fall (48). Hence, exercise strategies to improve both balance and bone health may serve as important adjuncts to best medical care. Despite the established role of exercise as an adjunct to best medical care for treatment of osteoporosis (49), few studies have systematically examined the potential for exercise to improve balance and bone health after stroke (43). Three studies with positive outcomes on falls (50–52) used repetitive functional tasks which most likely improved motor coordination, movement speed, and strength (50).

Impairments in Peripheral Blood Flow. Findings of unilaterally impaired paretic leg blood flow in chronic stroke identify yet another clinical feature related to reduced

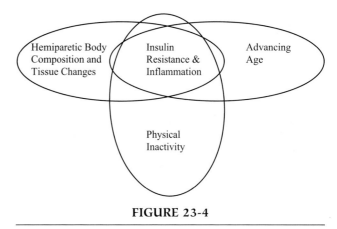

FIGURE 23-4

Interacting features in the stoke population that combine to produce elements of the Metabolic Syndrome.

cardiovascular fitness and enhanced CVD risk. When resting and post-ischemic reactive hyperemic blood flow was compared between the affected and unaffected legs of stroke patients, results showed 32% and 35% reductions, respectively (53).

Metabolic Consequences of Paretic-Side Tissue-Level Changes

The skeletal muscle, bone, and vasomotor regulatory abnormities on the paretic side may contribute to worsening cardiovascular risk by propagating physical inactivity, insulin resistance, and the metabolic syndrome. Kernan et al. (54) originally identified a high prevalence of insulin resistance during the sub-acute stroke recovery period . Subsequent findings in chronic stroke reveal an extremely high prevalence of abnormal glucose metabolism (55). In this chronic stroke study involving over 200 volunteers, 35% screened had documented diabetes by medical history. Additionally, fasting and post-load hyperglycemia were highly prevalent in those who were not identified as diabetic by medical history. Collectively, the findings suggest that the rate of abnormal glucose metabolism may be as high as 80% in chronic stroke (55). This is clinically relevant, given that impaired and diabetic glucose tolerance prospectively predict two- to threefold increased risk for recurrent cerebrovascular events (56). The above figure depicts some contributors to post-stroke metabolic syndrome and their interaction with one another (Figure 23-4).

PHYSIOLOGICAL AND FUNCTIONAL EFFECTS OF EXERCISE AFTER STROKE

The following section provides an overview of evidence that exercise can improve cardiovascular-metabolic fitness and function after stroke. Our focus is on exercise programs involving the lower extremities or whole body, consistent with the mission of improving mobility function, fitness, metabolic health, and countering the secondary body composition abnormalities that occur as a consequence of stroke and physical inactivity. In practical terms, this approach primarily engenders elements of aerobic training by incorporating larger muscle groups that are more effective to provide a cardiovascular exercise stimulus to improve metabolic health, consistent with consensus statements for exercise recommendations in high cardiovascular disease risk populations (13). Where such information is available, the specific exercise intensity and progression formula are described, as these may affect the nature and temporal profile of exercise mediated adaptations. We include recent advances in the application of resistance training in stroke survivors which provide evidence of strength gains and paretic leg performance capacity, without deleterious increases in spasticity. Finally, some attention is given to community feasible and home-based exercise models, which may afford opportunities to better disseminate health and function, promoting training programs to larger numbers of stroke survivors.

Exercise Training for Cardiovascular Fitness after Stroke

Several exercise modalities have proven to increase cardiovascular fitness in stroke survivors. A synthesis of these studies suggests that approaches to exercise training may necessarily vary as a function of neurologic deficit severity, baseline fitness levels, and the time phase of recovery after stroke (Table 23-2) (18). Moreover, differing elements of training prescriptions and their progression (e.g., aerobic intensity, training velocity, repetition) may further determine the nature of exercise-mediated outcomes. The following table summarizes some of the more widely cited exercise intervention studies measuring impacts on peak aerobic capacity.

Notably, a gain in peak fitness of as little as 1 MET (3.5 mLs/kg/min), prospectively predicts 17–29% lower non-fatal and 28–51% fatal cardiac events in men (59). Therefore, the importance of the gains observed in the studies involving stroke patients cannot be overstated from the standpoint of clinical relevance. Beyond goals of improving function after stroke, tertiary stroke prevention and cardiovascular disease risk factor modification should be a major objective of exercise in this population (13).

TABLE 23-2
Exercise Intervention Studies and Their Impact on Peak Aerobic Fitness Reprinted with Permission from NeuroRx.

STUDY	DESIGN/POPULATION	INTERVENTION	VO2 PEAK
Potempa et al.1995 (3)	Randomized/ Chronic Stroke	10 weeks cycle training 3x/wk. vs. passive range of motion	**Treatment: +13%**</br>Control: +1 %
Rimmer et al. 2000 (17)	Randomized/ Chronic Stroke	12 weeks on a variety of aerobic (30 min.) and strength equipment (20 min.) 3x/wk vs. delayed entry controls	**Treatment: +8%**</br>Control: −10%
Macko et al 2001 (57)	Noncontrolled/ Chronic Stroke	6 months treadmill exercise 3x/wk.	**Treatment: +10%***
Duncan et al 2003 (15)	Randomized/ Subacute Stroke	12 week in-home therapist supervised program emphasizing strength, balance, endurance (cycle) vs. usual care	**Treatment: +9%**</br>Control: +1%
Chu et al. 2004 (1)	Randomized/ Chronic Stroke	8 weeks water based aerobics up to 80%HRR vs. upper extremity functional exercise	**Treatment: +23%**</br>Control: +3%
Macko et al 2005 (16)	Randomized/ Chronic Stroke	6 month progressive treadmill training 3x/wk. vs. attention controls (stretching)	**Treatment: +17%**</br>Control: +3%
Pang et al. 2005 (58)	Randomized/ Chronic Stroke	Community-based UE vs. LE exercise 3x/wk. 19 weeks	**Treatment (LE): +11%**

**significant between groups across time. *significant within group.
LE= Lower Extremity, UE= Upper Extremity, HRR= Heart Rate Reserve

In high CVD risk non-stroke populations, exercise has been shown to improve a number of physiological factors linked to stroke and cardiac event risk, including insulin sensitivity (60), hemostatic and inflammatory markers (61, 62), and indices of vascular endothelial dependent vasomotor reactivity in coronary and peripheral circulations (63). Other health benefits include improved lipid profiles (64) and improved autonomic tone, which is linked to lower cardiac mortality (65). Exercise is established as an adjunct to best medical care in management of obesity, dyslipidemia, diabetes, and hypertension, strongly supporting a role for exercise to address cardiovascular comorbidities in stroke survivors. Recently, it has been shown that progressive treadmill aerobic exercise can reduce insulin resistance and improve diabetes status in chronic hemiparetic stroke survivors (65a).

Effects of Exercise on Sensorimotor Function after Stroke

Approximately 75% of stroke survivors are left with residual deficits that persistently impair function. In particular, sensorimotor deficits impairing gait and balance limit functional independence and promote a sedentary lifestyle with subsequent physical deconditioning. Until recently, the window for motor recovery with conventional rehabilitation was widely considered to be only three to six months, with little functional improvement thereafter (66). Seminal studies in rehabilitation of the paretic upper extremity now inform us that task-repetitive training can improve arm motor function in chronic stroke, and that the functional gains are associated with brain plasticity (67). A similar paradigm shift is taking place in our understandings of brain plasticity and lower extremity motor control.

Increasing clinical and experimental data provide evidence that exercise has the potential to improve selected motor performance outcomes, even years after stroke, and that the functional improvements are associated with mechanisms of neuroplasticity (67a). Table 23-3 presents some examples of exercise intervention studies producing significant improvements in basic ADL related functional parameters in sub-acute and chronic stroke patients (18).

Exercise Intervention Strategies after Stroke using Multiple Modalities

Although a comprehensive review of the exercise literature in stroke is beyond the scope of this chapter, details related to some of the more widely cited studies are provided in the following paragraphs. Efforts were made to select several representative studies that employ diverse training modalities including: cycle ergometry, water-based exercise, resistance (strength) training, treadmill training, partial body weight support treadmill training, multi-modal therapy, as well as home and community-based interventions. Clearly, much work remains in elucidating the optimal exercise form for producing maximal gains in fitness and function to delay disability and cardiovascular morbidity/mortality after stroke.

Cycle Ergometry. A seminal study conducted by Potempa et al. (3) compared 10 weeks of adapted bicycle ergometer exercise with a control intervention consisting of passive range of motion exercise in chronic stroke patients. Results showed a significant between-group difference in VO_2 peak change over time, with the bicycle ergometer group (n=19) achieving 13% gains compared to no change for controls (n=23). Though Fugl-Meyer sensorimotor scores were positively correlated with gains in peak VO_2, neither of the treatment groups showed significant differences in functional outcome scores. This study showed that aerobic exercise using cycle ergometry is feasible and improves fitness in chronic hemiparetic stroke, but provided no clear evidence that cycle exercise could improve neuromuscular function or functional mobility.

Water-Based Exercise. Chu et al. conducted a water based exercise study lasting 12 weeks (1). Those in the experimental group exercised for one hour, three days per week, in a swimming pool. The patients were progressed to 30 minutes of water aerobics at 80% HRR, with the remainder of time consisting of stretching and warm-up/cool down. Although this study had a very small sample size (7 treatment and 5 controls) the intervention produced the greatest relative gains in peak aerobic capacity shown to date (23%), perhaps arguing for strong consideration of this form of intervention for stroke survivors. A higher level of baseline fitness and function may have influenced results and confounded interpretation relative to other experiments in the field of post-stroke exercise rehabilitation.

Home-Based Therapy. Duncan et al. (69) were the first of the randomized studies to utilize a home-based intervention model. The program consisted of 36 sessions of 90-minute duration over 12–14 weeks. Subjects in the usual care group had services as prescribed by their physicians. All sessions for the exercise group were supervised by a physical or occupational therapist at home. Components of the program were range of motion and flexibility, strengthening, balance, upper extremity functional use, and endurance training (riding a stationary bike for 30 minutes). Both the intervention and usual care groups improved in strength, balance, upper- and lower-extremity motor control, upper-extremity function, and gait velocity. Gains for the intervention group exceeded those in the usual care group in balance, endurance, peak aerobic capacity, and mobility. The study was important in demonstrating the practical utility of home-based interventions compared to

TABLE 23-3

Exercise Intervention Studies and Their Impact on Selected Functional and Physical Performance Outcomes
Reprinted with Permission from NeuroRx

Study	Design/ Population	Intervention	Function
Hesse et al 1994 (68)	Noncontrolled/ Subacute and Chronic Stroke	5 weeks 5x/wk. off partial weight support treadmill walking	*Rivermead Mobility* **Treatment: +110%** *Gait velocity:* **Treatment: +250%**
Potempa et al 1995 (3)	Randomized/ Chronic Stroke	10 weeks cycle training 3x/wk. vs. passive range of motion	*Fugl-Meyer Index* **Treatment: No change** Control: No change
Duncan et al. 1998 (69)	Randomized/ Subacute Stroke	12 weeks home based. Theraband, walking or bike for 20 minutes vs. usual care	*10-m gait velocity* **Treatment: +37.3 %** Control: +12.3% *6-min walk* **Treatment: +28%** Control: +17%
Teixeira-Salmela et al. 1999 (70)	Noncontrolled/ Chronic stroke	10 weeks aerobic + strength training 3x/ wk.	*30-m gait speed (m/s)* **Treatment: +21.2%***
Rimmer et al. 2000 (17)	Randomized/ Chronic Stroke	12 weeks on a variety of aerobic (30 min.) and strength equipment (20 min.) 3x/wk vs. delayed entry controls	*Exercise Time* **Treatment: +29%** Control: +15%
Katz-Leurer et al. 2003 (71)	Randomized/ Acute Stroke	8 weeks cycle ergometer 2x/wk at 60%HRR vs. usual care	*Post-intervention walk distance* **Treatment: 143 m** Control: 108 m *Stair climbing* **Treatment: 26 n.** Control: 18 n
Eng et al. 2003 (72)	Noncontrolled/ Chronic Stroke	8 weeks community-based 3x/wk. aerobic stepping, stretching, functional LE strengthening (chair rise)	*12 min. walk* **Treatment: +9.5%** *10 m walk speed* **Treatment: +14.4% (self-selected) +9.3% (fastest)**
Duncan et al. 2003 (15)	Randomized/ Subacute Stroke	12 week in-home therapist supervised program emphasizing strength, balance, endurance vs. usual care	*10-m gait velocity* **Treatment: +25.7%** Control: +18 % *6-min walk distance* **Treatment: +26%** Control: +15%
Chu et al. 2004 (1)	Randomized/ Chronic Stroke	8 weeks water-based aerobics up to 80%HRR vs. upper extremity functional exercise	*Self-selected gait speed (m/s)* **Treatment: +16.1%** Control: +2.9%
Eich et al, 2004 (73)	Randomized/ Subacute Stroke	6 weeks 5x/wk harness-secured and minimally supported treadmill walking (30 min) plus physiotherapy (30 min) vs. physiotherapy alone (60 min)	*10-m walk* **Treatment: +78%** Control: +36%

TABLE 23-3
(Continued)

STUDY	DESIGN/ POPULATION	INTERVENTION	FUNCTION
			6-minute walk **Treatment: +84%** Control: +51%
Macko et al. 2005 (16)	Randomized/ Chronic Stroke	6-month progressive treadmill training vs. attention controls (stretching)	*6-mi nute walk* **Treatment: +30%** Control: +11% *WIQ Distance* **Treatment: +56%** Control: +12%
Pang et al. 2005 (58)	Randomized/ Chronic Stroke	Community-based UE vs. LE exercise 3x/wk. 19 weeks	*6-minute walk* **Treatment (LE): +19.7%**
Pang et al. 2006 (74)	Randomized/ Chronic Stroke	Community-based UE vs. LE exercise 3x/wk. 19 weeks	*Wolf Motor Function* LE: 0% UE: +7% *Fugl-Meyer Assessment* LE: +2% UE: +12% *Dynamometry (grip strength)* LE: +2% UE: 17%

the more frequently applied hospital-based intervention programs for improving fitness and function after stroke. However, it should be noted that there was still a high level of supervision despite the study being home-based.

Resistance (Strength) Training. A systematic review of outcomes related to progressive strength training after stroke (75) yields some important observations. Out of eight studies, three (6, 31, 49) were randomized controlled trials (RCT), with the remainder being single case time series analyses (76) or single group pre-post trials (77–80). Wide variation was found in the frequency and duration of the training programs, as well as type of equipment used. Studies had participants training anywhere from 2–5 sessions per week, with a total intervention period ranging from 4–12 weeks. Four of the studies used isokinetic dynamometers for training (Cybex or Kin-Com) (77–79, 81), with the remainder using weight machines, hand weights and a pupose-built static dynamometer. Training was primarily targeted to larger muscle groups of the lower limb, with the exception of one study exercising wrist extensors and upper limb flexors (76). Adherence among the trials was variable. All of the studies that measured strength reported significant increases with large effect sizes. Three of the single group pre-post studies (77–79) and one RCT (82) measured effects of the training on spasticity by Hoffman reflex, stretch reflex, Achilles tendon jerk,

the pendulum test during knee flexion, electromyography (EMG) in the quadriceps and hamstring groups, and the modified Ashworth scale. None of the studies reported increases in spasticity after a resistance training exercise program. All of the eight articles measured the effects of training on at least one functional outcome. Generally, walking speeds were significantly increased with this form of training, with effect sizes ranging from 0.5 to 1.5. The RCT with the largest walking speed effect size (82) focused training on the hip, knee, and ankle of each patient's paretic limb. Collectively, this small group of clinical trials provides preliminary evidence that progressive resistance strength training can be effectively used to improve strength and function without a concomitant increase in spasticity after stroke.

Multi-Modal Approach. A trial involving primarily African American stroke survivors utilized a multi-modal intervention (17). A delayed-entry controlled design was used to provide training to all 35 participants. Outcome testing included measures of peak VO_2, strength, flexibility, and body composition. The 3 times per week training protocol consisted of the following components: cardiovascular endurance (30 minutes), muscle strength and endurance (20 minutes), and flexibility (10 minutes). Results showed significant time by group interactions for the following measures during cycle ergometer fitness testing: VO_2 peak, time to exhaustion, and maximal workload. This was among the first randomized exercise studies in stroke to show significant between group effects for muscular strength and endurance as well as improvements in body composition (body weight, BMI, total skinfolds) (17). Other multi-modal exercise therapies have also been successful after stroke (50–52), particularly in the context of fall prevention.

Treadmill(TM)-Based Training Approaches. Based on pioneering studies of hindlimb stepping recovery in despinalized cats, variants of TM- based training have emerged to promote locomotor learning after stroke (83, 84). A biomechanical basis for this approach is supported by findings that TM walking improves reflexive gait patterning in hemiparetic patients (85, 86). The facilitation of gait patterning with TM is well-characterized for both body weight support (BWS) (85) and self-supported full weight bearing TM exercise conditions (86). TM produces a 50% improvement in inter-limb stance to swing symmetry ratios, 30% improvement in impulse symmetry, and improved timing of quadriceps activation compared to over-ground walking in hemiparetic stroke patients (87). TM-based training also provides task-repetition that animal and human studies suggest is requisite to mediate motor learning and neuroplasticity (88, 89). Randomized studies show benefits of TM training translate into improved over-ground walking, and can be extended to more severely impaired subjects using BWS strategies (90). TM-based training can also be combined with progressive aerobic exercise to improve both fitness and ambulatory function (16), as discussed in the following sections:

Partial body-weight support treadmill training: Partial body weight support treadmill (BWST) has received much investigation, particularly as a means to provide a physiological gait training stimulus to more impaired subjects across earlier phases of stroke recovery (85). This approach utilizes a suspensory harness to progress patients from 30–40% BWS to full weight-bearing TM walking, typically with one or two therapists facilitating stepping and truncal stability across 4–6 weeks. Early studies by Hesse et al. provide evidence that BWST may restore gait in severely affected non-ambulatory patients (85, 90). Subsequent randomized studies confirm BWST training is better tolerated and more effective than full weight bearing TM to improve gait and balance function in more severely hemiplegic patients, specifically that subset with lower gait velocities (<0.2 m/s), poorer balance (Berg Scores <15 points) (91, 92), and in advancing age. The latter finding may be explained by the significantly lower oxygen demands of BWST; a finding which brings into question whether BWS using current protocols provides adequate aerobic intensity for metabolic health benefits (93).

Despite some positive findings, a Cochrane Review finds no significant effects from BWST except greater walking speed in those already ambulatory (94). Whether BWST or other TM-based training strategies are more effective than conventional therapy to durably improve function or fitness after stroke remains unclear (95). However, few studies have systematically investigated the training parameters or conditions to BWST outcomes. One promising avenue is that BWST at higher velocities may be more efficacious to improve walking velocity during the sub-acute stroke period (96). These findings have spurred important clinical trials investigating the relative benefits of BWST across the sub-acute vs. chronic stroke phases.

Full body-weight support treadmill training Although partial body weight support TM training may be an effective means for initiating training, particularly for those with greater gait impairment (91), this form of training has not traditionally utilized aerobic progression formulas (93). Thus, based on studies of exercise rehabilitation in the frail elderly, we have studied the profile of fitness and mobility function gains across 6 months of progressive full body-weight support TM aerobic exercise training in stroke survivors with chronic hemiparesis (16, 19, 24, 57). This is a much longer therapeutic duration than is typical for most stroke rehabilitation programs. Our results show that the time profile of cardiovascular fitness gains with regular TM exercise training are progressive and nearly equal across the initial three months and third to sixth month of training (Figure 23-5) (16). There is no evidence of plateau, suggesting that training even beyond

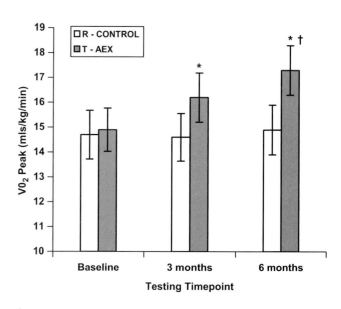

*p < 0.05 within group
†p < 0.01 between groups

FIGURE 23-5

Progression of improvement in VO2 peak across 6 months with progressive full BWS treadmill training in chronic hemiparetic stroke patients *Reproduced with permission from Stroke.*

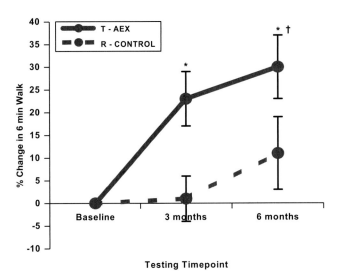

* < 0.05 within group
† < 0.05 between groups

FIGURE 23-6

Progression of improvement in 6 minute walk distance across 6 months with progressive full BWS treadmill training in chronic hemiparetic stroke patients *Reproduced with permission from Stroke.*

six months may produce further benefits in peak fitness levels. In addition, full body-weight support TM exercise also improves 6-minute walk performance and self-reported indices of functional mobility across six months, with greater gains in 6-minute walk occurring within the initial three months of training (Figure 23-6) (16). fMRI randomized studies also show that TM training result in activation of subcortical networks including cerebellum and midbrain during paretic knee movement, which predicts the growth in peak walking performance. This provides evidence of brain plasticity with task-oriented exercise to improve locomotor function in the chronic phase of strokes (96a).

Notably, prospective studies show a plateau in mobility recovery within three months after stroke in 95% of hemiparetic patients receiving conventional rehabilitation care (97). Our findings in a randomized study show that TM training improves both fitness and mobility function long after conventional rehabilitation care has ended, and that the duration of exercise therapy to optimize these outcomes is at least six months. These results support a rationale for long-term exercise after stroke, consistent with public health recommendations for sustained regular exercise to improve fitness and cardiovascular health for all Americans (13).

Community-Based Intervention Strategies. Numerous behavioral and psychosocial issues associated with chronic disability and aging influence exercise adherence and can serve as barriers to participation following stroke (98). Limited access and labor intensity of individualized conventional stroke therapies further constrain resources for exercise programs post-stroke. While both home- and rehabilitation center-based programs have been studied, the safest and most effective settings and behavioral strategies to best disseminate exercise programs to stroke survivors are unknown. Group exercise programs feasible for conduct in the community setting have recently been investigated to increase access, while providing a socially reinforced model for structured physical activity across the chronic stroke period.

A seminal Canadian study by Pang et al. (58, 74) was the first to examine effects of community-based exercise programs on bone health and mobility outcomes in older individuals with chronic stroke. Individuals with remote stroke (>1 yr) that could walk 10 meters independently (with or without walking aids) were randomized to 19 weeks of three one-hour session per week Arm Exercise Group or a fitness and mobility exercise (FAME) program that included brisk walking, sit-to-stand exercises, stepping onto low platforms, walking obstacle course, and partial squats and toe rises to improve strength. FAME significantly increased VO_2 peak by 9%, 6-minute walk distance by 20%, and improved paretic leg strength, but not Berg Balance Scores. However, most subjects had milder balance deficits, while that subset with moderate deficits did not successfully progress their exercise intensity. Notably, FAME intervention prevented the declines in femoral neck bone mineral density that occurred in the Arm Group, and increased distal tibial trabecular bone mineral content on the paretic side. This shows community-based exercise programs can improve fitness, walking capacity, leg strength, and bone health for older individuals with milder chronic deficits (58, 74).

Based on models of task-oriented exercise and social learning to facilitate exercise behaviors in frail elderly, an adaptive physical activity (APA) program with gymnasium and home components was designed to improve mobility and ADL function for chronic stroke patients (99). Group exercises targeting improved gait and balance were utilized to enhance social support, with a parallel home regimen to build self-efficacy for habitual physical activities. Two months APA improved Berg Balance, 6-minute walk distance, and Barthel Index Scores in 20 older subjects with chronic hemiparetic deficits (99). To date, Tuscany Regional Health Authorities have established APA programs at 11 community sites for 190 chronic stroke participants in a 30 x 30 km region of Italy where health services outcomes are tracked. These findings provide proof of the concept that community-based exercise programs improve mobility and basic ADL function, and can be implemented in geographically defined regions to improve outcomes for older chronic stroke patients.

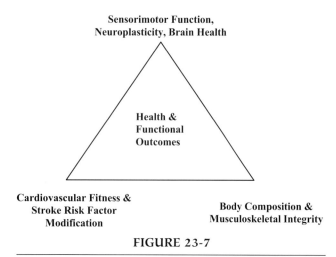

FIGURE 23-7

Multiple physiological systems that define the targets of exercise after stroke.

STRATEGIES FOR DESIGNING EXERCISE PROGRAMS IN STROKE SURVIVORS

Goals of Exercise Training

Structured exercise programs should be considered for all stroke survivors. As detailed in the prior section, a number of randomized studies now demonstrate that various exercise modalities can significantly improve cardiovascular fitness after stroke. While fundamental questions remain regarding how to optimize the exercise prescriptions, the magnitude of VO_2 peak gains that are attainable with exercise after stroke are considered clinically significant in terms of both functional capacity and cardiovascular health promotion (59). Risk factor modification is a second major objective of long-term exercise after stroke. Cardiovascular fitness and metabolic health are integrally linked and modifiable by exercise training, which may translate into reduced recurrent stroke risk and cardiovascular events in this population (13). Individuals aging with the chronic disability of stroke are further subject to body composition abnormalities that are propagated by sedentary lifestyle, worsening rehabilitation outcomes and cardiovascular risk. The inter-related goals for improving fitness and preventing the body composition complications of physical inactivity constitute a multiple physiological systems model defining the targets of exercise therapy after stroke (Figure 23-7).

Intrinsic to this model is an emerging recognition that exercise can improve function by leveraging principals of motor learning, even years after stroke. Emerging clinical and experimental data show that task-repetitive training can mediate functionally relevant motor learning, in both the paretic upper and lower extremity (85, 86). Conversely, lack of practice or "disuse" can propagate disability at a musculoskeletal and central nervous system level. Habitual daily physical activity patterns are a determinant of outcomes that warrant attention as an adjunct to any structured exercise program in the long-term care of stroke survivors. Hence, an objective of exercise therapy is improving sensorimotor function that translates into improved daily activity profiles and quality of life across the continuum of stroke care. As clinically appropriate, motor learning strategies can be combined with aerobic training to improve multiple physiological systems that determine functional and health outcomes (Figure 23-7).

Planning Exercise Programs across the Stages of Stroke Rehabilitation

The planning of exercise programs for stroke patients should be initiated early on, with specific education to participants and family regarding the clinical relevance of exercise to functional recovery, cardiovascular health, and stroke risk factor modification. Most stroke survivors and many health care providers outside the field of rehabilitation care are unaware that both lower and upper extremity motor function can be improved by structured motor learning based exercises, even years after the initial stroke event (16, 100). That physical inactivity is an independent risk factor for stroke, and "disuse" leads to deconditioning which worsens disability and stroke risk, are understated health concerns that need reinforcement across the phases of rehabilitation care. Patients should be informed that consensus statements strongly recommend exercise as an adjunct to medical treatment for optimal management of hypertension, dyslipidemia, obesity, insulin resistance, and diabetes, all of which are elements of the Cardio-Metabolic Syndrome and highly prevalent after stroke. Figure 23-8 lists some recommendations for planning exercise across the phases of stroke recovery.

Medical Evaluation & Safety Issues Related to Exercise

Due to the high incidence of medical and cardiovascular comorbid conditions that can influence exercise participation, evaluation for an exercise program should begin with a medical history, physical, and cardiopulmonary examination. Medical exclusions for exercise after stroke are consistent with American College of Sports Medicine (ACSM) criteria for high cardiovascular disease (CVD) risk subjects (101). In brief, exclusion criteria that have been systematically employed for exercise research include symptomatic heart failure, unstable angina, peripheral arterial occlusive disease, chronic pain syndromes, dementia or severe aphasia (operationally defined as incapacity to follow 2-point commands) (19)

Acute Stroke Phase
o   Patient/Family Education—Importance of exercise in stroke recovery & risk factor management.
o   Identify metabolic risk factors modifiable by exercise and coordinate care with medical team.
o   Establish outpatient/ongoing follow-up plans for exercise evaluation and program design.

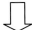

Sub-Acute Intensive Stroke Rehabilitation Period
o   Assess adequacy of usual rehabilitation care (physical therapy) to provide aerobic stimulus.
o   Evaluate medical safety & tolerance for supplemental regular low-intensity exercise.
o   Identify barriers and plan continuity of exercise programs and structured home physical activity.

Chronic Stroke Rehabilitation Period
o   Medical eligibility evaluation; optimally conduct exercise test for safety and HR training goals.
o   Evaluate neurologic status; select exercise modalities appropriate to deficits and recovery needs.
o   Design progressive exercise program with safety monitoring, fitness, and functional goals.

FIGURE 23-8

Strategies for implementing exercise across the phases of stroke rehabilitation.

and other medical conditions that preclude participation in low intensity aerobic exercise, consistent with ACSM guidelines (101). Using these eligibility criterion along with entry exercise tests, our safety data tracking across >10,000 TM aerobic training sessions and >400 peak exercise tests in chronic hemiparetic patients reveals no study-related serious adverse events. Analysis from a randomized study reveals only occasional minor musculoskeletal complaints reported by these deconditioned patients across six months progressive treadmill aerobic training at an expected rate not different from controls performing supervised stretching exercises and low intensity walking (16).

However, cumulative experience in safety of exercise after stroke is limited to research studies with very small sample sizes. These are inadequate to identify the full scope of medical or neurologic factors that could complicate different exercise training approaches in the diverse stroke population. In one study, Rimmer et al. reported transient stroke symptoms, a seizure, and a hypotensive response during exercise testing (17), whereas other analyses of full weight bearing treadmill exercise revealed no serious training-related adverse events (16). However, hemiplegic arm and major hemi-sensory deficits predicted higher non-injurious fall risk, prompting our use of safety harnesses for subjects with specific deficit profiles. A further consideration is that strenuous exertion, as that accompanying peak exercise testing, can precipitate arrhythmias and lower blood pressure in predisposed individuals with cardiac disease (101). Hence, exercise testing should be approached with caution in

subjects with hemodynamic carotid stenosis or recent large territorial brain infarction. While no exercise safety data yet exists, these conditions are known to markedly impair cerebral autoregulation, reducing capacity to compensate for drops in systemic blood pressure (13). Until more information is available, best clinical judgment and appropriate cardiopulmonary assessment should be used to guide the timing and design of exercise testing and training post-stroke.

Exercise in Sub-Acute Stroke Period

Structuring exercise programs after stroke presents unique safety and feasibility questions. Clinical research has not yet resolved basic questions regarding when to start structured exercise, as well as which training modality (or modalities) or dose-intensity are optimal across the phases of stroke recovery. Implementing exercise during the sub-acute stroke period is further complicated by the greater deficit profiles (85, 91, 97), high prevalence of cardiac comorbid conditions (102, 103), and medical problems such as autonomic deconditioning and pain syndromes that are common and known to affect rehabilitation care (20). These factors limit patients' activity tolerance, forcing clinicians to weigh the feasibility of adding further exercise to already demanding early-intensive rehabilitation. However, delay can be costly. Inactivity produces rapid declines in fitness and muscle mass that could worsen the functional aerobic impairment already present in the early stroke period (26).

Conventional rehabilitation does not likely provide adequate exercise intensity to reverse deconditioning after stroke (21, 104). However, practice patterns differ considerably, as can the physical efforts and cardiopulmonary response to exertion during rehabilitation in different stroke patients (103). One practical approach is to assess the exercise intensity of usual physical therapy, focusing on upright and transitional movements that produce greatest exertion (21). Heart rate monitoring and Ratings of Perceived Exertion (RPE) scales can be used for this purpose. If the aerobic component of usual rehabilitation care is considered deficient, therapists can consider adding low intensity exercise, based on the cardiopulmonary safety profile, tolerability, and rehabilitation needs for each patient. While the long-term benefits of starting specific exercise modalities early after stroke is not yet established, BWS TM is better tolerated by individuals with greater gait deficits (91), and can provide an aerobic stimulus if properly administered (68). Hence, BWS treadmill or other modalities to facilitate exercise in more disabled subjects warrant consideration early on.

Exercise Programs and Barriers to Participation in Chronic Stroke

In order for exercise programs to be successful across the chronic phase of stroke, a thorough pre-exercise entry evaluation including assessment of barriers to exercise is important (13). Numerous factors can interrupt the continuity of health- promoting exercise programs when transitioning from sub-acute to the chronic phase of stroke. While most stroke survivors desire and would participate in regular exercise if available, a number of common psychosocial and behavioral factors can become formidable barriers. Stroke patients have a poor self-efficacy for exercise, which predicts reduced free-living physical activity and exercise behaviors in chronic stroke patients (13, 98). An important and often ignored component of poor self-efficacy for exercise and ADL function after stroke is fatigue (8, 105). Nearly half of stroke survivors report fatigue is a factor that interferes with daily function and reduces confidence to participate in regular exercise (8). Hence, evaluation using validated instruments, such as the Fatigue Severity Scale (8), can be used to identify this common barrier in the pre-exercise evaluation. Similarly, depression after stroke is common and could impede exercise participation (66). Since some studies show exercise can improve mood after stroke, pre-exercise evaluation of depression and tracking using validated scales is advised. Another factor related to poor self-efficacy for exercise after stroke is inadequate outcome expectations. Most stroke patients are unaware that exercise can be undertaken to improve fitness, health, and function, even years after a disabling stroke. Further, physician recommendations influence exercise patterns in aging and disability

populations, and are historically under-utilized to promote exercise in the chronic stroke phase. Collectively, these findings are consistent with social learning theories to promote exercise behaviors in aging and chronic disease, and highlight the importance of education and behavioral strategies to overcome barriers.

Important additional barriers are lack of resources, social isolation, and limited family support to sustain successful exercise programs in the chronic phase of stroke. Assessment of family and psychosocial support in the context of resources for maintaining exercise programs is advised (69). In practical terms, most stroke patients have limited access to exercise facilities or community programs that can provide the social support and oversight to successfully implement evidence-based exercise programs. Moreover, the efficacy and viability of long-term home exercise programs after stroke is unknown. These issues underscore the importance of rehabilitation health professional partnering with primary medical care providers to jointly increase access to community and home services promoting exercise, health, and wellness after stroke.

Recent advances in home and community-based exercise programs supporting this model are promising (58, 69, 72, 99).

Selecting Exercise Training Formulas

By the time most individuals have reached the chronic phase of stroke, gait deficits are less pronounced, and subsequently, exercise-training capabilities are different. Most have achieved some degree of ambulatory function and may not require BWS or more dependent modalities for training. The gains in function often enable patients to participate in more rigorous and longitudinal exercise programs that have the potential to maintain and improve fitness and function while aging with the disability of stroke. Exercise modalities appropriate to deficit severity can optimally be implemented according to specific aerobic progression formulas based on cardiopulmonary exercise testing that can enhance safety and cardiovascular-metabolic health effects, as outlined in the following sections.

Exercise Testing Post-Stroke

Epidemiological studies show that 75% of stroke patients have cardiovascular disease (102, 103). While uncommon, exertion-related myocardial events are possible in individuals with pre-existing cardiac disease and sedentary lifestyle (101). Further, many stroke patients have marked activity intolerance, particularly older individuals and those with greater gait deficits, which predict lower fitness levels post-stroke. Exercise testing has revealed previously undiagnosed or asymptomatic coronary artery disease in 20–40% of stroke

TABLE 23-4
Treadmill Exercise Tests

TEST	PURPOSE
Zero-incline TM tolerance test	Acclimatize to TM; select speed for stress test
Screening TM exercise stress test	Identify cardiopulmonary response to strenuous exertion. Screen for underlying cardiac abnormalites
VO$_2$ peak exercise test	Measure peak oxygen consuming capacity with open circuit spirometry as an outcome variable on a separate day from the screening TM exerci se stress test

survivors (106), and provides information regarding the cardiopulmonary response to exertion that can be used to optimize safety and customize design of the aerobic exercise prescription. Therefore, submaximal effort or symptom-limited maximal effort exercise testing is recommended when clinically feasible, to evaluate the cardiopulmonary safety and tolerability of stroke patients to strenuous physical exertion before starting exercise training. Treadmill testing and training recommendations are summarized in Tables 23-4 and 23-5.

Which exercise testing modality is selected may be influenced by many clinical factors such as deficit profile, rehabilitation goals, or planned congruence with anticipated training modality. Since exercise testing can provide a reliable and valid means for quantifying fitness gains with training for both treadmill and bicycle testing modalities in hemiparetic stroke patients (3, 107), congruence

TABLE 23-5
Suggested Exercise Testing Protocol for Stroke Survivors

1. Start at 0.1 mph and increase to velocity determined from zero incline treadmill test.
2. Fastest comfortable walking velocity maintained at no incline for initial 2 minutes, then:
   - Milder gait deficits: advance to 4% incline for next 2 minutes, then increase incline 2% every minute thereafter (velocity constant) to peak volitional exertion.
   - Moderate-to-severe deficits: advance to 2% incline for next 2 minutes, then increase incline by 2% every 2 minutes thereafter, with velocity held constant.

in testing and training modalities is recommended. There are no studies in stroke patients to discriminate between choices of submaximal vs. symptom-limited peak effort exercise protocols. The term "peak effort," rather than maximal exercise test, is here employed because most stroke patients do not achieve full criterion for VO$_2$ max by open circuit spirometry testing (107). Peak exercise testing provides the most useful information for aerobic exercise in high-risk populations. Peak exercise heart rates are most accurate, and have proven useful to design HR training progression in accordance with the Formula of Karvonen. For high cardiac risk patients, training should be conducted at least 10 beats per minute below the exercise intensity that produces systolic blood pressures >250 mm Hg or diastolic blood pressure >115 mm Hg, ST segment depression >1 mm, or other significant ECG or clinical cardiopulmonary intolerance (101). These criteria may best be revealed using peak exercise protocols.

Little is published regarding use of submaximal exercise to design aerobic prescriptions after stroke, or exercise planning for stroke patients that cannot receive exercise tests. Peak exercise testing may not be feasible or desired for some patients, particularly those less than one month post-stroke, a period within which cerebral autoregulation is likely to be most impaired. In a seminal AHA consensus statement, submaximal exercise testing was recommended using predetermined endpoints of 70% of age predicted maximum HR, consistent with practice in post-myocardial infarction patients (13). A period of ECG telemetry monitoring is recommended for those stroke patients deemed at high cardiac risk and that cannot undergo any exercise testing (101). While no studies have yet established the efficacy in stroke, low intensity exercise at increased training duration and/or frequency has been recommended for cardiac patients without an entry exercise test. Such guidelines extrapolated from cardiac patients may be useful, until further data is available for stroke patients considered at high cardiac risk.

General Guidelines for Exercise Training and Progression

Treadmill Training. The target training parameters used in chronic stroke patients from our laboratory (16) consist of three 40–45 minute sessions per week of treadmill walking at 60% to 70% of Heart Rate Reserve (HRR), where Target Heart Rate is calculated with the Karvonen formula:

$$\text{Heart Rate Reserve (HRR)} = \text{Maximum Heart Rate} - \text{Resting Heart Rate}$$

$$\textbf{Target Heart Rate} = \textbf{(HRR x training \%)} + \textbf{Resting Heart Rate}$$

Creating a zone of 60–70% simply requires performing the calculation twice to come up with an upper and lower limit for the desired range. Training is initiated conservatively at 40% of HRR for durations of 10–15 minutes and advanced as tolerated. Discontinuous training epochs consisting of 3–5 minutes TM walking with similar duration interval rests are used in those highly deconditioned or more severely disabled patients incapable of continuous training. Total training duration is then advanced as tolerated toward the target. Handrail support is used, and 5-minute treadmill warm-up and cool-down periods at approximately 30% of HRR are phased into each workout as participants develop the necessary endurance for longer bouts of training. Regression analyses of clinical factors related to training safety reveal that arm hemiplegia (inability to grasp TM handrail for support) and presence of major sensory deficit is associated with increased risk of falls during TM training. While such events are uncommon and low impact, we use suspensory safety harnesses in a non–weight-bearing fashion (Biodex Medical, Shirley, NY) to eliminate the risk of fall injury in our patients. Heart rate is monitored continuously by two-lead ECG (Polar Electro, Woodbury, NY), and blood pressure recordings are taken before, at the mid-point, and at the conclusion of each exercise session to ensure safety and to document the intensity of the training session.

Progression of training workload is determined biweekly by monitoring each patient's gait, HR response, and patient-reported level of fatigue at the end of a training session. If no gait instability, exaggerated HR response (HRR >80%), or extreme fatigue is noted (Borg Perceived Exertion used as adjunct to rate tolerability), an increase in training speed by 0.1-mph increments is prioritized to reach the target training intensity. Increase in TM grade (1% increments) is utilized secondarily to achieve target aerobic intensity for those individuals who do not tolerate further TM velocity progression to meet this goal. Training duration is typically advanced approximately 5 minutes every 2 weeks, as tolerated, to arrive at a total 45 minutes training by the third month of training. For those completing intermittent bouts of exercise, only duration is altered in order to progress to one continuous bout of 15 minutes.

Bicycle Training.   Potempa et al. achieved aerobic fitness gains after stroke using a bicycle ergometer training protocol (3). In this case, subjects exercised on an adapted cycle ergometer for 30 minutes, three times per week. The intervention period lasted a total of 10 weeks. In the first four weeks, the training load was increased from 30–50% of maximal effort to the highest level attainable by the subject. The highest training load was then maintained for the final 6 weeks of training. Although this protocol resulted in fitness gains, sensoritmotor function was not improved using this adapted bicycle ergometry protocol.

SUMMARY AND FUTURE RESEARCH

In summary, most stroke patients have profound deconditioning and secondary body composition changes that can worsen disability and cardiovascular-metabolic risk profiles. Randomized studies now show that several different exercise training modalities can improve fitness and selected functional outcomes. In particular, locomotor-based training programs currently provide the strongest evidence base that task-repetitive exercise programs can improve mobility function, even years after stroke. Existing data suggests that exercise programs can be safely and successfully progressed using specific aerobic exercise formulas in selected stroke patients, with appropriate pre-exercise evaluation and safety monitoring. A small number of promising studies provide proof of the concept that structured exercise programs may be extended to the community to chronic stroke survivors, at least those with milder deficit profiles. There is evidence that exercise can improve bone health, and selected indices related to cardiovascular-metabolic risk including lipoprotein lipid profiles, body fat, insulin-glucose metabolism, blood pressure response to exercise, and left ventricular ejection fraction in those with cardiac disease.

These findings, largely generated over the last decade, provide a strong rationale for exercise to improve fitness, function, and cardiovascular health after stroke. However, there is a large practice gap, with many basic questions regarding the practice and effects of exercise after stroke left unanswered. The optimal training modalities and dose-intensity of exercise, and how these may relate to deficit profiles or time since stroke are unknown. While selected CVD risk markers are improved, there is no long-term data to determine whether exercise reduces recurrent stroke, cardiovascular events, or progression of insulin resistance to diabetes. Future research could consider the promising findings from bench and clinical studies in non-stroke populations that exercise improves cognitive function, depression, and alters neural growth factors that could improve brain health in aging and mediate brain plasticity linked to motor learning. In practical terms, many of the recommended safety and training approaches for stroke patients are borrowed from the cardiac literature. These need empirical testing in stroke patients; a population that in many ways is clinically and biologically unique. Further studies in community translation and systematic strategies to overcome barriers to longitudinal participation are needed to better realize the benefits of exercise after stroke.

References

1. Chu KS, Eng JJ, Dawson AS, Harris JE, Oakaplan A. Water-based exercise for cardiovascular fitness in people with chronic stroke: A randomized controlled trial. *Arch Phys Med Rehabil.* 2004; 85:870–874.
2. Ivey FM, Macko R.F, Ryan A.S., Hafer-Macko CE. Cardiovscular health and fitness after stroke. *Top Stroke Rehabil.* 2005; 12:1–16.
3. Potempa K, Lopez M, Braun LT, Szidon JP, Fogg L, Tincknell T. Physiological outcomes of aerobic exercise training in hemiparetic stroke patients. *Stroke* 1995; 26:101–105.
4. Corcoran PJ, Jebsen RH, Brengelmann GL, Simons BC. Effects of plastic and metal leg braces on speed and energy cost of hemiparetic ambulation. *Arch Phys Med Rehabil.* 1970; 51:69–77.
5. Fisher SV, Gullickson G, Jr. Energy cost of ambulation in health and disability: A literature review. *Arch Phys Med Rehabil.* 1978; 59:124–133.
6. Olney SJ, Monga TN, Costigan PA. Mechanical energy of walking of stroke patients. *Arch Phys Med Rehabil.* 1986; 67:92–98.
7. Michael KM, Allen JK, Macko RF. Fatigue after stroke: Relationship to mobility, fitness, ambulatory activity, social support, and falls efficacy. *Rehabil Nurs.* 2006; 31: 210–217.
8. Michael K. Fatigue and stroke. *Rehabil Nurs.* 2002; 27:89–94, 103.
9. Ryan AS, Dobrovolny CL, Smith GV, Silver KH, Macko RF. Hemiparetic muscle atrophy and increased intramuscular fat in stroke patients. *Arch Phys Med Rehabil.* 2002; 83:1703–1707.
10. De Deyne PG, Hafer-Macko CE, Ivey FM, Ryan AS, Macko RF. Muscle molecular phenotype after stroke is associated with gait speed. *Muscle and Nerve.* 2004; 30: 209–215.
11. Frontera WR, Grimby L, Larsson L. Firing rate of the lower motoneuron and contractile properties of its muscle fibers after upper motoneuron lesion in man. *Muscle Nerve.* 1997; 20:938–947.
12. Jakobsson F, Edstrom L, Grimby L, Thornell LE. Disuse of anterior tibial muscle during locomotion and increased proportion of type II fibres in hemiplegia. *J Neurol Sci.* 1991; 105:49–56.
13. Gordon NF, Gulanic M, Costa F, et al. Physical activity and exercise recommendations for stroke survivors: An American Heart Association Scientific Statement. *Circulation.* 2004; 109:2031–2041.
14. Ramnemark A, Nyberg L, Borssen B, Olsson T, Gustafson Y. Fractures after stroke. *Osteoporosis Int.* 1998; 8:92–95.
15. Duncan P, Studenski S, Richards L, et al. Randomized clinical trial of therapeutic exercise in subacute stroke. *Stroke.* 2003; 34:2173–2180.
16. Macko RF, Ivey FM, Forrester LW, et al. Treadmill exercise rehabilitation improves ambulatory function and cardiovascular fitness in patients with chronic stroke: A randomized, controlled trial. *Stroke* 2005; 36:2206–2211.
17. Rimmer JH, Riley B, Creviston T, Nicola T. Exercise training in a predominantly African-American group of stroke survivors. *Med Sci Sports Exerc.* 2000; 32:1990–1996.
18. Ivey FM, Hafer-Macko CE, Macko RF. Exercise rehabilitation after stroke. *NeuroRx.* 2006; 3:439–450.
19. Macko RF, Ivey FM, Forrester LW. Task-oriented aerobic exercise in chronic hemiparetic stroke: Training protocols and treatment effects. *Top Stroke Rehabil.* 2005; 12:45–57.
20. USDHHS. Post-Stroke Rehabilitation: Clinical Practice Guideline. 95-0662. 1995. AHCPR.
21. MacKay-Lyons MJ, Makrides L. Cardiovascular stress during a contemporary stroke rehabilitation program: Is the intensity adequate to induce a training effect? *Arch Phys Med Rehabil.* 2002; 83:1378–1383.
22. American College of Sports Medicine's guidelines for exercise testing and prescription. In: Lippincott WaW, ed. 6th ed. Baltimore: 2000.
23. Bruce RA, Kusumi F, Hosmer D. Maximal oxygen intake and nomographic assessment of functional aerobic impairment in cardiovascular disease. *Am Heart J.* 1973; 85:546–562.
24. Macko RF, DeSouza CA, Tretter LD, et al. Treadmill aerobic exercise training reduces the energy expenditure and cardiovascular demands of hemiparetic gait in chronic stroke patients. A preliminary report. *Stroke* 1997; 28:326–330.
25. Fujitani J, Ishikawa T, Akai M, Kakurai S. Influence of daily activity on changes in physical fitness for people with post-stroke hemiplegia. *Am J Phys Med Rehabil.* 1999; 78:540–544.
26. MacKay-Lyons MJ, Makrides L. Exercise capacity early after stroke. *Arch Phys Med Rehabil.* 2002; 83:1697–1702.
27. Kelly JO, Kilbreath SL, Davis GM, Zeman B, Raymond J. Cardiorespiratory fitness and walking ability in subacute stroke patients. *Arch Phys Med Rehabil.* 2003; 84: 1780–1785.
28. Jette M, Sidney K, Blumchen G. Metabolic equivalents (METS) in exercise testing, exercise prescription, and evaluation of functional capacity. *Clin Cardiol.* 1990; 13: 555–565.
29. Ainsworth BE, Haskell WL, Whitt MC, et al. Compendium of physical activities: An update of activity codes and MET intensities. *Med Sci Sports Exerc.* 2000; 32: S498–S504.
30. Ryan A.S., Dobrovolny L., Silver KH, Smith GV, Macko R.F. Cardiovascular fitness after stroke: Role of muscle mass and gait deficit severity. *J Stroke Cerebrovasc Disorders.* 2000; 9:1–8.
31. Chokroverty S, Reyes MG, Rubino FA, Barron KD. Hemiplegic amyotrophy. Muscle and motor point biopsy study. *Arch Neurol.* 1976; 33:104–110.
32. Hachisuka K, Umezu Y, Ogata H. Disuse muscle atrophy of lower limbs in hemiplegic patients. *Arch Phys Med Rehabil.* 1997; 78:13–18.
33. Landin S, Hagenfeldt L, Saltin B, Wahren J. Muscle metabolism during exercise in hemiparetic patients. *Clin Sci Mol Med.* 1977; 53:257–269.
34. Scelsi R, Lotta S, Lommi G, Poggi P, Marchetti C. Hemiplegic atrophy. Morphological findings in the anterior tibial muscle of patients with cerebral vascular accidents. *Acta Neuropathol.* 1984; 62:324–331.
35. Daugaard JR, Richter EA. Relationship between muscle fibre composition, glucose transporter protein 4 and exercise training: Possible consequences in non-insulin-dependent diabetes mellitus. *Acta Physiol Scand.* 2001; 171:267–276.
36. Huey KA, Roy RR, Baldwin KM, Edgerton VR. Temporal effects of inactivity on myosin heavy chain gene expression in rat slow muscle. *Muscle and Nerve.* 2001; 24:517–526.
37. Kandarian SC, Stevenson EJ. Molecular events in skeletal muscle during disuse atrophy. *Exerc Sport Sci Rev.* 2002; 30:111–116.
38. Hafer-Macko CE, Yu S, Ryan AS, Ivey FM, Macko RF. Elevated tumor necrosis factor-alpha in skeletal muscle after stroke. *Stroke.* 2005; 36:2021–2023.
39. de Alvaro C, Teruel T, Hernandez R, Lorenzo M. Tumor necrosis factor alpha produces insulin resistance in skeletal muscle by activation of inhibitor kappaB kinase in a p38 MAPK-dependent manner. *J Biol Chem.* 2004; 279:17070–17078.
40. Greiwe J, Cheng B, Rubin DC. Resistance exercise decreases skeletal muscle tumor necrosis factor alpha in frail elderly humans. *FASEB J.* 2001; 15:475–482.
41. Hunter RB, Stevenson E, Koncarevic A, Mitchell-Felton H, Essig DA, Kandarian SC. Activation of an alternative NF-kappaB pathway in skeletal muscle during disuse atrophy. *FASEB J.* 2002; 16:529–538.
42. Saghizadeh M, Ong JM, Garvey WT, Henry RR, Kern PA. The expression of TNF alpha by human muscle: Relationship to insulin resistance. *J Clin Invest.* 1996; 97: 1111–1116.
43. Eng J, Pang M, Ashe M. Balance, falls, and bone health: Role of exercise in reducing fracture in risk after stroke. *J Rehab Res Dev* 2008; 45:297–315.
44. Harris JE, Eng JJ, Marigold DS, Tokuno CD, Louis CL. Relationship of balance and mobility to fall incidence in people with chronic stroke. *Phys Ther.* 2005; 85: 150–158.
45. Pang M, Eng JJ, McKay HA, Dawson AS. Reduced hip bone mineral density is related to physical fitness and leg lean mass in ambulatory individuals with chronic stroke. *Osteoporos Int.* 2005; 16:1769–1779.
46. Browner WS, Pressman AR, Nevitt MC, Cauley JA, Cummings SR. Association between low bone density and stroke in elderly women. The study of osteoporotic fractures. *Stroke.* 1993; 24:940–946.
47. Jorgensen L, Engstad T, Jacobsen BK. Higher incidence of falls in long-term stroke survivors than in population controls: Depressive symptoms predict falls after stroke. *Stroke.* 2002; 33:542–547.
48. Forster A, Young J. Incidence and consequences of falls due to stroke: A systematic inquiry. *BMJ.* 1995; 311:83–86.
49. North American Menopause Society. Management of osteoporosis in postmenopausal women: 2006 position statement of The North American Menopause Society. *Menopause* 2007; 13:340–367.
50. Cheng PT, Wu SH, Liaw MY, Wong AM, Tang FT. Symmetrical body-weight distribution training in stroke patients and its effect on fall prevention. *Arch Phys Med Rehabil.* 2001; 82:1650–1654.
51. Marigold DS, Eng JJ, Dawson AS, Inglis JT, Harris JE, Gylfadottir S. Exercise leads to faster postural reflexes, improved balance and mobility, and fewer falls in older persons with chronic stroke. *J Am Geriatr Soc.* 2005; 53:416–423.
52. Vearrier LA, Langan J, Shumway-Cook A, Woollacott M. An intensive massed practice approach to retraining balance post-stroke. *Gait Posture* 2005; 22:154–163.
53. Ivey FM, Gardner AW, Dobrovolny CL, Macko RF. Unilateral impairment of leg blood flow in chronic stroke patients. *Cerebrovasc Dis* 2004; 18:283–289.
54. Kernan WN, Inzucchi SE, Viscoli CM, et al. Impaired insulin sensitivity among nondiabetic patients with a recent TIA or ischemic stroke. *Neurology* 2003; 60:1447–1451.
55. Ivey FM, Ryan A.S., Hafer-Macko CE, et al. High prevalence of abnormal glucose metabolism and poor sensitivity of fasting plasma glucose in the chronic phase of stroke. *Cerebrovasc Dis.* 2006; 22:368–371.
56. Vermeer SE, Sandee W, Algra A, et al. Impaired glucose tolerance increases stroke risk in nondiabetic patients with transient ischemic attack or minor ischemic stroke. *Stroke* 2006; 37:1413–1417.
57. Macko RF, Smith GV, Dobrovolny CL, Sorkin JD, Goldberg AP, Silver KH. Treadmill training improves fitness reserve in chronic stroke patients. *Arch Phys Med Rehabil.* 2001; 82:879–884.
58. Pang MY, Eng JJ, Dawson AS, McHay HA, Harris JE. A community-based fitness and mobility exercise program for older adults with chronic stroke. *J Am Geriatr Soc.* 2005; 53:1667–1674.
59. Laukanen JA, Kurl S, Salonen R, Rauramaa R, Salonen JT. The predictive value of cardiorespiratory fitness for cardiovascular events in men with various risk profiles: A prospective population-based cohort study. *Eur Heart J.* 2004; 25:1428–1437.
60. Holloszy JO. Exercise-induced increase in muscle insulin sensitivity. *J Appl Physiol.* 2005; 99:338–343.
61. Hjelstuen A, Anderssen SA, Holme I, Seljeflot I, Klemsdal TO. Markers of inflammation are inversely related to physical activity and fitness in sedentary men with treated hypertension. *Am J Hypertens.* 2006; 19:669–675.

62. Womack CJ, Nagelkirk PR, Coughlin AM. Exercise-induced changes in coagulation and fibrinolysis in healthy populations and patients with cardiovascular disease. *Sports Med.* 2003; 33:795–807.

63. Green DJ, Maiorana A, O'Driscoll G., Taylor R. Effect of exercise training on endothelium-derived nitric oxide function in humans. *J Physiol.* 2004; 561:1–25.

64. Buyukyazi G. Differences in blood lipids and apolipoproteins between master athletes, recreational athletes and sedentary men. *J Sports Med Phys Fitness.* 2005; 45:112–120.

65. Rosenwinkel ET, Bloomfield DM, Arwady MA, Goldsmith RL. Exercise and autonomic function in health and cardiovascular disease. *Cardiol Clin.* 2001; 19:369–387.

65a. Ivey FM, Ryan AS, Hafer-Macko CE, et al. Treadmill aerobic training improves glucose tolerance and indices of insulin sensitivity in disabled stroke survivors. *Stroke* 2007; 38:2752–2758.

66. Gresham GE, Phillips TF, Wolf PA, McNamara PM, Kannel WB, Dawber TR. Epidemiologic profile of long-term stroke disability: The Framingham study. *Arch Phys Med Rehabil.* 1979; 60:487–491.

67. Luft AR, McCombe-Waller S, Whitall J, et al. Repetitive bilateral arm training and motor cortex activation in chronic stroke: A randomized controlled trial. *JAMA* 2004; 292:1853–1861.

67a. Forrester L, Wheaton, L, Luft A. Exercise-mediated locomotor recovery and lower-limb neuroplasticity after stroke. *J Rehab Res Dev* 2008; 45:205–221.

68. Hesse S, Bertelt C, Jahnke MT et al. Treadmill training with partial body weight support compared with physiotherapy in nonambulatory hemiparetic patients. *Stroke.* 1995; 26:976–981.

69. Duncan P, Richards L, Wallace D, et al. A randomized, controlled pilot study of a home-based exercise program for individuals with mild and moderate stroke. *Stroke.* 1998; 29:2055–2060.

70. Teixeira-Salmela L, Olney SJ, Nadeau S, Brouwer B. Muscle strengthening and physical conditioning to reduce impairment and disability in chronic stroke survivors. *Arch Phys Med Rehabil.* 1999; 80:1211–1218.

71. Katz-Leurer M, Shochina M, Carmeli E, Friedlander Y. The influence of early aerobic training on the functional capacity in patients with cerebrovascular accident at the subacute stage. *Arch Phys Med Rehabil.* 2003; 84:1609–1614.

72. Eng JJ, Chu KS, Kim CM, Dawson AS, Carswell A, Hepburn KE. A community-based group exercise program for persons with chronic stroke. *Med Sci Sports Exerc.* 2003; 35:1271–1278.

73. Eich HJ, Mach H, Werner C, Hesse S. Aerobic treadmill plus Bobath walking training improves walking in subacute stroke: A randomized controlled trial. *Clin Rehabil.* 2004; 18:640–651.

74. Pang MY, Harris JE, Eng JJ. A community-based upper-extremity group exercise program improves motor function and performance of functional activities in chronic stroke: A randomized controlled trial. *Arch Phys Med Rehabil.* 2006; 87:1–9.

75. Morris SL, Dodd KJ, Morris ME. Outcomes of progressive resistance strength training following stroke: A systematic review. *Clin Rehabil.* 2004; 18:27–39.

76. Butefisch C, Hummelsheim H, Denzler P, Mauritz KH. Repetitive training of isolated movements improves the outcome of motor rehabilitation of the centrally paretic hand. *J Neurol Sci.* 1995; 130:59–68.

77. Engardt M, Knutsson E, Jonsson M, Sternhag M. Dynamic muscle strength training in stroke patients: Effects on knee extension torque, electromyographic activity, and motor function. *Arch Phys Med Rehabil.* 1995; 76:419–425.

78. Karimi H. *Isokinetic Strength Training and Its Effect on the Biomechanics of Gait inSubjects with Hemiparesis as aResult of Stroke.* Kingston: Queens University, 1996.

79. Sharp SA, Brouwer BJ. Isokinetic strength training of the hemiparetic knee: Effects on function and spasticity. *Arch Phys Med Rehabil.* 1997; 78:1231–1236.

80. Weiss A, Suzuki T, Bean J, Fielding RA. High intensity strength training improves strength and functional performance after stroke. *Am J Phys Med Rehabil.* 2007; 79:369–376.

81. Giuliani C, Light KE, Rose D. The effect of an isokinetic exercise program on the performance of sit-to-stand in patients with hemiparesis. *Proceedings: Forum on Stroke Rehabilitation.* 1992; 4:49–54.

82. Bourbonnais D, Bilodeau S, Lepage Y, Beaudoin N, Gravel D, Forget R. Effect of force-feedback treatments in patients with chronic motor deficits after a stroke. *Am J Phys Med Rehabil.* 2002; 81:890–897.

83. Barbeau H, Rossignol S. Recovery of locomotion after chronic spinalization in the adult cat. *Brain Res.* 1987; 412:84–95.

84. Richards CL, Malouin F, Wood-Dauphinee S, Williams JL, Bouchard JP, Brunet D. Task specific physical therapy for optimization of gait recovery in acute stroke patients. *Archives of Physical Medicine and Rehabilitation* 1993; 74:612–620.

85. Hesse S, Konrad M, Uhlenbrock D. Treadmill walking with partial body weight support versus floor walking in hemiparetic subjects. *Arch Phys Med Rehabil.* 1999; 80: 421–427.

86. Silver KH, Macko RF, Forrester LW, Goldberg AP, Smith GV. Effects of aerobic treadmill training on gait velocity, cadence, and gait symmetry in chronic hemiparetic stroke: A preliminary report. *Neurorehabil Neural Repair.* 2000; 14:65–71.

87. Harris-Love ML, Forrester LW, Macko RF, Smith GV. Hemiparetic vastus lateralis activation patterns in overground compared with treadmill walking. *Neurorehabilitation and Neural Repair.* 2002; 16:379.

88. Dobkin BH, Firestine A, West M, Saremi K, Woods R. Ankle dorsiflexion as an fMRI paradigm to assay motor control for walking during rehabilitation. *Neuroimage.* 2007; 23:370–381.

89. Schmidt RA, Lee TD. *Motor Control and Learning: A Behavioral Emphasis.* 3rd ed. Champaign, IL: Human Kinetics, 1999.

90. Hesse S, Bertelt C, Schaffrin A, Malezic M, Mauritz KH. Restoration of gait in nonambulatory hemiparetic patients by treadmill training with partial body-weight support. *Arch Phys Med Rehabil.* 1994; 75:1087–1093.

91. Barbeau H, Visintin M. Optimal outcomes obtained with body-weight support combined with treadmill training in stroke subjects. *Arch Phys Med Rehabil.* 2003; 84: 1458–1465.

92. Visintin M, Barbeau H, Korner-Bitensky N, Mayo NE. A new approach to retrain gait in stroke patients through body weight support and treadmill stimulation. *Stroke* 1998; 29:1122–1128.

93. Danielsson A, Sunnerhagen KS. Oxygen consumption during treadmill walking with and without body weight support in patients with hemiparesis after stroke and in healthy subjects. *Arch Phys Med Rehabil.* 2000; 81:953–957.

94. Mosely AM, Stark A, Cameron ID, Pollock A. Treadmill training and body weight support for walking after stroke (Cochrane Review). Chichester, UK: John Wiley & Sons, Ltd. The Cochrane Library (Issue 2), 2004

95. Nilsson L, Carlsson J, Danielsson A, et al. Walking training of patients with hemiparesis at an early stage after stroke: A comparison of walking training on a treadmill with body weight support and walking training on the ground. *Clin Rehabil.* 2001; 15:515–527.

96. Sullivan KJ, Knowlton BJ, Dobkin BH. Step training with body weight support: Effect of treadmill speed and practice paradigms on poststroke locomotor recovery. *Archives of Physical Medicine and Rehabilitation* 2002; 83:683–691.

96a. Luft AR, Macko RF, Forrester LW, Villagra F, Ivey F, Sorkin JD, Whitall J, McCombe-Waller S, Katzel L, Goldberg AP, Hanley DF. Treadmill Exercise Activates Subcortical Neural Networks and Improves Walking After Stroke: A Randomized Controlled Trial. *Stroke.* 2008; Aug 28. [Epub ahead of print]

97. Jorgensen HS, Nakayama H, Raaschou HO, Vive-Larsen J, Stoier M, Olsen TS. Outcome and time course of recovery in stroke. Part II: Time course of recovery. The Copenhagen Stroke Study. *Arch Phys Med Rehabil.* 1995; 76:406–412.

98. Shaughnessy M, Resnick BM, Macko RF. Testing a model of post-stroke exercise behavior. *Rehabil Nurs.* 2006; 31:15–21.

99. Macko RF, Benvenuti F, Stanhope S, et al. Adaptive physical activity improves mobility function and quality of life in chronic hemiparesis. *J Rehab Res Dev* 2008; 45(2):323–329.

100. Wolf SL, Winstein CJ, Miller JP, et al. Effect of constraint-induced movement therapy on upper extremity function 3 to 9 months after stroke: The EXCITE randomized clinical trial. *JAMA* 2006; 296:2095–2104.

101. *American College of Sports Medicine's guidelines for exercise testing and prescription.* 7th ed. Baltimore: Lippincott, Williams & Wilkins, 2006.

102. Roth EJ. Heart disease in patients with stroke: Incidence, impact, and implications for rehabilitation. Part 1: Classification and prevalence. *Arch Phys Med Rehabil.* 1993; 74:752–760.

103. Roth EJ. Heart disease in patients with stroke. Part II: Impact and implications for rehabilitation. *Arch Phys Med Rehabil.* 1994; 75:94–101.

104. Hjeltnes N. Capacity for physical work and training after spinal injuries and strokes. *Scand J Soc Med Suppl.* 1982; 29:245–251.

105. Glader EL, Stegmayr B, Asplund K. Poststroke fatigue: A 2-year follow up study of stroke patients in Sweden. *Stroke.* 2001; 33:1327–1333.

106. Macko RF, Katzel LI, Yataco A, et al. Low-velocity graded treadmill stress testing in hemiparetic stroke patients. *Stroke* 1997; 28:988–992.

107. Dobrovolny CL, Ivey FM, Rogers MA, et al. Reliability of treadmill exercise testing in older patients with chronic hemiparetic stroke. *Arch Phys Med Rehabil* 2003 Sep; 84(9): 1308–1312.

24 Medical Complications after Stroke

Lalit Kalra

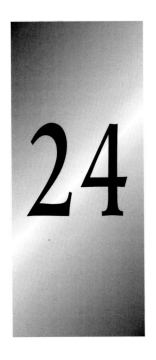

Patients with stroke are at risk of developing a wide range of medical complications that have the potential of causing death or delaying successful rehabilitation. Several studies have shown that medical complications may be the primary cause of hospital-related death in over 50% of stroke patients and contribute to death in an even larger proportion (1). The timing of deaths in stroke is bimodal, the first peak occurring in the first week, predominantly as a direct consequence of brain damage, and the second peak occurring several weeks later, mainly as a result of potentially preventable medical complications such as infection, venous thromboembolism, or cardiac disease(1–5). Medical complications not only increase mortality during inpatient care but have also been shown to have a significant effect on long-term mortality. A study in nearly 600 patients has shown that the presence of one or more medical complications during hospitalization was associated with a hazard ratio for mortality ranging from 2.67 in the initial cohort to 8.93 in patients who had survived three or more years, after adjusting for age, gender, initial stroke severity, stroke subtype, co-morbidity, and disability at the time of discharge from hospital (6).

Medical complications have also been associated with increased disability and poor functional outcome in stroke patients. The scope of intensive therapy is limited in patients suffering complications during rehabilitation, which may result in longer hospital stays, increased resource use, and institutionalization (4, 7). Mortality-adjusted data analysis from the RANTTAS trial, which excluded patients who were dead at three months, showed that serious medical events during hospitalization were associated with fourfold increase in residual severe disability, independent of stroke severity and other variables (5). The length of hospital stay for rehabilitation is directly proportional to the number of medical complications suffered by patients, and 7% to 17% of stroke patients undergoing rehabilitation need to be transferred back to acute-care settings, which further increases the overall cost of stroke management (4, 8). It is, therefore, both inaccurate and misleading to view inpatient stroke rehabilitation as a medically quiescent process that does not require ongoing medical input.

FREQUENCY AND TYPE OF MEDICAL COMPLICATIONS

Medical complications are known to be common in patients with stroke, but estimates of their prevalence in rehabilitation settings differ significantly, ranging from 27% to 96% in various studies, with a median of 75% (1–11). Complications appear to be more frequent in patients with severe strokes (94%) compared to patients with mild or moderate deficits (16% [7]). The prevalence of complications is higher (75–85%) in studies that include acute patients and in studies that have used rigorous and prospective methods for data collection. The type of medical complications also varies with patient characteristics and management settings. The commonest medical complications seen in rehabilitation settings are infections (particularly of the chest or bladder), falls, deep vein thrombosis and thromboembolism, pain, loss of skin integrity and/or pressure sores, and other mobility-related problems, such as musculoskeletal pain or limb edema. During rehabilitation, patients with stroke are more susceptible to exacerbations of pre-existing cardiac, vascular, and metabolic diseases, which are frequently present in this population. A list of frequently encountered medical complications is given in Table 24-1, which is by no means exhaustive.

The wide variation in estimating the frequency and types of medical complications that people with stroke experience during their rehabilitation reflects the methodological problems and inherent biases encountered in undertaking such studies (10, 11). Earlier studies have either incorporated a retrospective case ascertainment design (2–4, 10) or prospective analysis of patients selected for intervention studies (5, 7), with different criteria for patient selection, definition of complications, timing of assessments, and duration of follow-up. The retrospective identification of complications from case notes is further influenced by the diagnostic criteria used, interobserver bias, and the standard of note-keeping. Most studies have recorded only symptomatic complications that occurred during the inpatient stay, which will be influenced by reporting bias and duration of observation (11). Very few studies have investigated the prevalence of complications in a defined representative sample of stroke patients from a fixed time point early in the course of their disease, using prespecified objective criteria for identifying complications, prospective data-collection methods, and regular follow-up (8, 11).

THE DETERMINANTS OF MEDICAL COMPLICATIONS

The incidence and frequency of complications in stroke rehabilitation is influenced by several factors. Most studies show that the frequency of complications increases with age of patients and the severity of neurologic or functional deficits (Table 24-3). Prestroke disability, urinary incontinence, vascular risk factors such as diabetes and hypertension, markers of poor nutritional status (e.g. hypoalbuminaemia), and length of hospital stay also identify patients at higher risk of developing infections (8, 10, 11). Factors that predict transfer to acute medical facilities from rehabilitation settings include elevated admission

white blood cell counts, low admission hemoglobin levels, greater neurologic deficit, and a history of cardiac arrhythmia (8).

The relationship reported in some studies between increased length of hospital stay and increased prevalence of complications raises important issues. It remains unclear whether prolonged hospitalization is a cause or a result of stroke-related complications, but it is likely that complications are both a cause and an effect of prolonged hospitalization. The setting in which patients are managed also has an important influence on the frequency and type of complications. Kalra et al. (7) have shown that although there are no differences in the frequency of complications between generic and specialist settings, there is a significant difference in the type of complications between the two settings. This difference may be one of the reasons for better outcomes and shorter lengths of hospital stays reported in specialist settings. It is likely that patients cared for in a dedicated stroke unit are under more scrupulous observation by experienced staff and may experience fewer severe or life-threatening complications, whereas less-severe complications may appear to be more frequent simply because of better recognition and documentation in case records (10). This explanation is supported by a study on processes of care on specialist units, which showed that patients on a stroke unit were monitored more frequently than those in general units and that more patients received antipyretics, measures to reduce aspiration, and early nutrition. Complications were less common in the specialized setting, with fewer patients suffering from chest infection or dehydration, which was associated with reduced mortality, fewer instances of institutionalization, and shorter length of hospital stay (12). Similar findings have been reported from the most recent Stroke Unit Trialists Collaboration meta-analysis of medical complications data from seven trials, which included 3327 patients and showed significantly lower complications arising from immobility and infections, in patients managed on specialist units (13).

SPECIFIC MEDICAL COMPLICATIONS

Aspiration and Pneumonia

Aspiration and swallowing impairment are common after stroke; a recent meta-analysis has shown that incidence ranges from 51 to 55% on clinical tests and 64 to 78% on videofluoroscopy or other instrumental tests (5). Dysphagia is associated with a threefold increase in the risk of chest infections, which increases to elevenfold in those with definite aspiration. Large stroke registries across the world have shown pneumonia to be the single most important cause of death in the entire stroke population, accounting for 23% of deaths in the

TABLE 24-1

Frequency of Medical Complications Reported in Different Studies

	DOBKIN ET AL.[2] (N=200)	DROMERICK ET AL. [3] (N=100)	KALRA ET AL. [6] (N=245)	DAVENPORT ET AL. [9] (N=607)	JOHNASTON ET AL. [4] (N=279)	LANGHORNE ET AL. [10] (N=311)	ROTH ET AL. [8] (N=1029)	BAE ET AL. [5] (N=579)
Study design	retrospective	retrospective	retrospective	retrospective	prospective	prospective	prospective	prospective
Study setting	rehabilitation	rehabilitation	rehabilitation	rehabilitation	acute and rehabilitation	rehabilitation	rehabilitation	acute and rehabilitation
Centers	single center	single center	single center	single center	multi-center	multi-center	single center	
Complications								
Chest infection	2%	7%	12%	12%	10%	22%	4%	11%
Urinary tract infection	7%	44%	25%	16%	11%	24%	31%	8%
Deep vein thrombosis	2%	4%	5%	3%	2%	2%	4%	
Pulmonary embolism	2%	0%	1%	1%	1%	1%	1%	
Skin breaks/ pressure sores	2%		3%	18%	5%	21%	4%	1%
Falls		25%		22%		25%	11%	
Cardiac events					8%		5%	1%
GI bleeding					5%		3%	3%
Pain (excl. painful shoulder)			31%	8%		34%	14%	
Total	**40%**	**96%**	**60%**	**59%**	**85%**	**85%**	**75%**	**27%**

TABLE 24-2
Medical Complications Reported in Stroke Patients

Infections	Aspiration pneumonia, chest infections, urinary tract infection, sepsis, cellulitis, clostridium difficile enteritis
Mobility-related problems	Falls, fractures, musculoskeletal pain, edematous limbs, deep vein thrombosis in calf, thigh or axilla, pulmonary embolism, loss of skin integrity, breaking skin, pressure ulcers, urinary retention or incontinence, constipation, diarrhea
Co-morbidity	Angina, myocardial infarction, congestive cardiac failure, atrial or ventricular arrythmias, cardiac arrest, hypertension, hypotension, poor diabetic control, hypoglycemia, ischemic colitis, exacerbation of chronic lung disease, peripheral vascular disease
Others	Non-cardiac pulmonary edema, gastro-intestinal bleeding, dehydration and electrolyte imbalance, renal impairment, anemia, malnutrition

Japanese registry (15) and 31% in the German Stroke Registers Study (1). In addition, as many as two out of three stroke patients who appear to be able to swallow safely on clinical assessment have been shown to aspirate using instrumental diagnostic techniques. Aspiration is associated with a higher risk of chest infections and mortality (16).

Although aspiration is common after stroke, not all patients who aspirate will develop chest infections. It is likely that there are several mechanisms that protect the lower airways, ranging from physical processes that clear the airways of the aspirated material, to cellular and immunological processes that combat infection. Of these, voluntary expiration and cough are particularly important for maintaining the patency of airways. Cough, whether voluntary or reflex, generates high expiratory flows with laminar flow in the smaller airways, which dislodge and eject foreign material from the pulmonary system. The relationship between cough and aspiration has not been explored in detail, but the few studies available show that absent or weak cough in stroke patients is associated with a higher incidence of aspiration and chest infections (17, 18). It is also been shown that several aerodynamic measures of voluntary cough are impaired in stroke patients compared to non-stroke control subjects, and in aspirating compared to non-aspirating stroke patients (18). The final common pathway for the production of effective cough is the ability to generate high intra-abdominal pressure by strong contraction of the abdominal muscles. Recent studies have shown diaphragmatic involvement on the affected side, disruption of cortico-respiratory neuronal outflow, and decreased expiratory muscle excitation from the affected hemisphere in patients with stroke (19). It is quite likely, but remains unproven, that impairment of expiratory muscle function may impair voluntary cough efficacy and contribute to increased susceptibility to chest infections after stroke. In addition, stroke may induce an immunodeficient state

secondary to impairments of sympathetic autonomic activity. In a mouse model of focal cerebral ischemia, stroke induced an extensive apoptotic loss of lymphocytes with spontaneous septicemia and pneumonia in these animals (20). A catecholamine-mediated defect in early lymphocyte activation was found to underlie this impairment of antibacterial immune response, which was reversed by beta adrenoceptor blockade.

Despite several studies showing strong associations between dysphagia and chest infections, there are few intervention trials of antibiotics used to prevent chest infections. A randomized, double-blind, placebo-controlled study of antibiotic prophylaxis in 136 stroke patients showed no differences in the infection rates at one week or three months between treated and untreated patients (21). More recently, a prospective, randomized, placebo-controlled double-blind trial of selective decontamination of the digestive tract for prophylaxis against chest infection in 203 acute stroke patients showed that patients treated with 500 mg of oral gel containing colistin, polymyxin, and amphotericin four times a day for three weeks had significantly fewer aerobic gram negative organisms isolates and fewer pneumonias, but comparable mortality (22). Existing guidelines have evidence-based recommendations on the assessment, positioning, and feeding of acute stroke patients to prevent chest infections, but there is not enough evidence to support a clear strategy for antibiotic use for prevention (23). The current policy is to adopt a "wait and watch" approach to identifying early signs of chest infection and treat aggressively with appropriate antibiotics if any of these are present (23). For further reading on the management of dysphagia, see chapter 11.

Falls

Falls during rehabilitation are common, and a high prevalence has been reported in many studies (Table 24-1). In

TABLE 24-3
*Common Risk Factors for Post-Stroke
Complications*

RISK FACTOR	OR (95% C.I.)
Complications	
Age	2.4 (1.6–3.8)
Stroke severity	4.6 (2.7–7.9)
Premorbid disability	2.7 (1.7–4.3)
Urinary incontinence	8.5 (5.6–13.0)
Diabetes	1.9 (1.1–3.4)
Hypertension	1.8 (1.3–2.6)
Hypoalbuminemia	1.7 (1.2–2.5)
Length of stay >30 days	12.9 (7.7–22.0)
Specialist unit management	0.6 (0.4–0.9)
Transfer to acute facilities	
Elevated admission white blood cell counts	1.9 (1.3–2.8)
Low admission hemoglobin	1.9 (1.3–2.7)
Greater neurologic deficit	2.5 (1.4–4.4)
History of cardiac arrythmia	1.8 (1.2–2.7)

Data from Davenport et al. (10), Roth et al. (8), and SUTC (13)

the study by Davenport et al., falls were the most common individual complication and occurred in 22% of patients (10). An even higher proportion of falls during the hospital stay was reported by patients discharged from rehabilitation, with nearly 46% claiming to have fallen at least once during their hospital stay and 73% experiencing a fall within the first six months of discharge (24). In most instances, these falls are benign; soft-tissue damage or need for further investigations is seen in about 10% of fallers and only 1 to 3% of patients who fell suffered a fracture as a result of the fall. An important consideration is falls occurring in patients receiving anticoagulation for secondary-stroke prevention while undergoing rehabilitation. Stein et al. have shown that although falls in patients on anticoagulation were as frequent as in non-anticoagulated patients undergoing rehabilitation, the risk of injury, major bleed, or intracranial hemorrhage was comparable to those not receiving anticoagulation (25).

The great paradox of rehabilitation is that most therapy activity is geared toward increasing mobility in stroke patients, yet patients who have some ability to mobilize are most prone to falling. The main reason for falls reflects stroke-related disability with most patients losing balance while attempting to undertake basic activities such transferring, walking, or reaching. Factors associated with increased risk of falls include age, severity of stroke deficit, neglect, cognitive impairments, co-morbidity, and a tendency to "push" from the unaffected side (26). Patients who have one fall are at a greater risk of suffering further

falls. The Berg balance test has been suggested as a reliable, objective test for identifying potential fallers in rehabilitation settings, but its use in clinical practice remains to be validated (27).

The greatest risk of falling in rehabilitation settings is during unsupervised activity, but it may neither be feasible to monitor patients on a 24-hour basis, nor desirable to lower their optimism and perceptions of recovery by severely restricting activity. The answer may lie in effective therapy techniques and strategies to prevent falls, good communication with patients to provide a clear understanding of stroke-related problems and their abilities, safe environments, toileting programs, and use of aids and technology. However, there also needs to be acceptance, by both patients and professionals, of the small element of risk of falling, which is inherent to promoting independence and self-confidence in stroke patients undergoing rehabilitation.

Urinary Dysfunction

The most frequently occurring urinary problems associated with stroke are frequency, incontinence, retention, and infection. Urinary incontinence has a reported incidence ranging from 37% to 79% (28) and is one of the most commonly encountered medical complications in rehabilitation settings (8). Patients who are incontinent on admission to rehabilitation suffer additional complications and have greater morbidity, both during their hospital stay and at three months after stroke (29). Many stroke patients who are initially incontinent regain continence in two weeks, but 15–20% patients may have persisting problems at six months after stroke (30). The main predictors of incontinence in the 935 patients included in the Copenhagen Stroke Study were age, severity of stroke, diabetes, and pre-existing functional comorbidity (30). Factors associated with increased risk of urinary tract infections included older age, a history of prior stroke, greater stroke severity, use of beta blockers or antidepressants, and a post-void bladder residual of greater than 150 mL.

Several mechanisms contribute to incontinence in stroke patients. Patients may present with incontinence because of impairments of bladder function resulting from an "uninhibited bladder" and/or hyperreflexia from disrupted neuromicturition pathways. Other patients have normal bladder function but may still be incontinent because of stroke-related motor, cognitive, and language deficits. In some patients, incontinence may result from bladder hyporeflexia caused by concurrent neuropathy associated with age or diabetes or from concurrent medications, which are unrelated to the acute stroke. In addition, there may be many non-physiological factors that contribute to increased prevalence of reported incontinence in stroke patients. These include other stroke-related problems such as depression, apathy, confusion, or speech difficulties, which may affect the desire or the ability to communicate voiding needs. Some patients who are dependent on caregivers for transfers and mobility may find it difficult to void in a socially appropriate manner. Lack of caregiver support may also make it difficult to toilet stroke patients quickly enough. Medications (such as diuretics) can increase the frequency of the need to void, whereas others (such as those with anticolinergic effects, and beta blockers in particular) can increase confusion or affect the autonomic nervous system, leading to incontinence or retention.

There are few randomized controlled trials that evaluate the efficacy of interventions to treat urinary incontinence after stroke. A stepwise approach beginning with behavior intervention, progressing to medication only if these measures fail, and considering surgical interventions as a last resort has been recommended (28). There are a wide range of interventions, including bladder training, continence nurse practitioner care, pharmacological treatments, and sensory-motor biofeedback techniques, available to manage continence in stroke patients. Although evidence supports the use of many of these techniques, no single treatment has been shown to be superior to any other in improving continence.

The use of indwelling catheters in patients with incontinence is an important issue in stroke management. It is generally believed that early use of indwelling catheters will inhibit regaining continence in stroke patients, and that the use of indwelling catheters should be limited to patients with incontinence that cannot be treated with other means, patients with urinary-outlet obstruction, severely impaired patients with skin breakdown in whom frequent bed or clothing changes would be difficult or painful, and patients in whom incontinence interferes with monitoring of fluid and electrolyte balance (28). Chronic use of indwelling catheters also increases the risk of urinary tract infection and inflammatory bladder wall changes, which contribute further to incontinence and infection.

Deep Vein Thrombosis

There is wide variability in the reported incidence of deep vein thrombosis (DVT) following stroke. The overall incidence of clinically apparent and silent DVT may be as high as 45% in acute stroke patients. This rate falls to 10% or lower in patients in the sub-acute phase of stroke receiving rehabilitation (28, 31, 32). The incidence of pulmonary embolisms varies between 9 and 15% in patients who have DVT and, like DVT, is lower in those undergoing rehabilitation. DVT and pulmonary embolism account for 1 to 2% of mortality in stroke patients in rehabilitation settings (28), but pulmonary embolism has been implicated as a cause of death in 12 to 20%

of patients in acute settings and in up to 50% of stroke patients with sudden death (33, 34). Clinical symptoms of DVT (pain, swelling, erythema) may often be absent in stroke patients, even when diagnostic tests are positive. The risk of DVT and pulmonary embolism is high in patients with advanced age, more severe strokes, lower-limb plegia, reduced consciousness, obesity, history of a previous DVT, and longer duration of hospital stay (35). Many reports show that the prevalence of DVT appears higher in patients with hemorrhagic compared with ischemic strokes, which has partially been attributed to the use of anticoagulant medications in ischemic stroke patients (36).

Although anticoagulants are very effective in preventing DVT and pulmonary embolism in immobile patients, they can lead to serious complications, such as hemorrhagic transformation and intracranial bleeding, especially in patients with large infarcts or bleeds. Hence, there is a difference of opinion on their management, and guidelines for thromboprophylaxis in stroke vary between countries. North American guidelines strongly recommend early use of anticoagulants, heparin, or other antithrombotic measures to prevent DVT in immobilized stroke patients (37). In contrast, UK guidelines warn against the routine use of heparin or anticoagulation and recommend the use of aspirin and elastic compression stockings in stroke patients (23).

There is very strong, good-quality evidence in literature that anticoagulation significantly reduces the incidence of deep venous thrombosis (38). Literature also strongly supports the use of low molecular-weight over unfractionated heparin because of its greater effectiveness in preventing DVT and lower risks in hemorrhagic stroke patients (38). In contrast, evidence is unclear on the effectiveness of graded compression stockings in reducing the risk of developing DVT, and a large international clinical trial is currently ongoing (the CLOTS study).

Regardless of this debate, a major issue in stroke management is the translation of good research evidence into good clinical practice. In the Post-Stroke Rehabilitation Outcomes Project, Zorowitz et al. (31) showed that despite the strength of evidence and support from clinical guidelines, nearly 33% of patients without DVT and 1% of patients with DVT had no documented orders for anticoagulant medications. The study concluded that although much is known about the prevention and treatment of post-stroke DVT, clinicians need to learn to apply prevention protocols in order to prevent interruptions of the rehabilitation process.

Edematous Limbs

Swelling of the limbs on the affected side is common after stroke. A recent study in 88 stroke patients on a rehabilitation unit showed that some degree of hand swelling was present in 73%, and edema in 33%, of patients (39). These problems are more common in patients with hypertonic fingers and impaired sensation and have been associated with worse outcomes for arm and hand function. Limb edema also causes considerable discomfort and concern to stroke survivors, especially because it may never resolve in some patients. Elderly patients and those with more severe strokes are likely to suffer from these problems and have an increased risk of venous thrombosis.

The precise etiology of edema of the hand of the paralyzed arm is not known, but various mechanisms such as complex regional pain syndrome (reflex sympathetic dystrophy), posture, and lack of muscle activity have been suggested in the past. Geurts et al. (40) undertook an extensive review of studies on the etiology and treatment of post-stroke hand edema and shoulder-hand syndrome. This review included etiological studies on lymph scintigraphy in hand edema, bone scintigraphy, putative risk factors, and the existence of autonomic dysregulation or peripheral nerve lesions. Therapeutic studies included investigations of continuous passive motion and neuromuscular stimulation in hand edema, as well as oral corticosteroids, intramuscular calcitonin, and trauma prevention. They concluded that hand edema is not lymphedema but is rather associated with increased arterial blood flow, possibly resulting from autonomic dysregulation, and is probably worsened by trauma causing aseptic inflammation of the joints. Furthermore, there was no specific pharmacological treatment that had any advantage over physical methods for reducing hand edema (40). Available treatment modalities include elevation of the hand, massage, application of elastic bandages, immersion of the hand in cooled water, and pneumatic compression, all of which remain debatable.

MEDICAL MANAGEMENT IN REHABILITATION

The medical management of patients with stroke requires the skills of a well-coordinated multidisciplinary team because of the number of problems associated with stroke (e.g., impaired sensation or cognition, paresis, dysphagia), the high risk of stroke-related complications (e.g., aspiration pneumonia, venous thrombosis), the specialized needs of stroke patients (e.g., communication problems, visuospatial impairment), and patients' dependence on others for basic activities of daily living.

Most of the medical treatment during stroke rehabilitation is supportive, allowing time for neurologic injury to settle with minimization of further risk from potential complications. This includes maintaining stable respiratory and cardiovascular function, with particular attention to oxygenation and appropriate blood pressure; correcting fluid electrolyte imbalances and optimizing blood glucose levels; ensuring adequate nutrition; and preventing complications such as aspiration pneumonitis, urinary retention or infection, venous thromboembolism, pressure sores, and falls. Of particular importance is the maintenance of nutrition and hydration, because stroke is often associated with disturbances of water, glucose, and salt mechanisms. These conditions may be a result of impaired consciousness, inability to perceive or respond to hunger and thirst, or hypothalamic disturbances causing salt-losing or -retaining syndromes. Although stroke patients also have high metabolic needs, factors such as metabolic impairments, renal function, and glycemic status need to be taken into consideration while planning nutrition regimens. Poor nutrition, dehydration, and electrolyte imbalance are the precursors of many—and contribute to the severity and consequences of almost all—complications encountered in stroke (see also chapter 29). Meticulous attention to managing these often "silent" derangements is often rewarded by fewer complications, better participation in rehabilitation, and better functional and psychological outcomes.

The key message emerging from several research studies and years of clinical experience is that the best intervention to reduce stroke-related complications and optimize rehabilitation outcomes is to manage stroke patients on specialized dedicated units where staff, who are knowledgeable about stroke and stroke-related complications, monitor patients regularly and institute measures that can proactively prevent the occurrence of such complications or provide early aggressive interventions to mitigate consequences once complications occur.

RESEARCH FRONTIERS

Although there is considerable literature available on outcomes, rehabilitation, and service organization in stroke rehabilitation, research into the prevalence, management, and consequences of medical complications has merited relatively little attention. Studies that can measure the independent impact of complications on recovery and the benefits of prevention of individual complications are difficult to design because of the interactions between different processes of care in determining stroke outcome. There is still no satisfactory longitudinal representative cohort study with a large enough number of patients for accurate estimation of the incidence and prevalence of stroke-related medical complications and their temporal profile during various stages of stroke management. Similarly, there are no robust intervention studies on the prevention or treatment of these complications that can guide clinical practice for the specific management of these problems. There are several small ongoing studies that investigate various aspects of medical management of stroke patents, but small sample sizes and design heterogeneity will limit the impact of their findings and their potential for inclusion into meta-analyses.

References

1. Heuschmann PU, Kolominsky-Rabas PL, Misselwitz B, et al.; German Stroke Registers Study Group. Predictors of in-hospital mortality and attributable risks of death after ischemic stroke: The German Stroke Registers Study Group. *Arch Intern Med* 2004 Sep 13; 164(16):1761–1768.
2. Silver FL, Norris JW, Lewis AJ, Hachinski VC. Early mortality following stroke: a prospective review. *Stroke* 1984; 15:492–496.
3. Dobkin BH. Neuromedical complications in stroke patients transferred for rehabilitation before and after diagnostic related groups. *J Neurol Rehab* 1987; 1:3–7.
4. Dromerick A, Reding M. Medical and neurological complications during inpatient stroke rehabilitation. *Stroke* 1994 Feb; 25(2):358–361.
5. Johnston KC, Li JY, Lyden PD, et al. Medical and neurological complications of ischemic stroke: Experience from the RANTTAS trial. RANTTAS Investigators. *Stroke* 1998 Feb; 29(2):447–453.
6. Bae HJ, Yoon DS, Lee J, et al. In-hospital medical complications and long-term mortality after ischemic stroke. *Stroke* 2005 Nov; 36(11):2441–2445.
7. Kalra L, Yu G, Wilson K, Roots P. Medical complications during stroke rehabilitation. *Stroke* 1995 Jun; 26(6):990–994.
8. Roth EJ, Lovell L, Harvey RL, et al. Incidence of and risk factors for medical complications during stroke rehabilitation. *Stroke* 2001 Feb; 32(2):523–529.
9. Siegler EL, Stineman MG, Maislin G. Development of complications during rehabilitation. *Arch Intern Med* 1994 Oct 10; 154(19):2185–2190.
10. Davenport RJ, Dennis MS, Wellwood I, Warlow CP. Complications after acute stroke. *Stroke* 1996 Mar; 27(3):415–420.
11. Langhorne P, Stott DJ, Robertson L, et al. Medical complications after stroke: A multi-center study. *Stroke* 2000 Jun; 31(6):1223–1229.
12. Evans A, Perez I, Harraf F, et al. Can differences in management processes explain different outcomes between stroke unit and stroke team care? *Lancet* 2001; 358:1586–1592.
13. Govan L, Langhorne P, Weir CJ; Stroke Unit Trialists Collaboration. Does the prevention of complications explain the survival benefit of organized inpatient (stroke unit) care?: Further analysis of a systematic review. *Stroke*. 2007 Sep; 38(9):2536–2540.
14. Martino R, Foley N, Bhogal S, et al. Dysphagia after stroke: Incidence, diagnosis, and pulmonary complications. *Stroke* 2005; 36(12):2756–2763.
15. Kimura K, Minematsu K, Kazui S, Yamaguchi T; Japan Multicenter Stroke Investigators' Collaboration (J-MUSIC). Mortality and cause of death after hospital discharge in 10,981 patients with ischemic stroke and transient ischemic attack. *Cerebrovasc Dis* 2005; 19(3):171–178.
16. Ramsey D, Smithard D, Kalra L. Silent aspiration: What do we know? *Dysphagia* 2005; 20(3):218–225.
17. Addington WR, Stephens RE, Gilliland KA. Assessing the laryngeal cough reflex and the risk of developing pneumonia after stroke: An interhospital comparison. *Stroke* 1999; 30:1203–1207.
18. Smith-Hammond CA, Goldstein LB, Zajac DJ, et al. Assessment of aspiration risk in stroke patients with quantification of voluntary cough. *Neurology* 2001; 56:502–506.
19. Urban PP, Morgenstern M, Brause K, et al. Distribution and course of cortico-respiratory projections for voluntary activation in man: A transcranial magnetic stimulation study in healthy subjects and patients with cerebral ischaemia. *J Neurol* 2002; 249(6):735–744.
20. Prass K, Meisel C, Hoflich C, et al. Stroke-induced immunodeficiency promotes spontaneous bacterial infections and is mediated by sympathetic activation reversal by poststroke T helper cell type 1-like immunostimulation. *J Exp Med* 2003 Sep 1; 198(5):725–736.
21. Chamorro A, Horcajada JP, Obach V, et al. The Early Systemic Prophylaxis of Infection After Stroke study: a randomized clinical trial. *Stroke* 2005; 36(7):1495–1500.
22. Gosney M, Martin MV, Wright AE. The role of selective decontamination of the digestive tract in acute stroke. *Age Ageing* 2006; 35(1):42–47.
23. Intercollegiate Stroke Working Party. National clinical guidelines for stroke, second edition. Clinical Effectiveness & Evaluation Unit, Royal College of Physicians, 2004 London.
24. Forster A, Young J. Incidence and consequences of falls due to stroke: A systematic inquiry. *BMJ* 1995; 311:83–86.
25. Stein J, Viramontes BE, Kerrigan DC. Fall-related injuries in anticoagulated stroke patients during inpatient rehabilitation. *Arch Phys Med Rehabil* 1995; 76(9):840–843.
26. Suzuki T, Sonoda S, Misawa K, et al. Incidence and consequence of falls in inpatient rehabilitation of stroke patients. *Exp Aging Res* 2005 Oct–Dec; 31(4):457–469.
27. Andersson AG, Kamwendo K, Seiger A, Appelros P. How to identify potential fallers in a stroke unit: validity indexes of four test methods. *J Rehabil Med* 2006 May; 38(3):186–191.
28. Teasell R, Foley N, Bhogal S. Medical complications post stroke. Evidence-based review of stroke rehabilitation; sixth edition. Canadian Stroke Network, 2006. www.ebrsr.com
29. Gariballa SE. Potentially treatable causes of poor outcome in acute stroke patients with urinary incontinence. *Acta Neurol Scand* 2003 May; 107(5):336–340.
30. Nakayama H, Jorgensen HS, Pedersen PM, Raaschou HO, Olsen TS. Prevalence and risk factors of incontinence after stroke. The Copenhagen Stroke Study. *Stroke* 1997 Jan; 28(1):58–62.
31. Zorowitz RD, Smout RJ, Gassaway JA, Horn SD. Prophylaxis for and treatment of deep venous thrombosis after stroke: The Post-Stroke Rehabilitation Outcomes Project (PSROP). *Top Stroke Rehabil* 2005 Fall; 12(4):1–10.
32. Wilson RD, Murray PK. Cost-effectiveness of screening for deep vein thrombosis by ultrasound at admission to stroke rehabilitation. *Arch Phys Med Rehabil* 2005 Oct; 86(10):1941–1948.
33. Bounds JV, Wiebers DO, Whisnant JP, Okazaki H. Mechanisms and timing of deaths from cerebral infarction. *Stroke* 1981 Jul–Aug; 12(4):474–477.
34. Wijdicks EF, Scott JP. Pulmonary embolism associated with acute stroke. *Mayo Clin Proc* 1997 Apr; 72(4):297–300.
35. Imberti D, Prisco D. Venous thromboembolism prophylaxis in medical patients: future perspectives. *Thromb Res* 2005; 116(5):365–375.
36. Skaf E, Stein PD, Beemath A, et al. Venous thromboembolism in patients with ischemic and hemorrhagic stroke. *Am J Cardiol* 2005 Dec 15; 96(12):1731–1733.
37. Adams HP Jr, Adams RJ, Brott T, et al; Stroke Council of the American Stroke Association. Guidelines for the early management of patients with ischemic stroke: A scientific statement from the Stroke Council of the American Stroke Association. *Stroke* 2003 Apr; 34(4):1056–1083.
38. Andre C, de Freitas GR, Fukujima MM. Prevention of deep venous thrombosis and pulmonary embolism following stroke: A systematic review of published articles. *Eur J Neurol* 2007 Jan; 14(1):21–32.
39. Boomkamp-Koppen HG, Visser-Meily JM, Post MW, Prevo AJ. Poststroke hand swelling and oedema: prevalence and relationship with impairment and disability. *Clin Rehabil* 2005 Aug; 19(5):552–559.
40. Geurts AC, Visschers BA, van Limbeek J, Ribbers GM. Systematic review of aetiology and treatment of post-stroke hand oedema and shoulder-hand syndrome. Scand J Rehabil Med 2000 Mar; 32(1):4–10.

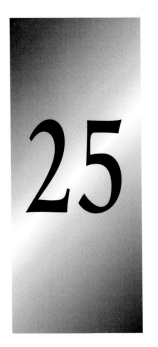

25 Physiology and Management of Spasticity after Stroke

Gerard E. Francisco
John R. McGuire

S pasticity is commonly defined as "a motor disorder characterized by a velocity-dependent increase in tonic stretch reflexes with exaggerated tendon jerks, resulting from hyperexcitability of the stretch reflex, as one component of the upper motor neuron syndrome"(1). It magnifies weakness and other motor abnormalities, and thus worsens the functional impairments commonly associated with stroke, such as difficulty with gait and upper limb use. In more severe states, it causes pain and leads to contractures and permanent joint deformities. Unfortunately, this often-quoted definition does not describe commonly-observed clinical findings, such as the intermittent nature of spastic hypertonia. It also does not consider the other abnormalities associated with the upper motor neuron syndrome (UMNS), of which spastic hypertonia is but one component: dystonia, co-contraction of agonists and antagonists, clonus, weakness, and incoordination (2–8). Lastly, this definition does not acknowledge the role of the sensory system in causing motor abnormalities. Thus, Pandyan proposed an alternate definition: spasticity is "a disordered sensorimotor control, resulting from an upper motor neuron lesion, presenting as intermittent or sustained involuntary contraction of muscles" (9).

Since spasticity is a multi-dimensional problem with various components, a thoughtful clinical assessment should take these factors into consideration in order to design a comprehensive treatment plan that will address all impairments that contribute to the functional problem. For instance, while pharmacologic interventions can effectively reduce hypertonia, they may either uncover or cause motor weakness and incoordination, which will need to be addressed through strengthening exercises.

The reported incidence of post-stroke hypertonia varies from to 19–70% depending on the sample population and method of assessment (10–12). A large study involving 106 stroke patients living in the community reported that 36% had spasticity, as measured by the Tone Assessment Scale, at 12 months' follow-up. Additionally, it was estimated that 20% had severe spasticity. Two other studies estimated the incidence of post-stroke spasticity. One included a cohort of 59 community-dwelling stroke survivors, 39% of whom had spasticity at 12 months post-stroke (11). Another study reported an incidence of only 19% among 99 stroke survivors, who were assessed using the modified Ashworth Scale (MAS) at three months post-stroke (10, 13). At around the same time point, only 67% were still hemiparetic, suggesting that the sample size had a cohort of stroke survivors with relatively mild severity of impairments. This may explain why the incidence of spasticity is quite different from our observation that up to about 70% of 189 hospitalized stroke survivors had abnormally increased muscle tone during their first admission to an acute rehabilitation unit (12). Many of the patients included in this investigation also had severe motor, language, and cognitive impairments, which may be related to more severe spastic hypertonia.

ASSESSMENT

When assessing post-stroke hypertonia, it is important to understand that spasticity is only one component of the muscle overactivity seen as part of the upper motor syndrome (Table 25-1).

Spastic co-contraction, spastic dystonia, synergistic limb patterns, weakness, and soft tissue contractures are important considerations in the assessment of post-stroke patients (2, 3, 7, 8, 14, 15). Upper motor neuron lesions cause motor dysfunction that result in a "convoluted mixture of obligatory and compensatory motor behaviors that are difficult to interpret" (16). Simple bedside testing is usually an inadequate determinant of an overall treatment strategy; a description of the problem in different circumstances is of far more value than a single examination (17). Assessments from physical, occupational, and speech therapists, as well as input from the patient and their caregivers, are essential for establishing patient-specific goals and an optimal treatment plan (18).

Clinical, electrophysiological, and biomechanical measures have been used to quantify post-stroke spasticity (Table 25-2).

The most commonly used clinical measures of post-stroke spasticity are the Ashworth scale (AS) and MAS. The AS grades muscle tone from 0 (normal) to 4 (severe) and is shown in 25-3 (19).

The MAS adds an additional intermediate grade (1+), but has less inter-rater reliability than the AS (13, 20, 21). Despite their widespread use, the AS and MAS have marginal intra-rater and inter-rater reliability (20–23).

TABLE 25-1
Upper Motor Neuron Syndrome

Positive Symptoms
Spasticity
Spastic co-contraction
Spastic dystonia
Flex/Ext synergistic muscle patterns
Reflex release phenomena

Negative Symptoms
Weakness, fatigue
Loss of dexterity, balance
Loss of selective muscle control

Rheologic changes
Contracture, fibrosis, atrophy

The reliability of the AS for upper limb spasticity can be improved if the examiner completes a standardized training program and testing is done in a similar format (22). Other limitations of the AS include a "clustering" effect of the patients in the middle grades, and the measure does not differentiate contracture from hyperexcitable stretch reflexes (23).

The Tardieu scale has advantages over the AS because it not only quantifies the muscles reaction to stretch, but it controls for the velocity of the stretch and measures the angle at which the catch, or clonus, occurs (24–26) (Table 25-4). The quality of muscle reaction to passive stretch at certain velocities is scored between 0 (no resistance with passive movement) and 4 (unfatigable clonus > 10 seconds). The spasticity angle is the difference between the angle at the end of passive range of motion (PROM) at slow speed (V1) and the angle of catch at fast speed (V2 or V3). The spasticity angle provides an estimation of the relative contribution of neural mechanisms (spasticity) and the mechanical restraint of the soft tissues. Grading is performed at the same time

TABLE 25-2
Measures of Spasticity and Motor Control

	MEASURES OF SPASTICITY	MEASURES OF MOTOR CONTROL
Clinical	Ashworth Scale Modified Ashworth Scale Tardieu Scale Oswestry Scale Spasm frequency scale Tone Assessment Scale	Fugl-Meyer Wolf Motor Function Test) Timed walk, Timed up & Go
Electrophysiological	H/M ratio	Dynamic EMG
Biomechanical	Servo-control device	Motion Analysis Systems

TABLE 25-3
Ashworth Scale and Modified Ashworth Scale

0. no increased tone
1. slight increase in muscle tone, manifested by a catch and release or by minimal resistance at the end of the range of motion when the affected part is moved in flexion or extension
(The Modified Ashworth Scale includes: 1+ –)
2. more marked increase in muscle tone through most of the range of motion, but affected part(s) easily moved
3. considerable increase in muscle tone, passive movement difficult
4. affected part(s) rigid in flexion or extension

---

of day and in a constant position of the body for a given limb (26). The Tardieu scale is a valid clinical measure of spasticity after stroke (27).

Electrophysiologic tests such as the H-reflex, H/M ratio, F-wave, and tonic vibration reflex (TVR) have been used to quantify spasticity in stroke patients (28, 29). Historically, these measures tend to correlate poorly with the degree of spasticity (30). Recently, Pizzi and colleagues demonstrated a positive correlation between the flexor carpi radialis H/M ratio and the MAS scores at the wrist in 65 post-stroke spastic hemiparetic patients (31). The correlation was strongest with the higher AS scores (3 and 4). The soleus H/M ratio can be used to confirm the effects of intrathecal baclofen (ITB) during the ITB trial, and potentially for trouble-shooting (29, 32). In a prospective case series involving nine stroke, 17 traumatic brain injury, and 4 anoxic brain-injured subjects treated with 50 μg intrathecal bolus of baclofen, there was a reduction of the H/M ratio from 62% ± 28% to 14% ± 19% and Ashworth scores from 2.4 ± 0.7 to 1.5 ± 0.6 on the more involved side five hours post-bolus

---

TABLE 25-4
Tardieu Scale

Quality of Muscle Reaction
0. No resistance
1. Slight resistance
2. Catch followed by a release
3. Fatigable clonus (<10 seconds)
4. Infatigable clonus (>10 seconds)

Angle of Muscle Reaction

Velocity of Stretch
V1. As slow as possible
V2. Speed of limb falling under gravity
V3. As fast as possible

---

(32). This study suggests that the soleus H/M ratio may be more sensitive than the AS score in detecting a physiologic response to ITB bolus.

Biomechanical measurements of spasticity using a servo-controlled motor-driven device can provide a more reliable measure of spasticity, but is limited to the research laboratory. The device can provide a controlled stretch of a limb while measuring torque, joint angle, and reflex EMG activity (33, 34). Large amplitude perturbations have been used to quantify spastic stretch reflexes at a joint (33–35). These reflex measures were shown to be reliable measures of elbow spasticity in 16 chronic stroke patients with upper limb spasticity (36). In this study, elbow stretch reflexes were assessed using a custom made manipulandum attached to a Biodex System. Movements into elbow flexion and extension were imposed at four speeds: 6, 30, 60, and 90 degrees per second. Ninety percent reliability in the measurement of peak torque, peak stiffness, and reflex threshold angle was obtained when at least two days of testing were performed. The biomechanical measures correlated well with the AS (Spearman $\rho=0.84$, $P<0.005$) (36).

The assessment of patients with post-stroke hypertonia should also include measures of motor control (Table 25-2). The Fugl-Meyer Scale (FMS) is a reliable and validated measure of upper and lower extremity motor impairment based on the natural progression of functional return after a stroke (37). The FMS has been demonstrated to have high intra-rater and inter-rater reliability, and can be completed in 10–20 minutes. Decline of function of the FMS has been shown to correlate closely with the severity of spasticity (38).

The Functional Test for the Hemiparetic Upper Extremity was developed at Rancho Los Amigos Hospital and consists of 17 graded tasks with seven levels of difficulty. The test is based on the Brunnstrom scale, and each task is timed and graded pass/fail (14, 39). The patient has three opportunities to try each task, and can work no longer than 3 minutes on each item. The test is functionally based, has good inter-rater reliability, and the timing of each task allows for detecting more subtle changes (40).

The Barthel Index (BI) is an ordinal scale of global function and mobility that may not be sensitive to the functional implications of spasticity (10, 41). Francis and colleagues proposed a "Composite Functional Index" (CFI) that was shown to correlate well with reduction of arm spasticity (42). The index (range 0–17) uses the dressing, grooming, and feeding sections of the BI, and adds three subjective measures: putting arm through sleeve, cleaning palm, and cutting finger nails. In a meta-analysis of two randomized controlled trials, 26 of 47 had improved arm function (CFI) and reduced spasticity (MAS) after injections of botulinum toxin (Dysport) (42). The Disability Assessment Scale (DAS) (range 0–12) developed to assess functional impairment in patients with post-stroke upper limb spasticity (i.e., dressing, hygiene, limb position, pain) and has shown good intra- and inter-rater reliability (22).

Dynamic polyelectromyographic (PEMG) recordings can be used to identify the timing and duration of muscle over activity in post-stroke spastic hypertonia. These EMG recordings can be helpful for understanding muscle involvement when assessing for treatment with chemodenervation, chemical neurolysis, or surgical release of individual muscles (43). For example, in the patient with a spastic flexed elbow, PEMG can be used to identify spastic co-contraction of the elbow flexors and extensors (43). By combining PEMG with kinematic data from a motion analysis lab, the primary upper or lower extremity motor dysfunction can be localized (44, 45). Quantitative gait analysis can differentiate quadriceps overactivity from hip flexor weakness or poor ankle mechanics as the cause of stiff-legged gait (46).

IMPACT ON REHABILITATION AND RECOVERY

Some investigators have suggested that the importance of spasticity may be overstated (10, 47). Despite a lack of good epidemiological data, most clinicians would agree that treating spasticity "just because it's there" as suggested by Landau is not the best practice (47). There are potential benefits of increased muscle tone. Increased extensor tone of the legs can assist with standing and transfers (48). Reflex muscle activity may preserve muscle bulk and slow osteoporosis (49).

When spasticity interferes with active or passive function, or becomes painful, then appropriate interventions need to be considered (50). Even though limb weakness may be the more important factor when considering active function, spasticity or spastic co-contraction can impede limb movement (8, 50). Upper limb spasticity, such as the adducted internally rotated shoulder or flexed elbow, can make activities such as reaching overhead more difficult. Spastic co-contraction of elbow flexors and extensors can limit active elbow extension and flexion (50).Increased tone of the wrist and finger flexors can interfere with releasing objects after grasping them. Lower extremity spasticity such as the adducted hip, flexed, or extended knee can interfere with standing, transfers, or walking. The inability to obtain a foot flat position during the stance phase of gait, as in the equinovarus foot, can lead to gait instability and make stair climbing more difficult.

Spasticity may play a more important role by interfering with passive function such as hygiene in the axilla, elbow, and palm of the hand. Finger flexor spasticity, as in

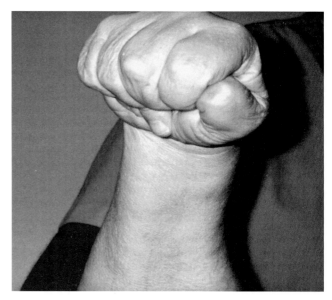

FIGURE 25-1

Finger flexor spasticity as shown in the "clenched fist" condition.

the "clenched fist" condition, can lead to skin breakdown and nail bed infections (43) (Figure 25-1).

Lower extremity passive function such as perineal care, bladder catheterization, toileting, and bathing can be more difficult with spasticity of the hip adductors. Overactivity of the hip flexors or extensors can interfere with wheelchair positioning.

Spasticity of the shoulder internal rotators is one of several causes of post-stroke shoulder pain. The prevalence of shoulder pain varies from 16% to 84%, of which 31% to 57% have spasticity (7, 51–57). In an uncontrolled observational study of 13 patients with spastic hemiplegia, subjects had reduced shoulder pain and improved ROM after phenol injection of the nerve to the subscapularis muscle (58). In a randomized double-blind placebo controlled study, ten spastic post-stroke patients had reduced spasticity, improved ROM, and decreased shoulder pain after BTX injections to the subscapularis muscle (59).

Early treatment of spasticity may lead to improved outcomes in motor recovery. Windows of opportunity may exist in the early management of spasticity (60). If one takes "a wait and see" approach, optimal treatment benefits may be lost. Twitchell noted that severe proximal spasticity at one month post-stroke was a predictor of poor motor recovery (61). In some stoke survivors, spasticity may be a constraint on motor recovery, and early treatment may improve their motor recovery. Although not all stroke survivors will have improved motor recovery, early spasticity treatment may impact the clinical course of the increased tone. A double-blind placebo controlled trial of three treatments for lower extremity spasticity in twenty-eight patients with acute TBI demonstrated improved ROM and reduced MAS in the patients treated with serial casting and saline or BTX, when compared to physical therapy alone (62). Despite the limited number of subjects, this study suggests that early intervention may have a beneficial effect on the long-term consequences of spastic hypertonia. Further investigation is needed to identify which patients may benefit most from early spasticity treatment.

ORAL MEDICATIONS

Stroke survivors generally have a poor tolerance for oral medications because of the central nervous system (CNS) side effects. Of the oral antispasticity medications currently available in the United States, only baclofen, tizanidine, valium, dantrium, and clonazepam have been evaluated in persons with stroke (63–66). In 2004, Montané et al. completed a systematic review of double-blind randomized controlled trials of antispastic oral medications for stroke and reviewed six trials (64, 65, 67–71). Because of the small numbers, lack of quality of life measures, and high incidence of adverse drug effects (drowsiness, sedation, and muscle weakness), they concluded that the evidence for the use oral antispastic medications in stroke is weak (65) (Table 25-5).

Baclofen is a structural analog of gamma-aminobutyric (GABA), which is one of the main inhibitory neurotransmitters in the CNS (72). The half-life of oral baclofen is 3.5 hours and is excreted primarily by the kidney, although 15% is metabolized in the liver (63). In a double-blind placebo controlled crossover trial of 20 stroke patients, those treated with up to 30 mg/d of baclofen for one month had reduced Ashworth scores, no functional improvement, and higher adverse events (50% vs. 15%) when taking baclofen vs. placebo (73). The most common adverse effects were sedation, dizziness, and weakness. In a retrospective review of 35 subjects with acquired brain injury that included seven stroke patients, those treated with an average dose of 57 mg/d of baclofen had reduced lower extremity spasticity and no change in the upper extremity (74). There were no functional measures reported, and 17% of the patients had sleepiness, which limited dose increases (74).

Dantrolene sodium is a hydantoin derivative that acts primarily on the muscle fiber by blocking the release of calcium from the sarcoplasmic reticulum, which reduces the force of the muscle contraction (63). The half-life of dantrolene sodium is 4 to 15 hours after oral dose and 12 hours after intravenous dose, and metabolized primarily by the liver (63). The most common side effects are drowsiness, nausea, paresthesias, and weakness. Even though the risk of hepatic toxicity is rare (1–2%), it is recommended to monitor liver function tests before and during treatment (63). In a double-blind placebo controlled crossover study of 31 stroke patients treated with 50-200 mg per day of dantrolene, subjects showed no change in AS or Barthel scores while reducing strength in the unaffected limb, but not the paretic limb, based on isokinetic testing (17). In a double-blind parallel study, 14 stroke patients who achieved reduced spasticity with dantrolene for 6 weeks were randomized to either placebo or continued dose of dantrolene for 6 more weeks (75). The placebo group noted increased deficits, and 13 of the 14 chose to continue dantrolene (average dose 165 mg/d) after the six week trial had ended. Side effects were mild and transient (75).

Tizanidine is an alpha-2 adrenergic agonist that binds to spinal and supraspinal imidazoline receptors and prevents the release of excitatory neurotransmitters(63). The half life of tizanidine is 2.5 hours, and it is metabolized by the liver. The most common side effects are drowsiness, dry mouth, weakness, hypotension, and elevated liver function tests (5%) (63). Because of this, liver function tests should be monitored before treatment, and at one, three, and six months and then annually after initiating treatment. In a small double-blind placebo controlled crossover study that included 9 stroke patients treated with 12-36 mg/d of tizanidine, subjects demonstrated dose-dependent reduced upper and lower extremity AS scores. No functional measures were reported. The most common adverse events were somnolence (41%), increased liver function tests (18%), and dry mouth (12%) (64). In a double-blind comparative study of thirty stroke patients treated with tizanidine (8-20mg/d) or baclofen (20-50mg/d), both groups had similar improvements in AS scores. The side effects in the tizanidine group were mild and transient, and no patients discontinued the study. For the baclofen, three patients discontinued the study due to severe side-effects (68). In an open label dose titration study of 47 chronic stroke patient treated with tizanidine (2-36 mg/d), total upper extremity AS score improved with no decline in strength. Pain intensity, quality of life, and physician assessment of also improved. The maximum average daily dose was 20 mg/d, and 10 out of 47 patients were able tolerate the maximum dose of 36 mg/d. The most frequent side effects were somnolence (62%), dizziness (32%), asthenia (30%), dry mouth (21%), hypotension (13%), and elevated liver function tests (4%) (76).

Despite limited evidence in the literature to support the use of oral antispasticity medications in stroke patients, and frequent adverse effects, there is a role for their use. Because somnolence is a common side effect of oral medications, low doses at night may be useful in select patients with difficulty sleeping because of muscle spasms. As with most medications in stroke survivors, it is suggested to "start low and go slow". Rather than higher

TABLE 25-5
Oral Spasticity Medications

Author (year)	Study Design	Subjects and Intervention	Results
Basmajian, 1984 (264)	Randomized, double-blind, placebo-controlled, crossover	24 stroke survivors out of 50 subjects, but only 19 completed study 3 treatment conditions: Ketazolam 10 and 20 mg/d (1 wk each) Diazepam 5 and 10 mg/d (1 wk each) Placebo (2 wks)	Ketazolam and diazepam conditions better than placebo on most outcomes (p<.05) but no significant difference between ketazolam and diazepam
Bes, 1988 (103)	Randomized, double-blind, Parallel group	N=105 hemiplegics (89 stroke, 16 cranial trauma) 2 groups well-matched for sex, age, height and body weight: Tizanidine (46 stroke) started at 6 mg/d and titrated up to maximum of 24 mg/d within 2 wks (mean dosage at week 8: 17.08 mg/d); Diazepam (43 stroke) started at 7.5 mg/d and titrated up to maximum of 30 mg/d (mean dosage at week 8: 19.52 mg/d)	15 subjects on tizanidine and 6 on diazepam dropped out due to side effects Tizanidine group improved walking distance on flat ground; 3 of 11 bedridden subjects on tizanidine, and 2 of 4 bedridden subjects on diazepam became ambulatory
Cocchiarella, 1967 (115)	Randomized, double-blind, placebo-controlled, multiple crossover	Mixed diagnoses; 16 stroke survivors out of 19, but were not identified in data analysis 5 treatment conditions: Placebo Diazepam 6 mg/d Diazepam 15 mg/d Phenobarbital 45 mg/d Phenobarbital 90 mg/d	No significant difference in leg drop and straight leg raise tests, and total steps taken Slower ambulation while on diazepam 15 mg/d compared to placebo
Glass, 1974 (266)	Double-blind, placebo-controlled, crossover	24 stroke survivors out of 62; 16/62 participated in crossover phase, but only 11/16 completed (Unknown number of stroke survivors in crossover phase or among drop-outs) 4 Treatment conditions: Dantrolene (100 mg qid) Diazepam (5mg qid) Dantrolene (100 mg qid) and Diazepam (5 mg qid) Placebo	Combined dantrolene and diazepam was superior to diazepam or dantrolene alone or placebo in clinical measures
Meythaler, 2001 (188)	Randomized, double-blind, placebo-controlled, crossover	9 stroke survivors among 17 subjects 2 Treatment conditions: Placebo; Tizanidine 4 mg qHS titrated to goal of 12-36 mg/d	Only 6 tolerated up to 9 pills of tizanidine (36 mg/d), while 11 tolerated all 9 placebo pills Somnolence in 41% on tizanidine and none in placebo
Meythaler, 2004 (189)	Retrospective	35 acquired brain injuries (7 stroke) Average oral baclofen dose 57 mg/day	Decreased lower, but not upper, limb spasticity 17% complained of sleepiness

Adapted from Francisco GE. Pharmacologic management of lower limb spastic hypertonia in stroke: What is the evidence? In: Condie E, ed. Report of a consensus conference on the orthotic management of stroke patients. Copenhagen: ISPO, 2004:137–147.

TABLE 25-6
Phenol, Alcohol, and Anesthetic Nerve Blocks

AUTHOR (YEAR)	STUDY DESIGN	SUBJECTS AND INTERVENTION	RESULTS
Albert, 2002 (268)	Case series	7 stroke survivors out of 12 subjects with hemiplegia disabled by quadriceps overactivity Etidocaine 1%, 2 cm³ was injected to block the branch of the femoral nerve to either the vastus intermedius or lateralis.	Decrease in quadriceps spasticity, but results were difficult to interpret, based on the data reported
Chua, 2000 (269)	Case series	5 stroke survivors out of 8 subjects with hemiplegia and severe knee flexor spasticity Ethyl alcohol 50–100% (with 1% lidocaine) injected to sciatic nerve using repetitive monopolar electric stimulation	MAS scores of knee flexors improved significantly at 1 ($p<.005$), 3 ($p<.01$), and 6 ($p<.02$) months post-injection
Kirazli, 1998 (63)	Randomized, double-blind (?), parallel group	N=20; Botulinum toxin-A (Botox®) 400 units injected to lower limb muscles using electromyographic guidance vs phenol 5% tibial nerve block	Significant improvement in AS in both groups ($p<.05$) for ankle plantarflexor; Toxin group had more improvement in AS of ankle invertors than phenol ($p>.05$); AS and clonus duration more improved in toxin group than phenol at weeks 2 and 4, but not at wks 8 and 12

From Francisco GE. Pharmacologic management of lower limb spastic hypertonia in stroke: What is the evidence? In: Condie E, ed. Report of a consensus conference on the orthotic management of stroke patients. Copenhagen: ISPO, 2004:137–147

doses of one medication, a combination of lowers doses of two medications may be better tolerated (77). Also, these medications should be tapered off slowly, especially with baclofen wherein abrupt withdrawal can result in seizures and other life-threatening situations.

NERVE BLOCKS

Neurolytic procedures using phenol or alcohol are effective in treating focal spastic hypertonia from various etiologies, including cerebral palsy, traumatic brain injuries, and stroke (58, 78–86) (Table 25-6).

In sufficiently high concentrations, phenol (5–6%) and alcohol (35–60%) work by denaturing proteins, leading to neurolysis, while at lower concentrations (i.e., 3% and lower), phenol acts as an anesthetic (87). Phenol appears to control muscle hypertonia as a result of denervation and degeneration of muscle spindles (88). Phenol injures afferent and efferent nerve fibers, and the damage to the axons and membranes can be extensive (89, 90).

Following injection of either agent, muscle relaxation is almost immediate due to the anesthetic effects. The neurolytic effect sets in about an hour after injection, and lasts for a few months. The effect may last for as long as a year or longer, depending on the degree of nerve blockade. Hypertonia usually recurs due to muscle reinnervation, but this recovery is incomplete (88). Common side effects include pain at the injection site, post-injection dysesthesia, localized swelling, and excessive weakness (87, 91). If inadvertently injected into vessels, or if systemic absorption occurs, central nervous system effects, such as tremor, convulsions, and CNS depression may result.

There is a paucity of well-designed studies on the use of phenol or alcohol in the treatment of spastic hypertonia. For one, these drugs are rarely used in the upper limb due to concerns with complications, most especially dysesthesia. Most reported treatment of spasticity of the finger flexors, elbow flexors, and other muscle groups in the traumatic brain injury population (82–84, 92). Hecht treated 11 patients with painful shoulder attributed to hypertonia of the subscapularis muscle (58). Three to

6 ml of aqueous phenol 6.7% was percutaneously injected into the subscapular nerve branches. This resulted in improvement in shoulder flexion, abduction, and external rotation, presumably due to a decrease in pain and hypertonia.

One investigation reported effective treatment of hip flexor spasticity by injecting up to 3.5 ml of phenol 5% into the belly of the psoas major and minor muscles under ultrasonic monitoring (85). Nine of the twelve patients had spasticity from stroke. In addition to increased range of motion, improvement in sitting position, standing and walking posture, and pain relief were noted. No complication occurred. Another study reported the beneficial effects of phenol in reducing spasticity of tibial-innervated muscles (93).

An investigation demonstrated significant reduction of quadriceps muscle tone with use of etidocaine 1%, 2 cm^3 after a femoral nerve block (94). This study's primary intent was to demonstrate an anatomical injection technique, and thus it used an anesthetic, whose effect on muscle tone was transient. Chua and Kong used ethyl alcohol of varying concentrations (50–100%) to block the sciatic nerve, and found that the decrease in hamstring muscle tone lasted up to 6 months post-intervention, and in some subjects, improved the quality of ambulation and facilitated wheelchair positioning (86).

The popularity of phenol and alcohol has been eclipsed by botulinum toxin chemodenervation. The latter is easier to administer and appears to have a better side effect profile, but phenol and alcohol are much less expensive and may last longer. While both treatments are effective, there has been no convincing evidence as to the superiority of one over the other in treating spastic hypertonia. Only one attempt has been made to compare the effects of phenol 5% and botulinum toxin type-A (BTX-type A) in controlling clonus and hypertonia. In the investigation, both phenol and BTX-type A improved muscle tone (as measured by AS scores) of ankle plantarflexors and invertors, but it appeared that the BTX group had superior efficacy over phenol (P<.05) both in decreasing muscle tone and ankle clonus at 2 and 4 weeks, but not at 8 and 12 weeks, post-treatment (95). The study result may have been affected by the relatively low dose of phenol used, since the amount injected was not adjusted based on clinical response after the first few injections, as is commonly done in clinical practice. Table 25-7 presents further comparison of the clinical characteristics of these two medications.

BOTULINUM TOXINS

Botulinum toxins (BTX) are arguably the most commonly used intervention for spastic hypertonia. Derived from the bacterium, *Clostridium botulinum*, it has seven types,

TABLE 25-7

Comparison of Phenol and Botulinum Toxin Treatment for Spasticity

	PHENOL	BTX
Effectiveness	✓✓✓	✓✓✓
Evidence of Efficacy	Lower Limb No RCT	Upper Limb ✓ RCT
Ease of Administration		✓✓✓
Onset	✓✓✓	
Duration	✓✓	
Pain and occurrence of other adverse events		✓✓✓
Cost	✓✓✓	

designated A through G, which are antigenically and serologically distinct but structurally similar (96). The toxin molecule is formed by heavy and light polypeptide chains that are linked by a disulphide bond. BTX act by binding on pre-synaptic cholinergic nerve terminals. Once in the nerve terminal, it blocks the release, but not the synthesis, of acetylcholine into the neuromuscular junction, thereby disallowing muscular contraction. In addition to its reduction of alpha motor neuron activity on extrafusal muscle fibers, BTX exert their effects on reduction of Ia afferent signal from muscle spindles at the gamma motor neuron level. The decreased signal from Ia afferents will then result in a reduction of feedback to alpha motor neurons, resulting in decreased muscle activity. The duration of clinical effect lasts three to four months, and is most likely due to axonal sprouting and muscle reinnervation when new neuromuscular junctions are established. DePaiva et al. suggested that previously blocked junctions undergo functional repair (97).

In the last decade, two BTX serotypes, A and B, have emerged as an important treatment for focal post-stroke spastic hypertonia. A recent consensus paper supported the use of BTX for focal spastic conditions in adults (98). Its popularity owes to the impressive clinical outcomes experienced by stroke survivors and clinicians, despite the relative lack of convincing scientific evidence of its effects on function. For a variety of reasons, such as study design limitations, sensitivity of outcome measures, and appropriateness of patient selection criteria, published literature has yet to demonstrate that BTX lead to functional enhancement, although significant improvement in muscle tone has been shown.

BTX also have the advantage of target treatment specificity (i.e., exerting significant changes only in injected muscles), as opposed to the systemic effects of oral medications, and have a better adverse event profile. For instance, the incidence of drowsiness and sedation, which are commonly associated with oral spasmolytics, are practically non-existent with toxins. BTX also appear to be favored by many clinicians over phenol and alcohol, which are more technically challenging and have a higher incidence of complications, such as dysesthesia.

Evidence of Efficacy of Botulinum Toxin Type A (BTX-A)

Upper Limb. Various studies have demonstrated significant improvement of upper limb post-stroke spastic hypertonia (Table 25-8). Simpson investigated the effect of three total doses of Botox® (Allergan, Inc., Irvine, CA) as compared to placebo in 39 subjects (99). Saline or one of three doses of Botox® (75u, 150u, or 300u) were injected to the biceps, flexor carpi radialis (FCR), and flexor carpi ulnaris (FCU). At 2, 4, and 6 weeks post-injection, all treatment groups had better outcome than placebo, but the group that received the highest dose had the most robust improvement in hypertonia reduction in the elbow and wrist flexors. The effects lasted for about 16 weeks. This dose-dependent effect of BTX was also demonstrated in a later study (100). Ninety-one stroke survivors received either Botox® or placebo to spastic finger, wrist, and elbow flexors. Participants were randomized to one of the following groups: placebo, 90, 120, and 360 u of Botox®. All treatment groups demonstrated improvement in MAS scores (P<0.05), but the group that received the highest dose also had the most improvement.

In the largest study on BTX for spastic hypertonia, Brashear et al. compared Botox® 200–240 units to placebo injected into the wrist, finger, and thumb flexors. At 4, 6, 8, and 12 weeks, the Botox® group had superior improvement in muscle tone over placebo (22). Additionally, this study also measured changes in various impairment and functional domains, including pain, deformity, hygiene, and orthotic fit, using the Disability Assessment Scale (DAS). At week 6, the treatment group had more significant improvement on the DAS in the principal target of treatment (P<0.001). As in the Simpson study, no major adverse event was reported (99).

Experience with the use of another preparation of BTX-type A (Dysport®; Ipsen, UK), has been similar. In one study, 59 subjects were randomized to receive either placebo or 1000 u of Dysport® divided between the biceps, flexor carpi radialis (FCR), flexor carpi ulnaris (FCU), flexor digitorum superficialis (FDS), and flexor digitorum profundus (FDP). At 4 weeks post-injection, the Dysport® group had a more significant improvement in muscle tone (as measured by MAS) when compared to placebo (p=0.004). The same investigators also conducted a dose-ranging investigation involving 83 stroke survivors, who were randomized to one of three Dysport®

doses (500, 1000, 1500 u) or placebo. Muscles injected included the biceps, FCR, FCU, FDS, and the FDP (101, 102). The treatment groups demonstrated more significant improvement in tone than placebo. Weakness was observed in the 1500 u group.

Another investigation compared the efficacy of Dysport® 500, 1000, and 1500 u, with placebo in treating spastic hypertonia of the biceps, wrist flexors, finger flexors, and thumb adductors/flexors (103). When compared to placebo at six weeks, improvement in muscle tone in the elbow and wrist flexors (p<0.05) and passive elbow range of motion (p<0.02) were noted in all treatment groups. Consistent with Bakheit et al.'s findings, the group that received higher doses had greater hypertonia reduction than placebo, but did not have an advantage in terms of duration of effect (103).

Lower Limb. A study on the effect of Dysport® involving 23 stroke survivors showed that 1000 u to various lower limb muscles was significantly superior to placebo in improving AS scores in the ankle plantarflexors (p<0.0002) and invertors (p=0.0002) (104). Muscles injected included the gastrocnemius, soleus, tibialis posterior, and flexor digitorum longus. Another investigation of the impact of Dysport® injected to both heads of the gastrocnemius and soleus showed similar results (105). In this study, 234 subjects were randomized to one of four groups (placebo, Dysport® 500, 1000, and 1500 u) (105). Similar to previous findings, the most significant improvement in spasticity was in the group that received the highest dose (1500u).

A randomized, double-blind, dose-ranging trial by Mancini et al. on 45 spastic feet due to stroke demonstrated the efficacy and safety of about 300 units of BTX-A injected in various lower limb muscles (106). Subjects were randomized into three groups: Groups 1 (mean total BTX dose: 167 u), 2 (mean total BTX dose: 320 u), and 3 (mean total BTX dose: 540 u). While all three groups improved on various outcome measures, including the modified AS, Medical Research Clinical Scale, Gait assessment, ankle clonus, and visual analog scales for gait and pain, groups 2 and 3 had more improvement at 4 months post-injection. Group 3 reported the highest incidence of adverse events 4 weeks post-treatment, suggesting a dose-response relationship.

Evidence of Efficacy of BTX Type B (BTX-B)

BTX-B (marketed as Myobloc® in the United States, and as Neurobloc® in Europe and elsewhere), has limited published research on its use for spastic hypertonia. An open-label study reported that Myobloc® (Solstice Neurosciences, Inc., Malvern, PA) effectively decreased upper limb tone in 10 subjects with acquired brain injuries (nine of whom had a stroke) (107). A total dose of 10,000 u

TABLE 25-8

Botulinum Toxin for Post-stroke Spastic Hypertonia

Author (Year)	Subjects	Intervention	Main Outcome Measure(s)	Results	Comments
Botox™ Simpson et al., 1996 (50)	N=39; ≥9 mo post-stroke (mean=3 yr); Average MAS≥2.5 in elbow and wrist flexors	Compared three total doses of Botox™ to placebo injected to BB, FCR, FCU, or placebo: Low – 75 u total Medium – 150 u total High – 300 u total	MAS	Improvement in elbow and wrist flexor MAS scores in High Dose (HD; 300 u) group at 2, 4, and 6 wks post-injection compared to placebo (P; p<0.05) MAS returned to near-baseline scores by wk 16 post-injection	No significant difference between placebo and treatment groups on other impairment and functional measures (FIM; FM; caregiver dependency; function and pain assessment; motor/function task rating scale)
Brashear et al., 2002 (51)	N=126; ≥6 mo post-stroke; AS≥3 in wrist flexors and AS≥2 in finger flexors; DAS≥2	Injected Botox™ to FCR, FCU, FDS, FDP ± FPL/FPB (total 200–240 u) or placebo	AS; DAS	Improvement in DAS scores in BTX group compared to placebo (P) at 4 and 6 (p≤0.001) wks and 8 and 12 wks (p=0.03):	DAS was meant to measure one target "functional disability" (hygiene, dressing, limb position, pain)

Simpson et al. results table:

Wk	MAS Change Elbow Flexor		MAS Change Wrist Flexor	
	P	HD	P	HD
2	0.3	1.4	0.3	1.4
4	0.3	1.4	0.2	1.5
6	0.6	1.5	0	1.4

Brashear et al. results table:

Wk	Change in DAS Scores		
	P	BTX	P value
6	−0.31	−0.94	<0.001
12	−0.46	−0.88	0.02

Childers et al., 2004 (49)

N=91; ≥6 wk post-stroke (mean 25.8 mo; range 0.9-226.9 mo); MAS≥3 in wrist flexor and MAS≥2 in elbow flexor

Up to two injections with either placebo or Botox™ (90, 180, 360 u total) to elbow, wrist, and finger flexors
Concurrent PT or splinting allowed but not changed during study participation

MAS

Improvement in wrist and finger, and thumb flexor AS scores at 4, 6, 8, and 12 wks post-injection:

	Change in AS Scores		
	P	BTX	P value
Wrist Flexors			
Wk 6	-0.48	-1.66	<0.001
Wk 12	-0.31	-1.07	<0.001
Finger Flexors			
Wk 6	-0.32	-1.34	<0.001
Wk 12	-0.12	-0.378	<0.001
Thumb Flexors			
Wk 6	-0.62	-1.31	0.09
Wk 12	-0.31	-0.92	0.02

Improvement in elbow, wrist and finger flexor MAS scores at various wks post-injection in Botox groups compared to placebo (p<0.05):

Wk	Change in DAS Scores of Wrist Flexors (primary outcome measure)		
	P	BTX 360 u	P value
3	-0.6	-1.5	<0.001
6	-0.7	-1.6	<0.001
9	-0.6	-1.4	<0.05

Similar improvement in MAS scores after repeated Botox™ injection
Dose-response pattern in MAS, but not FIM, global assessment, or SF-36 Health Survey

Wide range of stroke duration may have affected outcome
First study to show effect of repeated Botox™ injection in a blinded manner
14 subjects (15.3%) did not complete study (first injection)

TABLE 25-8
(Continued)

Author (Year)	Subjects	Intervention	Main Outcome Measure(s)	Results	Comments
Dysport™ Bakheit et al., 2000 (53)	N=83; ≥3 mo post-stroke; MAS≥2 in elbow, wrist, and finger flexors	Injected placebo or Dysport™ to BB, FCR, FCU, FDS, FDP: (500 u, 1000 u, or 1500 u total)	MAS	Improvement in summed MAS scores (elbow + wrist + finger flexors) at 4 wks post-injection in Dysport™ groups compared to placebo ($p<0.05$):	Optimal dose in those with residual voluntary upper limb movement is 1000 u

Summary of Best Change in Summed MAS Scores at 4 wks post-injection and Odds Ratio for Improvement in Dysport® Groups as compared to Placebo (P)

MAS score change from baseline	P	500u	1000u	1500u
−4	0	0	1	2
−3	0	4	7	4
−2	6	11	8	4
−1	7	5	4	5
0	6	2	1	4
1	0	0	1	0
Odds Ratio		0.246	0.134	0.245

Study	Population	Intervention	Outcome measures	Results	Comments
Smith et al., 2000 (52)	N=21 (19 stroke, 2 head injury), with "troublesome spasticity" in the upper limb; ≥1 yr post-stroke	Injected placebo or Dysport™ (500 u, 1000 u, or 1500 u total) 2/3 of total dose allotted to "above elbow" muscles, and 1/3 to "below elbow" muscles (divided equally between wrist and finger flexors)	MAS; PROM/AROM; FAT	No statistically significant improvement in active and passive ROM, pain, Barthel Index, MAS, and specific functional activities (cleaning palm of hand, cutting fingernails, putting arm through sleeve). Improvement in wrist and finger flexor MAS ($p<0.01$) and wrist PROM ($p=0.05$) at 6 wks in combined treatment groups compared to placebo	Mixed diagnostic groups. Injected muscles varied depending on "distribution of spasticity"; no clear criteria for muscle and dose selection. Nine of 17 subjects who received Dysport™ to the BB due to "associated flexor reaction" also had some improvement in various gait parameters
Bakheit et al., 2001 (54)	N=59; ≥3 mo post-stroke; MAS≥2 in at least two of the elbow, wrist, and finger flexors, and a score of 1+ in the remaining area	Injected placebo or Dysport™ 1000 u to BB, FCR, FCU, FDS, FDP	MAS	No significant change in AROM and FAT. Improvement in summed MAS scores (elbow + wrist + finger flexors) at 4 wks post-injection in Dysport™ group compared to placebo, but at 16 wks ($p=0.004$), individual muscle group MAS had significant differences only in wrist ($p=0.004$)	No significant difference in ROM, Barthel Index, muscle pain, and goal-attainment scale

Mean Change in MAS Scores at 6 wks post-injection (Smith et al., 2000):

Group	Elbow Flexor	Wrist Flexor	Finger Flexor
Placebo	1	0	2
500u	−1	−1*	−3
1000u	−2	−2	0
1500u	−1**	−2**	−1**
Combined	−1	−2¶	−2¶

*$p<0.05$; **$p<0.01$; ¶$p=0.06$

TABLE 25-8
(Continued)

AUTHOR (YEAR)	SUBJECTS	INTERVENTION	MAIN OUTCOME MEASURE(S)	RESULTS	COMMENTS
				and finger flexors (p=0.001) when compared to placebo	

MAS score change from baseline	Placebo	Dysport® 500u*
−4	0	2
−3	4	5
−2	3	7
−1	15	8
0	10	5

*p=0.004

AS – AS
BB – biceps brachii
DAS – Disability Assessment Scale
FAT – Frenchay Arm Test
FCR – flexor carpi radialis
FCU – flexor carpi ulnaris
FDS – flexor digitorum superficialis
FDP – flexor digitorum profundus
FIM – Functional Independence Measure
MAS – modified AS
PROM – passive range of motion
PT – physical therapy
RMAS – Rivermead Motor Assessment Scale
ROM – range of motion

Reprinted with permission from Francisco GE. Botulinum toxin for post-stroke spasticity. *Ann Acad Med* 2007; 36:22–30.

was injected into various muscles, including the biceps (3750 u), FCR (2500 u), FCU (2500 u), FDS (625 u), and FDP (625 u). AS scores improved significantly from baseline in the elbow (p=0.016), wrist (p=0.004), and finger flexors (p=0.02) at week 4. The most commonly reported adverse event was dry mouth.

Clinical Issues in the Use of BTX

In the United States, BTX dosing for spastic hypertonia is neither standardized nor based on scientific data. Instead, dosing is based on recommendation by experts and unique experience of clinicians (108). The optimal dose of BTX is the most effective amount required to achieve a pre-determined outcome, such as reduced hypertonia, increased range of motion, improved hygiene and function, without causing an adverse event (e.g., weakness). Several factors affect the outcome of BTX therapy and influence clinical decision regarding choice of dose. These are summarized in Tables 25-9, 25-10, and 25-11.

BTX is usually not administered more frequently than every three months, because of theoretical concern for antibody development (108). This cautionary measure is based on findings in earlier studies on the use of BTX in cervical dystonia, where frequent injection, administration of "booster" injections, and initial high doses appeared to contribute to the development of BTX antibodies (109, 110). It is estimated that the incidence of antibody to BTX in the spastic hypertonia population is less than 1%, but there is no published data yet based on a prospective investigation (111, 112). Repeated injection of BTX appears to be effective and safe (113, 114). Lagalla et al. studied the effects of repeated injections every three to five months over a two-year period to various upper limb muscles in 28 stroke survivors (113). Muscle tone, range of motion, and satisfaction

---

TABLE 25-9
Factors that Affect Dose Selection of BTX

Patient-related Factors
  Spastic hypertonia severity
  Muscle and limb involvement
  Spastic hypertonia duration
  Age and body mass
  Outcome of prior BTX treatment

Clinician-related Factors
  Experience, Knowledge, and Expertise

Other Factors
  Cost
  Availability of Adjunctive Therapy

Reprinted with permission from Francisco GE. Botulinum toxin for post-stroke spasticity. *Ann Acad Med* 2007; 36:22–30.

---

and functional measures (e.g., putting on gloves, axillary hygiene) improved after each treatment, and this response was sustained over time. Additionally, there was no significant increase in treatment doses, and treatment intervals increased from a mean of 3.9±1.2 months between the first two sessions to 6.4+1.7 months between the fourth and fifth doses.

The preparation of Botox® for injection has not been standardized, but a common practice is to dilute a 100-unit vial with 1-2 ml of preservative-free saline. A small prospective study comparing dilution of 100 u of Botox® with one and two ml of saline did not show a difference in improving hypertonia of wrist and finger flexors (115). Another small trial suggested that dilution of Botox® with 5 ml of preservative-free saline is superior to more concentrated solution for decreasing spastic hypertonia of elbow flexor muscles (116). This is not an issue with Myobloc®, which already comes in a solution. No published information is available regarding dilution of Dysport®.

Little has been published in the literature on the role of adjunctive therapy modalities with BTX. Small, uncontrolled trials claim that the combination of BTX and various therapy modalities enhance clinical outcome. These include electrical stimulation of muscles injected with Botox® or Dysport®, ankle taping, and casting (117–119). A "low dose" of Botox® plus casting resulted in improved ankle range of motion and foot positioning similar to that obtained with a "high dose" (190–320 u) but without subsequent taping. The combined effect of BTX and physiotherapy and other therapeutic modalities in the stroke population has yet to be systematically investigated.

The reviewed studies have demonstrated that BTX is an effective therapy for focal post-stroke spastic hypertonia, but there has been no persuasive published evidence on its impact on generalized spastic hypertonia and function. Only a few studies attempted to investigate the effect of BTX on the functionality of the upper limb (e.g. changes in hygiene and use of orthosis; decrease in caregiver burden) (22, 117, 120). The same observation is true for lower limb studies, which addressed spastic hypertonia reduction primarily. Only one study investigated gait as a main outcome measure (105). The lack of a systematic substantiation of BTX's influence on post-stroke recovery may be due to study design, patient selection, and choice of study outcome measures.

INTRATHECAL BACLOFEN

Intrathecal baclofen (ITB) therapy differs from the oral form of the medication in that it provides direct infusion of baclofen into the intrathecal space, thereby bypassing

TABLE 25-10

Recommended or Published Botox® Doses for Spastic Hypertonia due to Various Etiologies

UPPER LIMB MUSCLES	DOSE (UNITS)	REFERENCE
Subscapularis	50–100	108
Teres major	25–100	108
Latissimus Dorsi	50–150	108
Pectoralis complex	75–150	108
Triceps	50–200	Author's experience
Biceps	50–200	99, 100, 108, 116, 183, 184
Brachialis	40–100	108
Brachioradialis		108
Pronator teres	25–75	108, 185
Pronator quadratus	10–50	108
Flexor carpi radialis	25–100	22, 99, 100, 108, 115, 186, 187
Flexor carpi ulnaris	20–70	22, 99, 100, 108, 115, 186, 187
Flexor digotorum superficialis	20–60	22, 99, 100, 108, 115, 186, 187
Flexor digitorum profundus	20–60	22, 99, 100, 108, 115, 186, 187
Flexor pollicis longus	10–30	108, 186, 187
Opponens pollicis	5–25	186
Adductor pollicis	5–25	108
Lumbricals	5–15 per lumbrical	108, 188
LOWER LIMB MUSCLES		
Quadriceps mechanism	50–200	108
Hamstrings	50–200	108
Hip adductor group	200–400	108, 189
Gastrocnemius	50–250	95, 106, 108, 190
Soleus	50–200	95, 106, 108
Tibialis posterior	50–150	95, 106, 108
Tibialis anterior	50–150	108
Extensor hallucis longus	50–100	191, 192
Flexor hallucis longus	25–75	108, 192
Flexor digitorum longus	25–100	108, 192
Flexor digitorum brevis	20–40	108

Reprinted with permission from Francisco GE. Botulinum toxin for post-stroke spasticity. *Ann Acad Med* 2007; 36:22–30.

the blood-brain barrier. In contrast to oral baclofen, ITB is delivered in close proximity to the drug's site of action in the dorsal horn of the spinal cord. Therefore, only a small concentration of the drug is required to exert therapeutic effects without increasing the risk for side effects commonly associated with oral baclofen, such as sedation, drowsiness, and weakness. A programmable pump that infuses baclofen includes a small titanium disk containing a refillable reservoir for the drug and houses a computer chip that regulates the battery. A flexible silicone catheter, connected to the pump, delivers the drug into the intrathecal space. Prior to ITB pump implantation, a screening trial consisting of a bolus injection of 50–150 micrograms of baclofen is customarily performed to determine responsiveness of hypertonia to the medication.

ITB was initially used in persons with stroke and severe multi-limb spastic hypertonia (121, 122). Typical goals were facilitation of hygiene, positioning, and comfort. Lately, more clinicians have been utilizing ITB therapy chiefly to enhance upper limb function and gait (123, 124). When applied in the appropriate clinical setting and combined with a rehabilitation program, ITB therapy is an effective means of managing post-stroke spastic hypertonia in individuals of various functional levels.

TABLE 25-11
Published Dyport® Doses for Spastic Hypertonia

UPPER LIMB MUSCLES	DOSE (UNITS)	REFERENCE
Subscapularis	250	73
Biceps	100–400	57, 58, 61, 62
Brachialis	250	62
Brachioradialis	100	58
Flexor carpi radialis	150	58, 74
Flexor carpi ulnaris	100–150	57, 58, 74
Flexor digitorum superficialis	150–300	57, 58, 74
Flexor digitorum profundus	150–200	57, 58, 74
LOWER LIMB MUSCLES		
Hip adductor group	500–1000	83
Gastrocnemius	250–1000	60, 64, 92
Soleus	200–500	60, 64, 92
Tibialis posterior	200–500	60, 64. 92
Flexor digitorum longus	150–300	64

Reprinted with permission from Francisco GE. Botulinum toxin for post-stroke spasticity. *Ann Acad Med* 2007; 36:22–30.

The body of literature supporting the efficacy of ITB in post-stroke spastic hypertonia is limited. Thus far, no randomized, controlled study has been published. Much of what is known is based on a handful of open-label trials and case series (Table 25-12) and a consensus statement of experts (121–128). Two small investigations were conducted using a randomized, double-blind, placebo-controlled, crossover design, but only during the first part of the study (ITB bolus injection during the screening trial), and then assumed an open-label design during the continuous ITB infusion phase (121, 122). They showed a significant improvement in spastic hypertonia. A much larger series involving 94 subjects suggested that ITB therapy can positively enhance function and quality of life based on significant changes in Functional Independence Measure (FIM) and Sickness Impact Profile (SIP) scales, respectively (126). The limitation of study design and choice of outcome measures, however, prevent interpretation of the results and correlation with clinically significant functional changes. Thus far, only three investigations have suggested actual functional improvement. Two small case series demonstrated significant improvement in gait speed, while one demonstrated increased upper limb use following ITB and physical or occupational therapy (124, 127).

A consensus statement suggested that ITB therapy be considered in stroke survivors whose spastic hypertonia did not respond adequately to other pharmacologic and non-pharmacologic management interventions (128). ITB should also be considered regardless of the severity of hypertonia, as long as the spastic condition is significant enough to cause other problems, such as pain, joint deformities, postural abnormalities, and functional deficits, such as impairment in gait and inability to adequately perform activities of daily living. It should also be considered in persons whose progress in a rehabilitation program is hindered by spastic hypertonia that failed to respond to other treatment strategies. Table 25-13 summarizes typical goals for the application of ITB in stroke.

Concerns regarding the early use of ITB therapy after a stroke are based on animal studies, where early use of baclofen and other medications that mimic or enhance the effects of gamma-amino-butyric acid (GABA) after experimentally induced cerebral lesions slowed neurologic recovery (129, 130). Reports also suggest that certain drugs, including baclofen and other GABA agonists, may have a negative impact on cognitive and motor recovery after a stroke (131). However, it is widely acknowledged that delayed or inadequate treatment of spastic hypertonia may result in costly complications such as contractures, persistent pain, and failure to benefit from rehabilitation efforts. Thus the same consensus statement recommended that ITB therapy should be considered as early as three to six months post-stroke, whenever it causes significant functional impact or hinders progress in rehabilitation (128).

TABLE 25-12
Intrathecal baclofen in Post-stroke Spastic Hypertonia

STUDY/AUTHOR	SUBJECTS	STUDY DESIGN	OUTCOME
Meythaler et al., 1996 (316)	Stroke = 3; TBI = 3	Randomized, double-blind, placebo-controlled, crossover (screening phase only); open label after ITB pump implantation 3 mo follow-up	Improved AS, SFS, and reflex scores No effect on motor strength on the normal side
Meythaler et al., 2001 (317)	Stroke = 21	Randomized, double-blind, placebo-controlled, crossover (screening phase only); open label after ITB pump implantation 12 mo follow-up	Improved AS, SFS , and reflex scores No effect on motor strength on the normal side Three subjects recovered ability to ambulate
Francisco and Boake, 2003 (319)	Stroke = 10, all ambulatory	Open label Mean 8.9 months follow-up	Improved modified AS scores and gait speed. Preserved strength in unaffected limbs.
Remy-Neris et al., 2003 (310)	Stroke = 4 TBI = 3	Case series, open-label; bolus intrathecal baclofen only	Improved AS scores and maximal walking speed , but preferred walking speed was unchanged Minimal knee extension and maximal ankle flexion were the only kinematic data that significantly improved
Horn et al., 2005 (311)	Stroke = 13 TBI = 12 HE = 3	Case series; open-label 2, 4, and 6 hours post-ITB bolus injection	Improved AS scores and gait velocity Significant correlation between baseline gait velocity and peak change in velocity after ITB bolus No significant correlation between AS and change in temporospatial outcome gait measures
Ivanhoe et al., 2006 (307)	Stroke = 74	Open-label Post-ITB follow-up at 3 and 12 months	Significant improvement in AS, FIM, and SIP scores at both follow-ups No effect on muscle strength on unaffected side Largest study in stroke

AS – Ashworth Scale

FIM – Functional Independence Measure

HE – Hypoxic encephalopathy

ITB – Intrathecal Baclofen Therapy

SFS – Spasm Frequency Scale

SIP – Sickness Impact Profile

TBI – Traumatic brain injury

Used with permission from, *Topics in Stroke Rehabilitation* 2006; 13(4):74, Thomas Lund Publishers.

TABLE 25-13
Goals for ITB Therapy in Post-Stroke Hypertonia

High Level Patient
Mobility
    Increased speed of gait
    Increased safety of gait
    Improved quality of gait
    Prevent long-term injury due to alteration in joint
        biomechanics
Activities of Daily Living (ADL)
    Dressing
    Independence in hygiene
    Decreased time to accomplish ADL
Others
    Discontinuation of oral spasmolytic drugs (and
        avoidance of drug side effects)
    Decreased time spent on stretching as part of an
        exercise program

Low-level Patient
    Improved positioning
    Facilitation of hygiene
    Decreased caregiver burden and time
    Prevention of complications (i.e. contractures and
        non-use of paretic limb)
    Increased orthotic fit and compliance
    Decreased pain due to nighttime spasms
    Improved quality and duration of sleep

Used with permission from, *Topics in Stroke Rehabilitation*
2006; 13(4):74, Thomas Lund Publishers.

Although not unique to persons with stroke, certain clinical issues warrant thoughtful consideration prior to instituting ITB therapy, such as concomitant use of blood-thinning agents. There is insufficient evidence regarding the risk of withdrawing anti-platelets and anticoagulants prior to ITB screening or implantation to guide treatment. Thus, the decision whether to withdraw anti-platelet and anticoagulation treatment, its timing, and re-institution, will need to be made in consultation with the implanting surgeon and other specialists (cardiologists, hematologists, neurologists) involved in patient's care. Seizures are also known to occur during ITB therapy in other patient populations, but their occurrence among stroke survivors with ITB is not known (132, 133). Changes in gastrointestinal motility associated with ITB therapy have also been described (134). This may aggravate constipation, which commonly occurs during the acute and sub-acute phases of recovery from a stroke, when individuals are relatively immobile. Sexual dysfunction associated with ITB has been reported in the spinal cord injury population, but has yet to be reported in stroke survivors (135).

The impact of BTX and ITB on functional recovery

BTX and ITB therapies are effective treatments for post-stroke spastic hypertonia; yet their influence on function has not been fully demonstrated indubitably by well-designed studies. While it is tempting to dismiss their therapeutic impact on functional recovery due to the dearth of published evidence, common clinical experiences dictate otherwise. Perhaps the lack of scientific evidence does not accurately reflect BTX and ITB's effect on function, but rather, results from limitations in study design and methods. Likewise, it is also possible that it is incorrectly assumed that spastic hypertonia is the chief cause of a functional deficit, where in fact, other abnormalities associated with the UMNS, such as incoordination and co-contraction of agonist and antagonist muscles, are the primary reason for impaired function. Many times, an erroneous assumption is made that a decrease in spastic hypertonia alone will automatically translate to enhanced function. Doing so oversimplifies function, which is a complex and multifaceted phenomenon that depends not only on muscle tone, but also on muscle strength, coordination, and endurance, in addition to the influence of behavior of cognition. In fact, some have suggested that tonic stretch reflex activity does not meaningfully contribute to active motor function after stroke (6).

Inappropriate patient selection may also explain poor functional outcomes in BTX and ITB studies. Subjects with no or poor potential for motor and functional recovery could not be expected to demonstrate further functional improvement despite significant reduction of spastic hypertonia. Moreover, BTX injections and ITB therapy may worsen residual function by transiently inducing or uncovering latent weakness if too high a dose is used. Sheehan and Francis et al. have discussed this issue in greater detail in their excellent reviews (42, 136).

ROLE OF SURGICAL INTERVENTION

Surgical procedures are typically reserved for those stroke patients with muscle or tendon shortening who have not responded to the less invasive procedures, or as a "last resort". Tendon transfer, release, or lengthening are the most common orthopedic procedures (137). The split anterior tibial tendon transfer (SPLATT) and tendon Achilles lengthening (TAL) have been used in to manage the spastic equinovarus foot (138–142). In a retrospective review of 73 operated feet in patients with stroke, cerebral palsy, and brain injury, there was improved ability to ambulate, decreased need to wear orthosis, and increased ability to wear normal shoes with minimal complications (143). In a study of 21 stroke patients one year after a SPLATT, 83% report good or excellent results. All ambulatory patients had improved gait,e and 35% were able to discontinue their orthosis. Poor surgical outcomes were associated with nonambulatory status (144). The additional transfer of the flexor hallucis longus and flexor digitorum longus to the os calcis with the SPLATT and TAL improved calf strength, and patients had less reliance on orthotics (70% vs. 40%) (145). Pinzur et al. reported improved prehension after brachioradialis to finger extensor tendon transfer in four patients with spastic hemiplegia (146). Eighteen patients with spastic hand deformities had improved prehension after release of the flexor-pronator origin and step-cut lengthening of flexor pollicis longus (147). Polyelectromyography may be useful in identifying which patients would benefit most from orthopedic procedures (148). Other procedures, such as neurotomy, have also been shown to benefit spastic conditions (70, 81, 149).

NON-PHARMACOLOGIC MODALITIES

Collaboration with physical and occupational therapists is critical to the effective management of post-stroke spasticity (60). The therapist can help with patient evaluations, education, and establishing patient-specific goals (18). A number of conventional therapies have been used to manage spasticity and improve function (18, 150) (Table 25-14). The primary focus of these therapies is aimed at providing prolonged stretch to shortened muscles and tendons, reducing muscle overactivity, strengthening weak muscles, and improving motor control (151). Unfortunately, there is a significant variation in the use of these therapies, and lack of controlled trials (152). The reader is referred to three reviews on the benefits of stretch and physical modalities in the management of spasticity (152–154). In a randomized controlled study of 44 stroke patients, those treated with 20 sessions of Bobath treatment for four weeks had improved motor

---

TABLE 25-14
Rehabilitation Interventions for Spasticity

Inhibitory/serial casting
Weight bearing
Cryotherapy
Neurofacilatory techniques
Electrical stimulation
Aquatic therapy
EMG biofeedback
Constraint induced movement therapy
Robotic training
Partial weight support treadmill training

---

function and reduced spasticity, compared with the orthopedic treatment group (155, 156).

Surface electrical stimulation in stroke survivors has been shown to reduce atrophy, enhance strength, and possibly reduce spasticity (4, 157–164). Unfortunately, these studies have shown limited functional improvement, and many patients are unable to tolerate the electrical stimulation (163, 165). Initial work with an upper limb neuroprosthesis used to improve function was limited to the laboratory, and stimulation was limited to hand opening (54, 158).

A new approach is a device that combines a wrist-hand orthosis with neuromuscular electrical stimulation (NMES) of wrist and finger flexors and extensors during a repeated prehension exercise paradigm. The NESS H200™ is a neuroprosthesis that is well tolerated and has been shown to reduce impairments and improve function (164, 166–168). The major advantage of this system is that the device is custom fitted to the patient's forearm, assuring that the electrodes always stay in the correct place and provide consistent activation of the targeted muscles. The device is easy to don and doff and activate with one hand. The integrated NMES system provides reproducible stimulation of both wrist and finger flexors and extensors. The NESS 200 is intended to be self-administered, and allows NMES-assisted exercises involving prehension. The simplicity of using the system improves compliance with the treatment program (167). Improved function can be obtained when NMES is combined with a home exercise program. In a multi-center, multi-country non-randomized study, 77 stroke survivors completed a five-week daily home training program with the NESS H200. Subjects trained two to three times each day for seven days a week, and all enrolled subjects completed the study. The Jebsen-Taylor simulated feeding time improved 35%, the light object lift improved 45%, and the nine-hole peg test improved 59%. Mean spasticity reduction was 0.87 at the elbow and 0.78 at the wrist as measured by the AS. Thirty-three of the 77 patients had persistent upper limb pain with mean reduction 3.5 to 1.9 (167). Although this study is promising, it did not include a control group, so it is difficult to determine whether the benefits result from the NMES or from the regular exercise program.

LOOKING AHEAD: THE FUTURE OF SPASTIC HYPERTONIA MANAGEMENT

Spastic hypertonia and the UMNS, being complex and multifaceted conditions, create opportunities for innovative therapies for the future. Drugs that have been used for indications other than stroke have the potential to alleviate spastic hypertonia and other abnormalities. 4-amino-pyridine, an orally-administered medication touted to alleviate symptoms in multiple sclerosis by improving impulse conduction along damaged nerve fibers, has been reported to have anti-spasticity properties (169). Clonidine, already used as an adjunctive oral therapy for spastic hypertonia, can also be delivered intrathecally (170, 171). Its use is more common in Europe than in the United States. The use of intrathecal tizanidine has also been described in painful conditions, although its effect on spasticity similar to that of the oral preparation is yet to be shown (172). Another intrathecally-administered drug, ziconotide, a neurotoxin that is an emerging treatment for severe pain, has been shown to have spasmolytic properties in the spinal cord injury population (173). An ancient therapy, acupuncture, has been used to treat spastic hypertonia, but its efficacy has yet to be established (see chapter 41) (174–177) Earlier studies have suggested that spinal cord stimulation decreases spasticity, but clinical application of this modality has become more common for pain (178, 179). Interest in the use of direct motor nerve stimulation appears to be revived, judging by the recent publication of the results of animal investigations (180, 181). A promising avenue for the future treatment of spastic hypertonia is gene therapy (182). Being able to control muscular overactivity through genes capable of specifically inducing synaptic inhibition and suppressing neuromuscular transmission offers the advantage of addressing the root of the neuromuscular dysfunction (182).

Decisions on the treatment of spasticity after stroke depend on the severity of spastic hypertonia and its impact on function and well-being. Other factors to consider include disease etiology and duration, previous response to therapies, topographical involvement, response to medication side effects, and cost. Therapeutic efforts have focused on peripheral (e.g., altering muscle properties through physical techniques) and central (e.g., influencing neurotransmission through GABA-mediated medications, and modifying reciprocal inhibition through chemodenervation) strategies. Spastic hypertonia and the other UMNS signs and symptoms result in physical deformities and performance deficiencies. Thus, it is logical for interventions to target not only the underlying central nervous system pathology, but also the ensuing physical abnormalities. Consequently, it is a widely held belief that concurrent use of various pharmacologic and non-pharmacologic treatment modalities results in a more optimal management outcome.

Reference List

1. Lance J. Symposium synopsis in spasticity. In: Feldman RG, Young R, Koella WP, eds. *Disordered Motor Control*. Chicago: Year Book Medical Publishers, 1980.
2. Denny-Brown D. *The cerebral control of movement*. Liverpool: Liverpool University Press, 1966.
3. Fahn S, Bressman SB, Marsden CD. Classification of Dystonia. *Advances in Neurology* 1998; 78:11–25.
4. Levin MF, Hui-Chan CWY. Relief of hemiparetic spasticity by TENS is associated with improvement in reflex and voluntary motor function. *Electroencephalogr Clin Neurophysiol*. 1992; 85:131–142.
5. Sgouros S, Seri S. The effects of intrathecal baclofen on muscle co-contraction in children with spasticity of cerebral origin. *Pediatr Neurosurg*. 2002; 37:225–230.
6. Ada L, Vattanasilp W, O'Dwyer NJ, et al. Does spasticity contribute to walking dysfunction after stroke? *J Neurol Neurosurg Psychiatry*. 1998; 64:628–635.
7. Gracies JM. Pathophysiology of spastic paresis. I: Paresis and soft tissue changes. *Muscle & Nerve* 2005; 31:535–551.
8. Gracies JM. Pathophysiology of spastic paresis. II: Emergence of muscle overactivity. *Muscle & Nerve* 2005; 31:552–571.
9. Pandyan AD, Gregoric M, Barnes MP. Spasticity: Clinical perceptions, neurological realities and meaningful measurement. *Disabil Rehabil*. 2005; 27:2–6.
10. Sommerfield DK, Eek E, Svensson AK, et al. Spasticity after stroke: Its occurrence and association with motor impairments and activity limitations. *Stroke* 2004; 35:134–139.
11. Watkins CL, Leathley MJ, Gregson JM, Moore AP, Smith TL, Sharma AK. Prevalence of spasticity post stroke. *Clinical Rehabilitation* 2002; 16:515–522.
12. Francisco GE. How common is spastic hypertonia after stroke? *Arch Phys Med Rehabil*. 2002; 83:1644.
13. Bohannon RW, Smith MB. Interrater reliability on a modified Ashworth scale of muscle spasticity. *Phys Ther*. 1987; 67:206–207.
14. Brunnstrom S. *Movement Therapy in Hemiplegia a Neurophysiological Approach*. New York: Harper & Row, 1970.
15. Colebatch JG, Gandevia SC. The distribution of muscular weakness in upper motor neuron lesions affecting the arm. *Brain* 1989; 112:749–763.
16. Mayer N. Clinicophysiologic concepts of spasticity and motor dysfunction in adults with an upper motoneuron lesion. *Muscle & Nerve* 1997; 6:S1–S13.
17. Barnes M. An overview of the clinical management of spasticity. In: Barnes M, Johnson G, eds. *Upper Motor Neurone Syndrome and Spasticity*. New York: Cambridge University Press, 2001:1–11.
18. Scanlan S, McGuire J. Effective collaboration between physician and occupational therapist in the management of upper limb spasticity after stroke. *Top Stroke Rehabil*. 1998; 4:1–13.
19. Ashworth B. Preliminary trial of carisoprodol in multiple sclerosis. *Practitioner* 1964; 192:540–542.
20. Pandyan AD, Price CIM, Barnes M, et al. A review of the properties and limitations of the Ashworth and modified Ashworth Scales as measures of spasticity. *Clinical Rehabilitation* 1999; 13:373–383.
21. Blackburn M, van Vliet P, Modkett SP. Reliability of measurements obtained with the modified Ashworth Scale in the lower extremities of people with stroke. *Phys Ther*. 2002; 82:25–34.
22. Brashear A. Gordon MF, Elovic E, Kassicieh D, Marciniak C, Do M, Lee, Chia-Ho, Jenkins SW, Turkel C. Intramuscular injection of botulinum toxin for the treatment of wrist and finger spasticity after stroke. *N Engl J Med* 2002; 347: 395–400.
23. Nielsen JF, Sinkjaer T. A comparison of clinical and laboratory measures of spasticity. *Multiple Sclerosis* 1996; 1:296–301.
24. Tardieu C, Shentoub S, Delarue R. A la recherche d'une technique de mesure de la spasticite. *Rev Neurol*. 1954; 91:143–144.
25. Held JP, Pierrot-Deseilligny E. Reeducation motrice des affections neurologiques. *Baillie*. 1969; 31–42.
26. Gracies JM, Renton R, Sandanam J, et al. Short-term effects of dynamic Lycra splints on upper limb in hemiplegic patients. *Arch Phys Med Rehabil*. 2000; 81:1547–1555.
27. Patrick E, Ada L. The Tardieu Scale differentiates contracture from spasticity whereas the Ashworth Scales is confounded by it. *Clinical Rehabilitation* 2006; 20:173–182.
28. Sehgal N, McGuire JR. Beyond Ashworth. Electrophysiologic quantification of spasticity. *Phys Med & Rehabil Clinics of North America* 1998; 9:949–979.
29. Yablon SA, Stokic DS. Neurophysiologic evaluation of spastic hypertonia. *Am J Phys Med Rehabil* 2004; 83:S10–S18.
30. Delwaide PJ. Electrophysiological testing of spastic patients: Its potential usefulness and limitations. In: Delwaide PJ, Young RR, eds. *Clinical Neurophysiology in Spasticity: Contributions to Assessment and Pathophysiology*. Amsterdam: Elsevier, 1985.
31. Pizzi A, Carlucci G, Falsini C, et al. Evaluation of upper-limb spasticity after stroke: A clinical and neuropathophysiologic study. *Arch Phys Med Rehabil* 2005; 86:410–415.
32. Stokic DS, Yablon S, Hayes A. Comparison of clinical and neurophysiologic responses to intrathecal baclofen bolus administration in moderate-to-severe spasticity after acquired brain injury. *Arch Phys Med Rehabil* 2005; 86:1801–1806.
33. Schmit BD, Dhaher Y, Dewald JP, et al. Reflex torque responses to constant velocity movements in spastic elbow muscles: Theoretical analyses and implications for quantification of spasticity. *Ann Biomed Engineering* 1999; 27:815–829.
34. Schmit BD. Mechanical measures of spasticity. *Top Stroke Rehabil* 1999; 8:13–26.
35. Powers RK, Campbell DL, Rymer WZ. Stretch reflex dynamics in spastic elbow flexor muscles. *Ann Neurol* 1989; 25:32–42.

36. Starsky AJ, Sangani SG, McGuire JR, et al. Reliability of biomechanical spasticity measurements at the elbow of people poststroke. *Arch Phys Med Rehabil* 2005; 86:1648–1654.

37. Fugl-Meyer AR, Jaasko L, Leyman I, et al. The post-stroke hemiplegic patient. *Scand J Rehabil Med* 1975; 1975:7–13.

38. Katz RT, Rovai GP, Brait C, Rymer WZ. Objective quantification of spastic hypertonia: Correlation with clinical findings. *Arch Phys Med Rehabil* 1992; 73:339–347.

39. Wilson DJ, Baker LL, Craddock JA. Functional test for the hemiparetic upper extremity. *Occupational Therapy* 1984; 38:159–164.

40. Okkema KA, Culler KH. Functional evaluation of upper extremity use following stroke. *Top Stroke Rehabil* 1998; 4:54–75.

41. Mahoney FI, Barthel DW. Functional evaluation: Barthel Index. *Md State Med J* 1965; 14:61–65.

42. Francis HP, Wade DT, Turner-Stokes L, et al. Does reducing spasticity translate into functional benefit? An exploratory meta-analysis. *J Neurol Neurosurg Psychiatry* 2004; 75:1547–1551.

43. Mayer N, Esquenazi A. A muscle overactivity and movement dysfunction in the upper motoneuron syndrome. *Phys Med & Rehabil Clinics of North America* 2003; 14:855–883.

44. Hingtgen B, Wang M, McGuire J, et al. Au upper extremity kinematic model for evaluation of hemiparetic stroke. *J Biomech* 2006; 39:681–688.

45. Kerrigan DC, Karvosky ME, Riley PO. Spastic paretic stiff-legged gait: Joint kinetics. *Am J Phys Med Rehabil* 2001; 80:244–249.

46. Kerrigan DC, Bang M-S, Burke DT. An algorithm to assess stiff-legged gait in traumatic brain injury. *J Head Trauma Rehabil* 1999; 14:136–145.

47. Laudau WM, Sommerfield DK, Eek E, et al. Spasticity after stroke: Why bother? *Stroke* 2004; 35:1787–1788.

48. McGuire J, Rymer WZ. Spasticity: Mechanisms and management. In: Green D, ed. *Medical Management of Long-Term Disability*. Newton: Butterwoth-Heinemann,, 1996:277–288.

49. Glenn M. Nerve blocks. In: Glenn M, Whyte J, eds. *Practical Management of Spasticity in Children and Adults*. Philadelphia: Lea and Febiger, 1990:227–258.

50. Mayer N. Choosing upper limb muscles for focal intervention after traumatic brain injury. *J Head Trauma Rehabil* 2004; 19:119–142.

51. Snels IAK, Dedder JHM, Van Der Lee JH, et al. Treating patients with hemiplegia shoulder pain. *Am J Phys Med Rehabil* 2002; 81:150–160.

52. Bohannon RW, Larkin PA, Smith MD, Horton MG. Shoulder pain in hemiplegia: Statistical relationship with five variables. *Arch Phys Med Rehabil* 1986; 67:514–516.

53. Griffin JW. Hemiplegic shoulder pain. *Phys Ther* 1986; 66:1884–1893.

54. Rebersek S, Vodovnik L. Proportionally controlled functional electrical stimulation of hand. *Arch Phys Med Rehabil* 1973; 54:378–382.

55. Roy CW, Sands MR, Hill LD. Shoulder pain in acutely admitted hemiplegics. *Clinical Rehabilitation* 1994; 67:23–26.

56. Wanklyn P, Forster A, Young J. Hemiplegic shoulder pain (HSP): Natural history and investigation of associated features. *Disabil Rehabil* 1996; 18:497–501.

57. Van Ouwenaller C, Laplace PM, Chantraine A. Painful shoulder in hemiplegia. *Arch Phys Med Rehabil* 1986; 67:23–26.

58. Hecht JS. Subscapular nerve block in the painful hemiplegic shoulder. *Arch Phys Med Rehabil* 1992; 73:1036–1039.

59. Yelnik AP, Colle FM, Bonan I, et al. Treatment of shoulder pain in spastic hemiplegia by reducing spasticity of the subscapular muscle: A randomized, double-blind, placebo-controlled study of botulinum toxin A. *J Neurol Neurosurg Psychiatry* 2006.

60. McGuire J, Harvey RL. The prevention and management of complications after stroke. *Phys Med & Rehabil Clinics of North America* 1999; 10:857–874.

61. Twitchell TE. The restoration of motor function following hemiplegia in man. *Brain* 1951; 74:443–480.

62. Verplancke D, Snape S, Salisbury CF, Jones PW, Ward AB. A randomized controlled trial of botulinum toxin on lower limb spasticity following acute acquired severe brain injury. *Clinical Rehabilitation* 2005; 19:117–125.

63. Gracies JM, Nance P, Elovic E, McGuire JR. Traditional pharmacological treatments for spasticity. Part II. General and regional treatments. *Muscle & Nerve* 1997; Suppl 6: S92–S120.

64. Meytheler JM, Guin-Renfroes, Johnson A, et al. Prospective assessment of tizanidine for spasticity due to acquired brain injury. *Arch Phys Med Rehabil* 2001; 82:1155–1163.

65. Montane A, Vallano, Laporte JR. Oral antispastic drugs in nonprogressive neurologic diseases. *Neurology* 2004; 63:1357–1363.

66. Zafonte R, Lombard L, Elovic E. Antispasticity medications: Uses and limitations of enteral therapy. *Am J Phys Med Rehabil* 2004; 83:S50–S58.

67. Bes A, Eyssette M, Pierrot-Deseilligny E, et al. A multi-centre, double blind trial tizanidine, a new antispastic agent, in spasticity associated with hemiplegia. *Curr Med Res Opin* 1988; 10:709–718.

68. Mediai M, Pebet M, Ciblis D. A double-blind, long term study of tizanidine ("Sirdalud") in spasticity due to cerebrovascular lesions. *Curr Med Res Opin* 1989; 11:398–407.

69. Ketel WB, Kolb ME. Long-term treatment with dantrolene sodium of stroke patients with spasticity limiting the return to function. *Curr Med Res Opin* 1984; 9:161–169.

70. Hassan N, McLellan DL. Doubles-blind comparison of single doses of DS103–282, baclofen, and placebo for suppression of spasticity. *J Neurol Neurosurg Psychiatry* 1980; 1132–1136.

71. Katrak PH, Cole AMD, Poulos CJ, et al. Objective assessments of spasticity strength and function with early exhibition of dantrolene sodium after cerebrovascular accident: A randomized double-blind controlled study. *Arch Phys Med Rehabil* 1992; 73:4–9.

72. Davidoff RA. Antispasticity drugs: Mechanisms of action. *Ann Neurol* 1985; 17:107.

73. Medear R, Hellebuyk H, Van Den Brande E, et al. Treatment of spasticity due to stroke. A double-blind, cross-over trial comparing baclofen with placebo. *Acta Therapeutica* 1991; 17:323–331.

74. Meytheler JM, Clayton W, Davis LK, et al. Orally delivered baclofen to control spastic hypertonia in acquired brain injury. *J Head Trauma Rehabil* 2004; 19:101–208.

75. Chyatte SB, Birdsong JH, Bergman BA. The effects of dantrolene sodium on spasticity and motor performance in hemiplegia. *South Med J* 1971; 64:180–185.

76. Gelber DA, Good D, Dromerick A, et al. Open label dose-titration safety and efficacy study of tizanidine hydrochloride in the treatment of spasticity assocaited with chronic stroke. *Stroke* 2001; 32:1841–1846.

77. Nance P. Alpha adrenergic and serotonergic agents in the treatment of spastic hypertonia. *Phys Med & Rehabil Clinics of North America* 2001; 12:889–905.

78. Trainer N, Bowser BL, Dahm L. Obturator nerve block for painful hip in adult cerebral palsy. *Arch Phys Med Rehabil* 1986; 67:829–830.

79. Yadav SL, Singh U, Dureja GP, et al. Phenol block in the management of spastic cerebral palsy. *Indian J Pediatr* 1994; 61:249–255.

80. Carpenter EB. Role of nerve blocks in the foot and ankle in cerebral palsy: Therapeutic and diagnostic. *Foot Ankle* 1983; 4:164–166.

81. Khalili AA, Betts HB. Peripheral nerve block with phenol in the management of spasticity. Indications and complications. *JAMA* 1983; 200:1155–1157.

82. Botte MJ, Abrams RA, Bodine-Fowler SC. Treatment of acquired muscle spasticity using peripheral nerve blocks. *Orthopedics* 1995; 18:151–159.

83. Garland DE, Lilling M, Keenan MA. Percutaneous phenol blocks to motor points of spastic forearm muscles in head-injured adults. *Arch Phys Med Rehabil* 1984; 65:243–245.

84. Keenan MA, Tomas ES, Stone L, Gersten LM. Percutaneous phenol block of the musculocutaneous nerve to control elbow flexor spasticity. *J Hand Surg* 1990; 15:340–346.

85. Koyama H, Murakami K, Suzuki T, Suzaki K. Phenol block for hip muscle spasticity under ultrasonic monitoring. *Arch Phys Med Rehabil* 1992; 73:1040–1043.

86. Chua KSG, Kong K-H. Alcohol neurolysis of the sciatic nerve in the treatment of hemiplegic knee flexor spasticity: Clinical outcomes. *Arch Phys Med Rehabil* 2000; 81:1432–1435.

87. Gracies JM, Elovic E, McGuire J, Simpson DM. Traditional pharmacological treatments for spasticity. Part I: Local treatments. *Mucle Nerve Suppl* 1997; 6:S61–S91.

88. Wolf JH, English AW. A muscle spindle reinnervation following phenol block. *Cell Tissue Organs* 2000; 166:25–329.

89. Bodine-Fowler SC, Allsing SS. Time course of muscle atrophy and recovery following a phenol-induced nerve block. *Muscle & Nerve* 1996; 19:497–504.

90. Burkel W, McPhee M. Effect of phenol injection into peripheral nerve of rat: Electron microscope studies. *Arch Phys Med Rehabil* 1970; 50:391–397.

91. Zafonte R, Munin MC. Phenol and alcohol blocks for the treatment of spasticity. *Phys Med & Rehabil Clinics of North America* 2001; 12:817–832.

92. van Kuijk AA, Geurts ACH, Bevaart BJW, van Limbeek J. Treatment of upper extremity spasticity in stroke patients by focal neuronal or neuromuscular blockade: A systematic review of the literature. *J Rehab Med* 2002; 34:51–61.

93. Petrillo CR, Knowploch S. Phenol block of the tibial nerve for spasticity: A long-term follow-up study. *Int Disab Stud* 1998; 10:97–100.

94. Albert TA, Yelnik A, Colle FM, et al. Anatomic motor point localization for partial quadriceps block in spasticity. *Arch Phys Med Rehabil* 2000; 81:285–287.

95. Kirazli Y, On AY, Kismali B. Comparison of phenol block and botulinus toxin type A in the treatment of spastic food after stroke. *Am J Phys Med Rehabil* 1998; 77:510–515.

96. Aoki KR. Pharmacology and immunology of botulinum toxin serotypes. *J Neurol* 2001; 248:1–3.1/10.

97. dePaiva A, Meunier FA, Molgo J, Aoki KR, Dolly JO. Functional repair of motor endplates after botulinum neurotoxin type A poisoning: Byphasic switch of synaptic activity between nerve sprouts and their parent terminals. *Proc Natl Acad Sci* 1999; 96:3200–3205.

99. Davis TL, Brodsky MA, Carter VA, et al. Consensus statement on the use of botulinum neurotoxin to treat spasticity in adults. *P&T* 2006; 31:666–682.

99. Simpson DM, Alexander DN, O'Brian CF, Tagiati M, Aswad AS, Leon JM, Gibson J, et al. Botulinum toxin type A in the treatment of upper extremity spasticity: A randomized, double-blinded, placebo-controlled trial. *Neurology* 1996; 46:1306–1310.

100. Childers MK, Brashear A, Jozefczyk P, Reding M, Alexander D, Good D, Walcott JM, Jenkins SW, Turkel C, Molloy PT. Dose-dependent response to intramuscular Botulinum Toxin Type A for upper-limb spasticity in patients after stroke. *Arch Phys Med Rehabil* 2004; 85:1063–1069.

101. Bakheit AMO, Pittock S, Moore AP, Wurker M, Otto S, et al. A randomized, double-blind, placebo-controlled study of the efficacy and safety of botulinum toxin type A in upper limb spasticity in patients with stroke. *European J of Neurol* 2001; 8:559–565.

102. Bakheit AMO, Thilmann AF, Ward AB, Poewe W, et al. A randomized, double-blind, placebo-controlled, dose-ranging study to compare the efficacy and safety of three doses of botulinum toxin type A (Dysport) with placebo in upper limb spasticity after stroke. *Stroke* 2000; 31:2402–2406.

103. Smith SJ, Ellis E, White S, Moore AP. A double-blind placebo-controlled study of botulinum toxin in upper limb spasticity after stroke or head injury. *Clinical Rehabilitation* 2000; 14:5–13.

104. Burbaud P, Wiart L, Dubos JL, et al. A randomized, double blind, placebo controlled trial of botulinum toxin in the treatment of spastic foot in hemiparetic patients. *J Neurol Neurosurg Psychiatry* 1996; 61:265–269.

105. Pittock S, Moore A, Hardiman O, et al. A double-blind randomised placebo-controlled evaluation of three doses of botulinum toxin type A (Dysport) in the treatment of spastic equinovarus deformity after stroke. *Cerebrovasc Dis* 2003; 15:289–300.

106. Mancini F, Sandrini G, Moglia A, Nappi G, Pacchetti C. A randomised, double-blind, dose-ranging study to evaluate efficacy and safety of three doses of botulinum toxin type A (Botox) for the treatment of spastic foot. Neurol Sci 2005; 26:26–31.

107. Brashear A, McAfee AL, Kuhn ER, Ambrosius WT. Treatment with botulinum toxin type B for upper-limb spasticity. Arch Phys Med Rehabil 2003; 84:103–107.

108. We Move Spasticity Study Group. Dose, administration, and a treatment algorithm for use of botulinum toxin type A for adult-onset muscle overactivity in patients with an upper motoneuron lesion. A We Move Self-Study CME Activity 2002:154–165.

109. Green P, Fahn S, Diamond B. Development of resistance to botulinum toxin type A in patients with torticollis. Mov Disord 1994; 9:213.

110. Zuber M, Sebald M, Bathien N, et al. Botulinum toxin antibodies in dystonic patients treated with type A botulinum toxin. Neurology 1993; 43:1715.

111. Yablon SA, Daggett S, Brin MF. Toxin neutralizing antibody formation with botulinum toxin type A (BoNTA) treatment. Am Academ Neurol [57th Annual Meeting], 153. 2005.

112. Turkel C, Dru RM, Daggett S, Brin MF. Neutralizing antibody formation is rare following repeated injections of a low-protein formulation of botulinum toxin type A (BTX-A) in patients with post-stroke spasticity. Neurology 2002; 58:P04.148; A316.

113. Lagalla D, Danni M, Reiter F, et al. Post-stroke spasticity management with repeated botulinum toxin injections in the upper limb. Am J Phys Med Rehabil 2000; 79:377–384.

114. Nauman M, Albanese A, Heinen F, Molenaers G, Relja M. Safety and efficacy of botulinum toxin type A following long-term use. Eur J Neurol 2006; 13:35–40.

115. Francisco GE, Boake C, Vaughn A. Botulinum toxin in upper limb spasticity after acquired brain injury. A randomized trial comparing dilution techniques. Am J Phys Med Rehabil 2002; 81:355–363.

116. Gracies JM, Weisz DJ, Yang BY, Flanagan S, Simpson D. Impact of botulinum toxin type A (BTX-A) dilution and endplate targeting technique in upper limb spasticity. Ann Neurol 2002; 52:Suppl 1:S87.

117. Hesse S, Reiter F, Konrad M, Mathias JT. Botulinum toxin type A and short-term electrical stimulation in the treatment of upper limb flexor spasticity after stroke: A randomized, double-blind, placebo-controlled trial. Clinical Rehabilitation 1998; 12:381–388.

118. Reiter F, Maura D, Lagalla D, et al. Low-dose botulinum toxin with ankle taping for the treatment of spastic equinovarus foot after stroke. Arch Phys Med Rehabil 1998; 79:532.

119. Hesse S, Jahnke TM, Lucke D, Mauritz KH. Short-term electrical stimulation enhances the effectiveness of botulinum toxin in the treatment of lower limb spasticity in hemiparetic patients. Neurosci Letters 1995; 201:37–40.

120. Bhakta BB, Cozens JA, Bamford JM, Chamberlain MA. Use of botulinum toxin in stroke patients with severe upper limb spasticity. J Neurol Neurosurg Psychiatry 1996; 61:30–35.

121. Meytheler JM, Devivo M, Hadley M. Prospective study on the use of bolus intrathecal baclofen for spastic hypertonia due to acquired brain injury. Arch Phys Med Rehabil 1996; 77:461–466.

122. Meytheler JM, Guin-Renfroe S, Brunner RC, Hadley M. Intrathecal baclofen for spastic hypertonia from stroke. Stroke 2001; 32:2099–2109.

123. Schiess MC, Acosta F, Izor R, Fischer S, Furr E, Simpson R. Functional motor control improvement after intrathecal baclofen pump therapy in stroke related spastic hemiplegia. Neural Repair 2006; 66.

124. Francisco GE, Boake C. Improvement in walking speed in post-stroke spastic hemiplegia after intrathecal baclofen therapy: A preliminary study. Arch Phys Med Rehabil 2003; 84:1194–1199.

125. Remy-Neris O, Tiffreau V, Bouilland S, Bussel B. Intrathecal baclofen in subjects with spastic hemiplegia: Assessment of the antispastic effect during gait. Arch Phys Med Rehabil 2003; 84:643–650.

126. Ivanhoe C, Francisco GE, McGuire J. Intrathecal baclofen (ITB) management of post-stroke spastic hypertonia following stroke: Implications for function and quality of life. Arch Phys Med Rehabil 2006; 87:1509–1515.

127. Horn TS, Yablon SA, Stokic DS. Effect of intrathecal baclofen bolus injection on temporospatial gait characteristics in patients with acquired brain injury. Arch Phys Med Rehabil 2005; 86:1127–1133.

128. Francisco GE, Yablon S, Schiess MC, et al. Consensus panel guidelines on the use of intrathecal baclofen (ITB) therapy for post-stroke spastic hypertonia. Top Stroke Rehabil 2006; 13:74–85.

129. Brailowsky S, Knight RT, Blood K, Scabini D. Gamma-aminobutyric acid-induced potentiation of cortical hemiplegia. Brain Research 1986; 362:322–330.

130. Schallert T, Hernandez TD, Barth TM. Recovery of function after brain damage: Severe and chronic disruption by diazepam. Brain Research 1986; 379:104–111.

131. Goldstein LB. Potential effects of common drugs on stroke recovery. Arch Neurol 1998; 55:454–456.

132. Kofler M, Kronenberg MF, Rifici C, Saltuari L, Bauer G. Epileptic seizures associated with intrathecal baclofen application. Neurology 1994; 44:25–27.

133. Schuele SU, Kellinghaus C, Shook SJ, Boulis N, Bethoux F, Lodenhemper T. Incidence of seizures in patients with multiple sclerosis treated with intrathecal baclofen. Neurology 2005; 64:1086–1087.

134. Kofler M, Matzak h, Saltuari L. The impact of intrathecal baclofen in gastrointestinal function. Brain Inj 2002; 16:825–836.

135. Denys P, Mane M, Azouvi P, Chartier-Kastler E, Thibaut JB, Bussel B. Side effects of chronic intrathecal baclofen on erection and ejaculation in patients with spinal cord lesions. Arch Phys Med Rehabil 1998; 5:494–496.

136. Sheean GL. The pathophysiology of spasticity. Eur J Neurol 2002; 9:3–9.

137. Izzo KL, Aravabhumi S. Cerebrovascular accidents. Clin Podiatr Med Surg 1989; 6:745–759.

138. Keenan MA. The orthopedic management of spasticity. J Head Trauma Rehabil 1987; 2:62–71.

139. Botte MJ, Keenan MA, et al. Orthopaedic management of the stroke patient: Part II—Treating deformities of the upper and lower extremities. Orthop Rev 1988; 17:891–910.

140. Botte MJ, Waters RL, Keenan MA, et al. Orthopaedic management of the stroke patient. Orthop Rev 1988; 17:637.

141. Chambers H. The surgical treatment of spasticity. Muscle & Nerve 1997; 6:S121–S128.

142. Anmuth C, Esquenazi A, Keenan M. Lower extremity surgery for the spastic patient. Phys Med & Rehabilitation: State of the Art Reviews 1994; 8:547–577.

143. Vogt JC. Spit anterior tibial transfer for spastic equinovarus foot deformity: Retrospective study of 73 operated feet. J Foot Ankle Surg 1998; 37:2–7.

144. Edwards P, Hsu J. SPLATT combined with tendo Achilles lengthening for spastic equinovarus in adults: Results and predictors of surgical outcome. Foot Ankle 1993; 14:335–338.

145. Keenan MA, Lee GA, Tuckman AS, et al. Improving calf muscle strength in patients with spastic equinovarus deformity by transfer of the long toe flexors to the Os calcis. J Head Trauma Rehabil 1999; 14:163–175.

146. Pinzur MS, Wehner J, Kett N, et al. Brachioradialis to fingers extensor tendon transfer to achieve hand opening in acquired spasticity. J Hand Surg 1998; 13:549–552.

147. Pinzur MS. Flexor origin release and functional prehension in adult spastic hand deformity. J Hand Surg 1991; 16:133–136.

148. Keenan MA, Fuller DA, Whyte J, et al. The influence of dynamic polyelectromyography in formulating a surgical plan in treatment of spastic elbow flexion deformity. Arch Phys Med Rehabil 2003; 84:291–296.

149. Decq P, Cuny E, Filipetti P. Peripheral neurotomy in the treatment of spasticity: Indications, techniques and results in the lower limbs. Neurosurgie 1998; 44:175–182.

150. Albany K. Physical and occupational therapy considerations in adult patients receiving botulinum toxin injections for spasticity. Muscle & Nerve 1997; 6:S221–S231.

151. Boyd R, Ada L. Physiotherapy management of spasticity. In: Barnes M, Johnson G, eds. Upper Motor Neurone Syndrome and Spasticity. New York: Cambridge University Press, 2001:96–121.

152. Watanabe T. The role of therapy in spasticity management. Am J Phys Med Rehabil 2004; 83:S45–S49.

153. Gracies JM. Pathophysiology of impairment in patients with spasticity and use of stretch as a treatment of spastic hypertonia. Phys Med & Rehabil Clinics of North America 2001; 12:747–768.

154. Gracies JM. Physical modalities other than stretch in spastic hypertonia. Phys Med & Rehabil Clinics of North America 2001; 12:769–792.

155. Bobath B. Evaluation and Treatment. 3rd ed. London: William Heinemann Medical Books, 1990.

156. Wang RY, Chen HI, Chen CY, et al. Efficacy of Bobath versus orthopedic approach on impairment and function at different motor recovery stages after stroke: a randomized controlled study. Clinical Rehabilitation 2005; 19:155–164.

157. Alfieri V. Electrical treatment of spasticity. Scan J Rehabil Med 1982; 14:177–182.

158. Merletti R, Zelaschi F, Latella D, et al. A control study of muscle force recovery in hemiparetic patients during treatment with functional electrical stimulation. Scand J Rehabil Med 1978; 10:147–154.

159. Baker LL, Yeh C, Wilson D, et al. Electrical stimulation of wrist and fingers for hemiplegic patients. Phys Ther 1983; 59:1495–1500.

160. Vodovnik L, Rebersek S, Stefanovska A. Electrical stimulation for control of paralysis and therapy of abnormal movements. Scand J Rehabil Med Suppl 1988; 17:91–97.

161. Faghri PD, Rodgers MM, Glaser RM, et al. The effects of functional electrical stimulation on shoulder subluxation, arm function recovery, and shoulder pain in hemiplegic stroke patients. Arch Phys Med Rehabil 1994; 75:73–79.

162. Kraft GH, Fitts SS, Hammond MC. Techniques to improve function of the arm and hand in chronic hemiplegia. Arch Phys Med Rehabil 1992; 73:220–227.

163. Chae J, Bethoux F, Bohine T, et al. Neuromuscular stimulation for upper extremity motor and functional recovery in acute hemiplegia. Stroke 1998; 29:945–979.

164. Weingarden H, Zelig G, Heruti R, et al. A new hybrid FES-orthosis system for the upper limb-use in chronic stable hemiplegia. Am J Phys Med Rehabil 1998; 77:276–281.

165. Yu DT, Chae J, Walker ME, et al. Comparing stimulation-induced pain during percutaneous (intramuscular) and transcutaneous neuromuscular electric stimulation for treating shoulder subluxation in hemiplegia. Arch Phys Med Rehabil 2002; 82:756–760.

166. Alon G, McBride K, Ring H. Improving selected hand functions using a noninvasive neuroprosthesis in persons with chronic stroke. J Stroke Cerebrovascular Diseases 1996; 11:99–106.

167. Alon G, Stibrant K, Geurts CH, et al. A home based, self-administered stimulation program to improve selected hand functions in chronic stroke. Neuro Rehabilitation 2003; 18:215–225.

168. Hendricks HT, MJ IJ, de Kroon JR, et al. Functional electrical stimulation by means of the Ness Handmaster Orthosis in chronic stroke patients: An exploratory study. Clinical Rehabilitation 2001; 15:217–220.

169. Graziani V, Ditunno JF, Lammertse D, et al. Two multi-center trials demonstrate potential efficacy of sustained-release 4-amino-pyridine for spasticity management in subjects with spinal cord injury. Arch Phys Med Rehabil 2002; 83:1689.

170. Middleton JW, Siddall PJ, Walker S, et al. Intrathecal clonidine and baclofen in the management of spasticity and neuropathic pain following spinal cord injury. A case study. Arch Phys Med Rehabil 1996; 77:824–826.

171. Remy-Neris O, Barbea H, Daniel O. Effects of intrathecal clonidine injection on spinal reflexes and human locomotion in incomplete paraplegic subjects. Exp Brain Res 1999; 129:433–440.

172. Kroin JS, McCarthy RJ, Penn RD. Continuous intrathecal Clonidine and Tizanidine in conscious dogs: Analgesic and Hemodynamic effects. *Anesth Analg* 2003; 96:776–782.

173. Ridgeway B, Wallace M, Gerayli A. Ziconotide for the treatment of severe spasticity after spinal cord injury. *Pain* 2000; 85:287–289.

174. Mukherjee M, McPeak LK, Redford JB, Sun C, Liu W. The effect of electro-acupuncture on spasticity of the wrist joint in chronic stroke survivors. *Arch Phys Med Rehabil* 2007; 88:159–166.

175. Moon S-K, Whang Y-K, Park S-U, Ko C-N, Kim Y-S, et al. Antispastic effect of electroacupuncture and moxibustion in stroke patients. *Am J Chinese Med* 2003; 31:467–474.

176. Wayne PM, Krebs DE, Macklin EA, Schnyer R, Kaptchuck TJ, et al. Acupuncture for upper extremity rehabilitation in chronic stroke: A randomized Sham-controlled study. *Arch Phys Med Rehabil* 2005; 86:2248–2255.

177. Fink M, Rollnick JD, Bijak M, Borstadt C, Dauper J, et al. Needle acupuncture in chronic poststroke leg spasticity. *Arch Phys Med Rehabil* 2004; 85:667–672.

178. Campos RJ, Dimitrijevic MR, Sharkey PC, Sherwood AM. Epidural spinal cord stimulation in spastic spinal cord injury patients. Meeting of the American Society for Stereotactic and Functional Neurosurgery. *Appl Neurophysiol* 1987; 50:453–454.

179. Cioni B, Meglio M, Prezioso A, Talamonti G, Tirenti M. Spinal cord stimulation (SCS) in spastic hemiparesis. PACE 1989; April, Part II:739–742.

180. Bhadra N, Kilgore K. Block of mammalian motor nerve conduction using high frequency alternating current. 2nd International IEEE EMBS Conference. *Neural Engineering* [March 16-19], 479–481. 2005.
Ref Type: Conference Proceeding

181. Kilgore KL, Bhadra N. Nerve conduction block utilizing high frequency alternating current. *Med & Biol Eng & Comput* 2004; 42:394–406.

182. McClelland SI, Teng Q, Benson LS, Boulis NM. Motor neuron inhibition-based gene therapy for spasticity. *Am J Phys Med Rehabil* 2007; 86:412–421.

183. Pavesi G, Brianti R, Medici D, Mammi P. Botulinum toxin type A in the treatment of upper limb spasticity among patients with traumatic brain injury. *J Neurol Neurosurg Psychiatry* 1998; 64:419–420.

184. Wang HC, Hsieh LF, Chi WC, Lou SM. Effects of intramuscular botulinum toxing injection in upper limb spasticity in stroke patients. *Am J Phys Med Rehabil* 2002; 81:272–278.

185. Panizza M, Castagna M, diSumma A, et al. Functional and clinical changes in upper limb spastic patients treated with botulinum toxin (BTX). *Funct Neurol* 2000; 15:147–155.

186. Sampaio C, Ferreira J, Pinto AA. Botulinum toxin type A for the treatment of arm and hand spasticity in stroke patients. *Clinical Rehabilitation* 1997; 11:3–7.

187. Girlanda P, Quartarone A, Sinicropi S, et al. Botulinum toxin in upper limb spasticity: Study of reciprocal inhibition between forearm muscles. *NeuroReport* 1997; 8:3039–3044.

188. Palmer D, Horn LJ, Harmon R. Botulinum toxin treatment of lumbrical spasticity: A brief report. *Am J Phys Med Rehabil* 1998; 77:348–350.

189. Snow BI, Tsui JKC, Bhatt MH, et al. Treatment of spasticity with botulinum toxin: A double-blind study. *Ann Neurol* 1990; 28:512.

190. Childers MK, Stacy M, Cooper PR. Comparison of two injection techniques using botulinum toxin in spastic hemiplegia. *Am J Phys Med Rehabil* 1996; 75:462–469.

191. Yelnik A, Colle FM, Bonan I, Lamotte DR. Disabling overactivity of the extensor hallucis longus after stroke clinical expression and efficacy of botulinum toxin type A. *Arch Phys Med Rehabil* 2003; 84:147–149.

192. Suputtitada A. Botulinum toxin type A injections in the treatment of spastic toes. *Am J Phys Med Rehabil* 2002; 81:770–775.

26 Shoulder Pain and Other Musculoskeletal Complications

David Tzehsia Yu

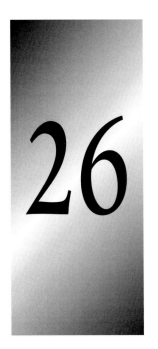

Musculoskeletal complications are common after stroke, occurring in approximately one-third of stroke survivors during inpatient rehabilitation (1, 2). The cumulative incidence of musculoskeletal pain among stroke survivors and the prevalence of musculoskeletal pain during various phases of recovery after stroke have not been well documented, with the exception of shoulder pain. Among musculoskeletal complications due to stroke, shoulder pain has been by far the most studied. Thus, though this chapter seeks to discuss the spectrum of musculoskeletal complications due to stroke, the bulk of the chapter discusses shoulder pain. It should also be noted that this chapter only addresses musculoskeletal complications that result directly from stroke. Musculoskeletal complications that are an indirect consequence of stroke, such as traumatic fractures that may occur due to the increased risk of falls experienced by many stroke survivors, are not included.

The quantity of musculoskeletal complications after stroke, particularly shoulder pain, that are refractory to available treatments and become chronic testifies to the current standards of care and state of research, and underlines the need for further work. Where data are available, an evidence-based approach to diagnosis and management of specific conditions is outlined. Where the data are equivocal, the author has often tried to provide a concise review for the reader's interpretation. Where the data are insufficient, the author has attempted to make recommendations based on expert opinion. Though a formal evaluation system was not used, the strength of the evidence for given recommendations is discussed.

SHOULDER PAIN

While the pathogenesis of shoulder pain and diagnoses causing shoulder pain after stroke remain controversial, shoulder pain is clearly a common complication after stroke that can inhibit functional recovery and reduce quality of life. Although the shoulder is technically comprised of three joints (glenohumeral joint, acromioclavicular joint, and sternoclavicular joint) and one articulation (scapulothoracic articulation), post-stroke shoulder pain by convention refers to pathology affecting the glenohumeral joint (Figure 26-1). Many types of shoulder pathology after stroke have been reported in the literature, including shoulder subluxation, impingement syndrome, rotator cuff injury, tendonitis, bursitis, capsulitis, peripheral nerve injuries, complex regional pain syndrome, spasticity, and contractures. No single type of pathology accounts for all shoulder pain after stroke. Conversely, it is important to recognize that more than one type of shoulder pathology may cause pain within an individual.

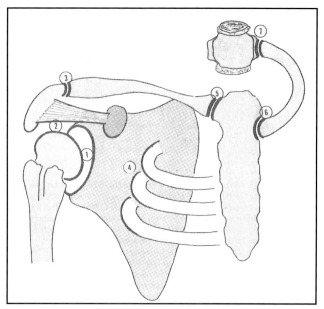

FIGURE 26-1

The joints of the shoulder girdle: (1) Glenohumeral; (2) Suprahumeral; (3) Acromioclavicular; (4) Scapulothoracic; (5) Sternoclavicular; (6) Costosternal; (7) Costovertebral *Reproduced with permission from Caillet R. Shoulder Pain. Philadelphia PA: F.A. Davis Co., 1981, p. 2.*

Among potential risk factors cited in the literature, shoulder pain after stroke has been most consistently correlated with severity of motor impairment (3–5). Less evidence is available for other reported risk factors, including duration of motor impairment (6), sensory impairment (3, 5), reduced range of motion (6), spasticity (7), and comorbidities such as diabetes mellitus. Thus, the prevalence of shoulder pain is higher for hemiplegic stroke survivors when compared to all stroke survivors. Because of the association between shoulder pain and motor impairment, shoulder pain as a complication of stroke is often referred to as hemiplegic shoulder pain (HSP). Langhorne et al. reported a 15% peak prevalence of shoulder pain between hospital discharge and 6 months after stroke among all stroke survivors (with or without hemiplegia) admitted to the hospital. In this prospective study, 9%, 15%, 11% and 12% of all stroke survivors had shoulder pain during hospitalization, from discharge to 6 months, from 6 to 18 months, and from 18 to 30 months, respectively (8). Among hemiplegic stroke survivors, the reported prevalence of shoulder pain ranges from 34% (9) to 84% (10). A study of one of the largest cohorts of hemiplegic subjects followed prospectively for an average of 11 months probably provides the best estimate of the incidence of shoulder pain in hemiplegic stroke survivors. In this study, shoulder pain occurred in 72% of hemiplegic stroke survivors (7).

The association between motor impairment and shoulder pain after stroke at first appears intuitive, but becomes more enigmatic as the data are reviewed. The glenohumeral joint is inherently unstable, seemingly designed for mobility while sacrificing stability, a design that permits individuals to utilize the hand within a large work volume. As a ball and socket joint, its mechanics contrast with the hip, a ball and socket joint that seems to have been designed for stability while sacrificing mobility. The shoulder socket, or glenoid fossa, is relatively shallow and contacts only about 10% of the surface area of the ball or humeral head. The articulating surface area is increased by 75% with the addition of the glenoid labrum, a cartilaginous ring that lines the periphery of the glenoid fossa. The glenohumeral joint is enveloped by a fibrous capsule and ligaments that are essentially thickened regions of the joint capsule. Though the capsule and ligaments provide passive restraint in multiple directions, they are not sufficient to provide joint stability, particularly during movement. Rather, it is the active restraints or muscles around the shoulder, including but not limited to the rotator cuff, that convey stability to the joint. Considering the mechanics of the glenohumeral joint, it seems intuitive that shoulder pathology after stroke would correlate with the degree of motor impairment in light of the essential role of active restraints (i.e. shoulder muscles) in maintaining joint stability. However, a cause and effect relationship between motor impairment and pain via joint instability comes into question, because studies evaluating the relationship between shoulder instability (measured in most studies in the inferior direction only) and pain have not consistently demonstrated a correlation. The role of shoulder subluxation in the genesis of shoulder pain after stroke remains controversial. Studies that evaluate this relationship will be discussed in the section on shoulder subluxation. To evaluate the relationship further, a critical review of the studies, methods, and recommendations for further research will be discussed in the section on research frontiers.

Although the pathogenesis and natural history of shoulder pain after stroke remain controversial, the literature evaluating the presence of shoulder pain over time is more consistent. It is clear that shoulder pain can be present during various periods after stroke. Although a significant number of cases occur during initial hospitalization, the prevalence of shoulder pain increases after hospital discharge, reaching a peak between hospital discharge and 6 months, and tending to decline after 6 months (4). Gamble et al. reported resolution of pain in 80% of cases when management included prompt diagnosis and early, appropriate intervention (5). However, studies consistently report a significant number of cases that do not resolve, with 12% of all stroke survivors reporting shoulder pain at 30 months post-stroke (8), and 20% of moderately to severely impaired stroke survivors

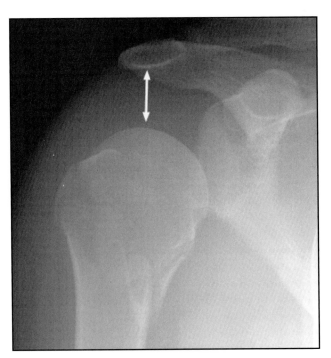

FIGURE 26-2

An anteroposterior radiograph of a inferiorly subluxed shoulder.

reporting pain four years post-stroke (4). The data suggest that post-stroke shoulder pain can improve in many cases with prompt diagnosis and appropriate intervention, but that a significant number of cases become chronic and refractory to available treatments.

SHOULDER SUBLUXATION

Subluxation is defined as partial dissociation or increased translation between two articulating surfaces of a joint (11) (Figure 26-2). Subluxation may be contrasted to dislocation, defined as complete dissociation between two articulating surfaces of a joint. By convention, shoulder subluxation due to hemiparesis after stroke refers to increased translation of the humeral head relative to the glenoid fossa. Generally, in clinical practice and in research, shoulder subluxation after stroke is measured in the inferior direction, with the upper limb in a dependent position allowing the weight of the limb to distract the humeral head from the glenoid fossa (6, 7, 12–24). Though these methods have become the standard by convention, the content validity of measuring only inferior subluxation is questionable and may contribute to the inconsistent correlation between subluxation and pain reported in the literature. Inferior subluxation as the most clinically relevant measure of glenohumeral instability after stroke will be critically evaluated in the "Research Frontiers" section of this chapter.

Shoulder subluxation is common in hemiplegia. Though subluxation has been reported to occur in up to 81% of cases (19), several studies, including one of the largest cohorts of hemiplegic subjects followed over months, suggest that the best estimate of the incidence of inferior shoulder subluxation in hemiplegia may be approximately 50% (7). Though shoulder subluxation is one of the most commonly cited causes of shoulder pain in the literature, the relationship between subluxation and pain remains controversial. While a number of studies suggest a correlation between subluxation and pain (7, 10, 25), others have demonstrated no correlation (24, 26–28). When considering the role of subluxation in the pathogenesis of pain, two questions must be considered. First, does subluxation directly cause pain? The lack of correlation between subluxation and pain in several studies strongly suggests that subluxation is not a direct cause of pain in many cases. However, on an individual basis, painful subluxation is difficult to refute when shoulder pain decreases during manual reduction of a subluxed joint, particularly in the absence of other pathology. Second, does subluxation cause pain by predisposing the shoulder to other types of painful pathology? Several studies have corroborated this notion by demonstrating a correlation between shoulder subluxation after stroke and the development of other causes of shoulder pain including complex regional pain syndrome, peripheral neuropathies, and rotator cuff injury(10, 29–31).

Shoulder subluxation in hemiplegia occurs due to the paralysis of active restraints that play a critical role in maintaining glenohumeral stability (32–35). Shoulder subluxation tends to occur early after stroke, with most cases occurring within the first three weeks, particularly in patients with flaccid hemiplegia (13). Spasticity develops in most hemiplegic patients and may have an effect on reducing shoulder subluxation. An inverse correlation between shoulder subluxation and spasticity has been reported in two studies where authors attribute the reduction of subluxation to return of muscle tone or volitional activation (13, 16). In another study, subluxation was reduced only when shoulder muscles became spastic within the first week post-stroke, but was not reduced when spasticity occurred three weeks or later post-stroke. This suggests that there may be a critical, brief time window for spasticity to have an effect on reducing subluxation (13). The results of this study also suggest that the passive restraints of the shoulder may only be sufficient for maintaining joint stability for a short period of time. Stretching of the joint capsule and ligaments may not be reversible after a point. In only one study, a higher incidence of shoulder subluxation was found when spastic and flaccid hemiplegic subjects were compared (7). Studies of functional electric stimulation (FES) of shoulder muscles to reduce subluxation after stroke also suggest that changes in muscle properties can reduce subluxation.

However, it is not clear whether relevant changes in muscle properties are due to the improvement in muscle tone, improvement in purely passive mechanical properties, or less likely, improvement in voluntary muscle contraction. The majority of FES studies have shown that stimulation-induced muscle contraction can reduce subluxation. Several of these studies have shown that the reduction of subluxation is maintained for months after muscle stimulation has been discontinued, suggesting an effect of passive muscle properties(12, 15, 23, 36). Though a few studies have shown that subluxation can be reduced in chronic stroke patients, a 2002 meta-analysis of the data suggests that FES for reducing post-stroke shoulder subluxation is most effective when applied early after stroke (37).

The clinical diagnosis of shoulder subluxation can be made without imaging studies. The most commonly used clinical measure of shoulder subluxation in hemiplegia quantifies inferior subluxation by determining the number of fingerbreadths that can be inserted between the inferior border of the acromion and the superior border of the humeral head while the patient is seated with the upper limbs hanging passively. The patient is seated because muscle tone may increase in the standing position, reducing the subluxation. Comparison to the unaffected shoulder is recommended, but care should be taken to palpate only the bony landmarks in order to avoid misinterpreting a unilateral flaccid or atrophied deltoid muscle as the difference between shoulders. The clinical fingerbreadth measure detects abnormal translation in the inferior direction only. This clinical measure has a resolution of a half fingerbreadth, and does not detect small changes in glenohumeral displacement that may be significant. Despite anatomical variability in finger widths, the reliability of the fingerbreadth measure has been established (38). The reliability of this technique may be in part a function of its limited resolution. Imaging studies such as plain radiographs, computed tomography, ultrasound, and magnetic resonance imaging will also show subluxation, often with greater resolution and the ability to detect abnormal translation in other dimensions. Because the clinical significance of subluxation in multiple dimensions is not known, the significance of small amounts of subluxation is not known. Because the role of subluxation as a cause of pain is controversial, these additional studies are not currently standards for diagnosing shoulder subluxation.

Despite the controversial relationship between shoulder subluxation and pain, treatment of subluxation continues to be the standard of care in rehabilitation facilities for several reasons. First, shoulder subluxation may be painful in some cases, particularly when manual reduction of the subluxed joint diminishes pain. Second, shoulder subluxation may predispose hemiplegic patients to the development of other painful conditions. If chronic shoulder pain develops, it is often refractory to available treatment, warranting prevention for at-risk patients and prompt treatment in patients with subluxation. Third, subluxation may inhibit functional recovery by limiting range of motion. Support of the hemiplegic upper limb in the seated and standing positions remains the standard of care for stroke survivors with shoulder subluxation, and those with flaccid paralysis of shoulder muscles who are at risk for developing shoulder subluxation. Upper limb support includes the use of wheelchair adaptations and judicious use of selected slings. When seated in the wheelchair, hemi-trays are appropriate for patients with sufficient motor function to maintain the upper limb in a resting position on the tray. Whereas a trough, in some cases with Velcro enclosures, attached to the wheelchair is suited for patients who lack sufficient motor control to prevent the upper limb from sliding from a tray. It should be mentioned, however, that wheelchair arm troughs and trays have not been shown to reduce subluxation or pain, and occasionally have been thought to predispose the affected shoulder to impingement syndromes (39, 40). Selected slings may be used to support the affected upper limb during transfers and ambulation. A neoprene cuff-type hemisling is recommended (Figure 26-3). Slings that place bulky material, such as a roll, under the axilla may cause lateral subluxation. Swath-type slings that hold the shoulder in adduction and internal rotation and the elbow in flexion should be avoided because they can rapidly lead to capsulitis, cause contractures over time, and promote

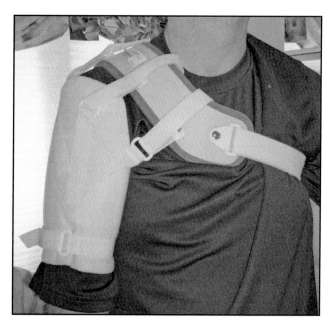

FIGURE 26-3

A neoprene cuff-type hemisling used to treat shoulder subluxation.

undesirable synergistic patterns of muscle activation (40). The use of tape to support the subluxated glenohumeral joint, known as strapping, has been evaluated in randomized, controlled trials with mixed results (41, 42). A Cochrane review of external supports suggests that strapping may delay the onset of shoulder pain, but does not reduce pain severity or associated disability (43). The limitations of orthotic applications such as strapping, slings, and wheelchair adaptations have prompted investigators to evaluate the efficacy of FES for reducing post-stroke shoulder subluxation and pain. The stimulation is most commonly delivered through electrodes placed on the skin surface (i.e. transcutaneous FES.) Electrodes are typically placed over the posterior deltoid and supraspinatus muscles. Baker et al. proposed that placing the cathode over the deltoid and the anode over the supraspinatus would reduce undesirable stimulation to the upper trapezius and resultant shoulder shrugging (12). Stimulation is typically delivered for 6 hours daily for 6 weeks. Transcutaneous FES reduces shoulder subluxation when applied within weeks of stroke onset (14, 15, 37). Clinical trials evaluating the efficacy of transcutaneous FES for reducing subluxation in chronic hemiplegia (12) and for reducing shoulder pain have yielded mixed results (14, 15). Clinical application of transcutaneous FES has been limited for several reasons. First, stimulation of cutaneous nociceptors results in stimulation-induced pain. Pain with transcutaneous FES is a well-recognized entity, and methods to improve tolerance to treatment have been described. Basically, stimulation time or intensity can be gradually increased until tolerance for therapeutic stimulation is achieved (12, 44). However, this strategy does not promote tolerance in all cases. Furthermore, it is time-consuming for the therapist and patient, and may not be practical under economic pressures to reduce cost. Approximately 30% of hemiplegic patients do not tolerate transcutaneous FES even when methods to enhance tolerance are employed (17). Second, activation of deep muscles cannot be achieved without stimulation of more superficial muscles. Third, clinical skill is required to place the electrodes and adjust stimulation parameters to provide optimal treatment. Treatment is typically administered daily by a skilled therapist. Few patients are able to administer treatments at home by themselves or with the assistance of a caregiver. Fourth, transcutaneous FES may interfere with the user's daily activities. Surface electrodes can be displaced from the skin during movement, and connecting leads can be accidentally pulled during activity. The significance of this limitation is obvious when considering that most treatment regimens require stimulation over hours, daily, for weeks.

Newer technologies permit direct stimulation of target peripheral nerve or motor points through percutaneously-placed electrodes (Figure 26-4). FES delivered through electrodes implanted near target nerve has several potential advantages over transcutaneous FES. First, percutaneous FES is less painful than transcutaneous FES for reducing shoulder subluxation after stroke (45). The stimulating surface of the electrode is placed near the peripheral nerve or muscle motor point so that stimulation of cutaneous nociceptors can be avoided, and lower stimulus intensities are required. Undesirable stimulation of adjacent muscles not intended for stimulation can be avoided. Second, implanted electrodes are optimally placed at the beginning of treatment and remain in place for the treatment duration. Thus, the system is more reliable, can be administered by the user or caregiver at home, and obviates the need for daily application by a therapist. At home, donning and doffing of a partially-implanted system comprised of electrodes implanted near motor points with external leads and an external stimulator required less than five minutes daily. This partially-implanted system also permitted users to perform typical daily activities while receiving treatment. The efficacy of electric stimulation delivered directly to peripheral nerve using this partially-implanted system for treating shoulder pain in chronic stroke patients with hemiparesis and subluxation was demonstrated in a multicenter randomized clinical trial. In this trial, pain reduction remained significant for at least one year after completing treatment. Of note, the reduction of subluxation between treatment and controls was not significant, calling into question the mechanism of pain reduction (46–48). Other partially-implanted systems comprised of fully-implanted electrodes and external stimulators requiring bulky metal coils to provide radio-frequency links between stimulator and electrode have been evaluated in non-randomized clinical trials. These trials suggest efficacy for reducing shoulder subluxation, but pain was not measured. A fully-implanted FES system comprised of a percutaneously injected microstimulator, battery, and electrode housed within a titanium and ceramic cylinder is currently under clinical investigation. The potential advantages of this fully-implanted system are numerous. It obviates the need for users to wear external components, making it easier to use, reliability is improved, infection risk posed by percutaneous hardware is avoided, and the risk of accidental electrode displacement is reduced. The system is designed to remain in the body for the life of the user. Thus, chronic or repetitive treatment is facilitated.

In summary, shoulder subluxation tends to occur early after stroke in patients with flaccid hemiplegia, and may be reversible through facilitation of muscle tone, motor recovery, or stimulated muscle contraction. There may be a brief, critical time window for reducing subluxation during the acute phase after stroke. The use of external upper limb support, including judicious use of slings and wheelchair adaptations, is indicated for patients with subluxation or those with flaccid hemiparesis who are at risk. FES reduces subluxation in acute stroke, but

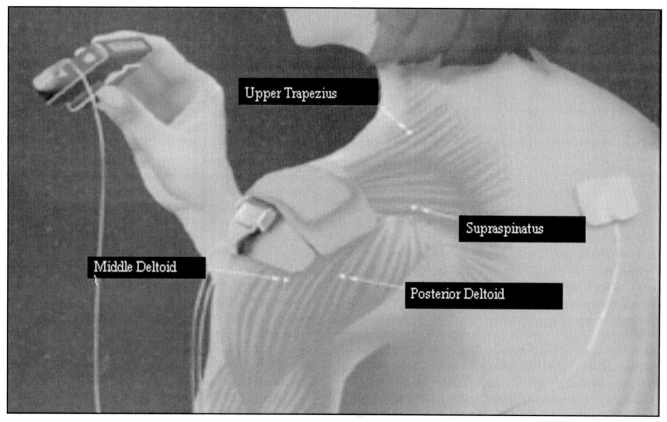

FIGURE 26-4

A percutaneous system of electrical stimulation for the shoulder. The system consists of a percutaneously injected microstimulator, battery and electrode housed within a titanium and ceramic cylinder.

the effect on subluxation in chronic stroke and the effect on reducing shoulder pain have not been established. The role of FES in treating shoulder dysfunction after stroke is evolving rapidly, with new technology under investigation that improves the clinical practicality and effectiveness of FES for treating post-stroke shoulder dysfunction.

CAPSULITIS AND RELATED CONDITIONS

Capsulitis, also known as *adhesive capsulitis* or *frozen shoulder*, is a common complication after stroke, and refers to shortening of the glenohumeral joint capsule and ligaments that are largely thickenings of the capsule. Several studies suggest that capsulitis may be one of the most significant causes of shoulder pain after stroke (6, 49, 50). The inflammatory response seen in this condition probably results from irritation and injury to shortened capsular fibers. The term "adhesive" refers to adhesions of the capsule found by Neviaser et al. during surgery (51). Other authors report fibrosis of the capsule but no adhesions found at the time of surgery (52). Fibrosis most likely

occurs in the chronic phase of this condition if inadequately treated.

On physical examination, decreased shoulder external rotation and abduction associated with pain is the hallmark of capsulitis. Because many patients with spastic hemiparesis have tonic adduction and internal rotation of the shoulder, shortening of shoulder internal rotators is common. Thus, palpation of these muscles during the exam is useful to determine whether musculotendinous shortening contributes to decreased range of motion and pain. It is also useful to measure passive shoulder rotation with the shoulder in adduction, because shoulder internal rotators have more slack than in abduction. In practice, shortening of capsular fibers often coexists with spasticity and shortening of the internal rotators of the shoulder (i.e. subscapularis, pectoralis, anterior deltoid, teres major, and latissimus muscles.) In such cases, treatment of all contributing entities affords better and longer-lasting outcomes than treatment of only one. In the stroke literature, decreased shoulder abduction and external rotation due to end range of motion or pain is often considered diagnostic of capsulitis, making it difficult to assess the relative contribution of spastic or shortened shoulder muscles in many published studies.

Keeping in mind the potential contribution of spastic shoulder muscles, the diagnosis of capsulitis can, in most cases, be made by physical exam alone. Occasionally, intra-articular injection of an anesthetic agent can corroborate the diagnosis or help to evaluate the relative contribution to shoulder pain when multiple diagnoses are suspected. Usually, there is already a high index of suspicion and the diagnostic injection is combined with therapeutic steroids. Arthrography can also be diagnostic, but usually is not warranted. Typical findings on arthrography include a scalloped appearance of the joint space border or a capsule that accommodates significantly less than the expected 12 ml of contrast. Contrast seen in the subacromial bursa after intra-articular injection typically indicates a rotator cuff tear.

Treatment of capsulitis is comprised of restoration of range of motion and reduction of inflammation. If spasticity or shortening of shoulder muscles contributes to pain, limits function, or predisposes to recurrent capsulitis, additional measures may be indicated. When possible, management of inflammation, spasticity, and pain should be performed concurrently with restoration of motion. Oral anti-inflammatory medications are sometimes useful, but in this author's experience, intra-articular injection of moderate to long acting steroids yields better results. It should be noted that intra-articular steroid injection did not yield statistically significant shoulder pain reduction after stroke in one randomized clinical trial. However, enrolled subjects were not selected based on a diagnosis of capsulitis without other pathology. Thus, a dilutional effect is likely. Moreover, the sample size was inadequate. A power calculation was performed based on the results from a preliminary case series, revealing a power of only 50%. Overall, the study demonstrated a mean pain reduction of 2.3 and 0.2 (p=.06) using a 10cm visual analogue scale in the treatment and control groups, respectively. No adverse events were reported(53). Thus, the study suggests that intra-articular steroid injection is safe, but conclusions with respect to efficacy cannot be made due primarily to the unacceptably high risk of type II error.

Restoring range of motion is best accomplished under the supervision of a therapist, with close communication between therapist and physician. Changes in range of motion should be monitored for progress. Improvement in range of motion provides important feedback to patients and caregivers. More importantly, if range of motion does not improve as expected, underlying biomechanical barriers, such as spasticity or medical barriers, such as pain, may need to be addressed. Care should be taken to avoid impingement problems caused by excessive shoulder abduction without concomitant external rotation. As mentioned previously, swath-type slings

that hold the shoulder in adduction and internal rotation should be avoided. Caregiver training and home supervision are important in most cases, because stroke survivors with hemiplegia often have some degree of neglect that may require cues for performing the appropriate range of motion exercises and promote attention to upper limb positioning in bed. Caregivers are often able to assist with range of motion exercises that patients have difficulty performing independently. Caregiver involvement becomes more critical in the setting of more pronounced unilateral neglect or cognitive impairment.

If spasticity or contracture of shoulder muscles contributes to reduced range of motion and capsulitis, oral spasmolytic medications, neuromuscular blockade with botulinum toxin, or neurolysis should be considered. Though use of spasmolytic medications is discussed in Chapter 27, it is worth noting that the systemic effect of spasmolytic medications on other functions must be considered (e.g. is the extensor tone in the lower limb required for weight bearing?) Several studies have evaluated the effect of botulinum toxin or chemical neurolysis on various muscles around the shoulder with mixed results. In a double-blind, randomized trial, botulinum toxin to the subscapularis muscle in selected patients resulted in less pain and improved range of motion(54). A case series evaluating phenol neurolysis to the subscapularis muscle yielded similar results. The author described a technique using a medial approach and emphasized the need to block at least two motor points of the muscle (50). Though neuromuscular blockade or neurolysis may benefit selected patients, the selection criteria for these procedures need to be further elucidated. At this time, it is recommended that use of neuromuscular blockade or neurolysis be considered only after careful evaluation of the effect on individual muscles on a patient-by-patient basis.

IMPINGEMENT SYNDROME AND ROTATOR CUFF INJURY

Impingement syndrome refers to injury to the supraspinatus muscle or tendon resulting from repetitive compression between the inferior border of the acromion and the greater tuberosity of the humerus. The greater tuberosity of the humerus rotates under the acromion with internal shoulder rotation, diminishing space for the supraspinatus muscle and tendon during shoulder abduction. Repetitive compression of the supraspinatus muscle occurs when the shoulder is abducted greater than 90 degrees without concomitant shoulder external rotation. Though not adequately studied, biomechanical changes after stroke such as laxity of passive restraints due to subluxation, weakness of muscles that stabilize the joint, abnormal muscle tone, and motor recovery in a proximal to distal gradient may place stroke survivors at greater risk for impingement syndrome. Inflammation of the supraspinatus muscle and tendon, and the surrounding subacromial bursa, are common sequelae. Though rotator cuff injury can occur due to trauma and may include any of the four rotator cuff muscles, after stroke, rotator cuff injury generally refers to injury to the supraspinatus muscle or tendon that occurs as a result of impingement that has not been adequately addressed (10, 55) (Figure 26-5).

The roles of impingement syndrome and rotator cuff injury have not been rigorously studied as a cause of shoulder pain after stroke. In some circles, their contribution to post-stroke shoulder pain is well accepted, while in others it remains controversial. Joynt et al. were able to produce moderately or markedly reduced pain in half of 28 subjects with chronic hemiplegia and functionally limiting shoulder pain by injecting lidocaine near the subacromial region of the affected shoulder. These results indirectly suggest that impingement syndrome, supraspinatus tendonitis, or subacromial bursitis are common causes of pain in hemiplegic stroke patients. Najenson

et al. found arthrographic changes diagnostic of rotator cuff tear in 40% of 32 subjects on the hemiplegic side, compared with 16% on the unaffected side. In all cases, evidence of rotator cuff rupture was accompanied by moderate to severe shoulder pain. The authors postulated that "pinching of the tuberosity cuff ligament insertion zone against the acromian which occurs when the arm is forcibly abducted without concommitant external rotation" served as the common mechanism of injury. The authors emphasize avoidance of injury by externally rotating the shoulder during passive shoulder abduction (10). In contrast, Hakuno et al., also using arthrography, did not find a difference in the incidence of rotator cuff tears between the affected and unaffected sides of 77 hemiplegic subjects (56). No rotator cuff tears were diagnosed by arthrography among 30 spastic, hemiplegic subjects in another study (49).

Prevention is the critical component of managing impingement syndrome and includes measures to prevent the syndrome from occurring as well as preventing further injury once it exists. Shoulder flexion or abduction, whether during passive or active exercise, should always be accompanied by external rotation. Altered biomechanics of the shoulder in hemiplegia resulting in displacement of the arc of the humeral head and tubercle may predisposed to impingement (57). Overhead passive range of motion exercises with shoulder internal rotation and the use of overhead pulleys that promote similar movement have been implicated as causes of impingement syndrome (10). Wheelchair arm supports have also been implicated (40). Care should also be taken to ensure that inadequate trunk control does not result in weight bearing through the elbow to the glenohumeral joint, particularly when it causes shoulder pain or occurs in the presence of hemisensory loss, unilateral neglect, or severe cognitive impairment. Inflammation may be reduced with oral anti-inflammatory medications or steroid injection to the subacromial bursa. Ultimately, as in able-bodied patients, treatment should attempt to enhance shoulder posture, particularly in retraction and elevation, and restore active restraints by strengthening the external and internal rotators of the shoulder. However, an adequate strengthening regimen may not be possible due to severity of hemiparesis. Theoretically, electrically stimulated exercise of appropriate muscles may be an alternative, but the efficacy of FES for impingement syndrome has not been investigated.

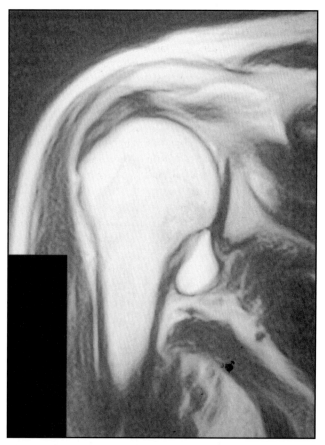

FIGURE 26-5

An example of a full-thickness tear of the rotator cuff with tendon retraction.

COMPLEX REGIONAL PAIN SYNDROME

Much of the literature discussing complex regional pain syndrome (CRPS) after stroke predates the recent nomenclature and refers to reflex sympathetic dystrophy (RSD) or shoulder hand syndrome. Generally, CRPS after stroke refers to type I, because it follows central nervous system injury. However, as discussed later in this section, root level injury or peripheral nerve injury may result from traction to neural tissue from persistent shoulder subluxation or possibly compression of nerve between bones. Thus, it is possible that *causalgia* or *complex regional pain syndrome type II* may also occur, but has not been specifically discussed in the stroke literature to date. Agreement among clinicians and scientists regarding the definitions and diagnostic criteria for CRPS have improved greatly over the past decades. By the same token, variability in the definitions and diagnostic criteria of CRPS are common in the earlier literature, and often complicate the evaluation of CRPS as a cause of shoulder pain after stroke. Vasomotor changes, edema, temperature changes, limited range of motion, limb pain, and eventual bony changes are the hallmarks of CRPS I that result from dysregulation of the autonomic nervous system.

The reported prevalence of CRPS I in hemiplegia ranges from 12.5% (58) to 70% (59). The variability in reported prevalence of CRPS I may result from differences in the diagnostic criteria used. Tepperman documented increased radionuclide uptake in the wrist, metacarpophalangeal (MCP) or interphalangeal joints of the hemiplegic upper limb on delayed images using scintigraphy in 25% of 85 hemiplegic subjects. The incidence of shoulder pain in these subjects was not reported. In their study group, the authors reported 100% sensitivity and specificity for MCP tenderness relative to their scintigraphic diagnostic criteria for CRPS I (60). VanOuwenaller found that 50 (23%) of 157 hemiplegic subjects with shoulder pain had physical findings of CRPS I. The majority of these subjects had radiographic evidence of shoulder subluxation (92%) or spasticity (94%), suggesting that they may have played a role in the pathogenesis of the CRPS I (7). Other studies of stroke cohorts over time also correlate early subluxation with the development of CRPS, suggesting traction injury to vasonervorum as a possible etiology (7, 31).

The diagnosis of CRPS I after stroke often can be made clinically. Triple-phase bone scan remains the diagnostic gold standard, and may be indicated when the diagnosis is unclear or response to treatment is inadequate. The typical presentation includes pain and limited range of motion at the shoulder, wrist, and hand, sparing the elbow. These findings are often accompanied by edema, warmth, and redness, primarily involving the wrist and hand. CRPS I typically evolves through three phases: 1) a primary inflammatory phase characterized by painful range of motion, edema, warmth, and erythema of the hand and wrist; 2) a secondary atrophic phase characterized by atrophic skin changes, progressive loss of range of motion, reduced skin temperature, and occasionally pain reduction; and 3) a final phase characterized by irreversible skin and muscle atrophy, variable pain,

severe loss of range of motion, and extensive osteoporosis. Triple-phase bone scan reveals radionuclide uptake in the pooling phase in a typical pattern involving the shoulder, wrist, and hand, particularly in the carpal and metacarpal joints.

Early diagnosis and treatment are paramount. Thus, bone scan is warranted when the decision to begin treatment remains unclear after careful exam. Oral prednisone and exercise usually comprise the initial treatment. Failing initial treatment, a host of pharmacological approaches have been investigated with variable results. The specifics of these studies are beyond the scope of this chapter, and additional literature review is recommended if these treatments are pursued. More invasive measures such as cervical sympathetic ganglia blocks, Bier blocks, and cervical sympathectomy may be warranted in cases that are refractory to medications and physical therapy.

BRACHIAL PLEXOPATHY AND AXILLARY NERVE INJURY

Brachial plexus injury and other peripheral nerve injuries as causes of shoulder pain after stroke are controversial, due primarily to the lack of a diagnostic gold standard. While electromyography (EMG) is considered the diagnostic gold standard for brachial plexus injuries, electrodiagnosis of brachial plexopathy in hemiplegia is confounded by loss of motor units that result from loss of descending input from upper motor neurons after central nervous system injury (61). Further, proximal nerve conduction studies lack reliability, because volume conducted potentials from non-target muscles affect recorded potentials from target muscles. The use of advanced imaging techniques to evaluate nerve injury has yet to be reported.

Prolonged nerve conduction latencies in the proximal upper limb of hemiplegic subjects have been reported by several investigators (29, 30, 62). Interpretations of these findings differ based on the diagnostic criteria used. Chino documented significantly delayed latencies of the suprascapular, axillary, musculocutaneous, and radial nerves compared with published normative values, and evidence of denervation on needle EMG in 21 hemiplegic subjects with shoulder subluxation. He postulated that shoulder subluxation may lead to traction injury to the brachial plexus (29). Kingery et al. documented delayed mean central latencies across the brachial plexus and spontaneous activity during needle EMG in hemiplegic subjects when compared with the unaffected limb. Subjects also had to meet strict physical examination criteria for brachial plexus injury. Though the findings in both studies were similar, in contrast to Chino, Kingery interpreted his results to reflect loss of motor units secondary to cortical injury rather than injury to the brachial plexus (62).

Based on available data, brachial plexopathy or peripheral nerve injury should be considered in the diagnosis of hemiplegic shoulder pain when (1) a mechanism for brachial plexus injury exists or (2) muscle tone, reflex changes, weakness, or sensory loss are not consistent with a CNS lesion, especially in the setting of pronounced shoulder subluxation. Because shoulder subluxation has been postulated as the cause of nerve injury, measures to prevent and reduce shoulder subluxation are warranted.

BICIPITAL TENDONITIS

Bicipital tendonitis has not been well described in the stroke literature. However, it bears inclusion in the differential diagnosis of hemiplegic shoulder pain. The prevalence is unknown. In this author's experience, it is rarely the only cause of shoulder pain within an individual. Bicipital tendonitis should be suspected particularly in hemiplegic patients with spasticity or movement synergies that result in over-activation of the biceps as elbow flexors or forearm supinators.

The diagnosis is suggested when there is greater tenderness to palpation of the long head of the biceps as it originates from the anterior glenoid labrum on the affected side compared to the unaffected side. Provocative maneuvers, such as Yergason's test that provokes pain at the biceps origin with resisted forearm supination, are useful when cognition and motor abilities are adequate. Injection of an anesthetic agent, often combined with a therapeutic steroid, on each side of the tendon can corroborate the diagnosis. As with all para-tendon injections, care must be taken to avoid injecting steroid directly into the tendon. Long-term benefit usually requires alleviation of the underlying biomechanical stresses through use of spasmolytic medications, botulinum toxin, chemical neurolysis, or rarely, tendon release, depending on the clinical scenario.

MYOFASCIAL PAIN

Myofascial pain has not been well documented in the stroke literature, possibly because it has only relatively recently gained wide acceptance within the medical and scientific communities. However, it bears inclusion in the differential diagnosis of hemiplegic shoulder pain. In this author's experience, it is never the only cause of shoulder pain within an individual, and seems to occur as a secondary phenomenon in the context of chronic pain and biomechanical abnormality. Due to the lack of interventional trials in stroke, treatment of myofascial pain should follow the same guidelines for its treatment in neurologically intact patients. In this author's experience, trigger points and tender points are often found in the upper trapezius, posterior deltoid, rhomboids, and

anterior deltoid. Dry needling or lidocaine injection to these regions often confers temporary benefit. Long-term benefit most likely requires treatment of other existing painful diagnoses and ultimately, restoration of normal biomechanics. While the latter may not be possible, there may be some critical biomechanical abnormalities, such as spasticity and contractures involving specific muscles, which can be addressed with available clinical tools.

CONTRACTURES

As with all upper motor neuron syndromes, contractures are common complications after stroke that result from the combined effects of immobility, spasticity, paralysis, and muscle imbalance. Prolonged joint immobilization results in collagen deposition and organization of fibrous structures in surrounding soft tissues, affecting muscle belly rather than tendon (63, 64). A number of deleterious effects can result, including loss of functional movement, pain, interference with hygiene, and development of pressure sores (65). In general, the clinical goal is prevention of permanent muscle shortening or contracture. In some cases, reversal of contracture can be accomplished with surgical or non-surgical interventions, but restoration of movement and function are often challenging and incomplete. As with all rehabilitation interventions, management must be considered within the context of functional restoration for the individual patient. After stroke, contractures can involve any joint affected by spastic paralysis.

Prevention of contractures requires prompt initiation of daily management, beginning 24 to 48 hours after stroke onset. Spasticity evolves in the majority of hemiplegic patients within one week of stroke onset (13). Assessment of joint range should also be performed daily so that more aggressive treatment can be initiated if range of motion declines. Passive range of motion exercises, splinting, and positioning are the mainstays of contracture prevention. After stroke, voluntary and involuntary muscle activation fall generally into extensor or flexor patterns or synergies (Figure 26-6). Preventative measures must consider these muscle synergies in assessing contracture risk for a given joint, and efforts should be apportioned according to risk. Joints should be moved through their complete range at least daily, and ideally several times daily. Adherence to a consistent regimen of aggressive stretching prevents contractures in the majority of cases (66, 67). If pain occurs during passive range of motion, analgesic medications should be given to minimize pain during exercise. Splinting should be considered in joints that are at high risk for contracture, or when passive range of motion exercises are insufficient to maintain range. Wrist and finger flexion contractures (Figures 26-7,b,c) and ankle plantar flexion contractures (Figure 26-8) are common. Thus preventative

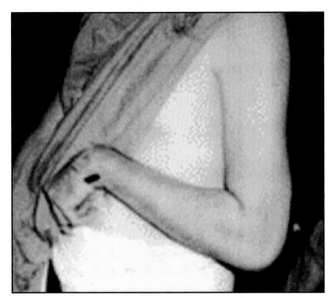

FIGURE 26-6

The adducted shoulder. This contracture consists of an adducted and internally rotated shoulder, and flexed elbow and wrist *Reproduced with permission from WE MOVE, www. wemove.org.*

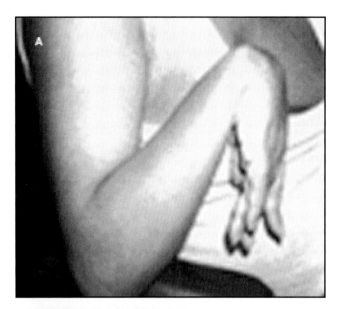

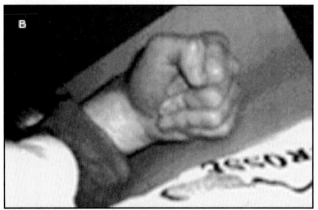

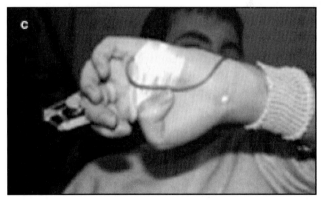

FIGURE 26-7

Contractures of the wrist and fingers a. The flexed wrist b. The clenched fist c. Thumb in palm *Reproduced with permission from WE MOVE, www.wemove.org.*

splinting of these joints in a neutral position is recommended when abnormal muscle tone or movement synergies put them at risk. Serial casting can be used to regain passive range of motion that has been lost. Positioning in bed is particularly important for the shoulder. Placement of a pillow between the impaired upper limb and trunk can help to offset common patterns of shoulder adduction and internal rotation (67). Care should be taken to prevent patients from lying on the impaired shoulder, particularly when the patient is unable to reposition the limb independently, or in the presence of hemi-neglect. Prone positioning, when possible, can be effective in reducing hip flexion contractures.

When range of motion declines despite optimal passive range of motion exercises, splinting, and positioning, more aggressive interventions are warranted in combination with passive range of motion, splinting, and positioning. Spasmolytic medications also can be considered, but their effectiveness is limited by several factors. First, titration to the optimal dose can take time. Second, sedative side effects can limit use, particularly in the acute phase after stroke and in elderly patients. Temporary neurolysis with short-acting local anesthetic agents have been advocated to facilitate passive range of motion exercises (68), but the need for repeated injections or multiple injections when several muscle groups require reduction of tone can be impractical. Focal neurolysis using injected botulinum toxin may be a more practical approach. However, the potential effects of weakening voluntary muscle on motor recovery should be considered carefully. The major advantages of botulinum toxin are that individual muscles can be targeted, the effect lasts for about three months, and sensory innervation is not

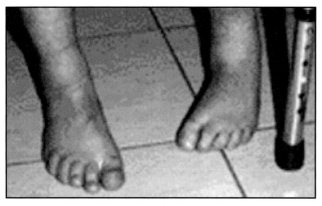

FIGURE 26-8

Contracture of ankle plantarflexion Reproduced with permission from WE MOVE, www.wemove.org.

affected. The use of botulinum toxin has a significant role in promoting functional movement in the upper limb (see Chapter 27), and a role in preventing contactures and their sequelae in the upper limb. In general, permanent neurolysis using phenol should only be considered after motor recovery has reached a plateau, when there is a very high level of confidence that paralyzing the muscle(s) will not have any negative consequences on functional movement at that time or in the future, and that effects on sensation will not reduce function or increase the risk of pressure sores. That said, permanent neurolysis can be effective in improving hygiene, reducing the risk of pressure sores, and improving functional movement. Muscle groups innervated by a single nerve, such as the hip adductor group innervated by the obturator nerve, are particularly amenable to neurolysis. Obturator neurolysis most often is performed to improve perineal hygiene or to reduce pressure sores at the medial knee, but have also been used to improve gait by reducing scissoring. When innervation of target muscles cannot be isolated to a single nerve, or when the sensory component of the nerve should not be sacrificed, motor point blocks can be considered.

Like permanent neurolysis, surgery, in general, should only be considered when no further motor recovery is anticipated. Further, surgery should only be considered after other less invasive management options have failed. The pre-operative objectives should be clear to the clinicians, caregivers, and patients, and are broadly directed at improving function or reducing the risk of medical complications. The physiologic objective is typically restoration of muscle balance. Successful outcomes require close attention to rehabilitation management following surgery. Clinical benefits have been reported in non-randomized clinical trials in stroke patients for a number of procedures, including release or lengthening of tight adductor tendons

for hip adduction contractures (69), selective release or fractional tendon lengthening for knee flexion contractures (66), Achilles tendon lengthening for ankle equinus deformities, split tibialis anterior tendon transfer combined with Achilles tendon lengthening for ankle equinovarus deformities (70), and capsular release plus resection of subscapularis and pectoralis tendons for shoulder capsulitis (71).

RESEARCH FRONTIERS

The need for further research to reduce musculoskeletal complications following stroke is best illustrated by the significant proportion of musculoskeletal complications, particularly shoulder pain, that are refractory to currently available treatments and become chronic. Among all stroke survivors, the prevalence of shoulder pain varies by only a few percent from acute hospitalization, through the recovery phase, and into the chronic phase, with 12% of all stroke survivors having shoulder pain at 18–30 months post-stroke (8). Among moderately to severely impaired stroke survivors, one-third have shoulder pain 6 months after stroke, and 20% continue to have shoulder pain at four years (4). Though obvious and applicable to all stroke sequelae, it bears mentioning that research leading to prevention of stroke or enhancement of recovery following stroke, particularly enhancement of motor recovery for musculoskeletal conditions, would reduce the impact of musculoskeletal complications following stroke. Short of stroke prevention and recovery, research should be directed at developing new, effective interventions to prevent and treat specific musculoskeletal conditions after stroke. Development of such treatments relies heavily on understanding the pathogenesis of individual conditions, including their causes, natural history, and pathophysiology. Though the basic goals of researchers tend to be universal, clinical research is unfortunately often fragmented, leaving gaps in fundamental knowledge. This section of the chapter seeks to highlight some of the more significant gaps in the current research methodology and the fund of knowledge.

Shoulder subluxation is one of the most commonly cited, yet controversial, causes of post-stroke shoulder pain in the literature. In most studies, subluxation is measured by quantifying abnormal translation of the humeral head in the inferior direction under the weight of the unsupported upper limb. The content validity of this measure has not been established. After traumatic shoulder dislocation, abnormal translation in the anterior direction is both common and clinically relevant. Further, because the ligaments of the glenohumeral joint provide stability in multiple directions, instability due to injury to passive restraints tends to be multidimensional (11).

Some investigators have correlated post-stroke shoulder pain with anterior but not inferior subluxation (72). Until the content validity of abnormal glenohumeral translation exclusively in the inferior dimension is established, measures of joint instability should be quantified in multiple dimensions, particularly the anterior-posterior dimension.

Further, measures of abnormal joint translation should account for changes in scapular and glenoid orientation after stroke. In flaccid paralysis, the scapula tends toward external rotation and depression. Recovery of muscle tone and voluntary activation often occurs in a proximal to distal gradient after stroke. When spasticity is present, the scapula tends toward internal rotation, elevation, and protraction. All of these changes in scapular position have an effect on the position and version of the glenoid fossa. Thus, abnormal translation of the humeral head should be referenced to the glenoid fossa rather than typically used bony landmarks such as the inferior border of the acromion.

While studies demonstrating a lack of correlation between shoulder subluxation and pain strongly suggest that painless shoulder subluxation can occur after stroke, these studies do not evaluate shoulder instability as an indirect cause of pain. Does shoulder subluxation serve as a common denominator in the pathogenesis of other painful conditions? Because shoulder subluxation tends to occur during the flaccid phase of hemiplegia and can remit with recovery of muscle tone (73), data collected in a cross-sectional manner cannot evaluate this potential relationship. Rather, the presence of subluxation should be correlated with the development of pain and specific painful conditions over time. Some authors have correlated post-stroke shoulder subluxation with the development of CRPS (31), peripheral nerve injury (29, 30), and rotator cuff tears (10). Research that can identify common denominators in the pathogenesis of post-stroke shoulder pain can play a critical role in developing effective interventions. Further, it is likely that varied combinations of basic abnormal physiologic processes seen after stroke, that is paralysis, spasticity, impaired motor control and, in some cases, sensory loss, act synergistically, resulting in the development of painful pathology. For example, it has been postulated that early subluxation resulting in joint instability predisposes to impingement syndrome when muscle tone returns in a proximal to distal gradient. Thus, the synergistic effects of abnormal physiologic processes should be considered in the evaluation of common denominators leading to shoulder pain.

Industry-sponsored research can facilitate the development of new interventions. Such research has demonstrated the efficacy of electric stimulation of various shoulder muscles delivered via percutaneously-placed electrodes for treating chronic shoulder pain after stroke (47, 48). The reduction of shoulder subluxation was not statistically significant, suggesting that it may not have been the primary mechanism of action. Pain reduction persisted for at least one year after discontinuation of treatment, suggesting that neuromodulation of pain may not be the primary mechanism of action. Studies evaluating the mechanism of action of efficacious treatments are warranted. They have the potential to teach us more about the factors that contribute to shoulder pain after stroke. Further, studies evaluating mechanisms can further optimize treatments with respect to the resulting clinical benefits.

Spasticity is a critical factor in the development of many musculoskeletal complications after stroke. Shoulder pain is more prevalent in spastic compared to flaccid hemiplegia (7). Specific types of shoulder pathology, such as capsulitis and impingement syndrome, are not likely to develop without spasticity. Contractures can affect any joint affected by spastic paralysis. Available methods to modulate spasticity are often inadequate. Oral spasmolytic medications have limited efficacy and adverse effects that may be more prevalent in stroke survivors. Intrathecal delivery of baclofen is invasive and affects lower limb tone more than upper limb tone. Botulinum toxin provides intermediate acting, focal, neuromuscular blockade without affecting sensory innervation. However, the effects of botulinum toxin are limited in larger muscles in the lower limb when given intramuscularly, due to the limits imposed by maximum dosages. Research to develop more effective methods to modulate spasticity would significantly impact musculoskeletal complications after stroke. In turn, more effective methods to modulate spasticity could further serve as research tools in interventional experiments that seek to evaluate the synergistic effects of spasticity and other abnormal physiologic processes seen after stroke.

SUMMARY

Musculoskeletal conditions are common complications in post-stroke hemiplegia that have significant impact on functional recovery and quality of life. The most common conditions include shoulder pain and contractures that can affect any joint affected by spastic paralysis. Of musculoskeletal complications after stroke, shoulder pain has been by far the most studied. Many types of shoulder pathology have been suggested as causes of shoulder pain in hemiplegia including shoulder subluxation, capsulitis, tendonitis, rotator cuff injury, bursitis, impingement syndrome, spasticity, CRPS, brachial plexus injury, and proximal mononeuropathies. More than one type of pathology may exist in a given patient. Shoulder pain improves in a significant proportion of cases with prompt diagnosis and appropriate management (5). Although the relationship between subluxation and pain remains controversial, upper limb support to reduce subluxation is the standard of care and may prevent the development of pain and secondary complications. Further work is needed to elucidate the causes and natural history of shoulder pain in hemiplegia, including the identification of physiologic common denominators that can lead to improved strategies for treatment and prevention.

References

1. Kalra L., et al. Medical complications during stroke rehabilitation. *Stroke* 1995; 26:990–994.
2. Dromerick A, Reding M. Medical and neurological complications during inpatient stroke rehabilitation. *Stroke* 1994; 25:358–361.
3. Ratnasabapathy Y, et al. Shoulder pain in people with a stroke: A population-based study. *Clinical Rehabil* 2003; 17:304–311.
4. Wanklyn P, Forster A, Young J. Hemiplegic shoulder pain (HSP): Natural history and investigation of associated features. *Disability and Rehabilitation* 1996; 18:497–501.
5. Gamble GE, et al. Poststroke shoulder pain: A porspective study of the association and risk factors in 152 patients from a consecutive cohort of 205 patients presenting with stroke. *European J Pain* 2002; 6:467–474.
6. Bohannon RW, et al. Shoulder pain in hemiplegia: Statistical relationship with five variables. *Arch Phys Med Rehabil* 1986; 67:514–516.
7. VanOuwenaller C, Laplace PM, Chantraine A. Painful shoulder in hemiplegia. *Arch Phys Med Rehabil* 1986; 67:23–26.
8. Langhorne P, et al. Medical complications after stroke: A multicenter study. *Stroke* 2000; 31:1223–1229.
9. Pesczynski M, Rardin TE. The incidence of painful shoulder in hemiplegia. *Bulletin of Polish Medical History and Science* 1965; 8:21–23.
10. Najenson T, Yacubovich E, Pikielni SS. Rotator cuff injury in shoulder joints of hemiplegic patients. *Scan J Rehab Med* 1971; 3:131–137.
11. Skyhar MJ, Warren RF, Altchek DW. Instability of the shoulder. In Nicholas J Hershman EB, eds. *The Upper Extremity in Sports Medicine.*St. Louis:C.V. Mosby Co., 1990:181–212.
12. Baker LL, Parker K. Neuromuscular electrical stimulation of the muscles surrounding the shoulder. *Physical Therapy* 1986; 66:1930–1937.
13. Chaco J, Wolf E. Subluxation of the glenohumeral joint in hemiplegia. *Amer J Phys Med* 1971; 50:139–143.
14. Chantraine A, et al. Shoulder pain and dysfunction in hemiplegia:Effects of functional electrical stimulation. *Arch Phys Med Rehabil* 1999; 80:328–331.
15. Faghri PD, et al. The effects of functional electrical stimulation on shoulder subluxation, arm function recovery, and shoulder pain in hemiplegic stroke patients. *Arch Phys Med Rehabil* 1994; 75:73–79.
16. Ikai T, et al. Evaluation and treatment of shoulder subluxation in hemiplegia:Relationship between subluxation and pain. *Am J Phys Med Rehabil* 1998; 77:421–426.
17. Kobayashi H, et al. Reduction in subluxation and improved muscle function of the hemiplegic shoulder joint after therapeutic electrical stimulation. *J Electromyography and Kinesiology* 1999; 9:327–336.
18. Linn SL, et al. Prevention of shoulder subluxation after stroke with electrical stimulation. *Stroke* 1999; 30:963–968.
19. Najenson T, Pikielny SS. Malalignment of the gleno-humeral joint following hemiplegia (A review of 500 cases). *Ann Phys Med* 1965; 8:96–99.
20. Shai G, et al. Glenohumeral malalignment in the hemiplecgic shoulder. *Scand J Rehab Med* 1984; 16:133–136.
21. Yu DT, et al. Muscular factors preventing inferior subluxation of the shoulder in hemiplegia. *Arch Phys Med Rehabil* 1998; 79:1151 (Abstract).
22. Yu DT, et al. Pain associated with percutaneous versus surface neuromuscular electrical stimulation for treating shoulder dysfunction in hemiplegia. *Arch Phys Med Rehabil* 1998; 79:1151 (Abstract).
23. Yu DT, et al. Percutaneous neuromuscular electrical stimulation for treating shoulder subluxation. *Arch Phys Med Rehabil* 1998; 79:1189.
24. Zorowitz RD, et al. Shoulder pain and subluxation after stroke:Correlation or coincidence. *Am J Occ Therapy* 1996; 50:194–201.
25. Griffin JW. Hemiplegic shoulder pain. *Phys Therapy* 1986; 66:1884–1893.
26. Bohannon RW, Andrews AW. Shoulder subluxation and pain in stroke patients. *Amer J Occ Therapy* 1989(October 3):507–509.
27. VanLangenberghe H,Hogan BM. Degree of pain and grade of subluxation in the painful hemiplegic shoulder. *Scand J Rehab Med* 1988; 20:161–166.
28. Arsenault AB, et al. Clinical significance of the V-shaped space in the subluxed shoulder of hemiplegics. *Stroke* 1991; 22:867–871.
29. Chino N. Electrophysiological investigation on shoulder subluxation in hemiplegics. *Scand J Rehab Med* 1981; 13:17–21.
30. Ring H, et al. Temporal changes in electrophysiological, clinical and radiological parameters in the hemiplegic's shoulder. *Scand J Rehab Med Suppl* 1985; 12:124–127.
31. Dursun E, et al. Glenohumeral joint subluxation and reflex sympathetic dystrophy in hemiplegic patients. *Arch Phys Med Rehabil* 2000; 81:944–946.
32. Aronen JG, Regan K. Decreasing the incidence of recurrence of first time anterior shoulder dislocations with rehabilitation. *Am J Sports Med* 1984; 12:283.
33. Glousman R. Dynamic EMG:analysis of the throwing shoulder with glenohumeral instability. In *Society of American Shoulder and Elbow Surgeons Third Open Meeting.* 1987. San Francisco.
34. Cain PR. Anterior stability of the glenohumeral joint:A dynamic model. *Am J Sports Med* 1987; 15:144.
35. Symeonides PP. The significance of the subscapularis muscle in the pathogenesis of recurrent anterior dislocation of the shoulder. *J Bone Joint Surgery* 1972; 54B:476.
36. Wang Y, et al. Functional electrical stimulation for treatment of shoulder subluxation of stroke patients. *Arch Phys Med Rehabil* 1996; 77:977 (Abstract).
37. Ada L, Foonghchomcheay A. Efficacy of electrical stimulation in preventing or reducing subluxation of the shoulder after stroke:A meta-analysis. *Aust J Physiother* 2002; 48:257–267.
38. Prevost R, et al. Shoulder subluxation in hemiplegia:A radiologic correlational study. *Arch Phys Med Rehabil* 1987; 68:782–785.
39. Moodie N, Brisbin J, Margan A. Subluxation of the glenohumeral joint in hemiplegia: evaluation of supportive devices. *Physiother Can* 1986; 38:151–157.
40. Brooke MM, et al. Shoulder subluxation in hemiplegia: Effects of three different supports. *Arch Phys Med Rehabil* 1991; 72:582–586.
41. Griffin A,Bernhardt J. Strapping the hemiplegic shoulder prevents development of pain during rehabilitation: A randomized controlled trial. *Clin Rehabil* 2006; 20:287–295.
42. Hanger HC, et al. A randomized controlled trial of strapping to prevent post-stroke shoulder pain. *Clin Rehabil* 2000; 14:370–380.
43. Ada L, Foongchomcheay A, Canning C. Supportive devices for preventing and treating subluxation of the shoulder after stroke. *Cochrane Database Syst Rev* 2005; 1: CD003863.
44. Baker LL,Bowman BR, McNeal DR. Effects of waveform on comfort during neuromuscular electrical stimulation. *Clinical Orthopaedics & Related Research* 1988; 233:75–85.
45. Yu DT, et al. Comparing stimulation-induced pain during percutaneous (intramuscular) and transcutaneous neuromuscular electrical stimulation for treating shoulder subluxation in hemiplegia. *Arch Phys Med Rehabil* 2001; 82:756–760.
46. Yu DT,Chae J. Neuromuscular stimulation for treating shoulder dysfunction in hemiplegia. *Crit Rev Phys Rehabil Med* 2002; 14:1–23.
47. Yu DT, et al. Intramuscular neuromuscular electric stimulation for poststroke shoulder pain: A multicenter randomized clinical trial. *Arch Phys Med Rehabil* 2004; 85:695–704.
48. Chae J, et al. Intramuscular electrical stimulation for hemiplegic shoulder pain: A 12-month follow-up of a multiple-center, randomized clinical trial. *Am J Phys Med Rehabil* 2005; 84:832–842.
49. Rizk TE, et al. Arthrographic studies in painful hemiplegic shoulders. *Arch Phys Med Rehabil* 1984; 65:254–256.
50. Hecht JS. Subscapular nerve block in the painful hemiplegic shoulder. *Arch Phys Med Rehabil* 1992; 73:1036–1039.
51. Neviaser JS. Adhesive capsulitis of the shoulder. *Med Times* 1962; 90:783.
52. Lundberg BJ. The frozen shoulder. *ACTA Orthop Scand Suppl* 1969; 19.
53. Snels IA, et al. Effect of triamcinolone acetonide injections on hemiplegic shoulder pain : A randomized clinical trial. *Stroke* 2000; 31:2396–401.
54. Yelnik AP, et al. Treatment of shoulder pain in spastic hemiplegia by reducing spasticity of the subscapular muscle: A randomised, double blind, placebo controlled study of botulinum toxin A. *J Neurol Neurosurg Psychiatry* 2007; 78:845–848.
55. Joynt RL. The source of shoulder pain in hemiplegia. *Arch Phys Med Rehabil* 1992; 73:409–413.
56. Hakuno A, et al. Arthrographic findings in hemiplegic shoulders. *Arch Phys Med Rehabil* 1984; 65:706–711.
57. Cailliet R. *The Shoulder in Hemiplegia.* F.A. Davis Company: Philadelphia:, 1980.
58. Davis SW, et al. Shoulder-hand syndrome in a hemiplegic population: A 5-year retrospective study. *Arch Phys Med Rehabil* 1977; 58:353–356.
59. Perrigot M, Bussel B, Pierrot DE. L'epaule de l'hemiplegique. *Ann Med Phys* 1975; 18:176–187.
60. Tepperman PS, et al. Reflex sympathetic dystrophy in hemiplegia. *Arch Phys Med Rehabil* 1984; 65:442–447.
61. Aisen ML,Brown W, Rubin M. Electrophysiologic changes in lumbar spinal cord after cervical cord injury. *Neurology* 1992; 42:623–626.
62. Kingery WS, Date ES, Bocobo CR. The absence of brachial plexus injury in stroke. *Am J Phys Med Rehabil* 1993; 72:127–135.
63. Roper BA. Rehabilitation after a stroke. *J Bone Joint Surg Br* 1982; 64:156–163.

64. Halar EM, et al. Gastrocnemius muscle belly and tendon length in stroke patients and able bodied persons. *Arch Phys Med Rehabil* 1978; 59:476–484.

65. Lusskin R, Grynbaum BB, Dhir RS. Peripheral surgery after stroke: An orthopedic-rehabilitative effort. *Geriatrics* 1971; 26:65–74.

66. Botte MJ, et al. Orthopedic management of the stroke patient: Part II treating deformities of the upper and lower extremeties. *Orthop Rev* 1988; 17:891–910.

67. McCollough NC. The role of the orthopedic surgeon in the treatment of stroke. *Orthop Clin North Am* 1978; 9305–324.

68. Gardner MJ, et al. Orthopedic issues after cerebrovascular accident. *Am J Orthop* 2002:559–568.

69. Mooney V, Perry J, Nickel VL. Surgical and nonsurgical orthopaedic care of stroke. *J Bone Joint Surg Am* 1967; 49:989–1000.

70. Waters RL, Montgomery J. Lower extremity management of hemiparesis. *Clin Orthop* 1974:102–133.

71. Caldwell CB, Wilson DJ, Braun RM. Evaluation and treatment of the upper extremity in the hemiplegic stroke patient. *Clin Orthop* 1969; 63:69–93.

72. Lee C, Han S. Evaluations of anterior displacement of humeral head in hemiplegic shoulder subluxation patients. *Arch Phys Med Rehabil* 2000; 81:1300 (abstract).

73. Ikai T, Yonemoto K, Miyano S. Interval change of the shoulder subluxation in hemiplegic patients. *J Rehabil Med* 1992; 29:569–575.

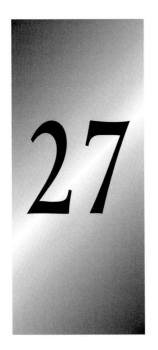

27 Depression and Other Neuropsychiatric Complications

Gianfranco Spalletta
Carlo Caltagirone

T he neuropsychiatric disorders associated with stroke have been recognized for more than 100 years. Neurologists and psychiatrists, such as Hughlings-Jackson (1) and Adolph Meyer (2), have recognized that emotional disorders after cerebral infarction constitute an important sequelae of stroke. The long-term nature of depressions following stroke was noted by Bleuler (3), who stated "melancholy mood lasting for months and sometimes longer appear frequently." Goldstein (4) described the abrupt onset of emotional symptoms of frustration, depression, and embarrassment in acute stroke patients, and defined them as a catastrophic reaction. Ironside (5) reported pathological emotions referred to as pseudobulbar affect because the disorder was often associated with bilateral lesions affecting the cortico bulbar pathways, producing dysphasia, dysarthria, or paralysis of the voluntary facial muscles. Babinski was the first to describe apathetic symptoms, calling them the "indifference reaction," and to use the term *anosognosia* to define unawareness of deficits in stroke patients (6).

Thus, for more than 100 years, clinicians have recognized emotional disorders as the result of stroke. While depression, mania, anxiety, and personality disorders are not specific of brain injury, other disorders such as catastrophic reaction, anosognosia, or pseudobulbar affect are neuropsychiatric disorders specifically associated with brain injury. This chapter will summarize these findings beginning with the most common emotional disorder associated with stroke, that is, post-stroke depression.

POST-STROKE DEPRESSION

Epidemiology

The epidemiological investigation of post-stroke depression indicates that stroke patients are at high risk of developing depressive disorders. Indeed, it is estimated that about one-third of stroke patients develop one of the different types of depressive disorders (7, 8). Conversely, in the community setting, the rate of depression in elderly people without stroke is many times lower than that found in stroke survivors in the same age range (9).

Overall, epidemiological results are highly discordant, but we are now aware that methodological issues of diagnosis of depression, time of assessment, and patient setting may be responsible for this lack of concordance (Table 27-1).

Thus, when we considered only studies using psychiatric interview for assessing diagnostic criteria for mood disorders, according with the *Diagnostic and Statistical Manual for Mental Disorders* (DSM) (11), which is

TABLE 27-1
Methodological Procedures on Post-Stroke Depression

	METHODS	
CHARACTERISTICS	**GOLD STANDARD PROCEDURES**	**PROBLEMATIC PROCEDURES**
Diagnosis	Structured clinical interview have to be used.	Usage of cutoff scores of rating scales should be avoided for diagnostic purposes.
Diagnostic typology	Diagnosis of MDD and MIND should be recognized separately because they are associated with different clinical expression, biological correlates, and outcome.	
Symptom severity	Rating scales validated and commonly used in PSD have to be used.	Rating scales that are not validated and not used in PSD should not be used.
Cognitive impairment	This should not be an exclusion criterion per se if it does not impair language comprehension or neuropsychiatric symptom assessment.	To exclude patients with mild or moderate cognitive deficit may produce a selection bias.
Aphasia	Only patients with severe language comprehension that impairs diagnosis and symptom assessment should be excluded from the studies. Language comprehension should be carefully assessed with specific tests, such as the token test (10)	To exclude all the patients with aphasia, independently from its severity may produce a selection bias.
Medical comorbidity	Major medical illnesses such as unstabilized diabetes, obstructive pulmonary disease, or asthma, oncological disorders, as well as clinically significant and unstable active hematological, gastrointestinal, renal, hepatic, endocrine, or cardiovascular system diseases, should be considered as exclusion criteria.	Including patients with major medical illnesses could confuse the role of the stroke on symptom expression.
Personal or familiar psychiatric anamnesis	A complete psychiatric anamnesis should be assessed in all studied patients. A positive anamnesis for previous psychiatric disturbances in stroke patients with depression could indicate a reactive phenomenon.	Does not consider this characteristic makes impossible to recognize if depression is a direct consequence of the brain lesion
Time from the acute stroke	It is important because the phenomenology of PSD changes over time elapsed from the acute stroke.	
Lesion location	When possible, it should be studied with MRI. Furthermore, time elapsed from the acute stroke should be always and carefully taken into consideration. This is because there is a strict relationship between these two characteristics.	

considered to be the most valid method for identifying depression after stroke, we found rates between 11–15% for post-stroke major depression and between 8–12% for post-stroke minor depression in the community setting. In the acute hospital, rates varied from 16–27% and from 13–20% for major and minor depression, respectively. Considering the rehabilitation hospital, patients suffering from major depression range from 9–41%, and rates varied from 17–44% for patients with minor depression. Finally, rates in the outpatient setting ranged from 20–31% for major depression and from 13–14% for minor depression. These prevalence rates were high both in community samples and hospital samples. However, the greater severity of stroke in patients assessed in the treatment setting, such as acute or rehabilitation hospitals, may explain the higher severity of depression symptoms and the higher prevalence of depressive disorders.

About 50% of studies on post-stroke depression have been conducted using cutoff scores of different rating scales for depression. Although the global prevalence rate for depression is quite similar to that found with DSM criteria (that is, 30%), using this method of assessment, we cannot discriminate between major and minor depression, two very different forms of depression regarding prevalence rate, biological correlates, as well as possible treatment response and outcome (7). Therefore, use of rating scales must be limited to the investigation of severity of depressive symptoms only, particularly during outcome studies, while structured interviews may be used to assess presence or absence of categorical mood disorders.

Diagnosis

Description of post-stroke depression diagnosis across studies varies in terms of diagnostic criteria definition and structured interview used. Two terms commonly used in post-stroke depression research are major and minor depression. While major depression usually defines "depression due to stroke with a DSM major depressive like episode," definitions of minor depression are sparse and sometimes confusing. They may vary from dystymic disorder with a modified temporal criteria of two weeks (changed in comparison to the standard criteria of two years), to some kind of subsyndromal major depression according to International Classification of Diseases (ICD) criteria, to minor depressive disorder according to DSM research criteria. Also, many structured interviews have been used to diagnose mood disorders in stroke patients. They are Present State Examination (PSE), Schedule for Affective Disorders and Schizophrenia (SADS), Structured Clinical Interview for DSM (SCID), and Composite International Diagnostic Interview (CIDI). These different interviews may have influenced the different rates of major and minor depression across studies.

Diagnosis of depression associated with physical illnesses is a challenge for both clinicians and researchers. Over the past years, many approaches have been used to resolve this issue in stroke patients (7):

1. An inclusive approach in which depressive symptoms are considered, even if they are related to the physical illness
2. An etiologic approach that considers symptoms of depression only if they are not the result of the physical illness
3. A substitutive approach that considers only the psychological dimension of depression
4. An exclusive approach that considers only those symptoms that are more frequent in depressed than in nondepressed patients

The effect of the four proposed methods was partially analyzed by Federoff et al. (12), Paradiso et al. (13) and Spalletta et al (14), and all studies are concordant that no reason exists to conclude that DSM criteria for mood disorders have to be modified for diagnosing categorical depression in stroke patients. In particular, in the Spalletta et al. (14) study, all vegetative and cognitive symptoms were more prevalent in patients with depression in comparison with patients without depression. Thus, there is evidence that, during the diagnostic procedure for depressive disorders in stroke patients, clinicians should consider equally important vegetative, cognitive, and psychological depressive symptoms, despite their nature.

Course of Depressive Disorders after Stroke

Comorbid depression in stroke patients is very frequent, but its rate may vary during the post-stroke period, depending on the type of depressive disorder and whether it is of early onset or late onset following the acute stroke event.

On the one hand, the frequency of major depression in stroke patients tends to decrease over the first two years after the stroke (15, 16, 17). In particular, there is a peak of frequency at three to six months and a decline one year after the acute stroke, where one out of two of patients tend to recover almost spontaneously (17). Astrom et al. (15) also suggest that the frequency of major depression may increase again at the initial levels three years after the acute stroke. A longitudinal study from the Iowa Group (18) described that about 30% of patients, who are not depressed at the initial evaluation after the acute stroke, will develop depression six months later. Astrom et al. (15) reported that only 60% of patients with early depression, that is, those who developed depression in the first three months from the stroke, had recovered at one year. Furthermore, Wade et al. (19) reported 50%

of recovery rate in their patients depressed after three weeks from the stroke. This means that a high percentage of these patients tended to develop chronic depression. However, it appears that patients with very early onset of depression, within the first days from the stroke, tend to have a spontaneous remission, while the onset of depression after seven weeks is associated with a lower rate of spontaneous recovery (20).

On the other hand, the frequency of minor depression is stable or increases during time after the stroke both in the community setting (21) and in patients seen firstly in acute hospital setting (22).

Thus, the major and minor forms of depression seem to describe two independent types of mood disorders not only in terms of severity of depressive symptoms but also in terms of natural course.

Relationship to Functional and Cognitive Impairment

There is a strict relationship between post-stroke depression and functional or cognitive impairment.

The literature is strongly concordant on the association between severity of depression and severity of functional impairment or failure of rehabilitation. Robinson et al. (23), in the first study analyzing this issue, described a significant correlation between physical/functional impairment and severity of depression at three- and six-month periods following the acute stroke. In addition, a convergence between depression and functional improvement at the two-year follow-up period has been reported in patients with major depression only, and no improvement in depression severity and functional impairment was described in patients with diagnosis of dysthymia (17). All other studies conducted in the following years in North America (24–27) and Europe (28–31) confirmed results found for the first time in the 80 years by the Robinson's group on mood/functional relationship.

Recently, some studies focused on the functional outcome in patients with post-stroke depression. Chemerinski et al. (32) described a group of inpatients with acute stroke suffering from major or minor depression at the initial evaluation who experienced a significant functional improvement at three- and six-month follow-ups only if they had 50% reduction of depression severity. The improvement was independent from demographic, lesion, and neurologic characteristics. Narushima and Robinson (33) clarified that an early antidepressant treatment within the first month from the acute stroke is more effective on improving the functional impairment in comparison with a late treatment started after the first month from the acute event. Thus, there is evidence that antidepressant treatment may influence the outcome of functional impairment and rehabilitation in stroke patients suffering from depression, particularly in patients who are treatment-responders (34).

A relationship between cognitive impairment and depression in stroke patients has been recognized from many years (35). This relation paralleled that found in elderly people without brain damage with a disorder defined as pseudodementia, or dementia of depression. However, in stroke victims, dementia of depression was described mainly in patients with diagnosis of major depression and left hemisphere laterality of lesion (36–37). Also, House et al. (38), Morris et al. (39), and Andersen et al. (40) found a relationship between depression severity and cognitive impairment in left hemisphere stroke patients only. Thus, dementia of depression is a problem accompanying a predefined subgroup of stroke patients only. On the other hand, stroke patients with major depression and right hemispheric stroke may suffer from a particular kind of unawareness of emotions called alexithymia (41–42).

There is evidence that both cognitive deficit and unawareness of emotions may respond to antidepressant treatment. In reality, the first studies on the treatment of post-stroke depression in which cognitive outcome was taken into consideration did not find any effect of antidepressant treatment on cognitive impairment (40, 43–45). However, subsequent, more focused studies clearly demonstrated that cognitive impairment improves in patients who respond to the treatment, independently from the type of treatment (that is, active or placebo) (46), and that cognitive recovery after treatment of post-stroke depression may remain stable for a long period (47).

Mechanisms

Laboratory studies in rats have identified that injury to axonal projections of biogenic amine containing neurons led to a shutdown of neurotransmitter production (48). Robinson et al. (49) first hypothesized that lesions of the left dorsal lateral frontal cortex or left basal ganglia may interrupt the biogenic amine containing axons as they course through the basal ganglia to the cortex. Injury to these ascending axonal projections may lead to a subsequent decrease in the production of norepinephrine and/or 5-hydroxytryptophan (5-HT) in order to facilitate the production of protein for neuronal regeneration or sprouting. The experimental evidence to support this hypothesis included the finding that post-stroke patients with depression had significantly lower concentrations of 5-hydroxy indoleacetic acid (5-HIAA), a metabolite of serotonin in CSF, compared to the age, gender, and hemispheric lesion location matched with nondepressed stroke patients (50) and that patients with left hemisphere stroke showed a significant inverse correlation between serotonin

5-HT$_2$ receptor binding as measured by ^{11}C N-methyl spiperone in their left temporal cortex and Hamilton Depression score (51).

In accordance with these observations, Robinson and Szetela (52) found a significant inverse correlation between the severity of depression following brain injury and the distance of the anterior border of the lesion from the left frontal pole. In subsequent studies, Starkstein et al. (53), Astrom et al. (15), Morris et al. (54), Herrmann et al. (55–56), and Vataja et al. (57–58) all found significant associations between left frontal and/or left basal ganglia lesions and post-stroke depression. However, some authors (59) criticized the evidence that left hemisphere lesions are associated with an increased risk of post-stroke depression. A meta-analysis (59) identified problems of sample heterogeneity (that is, exclusion of aphasic patients or study settings) as potential biases affecting results of studies measuring lesion location associated with post-stroke depression.

A systematic review of the literature and meta-analysis by Bhogal et al. (60) further clarified the complexity of this issue and described that patients with left anterior lesions had a significantly increased likelihood of having major depressive disorder if they were inpatients compared to community patients or if they were in the acute stroke period compared to the chronic stroke period. Thus, there is strong evidence that lesion location affecting the prefrontal-subcortical circuits, especially on the left side, is strictly connected with the phenomenology of depression. This association is present early after the stroke and tends to disappear during the first months following the acute event. Therefore, it is conceivable that the identification of biological substrates specifically contributing to the damage of this area could further clarify the pathogenetic basis of such observation.

However, based on the fact that both lesion variables and impairment variables have been correlated with the existence of post-stroke depression, it seems reasonable to conclude there are several kinds of depression following stroke, starting from those of secondary psychological reaction origin but also including those biologically based.

Recently, a second hypothesis has been proposed regarding the role of inflammatory cytokines in the production of post-stroke depression. According to this hypothesis, the increased production of proinflammatory cytokines, such as IL-1β, IL-6, TNF-α or IL-18, resulting from stroke may lead to an amplification of the inflammatory process, particularly in limbic areas. This inflammatory process could also lead to the widespread activation of indolamine-2-3-dioxygenase (IDO). The increased activation of IDO might then lead to the subsequent depletion of serotonin in paralimbic regions, such as the ventral lateral frontal cortex, polar temporal cortex, and basal ganglia, with the resultant physiological dysfunction leading to post-stroke depression (61).

Treatment

Drugs used in the prevention of post-stroke depression and the treatment of mood disorders after stroke modulate serotonergic and/or noradrenergic systems. The rationale of this treatment is based on the concept that stroke may cause lesions of the serotonergic and noradrenergic fibers ascending from the brain stem, thus causing impaired monoamine transmission within the brain.

The fact that depressive disorders have a high prevalence rate in stroke patients (7) cause negative outcome during rehabilitation (29) and increase risk for mortality (62–64) induced some research to focus on the issue of prevention of depressive disorders after acute stroke. In particular, five double-blind, placebo-controlled studies and one open study have been conducted on the post-stroke depression prevention issue. Results of the Palomaki et al. (65) study indicate that mianserin 60 mg/day does not prevent depression in stroke patients. The efficacy analysis of the Narushima et al. (66) study indicates that fluoxetine 40 mg/day and nortriptyline 10 mg/day groups had a lower rate of depression in comparison with the placebo group during the 12-week treatment period. However, after nine months of the treatment discontinuation, patients included in the treatment groups experienced a higher rate of depressive disorders, suggesting that the prophylactic treatment should be extended for a longer period and that patients should be monitored carefully. Results of the two sertraline studies are conflicting. While the Rasmussen et al. (67) study indicates that sertraline administered for 12 months showed superior prophylactic efficacy in comparison with placebo and that the active drug was well-tolerated, the Almeida et al. (68) study describes no difference in the incidence of depressive symptoms in a 24-week study. In the latter study, about one out of two patients of both groups discontinued the treatment, and this could be a possible explanation for the failure in preventing depression after stroke. Recently, Robinson et al. (69) demonstrated, with a well conducted randomized controlled trial for prevention of depression among 176 nondepressed patients assessed within three months following acute stroke, that escitalopram (5–10 mg/day) and problem-solving therapy were superior to placebo in preventing depressive (major or minor) episodes. However, using a more conservative method of data analysis problem solving therapy was not significantly better than placebo, but escitalopram remained superior to placebo. Finally, results of the one-year, open, randomized study with mirtazapine 30 mg/day or no treatment (70) suggest that mirtazapine may be useful in the prevention of depression after acute stroke. Indeed, 40% of the untreated patients and 6% of the treated patients developed post-stroke depression. Thus, from the published studies, there is a suggestion that antidepressant treatment may be efficacious in the prevention of post-stroke depression and that prophylactic treatment should last for at least one year. However, more studies are needed to confirm these suggestions.

Heterocyclic, SSRI, SNRI, and psychostimulant drugs have been used as active treatment of post-stroke depression in many randomized controlled and open studies. So far, three double-blind, controlled studies analyzed the efficacy of heterocyclic drugs. Lypsey et al. (43) found that nortriptyline 100 mg/day was superior to placebo in improving depressive symptoms in post-stroke depression patients. Robinson et al. (44) confirmed the superiority of nortriptyline 100 mg/day in comparison to placebo or to the SSRI fluoxetine 40 mg/day as treatment for post-stroke depression. In the same study, there was no significant difference between fluoxetine and placebo in improving depressive symptoms. Lauritzen et al. (71) described a superiority of Imipramine 50–150 mg/day plus mianserin 10–30 mg/day over desipramine 50–50 mg/day plus mianserin 10–30 mg/day in improving depressive symptoms in stroke patients. Thus, heterocyclic treatment of post-stroke depression may be considered efficacious. However, caution is needed because of the relatively high incidence of side effects in elderly patients.

Six randomized, controlled trials have been conducted in an attempt to measure the efficacy of SSRIs in the treatment of mood disorders after stroke. Results of the study of Andersen et al. (20) clearly demonstrated the superiority of citalopram 20–40 mg/day versus placebo (Table 27-2). The remaining trials conducted with sertraline and fluoxetine describe inconclusive or conflicting results. Murray et al. (72), in a study on patients with minor depression or a mild form of major depression, described no difference between sertraline 50–100 mg/day and placebo. Indeed, both groups of patients showed significant depression improvement. However, quality of life improvement was greater in the sertraline group in comparison with the placebo group. The remaining trials detected the possible superiority of fluoxetine over placebo treatment. Robinson et al. (44) and Choi-Kwon et al. (73) failed in demostraiting the superiority of fluoxetine in improving depressive symptoms. On the contrary, Wiart et al. (45) showed that fluoxetine (20 mg/day) was superior to placebo in improving depressive symptoms, and Fruehwald et al. (74) described improvement of depressive symptoms in the fluoxetine group (20–40 mg/day), but only after the 12-week period of double-blind treatment. The superiority of fluoxetine remained stable at the 18-month follow-up period. Thus, the issue of the efficacy of SSRIs in post-stroke depression patients is conflicting and further double-blind placebo controlled studies are strongly needed.

With a randomized, controlled trial, only the Rampello et al. (75) study examined the efficacy of the NARI reboxetine 4 mg in two daily doses in comparison with placebo in the treatment of the subtype of post-stroke depression called "retarded depression" with symptoms of anergia, hypokinesia, hypersomnia, slowness, hypomimia, and reduction of sexual activity. This form of depression may be secondary to a dopaminergic-noradrenergic dysfunction. They reported a superiority of reboxetine over placebo in improving depressive symptoms and a good tolerability of the active treatment. Thus, there is a suggestion that reboxetine may be a good alternative to the most commonly used SSRI in the treatment of patients with the retarded form of post-stroke depression, but a larger number of controlled trials are necessary to confirm this indication.

There is only a randomized, controlled study using the psychostimulant methylphenidate in patients with stroke and no definite depression diagnosis in a rehabilitation setting (76). A higher improvement in depressive symptoms was found in the active treatment group in comparison to the placebo group. There are also open studies using methylphenidate in patients with post-stroke depression that suggest about a 50% rate of complete recovery during treatment (77–79). Even though methylphenidate may have a good pharmacological profile for post-stroke depression treatment because of its effect on cortical and subcortical structures, its properties of neurotransmitter reuptake blocker, and its fast action on depressive symptoms, no final evidence of its efficacy in improving depression in stroke patients exists.

Finally, electroconvulsive (81–82) and repetitive transcranial magnetic stimulation (83) treatments have been proposed as promising in improving depressive symptoms after stroke in small trials with a limited numbers of patients.

ANOSOGNOSIA AND DENIAL OF ILLNESS

History and Definition

Anosognosia is commonly defined as the condition of a patient affected by a brain dysfunction who does not recognize the presence or appreciate the severity of deficits in sensory, perceptual, motor, affective, or cognitive functioning evident to clinicians and caregivers. Anosognosia must be distinguished from the defensive mechanism of denial of illness, which is characterized by different pathogenetic processes and behavioral manifestations (84–86).

At the end of the nineteenth century, Anton (87) and Pick (88) described cases of patients unable to recognize hemiparesis, visual loss, and aphasia (85, 89). However, in a later study by Babinski (6), for the first time, we will find the term *anosognosia* indicating specifically the lack of awareness of a motor deficit.

Anosognosia is studied mostly in stroke patients with hemiplegia. These subjects deny their deficit or overestimate their abilities, refer that they are moving their handicapped limb, or partially admit difficulties ascribing them to other causes, for example, arthritis, tiredness, and so forth. Often, their false belief persists despite contradictory evidence, and they even produce bizarre explanations to defend their conviction. Anosognosics usually do not show a catastrophic reaction or desperate feelings about their condition, and they are unduly optimistic about their prognosis and medical course. Notably, they do appear aware of all the other fields of their lives or admit other actual symptoms. Other subjects show various forms of bodily delusions called somatoparaphrenias, that is they can disclaim ownership of the limb (90). Other manifestations are a lack of concern about the deficit (anosodiaphoria) or hatred toward it (misoplegia).

Epidemiology and Course

Epidemiologic data are not concordant because of the variety of measures and criteria applied in different researches, and, at times, because of inaccuracy in reporting results and methods. In the first studies, rates of anosognosia were very high and ranged from 33–58% in stroke victims (91–92). In other more recent studies, they ranged from 10–17% (93–94). Most of the cases tend to recover within three months from the onset of the cerebral damage (90–91, 95). However, one-third of hemiplegic patients still show anosognosia during the chronic phase of the illness. Frequently, anosognosia co-occurs with the neglect syndrome, though the event of a co-diagnosis seems to depend on the extent of the neurologic damage because they would be related to different components of a unique neurologic network (96).

Diagnosis

The diagnosis of anosognosia is done mostly on the basis of clinical observations, but the need of more specific tools to detect and to investigate anosognosic phenomena in hemiplegia is more and more evident. In the field of the diagnostic measures we cite:

- The Bisiach's scale (91), which evaluates anosognosia on a four-level scale (absent, mild, moderate, severe)
- The Structured Awareness Interview (90), a questionnaire consisting of rather specific and discriminative items that can be integrated by asking the patient to estimate his or her ability to perform some unimanual, bimanual, and bipedal activities,

for example, combing hair, tying a knot, jumping, and so forth
- The Patient Competency Rating Scale (PCRS) (97), which consists of 30 questions addressed both to the patient and to the caregiver. On each item, ratings are made as to "how much of a problem" the subject would have in completing various activities on a five-point Likert scale. The items cover a wide range of functional abilities, interpersonal skills, and emotional status.
- The Awareness Questionnaire (98–99), a three-form interview to administer to the patient, a caregiver, and the clinician. On each form, the abilities of the brain injury patient to perform various tasks after the injury as compared to before the injury are rated on a five-point scale ranging from "much worse" to "much better."

Mechanisms

The vast majority of anosognosics show a lesion involving the right hemisphere (89, 94, 100–103). Various hypotheses were formulated to account this evidence. For instance, Geschwind's disconnection hypothesis (104) postulated that the lesion would isolate the dominant hemisphere (left) from the nondominant one (right), monitoring the integrity of the left side of the body. Thus, the verbal hemisphere could not be aware of the impairment, could not report it verbally, and would produce implausible explanations (confabulation). In the same years, Friedlander's handedness hypothesis (105) suggests anosognosia to be associated with handedness. The dominant side should be more extended in cortical representations, and, as a consequence, anosognosia would be less probable following lesions in the left hemisphere, as the corresponding (controlateral) body percept would be less damaged. On the contrary, an analogous damage in the right hemisphere would destroy a wider portion of the left body representation. However, up to date, no valid empirical evidence supports both these hypotheses (89). More recently, Ramachandran (84) suggested that, in normal conditions, the left hemisphere is concerned with managing small discrepancies in perception and thought in order to make daily life consistent and predictable. When the discrepancies are so prominent that they cannot be ignored or adjusted, the right hemisphere creates new mental schemata or modifies the existing ones. In this view, anosognosia would be a failure in this functional balance between the two hemispheres.

Modern neuroimaging techniques cast light on the involvement of some specific cerebral areas in anosognosia (Table 27-3). In particular, anosognosia emerges more frequently following lesions of the prefrontal cortex, specifically of the dorso-lateral and medial regions as well as of the right parieto-temporal areas. At a subcortical level,

TABLE 27-2

Results of Placebo-Controlled, Randomized, Double-Blind Studies on the Efficacy of Antidepressant Treatment of Post-stroke Depression

Treatment	Reference	Number (ITT Population or Completers)	Mean Age	Females %	Depression Diagnosis at Entry	Dose (mg/d)
Nortriptyline	Lipsey et al. (1984) (43)	17	62	36	DSM-III (50% with MDD)	20–100 increasing
Placebo		22	60	35		
Trazodone	Reding et al. (1986) (80)	11	68	34	Clinical diagnosis of depression and abnormal ZDS	50–200 increasing
Placebo		6	68	27		
Citalopram	Andersen et al. (1994) (20)	33	68	64	PSD according with DSM-III-R and HDRS > 12	10 mg in older patients; 20 mg in younger patients (doubled after 3 weeks in nonresponders)
Placebo		33	66	58		
Nortriptyline	Robinson et al. (2000) (44)	16	64	69	DSM-IV MDD or MIND and HDRS-28 items > 11	25–50–100 increasing
Fluoxetine		23	65	26		10–20–40 increasing
Placebo		17	73	47		
Fluoxetine	Wiart et al. (2000) (45)	16	66	44	ICD-10 MDD and MADRS > 19	20
Placebo		15	69	60		
Fluoxetine	Fruehwald et al. (2003) (74)	26	65	54	HDRS > 15	20–40 (40 mg in nonresponders after 4 weeks)
Placebo		24	64	29		
Sertraline	Murray et al. (2005) (72)	62	71	48	DSM-IV MDD or MIND and MADRS > 9	50–100 (100 mg in nonresponders after 4 weeks)
Placebo		61	71	56		
Reboxetine	Rampello et al. (2005) (75)	16	77	56	DSM-IV MDD or MIND and HDRS > 20; Retarded depression	4
Placebo		15	77	53		
Fluoxetine	Choi-Kwon et al. (2006) (73)	19	Not available	Not available	BDI>13; DSM-IV Criteria for PSD	20
Placebo		32	Not available	Not available		

ITT = Intent to Treat; PSD = Post-stroke Depression; ICD = International Classification of Disease; DSM = Diagnostic and Statistical Manual of Mental Disorder; MIND = Minor Depressive Disorder; MDD = Major Depressive Disorder; ZDS = Zung Depression Scale; BDI = Beck Depression Inventory; HDRS = Hamilton Rating Scale of Depression; MADRS = Montgomery Åsberg Depression Rating Scale

Time from Acute Stroke	Duration (Weeks)	Response % (>50% Decrease in Depression Severity)	Results	Side Effects (Most Important)
Not available	6	Not available	There was a significantly greater improvement in depression in patients treated with nortriptyline than in placebo-treated patients.	Delirium, confusion, drowsiness, and agitation
6 weeks (mean)	4	Not available	Patients with stroke and evidence of depression are likely to benefit from treatment with tradozone.	Not available
		Not available		Not available
< 52 weeks	6	59	Significantly greater improvement was seen in patients treated with citalopram.	Nausea, vomiting, fatigue, rash, and headache
		28		
< 6 months	12	77	Nortriptyline was associated with more consistently improving depression severity compared with either the fluoxetine or placebo groups.	Sedation
		14		Weight loss, gastrointestinal symptoms, anxiety, and insomnia
		31		
< 3 months	6	62.5	The fluoxetine-treated patients compared with placebo-treated patients demonstrated significant improvement in mean MADRS scores at end point.	Well-tolerated
		33.3		
2 weeks	12	Not available	HDRS scores improved significantly in fluoxetine and placebo groups with no difference between the two groups.	Dizziness, nausea and cephalalgia
		Not available		
< 12 months	26	76	The MADRS score decreased substantially in both treatment groups, with no significant differences between them at 6 and 26 weeks.	Dry mouth, diarrhea, nausea, dyspepsia, weight loss, increased sweating, and weight gain
		78		
< 12 months	16	Not available	Significant reduction of HDRS and BDI scores in the group treated with reboxetine.	Dryness of fauces, constipation, hyperperspiration
		Not available		
14 months (mean)	12	70.6	No significant difference in the mean BDI scores at any of the follow-up periods.	Not available
		46		Not available

TABLE 27-3
Pathogenetic Hypothesis for Anosognosia Modified by Orfei et al. Brain 2007 (106)

AUTHORS	HYPOTHESIS
	Neuropsychology
Levine et al. (1991) (107)	Hemisensorial deficits and general cognitive impairment
Starkstein et al. (1992) (100)	Relationship with impaired attentional and arousal mechanisms
Ramachandran (1996) (84)	Impairment of the right hemisphere's anomalies detector in self-perception deputed to set up new schemata for new data contrasting with old self-knowledge
Adair et al. (1997) (101); Heilman et al. (1998) (108)	Failure to compare planning and execution of an action
Vallar et al. (2003) (102)	Unawareness of a deficit of intention or movement planning component
Marcel et al. (2004) (90)	Failure to integrate awareness of episodic instances of the deficit in the long-term bodily representation
Coslett (2005) (89)	Failure of intention to act in addition to a disruption of sensorial feedback
	Hemispheric
Bisiach et al. (1986) (92); Starkstein et al. (1992) (100); Coslett (2005) (89); Baier et al. (2005) (94); Turnbull et al. (2005) (103)	Right hemisphere damage
Geschwind (1965) (104)	Disconnection
Friedlander (1964) (105)	Handedness
Turnbull et al. (2005) (103)	Failure of emotional perception and expression
	Key Cerebral Areas in Anosognosia
Starkstein et al. (1992) (100)	Superior temporal and inferior parietal cortex, basal ganglia, thalamus
Ramachandran (1996) (84)	Right parietal lobe
Berti et al. (2005) (96)	Frontal cortex (BA 6, BA 44, primary motor cortex, somatosensory area)
Baier et al. (2005) (94)	Right posterior insula
Prigatano (2005) (86)	Anterior medial prefrontal and posterior cingulate areas and thalamus (areas frequently activated when accessing information about the self)

an involvement of thalamus, insula, and basal ganglia was noted frequently.

From a neuropsychological perspective, it was hypothesized that anosognosia might be a manifestation of a global cognitive impairment, but this statement is not supported by significant evidence (90, 109). Likewise, the "theory of discovery" (107), which blames the loss of awareness of illness on a proprioceptive deficit, is not fully reliable because this kind of defect is not present in all the anosognosic patients. Other researchers suggest that anosognosia may be considered as secondary to memory deficits, and it would consist in a failure in the integration of new information into the body self-image that is stored in long-term memory (100). Currently, the more believable model is that which postulates a defect in the process of comparison between the planning of an action and its actual execution. In other words, the brain damage would cause an error in the comparison between the expectations of the movement and the sensorial feedback during the execution (108,110), which usually determines the awareness of the actions.

POST-STROKE APATHY

Definition and Epidemiology

Apathy is a frequent neuropsychiatric disorder observed in patients after stroke. Reduced motivation or interest, lack of initiative, little spontaneous speech, lack of feeling and emotion, and lack of concern are the phenomenological expressions characterizing apathy.

Sometimes, apathetic patients are diagnosed as depressed. Despite the fact that apathy is also a symptom of depressive disorders and that apathy and depression may overlap in the same patient, it is a disorder that has to be considered independent from depression. This is because different mechanisms, clinical outcome, rehabilitation program adherence, and response to the treatment have been described in the two disorders.

Apathy rate in acute stroke patients may vary from 23–50% (111–113). This range of apathy rate depends on sparse sociodemographic and clinical characteristics as well as possibly on the different types of assessment used.

Thus, apathy is a very frequent complication after stroke, and clinicians must pay attention to this disorder.

Clinical Outcome and Correlates

It has been described that patients with apathy frequently suffer from major but not minor depression (111) and that apathy is correlated with self- reported depression (113–114). However, depression and apathy should be considered independent phenomena. In addition, two recent published studies reported that apathy was not associated with depression in stroke patients (112, 115). Apathy is also associated with older age and impairment in functional activities of daily living and cognitive performances (111, 113, 115). In particular, reduced attention and speed of information processing and impaired verbal fluency have been described in apathetic patients (113, 115). Finally, caregivers of patients with stroke frequently complain of patients' apathy because of their increased functional dependence in daily living activity (116).

Mechanisms and Treatment

Apathy has been usually associated with hypofunction of dopaminergic transmission (117) as well as frontal functional and structural impairment (118). In particular, patients with right hemispheric stroke suffer frequently from apathy. However, there is no individual cerebral area for this disorder. Indeed, patients with apathy may have a reduced regional cerebral blood flow in the right dorsolateral frontal and left frontotemporal regions (114). Also, anterior thalamic infarct (119), bilateral amygdale, and anterior temporal lobe lesions (120) are associated with persistent apathy and Kluver-Bucy syndrome.

Differently from post-stroke depression, where available treatment is efficacious and safe, in post-stroke apathy, no treatment is available so far. It is possible to hypothesize that dopaminergic and perhaps serotonergic agents could be used for the treatment of this disorder, but, unfortunately, no studies have been conducted to demonstrate their efficacy.

OTHER NEUROPSYCHIATRIC COMPLICATIONS

Anxiety

There is a strong comorbidity between post-stroke anxiety disorder and post-stroke depression (PSD). In acute stroke patients (121), only 10% met DSM-IV criteria for generalized anxiety disorder (GAD), while 12% met criteria for GAD and comorbid major depression. About three out of four patients meeting criteria for GAD have either major or minor depression.

Astrom (122) also described that the GAD rate was 28% in acute stroke patients, with no significant decrease in prevalence throughout the three-year follow-up. Of all patients with GAD, about 50% had GAD alone, and 50% had GAD plus major depression. During the three-year follow-up, 85% of patients who met criteria for GAD also met criteria for major depression at some time point. Finally, Leppavouri (123) found that 21% of stroke patients met DSM-IV diagnostic criteria for GAD, with 17% having GAD associated with depression.

A study (124) described a higher frequency of cortical lesions among patients with GAD and depression in comparison with patients with depression who only showed a significantly higher frequency of subcortical lesions. Two studies (121–122) consistently found that, among acute stroke patients, those suffering from GAD and comorbid major depression had more left hemisphere lesions. On the contrary, right hemisphere lesions were more frequent in patients with GAD alone.

It is important to highlight that functional recovery of stroke patients is impaired by the presence of GAD (122, 125). Thus, treatment of anxiety disorders is a fundamental feature for post-stroke recovery and good rehabilitation outcome.

Despite benzodiazepines are the most commonly prescribed medications for the treatment of GAD, they may accumulate in older people, thus increasing the likelihood of falls, disinhibited behaviors, or delirium. One study has investigated the treatment of GAD in stroke patients (126). Nortriptyline treatment (increased 50–75–100 mg/day) induced significantly greater improvement than placebo on the patients' anxiety symptoms during six to nine weeks of treatment.

Mania

Mania rarely occurs following stroke. Even if case reports and empirical studies document that stroke is associated with mania, a large study of the Iowa group (127) described a 1% rate of mania in acute stroke patients.

Frequency of right hemisphere lesion is reported to be high in patients with post-stroke mania (128), and lesions associated with mania may be either cortical (basal-temporal cortex or orbitofrontal cortex) or subcortical (frontal white matter, basal ganglia, or thalamus).

There are no published double-blind, controlled studies in post-stroke mania. A retrospective study described positive response to lithium treatment or to a combination of carbamazepine and lithium (129), and a study on a single patient with mania following brain injury reported efficacy of Clonidine 0.6 mg/day (130). Taking into consideration their mechanisms of action, valproate, ziprasidone, or aripiprazole need to be evaluated in controlled trials.

Involuntary Emotional Expression Disorder (IEED)

Involuntary emotional expression disorder (IEED) (131) has previously been named pseudobulbar affect and defines emotionalism with pathological laughing and crying that are unrelated to or out of proportion to the elicited stimulus. This disorder is quite common among patients with acute stroke. In a community based study of 128 first-ever stroke patients (132), the reported prevalence of IEED was 15% at one month and 11% at one year following stroke. In another study (133), 12 (18%) of 66 patients had IEED. The largest study (134), conducted in 448 patients without severe cognitive impairment who were within one month of stroke, demonstrated IEED in a total of 101 (22.5%) subjects.

Morris et al. (135) found that patients with frontal or temporal lesions in either hemisphere had significantly greater frequency of IEED than patients with lesions in any other brain region. Andersen et al. (136) described that, among 12 selected patients with IEED, the group with the most frequent episodes of crying had bilateral, relatively large pontine lesions. Thus, post-stroke IEED may be a consequence of the injury of serotonergic nuclei and/or fibers.

There are four controlled trials assessing the treatment of IEED in stroke patients. Results demonstrated that nortriptyline is superior to placebo at both four and six weeks of treatment (137), that citalopram is superior to placebo in thirteen patients treated for nine weeks (136), that fluoxetine is superior to placebo in diminishing tearfulness among nineteen patients treated for ten days (138), and that sertraline produced a significant reduction in the frequency of crying episodes among twenty-eight patients treated for eight weeks (139).

Psychosis

Psychotic symptoms of delusions or hallucinations are rarely described in stroke victims (140–141). Right parietal lesions, subcortical atrophy, and seizures may be risk factors for developing psychosis after stroke (140, 142).

Generally, anecdotal case reports indicate that patients respond to treatment with typical neuroleptic medications. Some patients, however, have been treatment-resistant, and anticonvulsant medications have sometimes been reported to be useful (141). Currently, there are no studies examining treatment response to the atypical antipsychotics.

Aggression

Aggressive behavior is described as a quite frequent complication in stroke patients. However, the described level of aggression is generally not very severe. Paradiso et al. (143) described a 5.8% rate of aggression in a sample of 308 patients with acute stroke when the threshold for aggression was high. The same research group in a later study (144) described 25% rate of aggression using a milder level of aggression. This last frequency of aggressive behavior was described in other recently published studies. Indeed, Kim et al. (145) reported a 32% rate in their sample study, Aybek et al. (146) described a 17% rate of aggressiveness, and Santos et al. (147) detected anger in 35% of their acute stroke patients, 13% of whom were severely angry. Thus, about one out of four patients with acute stroke may experience mild symptoms of aggressiveness, and 5-10% of stroke patients may suffer from severe angry outburst. These aggressive symptoms have to be detected and properly treated because they cause severe stress for caretakers, poorer quality of life, and negative outcome during rehabilitation (148–149).

There is a correlation between aggressiveness and cognitive impairment or affective symptoms of depression and anxiety in stroke patients seen both in acute hospital (143–144) or rehabilitation hospital (37). In addition, correlation between aggressive behavior and cognitive impairment has been described as a phenomenon particularly affecting left hemispheric stroke patients (37, 143).

From a biological point of view, depression and aggression are linked by serotonin metabolism dysregulation, and decreased cerebrospinal fluid level of the serotonin metabolite 5-hydroxyindoleacetic acid has been persistently described in both disorders (150–151). Also, decreased brain 5-HT2 receptors in the homolateral temporal areas after left hemispheric lesions may contribute to serotonergic system impairment (51).

Studies aimed at clarifying brain areas implicated in aggressiveness in stroke patients suggest that frontal areas, or at least areas closer to the frontal pole of the brain, may have a crucial role in the pathophysiology of aggression (143–145). This result is very plausible considering that there is a large amount of papers indicating dysfunction in the frontal areas, particularly in the inferior orbital frontal cortex, anterior cingulate, and the interconnected areas, as the main determinants of aggressive behavior (152).

At last, cognitive impairment has been consistently associated with aggression in many different neuropsychiatric disorders (153). A mixture of biological and environmental factors may contribute to this association in stroke as in other neuropsychiatric patients. Frontal lesions with associated impaired executive functions, impaired ability to communicate, and misinterpretation of others' actions are the main explanations of this relationship.

There is a very recent double-blind, controlled study with fluoxetine 20 mg/day versus placebo (73) on the pharmacological management of anger proneness in stroke victims. This study documented an efficacy of fluoxetine after one, three, and six months from the baseline. Furthermore, results of a secondary analysis of a double-blind treatment study with antidepressants for recovery after stroke (144) indicated that aggressive patients with more than 50% reduction of depression severity after antidepressant treatment experienced a significant reduction in aggression severity in comparison with those patients who did not respond to antidepressant treatment. In the last group, aggressiveness did not improve at all. Thus, anger seems to be treatable in stroke patients, and response to antidepressant treatment is strongly required in stroke patients with depression and aggressive symptoms.

CONCLUSION

There are numerous neuropsychiatric disorders that may occur following stroke. Depression and anxiety are the most common, and they frequently occur as comorbid conditions. In addition to producing significant degrees of psychological distress, depression and anxiety disorders have been shown to be associated with particular lesion locations and to adversely affect both physical and cognitive recovery from stroke and to increase mortality. Similarly, anosognosia, apathy, IEED, and irritability are disorders that may occur following stroke and will probably influence the course and recovery as well as quality of life following stroke.

Although there are no genetic studies that have identified the basis for any of these neuropsychiatric

disorders, animal and imaging studies have identified those lesion locations that are frequently associated with an increased frequency of these disorders. Post-stroke depression within the first two months following stroke is significantly associated with left frontal and left basal ganglia lesions, while mania is associated with lesions in the right hemisphere of limbic connected cortical regions, such as the oribitofrontal and temporal cortex, as well as subcortical limbic-connected regions, including the basal ganglia and thalamus. Apathy has been associated with mixed lesions in the right hemisphere, right dorsolateral frontal, left frontotemporal regions, anterior thalamus, amygdale, and anterior temporal lobe. Psychosis has been associated with lesions involving the right hemisphere at the intersection of the occipital parietal and temporal lobes, as well as permissive factors such as seizure disorder or subcortical atrophy. Damages in the frontal areas are implicated in aggressiveness in stroke patients. Finally, IEED has been associated with bilateral lesions of the frontal and temporal regions as well as of the pons.

Numerous well-controlled studies have demonstrated that pharmacological treatment with antidepressants can effectively improve post-stroke depression and post-stroke IEED. Psychological treatments that have not yet been demonstrated to be effective in prevention (69) and treatment (154) of post-stroke depression may nevertheless be useful in helping patients adjust and cope with losses and impairments following stroke. Future research will hopefully identify the most effective treatments in post-stroke depression and other neuropsychiatric disorders following stroke.

References

1. Hughlings-Jackson J. On affections of speech from disease of the brain. *Brain* 1915; 38:106–174.
2. Meyer A. The anatomical facts and clinical varieties of traumatic insanity. *Am J Insanity* 1904; 60:373–442.
3. Bleuler EP. *Textbook of Psychiatry*. New York: Macmillan, 1951.
4. Goldstein K. *The Organism: A Holistic Approach to Biology Derived from Pathological Data in Man*. New York, American Books, 1939.
5. Ironside R. Disorders of laughter due to brain lesions. *Brain* 1956; 79:589–609.
6. Babinski J. Contribution à l'étude de troubles mentaux dans l'hémiplegie organique cérébrale *Rev Neurol* 1914; 27:845–847.
7. Robinson RG. Post-stroke depression: Prevalence, diagnosis, treatment, and disease progression. *Biol Psychiatry* 2003 Aug 1; 54(3):376–387.
8. Hackett ML, Yapa G, Parag V, Anderson CS. Frequency of depression after stroke. a systematic review of observational studies. *Stroke* 2005 Jun; 36(6):1330–1340.
9. Whyte EM, Mulsant BH, Vanderbilt J, et al. Depression after stroke: A prospective epidemiological study. *J Am Geriatr Society* 2004 May; 52(5):774–778.
10. De Renzi E, Faglioni P. Normative data and screening power of a shortened version of the Token Test. *Cortex* 1978; 14(1):41-49.
11. American Psychiatric Association. *Diagnostic and Statistical Manual of Mental Disorders*. 4th ed. Washington DC, 1994.
12. Fedoroff JP, Starkstein SE, Parikh RM, et al. Are depressive symptoms nonspecific in patients with acute stroke? *Am J Psychiatry* 1991 148(9):1172–1176.
13. Paradiso S, Okubo T, Robinson RG. Vegetative and psychological symptoms associated with depressed mood over the first two years after stroke. *Int J Psychiatry Med* 1997; 27(2):137–157.
14. Spalletta G, Ripa A, Caltagirone C. Symptom profile of DSM-IV major and minor depressive disorders in first-ever stroke patients. *Am J Geriatr Psychiatry* 2005; 13(2):108–115.
15. Astrom M, Adolfsson R, Asplund K. Major depression in stroke patients: A three-year longitudinal study. *Stroke* 1993; 24(7):976–982.
16. Verdelho A, Henon H, Lebert F, et al. Depressive symptoms after stroke and relationship with dementia: A three-year follow-up study. *Neurology* 2004; 62(6):905–911.
17. Robinson RG, Bolduc P, Price T. Two–year longitudinal study of post-stroke mood disorders: Diagnosis and outcome at one and two years. *Stroke* 1987; 18(5):837–843.
18. Robinson RG, Starr L, Price T. A two-year longitudinal study of mood disorder following stroke: Prevalence and duration at six months follow-up. *Br J Psychiatry* 1984; 144:256–262.
19. Wade DT, Lengh-Smith J, Hewer RA. Depressed mood after stroke: A community study of its frequency. *Br J Psychiatry* 1987; 151:200–205.
20. Andersen G, Vestergaard K, Lauritzen L. Effective treatment of post-stroke depression with the selective serotonin reuptake inhibitor citalopram. *Stroke* 1994; 25:1099–1104.
21. Burvill PW, Johnson GA, Jamrozik KD, et al. Prevalence of depression after stroke. The Perth Community Stroke Study. *Br J Psychiatry* 1995; 166:320–327.
22. Berg A, Palomaki H, Lehtihalmes M, et al. Post-stroke depression: A 18-month follow-up. *Stroke* 2003; 34:138–143.
23. Robinson RG, Starr LB, Kubos KL, Price TR. A two-year longitudinal study of post-stroke mood disorders: Findings during the initial evaluation. *Stroke* 1983; 14:736–741.
24. Parikh RM, Robinson RG, Lipsey JR, et al. The impact of post-stroke depression on recovery in activities of daily living over a two-year follow-up. *Arch Neurol* 1990; 47:785–789.
25. Morris PL, Raphael B, Robinson RG. Clinical depression is associated with impaired recovery from stroke. *Med J Aust* 1992; 157:239–242.
26. Hermann N, Black SE, Laurence J, et al. The Sunnybrook stroke study: A prospective study of depressive symptoms and functional outcome. *Stroke* 1998; 29:618–624.
27. Gillen R, Tennen H, McKee TE, et al. Depressive symptoms and history of depression predict rehabilitation efficiency in stroke patients. *Arch Phys Med Rehabil* 2001; 82:1645–1649.

28. Kotila M, Numminen H, Waltimo O, Kaste M. Post-stroke depression and functional recovery in a population-based stroke register. *The Finnstroke Study* 1999; 6:309–312.

29. Paolucci S, Antonucci G, Pratesi L, et al. Post-stroke depression and its role in rehabilitation of inpatients. *Arch Phys Med Rehabil* 1999; 80:985–990.

30. Wan de Weg FB, Kuik KJ, Lankhorst GJ. Post-stroke depression and functional outcome: A cohort study investigating the influence of depression on functional recovery from stroke. *Clinical Rehabilitation* 1999; 13:268–272.

31. Gainotti G, Antonucci G, Marra C, Paolucci S. Relation between depression after stroke, antidepressant therapy, and functional recovery. *J Neurol Neurosurg Psychiatry* 2001; 71:258–261.

32. Chemerinski E, Robinson RG, Kosier JT. Improved recovery in activities of daily living associated with remission of post-stroke depression. *Stroke* 2001a; 32:113–117.

33. Narushima K, Robinson RG. The effect of early versus late antidepressant treatment on physical impairment associated with post-stroke depression: Is there a time-related therapeutic window? *J Nerv Ment Dis* 2003; 191:645–652.

34. Chemerinski E, Robinson RG, Arndt S, Kosier JT. The effect of remission of post-stroke depression on activities of daily living in a double-blind randomized treatment study. *J Nerv Ment Dis* 2001b; 189:421–425.

35. Robinson RG, Bolla-Wilson K, Kaplan E, et al. Depression influences intellectual impairment in stroke patients. *Br J Psychiatry* 1986; 148:541–547.

36. Bolla-Wilson K, Robinson RG, Starkstein SE, et al. Lateralization of dementia of depression in stroke patients. *Am J Psychiatry* 1989; 146:627–634.

37. Spalletta G, Guida G, De angelis D, Caltagirone C. Predictors of cognitive level and depression severity are different in patients with left and right hemispheric stroke within the first year of illness. *J Neurol* 2002; 249:1541–1551.

38. House A, Dennis M, Warlow C, et al. The relationship between intellectual impairment and mood disorder in the first year after stroke: *Psychol Med* 1990; 20:805–814.

39. Morris PL, Robinson RG, Raphael B. Prevalence and course of depressive disorders in hospitalized stroke patients. *Int J Psychiatry Med* 1990; 20:349–364.

40. Andersen G, Vestergaard K, Riis JO, Ingeman-Nielsen M. Dementia of depression or depression of dementia in stroke? *Acta Psychiatr Scand* 1996; 94:272–278.

41. Spalletta G, Pasini A, Costa A, et al. Alexithymic features in stroke: Effect of laterality and gender. *Psychosom Med* 2001; 63:944–950.

42. Spalletta G, Ripa A, Bria P, et al. Response of emotional unawareness after stroke to antidepressant treatment. *Am J Geriatr Psychiatry* 2006; 14:220–227.

43. Lipsey JR, Robinson RG, Pearlson GD, et al. Nortriptyline treatment of post-stroke depression: A double-blind study. *Lancet* 1984; 1:297–300.

44. Robinson RG, Schultz SK, Castillo C, et al. Nortriptyline versus fluoxetine in the treatment of depression and in short-term recovery after stroke: A placebo-controlled, double-blind study. *Am J Psychiatry* 2000; 157:351–359.

45. Wiart L, Petit H, Joseph PA, et al. Fluoxetine in early post-stroke depression: A double-blind, placebo-controlled study. *Stroke* 2000; 31:1829–1832.

46. Kimura M, Robinson RG, Kosier JT. Treatment of cognitive impairment after post-stroke depression: A double-blind treatment trial. *Stroke* 2000; 31:1482–1486.

47. Narushima K, Chan K-L, Kosier JT, Robinson RG. Does cognitive recovery after treatment of post-stroke depression last: A 2-year follow-up of cognitive function associated with post-stroke depression. *Am J Psychiatry* 2003; 160:1157–1162.

48. Ross RA, Joh TH, Reis DJ. Reversible changes in the accumulation and activity of tyrosine hydroxylase and dopamine B hydroxylase in neurons of the locus coeruleus during the retrograde reaction. *Brain Res* 1975; 92:57–72.

49. Robinson RG. Differential behavioral and biochemical effects of right and left hemispheric cerebral infarction in the rat. *Science* 1979:105:707–710.

50. Bryer JB, Starkstein SE, Votypka V, et al. Reduction of CSF monoamine metabolites in post-stroke depression. *J Neuropsychiatry Clin Neurosci* 1992; 55:377–382.

51. Mayberg HS, Robinson RG, Wong DF, et al. PET imaging of cortical S_2-serotonin receptors after stroke: Lateralized changes and relationship to depression. *Am J Psychiatry* 1988; 145:937–943.

52. Robinson RG, Szetela B. Mood change following left hemispheric brain injury. *Ann Neurol* 1981; 9:447–453.

53. Starkstein SE, Robinson RG, Price TR. Comparison of cortical and subcortical lesions in the production of post-stroke mood disorders. *Brain* 1987; 110:1045–1059.

54. Morris PLP, Robinson RG, Raphael B, Hopwood MJ. Lesion location and post-stroke depression. *J Neuropsychiatry Clin Neurosci* 1996; 8:399–403.

55. Herrmann M, Bartles C, Wallesch C-W. Depression in acute and chronic aphasia: Symptoms, pathoanatomical-clinical correlations, and functional implications. *J Neurol Neurosurg Psychiatry* 1993; 56:672–678.

56. Herrmann M, Walesch C-W. Depressive changes in stroke patients. *Disabil Rehabil* 1993; 15:55–66.

57. Vataja R, Leppavuori A, Pohjasvaara T, et al. Post-stroke depression and lesion location revisited. *J Neuropsychiatry Clin Neurosci* 2004; 16:156–162.

58. Vataja R, Pohjasvaara T, Leppavuori A, et al. Magnetic resonance imaging correlates of depression after ischemic stroke. *Arch Gen Psychiatry* 2001; 58:925–931.

59. Carson AJ, MacHale S, Allen K, et al. Depression after stroke and lesion location: A systematic review. *Lancet* 2000; 356(9224):122–126.

60. Bhogal SK, Teasell R, Foley N, Speechley M. Lesion location and post-stroke depression. Systematic review of the methodological limitations in the literature. *Stroke* 2004; 35:794–802.

61. Spalletta G, Bossu P, Ciaramella A, et al. The etiology of post-stroke depression: A review of the literature and a new hypothesis involving inflammatory cytokines. *Mol Psychiatry* 2006; 11(11):984–991.

62. Morris PL, Robinson RG, Andrzejewski P, et al. Association of depression with 10-year post-stroke mortality. *Am J Psychiatry* 1993; 150:124–129.

63. Everson SA, Roberts RE, Goldberg DE, Kaplan GA. Depressive symptoms and increased risk of stroke mortality over a 29-year period. *Arch Intern Med* 1998; 158:1133–1138.

64. House A, Knapp P, Bamford J, Vail A. Mortality at 12 and 24 months after stroke may be associated with depressive symptoms at one month. *Stroke* 2001; 32:696–701.

65. Palomaki H, Kaste M, Berg A, et al. Prevention of post-stroke depression: One year randomized placebo-controlled, double-blind trial of mianserin with six-month follow-up after therapy. *J Neurol Neurosurg Psychiatry* 1999; 66:490–494.

66. Narushima K, Kosier JT, Robinson RG. Preventing post-stroke depression: A 12-week double-blind, randomized treatment trial and 21-month follow-up. *J Nerv Ment Dis* 2002; 190:296–303.

67. Rasmussen A, Lunde M, Poulsen DL, et al. A double-blind placebo-controlled study of sertraline in the prevention of depression in stroke patients. *Psychosomatics* 2003; 44:216–221.

68. Almeida OP, Waterreus A, Hankey GJ. Preventing depression after stroke: Results from a randomized, placebo-controlled trial. *J Clin Psychiatry* 2006; 67:1104–1109.

69. Robinson RG, Jorge RE, Moser DJ, et al. Escitalopram and problem-solving therapy for prevention of poststroke depression. *JAMA* 2008; 299(20):2391–2400.

70. Niedermaier N, Bohrer E, Schulte K, et al. Prevention and treatment of post-stroke depression with mirtazapine in patients with acute stroke. *J Clin Psychiatry* 2004; 65:1619–1623.

71. Lauritzen L, Bendsen BB, Vilmar T, et al. Post-stroke depression combined treatment with imipramine or desipramine and mianserin: A controlled clinical study. *Psychopharmacology* 1994; 114:119–122.

72. Murray V, von Arbin M, Bartfai A, et al. Double-blind comparison of sertraline and placebo in stroke patients with minor depression and less severe major depression. *J Clin Psychiatry* 2005; 66:708–716.

73. Choi-Kwon S, Han SW, Kwon SU, et al. Fluoxetine treatment of post-stroke depression, emotional incontinence, and anger proness: A double-blind, placebo-controlled study. *Stroke* 2006; 37:156–161.

74. Fruehwald S, Gatterbauer E, Rehak P, Baumhackl U. Early fluoxetine treatment of post-stroke depression: A three-month double-blind, placebo-controlled study with an open-label, long-term follow-up. *J Neurol* 2003; 250:347–351.

75. Rampello L, Alvano A, Chiechio S, et al. An evaluation of efficacy and safety of reboxetine in elderly patients affected by "retarded" post-stroke depression: A random, placebo-controlled study. *Arch Gerontol Geriatr* 2005; 40:275–285.

76. Grade C, Redford B, Chroslowski J, et al. Methylphenidate in early post-stroke recovery: A double-blind, placebo-controlled study. *Arch Phys Med Rehabil* 1998; 79:1047–1050.

77. Lingam VR, Lazarus LW, Groves L, Oh SH. Methylphenidate in treating post-stroke depression. *J Clin Psychiatry* 1988; 49:151–153.

78. Masand P, Murray GB, Pickett P. Psychostimulant in post-stroke depression. *J Neuropsychiatry Clin Neurosci* 1991; 3:23–27.

79. Lazarus LW, Moberg PJ, Langsley PR, Lingam VR. Methilphenidate and nortriptyline in the treatment of post-stroke depression: A retrospective comparison. *Arch Phys Med Rehabil* 1994; 75:403–406.

80. Reding MJ, Orto LA, Winter SW, et al. Antidepressant therapy after stroke: A double-blind trial. *Arch Neurol* 1986 Aug; 43(8):763–765.

81. Murray GB, Shea V, Conn DK. Electroconvulsive therapy for post-stroke depression. *J Clin Psychiatry* 1986; 47:258–260.

82. Currier MB, Murray GB, Welch CC. Electroconvulsive therapy for post-stroke depressed geriatric patients. *J Neuropsychiatry Clin Neurosci* 1992; 4:140–144.

83. Jorge RE, Robinson RG, Tateno A, et al. Repetitive transcranial magnetic stimulation as treatment of post-stroke depression: A preliminary study. *Biol Psychiatry* 2004; 55:398–405.

84. Ramachandran VS. The evolutionary biology of self-deception, laughter, dreaming, and depression: Some clues for anosognosia. *Med Hypotheses* 1996; 47(5):347–362.

85. Prigatano GP, Klonoff PS. A clinician's rating scale for evaluating impaired self-awareness and denial of disability after brain injury. *Clin Neuropsychol* 1998; 12(1):56–67.

86. Prigatano GP. Disturbances of self-awareness and rehabilitation of patients with traumatic brain injury: A 20-year perspective. *J Head Trauma Rehabil* 2005; 20(1):19–29.

87. Anton G. Uber die Selbstwahrnehmung der herderkrankungen des gehirns durch den kranken bei Rindbenbindheit und Rindentaubheit. *Archiv Fr Psychiatrie* 1899; 32:86–127.

88. Pyck A. *Beitrage zur Pathologie und Pathologische Anatomie des Centralnervensystems mit Bemerkungen zur normalen Anatomie desselben Karger.* Berlin, 1898:168–185.

89. Coslett BH. Anosognosia and body representations forty years later. *Cortex* 2005; 41(2):263–270.

90. Marcel A, Tegnér R, Nimmo-Smith I. Anosognosia for plegia: Specificity, extension, partiality, and disunity of bodily unawareness. *Cortex* 2004, 40(1):19–40.

91. Cutting J. Study of anosognosia. *J Neurol Neurosurg Psychiatry* 1978; 412(6):548–555.

92. Bisiach E, Vallar G, Perani D, et al. Unawareness of disease following lesions of the right hemisphere: Anosognosia for hemiplegia and anosognosia for hemianopia. *Neuropsychologia* 1986; 24(4):471–482.

93. Appelros P, Karlsson GM, Seiger A, Nydevik I. Prognosis for patients with neglect and anosognosia with special reference to cognitive impairment. *J Rehabil Med* 2003a; 35(6):254–258.

94. Baier B, Karnath HO. Incidence and diagnosis of anosognosia for hemiparesis revisited. *J Neurol Neurosurg Psychiatry* 2005; 76:358–361.

95. Jehkonen M, Ahonen JP, Dastidar P, et al. Unawareness of deficits after right hemisphere stroke: Double dissociations of anosognosia. *Acta Neurol Scand* 2000; 102(6):378–384.

96. Berti A, Bottini G, Gandola M, et al. Shared cortical anatomy for motor awareness and motor control. *Science* 2005:309:488–491.

97.   Prigatano GP, Fordyce D, Zeiner H, et al. Neuropsychological rehabilitation after brain injury. Johns Hopkins University Press, 1986.

98.   Sherer M, Bergloff P, Boake C, et al. The awareness questionnaire: Factor structure and internal consistency. *Brain Inj* 1998; 12(1):63–68.

99.   Sherer M, Hart T, Nick TG. Measurement of impaired self-awareness after traumatic brain injury: A comparison of the patient competency rating scale and the awareness questionnaire. *Brain Inj* 2003; 17(1):25–37.

100. Starkstein SE, Fedoroff JP, Price TR, et al. Anosognosia in patients with cerebrovascular lesions: A study of causative factors. *Stroke* 1992; 23(10);1446–1453.

101. Adair JC, Schwartz RL, Na DL, et al. Anosognosia: Examining the disconnection hypothesis. *J Neurol Neurosurg Psychiatry* 1997; 63(6):798–800.

102. Vallar G, Bottini G, Sterzi R. Anosognosia for left-sided motor and sensory deficits, motor neglect, and sensory hemiinattention: Is there a relationship? *Prog Brain Res* 2003; 142:289–301.

103. Turnbull OH, Evans CE, Owen V. Negative emotions and anosognosia. *Cortex* 2005; 41(1):67–75.

104. Geschwind N. Disconnection syndromes in animals and man. *Brain* 1965; 88(2): 237–294.

105. Friedlander WJ. Body percept, handedness, and anosognosia. *Cortex* 1964; 1:198–205.

106. Orfei MD, Robinson RG, Prigatano G, et al. Anosognosia for emiplegia after stroke is a multifaceted phenomenon: A systematic review of the literature. *Brain* 2007; 130(12):3075–3090.

107. Levine DN, Calvanio R, et al. The pathogenesis of anosognosia for hemiplegia. *Neurology* 1991; 41(11):1770–1781.

108. Heilman KM, Barrett AM, Adair JC. Possible mechanisms of anosognosia: A defect in self-awareness. *Philos Trans R Soc Lond B Biol Soc* 1998; 353(1377):1903–1909.

109. Vuillemier P. Anosognosia: The neurology of beliefs and uncertainties. *Cortex* 2004; 40(1):9–17.

110. Heilman KM, Valenstein E. Mechanisms underlying hemispatial neglect. *Ann Neurol* 1979; 5:166–170.

111. Starkstein SE, Fedoroff JP, Price TR, et al. Apathy following cerebrovascular lesions. *Stroke* 1993; 24:1625–1630.

112. Carota A, Berney A, Aybeck S, et al. A prospective study of predictors of post-stroke depression. *Neurology* 2005; 64:428–433.

113. Brodaty H, Sachdev PS, Withall A, et al. Frequency and clinical, neuropsychological, and neuroimaging correlates of apathy following stroke: The Sydney Stroke Study. *Psychol Med* 2005; 35:1707–1716.

114. Okada K, Kabayashi S, Yamagata S, et al. Post-stroke apathy and regional cerebral blood flow. *Stroke* 1997; 28:2437–2441.

115. Yamagata S, Yamaguchi S, Kobayashi S. Impaired novelty processing in apathy after subcortical stroke. *Stroke* 2004; 35:1935–1940.

116. House A, Dennis M, Mogridge L, et al. Mood disorders in the year after first stroke. *Br J Psychiatry* 1991; 158:83–92.

117. Marin RS. Apathy: Concept, syndrome, neural mechanisms, and treatment. *Seminar Clin Neuropsychiatry* 1996; 1:304–314.

118. Carota A, Staub F, Bogousslavsky J. Emotions, behaviours, and mood changes in stroke. *Curr Opin Neurol* 2002; 15:57–69.

119. Ghika-Schmid F, Bogousslavsky J. The acute behavioural syndrome of anterior thalamic infarction: A prospective study of 12 cases. *Ann Neurol* 2000; 48:220–227.

120. Lilly R, Cummings JL, Benson DF, Frankel M. The human Kluver-Bucy syndrome. *Neurology* 1983; 33:1141–1145.

121. Castillo CS, Starkstein SE, Fedoroff JP, et al. Generalized anxiety disorder following stroke. *J Nerv Ment Dis* 1993; 181:100–106.

122. Astrom M. Generalized anxiety disorder in stroke patients: A three-year longitudinal study. *Stroke* 1996; 27:270–275.

123. Leppavuori A, Pohjasvaara T, Vataja R, et al. Generalized anxiety disorders three to four months after ischemic stroke. *Cerebrovasc Dis* 2003; 16(3):257–264.

124. Starkstein SE, Cohen BS, Fedoroff P, et al. Relationship between anxiety disorders and depressive disorders in patients with cerebrovascular injury. *Arch Gen Psychiatry* 1990; 47:785–789.

125. Shimoda K, Robinson RG. Effect of anxiety disorder in impairment and recovery from stroke. *J Neuropsychiatry Clin Neurosci* 1998; 10:34–40.

126. Kimura M, Robinson RG. Treatment of post-stroke generalized anxiety disorder comorbid with post-stroke depression: Merged analysis of nortriptyline trials. *Am J Geriatr Psychiatry* 2003; 11(3):320–327.

127. Robinson RG. *The Clinical Neuropsychiatry of Stroke*. Cambridge: Cambridge University Press, 2006.

128. Robinson RG, Boston JD, Starkstein SE, Price TR. Comparison of mania with depression following brain injury: Causal factors. *Am J Psychiatry* 1988; 145:172–178.

129. Starkstein SE, Fedoroff JP, Berthier MD, Robinson RG. Manic depressive and pure manic states after brain lesions. *Biol Psychiatry* 1991; 29:149–158.

130. Bakchine S, Lacomblez L, Benoit N, et al. Manic-like state after orbitofrontal and right temporoparietal injury: Efficacy of clonidine. *Neurology* 1989; 39:778–781.

131. Cummings JL, Arciniegas DB, Brooks BR, et al. Defining and diagnosing involuntary emotional expression disorder. *CNS Spectr* 2006; 11(6):1–7.

132. House A, Dennis M, Molyneau A, et al. Emotionalism after stroke. *Br Med J* 1989; 298(6679):991–994.

133. Morris PU, Robinson RG, Raphael B. Emotional lability following stroke. *Aust N Z J Psychiatry* 1993; 27:601–605.

134. Calvert T, Knapp P, House A. Psychological associations with emotionalism after stroke. *J Neurol Neurosurg Psychiatry* 1998; 65(6):928–929.

135. Morris PU, Robinson RG, Raphael B. Emotional lability following stroke. *Aust N Z J Psychiatry* 1993; 27:601–605.

136. Andersen G, Vestergaard K, Riis J. Citalopram for post-stroke pathological crying. *Lancet* 1993; 342(8875):837–839.

137. Robinson RG, Parikh RM, Lipsey JR, et al. Pathological laughing and crying following stroke: Validation of measurement scale and double-blind treatment study. *Am J Psychiatry* 1993; 150:286–293.

138. Brown KW, Sloan RL, Pentland B. Fluoxetine as a treatment for post-stroke emotionalism. *Acta Psychiatr Scand* 1998; 98(6):455–458.

139. Burns A, Russell E, Stratton-Powell H, et al. Sertraline in stroke: Associated lability of mood. *Int J Geriatr Psychiatry* 1999; 14(8):681–685.

140. Rabins PV, Starkstein SE, Robinson RG. Risk factors for developing atypical (schizophreniform) psychosis following stroke. *J Neuropsychiatry Clin Neurosci* 1991; 3:6–9.

141. Levin DN, Finkelstein S. Delayed psychosis after right temporoparietal stroke or trauma: Relation to epilepsy. *Neurology* 1982; 32:267–273.

142. Price BH, Mesulam M. Psychiatric manifestations of right hemisphere infarctions. *J Nerv Ment Dis* 1985; 173:610–614.

143. Paradiso S, Robinson RG, Arndt S. Self-reported aggressive behavior in patients with stroke. *J Nerv Mental Dis* 1996; 184:746–753.

144. Chan K-L, Campayo A, Moser DJ, et al. Aggressive behavior in patients with stroke: Association with psychopathology and results of antidepressant treatment on aggression. *Arch Phys Med Rehabil* 2006; 87:793–798.

145. Kim JS, Choi S, Kwon SU, Seo YS. Inability to control anger or aggression after stroke. *Neurology* 2002; 58:1106–1108.

146. Aybek S, Carota A, Ghika-Schmid F, et al. Emotional behavior in acute stroke: The Lausanne emotion in stroke study. *Cogn Behav Neurol* 2005; 18:37–44.

147. Santos CO, Caeiro L, Ferro JM, et al. Anger, hostility, and aggression in the first days of acute stroke. *Eur J Neurol* 2006; 13:351–358.

148. Williams A. What bothers caregivers of stroke victims? *J Neurosci Nurs* 1994; 263: 155–161.

149. Angeleri F, Angeleri VA, Foschi N, et al. The influence of depression, social activity, and family stress on functional outcome after stroke. *Stroke* 1993; 24:1478–1483.

150. Van Praag HM, Plutchik R, Conte H. The serotonin hypothesis of (auto)aggression: Critical appraisal of the evidence. *Ann N Y Acad Sci* 1986; 487:150–167.

151. Coccaro EF, Siever LJ, Klar HM, et al. Serotonergic studies in patients with affective and personality disorders: Correlates with suicidal and impulsive aggressive behavior. *Arch Gen Psychiatry* 1989; 46:587–599.

152. Davidson RJ, Putnam KM, Larson CL. Dysfunction in the neural circuitry of emotion regulation: A possible prelude to violence. *Science* 2000; 289:591–594.

153. Blair RJ. Neurocognitive models of aggression: The antisocial personality disorders and psychopathy. *J Neurol Neurosurg Psychiatry* 2001; 71:727–731.

154. Lincoln NB, Flannaghan T. Cognitive behavioral psychotherapy for depression following stroke: A randomized, controlled trial. *Stroke* 2003; 34(1):111–115.

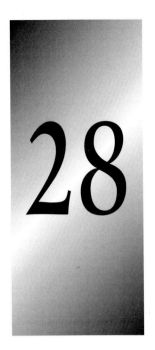

28 Fatigue and Sleep Disturbances after Stroke

Kathleen Michael

INTRODUCTION

Though implicated as a major disabling symptom in several chronic neurologic conditions (1–2), fatigue remains virtually unstudied in individuals with stroke (3–6). We know little about the nature and persistence of fatigue after stroke and even less about the consequences of fatigue on function, independence, and quality of life (4). For many individuals with stroke, fatigue ranks among their most distressing and limiting symptoms (3, 6). The relationship of fatigue and sleep disturbances with stroke is important, not only for the implications in cardiovascular risk, but also for the complex symptom patterns that influence everyday life.

In this chapter, we describe what is currently known about fatigue and sleep disorders after stroke. We develop a working definition and discuss theories and mechanisms of post-stroke fatigue. We characterize physiologic and biochemical dimensions, work performance and behavioral components, and symptom/sensory elements. Sleep disturbances related to stroke are explored, with specific discussion of the contribution of disordered sleep patterns to symptomatic fatigue. We outline the assessment of fatigue in individuals with stroke, along with management strategies to promote function and well-being. We discuss the evaluation and management of stroke-associated sleep disorders. Finally, we suggest research directions to

further develop knowledge about the mechanisms and features of post-stroke fatigue that may lead to effective rehabilitation interventions to reduce its impact.

Few studies have specifically measured fatigue in individuals with stroke. However, clinical experience and related studies point to the commonality of fatigue in this patient population. A substantial proportion of individuals with stroke (ranging from 39–76%) report significant and persistent fatigue affecting their daily lives (3–4, 6–7). In one of the few studies to examine fatigue in large numbers of individuals with stroke (3), self-reported fatigue was identified as an independent predictor for having to move into an institutional setting after stroke. Fatigue was also an independent predictor for being dependent in primary activities of daily living. This suggests that fatigue may reflect a decline in general health status and that fatigue accompanies reductions in functional independence.

Fatigue is frequent, often severe, and persists for months and even years after stroke (3). The frequency of self-reported fatigue is roughly twice as high in individuals with stroke as in matched controls, and it is not related to time post-stroke, stroke severity, or lesion location (4). Significant numbers of individuals with stroke report that fatigue is either their worst or one of their worst symptoms (3). Ingles and colleagues (4) found that individuals with stroke attributed more functional limitations to their fatigue than control subjects with fatigue did. Fatigue is also known to continue over time. Stein and colleagues (7) showed that 76% of individuals at eight months post-stroke complained of fatigue. At two years post-stroke, the number of individuals reporting that they are "always" or "often" fatigued was approximately 40% (2–4, 8). The observation that fatigue persists over time in individuals with stroke further increases the likelihood that fatigue is an important clinical feature of a progressively disabling pattern of inactivity. Patients who continue to experience subjective feelings of fatigue are less likely to be physically active. In studies of patients with neurologic conditions other than stroke, evidence was found for a negative relationship between subjective fatigue severity and physical activity (1, 9–11).

There is also a clear association of stroke with sleep disturbances and the likelihood that disruptions in continuity and architecture of sleep produce subjective fatigue by preventing adequate nightly restoration of physiologic and psychological resources. For example, obstructive sleep apnea is found in over half of individuals with stroke (12). The connection between sleep-disordered breathing and stroke is complex. While commonly viewed as a precursor to stroke because of its promotion of atherosclerosis and hypercoagulability as well as adverse effects on cerebral hemodynamics, sleep-disordered breathing persists after the stroke and is associated with poor outcomes (12). Diffuse cerebral symptoms, including fatigue, match the symptoms found in patients with sleep apnea alone (13). In a univariate analysis of the predictors of fatigue after stroke, sleep disturbances were identified as an important determinant (14).

Combined with motor deficits, cardiovascular and metabolic deconditioning, sleep disorders, and social isolation that often accompany neurologic impairment, post-stroke fatigue is associated with disruptions in physical, occupational, and social functions (15). Fatigue may impede full participation in a rehabilitation program (3) and promote and reinforce sedentary behaviors that contribute to learned patterns of disuse. The functional activity necessary to restore and maintain mobility and independence may be impacted negatively by fatigue (5). Even though fatigue has been associated with profound deterioration of activities of daily living in individuals with stroke, the symptom has received relatively little attention (3).

There are many reasons unique to stroke that might explain the pervasiveness of fatigue. First, there is the damage to brain tissue. Right hemispheric strokes in particular have been implicated in fatigue because of disconnection between the right insula and the frontal lobe or anterior cingulate cortex (16). Fatigue has also been associated with damage to the brain stem and thalamic regions, affecting the reticular activating system that regulates wakefulness (9). However, these physical associations with fatigue are inconsistent (4) and do not explain the widespread prevalence of fatigue in this population.

Second, fatigue may be linked with other consequences of stroke, such as depression (2, 6, 17–20), or other underlying disease states (3, 15). The association of sleep-disordered breathing and stroke risk is well-established (12, 21–24), and the persistence of sleep disturbances after stroke may further contribute to subjective symptoms of fatigue. Alterations of energy expenditure associated with hemiparetic gait also may be associated with fatigue (25), as may activity-associated cardiovascular/metabolic deconditioning (8). Deficits associated with stroke may impose limitations on social function and self-efficacy and may contribute to isolation and the subjective experience of fatigue (8). Understanding how fatigue relates to underlying pathology and impairment as well as how it is manifested in functional outcomes may hold the key to preventive and remedial strategies in stroke rehabilitation.

DEFINING FATIGUE

The symptom described as fatigue is common to many medical conditions and is recognized to have serious functional and emotional consequences (1, 4, 20, 26–29). To define fatigue, one may try to explain what it is, what it is caused by, or what it does. Most definitions describe fatigue's multidimensionality and frequently include a behavioral or work performance decrement, a physical or biochemical dimension, and a subjective or symptom/sensory aspect (30–33).

One definition by Aaronson and colleagues pertains to post-stroke fatigue especially well. Fatigue is depicted as "the awareness of a decreased capacity for physical and/or mental activity caused by an imbalance in the availability, utilization, and/or restoration of resources needed to perform activity" (34: 46). This definition affirms that fatigue occurs when systems are out of balance and there are insufficient resources, either because of excess demand or deficient supply. Fatigue is a symptom of imbalance.

Stroke imposes serious restrictions on the ability to activate, use, maintain, and restore physiologic and psychosocial resources, thereby promoting the imbalance that is felt as subjective fatigue. For example, the increased energy expenditure of hemiparetic gait results from the inability to activate normal movement patterns. There is a disproportionately large demand of cardiovascular/metabolic to produce hemiparetic ambulation (35), often compounded by the existence of deconditioning, underlying disease, and changes associated with aging. Because individuals with hemiparetic stroke have very little margin of unexpended reserves, their ability to restore physiologic resources is diminished. Add to this the sleep disturbances associated with stroke, and the balance of demands and reserves is further threatened.

Fatigue is characterized by distress and decreased functional status related to reduced energy (36) and behavioral adaptations to reduce symptom distress (8). Persons experiencing fatigue might describe it as "a sense of weakness . . . exhaustion, tiredness, lack of pep and energy, and/or low vitality" (37). Other descriptions of fatigue include feeling drained of energy, feeling more susceptible to pain, experiencing helplessness or loss of control, having difficulty with concentration, and irritability (9). Individuals may use terms such as tired, weak, exhausted, weary, worn-out, heavy, or slow. In whatever way it is described, fatigue is a multicausal, multidimensional sensation that affects sensory, affective, behavioral, and physiologic realms (27).

THEORIES AND MECHANISMS OF POST-STROKE FATIGUE

In defining fatigue, much attention has been paid to describing its source. Sources of fatigue differ from person to person and from time to time. They may include physical causes, such as pain, disease, anemia, inactivity, and other health problems (33, 38, 39–41). Fatigue may be associated with depression, overdoing, or trying to compensate for or hide a disability (42). Erratic sleep and too much stress may contribute to the development of fatigue (28). Environmental surroundings may add to fatigue, such as noise, air quality, stairs, warm weather, and uncomfortable furniture (38).

Out of this line of thought came the idea that there are specific types of fatigue and that their mechanisms of development and action are distinct. Dichotomous theories materialized in the attempt to organize and explain the complex and elusive nature of fatigue. One theory distinguished physical and psychological fatigues as two separate types (43–44). Another theory attempted to differentiate the fatigue associated with disease from that associated with exertion (45–46). Piper (27) proposed that there were two types of fatigue: acute and chronic. Acute fatigue occurs as a natural and protective response to a single cause; chronic fatigue comes from multiple, additive, or unknown causes and is deemed abnormal.

Each of these theories characterized fatigue as falling into two, discreet categories. Describing fatigue by such contrast and comparison was a necessary step in the development of constructed models. As the body of fatigue-related research expanded over the past decade, multidimensional factors were incorporated into the description and measurement of fatigue. Fatigue could no longer be completely and accurately categorized by types. The contributions of physiological and psychological functioning

as well as social and cultural factors had to be acknowledged (34), as did the outcomes of fatigue (47–49) and the interactions of an assortment of variables (50–51).

Physiologic and Biochemical Dimensions of Fatigue

There are a number of physiologic and biochemical issues associated with stroke that increase likelihood that fatigue will develop. A neurophysiologic model explains fatigue in terms of central and peripheral nervous system components (52). Impairment of the central component leads to decreased motivation and transmission of messages from brain and spinal cord as well as exhaustion of brain cells in the hypothalamic region. Impairment of the peripheral component can alter complex biochemical interactions between nerve and muscle that generate the force and power of movement. In individuals who have experienced strokes, there may be significant damage to the central components (16) and concomitant effects on peripheral components because of immobility, weakness, or spasticity (53). Post-polio research about fatigue has explored the effects of viral damage to the neurons of the reticular activating system, which may be pertinent to certain types of stroke. Damage to the reticular activating structures impairs the ability to maintain attention and leads to experiences of diminished concentration and drowsiness that polio survivors have aptly called "brain fatigue" (38). Strokes create impairments of the central nervous system caused by direct damage. The peripheral components are likewise compromised because of lack of innervation and the inability to recruit motor units. Some anticonvulsants and analgesics used to manage stroke-associated sequelae may further exert their effects on the central nervous system, and can compound the symptom of fatigue for stroke patients.

Another physiologic model of fatigue showed that changes in concentrations of metabolites interfered with force produced by muscle contractile proteins, leading to reduced muscle function and feelings of fatigue (41). The accumulation of lactic acid in working muscle is also implicated in the development of fatigue, which signals the body to rest in order to restore biochemical equilibrium. Cancer research has brought forth a number of biochemical mechanisms related to both disease and treatment that produce fatigue (45, 54–57).

Other explanations of the organic etiologies of fatigue have included looking at the causal role of decreased pulmonary function (58), decreased muscle strength and endurance (20), and increased oxygen consumption demands (59). Very important fatigue-related issues after stroke are the prevalence of sleep-wake disturbances, disruptions in circadian patterns, and sleep-disordered breathing, which are discussed later in this chapter.

Another physiologic model of fatigue that warrants discussion in the context of chronic stroke is that of the stress response and the activation of corticotrophin-releasing hormone and the sympathetic nervous system. Persons with chronic disease of any kind can be expected to experience a high degree of stress (52), springing from a variety of social, psychological, and physical sources. The stress response triggers the release of hormones (ACTH and corticotrophin) that act upon specific areas of the brain to coordinate behavioral responses. It is thought that, in the presence of chronic disease, the sustained stress response may lead to defective releases of corticotrophin, giving rise to behavioral depression and subjective fatigue (52, 60). Sources of chronic stress in this patient population might include physical issues such as immobility, gait problems, pain, spasticity, perceptual and communication deficits, and unaccustomed energy expenditures. The stress response might also relate to psychological, social, and role adjustment issues.

Work Performance and Behavioral Components of Fatigue

In the many definitions of fatigue, one common observation is its negative effect on work performance. When fatigued, people are less able to engage in physical, mental, or social activity. In the case of hemiparetic stroke, there appears to be a two-way relationship between fatigue and the work performance decrement. Subjective fatigue reduces activity levels, and reduced activity levels contribute to deconditioning and loss of function. Using ambulation as an example, one can discern the multiple triggers for the development of fatigue. First, there is the increased workload and energy expenditure in hemiparetic gait, stemming from the inability to control the functional and efficient manipulation of body segments through space (61). Adjustment of gait in hemiparesis includes reductions in walking speed, cadence, and step length (62) as well as musculoskeletal adjustments that shift the center of gravity and produce decreased velocity, decreased support time on the affected limb, and decreased weight transfer through the limb, all resulting in increased energy costs (61).

The greater the deficits and movement difficulties, the more body systems are involved in compensation, including neurologic, motor control, musculoskeletal, ligamentous, and cardiopulmonary. The increased recruitment of other systems to compensate for missing function leads to increased energy demand and fatigue, which can be seen with ambulation as decreased velocity and increased heart rate (63).

The development of fatigue in the face of mobility impairment and cardiovascular deconditioning is logical when one considers that reduced physical activity can be both an antecedent and a consequence of fatigue. A reciprocal and perpetuating association may exist between impairments in functional ability and fatigue. For example, neurologic deficits that compromise gait and balance increase energy expenditure and cardiovascular-metabolic demand for mobility-related activities of daily living (ADL) tasks, and cause patients to use a greater proportion of their physiologic fitness reserve to ambulate (61, 64–65). The depletion of energy may result in subjective fatigue, and patients may respond to symptom distress by limiting their activity. Inactivity further disrupts gait and balance through losses of muscle strength and lowered cardiovascular/metabolic fitness (53). Inactivity may also contribute to social isolation and loss of confidence in the performance of ADLs. Thus, a cycle of reduced activity and loss of fitness and mobility is propagated in the presence of fatigue.

There are also behavioral components of the work performance dimension that perpetuate the fatigue experience in individuals with stroke. Many individuals experience reduced motivation when their functional recoveries are slow or absent (61). This may contribute to social isolation and a disinclination to participate in household or community activities. The need to navigate architectural barriers may confine individuals to their homes. Fear of falling is also implicated as a behavioral limitation that has effects on the amount of activity in which individuals with stroke engage (66–67). With increasingly sedentary behavior patterns, individuals with stroke are at risk for fatigue, associated not only with energy costs of hemiparetic gait, but also with cardiovascular/metabolic deconditioning (8).

Subjective or Symptom/Sensory Dimensions of Fatigue

Several dimensions are common among all symptoms and all patient populations, including intensity, timing, level of perceived distress, and quality (68). In the case of fatigue in individuals with stroke, very little is known about the specific dimensions of the symptom. Intensity has been measured using scales that were developed for other populations, but they may not capture the distinct characteristics of stroke-related fatigue. The timing of fatigue in individuals with stroke is only known in terms of its persistence (3, 6–7) and has not been measured according to situational or temporal fluctuations. Rough estimates of the level of distress have been made based on how much patients report that fatigue affects their function and how often they describe fatigue as their worst or one of their worst symptoms (4). More work is needed to fully describe the symptom of fatigue in the stroke population.

Multidimensionality of Fatigue

Theories that address only the physiologic, work performance, or symptom effects do not adequately capture the multidimensional nature of fatigue. There are numerous features that can be observed or measured in a person who is experiencing fatigue. Manifestations of fatigue include perceptual, physiologic, biochemical, and behavioral signs. Contributors to fatigue may include innate host factors, such as age or gender. They may also reflect the accumulation of certain metabolites, for example, in muscle fatigue with the rise in lactic acid that follows strenuous work. There may also be pattern changes in energy and energy substrates, which can be seen in the mismatch of energy expenditure-to-reserve in hemiparetic gait. Disturbances in regulation and transmission patterns may result from injury to brain tissue and lead to subjective fatigue. Changes in activity and rest patterns may contribute to the experience of fatigue, as can disruptions in sleep and wake cycles, the presence of disease, or certain treatment effects. Psychology, social, and life events also have a role in the development of fatigue. Because the physical environment assumes greater importance in the presence of functional impairments, it must not be overlooked as another dimension of fatigue. For individuals with stroke, fatigue-inducing disruptions may occur in many areas and at many levels simultaneously.

Fatigue and Adaptation

Another way to look at fatigue is in the context of adaptive response. In response to a condition or stimulus, fatigue might actually serve a protective purpose (34). For example, in severely deconditioned patients, the perception of fatigue might curtail activity that would otherwise exceed their physiologic reserves. In individuals with stroke, the loss of cardiovascular/metabolic fitness results in reduction of exercise capacity. Individuals with stroke use a greater proportion of their physiologic reserve to perform everyday activities. This energy expenditure is compounded when gait and balance deficits increase the workload of functional ambulatory activity. Fatigue may be a warning sign of reaching the limits, causing patients to slow down or stop their actions, thereby protecting their diminished energy reserves and maintaining balance.

Fatigue and Psychosocial Factors

Psychosocial and behavioral factors may be as important as physical health variables in affecting stroke survivors' ability to function normally in their everyday life. Social support appears to play a significant role in explaining differences in subjective functioning (69). After stroke, high levels of family support, instrumental and emotional, are associated with progressive improvement of functional status (70). Peer influence is powerful. Social networks may subtly or directly influence physical activity and simultaneously reinforce a sense of belonging, purpose, and self-worth, thereby promoting mental health that may be reflected in low self-perceived fatigue and positive activity levels (71). Social support may also be influential in reducing the impact of depression and perceived disability (72). For example, in patients experiencing chronic fatigue, lack of social support was identified as a perpetuating factor of fatigue severity and functional impairment (73). In evaluating the relationships of mobility deficit severity, cardiovascular fitness, ambulatory activity and the effects of fatigue, inclusion of social measures adds a valuable dimension.

SIGNIFICANCE

With the evidence of fatigue's prevalence and persistence in the lives of persons living with stroke and its potential contribution to negative functional outcomes and disability, finding ways to prevent, manage, or respond to fatigue is imperative. The causes of fatigue in the chronic stroke population are many. Attention needs to be directed toward understanding the link between fatigue and the ability to engage in activities (11) as well as toward appreciating fatigue's relationship to specific functional outcomes such as ambulatory activity patterns. By building knowledge about fatigue after stroke, it may be possible to identify strategies for prevention, remediation, and/or compensation, thereby improving and preserving function, independence, and quality of life.

Fatigue and the Disabling Process

Individuals with stroke are at high risk for developing disability. As defined by the Institute of Medicine (74), the disabling process has four major components: pathology, impairment, functional limitation, and disability. Pathology refers to interruption or interference with normal body processes at the level of cells or tissues. Pathology in individuals with stroke exists on several planes, including direct damage and loss of brain tissue, lack of innervation to muscles, and other atrophic and metabolic changes on a cellular level. When the messages to and from the brain can no longer be transmitted or responded to normally, impairment results. Subjective fatigue in stroke patients may reflect disruptions to specific neural circuits in the brain and periphery, biochemical imbalances (41), circadian pattern problems (75), or physiologic responses to stress (52).

Impairment describes loss or abnormality of structure or function at the level of organs or organ systems and can include mental, emotional, physiological, or anatomical problems. Individuals with stroke experience a number of impairments not only as a result of damage to the brain, but also caused by changes in muscle structure and function, and changes in the use of the body. An example of this is hemiparesis. Changes in patterns of use may lead to such impairments as gait and balance disruption or cardiovascular/metabolic deconditioning. The workload of walking is magnified.

Functional limitation characterizes the restriction or lack of ability to perform an action or activity within the normal range and refers to the experience of the whole human organism. Restrictions on the ability to perform normal activities are evident when gait and balance deficits as well as deconditioning prevent stroke patients from participating fully and independently in activities of daily living and role functions. Other body systems are recruited at higher energy costs, and patients exhaust a greater proportion of their physiological capacity for activity. The imbalance of physiologic resources to energy consumption leads to the protective response of subjective fatigue (34).

Such limitations go beyond the individual and may be measured in terms of burdens and societal concerns, including the need for personal assistance with activities of daily living, the costs of health care, or the impact on family integrity and roles (74). Disability reflects the resultant inability to perform defined activities and roles in the social and physical environment because of functional limitations (74). For individuals with stroke, fatigue may be a very important component of the disabling process.

ASSESSMENTS/MEASURES OF FATIGUE

In individuals who have had strokes, the assessment of fatigue is complex. Its presence as a distinct symptom may emerge in the evaluation of other issues, such as weakness or depression. Individuals may experience significant weakness as a result of stroke, yet not describe themselves as fatigued. But when individuals are fatigued, their weakness may be more pronounced (4). Studies have found that, in individuals with stroke, somatic signs of depression may not always be accompanied by depressed mood and, in fact, may be more indicative of fatigue (17). Even when individuals do not have feelings of depression, the presence of fatigue may have a negative effect on their recovery (4). For individuals with stroke, fatigue should be recognized, evaluated, monitored, documented, and managed at all stages, from acute event through treatment and rehabilitation, to long-term recovery.

Because fatigue is multidimensional, its assessment must also be multidimensional. Patient report of fatigue symptoms is the starting point. Common across all symptoms and clinical populations are the dimensions of intensity, timing, level of perceived distress, and quality (68). A careful history should be gathered to characterize the individual's fatigue experience and to identify contributing factors. Assessments of fatigue in individuals with stroke should include evaluation of:

- Onset, Duration, and Intensity of Fatigue: How does the patient describe and interpret the fatigue? How has it impacted desired activities, independence, and function?
- Aggravating and Alleviating Factors
- Disease Process: Which area of the brain has been affected by the stroke? How long has it been since the event? What has the course of recovery been like? Have there been any complications?
- Current Medications: In particular, does the patient take anticonvulsants, antispasmodics, or pain medications?
- Sleep/Rest Patterns, Relaxation Habits, Rituals, and Customs
- Nutritional Status
- Effects of Fatigue on Functional Status: This includes mobility, activities of daily living, cognitive and social activities, as well as job and role performance. Has the patient had any falls?
- Presence of Depression or Other Psychiatric Condition
- Complete Physical Examination: Are there other disease processes, such as anemia, inflammatory disease, or cardiac or respiratory disease?
- Adherence to Treatment Plan: This includes therapy, use of adaptive devices, and precautions.

Fatigue may be measured in a variety of ways. In order to judge the presence and severity of fatigue or to determine if our interventions have had any effect on that experience, we may use measurement tools in conjunction with patient report, history, and observation of signs. Table 28-1 offers a summary of selected instruments that may be useful in measuring fatigue in individuals with stroke. Figure 28-1 provides a profile of fatigue severity in stroke patients, as compared to patients with Parkinson's Disease and arthritis, two other medical conditions in which fatigue is also known to impact upon quality of life.

FATIGUE MANAGEMENT STRATEGIES

The contributions of physiological, cognitive, and affective changes underlying fatigue are variable, and treatment is largely symptomatic and rehabilitative (76). Because the etiology and mechanisms causing and contributing to fatigue are multidimensional and interrelated, it is not surprising to find a considerable range of options for fatigue management. These may include education/counseling, cause-specific treatments, nonpharmacologic, and pharmacologic interventions.

TABLE 28-1
Selected Instruments for Measuring Fatigue after Stroke

NAME OF INSTRUMENT	DOMAINS MEASURED	COMMENTS
Piper Fatigue Scale (30)	Severity, temporal, affective, and sensory	• Multidimensional • Complicated format • Presumes the presence of fatigue
POMS-F Profile of Mood States—Fatigue (105)	Intensity	• Measures only one aspect of fatigue
Fatigue Assessment Instrument (31)	Global severity, triggers, and situations that modify fatigue	• 1–7 Likert scale • Measures fatigue in the past two weeks
Fatigue Severity Scale (1)	Physical and psychological function	• Patients select rating from 1–7 to signify agreement with statements • Functional impact of fatigue
FACT—F (106)	Fatigue in relationship to cancer treatment	• Specific to cancer patients
Multidimensional Fatigue Inventory (MFI) (107)	General, physical, mental, motivation, and activity	• Multidimensional
Rhoten Fatigue Scale (36)	Single item 10-point Likert rates	• Rates current level of fatigue • Cannot be evaluated by many forms of statistical analysis
Visual Analog Scale (VAS) (108)	Single item	• Simple, real-time measure • Cannot be evaluated by many forms of statistical analysis

Patient/Family Education

The most important rehabilitation intervention for the management of stroke-related fatigue is patient and family education and counseling. Providing anticipatory guidance about fatigue may diminish distress and

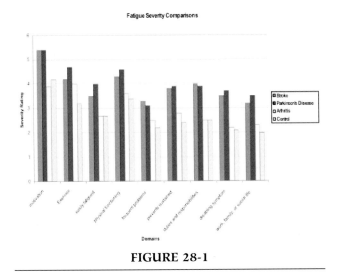

FIGURE 28-1

Comparisons between stroke, Parkinson's disease, arthritis, and control ratings of fatigue severity.
From Michael et al., adapted from Herlofson and Larsen, used with permission (8).

misunderstanding if it occurs as well as help individuals and families maintain feelings of control. Identifying fatigue-provoking activities, problem-solving to modify these activities, and suggesting individualized environmental changes empowers individuals and families to take concrete actions for symptom management.

Persons with strokes may benefit from learning energy conservation strategies that include prioritizing, pacing, delegating, or scheduling activities for periods of highest energy. They may also do well with structured daily routines that allow them to attend to one activity at a time and support scheduled rest times. Family members play an important part in helping to identify and reinforce successful compensatory strategies.

Cause-specific Treatments

The literature suggests that the diagnosis of fatigue is one of exclusion and that, even though it is seen very often in clinical practice, fatigue should not be presumed to be a natural consequence of brain injury (37). Individuals with stroke who have been ill and inactive for periods of time may have nutritional and metabolic deficits resulting in abnormal blood counts, which, in turn, can contribute to reduced oxygen-carrying capacity of the blood, and fatigue occurs as an adaptation to loss of energy. Treating anemias and supporting nutrition may make a positive difference for these individuals. Correcting fluid and electrolyte imbalances may dramatically restore feelings of energy.

Because individuals who have strokes are more likely to be in advanced years, they may have comorbidities that contribute to fatigue, such as arthritis, changes in thyroid function, alterations in glucose metabolism, and respiratory or cardiovascular disease (37). Alleviating acute inflammatory processes and correcting physiologic imbalances also may lessen symptoms of fatigue (42).

Nonpharmacologic Interventions

Reestablishing activity levels that maximize independence and function is a goal of rehabilitation. Many patients could benefit from an exercise program, which supports regular physical activity despite disability. For individuals with stroke, the use of appropriate adaptive devices and equipment may enhance participation in a regular exercise program as well as yield physical and psychological benefits (42, 77–79). Treadmill training, among other treatments, improves fitness reserve and lowers the energy cost of hemiparetic gait, which could be useful in relieving fatigue (80).

Restorative activities offer dividends for individuals with stroke. Time spent in natural environments, contemplation, and social activities may ameliorate the effects of fatigue. Some complementary therapies may be especially useful in managing stroke-related fatigue, such as biofeedback (81), relaxation techniques, meditation (82), music (83), and pet therapy (84). Such therapies offer multiple benefits through distraction and stress reduction as well as their inherent therapeutic effects.

Pharmacologic Interventions

For some stroke patients, the use of psychostimulants and antidepressants, particularly those with activating properties, may afford some relief from fatigue symptoms. When the damage from a stroke results in low initiation and psychomotor retardation, drugs such as methylphenidate have been used successfully (85). Fatigue is so often intermingled with depression that treatment of the latter may yield improvement in the former.

There have been no randomized, controlled studies of pharmacologic management of fatigue in individuals with stroke; however, anecdotal evidence from other neurologic conditions such as multiple sclerosis and Parkinson's disease suggests that some drugs may be helpful in treating fatigue when other contributing causes are eliminated. Depression and other organic conditions (anemia, cardiovascular disorders, kidney diseases, or hypothyroidism) should be treated first.

Physical activity, rehabilitation, psychotherapy, and avoidance of factors that may increase fatigue (fever, anxiety, depression, pain, and sleep disturbances) as well as avoiding some drugs like opioids and benzodiazepines are all interventions that may reduce post-stroke fatigue. If these measures do not reduce fatigue, in some circumstances, pharmacological treatment may lead to improvement. Amantadine, modafinil, and pemoline have been administered to such patients, but it is important to recognize that the evidence of their efficacy in reducing fatigue has not been established after stroke (86).

Future Research Directions

Rehabilitation research activities pertaining to stroke-related fatigue may help to substantiate its roots and remedies, determine its impact on function and independence, and strengthen the case for fatigue prevention and management as a worthy part of stroke rehabilitation. Growing from the knowledge that has been gained in the study of persons with cancer-related fatigue (27, 36, 40–41, 77–78, 87–90), fatigue assessments and interventions specific to individuals with stroke might be developed and refined. There is also a need for tools that measure the impact of fatigue on function, such as merging fatigue scales with functional independence measures (91). Instruments that can be used with individuals who have cognitive or communication impairments would also be useful.

SLEEP DISTURBANCES AFTER STROKE

Introduction

Sleep-wake disorders (SWDs) are commonly associated with stroke. About 20 to 40% of stroke patients have SWDs, mostly in the form of insomnia, excessive daytime sleepiness/fatigue, or hypersomnia (increased sleep needs) (92). Patients with stroke are also reported to have abnormal sleep architecture with significantly reduced slow-wave sleep (SWS) and rapid eye movement (REM) sleep when compared with controls (13).

Disruption of sleep-wake patterns may be attributed to the effects of direct damage to specific areas of the brain, sleep-disordered breathing (SDB), or other environmental and behavioral factors. The restorative features of sleep are critical to developing and processing motor learning and may strongly influence the outcomes of stroke rehabilitation and recovery (93). Growing evidence indicates a role for sleep in memory processing, specifically in post-training memory consolidation (94). Work by Walker and colleagues (94) affirmed that an overnight, systems-level change in the representation of a motor memory occurs with sleep and has important implications for acquiring real-life skills and in clinical rehabilitation following stroke. Given the importance of sleep in the cardiovascular risk profile, motor learning, and its contribution to the development of fatigue, efforts should be made to promptly evaluate and effectively treat sleep disorders after stroke.

Sleep-disordered Breathing and Stroke

A very important sleep disorder that deserves special attention in the context of stroke is obstructive sleep apnea (OSA). Not only does sleep-disordered breathing (SDB) lead to poor sleep quality, several studies have demonstrated an increased prevalence of OSA in stroke patients, and prospective studies suggest that sleep apnea is a risk factor for stroke, independent of other common cardiovascular risks (95). In individuals with stroke, sleep is reported to be often fragmented because of the presence of respiratory disturbances (13). SDB is a common condition, found in over half of patients with stroke (12). A measure of SDB recorded during a polysomnogram (PSG) is the apnea hypopnea index (AHI), which is the average number of disordered breathing events per hour that are seen during sleep. Between 44% and 95% of individuals with stroke are reported to have AHIs congruent with SDB (usually an AHI >10) (96).

SDB may be described as an absence or reduction of airflow through the respiratory passages during sleep (97). SDB that interrupts breathing, or apneas, fall into three major types: obstructive, central, and mixed. Obstructive apnea occurs when there is a complete absence of respiratory flow for 10 seconds or more, but with continued respiratory effort (97). Partial obstruction reduces the amount of airflow, usually by 30% or more, and is termed a hypopnea. Central apnea is both an absence of respiratory flow and respiratory (ventilatory) effort. A form of central apnea that is often seen following stroke is Cheyne-Stokes breathing (CSB). This form of central apnea appears as periodic central apneas followed by a respiratory effort in a crescendo-decrescendo pattern and can be seen during wakefulness as well (97). Some events start as obstructive, but then respiratory effort also stops, resulting in a combination of obstructive and central apnea. This is described as mixed apnea.

Both upper airway structure and neural control are implicated in the development or exacerbation of OSA after stroke. Some individuals may have preexisting narrowing of the upper airway. There may be increased compliance of the upper airway tissue caused by stroke-related weakness. Abnormal reflexes affecting the caliber of the upper airway (97) and pharyngeal inspiratory muscle function (97) further increase the likelihood of OSA after stroke. Symptoms of OSA typically include increased daytime sleepiness, fatigue, and lack of concentration (98). Other symptoms are habitual snoring, gasping and choking at night, irritability, anxiety, depression, morning headaches, and loss of sexual interest (99).

SDB represents both a risk factor and a consequence of stroke (92). For a variety of reasons, there is a strong association between moderate to severe SDB and prevalent stroke, independent of confounding factors (12, 100). Data from the Sleep Heart Health Study showed a dose-response association between OSA severity and the presence of hypertension four years later (101), placing individuals at greater risk of stroke. In normal sleep, blood pressure fluctuates, increasing with REM sleep and dropping during non-REM sleep, a pattern known as "dipping" (97). SDB causes increases in blood pressure during sleep as a response to the apnea-hypopnea pattern, without the normal decrease that occurs with non-REM sleep. Losing the nightly dipping pattern leads to a higher risk of cardiovascular morbidity (102).

Further, SDB may contribute to increased stroke risk by promoting atherosclerosis, hypercoagulability, and adverse effects on cerebral hemodynamics (12). OSA is not only a risk factor for hypertension, but it is also likely for atrial fibrillation and diabetes, conditions that, in turn, elevate risk for stroke (12).

SDB is more common during the acute and subacute recovery phases after stroke, as many recover during the chronic phase. While some individuals with stroke have preexisting problems with SDB, others may develop it caused by stroke-related weakness and disruptions of neural control. In some individuals, stroke recovery is accompanied by a concurrent improvement of SDB (93). Some will resolve with time and therapy. For example, in patients with transient pharyngeal muscle alterations secondary to the neurologic lesion, significant improvement in the number of obstructive apneic events is reported in the stable phase of a first-ever ischemic stroke (103).

RELATED FACTORS

Disruption of sleep and patterns of SDB may be associated with other stroke-related issues. The association of sleep disturbance and fatigue is apparent, but other factors such as depression, apathy, and cognitive issues may also implicate sleep problems. Nocturnal movement-related disorders may accompany stroke, and result in sleep disruption. In evaluating sleep problems and fatigue after stroke, it may be important to consider related factors, including not only sleep-related breathing disorders, but also other respiratory disorders, dysphagia, narcolepsy, parasomnias, sleep-related seizure disorders, restless leg syndrome, and periodic limb movement sleep disorder (104).

TABLE 28-2
Criteria and Evaluation of Sleep-disordered Breathing after Stroke

CRITERIA	EVALUATION
Obstructive Sleep Apnea: • BMI >25kg/m² • Neck circumference >40 cm • Loud nightly snoring • Witnessed apneas • Daytime sleepiness (Epworth Sleepiness Scale score >10) • Nocturnal oxygen desaturations Central apnea: • Witnessed apneas • Nocturnal oxygen desaturations • Associated congestive heart failure • Bilateral strokes or brain stem strokes	• Patient cardiovascular and medical profile • Sleep history; fatigue • Observations by hospital staff and family members • If strong clinical suspicion of OSA because of loud snoring, elevated BMI, and daytime sleepiness, proceed with an in-lab polysomnogram. • Because of the possibility of other related disorders, including periodic limb movement disorder, central sleep apnea, and parasomnias, home sleep studies are not recommended. • If the diagnosis is unclear, nocturnal pulse oximetry may be done to look for recurrent episodes of desaturations by 3–4% overnight. • If desaturations are noted, proceed with polysomnogram.

ASSESSMENT OF SLEEP DISORDERED BREATHING AFTER STROKE

The possibility of SDB or other sleep-related disorders after stroke is significant and carries important clinical consequences. Therefore, careful assessment of the risk factors, the diagnostic criteria, and the measurements to evaluate sleep-related issues must be included in post-stroke care. Further, by clearly identifying the features of sleep disorders, appropriate treatment and management can be determined. Table 28-2 provides a list of criteria associated with sleep disorders after stroke, along with recommended evaluation methods.

TREATMENT STRATEGIES

Following evaluation of fatigue and sleep disorders, the first line of management is to address potentially treatable contributing factors. Depression, anxiety, breathing disorders, stroke complications (nocturia, dysphagia, and urinary or respiratory infections), and drugs may contribute to sleep-wake disruptions and should be addressed first therapeutically (93). Spontaneous improvement of sleep disorders after stroke may reflect the resolution of other stroke-related medical and functional conditions.

Treating individuals with stroke who demonstrate OSA with continuous positive airway pressure (CPAP) can prevent or improve hypertension, reduce abnormal elevations of inflammatory cytokines and adhesion molecules, reduce excessive sympathetic tone, avoid increased vascular oxidative stress, reverse coagulation abnormalities, and reduce leptin levels (101). However, adherence to the use of CPAP apparatus is often very low. There is need to further evaluate the factors that influence compliance with CPAP treatment and to determine useful strategies to increase the consistent use of this effective intervention.

Clearly, sleep disorders after stroke warrant further investigation. There is much more to be learned about the symptoms and clinical outcomes associate with sleep disruption as well as the particular risks faced by individuals with stroke. Practical approaches to the management and treatment of sleep disorders after stroke are especially challenging, but they may have far-reaching consequences in terms of recovery, function, and quality of life. Rehabilitation professionals caring for individuals with stroke should actively evaluate fatigue and sleep disorders as well as integrate symptom management strategies into individualized therapeutic plans of care.

SUMMARY

This chapter presented some key information about fatigue and sleep disorders after stroke, using a relevant working definition of fatigue, with discussion of theories and mechanisms that may account for post-stroke fatigue. Stroke-specific assessment of fatigue was outlined, along with management strategies to promote function and well-being. SWDs associated with stroke were discussed, with suggestions for identifying risk, determining related conditions, evaluating sleep features, and developing treatment strategies.

Much of what is known about fatigue and sleep disorders has come from research in non-neurologic populations. Further fatigue- and sleep-related research is needed specific to stroke in order to fully elucidate the symptoms, mechanisms, and unique features of post-stroke fatigue and sleep disorders. With this knowledge, providers may more effectively design and implement rehabilitation interventions to reduce symptom distress, control risk factors, enhance recovery, and promote function, independence, and quality of life for individuals living with stroke.

References

1. Krupp LB, LaRocca NG, Muir-Nash J, Steinberg AD. The fatigue severity scale: Application to patients with multiple sclerosis and systemic lupus erythematosus. *Arch Neurol* 1989; 46(10):1121–1123.

2. van der Werf SP, van den Broek HL, Anten HW, Bleijenberg G. Experience of severe fatigue long after stroke and its relation to depressive symptoms and disease characteristics. *Eur Neurol* 2001; 45(1):28–33.

3. Glader EL, Stegmayr B, Asplund K. Post-stroke fatigue: A two-year follow-up study of stroke patients in Sweden. *Stroke* 2002; 33(5):1327–1333.

4. Ingles JL, Eskes GA, Phillips SJ. Fatigue after stroke. *Arch Phys Med Rehabil* 1999; 80(2):173–178.

5. Michael K. Fatigue and stroke. *Rehabil Nurs* 2002; 27(3):89–94, 103.

6. Staub F, Bogousslavsky J. Fatigue after stroke: A major but neglected issue. *Cerebrovasc Dis* 2001; 12(2):75–81.

7. Stein P, Sliwinski M, Gordon W, Hibbard M. Discriminative properties of somatic and non-somatic symptoms for post-stroke depression. *Clin Neuropsychol* 1996; 10:141–148.

8. Michael KM, Allen JK, Macko RF. Fatigue after stroke: Relationship to mobility, fitness, ambulatory activity, social support, and falls efficacy. *Rehabil Nurs* 2006; 31(5):210–217.

9. Belza BL. Comparison of self-reported fatigue in rheumatoid arthritis and controls. *J Rheumatol* 1995; 22(4):639–643.

10. Krupp LB, Christodoulou C. Fatigue in multiple sclerosis. *Curr Neurol Neurosci Rep* 2001; 1(3):294–298.

11. Packer TL, Sauriol A, Brouwer B. Fatigue secondary to chronic illness: Post-polio syndrome, chronic fatigue syndrome, and multiple sclerosis. *Arch Phys Med Rehabil* 1994; 75(10):1122–1126.

12. Brown DL. Sleep disorders and stroke. *Semin Neurol* 2006; 26(1):117–122.

13. Mohsenin V, Valor R. Sleep apnea in patients with hemispheric stroke. *Arch Phys Med Rehabil* 1995; 76(1):71–76.

14. Appelros P. Prevalence and predictors of pain and fatigue after stroke: A population-based study. *Int J Rehabil Res* 2006; 29(4):329–333.

15. Bennett JA, Stewart AL, Kayser-Jones J, Glaser D. The mediating effect of pain and fatigue on level of functioning in older adults. *Nurs Res* 2002; 51(4):254–265.

16. Sisson RA. Cognitive status as a predictor of right hemisphere stroke outcomes. *J Neurosci Nurs* 1995; 27(3):152–156.

17. Fedoroff JP, Starkstein SE, Parikh RM, et al. Are depressive symptoms nonspecific in patients with acute stroke? *Am J Psychiatry* 1991; 148(9):1172–1176.

18. Dalakas MC, Mock V, Hawkins MJ. Fatigue: Definitions, mechanisms, and paradigms for study. *Semin Oncol* 1998; 25(1 Suppl 1):48–53.

19. Staub F, Bogousslavsky J. Post-stroke depression or fatigue. *Eur Neurol* 2001; 45(1):3–5.

20. Walker G, Cardenas D, Guthrie M, et al. Fatigue and depression in brain-injured patients correlated with quadriceps strength and endurance. *Arch Phys Med Rehabil* 1991; 72:469–472.

21. Ferini-Strambi L, Fantini ML. Cerebrovascular diseases and sleep-disordered breathing. *Clin Exp Hypertens* 2006; 28(34):225–231.

22. Hsu CY, Vennelle M, Li HY, et al. Sleep-disordered breathing after stroke: A randomized, controlled trial of continuous positive airway pressure. *J Neurol Neurosurg Psychiatry* 2006.

23. Plante GE. Sleep and vascular disorders. *Metabolism* 2006; 55(10 Suppl 2):S45–49.

24. Wierzbicka A, Rola R, Wichniak A, et al. The incidence of sleep apnea in patients with stroke or transient ischemic attack. *J Physiol Pharmacol* 2006; 57 Suppl 4:385–390.

25. Michael KM, Allen JK, Macko RF. Reduced ambulatory activity after stroke: The role of balance, gait, and cardiovascular fitness. *Arch Phys Med Rehabil* 2005; 86(8):1552–1556.

26. Fisk JD, Ritvo PG, Ross L, et al. Measuring the functional impact of fatigue: Initial validation of the fatigue impact scale. *Clin Infect Dis* 1994; 18 Suppl 1:S79–83.

27. Piper B, Lindsey A, Dodd M. Fatigue mechanisms in cancer patients: Developing nursing theory. *ONF* 1987; 14(6):17–23.

28. Schwartz CE, Coulthard-Morris L, Zeng Q. Psychosocial correlates of fatigue in multiple sclerosis. *Arch Phys Med Rehabil* 1996; 77(2):165–170.

29. Vercoulen JH, Hommes OR, Swanink CM, et al. The measurement of fatigue in patients with multiple sclerosis: A multidimensional comparison with patients with chronic fatigue syndrome and healthy subjects. *Arch Neurol* 1996; 53(7):642–649.

30. Piper BF, Dibble SL, Dodd MJ, et al. The revised Piper Fatigue Scale: Psychometric evaluation in women with breast cancer. *Oncol Nurs Forum* 1998; 25(4):677–684.

31. Schwartz A. The Schwartz Cancer Fatigue Scale: Testing reliability and validity. *ONF* 1998; 25(4):711–717.

32. Ferrell B, Grant M, Dean G, et al. Bone-tired: The experience of fatigue and its impact on quality of life. *ONF* 1996; 23(10):1539–1547.

33. Carrieri-Kohlman V, Lindsey AM, West CM. *Pathophysiological Phenomena in Nursing: Human Responses to Illness.* 2nd ed. Philadelphia: Saunders, 1993.

34. Aaronson LS, Teel CS, Cassmeyer V, et al. Defining and measuring fatigue. *Image J Nurs Sch* 1999; 31(1):45–50.

35. Macko RF, Smith GV, Dobrovolny CL, et al. Treadmill training improves fitness reserve in chronic stroke patients. *Arch Phys Med Rehabil* 2001; 82(7):879–884.

36. Pickard-Holley S. Fatigue in cancer patients: A descriptive study. *Cancer Nurs* 1991; 14(1):13–19.

37. Zasler N. Brain Injury source at Ask the Doctor [electronic]. Accessed March 8, 2000.

38. Bruno RL, Galski T, DeLuca J. The neuropsychology of post-polio fatigue. *Arch Phys Med Rehabil* 1993; 74(10):1061–1065.

39. Glaus A, Crow R, Hammond S. A qualitative study to explore the concept of fatigue/tiredness in cancer patients and in healthy individuals. *Eur J Cancer Care (Engl)* 1996; 5(2 Suppl):8–23.

40. Irvine D, Vincent L, Graydon JE, et al. The prevalence and correlates of fatigue in patients receiving treatment with chemotherapy and radiotherapy: A comparison with the fatigue experienced by healthy individuals. *Cancer Nurs* 1994; 17(5):367–378.

41. St. Pierre BK, C. Fatigue mechanisms in patients with cancer: effects of tumor necrosis factor and exercise on skeletal muscle. *ONF.* 1992; 19(3):419–425.

42. Matsen F. Fatigue Management page at University of Washington Bone and Joint Source Website. Accessed March 8, 2000.

43. O'Dell MW, Meighen M, Riggs RV. Correlates of fatigue in HIV infection prior to AIDS: A pilot study. *Disabil Rehabil* 1996; 18(5):249–254.

44. Milligan R, Lenz ER, Parks PL, etc. Postpartum fatigue: Clarifying a concept. *Sch Inq Nurs Pract* 1996; 10(3):279–291.

45. Cella D, Lai JS, Chang CH, et al. Fatigue in cancer patients compared with fatigue in the general United States population. *Cancer* 2002; 94(2):528–538.

46. Stuifbergen AK, Rogers S. The experience of fatigue and strategies of self-care among persons with multiple sclerosis. *Appl Nurs Res* 1997; 10(1):2–10.

47. Bennett JA, Stewart AL, Kayser-Jones J, Glaser D. The mediating effect of pain and fatigue on level of functioning in older adults. *Nurs Res* 2002; 51(4):254–265.

48. Macko RF, Katzel LI, Yataco A, et al. Low-velocity graded treadmill stress testing in hemiparetic stroke patients. *Stroke* 1997; 28(5):988–992.

49. Schwartz AL. Fatigue mediates the effects of exercise on quality of life. *Qual Life Res* 1999; 8(6):529–538.

50. Breukink SO, Strijbos JH, Koorn M, et al. Relationship between subjective fatigue and physiological variables in patients with chronic obstructive pulmonary disease. *Respir Med* 1998; 92(4):676–682.

51. Given B, Given CW, McCorkle R, et al. Pain and fatigue management: Results of a nursing randomized clinical trial. *Oncol Nurs Forum* 2002; 29(6):949–956.

52. Swain MG. Fatigue in chronic disease. *Clin Sci (Lond)* 2000; 99(1):1–8.

53. Ryan A, Dobrovolny CL, Silver KH, et al. Cardiovascular fitness after stroke: Role of muscle mass and gait deficit severity. *Journal of Stroke and Cardiovascular Diseases* 2000; 9(4):185–191.

54. Nail LM. Fatigue in patients with cancer. *Oncol Nurs Forum* 2002; 29(3):537.

55. Piper BF, Dibble SL, Dodd MJ, et al. The revised Piper Fatigue Scale: Psychometric evaluation in women with breast cancer. *Oncol Nurs Forum* 1998; 25(4):677–684.

56. St Pierre BA, Kasper CE, Lindsey AM. Fatigue mechanisms in patients with cancer: Effects of tumor necrosis factor and exercise on skeletal muscle. *Oncol Nurs Forum* 1992; 19(3):419–425.

57. Woo B, Dibble SL, Piper BF, et al. Differences in fatigue by treatment methods in women with breast cancer. *Oncol Nurs Forum* 1998; 25(5):915–920.

58. Becker E, Bar-Or O, Mendelson L, Najenson T. Pulmonary functions and responses to exercise of patients following craniocerebral injury. *Scand J Rehabil Med* 1978; 10(2):47–50.

59. Richerson RL, Richerson ME. Energy expenditure in simulated tasks: Comparison between subjects with brain injury and able-bodied persons. *Arch Phys Med Rehabil* 1981; 62(5):212–214.

60. Clauw DJ, Chrousos GP. Chronic pain and fatigue syndromes: Overlapping clinical and neuroendocrine features and potential pathogenic mechanisms. *Neuroimmunomodulation* 1997; 4(3):134–153.

61. Fish DK, CS. Walking impediments and gait inefficiencies in the CVA patient. *Journal of Prosthetics and Orthotics* 1999; 11(2):33–37.

62. Lehmann JF, Condon SM, Price R, deLateur BJ. Gait abnormalities in hemiplegia: Their correction by ankle-foot orthoses. *Arch Phys Med Rehabil* 1987; 68(11):763–771.

63. Dettmann MA, Linder MT, Sepic SB. Relationships among walking performance, postural stability, and functional assessments of the hemiplegic patient. *Am J Phys Med* 1987; 66(2):77–90.

64. Fisher SV, Gullickson G, Jr. Energy cost of ambulation in health and disability: A literature review. *Arch Phys Med Rehabil* 1978; 59(3):124–133.

65. Macko RF, DeSouza CA, Tretter LD, et al. Treadmill aerobic exercise training reduces the energy expenditure and cardiovascular demands of hemiparetic gait in chronic stroke patients: A preliminary report. *Stroke* 1997; 28(2):326–330.

66. Tinetti ME, Powell L. Fear of falling and low self-efficacy: A case of dependence in elderly persons. *J Gerontol* 1993; 48:35–38.

67. Tinetti ME, Mendes de Leon CF, Doucette JT, Baker DI. Fear of falling and fall-related efficacy in relationship to functioning among community-living elders. *J Gerontol* 1994; 49(3):M140–147.

68. Lenz ER, Pugh LC, Milligan RA, et al. The middle-range theory of unpleasant symptoms: An update. *ANS Adv Nurs Sci* 1997; 19(3):14–27.

69. Koukouli S, Vlachonikolis IG, Philalithis A. Sociodemographic factors and self-reported functional status: The significance of social support. *BMC Health Serv Res* 2002; 2(1):20.

70. Tsouna-Hadjis E, Vemmos KN, Zakopoulos N, Stamatelopoulos S. First-stroke recovery process: The role of family social support. *Arch Phys Med Rehabil* 2000; 81(7):881–887.

71. Glass TA, Matchar DB, Belyea M, Feussner JR. Impact of social support on outcome in first stroke. *Stroke* 1993; 24(1):64–70.

72. Clarke PJ, Black SE, Badley EM, et al. Handicap in stroke survivors. *Disabil Rehabil* 1999; 21(3):116–123.

73. Prins JB, Bos E, Huibers MJ, et al. Social support and the persistence of complaints in chronic fatigue syndrome. *Psychother Psychosom* 2004; 73(3):174–182.

74. Brandt EN, Pope AM, Institute of Medicine (US), Committee on Assessing Rehabilitation Science and Engineering. *Enabling America: Assessing the Role of Rehabilitation Science and Engineering.* Washington DC: National Academy Press, 1997.

75. Richardson A, Ream E. The experience of fatigue and other symptoms in patients receiving chemotherapy. *Eur J Cancer Care (Engl)* 1996; 5(2 Suppl):24–30.

76. Chaudhuri A, Behan PO. Fatigue in neurological disorders. *Lancet* 2004; 363(9413):978–988.

77. Friendenreich CM, Courneya KS. Exercise as rehabilitation for cancer patients. *Clin J Sport Med* 1996; 6(4):237–244.

78. Mock V, Burke MB, Sheehan P, et al. A nursing rehabilitation program for women with breast cancer receiving adjuvant chemotherapy. *Oncol Nurs Forum* 1994; 21(5):899–907; discussion 908.

79. Winningham ML. Walking program for people with cancer: Getting started. *Cancer Nurs* 1991; 14(5):270–276.

80. Colle F, Bonan I, Gellez Leman MC, Bradai N, Yelnik A. Fatigue after stroke. *Ann Readapt Med Phys* 2006; 49(6):272–276, 361–364.

81. Glanz M, Klawansky S, Chalmers T. Biofeedback therapy in stroke rehabilitation: A review. *J R Soc Med* 1997; 90(1):33–39.

82. Harmon RL, Myers MA. Prayer and meditation as medical therapies. *Phys Med Rehabil Clin N Am* 1999; 10(3):651–662.

83. Snyder M, Chlan L. Music therapy. *Annu Rev Nurs Res* 1999; 17:3–25.

84. Wilkes CN, Shalko TK, Trahan M. Pet Rx: Implications for good health. *Health Educ* 1989; 20(2):6–9.

85. Grade C, Redford B, Chrostowski J, et al. Methylphenidate in early post-stroke recovery: A double-blind, placebo-controlled study. *Arch Phys Med Rehabil* 1998; 79(9):1047–1050.

86. Branas P, Jordan R, Fry-Smith A, et al. Treatments for fatigue in multiple sclerosis: A rapid and systematic review. *Health Technol Assess* 2000; 4(27):1–71.

87. Dean GE, Spears L, Ferrell BR, et al. Fatigue in patients with cancer receiving interferon alpha. *Cancer Pract* 1995; 3(3):164–172.

88. Hann D, Jacobsen, P, Azzarello, L, et al. Measurement of fatigue in cancer patients: Development and validation of the Fatigue Symptom Inventory. *Quality of Life Research* 1998; 7(4):301–310.

89. Nail LM, Winningham ML. Fatigue and weakness in cancer patients: The symptoms experience. *Semin Oncol Nurs* 1995; 11(4):272–278.

90. Winningham ML, Nail LM, Burke MB, et al. Fatigue and the cancer experience: The state of the knowledge. *Oncol Nurs Forum* 1994; 21(1):23–36.

91. Granger CV, Cotter AC, Hamilton BB, Fiedler RC. Functional assessment scales: A study of persons after stroke. *Arch Phys Med Rehabil* 1993; 74(2):133–138.

92. Bassetti CL. Sleep and stroke. *Semin Neurol* 2005; 25(1):19–32.

93. Hermann DM, Bassetti CL. Sleep apnea and other sleep-wake disorders in stroke. *Curr Treat Options Neurol* 2003; 5(3):241–249.

94. Walker MP, Stickgold R, Alsop D, et al. Sleep-dependent motor memory plasticity in the human brain. *Neuroscience* 2005; 133(4):911–917.

95. Yaggi HK, Concato J, Kernan WN, et al. Obstructive sleep apnea as a risk factor for stroke and death. *N Engl J Med* 2005; 353(19):2034–2041.

96. Cadilhac DA, Thorpe RD, Pearce DC, et al. Sleep-disordered breathing in chronic stroke survivors: A study of the long-term follow-up of the SCOPES cohort using home based polysomnography. *J Clin Neurosci* 2005; 12(6):632–637.

97. Richards KC, Hall KS, Shook D, et al. Sleep-disordered breathing and stroke. *J Cardiovasc Nurs* 2002; 17(1):12–29.

98. Norton PG, Dunn EV. Snoring as a risk factor for disease: An epidemiological survey. *Br Med J (Clin Res Ed)* 1985; 291(6496):630–632.

99. Krug P. Snoring and obstructive sleep apnea. *Aorn J* 1999; 69(4):792–801.

100. Arzt M, Young T, Finn L, et al. Association of sleep-disordered breathing and the occurrence of stroke. *Am J Respir Crit Care Med* 2005; 172(11):1447–1451.

101. Grigg-Damberger M. Why a polysomnogram should become part of the diagnostic evaluation of stroke and transient ischemic attack. *J Clin Neurophysiol* 2006; 23(1): 21–38.

102. Pankow W, Lies A, Lohmann FW. Sleep-disordered breathing and hypertension. *N Engl J Med* 2000; 343(13):966, author reply 967.

103. Martinez-Garcia MA, Galiano-Blancart R, Soler-Cataluna JJ, et al. Improvement in nocturnal disordered breathing after first-ever ischemic stroke: Role of dysphagia. *Chest* 2006; 129(2):238–245.

104. Kushida CA, Littner MR, Morgenthaler T, et al. Practice parameters for the indications for polysomnography and related procedures: An update for 2005. *Sleep* 2005; 28(4):499–521.

105. Norcross JC, Guadagnoli E, Prochaska JO. Factor structure of the Profile of Mood States (POMS): Two partial replications. *J Clin Psychol* 1984; 40(5):1270–1277.

106. Cella DF, Tulsky DS, Gray G, et al. The functional assessment of cancer therapy scale: Development and validation of the general measure. *J Clin Oncol* 1993; 11(3):570–579.

107. Smets EM, Garssen B, Bonke B, De Haes JC. The Multidimensional Fatigue Inventory (MFI) psychometric qualities of an instrument to assess fatigue. *J Psychosom Res* 1995; 39(3):315–325.

108. Lee KA, Hicks G, Nino-Murcia G. Validity and reliability of a scale to assess fatigue [see comments]. *Psychiatry Res* 1991; 36(3):291–298.

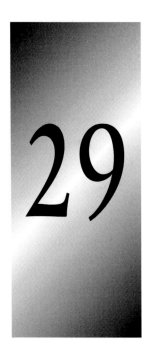

29 Malnutrition after Stroke

Hillel M. Finestone
Norine Foley
Linda S. Greene-Finestone

The nutritional status of patients who have had a stroke is vulnerable for a host of reasons. The presence of dysphagia is a key factor that may lead to eating difficulties and nutritional impairments, although other physical, cognitive, and perceptual issues often associated with advancing age may also contribute (Table 29-1). Awareness and proper management of the nutritional issues and problems contribute to better outcomes. It is important to identify and treat declines in nutritional status associated with stroke because of their negative impact on survival and functional recovery (2–4). Malnutrition and hypoalbuminemia have been associated with poorer functional outcomes (3, 5), higher complication rates (5), longer lengths of stay, and reduced functional improvement rates (3) in acute and rehabilitating stroke patients. In this chapter, methods of screening and assessing stroke patients' nutritional status as well as strategies for improving their food and fluid intake are addressed.

MALNUTRITION

The reported prevalence of malnutrition following stroke ranges widely, from 6 to 62% (2, 6–16). Table 29-2 presents the results from 12 studies that assessed the nutritional status of patients following stroke. Many factors may have influenced the precision of the estimate, such as method and timing of nutritional assessment, differences in stroke subtypes (infarction vs. hemorrhagic, large vs. small, and cortical vs. subcortical infarcts), comorbid conditions, and use of medication. Although many of these studies showed declines in nutritional indices and increases in malnutrition in the weeks following stroke, it is unclear whether this represents further declines superimposed on preexisting (prevalent) malnutrition or whether these were incident cases. Hama et al. (13) and Finestone et al. (12) reported that 57% and 49%, respectively, of stroke patients admitted to a rehabilitation unit were malnourished, which suggests that malnutrition develops as a consequence of stroke. The estimates of malnutrition assessed at admission to acute care hospitals are substantially lower, ranging from 8–19% (2, 6, 8–10, 14–16).

ENERGY REQUIREMENTS FOLLOWING STROKE

Hypermetabolism has been defined as an increase in metabolic rate associated with a diseased state above that predicted, using equations accounting for age, sex, height, and weight (17). Metabolic rates 140–200%

TABLE 29-1

Factors Contributing to Eating Difficulties and Nutritional Impairments after Stroke (1)

PRIMARY FACTOR	SECONDARY FACTORS
• Dysphagia	• Factors affecting ability to feed self (e.g., visuospatial perceptual deficits, upper extremity paralysis or paresis, and apraxia) • Cognitive changes affecting eating behaviors (e.g., attention-concentration deficit or forgetting to eat, combativeness or throwing food, eating too fast or too slowly, forgetting to swallow, and chewing constantly or overchewing food) • Right and left disorientation • Visual neglect or denial of the paralyzed extremity • Disturbance of sensory function • Depression • Agnosia

above predicted values have been described for burns, sepsis, and head injury (17–18), reflecting increased oxygen consumption associated with severe injury. However, it is unclear whether stroke results in similar metabolic perturbations. Only two studies have been conducted to measure the resting energy expenditure of patients following stroke (19–20). The authors found that energy expenditure was elevated by 110–115% above predicted values, which suggests that stroke patients are not at increased risk for malnutrition caused by the effects of hypermetabolism in the early post-stroke period. Weekes and Elia (20) found that patients were not hypermetabolic in the acute recovery period after stroke. Finestone et al. (19) studied normally nourished patients recovering from stroke over a three-week period, and, while much individual variation existed, patients were not noted to be hypermetabolic. Their resting energy expenditure during the study period was, on average, approximately 10% higher than the values obtained using a standard prediction equation developed by Harris-Benedict (a regression formula using height, weight, age, and sex to estimate basal metabolic rate in noninjured or nondiseased states) (21). In fact, the energy expenditures of subjects with stroke were similar to those of control subjects who had not experienced a stroke. The authors concluded that a "stress factor" specific to stroke was not evident, but the nutritional state of stroke patients should be evaluated on an individual basis.

PROTEIN REQUIREMENTS FOLLOWING STROKE

Evidence of increased protein catabolism following acute stroke was noted by Mountokalakis and Dellos (22) when they compared nitrogen loss, expressed as urea:creatinine ratio, in stroke patients and in surgical patients before and after surgery. While the ratio rose significantly in both groups, it exceeded the upper limit of normal only in the stroke patients. The ratio reached its peak in that group between the fourth and tenth days. Chalela et al. (23) reported that, of 27 severe stroke patients (median National Institutes of Health Stroke Scale of five) receiving enteral nutrition because of depressed consciousness or at risk for aspiration or intubation, 44% were in negative balance while receiving 25–30 nonprotein Kcal/kg per day and 1.5–2.0 g of protein/kg per day (8). The authors concluded that "critically ill stroke patients are being underfed." However, while protein requirement can increase during times of metabolic stress or catabolism, the extent to which requirement associated with stroke increases need is not yet known. Protein requirements of 0.8 g/kg per day have been previously recommended for healthy adults aged 19 years or older, including elderly people, yet it may be insufficient to meet the needs of stroke patients, particularly in the presence of concomitant infections (24).

SCREENING AND ASSESSMENT OF NUTRITIONAL STATUS

Nutritional Screening

The purpose of nutritional screening is to identify individuals who are considered to be malnourished or those at nutritional risk. Patients with stroke should be screened within 24 to 48 hours of admission. Screening tools should include questions designed to identify recent weight loss and assess nutritional intake. Screening is most often performed by nurses or, if the patient is also suspected of being dysphagic, by members of a swallowing team (25–26). Patients with positive findings should be referred to a registered dietitian for nutritional assessment.

Kovacevich et al. (27) developed a nonstroke-specific nutrition screening tool in which patients were assessed to be at "low nutritional risk" or "nutritional risk" based on the patient's diagnosis, nutrition intake history (reduced intake, diarrhea, and vomiting), comparison to ideal body weight, and weight history. A simple screening tool has been developed specifically for use with patients following stroke by the Heart and Stroke Foundation of Ontario (28). The Nutrition Screening for Stroke Survivors queries the following:

- Appearance of undernourishment
- Unplanned weight loss

TABLE 29-2

Studies Assessing the Nutritional Status of Patients Following Stroke

Author/Year	Prevalence of Malnutrition and Timing of Assessment	Indicators and Cutoff points or Indices Used to Assess Nutritional Status	Criteria Used to Establish Malnutrition
Axelsson et al. (1988) (6)	16% at hospital admission 22% at hospital discharge	Serum albumin <38 g/L (male) or 37 g/L (female) Prealbumin <0.18 g/L Transferrin <1.7 g/L (male) or <1.5 g/L (female) Body weight <80% relative body weight, tricep skinfold thickness (four levels based on age), and arm muscle circumference (four levels based on age)	Two or more variables below reference limits
DePippo et al. (1994) (11)	6.1% at any point between rehabilitation hospital admission and discharge	Albumin <25 g/L, sustained ketonuria without glycosuria >2 wk	At least one variable below reference limits
Unosson et al. (1994) (15)	8% on admission to hospital	Weight <80% of reference value, tricep skinfold thickness <6 mm (male) or 12 mm (female), arm muscle circumference (four levels based on age and sex), delayed hypersensitivity skin testing (<10 mm induration),serum albumin <36 g/L, prealbumin <0.20 g/L (male) or 0.18 g/L (female)	Three or more variables below reference limits, including one of each of the anthropometric, serum protein, and skin test measurements
Finestone et al. (1995) (12)	49% on admission to rehabilitation unit 34% at 1 month, 22% at 2 month, and 19% at follow-up (2–4 months)	Serum albumin <35 g/L Transferrin <2.0 g/L Total lymphocyte count <1800/mm³ Body weight <90% of reference weight or <95% of usual weight or body mass index <20 Sum of four skinfold measurements <5th percentile of reference population Mid-arm muscle circumference <5th percentile of reference population	Two or more variables below reference limits
Davalos et al. (1996) (8)	16.3% at hospital admission, 26.4% after 1 week, and 35% after 2 weeks	Serum albumin <35 g/L Tricep skinfold or mid-arm muscle circumference <10th percentile of reference population	Any single indicator below reference limits
Choi-Kwon et al. (1998) (7)	25% among patients with ischemic stroke 62% among patients with hemorrhagic stroke Assessed in acute period of stroke 13% among control subjects	Lean body mass Abdominal skinfold thickness Subscapular skinfold thickness Triceps skinfold thickness (all <80% of reference values) Body mass index <20 Total lymphocyte count <1500/mm³ Hemoglobin <12 g/dL Serum albumin <35 g/L	More than one biochemical indicator and two or more anthropometric indicators below reference values

TABLE 29-2
(Continued)

Author/Year	Prevalence of Malnutrition and Timing of Assessment	Indicators and Cutoff points or Indices Used to Assess Nutritional Status	Criteria Used to Establish Malnutrition
Westergren et al. (2001) (16)	8% at admission (acute) 29% at 1 month 33% at 3 month	Body mass index <20 or body weight ≤ 80% of reference weight or weight loss >5% since admission Subnormal triceps skinfold and mid-upper-arm muscle circumference Serum albumin <36 g/L	One abnormal weight measurement and at least two other abnormal markers
Davis et al. (2004) (1)	16% at admission	Subjective global assessment	Defined by the instrument
Dennis et al. (FOOD I) (2005) (9)	7.8% at admission	Body mass index <20 (more comprehensive assessment may have also been carried out in a portion of the patients, although details not provided)	Underweight vs. normal vs. overweight
Dennis et al. (FOOD II) (2005) (10)	8.6% at admission	Same as FOOD I	Underweight vs. normal vs. overweight
Martineau et al. (2005) (14)	19.2% at acute admission	Patient-generated subjective global assessment	Defined by the instrument
Hama et al. (2005) (13)	22–57% at admission to rehabilitation depending on criteria used	Serum albumin <40 g/L Body mass index <19	Either marker below reference value

- Loss of appetite
- Difficulty chewing or swallowing
- Nausea, vomiting, or diarrhea
- Shortness of breath affecting eating
- Inability to buy or prepare foods
- Multiple food allergies or restrictions
- Selected comorbid conditions

This screen complements the routine dysphagia screen.

Nutritional Assessment

Interest in identifying and treating all patients perceived to be in a nutritionally compromised state was aroused during the early 1970s, when iatrogenic malnutrition was believed to be a significant cause of poor outcome and rising health care costs. During that period, a series of nutrition assessment methods, many of which are still in use today, were proposed and adopted. However, regardless of the patient population under study, nutritional assessment has never been fully standardized, and no consensus exists as to which method of assessment is best. Therefore, wide variations occur in clinical practice. The nutritional screening and assessment of patients can range from very elaborate methods relying on a variety of biochemical and anthropometric markers (measures of fat and muscle stores) to simple methods using only a single measurement, such as body weight.

The ideal nutrition assessment method applicable for use in the stroke patient would be sensitive to recent intake, unaffected by disease state, inexpensive, simple, and noninvasive. Unfortunately, no such measure exists. This limitation can affect not only the initial determination of nutritional status, but also subsequent efforts to evaluate the response to nutritional interventions. In the absence of an acute or chronic underlying disease and/or institutionalization, the identification of malnutrition is less complicated, and the condition is thought to be attributable to negative energy balance, whereby nutritional intake is lower than requirement. However, in most diseases, including stroke, other metabolic processes may influence the detection of malnutrition. This interaction between nutritional status and severity of illness was recognized by the Board of Directors of the American Association of Parenteral and Enteral Nutrition and the Clinical Guidelines Task Force:

> There is an inextricable relationship between nutritional status and the severity of illness. Severely ill patients, no matter what assessment tools are used, will be identified as being malnourished. Whether this assessment in fact truly indicates malnutrition (a state induced by dietary deficiency that may be improved solely by administration of nutrients) or is merely a reflection of the severity of metabolic derangement caused by the underlying illness is arguable. (29)

The International Classification of Diseases, 10th revision (30), recognizes malnutrition as a disease condition and uses measures of body weight in relation to a reference population as a means to both define and identify people who are mildly, moderately, or severely malnourished. Although the document mentions that single markers cannot be considered diagnostic and should be combined with other markers, it does not specify which additional markers should be used. In an effort to overcome the limitations of using single markers to determine nutritional status, a variety of composite indices and scales were developed, some of which are presented in Table 29-3. Ironically, while many of these indices have been shown to be good prognostic markers of clinical outcome because they include a measure of disease severity, they may be poor markers of nutritional status because they contain the same biochemical components that may be influenced by disease state.

While sophisticated measurements, such as bioelectrical impedance analysis of body composition, antigen skin testing, and muscle strength, are available to aid in the assessment of nutritional state, they are often impractical for use in clinical practice. More frequently, a traditional approach is used. This method combines the results of biochemical tests, such as serum albumin and transferrin levels, and measurement of skeletal muscle mass and subcutaneous fat stores, collectively referred to as anthropometric measures. Examples of anthropometric measurements include body weight, mid-arm muscle circumference, and skinfold thickness, which can be measured using skinfold calipers and a measuring tape. With a traditional approach, the identification of malnutrition is usually inferred, based on a single value or multiple values falling outside specific population reference ranges or below a given percentile within these ranges. Several examples of this approach to nutrition assessment in the stroke patient are presented in Table 29-2. With a system based on cutoff values, a patient's state can change abruptly from one of being well nourished to one of malnourishment. These designations may be somewhat artificial, and additional information, including that obtained from questionnaires designed to assess premorbid nutritional intake, mood, functional status, or comorbid conditions, may be necessary to identify the truly malnourished patient.

Table 29-4 presents some of the biochemical indicators more commonly used in nutrition assessment, their normal reference ranges, and their limitations. While declines in the serum levels of these indicators may be

---

TABLE 29-3
Composite Nutrition Assessment or Screening Tools

INDEX/INTERPRETATION	DESCRIPTION/CALCULATION
Prognostic Nutrition Index (31) Low risk: <40% Intermediate risk: 40–49% High risk: >50%	158–16.6 (albumin) 0.78 tricep skinfold (mm) 0.2 (serum transferrin) 5.8 (maximum skin reactivity, scored from 0 to 2)
Prognostic Inflammatory Nutrition Index (32) Correlates with death in critically ill patients when >30	A-acid glycoprotein (mg/L) × C-reactive protein (mg/mL)/ albumin (g/L) × prealbumin (mg/L)
Nutrition Risk Index (33) >100: no malnutrition 97.5 to 100: mildly malnourished 83.5 to <97.5: moderately malnourished <83.5: severely malnourished	(1.519 × albumin [g/L]) + 41.7 (present weight/usual weight)
Instant Nutrition Assessment (34) Four degrees of nutritional state	Serum albumin (SA) and total lymphocyte count (TLC) 1st degree: SA ≥ 35 g/L, TLC ≥ 1500/mm^3 2nd degree: SA ≥ 35 g/L, TLC < 1500/mm^3 3rd degree: SA < 35 g/L, TLC ≥ 1500/mm^3 4th degree: SA < 35 g/L, TLC < 1500/mm^3

TABLE 29-4
Biochemical Markers of Nutritional Status (35)

MEASURE	NORMAL REFERENCE RANGE	LIMITATION(S)
Serum albumin	>35 g/L	• Large body pool • Poor specificity to nutritional changes • Not specific to nutritional status • Decreased with acute illness
Serum transferrin	2.0–2.60 g/L	• Not specific to nutritional status • Decreased with acute illness
Thyroxin-binding prealbumin	1.6–3.0 g/L	• Not specific to nutritional status • Decreased with acute illness
Retinol-binding protein	0.3–0.8 g/L	• Not specific to nutritional status
Total lymphocyte count	2,000–3,500/mm^3	• Poor sensitivity and specificity

associated with the development of malnutrition, many are affected independently by factors associated with stroke or any other acute illness. For example, the hepatic production of albumin, transferrin, and prealbumin is down-regulated during periods of acute illness, resulting in depressed serum values (36–37). This effect is likely mediated by cytokines, such as tumor necrosis factor and interleukin-6, which have been reported to be elevated following stroke (38–43). The presence of concurrent infection or temperature elevation is also associated with depressed serum levels of the same proteins. With respect to albumin in particular, transcapillary escape resulting from systemic inflammation may be manifest as hypoalbuminemia (44–45). While serum albumin levels can fall abruptly, recovery of levels may take time, owing to its relatively long half-life of 14 to 21 days; therefore, response to nutritional interventions can be slow (46). Moreover, several reports failed to demonstrate an association between serum albumin levels and adequacy of protein and energy intake (47–49). Using serum albumin as one of two nutritional indicators, Davalos et al. (8) reported that early, appropriate enteral feeding did not prevent the development of malnutrition during the first week after hospital admission. Similarly, levels of serum transferrin as an acute-phase protein fall in response to physiological stress. While its half-life of eight days is shorter than that of albumin, its specificity as a nutritional marker is similar to that of albumin (50). Of all of the visceral proteins used for nutritional assessment, serum prealbumin has the shortest half-life, at two days; therefore, it is more sensitive to changes in both disease severity and nutritional intake than either albumin or transferrin. Prealbumin also correlates with nitrogen balance. A dramatic decrease in serum prealbumin level can occur following three to five days of inadequate protein and energy intake or after significant physiological

stress (50). Therefore, the serum concentration of prealbumin will normalize with resolution of the stressful insult if nutritional intake is adequate, but it will remain depressed in the presence of adequate intake if stress or inflammation persists.

There are also limitations associated with anthropometric measurements, which can remain static and may be insensitive to recent change in nutritional intake. Skeletal muscle losses may also occur over prolonged periods as a result of atrophy or secondary to immobility, and they can be difficult to distinguish from a nutritional cause (50–51). Specialized equipment, training, and practice are required to ensure that reproducible measurements of body composition are obtained, and appropriate reference population norms must be available to ensure proper interpretation.

Some clinical methods of nutritional assessment do not include biochemical or sophisticated anthropometric data. Subjective global assessment (52) is a technique for assessing nutritional status that relies exclusively on the physical examination and history to determine whether a patient is well-nourished or moderately or severely malnourished. This technique was originally validated in a population of surgical patients (52). Although it has become more widely used, including in other diseases such as kidney and liver disease and cancer, it has never been validated with stroke patients. Some of the components of the evaluation may be less applicable to this population because they were developed to identify malnutrition associated with progressive gastrointestinal conditions before surgical intervention, while stroke represents a distinct event. The more general items, such as weight and dietary intake history, are likely to be more useful to the clinician than items such as the presence of ascites or a history of nausea and vomiting, which pertain more specifically to patients with significant gastrointestinal disorders.

In summary, the nutritional assessment of stroke patients is imperfect, affected by the lack of a gold standard or consensus with respect to the most appropriate method of assessment. There are limitations associated with almost all routinely used indicators of nutritional status, whether used alone or in combination. When evaluating the nutritional state of a patient who has sustained a stroke, the clinician is advised to incorporate the history, physical examination and body weight, as well as objective and subjective biochemical and anthropometric data. The use of serial assessments is encouraged to monitor the nutritional status of patients over time (see Table 29-2 for examples) and evaluate the response to nutritional interventions.

NUTRITIONAL INTERVENTION STRATEGIES

The major diet strategies for patients undergoing rehabilitation for stroke are dysphagia diets, enteral feeding, high-energy (calorie) and high-protein diets, energy-reduced diets, diabetic diets, low-saturated-fat diets, and high-fiber diets.

Dysphagia Diets

The word dysphagia is derived from the Greek words *dys*, meaning "difficult," and *phagein*, meaning "to eat." If not diagnosed and treated, dysphagia can lead to loss of the basic pleasure of eating, impaired nutritional status, or death caused by aspiration pneumonia (53–54). The diagnosis and treatment of dysphagia in patients who have experienced a stroke are discussed in Chapter 11. This section outlines the various dietary—oral and enteral—options available to the stoke patient with dysphagia.

Prescription and Implementation. The approach to the treatment of dysphagia is often multidisciplinary, with the team including nurses, speech-language pathologists, dietitians, and occupational therapists (21, 25). Signs and symptoms of dysphagia observed during and between meals are given in Table 29-5. Stroke patients should be screened initially for swallowing difficulties by a nurse, and those suspected of being dysphagic should be referred to a speech-language pathologist for assessment. A bedside clinical assessment is usually performed first if the patient is alert and sufficiently conscious to participate. A videofluoroscopic examination (modified barium swallow) may be performed if there is uncertainty with respect to clinical management. Based on the results of these assessments, diet recommendations are made, which usually include modification of solids and liquids. A clinical dietitian is involved in the management of the dysphagic patient to help ensure adequacy of energy,

---

TABLE 29-5
Signs and Symptoms of Dysphagia During and Between Meals (21, 53)

- Drooling, excessive secretions
- Excessive tongue movement, tongue thrusting, or spitting food out of mouth
- Poor control of tongue
- Facial weakness
- Pocketing of food in cheek, under tongue, or on hard palate
- Slurred speech
- Coughing or choking while eating*
- Regurgitation through nose, mouth, or tracheostomy tube
- Wet, gurgly voice after eating or drinking, or frequent clearing of throat
- Hoarse or breathy voice
- Complaints of food getting stuck in throat
- Delay or absence of laryngeal (Adam's apple or thyroid cartilage) elevation with swallowing
- Recurrent pneumonia (due to aspiration)
- Prolonged chewing or eating time
- Reluctance to consume particular food consistencies or to eat at all

*Caveat: Aspiration very commonly occurs without coughing. The presence or absence of the gag reflex does not indicate whether the swallowing reflex is intact.

---

protein, and fluid. Nursing staff may assist or supervise the patient at mealtimes. Where possible, this can be done in a common dining room in order to enhance the social atmosphere and allow for monitoring of eating difficulties, such as coughing, choking, or food pocketing. The occupational therapist can provide recommendations for adaptive equipment to assist with mechanical aspects of feeding. The physical therapist, along with the occupational therapist, can help determine any requirements for external support during feeding.

Types of Dysphagia Diets. Dysphagia diets are characterized by modifications of the texture of food and viscosity of fluids. The goal of the diet is to reduce the risk of aspiration and its possible sequela (pneumonia) by facilitating a safer swallow. Dysphagia diets are individualized according to the degree and site of the oral-pharyngeal impairment. Solids may be puréed, ground/minced, or soft/easy to chew (21, 25). The puréed diet includes mashed or blenderized foods that are smooth, dense, and homogeneous, with a pudding-like consistency. The minced or ground texture includes soft foods that are chopped to pea size and moist enough to form a bolus (for example, shepherd's pie). The soft/easy-to-chew diet includes soft minced or diced meats. Foods that cannot be formed into a bolus are difficult for patients with dysphagia to control and should be avoided.

Examples of these foods include dry particulates such as crumbly cheese and raw vegetables. Bread products should be avoided as they may stick to the throat. Mixed consistencies, such as cereal with milk, should also be avoided as the different consistencies must be separated in the mouth and managed separately.

Thin fluids are difficult for the dysphagic patient to control as they can enter the pharynx prematurely and leak into the airway (25). Thicker fluids can be sensed more readily. Thickened fluid viscosities generally vary from those of nectar to honey to pudding (21, 25). Commercial prethickened products are available. Thin liquids are most often thickened with commercially prepared starch-based products, although other food ingredients such as skim milk powder, puréed fruit, or infant cereal may be used. It is important that food items maintain their thickness until swallowed. For example, ice cream must be held at a sufficiently cold temperature to maintain its thick consistency.

Dysphagia diets are nutritionally adequate, provided that patients consume sufficient quantities to meet their energy requirements. Because patient compliance and acceptance of the diet are known to be poor, many institutions provide thickened, high-calorie, high-protein supplements as a standard component of the dysphagia diet. For this reason, the diet should be as liberal as possible both for psychological reasons (55) and to enhance palatability. Swallowing status should be reassessed frequently enough to avoid needless dietary restrictions.

Enteral Feeding

In cases in which the patient is unable to meet his or her nutritional requirements by mouth for a prolonged period, regardless of diet type, or if the risk of aspiration is high owing to dysphagia, enteral nutrition should be considered. By far, the greatest number of patients receive enteral nutrition because of unsafe swallowing. During the transition from enteral to oral intake, both types of feeding may be provided, with the enteral portion gradually being decreased as the oral portion is increased. Non-oral feeding may be discontinued once the adequacy of oral intake has been established.

Although most patients recovering from stroke are potential candidates for non-oral feeding, it is contraindicated in those without a functional gastrointestinal tract (for example, because of gastric or intestinal obstruction or paralytic ileus) and those with intractable vomiting or severe diarrhea. The choice of feeding tube and the route of access are dictated by the patient's medical conditions and the expected length of use. An algorithm for determining the optimal type of feeding is given in Figure 29-1. This flowchart takes into account the adequacy of oral intake, anticipated duration of enteral support, and risk of aspiration.

Enteral Formulations. Although enteral formulas vary in their energy density, osmolality, and molecular form of the substrates, most stroke patients do well with a standard polymeric formula (1.0–1.2 Kcal/mL). These nutritionally complete formulas can be titrated to meet patients' energy and protein requirements. When required, specialized formulas are available for patients with impaired renal function, compromised pulmonary function, or diabetes. A clinical dietitian should be consulted to advise on the management of patients who are being fed enterally.

Routes of Access. Feeding tube access can be achieved through either nasoenteric and enterostomy routes. Figure 29-2 illustrates the location of these sites. Nasoenteric feeding includes nasogastric (tube from nose to stomach, which is, by far, the most common), nasoduodenal (tube from the nose through the pylorus and into the duodenum) and nasojejunal (tube from the nose through the pylorus and into the jejunum, usually placed radioscopically) (21). The latter two are seldom used in patients with stroke. Enterostomy tubes can be inserted percutaneously or, less frequently, surgically. Common routes include the prepyloric gastrostomy and postpyloric jejunostomy. A gastrostomy involves tube placement into the stomach. Tube size and techniques vary. Jejunostomy involves the creation of a jejunal stoma that can be catheterized intermittently via needle catheter placement or direct tube placement. This is performed only rarely in the stroke patient. The rationale for wanting to deliver tube feeding to the stomach is that it is more "physiologic." Patients with severe reflux, however, may benefit from postpyloric tube insertion to prevent tube feeding-related aspiration. Percutaneous endoscopic gastrostomy (PEG) and jejunostomy are procedures in which the feeding tube is inserted percutaneously under endoscopic guidance into the stomach or jejunum. The tube is secured by rubber bumpers or an inflated balloon catheter. These procedures are often performed with local anesthesia by a gastroenterologist. Percutaneous gastrojejunostomy involves the percutaneous insertion of a guidewire followed by a feeding catheter into the jejunum via the stomach. This procedure is usually performed by a radiologist under fluoroscopic control, and only local anesthetic is required. Often, local experience and expertise will determine which method of tube insertion is chosen.

Methods of Administration. Feeding formula can be delivered by gravity drip or, for better volume accuracy and tolerance, infusion pump set at a constant rate. Feeding may be provided on a continuous basis, usually over a 24-hour period. This method reduces the possibility of pulmonary aspiration.

Intermittent infusions are equally divided feedings infused at intervals four to six times throughout

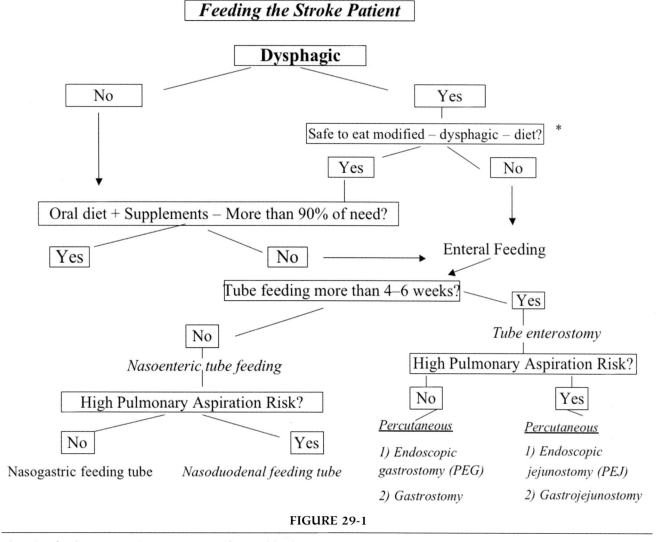

Feeding the Stroke Patient

Dysphagic

No

Yes

Safe to eat modified – dysphagic – diet? *

Yes

No

Oral diet + Supplements – More than 90% of need?

Yes

No

Enteral Feeding

Tube feeding more than 4–6 weeks?

Yes

Tube enterostomy

No

Nasoenteric tube feeding

High Pulmonary Aspiration Risk?

No

Yes

High Pulmonary Aspiration Risk?

No

Yes

Nasogastric feeding tube

Nasoduodenal feeding tube

<u>*Percutaneous*</u>

*1) Endoscopic
gastrostomy (PEG)*

2) Gastrostomy

<u>*Percutaneous*</u>

*1) Endoscopic
jejunostomy (PEJ)*

2) Gastrojejunostomy

FIGURE 29-1

Algorithm for determining the optimal type of enteral feeding.

the day (56). They can be given by gravity drip over 30 to 60 minutes or by infusion pump. This type of feeding frees patients from tube feeding equipment between feedings, so it is convenient for those undergoing active rehabilitation and those at home. It is also used in patients who are not critically ill. A cyclic method of intermittent infusion may be used wherein the tube feeding is administered at a high infusion rate over 8 to 20 hours. This may be helpful in the transition from tube feeding to oral diet, with tube feeding delivered at night and oral diet ingested by day (56).

Bolus feeding involves the rapid delivery of a feeding into the gastrointestinal tract by syringe or funnel. It is suited to rehabilitating patients who are receiving gastric feeding in a rehabilitation facility or at home. Feeding is completed over a short period, for example, 200–300 mL over 5 to 15 minutes, followed by a flush of 30 mL of water. The advantages are freedom

of movement and breaks from feeding. Disadvantages include risk of aspiration, volume intolerance, and delayed gastric emptying (56). Similar volumes of enteral feeding delivered into the jejunum are usually not tolerated by the stroke patient.

Feedings should begin with a full-strength formula, usually at a rate of 25 mL/h and advanced by 25-mL increments every four hours to goal rate, as tolerated (56). The residual gastric volume is often monitored every four hours when continuous feeds are administered. Occasional episodes of high-residual volume do not necessarily indicate that there is dysfunction. However, if a high volume (for example, 200 mL) occurs frequently and is associated with symptoms of cramping, the rate the formula administration should be reduced. Once the problem has resolved, rate increases are then slowly attempted. Diarrhea, a not uncommon problem, can be treated by slowing the rate of infusion or adding codeine

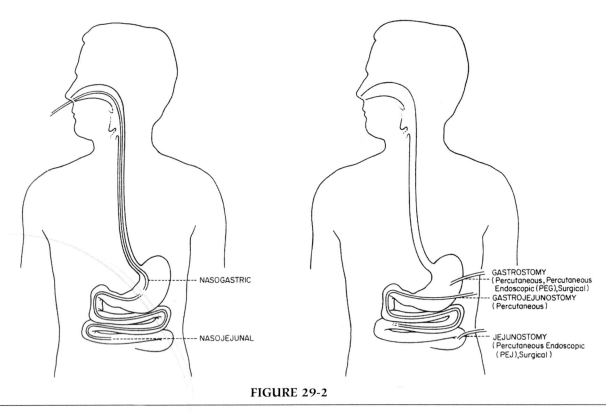

FIGURE 29-2

Common enteral feeding access routes. Reprinted from *Principles of Neurologic Rehabilitation,* edited by Richard B. Lazar, by permission of The McGraw-Hill Companies.

to the formula. In some cases, changing the formula proves effective.

Alternative methods of administering and/or delivering enteral feeding have been discussed in the recent literature. These include transnasal PEG placement without sedation (57), use of a novel nasal loop to better secure a nasogastric tube (58), and feeding intermittently via an oroesophageal tube, whereby enteral fluids, for example, are introduced into the esophagus, with the patient often placing the tube by himself or herself (59). These studies were small, and, although interesting, there are no apparent standards for the use of the methods described.

Complications. Complications associated with tube feeding can usually be detected and controlled through attentive monitoring. Complications largely fall into three categories: mechanical, gastrointestinal, and metabolic (56). Mechanical complications include tube blockage, local skin infection at the site of tube insertion, and inadvertent insertion in the trachea or lung parenchyma. Nasopharyngeal area erosion with prolonged nasogastric tube feeding can occur, especially if poor taping technique is practiced. PEG tube insertion can lead to burying of the bumper subcutaneously at the abdominal insertion site (buried bumper syndrome), causing local pain and swelling (56).

Gastrointestinal complications include peritonitis and free air in the abdomen. Gastrointestinal hemorrhage is also a potential complication of tube feeding. (9–10). Pathophysiological changes of the gastrointestinal tract in ischemic stroke have been recently reviewed (60). A few studies indicate increased incidence of hemorrhage or decreased transit time, but the area needs further study.

Metabolic complications in tube-fed populations are often related to fluid balance, electrolyte deficiencies, and hyperglycemia. Glycemic control in stroke rehabilitation patients being fed enterally can be difficult, especially when the patient requires insulin and enteral feeding is being provided largely at night to avoid interference with daytime rehabilitation activities. Carbohydrate-reduced formulas may prove useful for diabetic patients. The authors have found that the common practice of providing two-thirds of the subcutaneous insulin in the morning and the remaining one-third in the evening must be reversed. Kerr et al. (61) discussed a structured enteral feeding program for diabetic patients with a specific subcutaneous insulin regimen, which precedes three enteral feedings per day. Dehydration, another metabolic complication, may result if daily fluid requirements are not met. On average, standard polymeric formulas contain 85% free water; therefore, additional water must usually be provided to meet patients' needs. Water may be added directly to the feed or may be provided by way of tube flushes. If fluid losses are excessive because of fever, diarrhea, or vomiting, and fluids are not replaced, dehydration may also result. Patients who present with preexisting malnutrition resulting from a prolonged period of poor intake and those who have had food withheld for an extended period of time may be at risk for refeeding syndrome, a potentially life-threatening complication that can occur with rapid introduction of carbohydrate-containing feedings. In this syndrome, acute decreases in serum levels of potassium, magnesium, and phosphorous can appear, owing to intracellular shifts of electrolytes, with possible resultant cardiac, neuromuscular, and other dysfunction (62).

A comprehensive listing of potential adverse reactions to tube feeding together with potential causes and management is available from the American Society for Enteral and Parenteral Nutrition (56).

Home Tube Feeding (63).   Several factors should be considered before discharging a patient on a home tube-feeding program. The experience can prove overwhelming for patients and their families. The cognitive and functional ability of the patient or caregiver should be assessed to ensure that all tube feeding-related tasks can be carried out correctly and safely. The compatibility of tube feeding with the home-life schedule should also be considered. The availability of funding to cover, or partly cover, the cost of formula, infusion pump (if required), and associated supplies also needs to be explored. Finally, the availability of support personnel and a mechanism for home monitoring, follow-up, and support must be established.

Patient instructions should include the following, with written guidelines provided:

- Proper sanitation techniques for preparation
- Storage and infusion of formula
- Proper sanitation of equipment
- Rate and strength of feedings
- Time of administration
- Body position and length of time to remain in position
- Formula temperature
- Maximum hanging time
- Maximum time to keep open formula
- Amount of fluids to flush between feedings
- How to deal with complications
- Care of the tube and exit site

The reported incidence rates of death, aspiration pneumonia, and complications associated with home enteral nutrition vary among studies but are generally low (64–66). In time, most patients are able to resume a regular diet.

High-energy (calorie), High-protein Diet

Patients with preexisting malnutrition and those at nutritional risk owing to poor intake may benefit from a high-energy, high-protein diet. The rationale behind this diet is that the augmented protein intake supplies amino acids required for the building, maintenance, and repair of body tissue. Supplemental calories are needed to spare the protein from being used as a source of energy. At the same time, the energy level is increased to maintain body weight or promote weight gain.

High-energy, high-calorie supplements, which come in many forms (liquids, bars, and puddings) and flavors, may be offered. For dysphagic patients, liquid supplements can be thickened so that they can be consumed safely. Supplements may be given at mealtime along with reduced portions or between meals. The medication pass supplement program (med-pass), which provides a nutrient-dense supplement (60 mL four times daily), has been shown to be efficient (67–68). Most oral supplements contain approximately 250–300 Kcal and 8–13 g of protein per 250-mL serving. Efforts should be made to provide a pleasant atmosphere for inpatients and to offer appealing food that reflects the patient's food preferences. Six small meals per day, including snacks and nutritional supplements, may augment energy intake.

Energy-reduced Diet

While some patients may develop malnutrition following stroke, weight gain and obesity are encountered more frequently. Obesity, defined as body mass index greater than 30, adversely affects functions such as transfers and ambulation and places extra stress on caregivers. Furthermore, following stroke, patients' mobility and, consequently, energy requirements are often reduced.

Excess weight is treated by a reduction in total energy intake, while other nutrient requirements remain age-appropriate (24). Behavior modification, such as serving smaller portions, serving food on a smaller plate, instructing the patient to eat slowly (as it takes approximately 20 minutes to feel a sense of satiety), and increasing activity appropriate to the medical condition, may help the patient reduce energy intake. In addition, strategies to deal with contributing factors such as boredom and depression should be developed. Medications, for example, antidepressants and steroids, should also be evaluated, as increased appetite may be a side effect (68). Unfortunately, weight loss can be difficult to achieve following stroke. A collaborative team approach, which may include a psychologist and recreation therapist, may be helpful.

Diabetic Diet

Diabetes is a risk factor for stroke. Many patients enter the rehabilitation program with a diagnosis of diabetes and require special dietary attention. Promoting good glycemic control during the hospital stay will support the patient in his or her daily physical and mental activities. Stroke rehabilitation is also a good time to provide patients with additional diabetic education and to connect them with appropriate community resources.

Low-saturated-fat Diet

After a stroke, many patients are prescribed medication to lower their blood lipid levels. In conjunction, a diet low in fat, particularly saturated and trans fats, is introduced to maximize achievement of the blood lipid targets.

High-fiber Diet

Constipation may be associated with stroke. Reduced mobility, lack of dietary fiber, and inadequate fluid intake are the most common reasons. The degree of hydration should be assessed. Fluid intake should be recorded, and urine output and color noted. Fluid intake of at least 1,500 mL (six eight-ounce glasses) should be encouraged, provided there is no medical reason for fluid restriction (21, 68). When commercial fiber supplements, for example, psyllium, are used, additional fluid intake is recommended. Dietary sources of insoluble fiber are particularly effective in increasing fecal bulk (70), and the clinical dietitian can advise on this. Stool softeners, for example, docusate sodium, along with judicious use of oral and rectal laxatives are helpful adjuncts in the treatment of constipation. Exercise opportunities should be provided. Attention to the urge to defecate and the establishment of a routine schedule for toileting should be encouraged. Constipation may be a side effect of certain medications (69), such as antidepressants and narcotic preparations.

DEHYDRATION AND FLUID REQUIREMENTS

The risk of dehydration following stroke is often underappreciated, particularly in those with dysphagia who are receiving all their nutrition orally (71–72). For these patients, thin fluids, the most difficult food item to manipulate and control, are often restricted or replaced by those that are thickened. Dislike for the taste or texture of thickened fluids, dependence on others to provide and/or help consume fluids, and fatigue are all factors that increase the risk of dehydration (28).

For stroke rehabilitation inpatients, physicians should consider ordering overnight intravenous fluid administration, or hypodermoclysis. The fluid requirement for adults is 20–40 mL/kg of body weight, or 1.0–1.5 mL/Kcal of energy expended (73).

Although the fluid requirements of elderly people and those of younger adults are similar, elderly people

are particularly vulnerable to dehydration. Therefore, attention to intake and output data is critical in elderly people (73). Besides dysphagia, reasons for the underhydration of many elderly people include a blunted thirst mechanism, renal changes, and decreased mobility to reach a fluid source (73–74). In addition, loss of lean body mass with aging contributes to decreased total body water as a proportion of body weight, as lean muscle mass holds 40% of total body water (74).

THE FOOD TRIALS: FEEDING INTERVENTION STUDIES IN PATIENTS WITH STROKE

In 2005, *The Lancet* published the findings of the Feed or Ordinary Diet (FOOD) trials, a long-awaited series of three related large randomized controlled trials (9–10). The investigators attempted to provide definitive answers to three clinically relevant questions regarding the nutritional management of patients in the acute post-stroke period:

1. Does routine oral supplementation decrease the number of patients who have a poor outcome and patients requiring enteral feeding?
2. Do those who receive early feeding have better outcomes than patients whose feeding is delayed?
3. Do patients with PEG tubes have better outcomes than those with nasogastric tubes?

The trials enrolled 5,033 patients, but they were stopped before target numbers were reached owing to lack of funding.

Nondysphagic Patients (Trial One)

In this branch of the trial, patients were randomized to receive a daily oral supplement, which contained 540 Kcal/day and 22.5 g of protein daily until discharge, in addition to a regular diet or regular diet alone. There were no differences between the two groups in the proportion of patients who were dead or dead/disabled (defined as a Modified Rankin score of 3 to 5) at six months. The proportion of patients in each group who had experienced death or a poor outcome was identical (59%).

In subgroup analysis, patients who were undernourished at baseline, presumably those who would benefit the most from supplementation, had reduced odds of death or a poor outcome, although the results did not reach statistical significance. No indication of actual nutrient intake or its relationship to estimated nutrient requirement is provided, although the authors did note this as a limitation of the study. While the results from the FOOD trial suggest that routine supplementation does not reduce the odds of a poor outcome for all patients, regardless of nutritional state, supplementation is still recommended for malnourished patients and those perceived to be at nutritional risk.

Dysphagic Patients (Trials Two and Three)

In the second and third trials, patients with dysphagia who required non-oral feeding were allocated to early (within seven days of stroke) versus delayed enteral feeding and/or nasogastric versus PEG tube feeding groups. Although not statistically significant, the odds of death were slightly lower for patients in the early enteral group; however, survivors were more likely to be disabled. Patients could be enrolled in both parts of the study simultaneously.

In the PEG versus nasogastric tube trial, PEG feeding was associated with a statistically borderline increase in the risk of death or poor outcome and an insignificant increase in the risk of death. There was no difference between the early tube-feeding and the avoid tube-feeding groups in frequency of recurring stroke, worsening of neurologic impairment, or pneumonia, but there were significantly more gastrointestinal hemorrhages in the early group (10) than in the avoid group (33). Most hemorrhages occurred with the PEG or nasogastric tube in place, but a number occurred after the tube was removed. In the PEG versus nasogastric trial, significantly more hemorrhages occurred in the nasogastric group (11%) than in the PEG group (3%).

These unique data therefore suggest a greater risk of gastrointestinal hemorrhage with placement of any type of feeding tube, but particularly with the use of nasogastric tubes. However, these findings have limited clinical applicability. The use of a nasogastric tube for patients requiring long-term, that is, more than four to six weeks, enteral nutrition is not practical; thereafter, a PEG tube would be recommended.

CONCLUSION

The high prevalence of malnutrition in stroke patients on admission to a rehabilitation service (12–13) suggests that the decline in nutritional status develops as a consequence of stroke. In turn, malnutrition may adversely affect recovery from stroke. In malnourished stroke patients, poorer functional outcome and prolonged rehabilitation stay have been reported (2–4). Therefore, the clinical goal is to prevent or to identify and treat inadequate nutritional states.

The nutritional care of patients who have sustained a stroke is a relatively new field. Although much research in this area has occurred, there is room for further evaluation of the dietary needs of specific stroke diagnostic groups and of optimal methods of assessment, nutritional delivery, and therapy. Attending to nutritional issues is an important step toward helping stroke patients achieve their full rehabilitation potential.

ACKNOWLEDGEMENTS

The authors acknowledge the able editing of Ms. Gloria Baker, Élisabeth Bruyère Research Institute; the astute nutritional input of dietitians Ms. Julie Campagna and Ms. Patricia Giannantonio, Stroke Rehabilitation Service, Élisabeth Bruyère Health Centre; and the excellent search services provided by Ms. Mireille Éthier-Danis and Ms. Nathalie Lalonde, SCO Health Service library.

References

1. Davis JP, Wong AA, Schluter PJ, et al. Impact of premorbid undernutrition on outcome in stroke patients. *Stroke* 2004; 35(8):1930–1934.

2. Finestone HM, Greene-Finestone LS, Wilson ES, Teasell RW. Prolonged length of stay and reduced functional improvement rate in malnourished stroke rehabilitation patients. *Arch Phys Med Rehabil.* 1996; 77(4):340–345.

3. FOOD Trial Collaboration. Poor nutritional status on admission predicts poor outcomes after stroke: observational data from the FOOD Trial. *Stroke* 2003; 34(6):1450–1456.

4. Aptaker RL, Roth EJ, Reichhardt G, et al. Serum albumin level as a predictor of geriatric stroke rehabilitation outcome. *Arch Phys Med Rehabil* 1994; 75:80–84.

5. Buelow JM, Jamieson D. Potential for altered nutritional status in the stroke patient. *Rehabil Nurs* 1990; 15(5):260–263.

6. Axelsson K, Asplund K, Norberg A, Alafuzoff I. Nutritional status in patients with acute stroke. *Acta Med Scand* 1988; 224:217–224.

7. Choi-Kwon S, Yang YH, Kim EK, et al. Nutritional status in acute stroke: Undernutrition versus overnutrition in different stroke subtypes. *Acta Neurol Scand* 1998; 98(3):187–192.

8. Davalos A, Ricart W, Gonzalez-Huix F, et al. Effect of malnutrition after acute stroke on clinical outcome. *Stroke* 1996; 27(6):1028–1032.

9. Dennis MS, Lewis SC, Warlow C, FOOD Trial Collaboration. Routine oral nutritional supplementation for stroke patients in hospital (FOOD): A multicentre randomised controlled trial. *Lancet* 2005; 365:755–763.

10. Dennis MS, Lewis SC, Warlow C, FOOD Trial Collaboration. Effect of timing and method of enteral tube feeding for dysphagic stroke patients (FOOD): A multicentre randomised controlled trial. *Lancet* 2005; 365:764–772.

11. DePippo KL, Holas MA, Reding MJ, et al. Dysphagia therapy following stroke: A controlled trial. *Neurology* 1994; 44(9):1655–1660.

12. Finestone HM, Greene-Finestone LS, Wilson ES, Teasell RW. Malnutrition in stroke patients on the rehabilitation service and at follow-up: prevalence and predictors. *Arch Phys Med Rehabil* 1995; 76(4):310–316.

13. Hama S, Kitaoka T, Shigenobu M, et al. Malnutrition and nonthyroidal illness syndrome after stroke. *Metabolism* 2005; 54(6):699–704.

14. Martineau J, Bauer JD, Isenring E, Cohen S. Malnutrition determined by the patient-generated subjective global assessment is associated with poor outcomes in acute stroke patients. *Clin Nutr* 2005; 24(6):1073–1077.

15. Unosson M, Ek AC, Bjurulf P, et al. Feeding dependence and nutritional status after acute stroke. *Stroke* 1994; 25(2):366–371.

16. Westergren A, Ohlsson O, Rahm Hallberg I. Eating difficulties, complications, and nursing interventions during a period of three months after a stroke. *J Adv Nurs* 2001; 35(3):416–426.

17. Young B, Ott L, Yingling B, McClain C. Nutrition and brain injury. *J Neurotrauma* 1992; 9 Suppl 1:S375–S383.

18. Long CL. Nutritional assessment of critically ill patients. In: Wright RA, Hemsfield SB, eds. *Nutritional Assessment.* London: Blackwell Scientific Publications, 1984:15–24.

19. Finestone HM, Greene-Finestone LS, Foley NC, Woodbury MG. Measuring longitudinally the metabolic demands of stroke patients: Resting energy expenditure is not elevated. *Stroke* 2003; 34(2):502–507.

20. Weekes E, Elia M. Resting energy expenditure and body composition following cerebrovascular accident. *Clin Nutr* 1992; 11(1):18–22.

21. American Dietetic Association and Dietitians of Canada. *Manual of Clinical Dietetics.* 6th ed. Chicago: American Dietetic Association, 2000:667–693.

22. Mountokalakis T, Dellos C. Protein catabolism following stroke [letter]. *Arch Intern Med* 1984; 144:2285.

23. Chalela JA, Haymore J, Schellinger PD, et al. Acute stroke patients are being underfed: A nitrogen balance study. *Neurocrit Care* 2004; 1(3):331–334.

24. Trumbo P, Schlicker S, Yates AA, Poos M, Food and Nutrition Board of the Institute of Medicine, The National Academies. Dietary reference intakes for energy, carbohydrate, fiber, fat, fatty acids, cholesterol, protein, and amino acids. *J Am Diet Assoc* 2002; 102(11):1621–1630.

25. Heart and Stroke Foundation of Ontario. *Improving Recognition and Management of Dysphagia in Acute Stroke: A Vision for Ontario.* Toronto: Heart and Stroke Foundation of Ontario, 2002.

26. Pesce-Hammond K, Wessel J. Nutrition assessment and decision making. In: Merritt R, ed. *The A.S.P.E.N. Nutrition Support Practice Manual.* 2nd ed. Silver Springs, MD: American Society for Parenteral and Enteral Nutrition, 2005:3–26.

27. Kovacevich DS, Boney AR, Braunschweig CL, et al. Nutrition risk classsification: A reproducible and valid tool for nurses. *Nutr Clin Pract* 1997; 12:20–25.

28. Heart and Stroke Foundation of Ontario. Nutrition screening for stroke survivors. In: *Management of Dysphagia in Acute Stroke: Nutrition Screening for Stroke Survivors.* Toronto: Heart and Stroke Foundation of Ontario, 2005.

29. ASPEN Board of Directors and Clinical Guidelines Task Force. Guidelines for the use of parenteral and enteral nutrition in adult and pediatric patients. *JPEN J Parenter Enteral Nutr* 2002; 26(1 Suppl):1SA–138SA.

30. World Health Organization. *International Statistical Classification of Diseases and Health-related Problems.* 10th rev. Geneva: World Health Organization, 1992.

31. Mullen JL, Buzby GP, Waldman MT, et al. Prediction of operative morbidity and mortality by preoperative nutritional assessment. *Surg Forum* 1979; 30:80–82.

32. Ingenbleek Y, Carpentier YA. A prognostic inflammatory and nutritional index scoring critically ill patients. *Int J Vitam Nutr Res* 1985; 55(1):91–101.

33. Buzby GP, Mullen JL, Matthews DC, et al. Prognostic nutritional index in gastrointestinal surgery. *Am J Surg* 1980; 139(1):160–167.

34. Seltzer MH, Bastidas JA, Cooper DM, et al. Instant nutritional assessment. *JPEN J Parenter Enteral Nutr* 1979; 3(3):157–159.

35. Fleck A. Clinical and nutritional aspects of changes in acute-phase proteins during inflammation. *Proc Nutr Soc* 1989; 48(3):347–354.

36. Gabay C, Kushner I. Acute-phase proteins and other systemic responses to inflammation. *N Engl J Med* 1999; 340(6):448–454.

37. Beamer NB, Coull BM, Clark WM, et al. Interleukin-6 and interleukin-1 receptor antagonist in acute stroke. *Ann Neurol* 1995; 37(6):800–805.

38. Emsley HC, Smith CJ, Gavin CM, et al. An early and sustained peripheral inflammatory response in acute ischaemic stroke: Relationships with infection and atherosclerosis. *J Neuroimmunol* 2003; 139(1–2):93–101.

39. Ferrarese C, Mascarucci P, Zoia C, et al. Increased cytokine release from peripheral blood cells after acute stroke. *J Cereb Blood Flow Metab* 1999; 19(9):1004–1009.

40. Intiso D, Zarrelli MM, Lagioia G, et al. Tumor necrosis factor alpha serum levels and inflammatory response in acute ischemic stroke patients. *Neurol Sci* 2004; 24(6):390–396.

41. Smith CJ, Emsley HC, Gavin CM, et al. Peak plasma interleukin-6 and other peripheral markers of inflammation in the first week of ischaemic stroke correlate with brain infarct volume, stroke severity, and long-term outcome. *BMC Neurol* 2004;4(1):2.

42. Tarkowski E, Rosengren L, Blomstrand C, et al. Early intrathecal production of interleukin-6 predicts the size of brain lesion in stroke. *Stroke* 1995; 26(8):1393–1398.

43. Ballmer PE. Causes and mechanisms of hypoalbuminaemia. *Clin Nutr* 2001; 20(3):271–273.

44. Johnson AM. Low levels of plasma proteins: Malnutrition or inflammation? *Clin Chem Lab Med* 1999; 37(2):91–96.

45. Gibson RS. *Principles of Nutritional Assessment.* New York: Oxford University Press, 1990.

46. Akner G, Cederholm T. Treatment of protein-energy malnutrition in chronic nonmalignant disorders. *Am J Clin Nutr* 2001; 74(1):6–24.

47. Rosenthal AJ, Sanders KM, McMurtry CT, et al. Is malnutrition overdiagnosed in older hospitalized patients? Association between the soluble interleukin-2 receptor and serum markers of malnutrition? *J Gerontol A Biol Sci Med Sci* 1998; 53(2):M81–M86.

48. Sahyoun NR, Jacques PF, Dallal G, Russell RM. Use of albumin as a predictor of mortality in community dwelling and institutionalized elderly populations. *J Clin Epidemiol* 1996; 49(9):981–988.

49. Sullivan DH. What do the serum proteins tell us about our elderly patients? *J Gerontol A Biol Sci Med Sci* 2001; 56(2):M71–M74.

50. Deitrick JE, Whedon GD, Shorr E. Effects of mobilization upon various metabolic and physiological functions. *Am J Med* 1948; 4:3–36.

50. Ontario Dietetic Association and Ontario Hospital Association. *Nutrition Care Manual.* Don Mills, Ont: Ontario Hospital Association, 1989.

51. Schonheyder F, Heilskov NC, Olesen K. Isotopic studies on the mechanism of negative nitrogen balance produced by immobilization. *Scand J Lab Invest* 1954; 178–188.

52. Baker JP, Detsky AS, Wesson DE, et al. Nutritional assessment: A comparison of clinical judgment and objective measurements. *N Engl J Med* 1982; 306(16):969–972.

53. Pardoe EM. Development of a multistage diet for dysphagia. *J Am Diet Assoc* 1993; 93(5):568–571.

54. Sitzmann JV. Nutritional support of the dysphagic patient: Methods, risks, and complications of therapy. *JPEN J Parenter Enteral Nutr* 1990; 14:60–63.

55. Nelson RA, Millikan CH, Stollar C, Stone DB. Nutrition and the stroke patient. In: Gastineau CF, ed. *Dialogues in Nutrition.* vol. 3(4). Bloomfield, NJ: Health Learning Systems, 1979:1–6.

56. Lord L, Harrington M. Enteral nutrition implementation and management. In: Merritt R, ed. *The A.S.P.E.N. Nutrition Support Practice Manual.* 2nd ed. Silver Springs, MD: American Society for Parenteral and Enteral Nutrition, 2005:76–89.

57. Dumortier J, Lapalus MG, Pereira A, et al. Unsedated transnasal PEG placement. *Gastrointest Endosc* 2004; 59(1):54–57.

58. Nakajima M, Kimura K, Inatomi Y, et al. Intermittent oro-esophageal tube feeding in acute stroke patients: A pilot study. *Acta Neurol Scand* 2006; 113(1):36–39.

59. Schaller BJ, Graf R, Jacobs AH. Pathophysiological changes of the gastrointestinal tract in ischemic stroke. *Am J Gastroenterol* 2006; 101:1655–1665.

60. Kerr D, Hamilton P, Cavan DA. Preventing glycaemic excursions in diabetic patients requiring percutaneous endoscopic gastrostomy (PEG) feeding after a stroke. *Diabet Med* 2002; 19(12):1006–1008.

61. Solomon SM, Kirby DF. The refeeding syndrome: A review. *J Parenter Enteral Nutr* 2002; 26:39SA–41SA.

62. Chicago Dietetic Association Staff and South Suburban Dietetic Association Staff. *Manual of Clinical Dietetics.* 5th ed. Chicago: American Dietetic Association, 1996:293–298.

63. de Luis DA, Aller R, de Luis J, et al. Clinical and biochemical characteristics of patients with home enteral nutrition in an area of Spain. *Eur J Clin Nutr* 2003; 57(4):612–615.

64. Schneider SM, Raina C, Pugliese P, et al. Outcome of patients treated with home enteral nutrition. *JPEN J Parenter Enteral Nutr* 2001; 25(4):203–209.

65. Wicks C, Gimson A, Vlavianos P, et al. Assessment of the percutaneous endoscopic gastrostomy feeding tube as part of an integrated approach to enteral feeding. *Gut* 1992; 33(5):613–616.

66. Jukkola K, MacLennan P. Improving the efficacy of nutritional supplementation in the hospitalized elderly. *Australas J Ageing* 2005; 24(2):119–124.

67. Welch P, Porter J, Endres J. Efficacy of a medication pass supplement program in long-term care compared to a traditional system. *J Nutr Elderly* 2003; 22(3):19–28.

68. Consultant Dietitians in Health Care Facilities/American Dietetic Association. *Mental Status, Nutrition Care for Specific Diseases. Practical Interventions for the Caregivers of the Eating-disabled Older Adult.* Chicago: American Dietetic Association, 1994:109–122, 147–172.

69. Wrick KL, Robertson JB, Van Soest PJ, et al. The influence of dietary fiber source on human intestinal transit and stool output. *J Nutr* 1983; 113(8):1464–1479.

70. Finestone HM, Foley N, Woodbury MG, Greene-Finestone L. Quantifying fluid intake in dysphagic stroke patients: A preliminary comparison of oral and nonoral strategies. *Arch Phys Med Rehabil* 2001; 82:1744–1746.

71. Whelan K. Inadequate fluid intakes in dysphagic acute stroke. *Clin Nutr* 2001; 20(5):423–428.

72. Forchielli ML, Miller SJ. Nutritional goals and requirements. In: Merritt R, ed. *The A.S.P.E.N. Nutrition Support Practice Manual.* 2nd ed. Silver Springs, MD: American Society for Parenteral and Enteral Nutrition, 2005:38–53.

73. Garcia ME. Dehydration of the elderly in nursing homes. *Nutr Noteworthy* 2001; 4:1–8.

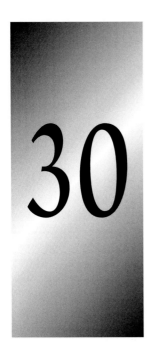

30 Bladder and Bowel Management after Stroke

Sylvia A. Duraski
Florence A. Denby
J. Quentin Clemens

O f all the functional deficits experienced by the survivor of a stroke, incontinence is often an overlooked consequence despite its huge impact on rehabilitation and recovery. Over the years, health care providers and researchers have concluded that those who experience urinary incontinence (UI) after stroke have a poorer prognosis, decreased functional outcomes, and an increased risk of institutionalization (1–6). This does not include other negative consequences that can result from urinary incontinence, such as depressed mood, social isolation, increased risk of skin breakdown, infection, and falls with or without injury.

BLADDER MANAGEMENT

Urinary Incontinence

Prevalence. The prevalence of UI after stroke varies depending upon when the survivor is assessed. In the acute stroke survivor, the prevalence of UI has been documented to range between 32%–83% (1–6). Brittain et al. (7) specifically looked at nine studies conducted to identify the prevalence of UI after stroke. The studies showed that between 32–79% of stroke patients at admission experienced some form of UI. The huge variance in prevalence could be the result of two factors. One is the varying times between the onset of stroke and when the survivor is first assessed for incontinence. Some studies assessed the stroke survivor within days of the onset of the stroke, while others assessed the survivor from three months to two years after stroke. Still other studies did not list the time from stroke onset. The second possible factor for the large variance in prevalence of UI after stroke is the lack of information about the presence of pre-stroke UI. Borrie et al. (8) conducted one of the few studies that identified that 17% of his subjects were incontinent prior to their stroke.

The prevalence of UI after stroke is significant even weeks after onset. Ween et al. (9) found that 41% of the post-stroke survivors were incontinent on admission to rehabilitation. However, the prevalence of post-stroke incontinence decreases over time. In 135 stroke survivors studied over a six-month period, Brockelhurst and his colleagues (10) showed that 51% of their subjects were incontinent of urine during the first year after stroke. Incontinence resolved eight weeks post-stroke in 55% of the subjects, and by six months, 80% of stroke survivors were continent. Borrie and his colleagues (8) had similar findings that show a downward trend in the number of incontinent survivors over time. In 151 patients with 154 strokes, 55% were incontinent after one week, 32% were incontinent after four weeks, and 21% were incontinent after twelve weeks. Brittain et al. (11) cited rates of UI in hospitalized stroke patients between 32–79% at the time of admission, 25–28% at discharge, and 12–19% several months after onset. Patel et al. (3) reported that in 235 stroke survivors, 40% were incontinent on initial assessment, 19% at three month follow up, 15% after one year, and 10% after two years. The method used to manage the incontinence was not identified in any study, therefore it is unknown if any particular intervention or if natural recovery led to the decrease in UI.

Prognostic Factors.   Numerous studies have reported on UI and its prognostic factors in stroke mortality and recovery. Wade and Hewer (12) showed that incontinence had an overall predictive value of 78% for death. Nakayama and his colleagues (5) looked at 935 acute stroke patients admitted to the hospital over a 19-month period. Of those with some degree of UI on admission, 68% died by discharge, and 25% died within six months of discharge. Brittain and her colleagues (7) concluded that 52% of the patients who experienced UI were dead within six months, compared to only 7% who were continent.

UI may impact on functional status and recovery in rehabilitation. Jongbloed (13) reviewed 33 studies conducted between 1950 and 1985 to identify factors predictive of improvement in stroke survivors. This author concluded that the presence of UI on admission was an adverse prognostic factor for functional outcome (13). Wade and Hewer (12) and Ween (9) also found that UI is an important prognostic factor impacting rehabilitation. In these studies, UI was associated with a more severe stroke, an inability to communicate, an inability to transfer, fecal incontinence (FI), and a greater risk of infection. Other studies confirm that UI is a strong predictor of functional recovery (5, 12). In stroke survivors younger than 75 years of age, UI was the best single predictor of disability at three months.

Risk Factors.   It is unclear whether UI results from time lost from therapeutic treatment, the survivor's advanced age, gender, severity, location, type of stroke, cognitive, language, or functional impairments (14). In 1987, Reding and his colleagues (14) documented possible co-morbid reasons for UI in the stroke survivor. This study concluded that there was an association between UI and the presence of aphasia, or the combination of hemiplegia, visual association, and cognitive impairment and incontinence. Gelber et al. (14)assessed 51 patients with unilateral ischemic hemispheric strokes admitted to a neurorehabilitation unit. They concluded that the presence of aphasia, cognitive impairments, and poorer functional status strongly correlated with incontinence in the stroke survivor (14).

Owen et al. (15) performed a retrospective review of 225 patients admitted to a rehabilitation center in a tertiary medical center during a 14-month period of time. Their findings compared characteristics of incontinent stroke survivors to those of continent stroke survivors. More than 90% of subjects that remained incontinent experienced dysphagia, lower Functional Independence Measure (FIM) scores, and significant impairments in orientation to time, memory, and problem solving. Nakayama et al. (5) found that patients with initial UI were older, female, and had more co-morbid conditions. Ween et al. (9) concluded that the incontinent group in his study had significantly lower admission average FIM scores (43 versus 75) when compared with that of the continent group. In a nonrandom sample of 45 continent and incontinent stroke survivors, Gross (16) found that the group that remained incontinent had significantly lower admission and discharge FIM scores. While the incontinent group showed improvement on all measures in this study, they still had lower mean FIM scores (16). All of these researchers agreed with previous studies that identified that stroke survivors who were incontinent experienced more disabling strokes. While incontinent stroke survivors do make functional gains, they are not as great as in the continent stroke survivor. This not only impacts functional outcomes, but also affects the length of hospital and rehabilitation stays, as well as discharge destination.

Discharge Destination.   Whether the result of UI alone, or combined with the severity of stroke or other medical co-morbidities, numerous studies have documented that discharge destination for stroke survivors is negatively affected. Van Kuijk et al. (17) performed a cohort study on 143 stroke survivors admitted for postacute rehabilitation. They showed that in the incontinent group, eight survivors went home and six went to nursing homes, while in the continent group, 119 went home and eight went to nursing homes. They found that the difference in discharge destination was statistically significant, suggesting an association between UI and admission to a long-term nursing facility (17). Ween et al. (9) found similar findings in his study. Of the patients with UI on discharge, 61% went to nursing homes, while only 18% of patients who were continent were discharged to nursing homes (9). Patel et al. (3) found that if the stroke survivor remained incontinent over time, institutionalization rates were even higher. In one study that did not find a correlation between incontinence and discharge destination, the majority of patients in both the continent and incontinent group were discharged to home (16).

Neural Control of the Lower Urinary Tract

Components of normal lower urinary tract function include the storage of urine at low pressure without leakage (storage phase), interrupted by the periodic, voluntary expulsion of urine (voiding phase). These processes involve the coordination of the peripheral autonomic,

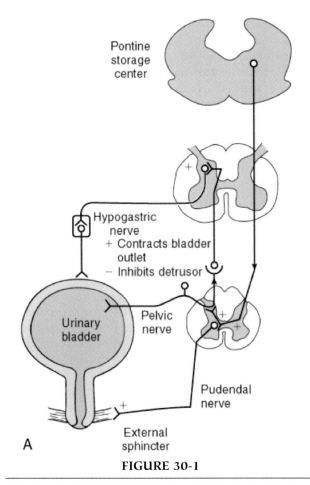

FIGURE 30-1

Storage Reflex
Afferent signals from the bladder wall to the spinal cord results in relaxation of detrusor muscle and contraction of the bladder neck and uretheral sphincter.

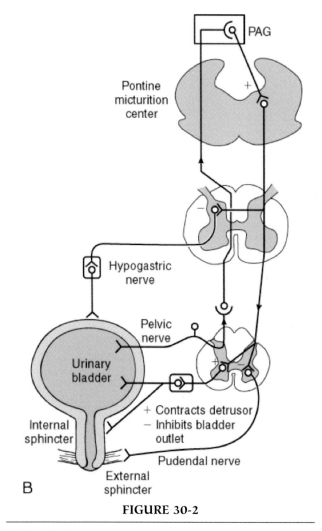

FIGURE 30-2

Voiding Reflex
Cortical signaling leads to relaxation of the urethral sphincter and contraction of the detrusor muscle.

somatic, and central nervous systems (18, 19).Sympathetic autonomic activity promotes urine storage, while parasympathetic activity promotes voiding.

Preganglionic parasympathetic efferent neurons exit the spinal cord at S2–4 and travel in the pelvic nerve to ganglia located in the bladder wall. These parasympathetic fibers modulate detrusor muscle contraction. Sympathetic efferent fibers exit the spinal cord at T10–L2 and travel in the hypogastric nerve. These fibers modulate contraction of the urethral smooth muscle and bladder outlet, and inhibit parasympathetic activity to the detrusor muscle. Somatic efferent fibers exit from S2–4 and travel in the pudendal nerve to the striated urethral sphincter. These fibers modulate voluntary urethral sphincter contractions. Afferent fibers from the urethra and bladder are distributed throughout the pelvis in the pelvic, hypogastric, and pudendal nerves. Coordination of the bladder and urethral sphincter appears to be accomplished in the pons, as experimental electrical stimulation of the pontine micturition center (PMC) causes detrusor contraction and

urethral relaxation (20). The PMC receives input from multiple areas, including the cerebellum, basal ganglia, thalamus, hypothalamus, and cerebral cortex. Signals from these areas provide inhibition of the PMC, and allow voluntary expulsion of urine when socially appropriate.

When the bladder fills, stretch receptors in the bladder wall cause afferent signal transmission to the spinal cord. These signals result in increased sympathetic activity (contraction of the urethral sphincter and bladder neck), and decreased parasympathetic activity (detrusor muscle relaxation) (Figure 30-1). When voiding is desired, cortical signaling triggers a switch from storage to voiding function. PMC activity then leads to a coordinated relaxation of the urethral sphincter (decreased sympathetic activity), and contraction of the detrusor muscle (increased parasympathetic activity) (Figure 30-2). After completion of voiding, the storage phase resumes.

Detrusor muscle contractions are mediated by muscarinic cholinergic receptors in the detrusor muscle cell wall (21). Parasympathetic neurons release acetylcholine, which binds to muscarinic receptors and triggers an increase in intracellular calcium. This in turn triggers downstream intracellular processes that cause muscle contraction.

Classification of Voiding Dysfunction after Stroke

Researchers have concluded that the degree of voiding dysfunction after stroke is dependent upon the size of the stroke, the location of the stroke, and the time from onset of stroke.

Early Phase.   After the onset of stroke, areflexia has been documented as the most common detrusor dysfunction. Detrusor areflexia presents clinically in the stroke survivor as urinary retention or overflow incontinence, a problem of bladder emptying. Often times referred to as "cerebral shock," this term is used to describe the loss of reflexes below the level of the lesion, much as "spinal shock" is used to describe what is experienced in someone with an acute spinal cord injury. The neurophysiology of "cerebral shock" is unclear (22). Some speculate that persistent areflexia in the stroke survivor may be the result of a lesion in an area of the brain that is responsible for voiding (23). Others believe that detrusor areflexia is due to an impaired level of consciousness or a temporary detrusor failure resulting in overdistention (24).

Whatever the cause, many studies of detrusor activity after stroke have concluded that detrusor hyporeflexia immediately after the onset of stroke is common. Reports of the incidence of urinary retention after stroke vary, and are estimated as high as 47% when survivors are assessed within 72 hours after the onset of stroke (25). Gelber and his colleagues followed 19 stroke survivors with unilateral ischemic stroke admitted to a neurorehabilitation unit. Urodynamic studies were performed on all of the survivors. Gelber concluded that bladder hyporeflexia occurred in the early phase of acute hemispheric stroke, with a gradual increase in bladder tone as the survivor recovered (14). In 1996, Burney and her colleagues followed 45 men and 15 women between the ages of 32 to 80 years of age only 3 days after the onset of stroke. Forty seven percent (47%) of patients that were evaluated presented with retention and overflow incontinence. The cause of the retention was concluded to be detrusor areflexia (26). This study correlated the increased frequency of detrusor areflexia with rapid assessment time from onset of stroke. Other studies varied in the amount of time from stroke onset to assessment. Those that assessed more

chronic stroke survivors found less detrusor areflexia in cystometric testing.

One study found that a large number of those who experienced detrusor areflexia were diagnosed with lesions of the cerebellum, but no other study has been able to duplicate these results (26). Other potential causes of the detrusor areflexia have been assessed. Several studies looked for other causes of urinary retention such as urinary tract infections, anticholinergic medications, diabetic neuropathy, and benign prostatic hypertrophy. Given the average age of the stroke survivor, other factors may contribute to the retention. It has been estimated that approximately 50% of men by the age of 60 years and 80% of men by the age of 80 years have benign prostatic hypertrophy (BPH) (27). Some of the potential problems that also cause retention such as BPH may have existed prior to the stroke, but it is not until the stroke occurs that the individual exhibits symptoms they can no longer manage. Most studies concluded that true detrusor areflexia with normal smooth sphincter function was common immediately after stroke. Smooth sphincter function is generally unaffected by stroke (22).

Late Phase.   Just days to weeks after the onset of stroke, the most common detrusor dysfunction observed is hyperreflexia. The cause for this change is thought to be the result of the release of spinal micturition reflexes secondary to injury to the cerebral inhibitory centers of voiding (23). During this phase, the stroke survivor generally has intact sensation and presents with urgency, frequency, and urge incontinence as a result of the inability to suppress bladder contractions even at low detrusor filling volumes. This is a problem that can be categorized as a failure to store, secondary to bladder overactivity. Some studies demonstrate on cystometric testing that stroke survivors who are incontinent may have symptoms of hyperreflexia, not urgency. Tsuchida et al. performed cystometric studies on 39 stroke survivors. The time of stroke onset ranged from 11 days to 13 years. They concluded that urinary frequency or urge incontinence were the most commonly observed symptoms in this population (28). Khan and his colleagues found that the most common cystometric finding in this group was detrusor hyperreflexia (29). Kong et al. studied 27 stroke survivors admitted to a rehabilitation center in a three-month period of time. The cystometric studies reported that 11 patients had detrusor hyperreflexia, one patient had detrusor areflexia, and 15 patients had normal results (1). Of interest, the one patient who had detrusor areflexia was only 12 days post-stroke.

While it is still not completely understood what part of the brain controls voiding, lesions of the cerebral cortex, particularly the frontal lobe, have been identified as impairing the stroke survivor's ability to suppress detrusor contractions. Several studies concluded that cerebral hemispheric lesions most commonly cause detrusor hyperreflexia (14, 26, 29). Sakakibara et al. followed the urinary history and cystometric test results of 72 acute hemispheric stroke patients. They concluded that voiding dysfunction is common in frontal lesions and infarctions of the anterior cerebral artery territory (30). Burney et al., Khan et al., and Tsuchida et al. concluded that stroke lesions in the cerebral cortex, internal capsule, and basal ganglia resulted in detrusor hyperreflexia (26, 28, 29). Other researchers also concluded that there was no difference between voiding dysfunction and dominant and nondominant hemisphere lesions.

Incontinence also has been documented in incontinent stroke survivors with normal cystometric testing of the detrusor muscle. Since there is no true voiding dysfunction in these stroke survivors, how is incontinence in this group explained? Health care professionals have concluded that neurologic deficits of the stroke contribute to incontinence. For example, motor deficits prevent the stroke survivor from getting to the bathroom for toileting. Sensory deficits interfere with the awareness of the need to void. Cognitive deficits interfere with remembering what to do to stay dry. Communication deficits interfere with the survivor asking for assistance with toileting.

Management

Initial management consists of supportive care and management of life-threatening sequelae of the stroke. It is common for an indwelling urethral catheter to be placed at this time. When the patient is medically stable, the catheter is removed and a voiding trial is begun. If the patient is able to void, post-void residual volumes should be obtained. If the residual volumes are acceptably low after 2–3 voids, no additional measurements are needed. In a patient with an unsuccessful voiding trial, a urine culture should be obtained, and any bacteriuria should be treated with 3–7 days of appropriate antibiotics.

Cerebral Shock Phase

During the cerebral shock phase (6–12 weeks), it is common for patients to fail decatheterization trials. When the catheter is removed, these patients may be unable to void, or they may void but only partially empty the bladder. Management of these patients consists of supportive care, medications, and catheterization.

Supportive Care. Intensive stroke rehabilitation is paramount, as immobility, polypharmacy, delirium, and pain may contribute to voiding dysfunction. As performance status improves, the ability to void also improves.

Therefore, the timing of catheter removal needs to be individualized, as it may not be appropriate to remove an indwelling catheter in patients who remain severely disabled (e.g. cannot get out of bed).

Medications. Medications to improve bladder contractility and to decrease bladder outlet resistance may be prescribed. These may help to decrease the duration of urinary retention. Bethanechol (Urecholine) is an oral cholinergic agonist that may theoretically improve bladder contractility by stimulating cholinergic receptors in the bladder wall. However, data to support its clinical efficacy are very limited. Potential side effects include diarrhea, nausea, and bronchospasm. Alternatively, therapy to reduce bladder outlet resistance may be instituted with alpha-adrenergic blockers such as tamsulosin (Flomax), alfuzosin (Uroxatral), doxazosin (Cardura) and terazosin (Hytrin). These agents are used to treat bladder outlet obstruction caused by benign prostatic hyperplasia (BPH), and are commonly used as initial therapy in men with urinary retention. As alpha-adrenergic receptors are located in the bladder neck as well as the prostate, these agents could theoretically be used in both men and women, although very limited data exist regarding the efficacy on the latter. Table 30.1 lists several medications that can be used to improve bladder contractility or reduce outlet resistance.

Catheterization. Intermittent or continuous bladder catheterization must be used in patients who are unable to empty their bladders spontaneously. The choice of which to use must be individualized to the patient. However, intermittent catheterization (IC) is often preferred, as it allows the clinician and patient to document voiding efficiency in an ongoing manner, and it appears to be associated with fewer infectious complications than indwelling catheterization (31). In the inpatient setting, nurses can perform the IC, and the patient can attempt to void prior to each catheterization so that post-void residual volumes can be assessed. Continuation of IC in the outpatient setting may not be possible, as the patient or caretaker may not be able or willing to perform the catheterization. If the patient is discharged with an indwelling catheter, arrangements must be made for follow-up visits for decatheterization trials.

Late Phase

Typically, the urinary retention associated with cerebral shock is replaced by urgency, urge incontinence, and complete bladder emptying. This is felt to be due to a loss of cortical inhibition of the voiding reflex (32). Therefore, the problem changes from a "failure to empty" to a "failure to store." The symptoms may be exacerbated by the loss of mobility that often occurs with a stroke, as more

TABLE 30-1
Medications Used to Treat Lower Urinary Tract Symptoms

GENERIC NAME	TRADE NAME	DOSE	INDICATION
Bethanechol	Urecholine	5, 10, or 25 mg po TID to QID	Increase bladder contractility
Tamsulosin	Flomax	0.4 mg po qD	Reduce bladder outlet resistance
Alfuzosin	Uroxatral	10 mg po qD	Reduce bladder outlet resistance
Doxazosin	Cardura	1, 2, 4, or 8 mg po qD (must be titrated)	Reduce bladder outlet resistance
Terazosin	Hytrin	1, 2, 5 or 10 mg po qD (must be titrated)	Reduce bladder outlet resistance
Tolterodine	Detrol	2 mg po bid	Decrease urgency, frequency, and urge incontinence
Tolterodine	Detrol LA	4 mg po qD	Decrease urgency, frequency, and urge incontinence
Oxybutynin	Ditropan	5–10 mg po tid	Decrease urgency, frequency, and urge incontinence
Oxybutynin	Ditropan XL	5, 10, or 15 mg po qD	Decrease urgency, frequency, and urge incontinence
Oxybutynin	Oxytrol patch	3.9 mg – change twice weekly	Decrease urgency, frequency, and urge incontinence
Solifenacin	Vesicare	5 or 10 mg po qD	Decrease urgency, frequency, and urge incontinence
Darifenacin	Enablex	7.5 or 15 mg po qD	Decrease urgency, frequency, and urge incontinence
Trospium	Sanctura	20 mg po BID	Decrease urgency, frequency, and urge incontinence

time may be required to get to the toilet. A moderate degree of urgency that is manageable for a healthy person may be quite troublesome for someone who requires more time to get to the toilet. Management of this problem is the same as for other patients with urgency and urge incontinence, although these treatments may be less effective following a stroke due to the more severe nature of the symptoms.

Behavioral Therapy. Simple measures (use of a bedside commode, timed/prompted voiding, and avoidance of bladder irritants such as caffeine) may be used on virtually all patients. Other therapies such as pelvic floor physical therapy, biofeedback, and electrical stimulation require a level of motivation and muscle control that may not be present in all patients. However, these measures may be quite effective in properly chosen patients (33).

Antimuscarinic Medications. These oral medications block the binding of acetylcholine to the muscarinic receptor, and result in decreased detrusor muscle contractile activity (34). Clinically, this receptor blockage causes a reduction in urinary urgency, frequency, and urgency incontinence. Examples of these medications include tolterodine (Detrol), oxybutynin (Ditropan, Oxytrol), solifenacin (Vesicare), darifenacin (Enablex), and trospium (Sanctura) (Table 30.1). Side effects (e.g., dry mouth, constipation, dry eyes) are common, and clinical response is variable and unpredictable. The outcome appears to be better if these medications are combined with behavioral therapy (35).

Additional Diagnostic Tests. At times, patients may demonstrate incomplete bladder emptying or urinary retention that persists longer than would be expected after the initial cerebral shock phase. This may be due to pre-existing voiding dysfunction that was present prior to the stroke. In such patients, further evaluation with urodynamic testing and cystoscopy can be useful to determine if there is evidence of underlying bladder outlet obstruction (27). If obstruction is present, treatment with prostate resection can allow resumption of voiding, but these patients should be counseled that they may experience urge incontinence postoperatively.

Research Frontiers

The urgency and urge incontinence that often occur following a stroke can be more severe and difficult to treat than similar symptoms that occur in the absence of neurologic pathology. Two relatively new treatments that may be applied to these patients include sacral neuromodulation and detrusor injections of botulinum toxin.

Sacral Neuromodulation. Sacral neuromodulation was approved by the US Food and Drug Administration in 1997 for the treatment of refractory urinary urgency and urge incontinence. Although the exact mechanism of action is not clear, the therapy appears to activate latent inhibitory reflexes to the bladder through stimulation of somatic afferent nerve fibers (36). The outpatient procedure is performed using sedation and local anesthesia, with the patient in the prone position. Under fluoroscopic guidance, a lead is placed percutaneously into one of the S3 sacral foramena. The lead is initially attached to an external battery, which is worn for a two- to three-week test period. If the stimulation results in a >50% improvement in incontinence episodes, a second outpatient procedure is performed in which the external portion of the lead is removed, and permanent subcutaneous battery is placed in the upper buttock. Multiple initial series demonstrated 70–80% success rates for the treatment of urgency and urge incontinence, although none of these focused exclusively on patients with these symptoms following a stroke (37). Potential complications include lead migration, pain at the stimulator site, and wound infection. No major neurologic complications have been reported to date. As with any metal implant, magnetic resonance imaging cannot be performed following the procedure. Most recently, in a series of 12 patients with refractory urge incontinence following stroke, Kuo found improvements in the grade of incontinence in 50% after detrusor injections of 200 units botulinum toxin type A (38).

Injection of Botulinum Toxin. The use of botulinum toxin for medical purposes is well established in physiatry, but its use for urologic applications has been a very recent development. In 2000, Schurch and colleagues first described the cystoscopic injection of botulinum toxin type A into the detrusor for the treatment of neurogenic detrusor overactivity in individuals with traumatic spinal cord injury (39). Since then, multiple other investigators have reported excellent results for the treatment of both idiopathic and neurogenic urge incontinence (40, 41). Significant improvements in incontinence episodes, pad use, and quality of life have been consistently demonstrated. Typical doses have been from 200–300 units injected at a random location into the bladder wall in 10-unit increments. To date, there have been no reports of *de novo* urinary retention. In those who respond to the treatment, the effects have been reported to last from 4–14 months. While this is exciting new technology with great promise, larger randomized clinical trials are needed to more completely assess its efficacy and safety.

BOWEL MANAGEMENT

Introduction

This portion of the chapter begins by describing the prevalence and prognosis of neurogenic bowel after stroke. Following this is an explanation of normal bowel function, the relationship of the central nervous system

and bowel function, and the effect stroke has on fecal elimination. The section ends with a practical approach to the assessment of neurogenic bowel, as well as a discussion of future research in neurogenic bowel in stroke survivors.

Fecal Incontinence. There is a natural relationship between urinary and bowel continence. In a survey of 18,000 Wisconsin nursing home residents, urinary incontinence was the greatest risk factor for developing fecal incontinence (FI), and FI was the greatest risk factor for developing UI. Decreased ability to perform activities of daily living, immobility, dementia, and specific diseases such as stroke and diabetes also are related to FI (42).

Bowel disturbances occur when the central nervous system is impaired. Uninhibited neurogenic bowel occurs when there is injury to the upper motor neurons located in the cerebral cortex, internal capsule, brain stem, or spinal cord. If cerebral control is interrupted, then the awareness of urge and ability to inhibit defecation are lost, resulting in FI. Sensory impulses travel through the sacral reflex arc to the brain, but the brain is unable to read the impulses, resulting in a decreased awareness of the need to defecate and a decrease in voluntary control of the anal sphincter. Involuntary elimination occurs when the sacral defecation reflex is activated, but if sensation is not impaired, incontinence is coupled with a sense of urgency. In the uninhibited neurogenic bowel, the pattern of incontinence is characterized by a poor awareness of the need to defecate (43). In the general population, FI is the involuntary loss of anal sphincter control leading to the release of stool at any inconvenient or inappropriate time. There are three subtypes of incontinence: passive (the involuntary discharge of stool or gas without knowing); urge (the failed attempt to hold bowel contents); and fecal seepage (stool seeping out after a normal bowel movement) (44). FI increases the vulnerability for poor hygiene, skin breakdown, infection, depression, and social isolation. The etiology of FI may be the result of neuro-sensory-motor dysfunction of anal sphincter or pelvic floor; abnormal colonic transit; loose or liquid stool consistency; or decreased intestinal capacity with overflow. Multiple factors, including impaired consciousness and/or physical disability, influence bowel control after stroke (45, 46).

Prevalence. In a survey of US households, 7.1 % of the population reported fecal leakage, while 0.7% of the population experience fecal straining for more than one month. In the practice guidelines for diagnosis and management of FI, Rao summarizes its prevalence as ranging between 1% and 7.4% in the well population, and up to 25% in the institutionalized (44).

The prevalence of FI in community-dwelling individuals is reported between 1.4 and 15% in the adult population, and between 3.1 and 16.9% in individuals over the age of 60. The Chicago Health and Aging Project (CHAP) study of older biracial, geographically defined residents described the prevalence of FI by race, age, sex, the presence of stroke and diabetes, and the use of certain psychoactive medications. FI was significantly higher among persons with a reported history of stroke (21.5%) than in those with no stroke (8.3%, p< 0.0001). FI has a high association with stroke and diabetes. In a study using multivariate logistic regression analyses adjusted for age, sex, and race, the odds of FI was 2.8 times greater for persons who reported stroke (95% CFIF: 2.2–3.5) compared to people without stroke. Users of anticonvulsant, antipsychotic, hypnotic, antidepressant, and antiParkinsonian medications found that users were two to three times more likely to have fecal incontinence (47).

According to the Copenhagen Stroke study, 40% of the 935 stroke patients had FI at time of admission, 18% at time of discharge, and 9% at six-month follow up. Secondary to multiple risk factors, 62% of stroke survivors became incontinent during the nine months after the three-month acute phase (5). FI affects 56% of acute stroke survivors, 11% at three months post-stroke, and less than 22% at 12 months (10, 48). In a descriptive study of the natural history and independent associations of new onset FI in patients three months after stroke, the prevalence of post stroke FI was 30% at 7–10 days, 11% at three months, 11% at one year, and 15% at three years. One-third of the patients with FI at three months were continent at one year. Sixty-five percent of those who had been continent at three months were incontinent at one year (49).

Prognosis. In patients who were incontinent of feces at the time of admission, 53% died by discharge, 27% had full FI, 6% had occasional incontinence, and 82% had no FI. At a six-month follow up, 5% of the responders had full FI, 4% had partial incontinence, and 91% had no FI (5).

Stroke patients who suffered total anterior circulation infarcts were more likely to be incontinent of feces at three months than those with partial anterior circulation infarct or posterior circulation or lacunar circulation infarct. There was no association noted between FI and cerebral or subarachnoid hemorrhage versus infarct. Even though they are coexisting maladies, FI is less prevalent than UI. The strongest association with UI occurs at three months, with only 8% of stroke survivors having double incontinence. Identifying FI as a public health problem will continue to increase as the oldest age groups continue to grow. FI is associated with the presence of certain conditions: stroke, diabetes, aging, and the use of certain medications. Therefore, new onset FI, common for stroke survivors, may be transient and treated. Drugs that cause constipation, fecal impaction or incontinence,

decreased mobility, impaired proprioception, neglect, and inability to perform toileting activities are treatable risk factors (49).

Discharge Destination. In the Copenhagen Stroke Study, of patients with complete FI, 53% died prior to discharge as compared to 24% with partial FI, and only 3% of continent patients (5). Thirty-six percent of patients with new onset FI died at three months post-stroke, as compared with the death of only 4% continent patients. Of stroke survivors in nursing homes, 20% of incontinent patients died within one year, compared with only 8% of continent patients (49). Regarding discharge destination, FI at three months increased the risk of long-term placement, 28% versus 6%. FI is one of the most common reasons for nursing home placement in the United States, even more than dementia. Often caregivers are unable to manage the challenges of toileting, changing, and cleaning a dependent stroke survivor in the home setting (44, 46). FI is directly related to functional disability after stroke, and is more a result of poor functional recovery than a risk factor for death or institutionalization at six months (48, 50). The more dependent the stroke survivor is on caregivers, the greater the loss of function, and the higher the rate of institutionalization or death.

For those patients returning home with FI, family training regarding bowel program management must be incorporated into the rehabilitation plan. Expensive disposable supplies, such as diapers, pads for bedding, and protective barrier creams are requirements for the incontinent patient.

Normal Bowel Function

This section describes how the normal bowel functions to digest and absorb nutrients and to eliminate waste in order to maintain a healthy human body, and how the gut's anatomy is organized to accommodate bowel function. There are explanations of the neural control (reflexes) and the unique relationship between the gut and the brain.

Physiology of the Bowel. The gastrointestinal (GI) system consists of several organs, each with specialized anatomical functions, divided by autonomic muscular sphincters that compartmentalize each organ yet link together into one functioning system. Other body systems such as the neural, lymphatic, endocrine, and vascular work with the gut in serving the needs of the human body (51, 52). The GI system transports food starting at the stomach and ending at the anus. Digestion of food occurs in the stomach, duodenum, jejunum, and ileum. Secretory glands positioned throughout the GI tract produce digestive enzymes and electrolytes that stimulate and contribute to digestion (43). The upper GI tract processes food by mixing it with pepsin and acid and breaking it down into smaller particles. The proximal stomach serves a storage function by relaxing to accommodate a meal. The distal stomach contracts and propels solid food remnants against the pylorus, where it is repeatedly propelled proximally for further mixing before it empties into the duodenum. The stomach also secretes intrinsic factor Vitamin B12 for absorption. The middle of the GI tract extends from the duodenal papilla to the midtransverse colon, where digestion is completed. Absorption occurs in the small intestine and the proximal half of the colon. The colon is shorter in length and larger in diameter than the small intestine (43, 51, 53).

The large intestine is anatomically composed of the cecum; the ascending, transverse, descending, and sigmoid colon; the rectum; and the anal canal. The colon absorbs water and electrolytes from food matter and stores fecal matter until it is convenient to be expelled. The colon is bounded by the ileocecal sphincter at its proximal end, and by the anal sphincter at the perineum (53, 54). Colonic mucosa prepares feces for evacuation by absorbing fluid from the stool, decreasing the daily fecal volumes from 1,000 to 1,500 ml delivered from the ileum to the 100 to 200 ml expelled from the rectum (51).

There are several layers in the wall of the colon: The inner layer of the mucosa is gut epithelium with subepithelial connective tissue. The mucosal musculature senses the stretch of the lumen wall. The submucosa layer is the submucosal plexus with stretch receptors between the mucosa and the middle circular layer. The circular musculature is the next layer and contracts the lumen,

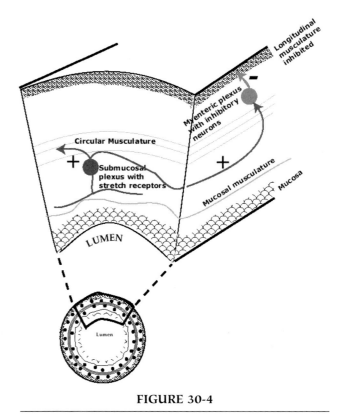

FIGURE 30-4

Cross Section of Colonic Wall
Large intestine musculature of intestinal wall.
Turner, B., Cowie, R. and Young, J. *The Functional Anatomy of Digestive and Urogenital Reflexes.*

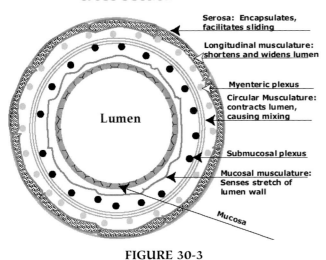

FIGURE 30-3

GI Wall Cross Section
Diagrammatic depiction of the layers of the wall of the colon.
Turner, B., Cowie, R. and Young, J. *The Functional Anatomy of Digestive and Urogenital Reflexes.*

causing mixing. The myenteric plexus is between the middle circular and the outer longitudinal muscle layers. The outer layer consists of the longitudinal muscle layers and the serosa, which encapsulates and facilitates sliding (53).

The Central Nervous System and Defecation. The colon's nervous system has two components: intrinsic and extrinsic. The colonic wall contains intrinsic elements that include the Auerbach's plexus and Meissner's plexus. Auerbach's plexus, also known as the *intramuscular myenteric plexus*, is located between the longitudinal and circular muscle layers and controls GI motility. Meissner's plexus, located in the submucosa, is referred to as *submucosa plexus* and controls GI secretion (55). The intrinsic component is actually the enteric nervous system, providing the basic control for propulsion and fluid regulation. It coordinates the colonic wall, mixing and advancing stool through the colon. The extrinsic neural input occurs through the autonomic nervous system's sympathetic and parasympathetic, pathway which provides volitional or involuntary control specific for each gut region (51, 53, 56).

Intestinal activity works with circular and segmental movements of the different sections of the intestinal tract. There are two types of movement in the colon. The propulsion of food matter, caused by a distended colonic segment forming a contractile ring around the colon to propel forward any material in front of it, is called peristalsis. The speed of peristalsis is greatest in the duodenum and jejunum, and is slowest in the ileum. To be effective, peristalsis requires an intact myenteric plexus. If peristalsis is weak, the myenteric plexus may be disturbed by disease or anticholinergic medication (53, 56). The second type of colonic movement, known as *haustrations,* is a mixing motion consisting of circular contractions digging into and rolling over the fecal material in the colon. Colonic movement depends on haustral contractions and mass movements. The gastroileal reflex stimulates the ileum to move semifluid contents into the cecum and gradually fill the ascending and transverse colon. Propulsion in the cecum and ascending colon is caused by the slow, haustral contractions. Movement of chyme from the ileocecal valve through the transverse colon requires 8 to 15 hours. Chyme evolves into a fecal, semisolid state as fluid is absorbed. This slows down the process for long intervals until a powerful mass movement of the transverse colon propels the contents into the lower colon. All of these processes remain involuntary (51, 53, 54).

Mass movements replace propulsion at the transverse colon and through the sigmoid colon. Gastrocolic and duodenocolic reflexes expedite mass movements that are strongest for about 15 minutes in the first hour after breakfast. In response to distention, usually in the transverse colon, a constrictive ring forms and mass movements begin. Twenty cm or more of colon distal to the constrictive ring lose the haustral contractions and move as a mass or unit. In response, fecal material in that colonic segment is forced down the colon to the rectum. Mass movements last for 10 to 30 minutes, but may return in 12 hours or 24 hours. As feces moves into the rectum, the need to defecate is felt (53).

Neurologic control (reflexes). The GI tract is unique from other organ systems, as the gut's function is influenced and altered by the outside environment. Most of its function is not under direct control of the brain. As mentioned previously, the GI tract functions with intrinsic and extrinsic neural components. Intrinsic nerves control most basic gut activities, while extrinsic nerves modulate visceral activity through sympathetic and parasympathetic functions (52). GI reflexes are mediated by extrinsic vagus or splanchic nerve pathways. The brain-gut axis alters function in regions not under voluntary regulation. Stress caused by external forces can alter GI motility as well as the gut's immune function (55).

The enteric nervous system and its relationship with the sympathetic and parasympathetic systems support three types of gastrointestinal reflexes essential to bowel control and defecation. The first group of reflexes occurs within the enteric nervous system and control GI secretion, peristalsis, and mixing contractions. The second group of reflexes travels from the gut to the prevertebral sympathetic ganglia and back to the GI tract. Gastrocolic reflexes transmit signals from the stomach to cause evacuation of the colon. Enterogastric reflexes from the colon and small intestine inhibit stomach motility and secretion. Colonoileal reflexes prevent the emptying of ileal contents into the colon. The third group of reflexes travels from the gut to the brain stem and then back to the GI tract. These include reflexes in the stomach and duodenum that control gastric motor and secretory activity. Pain reflexes can cause general inhibition of the entire GI tract. The defecation reflexes produce colonic, rectal and abdominal contractions needed for defecation (56).

Intrinsic neural control is altered by signals from the brain to the autonomic nervous system that innervates the gastrointestinal tract. The GI tract's enteric nervous system controls the automatic motor and secretory functions, and allows the gut to continue to function in isolation from its extrinsic nerve supply. Intestinal activity relies on the coordinated action of various parts of the nervous system, including the intramural plexus in the bowel wall, the autonomic nervous system, and the voluntary nervous system. The human brain can inhibit the sacral spinal center to decrease peristaltic activity by voluntarily increasing anal sphincter tone and relaxing the colon, causing the urge to defecate to disappear (53).

DEFECATION

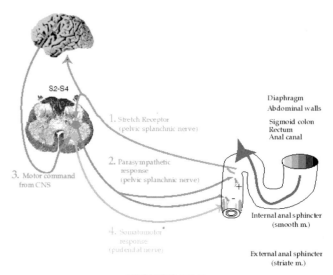

FIGURE 30-5

Defecation

Colonic spinal afferents contribute to fecal continence and defecation. The sympathetic nerve supply to the internal (involuntary) anal sphincter is excitatory as the parasympathetic is inhibitory. The pudendal nerve supplies the external anal sphincter, which is maintained in a state of tonic contraction.

Defecation requires the integration of the somatic nervous system (voluntary) and the autonomic nervous system (involuntary). Any interruption in the process can impair bowel function. The defecation reflex begins when mass movements propel fecal material forward, caused principally by the duodenocolic reflex that is initiated while the duodenum is filled. Feces enter the sigmoid colon and are kept there until right before defecation. The adult rectum is about four to six inches long and is usually empty of feces until defecation. Fecal bolus is propelled into the rectum by mass movement, causing distention and initiating the defecation reflex. The puborectalis muscle forms a sling around the rectoanal junction. To maintain continence, the puborectalis muscle must be contracted. The rectum contains vertical and transverse folds of tissue that help retain the feces. Each vertical fold contains an artery and vein. During defecation, sacral parasympathetic nerves relax this muscle and straighten the rectoangle. Rectal distention initiates temporary relaxation of the internal anal sphincter through intrinsic and reflex sympathetic innervation. The anal canal, which is about 1.5 inches long, contains an internal and external sphincter. Continual dribbling of fecal matter through the anus is prevented by tonic constriction of the internal sphincter, consisting of thick smooth muscle inside the anus. The external anal sphincter is composed of striated voluntary muscle that surrounds and extends distal to the internal sphincter. The external sphincter is controlled by nerve fibers in the pudendal nerve, which is part of the somatic (voluntary) nervous system (43, 52, 56). Reflexes to defecate are transmitted through the intramural nerve plexus, and intensified by parasympathetic system or overdistention of the colon. Feces enters the rectum, causing distention of the rectal wall and initiating afferent signals that spread through the myenteric plexus to start peristaltic waves in the descending colon, sigmoid, and rectum, forcing feces toward the anus. As the peristaltic wave moves toward the anus, the internal anal sphincter is relaxed by inhibitory signals from the myenteric plexus. As sigmoid and rectal contractions increase the pressure within the rectum, the rectosigmoid angle opens by greater than 15 degrees. The external sphincter relaxes voluntarily and permits fecal defecation. Voluntary increases in intra-abdominal pressure (i.e., Valsalva maneuver) can assist in defecation. If the intrinsic defecation reflex itself is too weak to be effective, it needs to be supported by a parasympathetic defecation reflex that involves the sacral segments of the spinal cord. Parasympathetic nerve fibers in the pelvic nerves intensify the peristaltic waves, relax the internal anal sphincter, and convert the intrinsic defecation reflex from a weak movement into a strong defecation process. In the continent person, relaxation of the internal sphincter and forward movement of feces toward the anus initiates an instantaneous contraction of the external sphincter, temporarily preventing defecation until an appropriate time (51, 56, 57).

The GI tract has dual innervation. The small intestine is rich with sensory fibers. Vagal and spinal afferent nerves to the CNS carry information from activated sensory receptors. The extrinsic supply is divided into efferent and afferent branches. Information is transported in parasympathetic and sympathetic nerve tracts, provided by the vagus and spinal nerves. Most efferent parasympathetic and sympathetic fibers terminate in the myenteric plexus and form connections in enteric ganglia. Some sympathetic axons terminate directly on sphincteric smooth muscles. GI activities are carried out independent of external neural control. Cell bodies of these efferent nerves reside predominantly in the brainstem. The vagus nerve contains three groups of efferent fibers: parasympathetic cholinergic, cholinergic, and sympathetic (55). Stimulation of efferent vagal cholinergic neurons principally activates nicotinergic receptors within enteric ganglia, exciting motor activity. The vagus nerve informs the brainstem about activities of the gut. In humans, the enteric nervous system contains up to 100 million neurons, compared with only 2,000 efferent fibers in the vagus. This suggests that the intrinsic nerves direct reflexes and control activities, and that extrinsic nerves serve as to modulate function (58, 59).

Effect of Stroke on Fecal Elimination

In order to improve the quality of life of patients with stroke, rehabilitation specialists need to have an understanding of how stroke may alter bowel function resulting in FI, diarrhea, and/or constipation. In addition to affecting speech and mobility, stroke can injure the cerebral areas responsible for bowel control. Ischemic stroke can result in secondary functional changes in the peripheral organs that communicate with the affected vascular areas of the brain (59).

Incontinence. People with stroke who experience UI often have problems with bowel irregularity including constipation, diarrhea, bowel impaction, and FI. Both UI and FI after stroke are frequently the result of immobility, decreased consciousness, and/or functional dependency rather than the impairment of neural pathways. FI in stroke is often temporary and may resolve, if the stroke survivor's recovery includes improved cognitive awareness and mobility (10).

Bowel problems in stroke patients often are not the result of one, but multiple issues. Needing help to use the toilet is one of the strongest predictors of FI after stroke. Poor mobility, impaired dexterity, changes in vision, decreased sensation, and communication can influence continence (60). Mobility and dexterity can be improved with physical and occupational therapy. The use of anticholintergic medications including antipsychotics, tricyclic antidepressants, oxybutynin, or antiemetics increase the risk of FI in stroke survivors by reducing contractility of smooth muscle of the gut by an antimuscarinic effect at acetylcholine receptor sites. In some cases, long-term use may induce chronic colonic dysmotility. As a comorbidity, stroke does not independently affect bowel continence in longer-term stroke survivors, but rather influences continence through associations with other clinical and functional factors. FI is not only a financial burden to caregivers and society, but also may cause the stroke survivor the additional cost of social isolation and dependence. The degree of disability is the most important factor causing FI in stroke, but using constipating drugs and functional difficulties with toileting strongly influence FI at three months post-stroke (49).

If incontinence is due to external factors such as medications or mobility, it can be managed through education and therapy. A randomized controlled trial of constipation and FI management showed that one year after a nursing intervention, subjects were more likely to alter their diet and fluid intake to control their bowels, and to receive different prescribed patterns of bowel agents. A single-encounter nurse-led intervention in stroke patients significantly improved measures of bowel dysfunction and changed bowel modifying lifestyle behavior. Findings promoted structured management of bowel problems in stroke patients and encouraged health education (48). In summary, FI is the involuntary evacuation of rectal contents and is most often caused by neuromuscular disorders or structural anorectal problems. FI may be aggravated by diarrhea or urgency, but their causes need to be identified separately (51).

Diarrhea. Diarrhea is defined as the passage of atypical liquid or unformed stool at rate of three or more bowel movements in 24 hours. Acute diarrhea lasts less than two weeks, persistent diarrhea lasts for longer than two weeks, and chronic diarrhea persists more than four weeks. When diarrhea occurs, it is harder for the anal sphincter to hold liquid stool, as compared to semi-solid state (62). Every 24 hours, the small intestine converts about 10 liters of fluid and digested food into 1.5–2 liters of ileal content. This volume is then converted into approximately 200 g of solid stool by fluid absorption in the colon. When the balance between the absorptive capacity in the intestine and its secretory function is disrupted, diarrhea occurs (63). Malnutrition, tube feedings, and debility put the stroke patient at risk for diarrhea.

Infectious agents cause more than 90% of acute diarrhea. The other 10% are caused by medications, toxic ingestions, and other conditions. Infections are transmitted through fecal-oral direct personal contact, or ingestion of food or water contaminated with pathogens. Diarrhea is one of the most common sources of nosocomial infections in hospitals and long-term care facilities. There are many microorganisms in the hospital setting. Currently, the most persistent microorganism is Clostridium difficile. Hospitalization predisposes stroke patients to nosocomial infections. Common outbreaks usually occur through food-borne epidemics, sharing toilets, or rooming with patients with infective diarrhea. Impaired cognition, decreased mobility, and functional ability contribute to decreased personal hygiene. Antibiotics disrupt the gut's normal flora and break down the colon's immunity. Side effects from drug therapy are the most common noninfectious cause of acute diarrhea, and can be easily determined by connecting the onset of symptoms with drug start date. In the stroke population, the most frequent diarrhea-causing drugs are antibiotics, cardiac antidysrhythmics, antihypertensives, nonsteroidal anti-inflammatories, antidepressants, antacids, and laxatives (63).

Constipation. According to the practice guidelines for the management of constipation published by the Rehabilitation Nursing Foundation, a proposed definition of constipation is "the passage of small amounts of hard, dry stool fewer than three times per week or a significant change in one's usual routine, accompanied by straining, and feelings of being bloated, or having abdominal fullness. Persistence of these symptoms for three months or longer is defined as chronic constipation" (53).

In the general population, the prevalence of constipation in North America is estimated to be between 2–27 %. Approximately 42 million people in the United States meet the defined criteria for functional constipation (53). Twice as many women as men complain of symptoms of constipation. It is more prevalent in the elderly (older than 65 years), non-whites, and individuals from lower socioeconomic or less educated groups. It is a serious problem in clinical practice, affecting up to 60% of those in stroke rehabilitation units (49, 63). Chronic constipation is associated with GI motility, sensory disorders including functional dyspepsia, heartburn, and gastroesophageal reflux disease (GERD). Twenty-nine percent of GERD patients also report functional constipation. Approximately 63 million people in North America meet the Rome II Criteria for constipation (64).

Constipation is linked to impairments of the central nervous system. In stroke, depending on the location of the lesion, weakness of the abdominal and pelvic muscles and hypomotility of the large bowel may occur (63). The rectum is bilaterally innervated on the motor cortex with asymmetric representation and unilateral dominance. It is uncertain if asymmetry accounts for difficulties in defecation after brain injury, or if unilateral pudendal nerve injury causes a disturbance of pelvic floor function (55). Lesions affecting the pontine defacatory center disrupt the sequencing of sympathetic and parasympathetic components of defecation, and impair the coordination of the peristaltic wave and relaxation of the pelvic floor and external sphincter. Drugs which contribute to constipation are diuretics, iron, antihypertensives, antipsychotics, anticholinergics, anticonvulsants, opioids, and ganglionic blockers (52, 63). Tricyclic antidepressants can cause constipation induced by blocking the reuptake of norepinephrine or serotonin. Antidepressants such as amitriptyline, as well as the selective serotonin reuptake inhibitors, affect visceral sensitivity and motility (47). Ninety-five percent of the patients on opioids are constipated. Verapamil, a calcium channel blocker, causes constipation by delaying GI transit time. Antacids that contain aluminum cause constipation due to the constricting agent. Diuretics causing fluid loss can constipate (52, 63).

In patients with ischemic stroke, colorectal dysfunction is caused by a combination of lesions of the central or peripheral nervous system, immobility, or altered dietary habits. Constipation in patients with stroke has been suggested to be disruption of the neuronal modulation of colonic motility. Colonic transit time is prolonged, especially in the right colon. The mechanism of intestinal pseudo-obstruction in stroke may be defective enteric neurons, smooth muscles, or both. The exact cause of constipation after stroke needs further study. Disruption to the modulation of colonic motility needs to be assessed. Because stroke is common in elderly patients, the aging affects of the GI tract need to be considered. GI changes with aging are very subtle (58, 59). In conclusion, ischemic stroke may disrupt neural control of GI motility by interrupting or altering the flow of information between the cortex and the GI system. Future research utilizing positron emission test scans and magnetic resonance imagining may be able to demonstrate a relationship between bowel dysfunction and stroke (59).

History. The first component of assessing bowel function is to obtain a history from the stroke survivor. Unfortunately, this may not always be possible secondary to cognitive or communication deficits. In these instances, the interviewer will need to rely on the family for information. In cases where the family is not present or unable to provide the necessary information, the nursing staff will need to be questioned.

Previous bowel habits. The assessment starts by obtaining information about the stroke survivor's previous bowel habits. Questions about previous bowel habits include: past problems with abdominal pain, bloating, discomfort, hemorrhoids, episodes of constipation, diarrhea or incontinence, frequency of occurrence, and use of medications for management. When asking questions about constipation or diarrhea, the interviewer should be specific. Often, misconceptions regarding normal bowel habits can interfere with obtaining accurate information. A

scale developed at the University of Bristol, the Stool Form Scale, can be used to help improve communication. The scale provides pictures and descriptions of different stool consistencies, so that the interviewer and stroke survivor are using the same terminology when discussing bowel habits. An incontinence problem that existed prior to the onset of stroke may make achieving continence more challenging.

Current bowel habits. Information regarding current bowel habits helps to contrast that of past bowel habits. Questions about current bowel habits include: the onset of FI; the number of incontinent and continent bowel movements; the consistency and size of the stool; the activity immediately preceding the incontinence; the ability to distinguish between passing of stool and gas; the presence of urgency, pain, or other symptoms; and the presence of blood in the stool. Changes in bowel habits may be due to stroke-related deficits, prolonged hospitalization, changes in diet, medications, or the development of a new medical problem.

Past medical history. The health care practitioner should obtain information about a previous history of small bowel obstruction, inflammatory bowel disease, malabsorption syndromes and treatment, GI surgery, trauma to the abdominal area, neurologic diseases that affect the central or peripheral nervous systems, diabetes that can effect gastric motility, antibiotic therapy, and urology problems. With male stroke survivors, the interviewer should ask about the presence of sexual dysfunction that may suggest impairment of pelvic floor innervation (65). With female stroke survivors, the interviewer should ask about the obstetrical history. In multiparous women, stretch injuries or lacerations of the pelvic floor are common causes of anorectal denervation and sphincter damage (65). All of these could likely contribute to FI after stroke.

Fluid and dietary intake. The examiner should determine the amounts, types, and timing of fluids consumed. Decreased fluid intake, or the intake of diuretic fluids, can increase the risk of constipation. Fluid intake should be spaced throughout the day to ensure adequate amounts are consumed. Stroke survivors drinking thickened liquids need to be encouraged to increase their fluid intake to prevent constipation. Inquiries about dietary intake should focus on the amount of dietary fiber consumed, potential dietary irritants, and food allergies. Fluid and oral caloric intake need to be monitored closely in stroke survivors on modified consistency diets or enteric feedings secondary to dysphagia. These individuals will have the same incontinence problems, but present a bigger challenge because of their swallowing impairment.

Medication review. In the hospitalized stroke survivor, it is much easier to monitor the medications he or she is taking, since rarely does one take anything other than that prescribed by the physician or administered by the nursing staff. In the stroke survivor who is at home, it is important to find out not only what prescription medications the person is taking, but also any over-the-counter medications, vitamins, and herbal supplements being taken. Not only can certain medications affect stool consistency and gastrointestinal motility, but also medications can affect a person's level of alertness, balance, or coordination, which can contribute to incontinence.

Functional status. Functional assessments performed by the rehabilitation team in all areas of mobility and activities of daily living are a necessary part of the bowel function assessment. Knowledge of the stroke survivor's cognitive status determines whether the person can identify the need to have a bowel movement and act upon it. It is important to know about the survivor's communication status. Aphasia or dysarthria may make it difficult for the survivor to communicate his or her needs for toileting. Sensory perceptual deficits may make it difficult to identify the bathroom, or to know what to do or where to go once in the bathroom. Visual deficits may make finding the bathroom difficult. Mobility or balance deficits will make it difficult to get to the bathroom, manage clothing, transfer to the toilet, and manage hygiene. If the environment is not wheelchair accessible, or if appropriate equipment is not available, establishing an effective program will be more difficult. For those stroke survivors who are home, it will be necessary to assess the environment and equipment available to assist with toileting.

Bowel diary. In cases where the stroke survivor is unable to provide information to the interviewer about current or previous bowel habits, it may be necessary to keep a bowel diary. The diary is a document that will provide the interviewer with information about current bowel function. Any rehabilitation treatment team member can develop a form to obtain the necessary information. The team or family member completing the diary should record fluid intake and timing, continent and incontinent bowel movements and timing, and consistency of stools. The diary can also assist the rehabilitation professional with documentation once a program has been put into effect.

Physical Examination   The next component of the assessment is the physical examination. The examiner always should explain to the stroke survivor what is to occur throughout the assessment. The first part of the physical examination begins with a visual inspection of the abdomen. The examiner should observe for surgical scars that might indicate past gastrointestinal surgery, or an enlarged, protuberant abdomen that may suggest gas, tumor, pregnancy, or fluid collection. The examiner then auscultates for bowel sounds. Hypoactive bowel sounds could be a sign of constipation, impaction, obstruction, paralytic ileus, or peritonitis. Hyperactive bowel sounds could be a sign of diarrhea or intestinal obstruction. The examiner then palpates the abdomen, assessing for tenderness, masses, and enlarged organs.

After examination of the abdomen, the stroke survivor should be asked or assisted to turn to his or her left side. The next portion of the physical examination is assessment of the anus and rectum. Using two hands, the examiner gently spreads the buttocks, looking for the presence of stool, hemorrhoids, fissures, skin breakdown, bulging, or gaping of the anal opening. These findings are suggestive of sphincter weakness and could help identify the potential cause of incontinence (44). Using a cotton-tip applicator, the examiner gently strokes the perianal area on either side of the anus. This should elicit a contraction of the external sphincter called the *anal wink.* The cotton-tip applicator can also be used to assess perianal sensation. The examiner then asks the stroke survivor to bear down gently, while looking for a bulging of the anus. A small amount of bulging is normal, but a large bulge, loss of stool, or organ prolapse is not. The examiner is now ready to perform a digital rectal examination. Using a lubricated, gloved index finger, the examiner gently checks the rectal vault for the presence of stool. At the same time, the examiner assesses anal tone. The examiner asks the stroke survivor to tighten the external sphincter around the gloved finger assessing for tone. The sphincter should tighten evenly around the gloved finger. Loss of rectal tone suggests that a significant neurologic problem is present.

Diagnostic Tests   There will be instances when some stroke survivors will require diagnostic testing. Diagnostic testing can provide additional information that will assist the healthcare practitioner determine the potential cause of FI. In stroke survivors with hypoactive bowel sounds, abdominal distention, or oozing of liquid stool upon examination, or the exact date of the last bowel movement is unknown, a simple abdominal radiograph can identify the presence of stool or impaction in the gastrointestinal tract. In the stroke survivor with hyperactive bowel sounds, abdominal discomfort, and large amounts of liquid stool, a stool culture can be obtained to rule out infection. Checking stool for occult blood also can help to rule out GI bleeding as a cause of incontinence or diarrhea.

Other diagnostic tests are available, but these are not performed frequently as part of an assessment. When there is a history of previous GI problems, neurologic complications, or the assessment does not help identify a problem, the stroke survivor should be referred to a gastroenterologist for further testing. Additional testing may include upper or lower GI tract endoscopy, balloon expulsion testing, anorectal manometry, colonic transit testing, endoanal ultrasound and magnetic resonance imaging, and defecography (66).

Treatment

The management of FI after stroke often is easier to address than UI. Depending upon the problem, stool may need to be softened for easier passage, or bulked up to increase sensory input. A regular toileting schedule may need to be devised. A combination of methods may need to be implemented. It is important to be realistic when establishing goals for the stroke survivor. It may take several months to achieve 100% continence. Initially, the goal may be to decrease the frequency of incontinence, or simply to regulate the individual with a program.

Nonpharmacologic Treatment. *Diet.* Increasing the fiber content in a diet can add bulk to stool to help increase size and improve rectal sensation. Fiber taken appropriately also can prevent constipation. Fibrous foods are poorly digested and remain in the lumen of the GI tract. They help form viscous, gel-like substances (53). The American Dietetics Association recommends 20–35 grams of fiber per day to maintain normal bowel function (67). This amount should be built up slowly in those who do not normally consume this amount of fiber, to prevent abdominal cramping. In those individuals who cannot ingest that amount of fiber in their diet, supplemental fiber can be used. Various supplements and recipes of bran, prune juice, and applesauce can help to increase dietary fiber intake (68). Bran, psyllium, guar gum ,and fiber concentrates also can be purchased to increase fiber intakes.

Fluids. The intake of fluid is very closely related to dietary intake. While increased fiber intake is effective in managing constipation, diarrhea, and FI in stroke survivors, an insufficient intake of fluids or fiber can actually be more harmful than beneficial. The American Dietetic Association recommends that the average person take in 2 liters of liquid or 10–12 glasses of fluids per day. The type of fluid should also be carefully monitored. The stroke survivor should avoid caffeinated and alcoholic fluids. These fluids are diuretics, and can worsen dehydration. In situations when the stroke survivor has an elevated temperature, diarrhea, and vomiting, fluid intake should be increased. Hot or warmed fluids help promote peristalsis and can be used to assist in achieving continence.

Activity/exercise. While research has been inconclusive regarding the effects of exercise and activity on bowel function, many health care practitioners will agree that remaining active helps improve appetite, shortens food transit time through the GI tract, and improves bowel function (53, 68). In those who have just suffered a stroke, activity and mobility is severely impaired. Participation in a rehabilitation program will help improve activity. Any activity that helps with re-establishing muscle tone can help return bowel function (43). Walking, leg lifts, stationary bicycling, turning in bed, hip lifts, or a home program are just some examples of exercises that have been tested, but none has been found to be more effective than another (53).

Positioning is also an important part of bowel function. As soon as the stroke survivor can tolerate it, sitting at 90 degrees will help gravity empty the rectal vault and decrease the risk of incontinence. The use of raised toilet seats or bedside commode chairs helps to improve compliance. Bedpans should be avoided whenever possible because gravity will not assist in emptying, and because of the increased risk of skin breakdown. In those with poor muscle tone, the use of a step stool under the stroke survivor's feet can help promote emptying. A squat position with the knees slightly higher than the hips improves the passage of stool by increasing abdominal pressure (43). If the person has sufficient trunk control, bending at the waist also can help increase abdominal pressure. Abdominal massage from right to left also can assist with emptying (68). The Valsalva maneuver or bearing down should be avoided in any stroke survivor with an unstable cardiac history.

Timing/privacy. A regular toileting schedule should be established to help decrease FI in the stroke survivor. When setting up a program in the hospital or for the home, the stroke survivor's schedule should be considered. Toileting after meals can help use the gastrocolic reflex to the survivor's advantage. Initially, the stroke survivor may need toileting after every meal, but morning toileting programs have been found to be more effective (69). The stroke survivor should also be provided with plenty of time and privacy for appropriate evacuation. If the person is rushed while having a bowel movement, inadequate emptying may occur. Over time, this can lead to constipation and impaction. Privacy should also be provided to avoid embarrassing odors or sounds. If the stroke survivor anticipates embarrassment from odors or sounds that could be made during toileting, the defecation reflex may be extinguished, which can lead to or worsen constipation or FI over time.

Education. In order for a program to remain effective, it is necessary that methods implemented are carried over by the stroke survivor. The individual should be taught about the importance of maintaining nonpharmacologic treatment methods in order to prevent constipation, diarrhea, or FI. Misconceptions regarding bowel habits should also be corrected. The stroke survivor should be educated on how to make changes to his or her program when ill, or as bowel habits change over time. Rehabilitation staff should be educated on how to explain the purpose of programs to stroke survivors and their families. Often stroke survivors and families do not understand the purpose of rectal medications and toileting programs to regulate the frequency of incontinent bowel movements. Education will help improve compliance and encourage family assistance. When the date of the last bowel movement is unknown, it will be difficult to establish if the stroke survivor is truly incontinent, or simply impacted. It will be necessary to give a rectal or oral laxative to "clean out" the stool before establishing a program. Stroke survivors and families should be made aware of this to prevent misunderstanding on the use of laxatives. The treatment team should be educated on the need to work together to ease the burden of care of a program. Physical therapists can help train staff and families to ease the effort needed for toilet transfers. Equipment should be issued to the stroke survivor that will improve toileting. Occupational therapists can help families or staff identify appropriate clothing to make management and hygiene less difficult. Speech language pathologists can work with staff and families on developing a communication system that will notify them when the stroke survivor feels the need to use the bathroom. Nursing staff can ensure a program is in place and can monitor the need for changes based on results.

Pharmacologic Treatment.   There will be cases when non-pharmacologic treatment alone is not effective in achieving continence. It will be necessary to combine nonpharmacologic and pharmacologic treatment in order to improve continence. When selecting a medication for the stroke survivor, careful attention should be paid to medical history, ease of administration, and availability of a caregiver. Those stroke survivors who use pharmacologic treatment should be monitored closely by a healthcare practitioner to ensure that the individual does not develop long-term problems.

Bulk forming/hydrophilic laxatives. This category of medications softens stool by increasing water content. This increases the frequency of stools. The site of action is the small and large intestine. As mentioned earlier, it is necessary that the stroke survivor should drink at least one eight ounce glass with each dose of medication. The onset of action can be as little as twelve hours, or up to three days. The most common side effect is abdominal bloating. Bulk forming agents should be avoided in those individuals with esophageal narrowing, intestinal adhesions, ulcers, or bowel stenosis (70). Several studies have used bulk forming agents to manage constipation or decrease fecal incontinence in stroke survivors (48, 71). Examples include psyllium, methylcellulose, and calcium polycarbophil.

Stool softeners/lubricant laxatives. This category of medications decreases the surface tension of stool by adding water and fatty substances. This medication does not induce defecation; it simply softens stool, making it easier to pass. The site of action is the small and large intestine. The onset of action is as little as six to eight hours, and can take up to three days (70). The most common side effect is loose stool that ceases when the medication is discontinued. Examples include docusate sodium, docusate calcium, and mineral oil. Tramonte, et al. cited multiple studies that used stool softeners and found them to be very effective in increasing the frequency of stools (71).

Stimulant laxatives. This category of medications alters water and electrolyte balance, thereby stimulating intestinal motor function. The site of action is the mesenteric plexus. This category of medications includes rectal and oral forms. The onset of action in the rectal forms is 15–60 minutes. The onset of action in the oral forms is six to twelve hours. The most common side effect is abdominal cramping. This category of medication is not recommended for long-term use (53). Examples include senna, bisacodyl, and cascara.

Hyperosmotic laxatives. This category of medications increases intraluminal pressure by increasing water content, thereby stimulating peristalsis. The site of action is the small and large intestine. This category of medications can be found in oral or rectal forms. The onset of action of the oral form is one to two days. The onset of action of the rectal form is 30–60 minutes. There are minimal side effects with the rectal preparations, but the oral preparations can cause abdominal cramps, diarrhea, and electrolyte imbalances. Examples include sorbitol, lactulose, sodium biphosphonate, and polyethylene glycol. Tramonte, et al. reviewed three studies that found an increase in bowel movement frequency and improvement in stool consistency when lactulose is used in long-term care and outpatient settings (71).

Research Frontiers

Future research needs to focus specifically on the management of fecal incontinence. There has been a great deal of work done on the management of constipation, but little on its management specifically after stroke. While many textbooks outline how to set up a bowel program, only Venn et al. (1992) (69) and Harari et al. (2004) (48) analyzed the use of nonpharmacologic and pharmacologic management and the effectiveness of bowel training. Even these authors recommended larger and longer longitudinal studies of patients who have effective bowel habits after discharge from rehabilitation. Traditionally, rehabilitation hospitals utilize rectal suppositories for the regulation of incontinent bowel movements, but this can be very distressing for the survivor and difficult for the family to understand. Research should also address the effectiveness of suppositories versus toileting programs, and whether stroke survivors achieve continence sooner with either or a combination of both interventions.

References

1. Kong KH, Chan KF, Lim AC, Tan ES. Detrusor hyperreflexia in stroke. *Ann Acad Med Singapore* 2004; 23(3):319–321.
2. Jorgensen L, Engstad T, Jacobsen BK. Self-reported urinary incontinence in noninstitutionalized long-term stroke survivors: A population-based study. *Arch Phys Med Rehabi*.2005; 86:416–420.
3. Patel M, Coshall C, Rudd AG, Wolfe CDA. Natural history and effects on 2-year outcomes of urinary incontinence after stroke. *Stroke* 2001; 32:122–127.
4. Dumoulin C, Korner-Bitensky N, Tannenbaum C. Urinary incontinence after stroke: Does rehabilitation make a difference? A systematic review of the effectiveness of behavioral therapy. *Top Stroke Rehabil* 2005; 12(3):66–76.
5. Nakayama H, Jorgensen HS, Pedersen PM, Raaschou, HO, Olsen TS. Prevalence and risk factors of incontinence after stroke: The Copenhagen stroke study. *Stroke* 1997; 28:58–62.
6. Brittain KR, Peet SM, Potter JF, Castleden CM. Prevalence and management of urinary incontinence in stroke survivors. *Age Aging* 1999; 28:509–511.

7. Brittain KR, Peet SM, Castleden CM. Stroke and incontinence. *Stroke* 1998; 29:524–528.

8. Borrie MJ, Campbell AJ, Caradoc-Davies TH, Spears GF. Urinary incontinence after stroke: A prospective study. *Age Aging* 1986; 15:177–181.

9. Ween JE, Alexander MP, D'Esposito M, Roberts M. Incontinence after stroke in a rehabilitation setting: Outcomes associations and predictive factors. *Neurology* 1996; 47:659–663.

10. Brocklehurst JC, Andrews K, Richards B, Laycock PJ. Incidence and correlates of incontinence in stroke patients. *J Amer Geriatr Soc* 1985; 33:540–542.

11. Brittain KR, Perry SI, Peet SM, et al. Prevalence and impact of urinary symptoms among community-dwelling stroke survivors. *Stroke* 1999; 31:886–898.

12. Wade DT, Hewer RL. Outlook after an acute stroke: Urinary incontinence and loss of consciousness compared in 532 patients. *Q J Med* 1985; 56(221):601–608.

13. Jongbloed L. Prediction of function after stroke: A critical review. *Stroke* 1986; 17(4):765–776.

14. Gelber DA, Good DC, Laven LJ, Verhulst SJ. Causes of urinary incontinence after acute hemispheric stroke. *Stroke* 1993; 24:378–382.

15. Owen DC, Getz PA, Bulla SA. Comparison of characteristics of patients with completed stroke: Those who achieve continence and those who do not. *Rehabil Nurs* 1995; 20(4):197–203.

16. Gross JC. Urinary incontinence and stroke outcomes. *Arch Phys Med Rehabil* 2000; 81:22–27.

17. VanKujik AA, van der Linde H,van Limbeek J. Urinary incontinence in stroke patients after admission to a postacute inpatient rehabilitation program. *Arch Phys Med Rehabil* 2001; 82:1407–1411.

18. Delancey J, Grosling J, Creed K, et al. Gross anatomy and cell biology of the lower urinary tract. In Abrahams P, Cardozo L, Khoury S, Wein A, eds. *Incontinence*. United Kingdom: Health Publications, Ltd., 2002:19–82.

19. Morrison J, Steers WD, Brading A, et al. Neurophysiology and neuropharmacology. In Abrams P, Khoury S, Wein A, eds. *Incontinence*. United Kingdom: Health Publications, Ltd., 2002:85–163.

20. Sugaya, K, DeGroat WC. Micturition reflexes in the in vitro neonatal rat brain stem-spinal cord-bladder preparation. *Am J Physiolog* 2004; 266:R658.

21. Andersson K-E, Arner A. Urinary bladder contraction and relaxation: Physiology and pathophysiology. *Physiol Rev* 2004; 84:935–986.

22. Wein AJ. Neuromuscular dysfunction of the lower urinary tract and its management. In Walsh PC, ed. *Campbell's Urology*, 8th ed. Philadelphia, Pa: Saunders, 2002:934–1025.

23. Staskin, DR. Intracranial lesions that affect lower urinary tract function. In Krane RJ, Siroky ME, eds. *Clinical Neuro-urology*. Boston: Little Brown, 1990:345–351.

24. Burney TL, Senapati M, Desai S, Choudhary ST, Badlani GH. Effects of cerebrovascular accident on micturition. *Urologic Clinics of North America* 1996; 23(3): 483–490.

25. Kong KH, Young S. Incidence and outcome of poststroke urinary retention: A prospective study. *Archives of Physical Medicine and Rehabilitation* 2000; 81:1464–1467.

26. Burney TL, Senapati M, Desai S, Choudhary ST, Badlani GH. Acute cerebrovascular accident and lower urinary tract dysfunction: A prospective correlation of the site of brain injury with urodynamic findings. *The Journal of Urology* 1996; 156(3): 1748–1750.

27. Nitti VW, Adler H, Combs AJ. The role of urodynamics in the evaluation of voiding dysfunction in men after cerebrovascular accident. *The Journal of Urology* 1995; 155:663–266.

28. Tsuchida S, Noto H, Yamaguchi O, Itoh M. Urodynamic studies on hemiplegic patients after cerebrovascular accident. *Urology* 1983; 21:315–320.

29. Khan Z, Starer P, Yang WC, Bhola A. Analysis of voiding disorders in patients with cerebrovascular accidents. *Urology* 1990; 35(3):265–270.

30. Sakakibara R, Hattori T, Yasuda K, Yamanishi T. Micturitional disturbance after acute hemispheric stroke: Analysis of the lesion site by CT and MRI. *Journal of the Neurological Sciences* 1996; 137:47–56.

31. Weld KJ, Dmochowski RR. Effect of bladder management on urological complications in spinal cord injured patients. *J Urol* 2000; 63:768–772.

32. Fowler, CJ. Neurologic disorders of micturition and their treatment. *Brain* 1999; 122:1213–1231.

33. Tibaek S, Gard G, Jensen R. Pelvic floor muscle training is effective in women with urinary incontinence after stroke: A randomized, controlled and blinded study. *Neurourol Urodyn* 2005; 56:232–236.

34. Sahai A, Khan MS, Arya M, John J, Singh, R, Patel HR. The overactive bladder: Review of current pharmacotherapy in adults. Part 1: Pathophysiology and anticholinergic therapy. *Expert Opin Pharmacother* 2006; 7:509–527.

35. Burgio KL, Locher JL, Goode PS. Combined behavioral and drug therapy for urge incontinence in older women. *J Am Geriatr Soc* 2000; 48:370–374.

36. Leng WW, Morrisroe SN. Sacral nerve stimulation for the overactive bladder. *Urologic Clinic NA* 2006; 33:491–506.

37. Brazzelli M, Murray A, Fraser C. Efficacy and safety of sacral nerve stimulation for urinary urge incontinence: A systematic review. *J Urol* 2006; 175:835–841.

38. Kuo HC. Therapeutic effects of suburothelial injection of botulinum A toxin for neurogenic detrusor overactivity due to chronic cerebrovascular accident and spinal cord lesions. *Urology* 2006; 56:232–236.

39. Schurch B, Schmid DM, Stohrer M. Treatment of neurogenic incontinence with botulinum toxin A. *N Engl J Med* 2000; 342:665.

40. Rapp DE, Lucioni A, Katx EE, O'Connor RC, Gerber GS, Bales GT. Use of botulinum-A toxin for the treatment of refractory overactive bladder symptoms: An initial experience. *Urology* 2004; 63:1071–1075.

41. Popat R, Apostolidis A, Kalsi V, Gonzalez G, Fowler CJ, Dasgupta P. A comparison between the response of patients with idiopathic detrusor overactivity and neurogenic detrusor overactivity to the first intradetrusor injection of botulinum-A toxin. *J Urol* 2005; 174:984–989.

42. Nelson RL. Epidemiology of fecal incontinence. *Gastroenterology* 2004; 126: S3–S7105.

43. Gender AR. Bowel regulation and elimination. In Hoeman SP, ed. *Rehabilitation Nursing Process and Application*. 2nd ed. St Louis, Mo: Mosby, 2006:452–475.

44. Rao SSC. Diagnosis and management of fecal incontinence. *American Journal of Gastroenterology* 2004; 1585–1804.

45. Chandler BJ. Continence and stroke. In: Barnes MP, Dobkin BH, Bogousslavsky J, eds. *Recovery after Stroke*. Cambridge, Ma: Cambridge University Press,2005: 415–435.

46. Nelson RL, Norton N, Cautley E, Furner, S. Community-based prevalence of anal incontinence. *JAMA* 1995; 274:559–561.

47. Quander CR, Morris MC, Melson J, Bienias JL, Evans DA. Prevalence of and factors associated with fecal incontinence in a large community study of older individuals. *Am J Gastroenterol* 2005; 100:905–909.

48. Harari D, Norton C, Lockwood L, Swift C. Treatment of constipation and fecal incontinence in stroke patients: Randomized controlled trial. *Stroke* 2004; 35:2549–2555.

49. Harari D, Coshall C, Rudd AG, Wolfe C. New-onset fecal incontinence after stroke prevalence, natural history risk factors and impact. *Stroke* 2003; 34:144–150.

50. Baztan JJ, Domenech JR, Gonzalez M. New onset fecal incontinence after stroke: Risk factor or consequences of poor outcomes after rehabilitation? *Stroke* 2003; 34:101–102.

51. Harrison's Internal Medicine. Disorders of the gastrointestinal system. McGraw-Hill's *Access Medicine*: http: //www.accessmedicine.com/ Accessed November 15, 2006.

52. Winge K, Rasmussen D, Werdelin LM. Constipation in neurological diseases. *J Neurol Neurosurg Psychiatry* 2003; 74:13–19.

53. Folden SL, Backer JM, Maynard F, et al. RNF practice guidelines for the management of constipation in adults. *Rehabilitation Nursing Foundation* 2002; Available at: http:// www.rehabnurse.org.

54. Weisbrodt NW. Motility of the large intestine. In: Johnson LR, ed. *Gastrointestinal Physiology*. 6th ed, St. Louis, Mo: Mosby, Inc.,2001:57–63.

55. Thompson DG. Neurogastroenterology: Imaging of the sensory and motor control of the GI tract. *Journal of Psychosomatic Research* 2006; 61:301–304.

56. Guyton AC. Regulation of gastrointestinal function, food intake, micturition, and body temperature. In: *Basic Neuroscience Anatomy and Physiology*. 2nd ed, Philadelphia, Pa: WB Saunders Co, 1991:348–364.

57. Prather CM, Ortiz-Camacho CP. Evaluation and treatment of constipation and fecal impaction in adults. *Mayo Clinic Proceedings* 1998; 881–887.

58. Krogh, K, Christensen P, Laurberg S. Colorectal symptoms in patients with neurological diseases. *Acta Neurol Scand* 2001; 103:335–343.

59. Schaller BJ, Graf R, Jacobs AH. Pathophysiological changes of the gastrointestinal tract in ischemic stroke. *American Journal of Gastroenterology* 2006; 101:1655–1665.

60. Barret JA, Akpan A. Fecal incontinence and constipation. British geriatrics society special approval article. *Geriatric Medicine* 2004; 6(3):99–108.

61. Bliss DZ, Norton CA, Miller J, Krissovich M. Directions for future nursing research on fecal incontinence. *Nursing Research* 2004; 53(6s):S15–S21.

62. Ahlquist Da Camilleri M . Diarrhea and Constipation. Ch35. In: *Harrison's Internal Medicine*. Available at: http://www.accessmedicine.com/ Accessed November 14, 2006.

63. Ratnaike RN. Constipation. In: *Practical Guide to Geriatric Medicine*. Roseville, Australia: McGraw-Hill;:505–519.

64. Brandt LJ, Prather CM, Quigley EM, Schiller LR, Shoenfeld P, Talley NJ. Systematic review on the management of chronic constipation in North America. *The American Journal of Gastroenterology* 2005; 100 (S1):s5–21.

65. MacLeod JH. Assessment of patients with fecal incontinence. In Doughty DB, ed. *Urinary and Fecal Incontinence: Nursing Management*. St. Louis, Mo: Mosby Year Book,1991:203–223.

66. Rogers RG, Abed H, Fenner DE. Current diagnosis and treatment algorithms for anal incontinence. *British Journal of Urology* 2006; 98(1):97–106.

67. American Dietetic Association. Position of the American Dietetic Association: Health implications of dietary fiber. *Journal of the American Dietetic Association* 2002; 102(7):993–1000.

68. Weeks SK, Hubbartt E, Michaels TK. Keys to bowel success. *Rehabilitation Nursing* 2000; 25(2):66–69.

69. Venn MR, Taft L, Carpentier B, Applebaugh G. The influence of timing and suppository use on efficiency and effectiveness of bowel training after stroke. *Rehabilitation Nursing* 1992; 17(3):116–120.

70. Lehman CA, Charles CV. Constipation management update. *Association of Rehabilitation Nurses Network Newsletter* 2005; 3–4.

71. Tramonte SM, Brand MB, Mulrow CD, Arnato MG, O'Keefe, ME, Ramirex G. The treatment of chronic constipation in adults: A systematic review. *Journal of General Internal Medicine* 1996; 12:15–24.

VI

OTHER REHABILITATION THERAPEUTICS

31 Orthotic Management in Stroke

Stefania Fatone

he word "orthosis" is derived from the Greek word *orthos*, meaning "to make straight." The International Standards Organization (ISO 8549-1, 1989) defines an orthosis or orthotic device as "an externally applied device used to modify the structural or functional characteristics of the neuro-musculo-skeletal system." The standardized nomenclature for orthoses is based on the principal joint or joints the orthosis encompasses. For example, an Ankle-Foot Orthosis (AFO) physically encompasses the ankle and foot and provides control principally at the ankle, whereas a Wrist-Hand Orthosis (WHO) encompasses the wrist and hand and provides control principally at the wrist. Often, orthoses are further described based on the control exerted on the joints they encompass. For example, a plantar flexion stop AFO or dorsiflexion assist AFO. Orthoses may allow free motion, resist or assist motion, stop motion, or provide an adjustable hold or lock (1). The basic functional goals of orthoses are to provide support, correct deformity, or modify motion occurring at a joint, either assisting motion where it is insufficient or substituting motion where it is absent. Overall, it is intended that orthoses aid function.

Generally, orthoses are designed based on biomechanical principles, working primarily through the application of force systems to relieve unwanted forces or moments from the body. However, the amount of force applied by orthoses is limited by tissue tolerances so as not to cause tissue injury (1). Orthoses affect normal movements by applying selective forces in relatively limited directions (1). Control of joint motion is generally achieved through the application of one or more three-point force systems, consisting of two counter (stabilizing) forces and one active (corrective) force applied proximally and distally to a joint to produce angular change in a specific plane (Figure 31-1). Generally, the more complex the impairment, the more three-point force systems are incorporated into the orthosis design. Orthoses may act directly or indirectly: an orthosis is acting *directly* if it surrounds the segment or joint it is attempting to influence, and *indirectly* if it attempts to modify the external forces acting on a joint beyond its physical boundaries (2). For example, during the stance phase of gait, an AFO acts directly on the ankle but indirectly on the knee by influencing the moments acting at the knee (Figure 31-2). Indirect action of the AFO at the knee is predicated on the closed kinetic chain occurring during stance phase, and hence is not applicable during swing phase.

With respect to neurologic conditions such as stroke, orthoses may also incorporate design modifications based on neurophysiologic principles. These principles are derived from neurodevelopmental therapies such as those developed by Bobath (3), and used in inhibitive

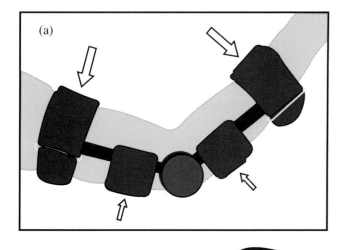

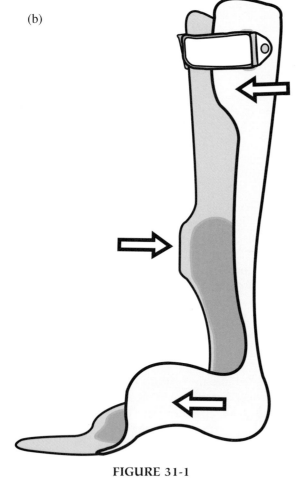

FIGURE 31-1

Two examples of three-point force systems used in orthoses for the hemiplegic limb: **(a)** static progressive contracture management of an elbow flexion contracture with stabilizing forces at each end of the orthosis and the net corrective force acting immediately proximal and distal to the posterior elbow; and **(b)** control of ankle inversion in spastic hemiparesis using an AFO with stabilizing forces acting on the medial arch and medial proximal calf, and the corrective force acting through a flange on the lateral distal tibia. Arrows indicate the application of forces.

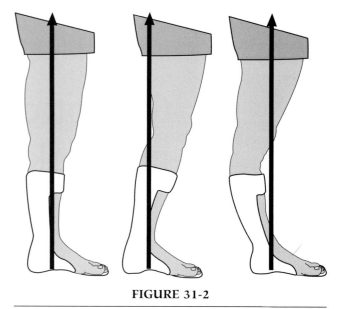

FIGURE 31-2

Indirect action of a non-articulated, rigid ankle-foot orthosis (AFO) on the knee during single limb stance: **(a)** AFO set at 90 degrees; **(b)** AFO set in 5 degrees dorsiflexion; and **(c)** AFO set in 5 degrees plantar flexion. Note the vertical ground reaction force vector (arrow), which is indicative of the external knee moment.

casting. Orthoses designed using neurophysiologic principles attempt to use sensory feedback (e.g., inhibition of reflexes, pressure over muscle insertions, active and static prolonged stretch, and orthokinetics—the physical effect of materials placed over muscle bellies) to decrease tone and improve isolated motor control, in particular facilitating movement patterns associated with decreased tone, while inhibiting movement patterns associated with increased tone (1, 4). Neurophysiologic devices tend to be considered "dynamic," as they typically allow greater freedom of movement than orthotic devices based on conventional biomechanical principles intended for use in the same given situation (1). Tone reducing modifications are commonly found in the foot-plate of lower limb orthoses or the palm area of upper limb orthoses. Table 31-1 describes some tone reducing modifications and their related reflexes. While there is some evidence to support the biomechanical effects of orthoses on joint motion and alignment (5, 6), there is little evidence to support the neurophysiologic effects of orthoses on tone and spasticity (4).

Orthotic management of the lower limb in stroke is intended to facilitate function, primarily the ability to stand and walk as safely and efficiently as possible. In the upper limb, orthotic management is intended mainly to avoid the development of orthopedic complications due to muscle weakness and abnormal tone (7).

Use of orthoses should be considered as part of an overall management plan during both the acute and chronic stages of stroke rehabilitation (8–10). Furthermore, since

TABLE 31-1
Tone Reducing Modifications and Their Related Reflexes (4, 63)

REFLEX	REFLEX FACILITATION	ORTHOTIC MODIFICATION
Toe (or plantar) grasp reflex	Stimulation or pressure over the ball of the foot results in toe flexion/clawing and ankle plantar flexion.	Eliminate stimulus of toe grasping reflex by bringing the orthosis foot-plate past the metatarsal heads and slightly extending the toes (approximately 20 degrees) (50) to decrease the potential development of equinus. Other AFO design features include spastic inhibitor bar (or toe crest), foam toe spreader/separators, and metatarsal arch supports to relieve weight from metatarsal heads.
Inversion reflex	Stimulation or pressure over the first metatarsal head and medial border of foot results in inversion of the foot.	Where there is a tendency toward inversion and/or varus, stimulate the antagonist (i.e., eversion) reflex to balance deformity by extending metatarsal pad of the foot to the lateral border.
Eversion reflex	Stimulation over the fifth metatarsal head and lateral border of foot results in eversion of the foot.	Where there is valgus of the hind foot and eversion of the forefoot, stimulate the antagonist (i.e., inversion) reflex to balance deformity by extending metatarsal pad of the foot to the medial border.
Dorsiflexion reflex	Stimulation of the central surface of the heel results in dorsiflexion of the foot.	Internal heel may serve to relieve weight from the ball of the foot and increase dorsiflexion, thus decreasing equinus tendency.
Palmar (flexion or grasp) reflex	Stimulation of palm results in flexion of the fingers and wrist.	Abduct fingers and avoid palm contact to decrease palmar reflex.

stroke recovery is a dynamic process, the use of orthoses should be intermittently reassessed in order to keep pace with the individual's changing abilities. Generally, the primary goal of orthoses during the acute phase is to maintain range of motion and prevent joint contractures that may interfere with eventual functional outcome. Prefabricated orthoses may be used initially during the acute phase as an interim measure while changes are occurring and a definitive prescription is unclear, or until a definitive, custom orthosis is ready. Adjustable orthoses are often preferred during the acute phase, because they can keep pace with the changes occurring with functional return. Individuals who demonstrate long-term need for orthotic treatment should receive custom orthoses to provide the necessary degrees of control, correction, and comfort, and have the highest degree of compliance in use (9, 10). Currently, there is no experimental evidence available regarding optimum timing of orthotic management (8). Hence, we do not know yet whether early orthotic management is superior to waiting until most natural recovery has occurred before making a decision about orthotic management (1). Determining the timing and magnitude of orthotic intervention is important, since over-bracing may prevent or delay the recovery of motor patterns, while under-bracing may lead to the development of undesirable deformities, compensatory movements and postures (11).

For orthoses to be successfully used in the management of stroke, they must be safe, and there must be realistic outcome expectations and appropriate follow-up to ensure proper fit and function. There must be adequate strength and stability of the orthosis to ensure that anatomical joints are protected from unnecessary damage. Orthoses must also minimize the pressure and friction applied to skin and bony prominences by careful fitting and padding. Furthermore, the axes of mechanical joints must be aligned with that of anatomic joints in order to avoid undesirable torques and motion between the orthosis and body (12, 13). It is also important to realize that most individuals require a period of adjustment or training when receiving an orthosis to achieve maximum benefit (1).

The objective of this chapter is to provide an overview of current practice in the orthotic management of stroke for both upper and lower limbs, describing different orthotic treatments, when and why they are provided, and how they work.

ORTHOTIC MANAGEMENT OF THE UPPER LIMB

Orthoses play a role in preventing or correcting upper extremity deformities in stroke that result from limited range of motion (14). After stroke, range of motion may be limited by, among other things, immobilization, paresis, increased muscle tone or spasticity, and myostatic contracture (14). Development of contracture is common in the hemiplegic limb, due to the presence of spasticity and abnormal muscle tone that is inherently resistant to passive stretch (15). Most commonly, the presence of spasticity after the onset of stoke prevents adequate range of motion and, if left untreated, leads to deformity. Although orthoses can be used to prevent deformity, it is often important to treat the underlying spasticity when it is severe, in order to use an orthotic device safely to effectively position the limb. Such treatments may include pharmacologic intervention, serial casting, and surgery, either in isolation or combination. If spasticity is not controlled, the forces required within the cast or orthosis to position the limb may be so great as to cause tissue breakdown. Where spasticity remains, orthoses may need to completely encompass the limb in order to adequately control position while minimizing the risk of skin breakdown (14).

Paresis following stroke can also contribute to the development of various abnormalities and deformities, especially when coupled with spasticity. Subluxation of the glenohumeral joint is common after stroke, with a reported incidence of 81–85% in individuals with spasticity following stroke, and may result in pain and decreased function (16, 17). Although shoulder pain is also very common in the hemiplegic upper limb, with a reported incidence of 38–84% of individuals with stroke, studies have been unable to establish a direct cause and effect relationship between shoulder pain and glenohumeral

subluxation (16–21). Despite a lack of evidence regarding whether shoulder subluxation is the primary cause of pain in individuals with stroke (7, 15), devices such as slings and wheelchair attachments may be prescribed to prevent subluxation and pain. Unfortunately, some of these devices also markedly restrict shoulder motion, which may diminish function and compromise hygiene. Furthermore, there is insufficient evidence to conclude whether devices such as slings and wheelchair attachments prevent subluxation, decrease pain, increase function, or adversely increase contracture in the shoulder after stroke (22).

Paresis, disuse, and poor positioning of the upper limb may also result in painful edema of the hand. Where possible, the arm is elevated at or above heart level to assist with venous return. In a wheelchair- or bed-bound individual, pillows or foam wedges placed on a lap board can be used to elevate the arm. In ambulatory individuals, compression gloves may be used to control edema of the hand and wrist. A sling may also be used to support the arm in a position that limits development of edema. However, slings also immobilize the arm and, depending on design, increase flexor tone (7) (Figure 31-3).

At the elbow, flexor spasticity and contracture are common and often severe. Flexion contractures are painful, and can lead to breakdown of the antecubital skin and place traction or pressure on the ulnar nerve in the cubital tunnel (14). Similarly, at the wrist, spastic forearm flexors typically cause wrist and finger flexion deformities. Carpal tunnel syndrome is a common orthopedic

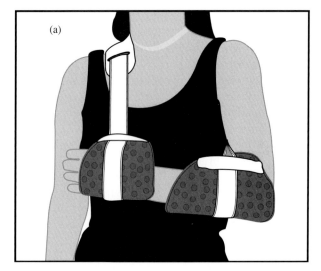
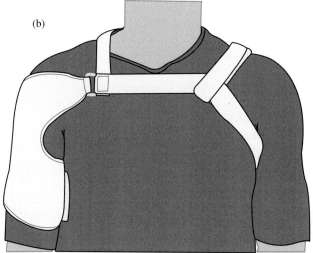

FIGURE 31-3

Examples of two slings: **(a)** the hemiplegic arm sling and **(b)** the vertical humeral cuff sling. Both slings attempt to reduce pain caused by shoulder subluxation by supporting the weight of the arm and reducing shoulder subluxation. However, they differ in the position that the arm is held, with the hemi sling encouraging a flexed posture.

problem in the hemiplegic arm (23). Orthotic treatment is primarily aimed at preventing wrist flexion so as to alleviate pressure on the median nerve.

Generally, upper limb assistive devices, including plaster casts, slings, wheelchair attachments, and orthoses, are used following stroke to prevent or correct contracture, maintain limb position, and to improve or assist function. Upper limb orthotic devices are regarded as either static or dynamic. Static orthoses hold the joints in optimum positions to reduce painful motions, prevent or correct deformity, and facilitate function. Dynamic orthoses provide mechanical assistance to joint motion where muscles are weak or paralyzed, or where muscle imbalance across joints is present (24). However, orthotic prescription for the upper limb remains primarily empirical, since few upper limb orthotic devices have been subjected to controlled analysis (7). Furthermore, compliance with use of orthoses is often poor in individuals with hemiplegia, due to the overall neglect of the involved limb and difficulty with donning and doffing of the orthosis. Many individuals simply use the uninvolved side for activities of daily living.

Contracture Management

Contracture management is important for both the upper and lower limb, since more than 50% of individuals develop contractures following stroke (25). Immobilization, muscle weakness or paralysis, and spasticity are the three main factors leading to the development of contractures that variously affect the joint, contractile tissue, and connective tissue (26). Along with other treatments, such as surgery, passive stretching, and Botulinum Toxin, casts and orthoses may be used to prevent and correct contractures. There are three main types of orthoses for contracture management: custom orthoses that hold the limb at the limit of range of motion but must be replaced when range of motion is gained; static progressive orthoses, which operate under the same principle as serial casting; and dynamic orthoses.

Casts. Three goals of casting for spasticity have been identified in the literature: increasing or preventing loss of passive range of motion by maintaining muscle fiber length, reducing hypertonicity by decreasing sensory input, and improving function. However, there is only evidence to support the use of casts to improve passive range of motion (27). Traditionally, different types of short-term plaster casts (or casts made from other materials such as fiberglass) have been used, sometimes in conjunction with other spasticity management, to prevent or correct contracture. Circular casts applied while an individual is immobile prevent contracture formation, while serial casts applied at frequent intervals (static progressive stretching) correct contractures. Types of casts

include long arm casts typically for elbow flexion contracture, short arm casts typically for wrist flexion contracture, thumb spica casts for thumb-in-palm deformity (Figure 31-4a), and finger casts for flexion contractures of the interphalangeal joints. By holding the muscle in a lengthened position, both types of casts increase sarcomeres (26). However, the limb is also immobilized, which may allow the antagonists to atrophy and shorten, or lead to fibrous adhesions within the joint space and connective tissue inextensibility (26). Therefore, the challenge is to apply the correct amount of load, and use it for the correct period of time, to remodel connective tissue without causing further immobility.

Drop out casts may be used when complete immobilization is unnecessary, as they allow movement into the desired range of motion but limit the progression of deformity by preventing motion in the opposite direction (14, 26). Bivalved or clamshell designs allow for casts

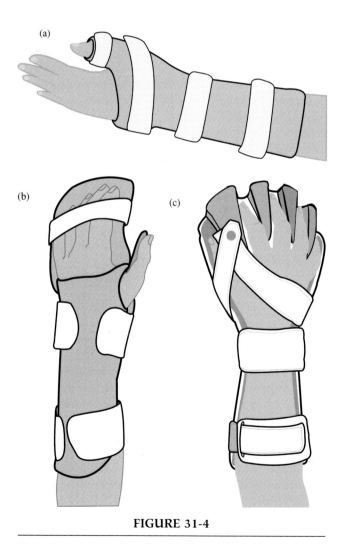

FIGURE 31-4

Examples of static wrist-hand orthoses (WHO): **(a)** thumb spica orthosis, **(b)** dorsal WHO and **(c)** rigid volar WHO.

to be removed for limb inspection, hygiene, or therapy, but should not be used in the presence of severe spasticity, as they do not provide sufficient immobilization of the limb to protect the skin from shearing and breakdown, nor should they be used where the limb is insensate or when cognition is impaired (14).

Static Progressive Orthoses. Orthoses can also be used to apply a static progressive stretch to joints with limited range of motion due to contracture (e.g., Joint Active System [JAS], Thera Tech Equipment, Inc.™, Bloomingdale, IL; Air Cast, Vista, CA; turnbuckle orthoses) (28–30). Similar to serial casting, static progressive orthoses allow for incremental changes in joint position, which are then held constant for a prescribed period of time. However, static progressive orthoses also allow for patient-directed therapy, since the stretch or force applied is typically increased by the patient in order to increase range of motion during the period of orthosis use. Static progressive stretch applied to contracted muscles is intended to restore lost range of motion through the biomechanical principle of stress-relaxation (26); soft tissues respond to mechanical loads in the same manner as a viscoelastic material, such that when stretched and then held at a constant length, the tendency to rebound gradually declines, leading to permanent plastic deformation rather than an elastic response (31). Static progressive orthoses are typically used for 30 minutes, two to three times per day, although it is possible for them to be applied for considerably longer periods (e.g., up to 6 to 12 hours). Unfortunately, there is scant evidence in the literature as to the most efficacious protocol for management of contracture in individuals with stroke. Joints that allow smoother incremental adjustment of joint position have replaced the use of ratcheting joints in static progressive orthoses, so that current orthotic technology allows the same degree of customization of joint position as casting.

Compared to serial casting, static progressive orthoses can be easily removed at regular intervals to allow for the inspection of the limb and maintenance of hygiene. Orthoses also reduce some of the risks of immobilization by allowing intermittent stretching of the antagonists, thus maintaining sarcomeres, and some normal activity that helps reduce connective tissue accumulation (26). However, despite maximizing lever arms and pressure distribution wherever possible, individuals with both contractures and spasticity are particularly at risk for skin breakdown, and may not tolerate a prolonged amount of time in a static progressive orthosis (15).

Dynamic Orthoses. Any technique that holds the joint in a fixed position, like static progressive stretching, will lose its stretching effect after a short period of time due to relaxation of the connective tissue. Hence, dynamic orthoses were developed that apply a continuous stretch to contracted tissue and are commonly used for 6 to 12 hours (32). Dynamic orthoses attempt to stimulate continuous lengthening by operating under a different biomechanical principle than static progressive orthoses: that of creep rather than stress-relaxation. Creep is a loading condition where a force or load is held constant over a long period of time while the displacement is allowed to vary (31).

Dynamic orthoses use a spring to generate torque at the contracted joint. There are three main types of springs used in dynamic orthoses, each with their own advantages and disadvantages: coil springs (e.g., Dynasplint®, Dynasplint Systems, Inc., Severna Park, MD), gas springs (e.g., ORLAU Contracture Correction Device, ORLAU, Oswestry, Shropshire, UK), and clockwork or flat springs (e.g., Advance Dynamic ROM®, Empi, St Paul, MN; Ultraflex Systems Inc., Pottstown, PA). Coil springs produce a linear force that is proportional to the change in length of the spring; in gas springs, the force produced depends on the gas pressure; and in clockwork springs, the torque produced is almost constant throughout the functional range (33). Since not all springs are capable of maintaining a constant torque throughout the joint range, they will need adjustment when range of motion improves if torque level is to be maintained (33). The advantages of spring mechanisms are that they provide an immediate dynamic response to activity by applying a controlled level of torque, and the spring tension can be set so that the user can overcome the stretching effect in the event of something like a spasm, but will return to the stretched position (33). In order for the applied forces to be tolerable, dynamic orthoses should incorporate large interface areas located as far distally as possible from the joint undergoing stretch to maximize the lever arm (33). It is important to be aware that the application of a mechanically-generated load to a joint will generate relatively static compressive forces across the joint surface compared to normal physiological activity, which is more dynamic and results in periodic unloading of pressure from the joint surface (34). Hence, prolonged use of orthoses should be undertaken with caution to limit compressive loading and its effect on cartilage (34). Although it has been reported that low-load prolonged stretch produces more increase in tendon length than a high-load stretch applied for a short time (35), the evidence is not definitively in favor of one protocol or the other.

To prevent contracture or maintain correction following resolution of contracture, static or fixed-position orthoses that hold the joint at the limit of its range of motion may be used (33). Such orthoses may be made from low- or high-temperature thermoplastics, depending on the expected life-span of the orthosis (see Management of Limb Position and Management of the Hemiplegic Hand, below).

Management of Limb Position

Various devices can be used to improve or assist function by positioning the limb adequately for use. At the shoulder, proper positioning and support of the weakened or subluxed upper extremity may help to decrease pain, prevent inferior subluxation, and avoid the development of secondary problems. Bed-bound individuals with paresis or spasticity of the shoulder tend to develop adduction and internal rotation contractures. In such cases, a foam abduction pillow can be used to position the shoulder in slight abduction and neutral rotation, preventing contracture, and facilitating care and hygiene.

For non-ambulatory individuals, the arm may be supported by a lap board placed over the arms of a wheelchair, or by wheelchair mounted slings and arm supports. Slings are the simplest and most common devices used with ambulatory individuals who require support of a flail arm to prevent inferior subluxation of the shoulder. Slings are inexpensive, lightweight, portable, and generally accepted by individuals. Examples include the hemi sling, figure-of-8 clavicular sling, the Bobath sling with axillary roll, the vertical humeral cuff sling, and the distal support sling that engages the thumb and wrist (Figure 31-3) (7). Although there are many different types of slings, no one type of shoulder support appears to be superior in reducing glenohumeral subluxation (7). The disadvantages of slings are that they immobilize the arm, have a tendency to increase flexor tone, and transfer of load may adversely affect the neck and contralateral shoulder.

Management of the Hemiplegic Wrist and Hand

Upper extremity orthoses are most commonly used distally in individuals with stroke (1). The main goals of orthotic management of the hemiplegic hand are to reduce flexor tone at the wrist and fingers, avoid flexion contractures and deformities (e.g., thumb-in-palm and Boutonniere deformities of the fingers—where the proximal interphalangeal joint [PIP] is flexed and the distal interphalangeal joint [DIP] is hyperextended), maintain the hand and wrist in a comfortable, anatomically neutral position, and avoid carpal tunnel syndrome and hand edema (7, 15). Avoidance of wrist and hand contractures not only serves a cosmetic purpose, it also allows adequate hygiene and skin care of the hand to be performed (7). Generally, rigid or static resting wrist-hand orthoses (WHO) are used to position the hand in a "functional position," with 20 to 30 degrees of wrist extension, 35 to 45 degrees of metacarpophalangeal (MCP) joint flexion, 20 to 45 degrees of PIP joint flexion, 10 to 20 degrees of DIP

joint flexion, and the thumb carpometacarpal joint partially abducted and opposed (36–38). While such orthoses provide support for weak wrists and hands, they limit range of motion and hence function. They are also constructed of rigid materials that are very unforgiving in the event of spasm or increased tone, especially if correction of the deformity is overly aggressive, and it has been suggested recently that they often contribute to deformity rather than prevent it (36). Hence, it has been proposed that use of more flexible materials that provide support but "give" a little in the event of increased flexor tone, as well as positioning of the MCP, PIP, and DIP joints in neutral to stretch flexor muscles, and better strap placement to more positively secure the fingers (e.g., SaeboStretch, Saebo Inc., Charlotte, NC) would result in less deformity and greater compliance with orthotic management (36). Unfortunately, research as to the relative benefits between particular WHOs in the management of individuals with stroke has not been extensively performed.

Dorsal and volar WHOs are lightweight thermoplastic devices that utilize three-point force systems to maintain the wrist, thumb, and fingers in a functional position. The dorsal WHO primarily contacts the posterior surface of the forearm, providing a platform for finger support (Figure 31-4b). The volar WHO primarily contacts the anterior surface of the forearm, maintaining the wrist, thumb, and fingers in a slightly extended position (Figure 31-4c). Volar wrist orthoses are most commonly indicated after surgical lengthening of spastic extrinsic finger flexor muscles in a hand with modest volitional motion, and are usually worn at night to maintain the hand in a corrected position (14). They should not be used in the presence of excessive spasticity, since they do not adequately control position and, if rigid, may cause skin breakdown or Boutonniere deformities of the fingers (14). Since the hemiplegic hand typically exhibits flexor tone, finger slings attached to the orthosis by springs (e.g., elastic bands or coiled wires) may be used within a dorsal WHO to create extension bias and a more dynamic device (7), where active contraction of the flexor muscles deforms the orthosis and the orthosis returns the joints to a predetermined resting (static equilibrium) position when muscles relax (Figure 31-5). WHOs may also incorporate neurophysiologic principles to inhibit flexor tone, such as abduction of the fingers and avoidance of palm contact, to eliminate facilitation of the grasp reflex.

Dynamic finger orthoses or spring splints are used to correct flexion contractures of the interphalangeal joints, but should not be used where flexor spasticity is present. The thumb abduction orthosis or thumb spica (Figure 31-4a) is a lightweight device that holds the thumb metacarpal in an abducted and slightly opposed position. It is used to avoid thumb-in-palm deformity and to improve thumb function, especially pinch. However, the traditional "C" position of the thumb may actually

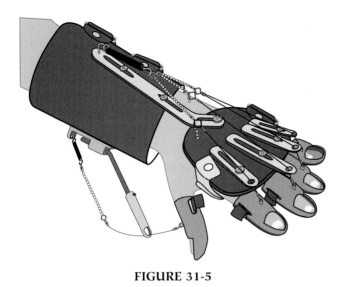

FIGURE 31-5

A dynamic finger extension WHO, the Saebo-flex (Saebo Inc., Charlotte, NC), for functional re-training of the hemiplegic hand. Springs on the dorsum provide resistance to finger flexion.

encourage deformity. A less opposed position, while less functional, would lengthen the thumb flexor and adductor muscles rather than shortening them.

Recently, a dynamic finger extension WHO (Saebo-Flex, Saebo Inc., Charlotte, NC) has been developed to aid in the re-training of function in the hemiplegic upper limb and hand (Figure 31-5). This device uses springs to assist in hand opening for individuals with flexor hypertonicity and/or weak wrist and finger extensors. Use of the device is predicated on the functional task approach (39, 40), wherein intensive, repetitive task-oriented training is used to improve function of the hand and upper limb by inducing long-term plasticity in the motor cortex (41–43). It has been suggested that this device potentially reduces tonicity/spasticity and improves range of motion and motor control through functional tone management, a process whereby spastic muscle activation followed by relaxation teaches individuals how to modulate forces or "turn off" spastic flexors and lengthen them eccentrically (44). In general, there is good evidence for the positive effect of repetitive function and strength training for the hand and upper limb (8), but the efficacy of functional tone management has yet to be assessed.

ORTHOTIC MANAGEMENT OF THE LOWER LIMB

Orthotic management of the lower limb is an important adjunct to the management and treatment of individuals with stroke during both the acute and the chronic

stages of rehabilitation (9). During the acute phase, the primary goals are similar to orthotic management of the upper limb, that is, to maintain range of motion and prevent joint contractures. Adjustable AFOs may be used at night to prevent or correct contracture of the plantar flexors, while knee orthoses, which may or may not include the ankle, are often used to prevent or correct flexion contracture of the hamstrings. Contracture management of the lower limb is based on the same principles as described for the upper limb (see Contracture Management, above). During both the acute and chronic phases, lower limb orthotic intervention is linked closely to the functional requirements of ambulation. Generally, lower limb orthotic devices provide lower extremity stability and safety by controlling limb alignment and eliminating excessive joint motion; enhance motion when muscle activity is not adequate in strength, timing, or coordination; and inhibit or decrease abnormal muscle tone or cutaneous and postural reflexes either by controlling range of motion or by incorporating neurophysiologic modifications (9).

Lower limb orthoses are ideally prescribed based on an assessment of walking to determine changes in limb alignment, motor control, and range of motion resulting from stroke that detrimentally affect function. The degree of sensation present (e.g., proprioception and touch) following recovery from stroke partly determines the ability to ambulate, since sensory deficits impair feedback with respect to limb position and placement (7). Therefore, decisions regarding orthotic prescription should also include assessment of sensation and cognitive status. Impaired balance, loss of trunk stability, proprioceptive loss, and/or loss of motor control may require use of additional supports for walking, such as a walker or quad cane (9). Individuals who are unlikely to ambulate may nevertheless require lower limb orthoses to prevent contracture that impedes transfers or the ability to wear shoes (9).

Although use of an orthosis may provide overall improvement in one functional task, it almost invariably also limits or resists other desirable movements, thereby hindering other tasks. Stroke affects not only the lower limb but half of the entire body, resulting in problems with proximal control and alignment of the trunk and pelvis. Proximal alignment affects distal function of the lower limb, and there are currently no lower limb orthoses that can influence alignment and function of the trunk and pelvis substantially (45).

Lower Limb Biomechanics and Function

Normal human walking is characterized by smooth, rhythmic patterns of motion that require relatively little effort by the individual. The functional requirements of able-bodied walking include: gait initiation and termination, balance and upright posture, stance phase stability, shock absorption, execution of the stepping motion, forward progression/propulsion, and energy conservation (46). These requirements are variably disrupted by stroke.

Although common gait patterns exist, there is great variability among individuals with hemiplegia. Generally, hemiplegic gait is asymmetrical, slow, and uncoordinated due to lack of selective motor control of muscles on the affected side (7, 47). Voluntary movement is often characterized by synergistic patterns corresponding to primitive extensor and flexor reflexes. Fortunately, these synergies are somewhat functional: by alternating synergy patterns, a hemiplegic person can walk, since stance phase requires predominantly extension to create stability and swing phase requires predominantly flexion to functionally shorten the limb for ground clearance. Unfortunately, following stroke, most individuals present with a predominant extensor synergy pattern in both swing and stance phase, leading to issues with limb clearance during swing and the adoption of compensatory gait patterns.

Compensatory gait patterns are commonly observed in individuals with hemiplegia. Inadequate knee flexion and dorsiflexion may require circumduction of the limb to prevent toe drag in swing (7). Circumduction, excessive posterior trunk bending, pelvic rotation, and hip hiking on the involved side, and vaulting on the sound side may be used to assist in swinging the involved leg (47). Disruption in normal motion and alignment, along with compensatory maneuvers and increased muscle activity, lead to greater than normal energy expenditure during walking and fatigue over short distances (48, 49).

Hemiplegic gait is generally characterized by shorter than normal step lengths bilaterally (with the uninvolved step length shorter than the involved), longer stance phase duration, and shorter swing phase duration during swing phase on the involved side (7, 47). Weight bearing on the involved limb is often decreased due to weakness, fear, perceptual or sensory impairments, and disorientation to midline. Persistent equinovarus of the ankle and foot during stance on the involved limb decreases the base of support, increasing instability. People with hemiplegia tend to walk with a retracted hemi pelvis, due primarily to perceptual and sensory deficits, and secondarily to altered muscle tone and weakness in the hip abductors, trunk, and abdominal muscles (47). Weak internal rotators and an inability to dissociate hip motion from a retracted pelvis leads to excessive external rotation of the hip during swing phase and excessive toe out distally. Pelvic retraction can also lead to hyperextension at the knee. Equinus of the ankle-foot may lead to initial contact with the forefoot or in a foot-flat position. Inability to achieve initial contact with the heel may result in an external extensor moment at the knee during early stance, leading to hyperextension. Forward flexion of the trunk is common, due to tight hip flexors or weak hip extensors, and will also contribute to an increased external extensor moment at the knee during stance. Forward flexion of the trunk may also be a compensation for lack of tibial advancement during stance resulting from tight plantar flexors. Weak knee extensors commonly result in knee instability and buckling, while weak dorsiflexors result in insufficient dorsiflexion and drop foot during swing (47).

Types of Lower Limb Orthoses

Shoe Modifications. Following stroke, shoe modifications may be used alone, or more likely in conjunction with lower limb orthoses to improve ankle-foot function (Figure 31-6). Velcro closures or elastic laces are commonly used to facilitate donning and doffing of shoes with one hand, since individuals with hemiplegia typically lack bilateral upper-limb function. Extra-depth footwear may be necessary to accommodate orthotic devices such as AFOs. When the stroke results in mild varus or valgus angulations of the ankle, a high top shoe may provide some control. Shoe modifications such as a cushion or beveled heel can be used to decrease loading of the limb at initial contact and during loading response. A cushion heel involves sandwiching a compressible material within the heel of a shoe, while a beveled heel involves beveling the posterior aspect of the existing heel (Figure 31-6a, b). Both modifications alter the position of the ground reaction force and serve to facilitate forward progression of the center of pressure, reducing the demand on the quadriceps by decreasing the external flexor moment acting at the knee during loading response. However, cushion and beveled heels are contraindicated in the presence of knee hyperextension unless a rigid, non-articulated AFO or an articulated AFO with plantar flexion stop is used to provide control at the knee (see Ankle-foot orthoses, below). Sole and heel wedges placed medially or laterally (Figure 31-6c, d) may be used to counteract undesirable coronal plane moments at the ankle and knee. Addition of a lateral border flare to the sole of the shoe increases the base of support and decreases the tendency for the foot to roll out laterally into varus during stance. Traditional metal AFOs often incorporate T-straps to control varus deformity at the ankle. It should be noted that if initial contact occurs with the fore-foot or with the foot flat, shoe modifications used in isolation of other orthoses are unlikely to be helpful.

Foot Orthoses. Foot orthoses (FO) encompass all or part of the foot, but terminate distal to the ankle joint. They may extend the length of the foot, or terminate at the toe sulcus or proximal to the metatarsal heads. FOs may be used to provide protection for insensate feet or corrective positioning (9). A rigid thermoplastic UCBL (University of California Biomechanics Laboratory) foot orthosis with neurophysiologic modifications may be used in the presence of stable subtalar and ankle

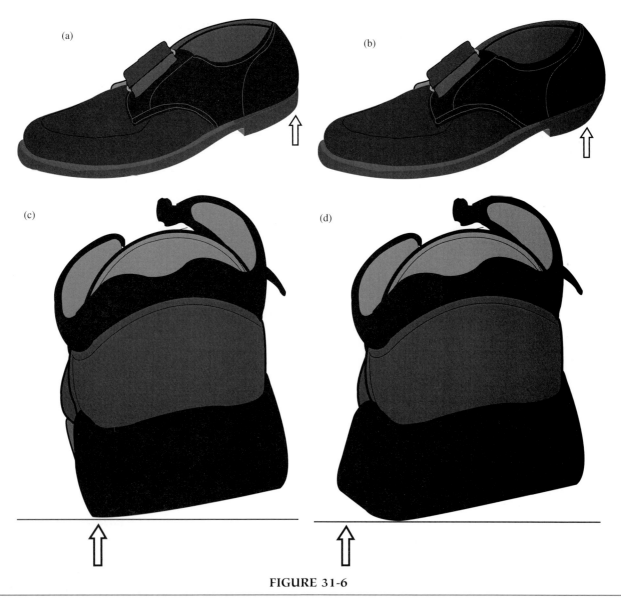

FIGURE 31-6

Examples of two shoe modifications: **(a, b)** side view of the beveled heel used to alter moments about the ankle in the sagittal plane, and **(c, d)** posterior view of the lateral border flare used to alter moments at the calcaneus in the coronal plane. Arrows indicate point of application of the ground reaction force at initial contact in the unmodified shoes (a, c) and the modified shoes (b, d).

joints to manage mild hypertonic foot reflex activity and toe clawing (Figure 31-7) (50). Since an FO such as the UCBL does not cross the ankle joint, it will not correct an equinus foot posture.

Ankle-foot Orthoses. Equinovarus positioning of the ankle-foot complex is the most common deformity observed in the lower limb following stroke (9), hence AFOs are the most commonly prescribed orthoses for management of gait abnormalities following stroke. AFOs may be made from a variety of materials such as metal, thermoplastics, thermosets, or a hybrid of metal and plastic, depending on their particular application. Plastic orthoses are popular because they provide

improved cosmesis and circumferential control compared with metal, although metal orthoses are indicated where fluctuating edema can not be controlled by compression garments or medication (Figure 31-8). Plastic AFOs are generally comprised of an intimate fitting, posterior shell typically made from homopolymer polypropylene or a polypropylene/polyethylene copolymer (1). Polyethylene homopolymer is more flexible than polypropylene, and typically used for circumferential or non-weight bearing orthoses such as upper limb orthoses. Fiber-reinforced thermoset laminations, such as those incorporating carbon graphite, are appropriate when transverse rotational forces need to be restricted. Despite resulting in stronger, stiffer, and lighter orthoses compared to polymers,

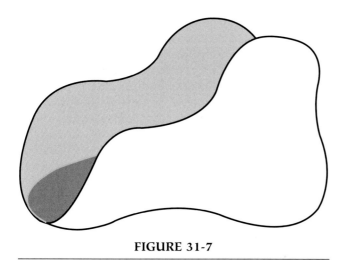

FIGURE 31-7

UCBL (University of California Biomechanics Laboratory) foot orthosis, side view with posterior aspect to the right.

thermosets are not used as widely because of their higher cost and more difficult fabrication process, although easier fabrication techniques using "prepreg composites" (i.e., fibrous material pre-impregnated with resin, partially cured and ready for molding) are emerging that allow for custom thermoset orthoses of varying flexibility and rigidity to be fabricated without the need for specialized facilities (51).

AFOs act directly at the ankle and indirectly on the knee and hip, although there is less evidence for the effect at the hip than there is at the knee (8, 52–55). The basic AFO design includes a proximal trim-line that terminates 20mm distal to the neck of the fibula, providing the longest possible lever arm for ankle motion control, which is particularly important if spasticity of the triceps surae muscle is present (24). AFOs differ substantially from ankle orthoses (AO). AOs are prefabricated orthoses intended to provide mediolateral stability at the ankle joint in the presence of ligamentous insufficiency. AOs provide only minimal support to prevent varus of the ankle-foot, but may be used transiently in mild cases until gait more fully improves (7). Generally, AOs are inappropriate for individuals with stroke, as they lack sufficient lever arm in the presence of hypertonicity to adequately control ankle motion. However, when worn AOs may have greater compliance than AFOs, as they are relatively inconspicuous and fit easily into regular footwear.

AFOs fall into two main categories: articulated and non-articulated (Figure 31-8). As the name implies, articulated AFOs incorporate mechanical joints at the ankle that allow control of sagittal plane motion. Articulated AFOs may be used to control joint range of motion (e.g., using adjustable joints), provide assistance to motion (e.g., with a dorsiflexion assist joint), or limit motion (e.g., with plantar flexion or dorsiflexion

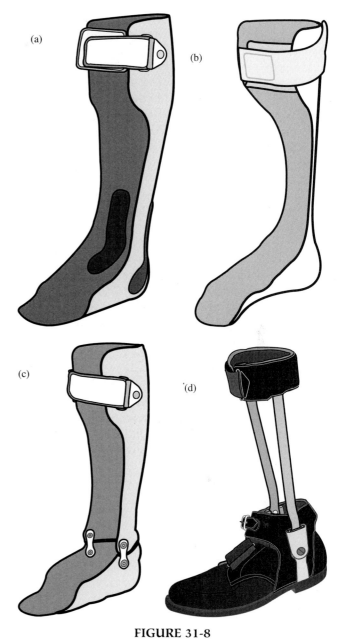

FIGURE 31-8

Four main types of AFO: **(a)** rigid non-articulated, **(b)** posterior leaf spring, **(c)** polymer articulated, and **(d)** metal articulated. The articulated polymer AFO incorporates a plantar flexion stop, whereas the metal articulated AFO has double action ankle joints that use combinations of pins and springs anterior and posterior to the joint to provide a plantar flexion stop (pin in posterior channel), dorsiflexion stop (pin in anterior channel), dorsiflexion assist (spring in posterior channel), and plantar flexion assist (spring in anterior channel).

stops). Although non-articulated AFOs do not incorporate joints, they may or may not allow motion at the ankle in the sagittal plane, depending on their flexibility. In a non-articulated polymer AFO, motion is determined by the rigidity of the orthosis about the ankle joint, which is usually a product of plastic thickness and geometry. Adding reinforcements about the ankle or an anterior shell may increase rigidity of the AFO. A non-articulated AFO is generally rigid if the trim-lines about the ankle are anterior to the malleoli, sometimes referred to as a solid or rigid AFO. The more posterior the trim-lines are to the malleoli, the more flexible the orthosis becomes, such as in a polymer posterior leaf spring AFO (PLS-AFO). In a PLS-AFO, motion occurs due to buckling or deformation of the plastic when a moment is applied. A PLS-AFO allows some plantar flexion at initial contact and dorsiflexion during mid-stance. It returns the ankle to neutral during swing phase when the only load acting on the orthosis is due to the weight of the foot. Hence, the PLS-AFO is contraindicated where there is spasticity, hypertonicity, or clonus of the plantar flexors, since the control of ankle position in swing is diminished if a plantar flexor moment is applied to the orthosis at that time (8).

AFOs may be either prefabricated or custom-made. Prefabricated or off-the-shelf AFOs are convenient, inexpensive, and may be adequate for some individuals. Although they may be used for training/evaluation or as interim devices, they are rarely recommended for long-term use due to their generic fit (8, 9), which also makes them unable to accommodate misalignment and deformity of the foot and ankle. Prefabricated PLS-AFOs are common because their limited biomechanical control easily allows for a more generic shape. A fundamental requirement of all orthoses is that they contour well to the body segment/s they encompass. Custom-made AFOs provide better biomechanical control than prefabricated orthoses because a more precise fit can be achieved, especially in the presence of complex deformities.

The primary indications for AFO use in stroke are: inadequate dorsiflexion in mid to terminal swing, resulting in foot clearance problems and compromising the ability to achieve initial contact with the heel; mediolateral ankle-foot instability in stance and swing; and insufficient tibial control in stance (9). Table 31-2 summarizes indications for the three basic types of AFOs (rigid non-articulated, articulated, and flexible non-articulated) as applied to individuals with stroke (8).

It is not uncommon for a person with stroke to require greater stability during the initial acute phase, but less stability as recovery occurs. In such cases, a progressive AFO, with biomechanical controls that can be altered as the individual's condition changes, may be useful. This can be a polymer AFO fabricated to include ankle joints, but that has yet to be "cut" to allow articulation. Similarly, a KAFO can be converted to an AFO as the individual's needs change (56). An AFO with adjustable ankle joints may also be useful during the acute phase, as it allows the ankle joint to be locked in any position from dorsiflexion to plantar flexion, or be free moving throughout the range. Dorsiflexion and plantar flexion stops can be used when partial range of motion is

---

TABLE 31-2

Summary of Indications for AFOs (from the International Society for Prosthetics and Orthotics Report of a Consensus Conference on the Orthotic Management of Stroke) (8).

Non-articulated AFOs (excluding leaf-spring AFOs) are indicated as follows:
- poor balance, instability in stance
- inability to transfer weight onto the affected limb in stance
- moderate to severe foot abnormality; equinus, valgus or varus, or a combination
- moderate to severe hypertonicity
- as above, but with mild recurvatum or instability of the knee
- to improve walking speed and cadence

Articulated AFOs are indicated as follows:
- dorsiflexor weakness only
- where passive or active range of dorsiflexion is present
- where dorsiflexion is needed for sit-to-stand or stair climbing
- to control knee flexion instability only; articulated AFO with dorsiflexion stop
- to control recurvatum only; articulated AFO with plantar flexion stop
- to improve walking speed and cadence

Posterior leaf spring AFOs are indicated as follows:
- isolated dorsiflexor weakness
- no significant problem with tone
- no significant mediolateral instability
- no need for orthotic influence on the knee or hip

required. Such adjustability allows the mechanical ankle joints to accommodate changes in range of motion as the individual progresses.

Where a rigid non-articulated AFO or an AFO with a plantar flexion stop is used, it is important to account for footwear heel height when casting, and keep the heel height of the shoe constant since changes in footwear heel height can alter the indirect effect of the AFO at the knee (57). Rigid devices may be used to maintain the ankle in a fixed position and prevent spasticity, since a spastic response tends to rapidly diminish when joints are immobile, but persists with even small amounts of motion (9). Although it has long been considered standard practice to cast the ankle at neutral (i.e., 90 degrees), recent literature suggests that the angular relationship between the shank and floor is more important for function, especially in a rigid non-articulated AFO (5), and that gastrocnemius length should be considered when deciding ankle alignment. The rationale for this conclusion is that controlling tibial progression in mid to late stance transfers forward momentum to the thigh, facilitating knee and hip extension in terminal stance if there is sufficient gastrocnemius length, and placing the limb in a more appropriate alignment for transfer of body weight to the contralateral limb, and commencing swing phase with the ipsilateral limb. There is some evidence that alignment of the orthosis at terminal stance and/or pre-swing will influence step length, gait symmetry, speed, and energy consumption (9). AFO alignment can also be used to enhance knee stability during stance where the knee extensors are weak and unable to support body weight during single support. Floor reaction or ground reaction AFOs (FRAFO or GRAFO) are rigid, non-articulated AFOs that hold the ankle in slight plantar flexion to create an external knee extension moment during stance. For these designs to be effective, they must provide good rotational control and should not be used in the presence of a knee hyperextension deformity.

AFOs that incorporate neurophysiologic modifications are sometimes referred to as dynamic or tone reducing AFOs. In these orthoses, control of muscle tone may be attempted by positioning the toes in extension, applying pressure points over strategic locations on the plantar surface of the foot and muscle insertions, providing static immobilization through total contact, and stimulation of antagonist muscle groups (9). For example, a toe spreader or toe separator may be used independently or in conjunction with an AFO to inhibit tonic foot reflexes such as the toe grasp reflex, which may cause excessive toe clawing, leading to pain and impeding forward advancement of the lower limb over the foot. Inhibition of abnormal tone in the toes allows the foot to become a better weight-bearing surface over which the body may progress during stance (1, 9). Function of toe spreaders/separators is based on the premise that abduction and extension of the toes releases intrinsic tone. Tone-reducing AFOs often incorporate total contact principles, with greater contact of the dorsal surface of the foot, to facilitate neutral alignment of the subtalar joint, which is purported to reduce tone in the foot but allow motion at the ankle joint (50). However, there is little evidence to support the ability of orthoses to reduce tone during ambulation.

Recently, it has been suggested that triplanar dynamic response orthoses may lead to greater functional improvements than conventional orthoses, through better control of segment alignment and motion (58) (Figure 31-9). These orthoses are made from thermosets, such as graphite composites, in order to provide sufficient rigidity to support body weight during stance and control forces in all three planes, yet allow sufficient flexibility to absorb and return energy. Unfortunately, there is as yet no evidence of their efficacy or applicability to individuals with spasticity and hypertonicity.

Knee-ankle-foot Orthoses. Knee-ankle-foot orthoses (KAFO) are used where a need exists for direct control of the knee joint in addition to the ankle and foot (24). A KAFO is also useful when there is lack of control of the hip extensor muscles (1). All KAFOs provide coronal plane knee stability by default, and the ankle section may

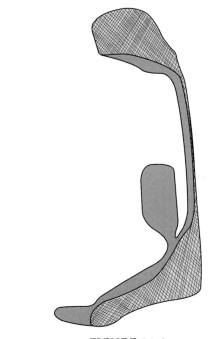

FIGURE 31-9

Graphite composite, triplanar control dynamic response AFO with lateral flange (Dynamic Bracing Solutions, San Diego, CA).

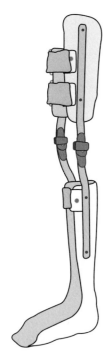

FIGURE 31-10

Hybrid metal and plastic knee-ankle-foot orthosis (KAFO) with drop-lock knee joints.

incorporate all the functions and designs of an AFO as needed (Figure 31-10).

Orthoses that encompass more than one joint, such as KAFOs, are usually bulky and cumbersome, and individuals with weakness, as often occurs in stroke, are unable to tolerate bulky, heavy devices (1). Traditionally, only two basic knee control options were available for use in KAFOs: unlocked or locked. A KAFO with unlocked knee joints provides coronal plane knee stability, with sagittal plane stability of the knee during stance predicated on geometric alignment. This may be achieved with a posterior offset knee joint where the mechanical axis of rotation is located posterior to the anatomical axis of rotation, supposedly resulting in an external knee extensor moment at the mechanical joints in early stance (24). These joints are not entirely reliable, especially on uneven terrain and slopes, and are indicated only where the individual retains adequate hip musculature strength and control, proprioception at the knee, and good balance to ensure stumble recovery should geometric stability not be achieved.

A KAFO with locked knees provides both coronal and sagittal plane control of the knee throughout stance, but also remains locked during swing phase, necessitating compensatory maneuvers during walking to achieve ground clearance of the extended limb during swing. As we progress proximally, immobilization

of lower limb joints increases energy expenditure during functional activities, with immobilization of the knee being particularly detrimental (59). Hence, KAFOs have been used infrequently, due to their increased weight and energy demands when walking.

Stance-control KAFOs. Stance-control orthoses incorporate knee joints that automatically stabilize the knee during stance phase, but release during swing phase to allow knee flexion. These new devices, and the availability of strong, lightweight materials, has renewed interest in the potential use of KAFOs with individuals with stroke (8, 56). It has been suggested that stance-control KAFOs may be particularly useful during the early rehabilitation phase post-stroke, as they may facilitate appropriate limb alignment and provide support of the weakened limb during gait training (60). This may decrease the development of abnormal postures, especially proximally, and lead to better long-term functional recovery. Stance-control orthoses may be of benefit both as a temporary post-stroke gait training aid, and as an on-going gait assist for individuals with permanent knee extensor weakness. Different stance-control knee mechanisms are commercially available (e.g., Stance-Control Orthosis™, Horton's Orthotic Lab. Inc., Little Rock, AK; UTX® and Model 9001 E-Knee™, Becker Orthopedic, Troy, MI; UltraSafeStep™, Ultraflex Systems Inc., Pottstown, PA; FreeWalk™, Otto Bock HealthCare, Minneapolis, MN; Swing Phase Lock, Fillauer LLC, Chattanooga, TN), which require different strategies to engage and disengage the knee joint. Hence, not all the available stance-control knee mechanisms may be appropriate for individuals following stroke.

RESEARCH FRONTIERS IN THE ORTHOTIC MANAGEMENT OF STROKE

Although orthoses are commonly used in the management of stroke and empirically have been found to be of benefit, a recent consensus conference concluded that evidence for the orthotic management of stroke is generally low, both in terms of quality and quantity (8). There exists the need to demonstrate efficacy more objectively, especially within the current medical paradigm of evidence-based practice. For example, there is no evidence in the literature regarding the most appropriate timing of lower limb orthotic management following stroke; the long-term or carry-over effect of lower limb orthoses has not been demonstrated; and the ability of an AFO to influence range of motion of the hip during gait is unconfirmed by experimental studies on stroke subjects (8). With regard to the upper limb, there is controversy over whether static, rigid WHOs prevent deformity or contribute to it; the long-term effects of contracture management, based on either stress-relaxation or creep are unknown;

and the optimal protocol for the application of stretch to spastic muscle is unclear. Furthermore, the interaction between orthoses and other therapies remains largely unexplored. Since much of the literature regarding the orthotic management of stroke is based on small numbers of subjects with the orthoses often poorly described, it has been recommended that well-controlled, multi-center trials involving large numbers of subjects are urgently needed (8).

In general, the science of orthotics is immature. Although orthotic technology continues to advance, especially with the application of new materials, microprocessors, and active elements such as pneumatic muscles (61,

62), our understanding of how best to apply that technology lags behind. In the past, most orthoses were passive, whereas today there is a growing interest in active orthoses that might, for example, power gait by providing propulsion at push-off (62). Active orthoses are currently limited in their clinical application by the size and weight of the devices, in large part as a result of the power sources required. While active devices may be applied to weak limbs in a reasonably safe manner, we need to develop a better understanding of how to safely apply active devices where spasticity and hypertonicity are present and there may be unpredictable resistance to the torque provided by the active orthosis.

References

1. Good D, Supan T. Basic principles of orthotics in neurological disorders. In: Aisen M, ed. *Orthotics in Neurological Rehabilitation.* New York, NY: Demos Publications, 1992:1–23.

2. Bowker P, Condie DN, Bader DL, et al. *Biomechanical Basis of Orthotic Management.* Oxford: Butterworth Heinemann, 1993.

3. Bobath K. *A Neurophysiological Basis for the Treatment of CerebralPpalsy.* Second ed. Oxford: Blackwell Scientific Publications, 1981.

4. Lohman M, Goldstein H. Alternative strategies in tone-reducing AFO design. *Journal of Prosthetics and Orthotics* 1993; 5(1):1–4.

5. Bowers RJ. Non-articulated ankle foot orthoses. In: Condie E, Campbell J, Martina J, eds. *Report of a Consensus Conference on the Orthotic Management of Stroke Patients.* Copenhagen, Denmark: International Society for Prosthetics and Orthotics, 2004:87–94.

6. Hoy D, Reinthal M. Articulated ankle foot orthoses designs. In: Condie E, Campbell J, Martina J, eds. *Report of a Consensus Conference on the Orthotic Management of Stroke Patients.* Copenhagen, Denmark: International Society for Prosthetics and Orthotics, 2004:95–111.

7. Rossi P. Stroke. In: Aisen M, ed. *Orthotics in Neurological Rehabilitation.* New York, NY: Demos Publications, 1992:45–61.

8. Condie E, Campbell J, Martina J, eds. *Report of a Consensus Conference on the Orthotic Management of Stroke Patients.* Copenhagen, Denmark: International Society for Prosthetics and Orthotics, 2004.

9. Fennell C, Yang A, Elson D. Orthoses for brain-injured patients. In: Goldberg B, Hsu J, eds. *Atlas of Orthoses and Assistive Devices.* Third ed. St Louis, MO: Mosby, 1997:379–389.

10. Veterans Health Administration, Department of Defense. *VA/DoD Clinical Practice Guideline for the Management of Stroke Rehabilitation in the Primary Care Setting.* Washington, D.C.: Department of Veteran Affairs, 2003.

11. Fish D. Orthotic management of the hip and knee for the post-cerebrovascular population. In: Condie E, Campbell J, Martina J, eds. *Report of a Consensus Conference on the Orthotic Management of Stroke Patients.* Copenhagen, Denmark: International Society for Prosthetics and Orthotics, 2004:162–170.

12. Bottlang M, Marsh J, Brown T. Articulated external fixation of the ankle: minimizing motion resistance by accurate axis alignment. *Journal of Biomechanics.* Jan 1999; 32(1):63–70.

13. Lehneis H. Brace alignment considerations. *Orthotic and Prosthetic Appliance Journal* June 1964; 18:110–114.

14. Keenan M. Upper extremity orthoses for the brain-injured patient. In: Goldberg B, Hsu J, eds. *Atlas of Orthoses and Assistive Devices.* Third ed. St Louis, MO: Mosby, 1997:281–289.

15. Parente N. Orthotic management of the upper limb. In: Condie E, Campbell J, Martina J, eds. *Report of a Consensus Conference on the Orthotic Management of Stroke Patients.* Copenhagen, Denmark: International Society for Prosthetics and Orthotics, 2004: 247–253.

16. Najenson T, Yacubovich E, Pikielni S. Rotator cuff injury in shoulder joints of hemiplegic patients. *Scandinavian Journal of Rehabilitation Medicine* 1971; 3(3):131–137.

17. Van Ouwenaller C, Laplace P, Chantraine A. Painful shoulder in hemiplegia. *Archives of Physical Medicine and Rehabilitation* 1986; 67(1):23–26.

18. Bender L, McKenna K. Hemiplegic shoulder pain: Defining the problem and its management. *Disability and Rehabilitation* 2001; 23(16):698–705.

19. Forster A. The painful hemiplegic shoulder: Physiotherapy treatment. *Reviews in Clinical Gerontology* 1994; 4:343–348.

20. Joynt R. The source of shoulder pain in hemiplegia. *Archives of Physical Medicine and Rehabilitation* 1992; 73(5):409–413.

21. Teasell R, Heitzner J. The painful hemiplegic shoulder. *Physical Medicine and Rehabilitation: State of the Art Reviews* 1998; 12:489–500.

22. Ada L, Foongchomcheay A, Canning C. Supportive devices for preventing and treating subluxation of the shoulder after stroke (Cochrane Review). *The Cochrane Database of Systematic Reviews* 2005(1):CD003863.

23. Dittmer D, McArthur-Turner D, Jones I. Orthotics in stroke. *Physical Medicine and Rehabilitation: State of the Art Reviews* 1993; 7(1):161–177.

24. Fatone S. Orthotics. In: Akay M, ed. *Wiley Encyclopedia of Biomedical Engineering.* Hoboken, NJ: John Wiley & Sons, Inc., 2006.

25. O'Dwyer N, Ada L, Neilson P. Spasticity and muscle contracture following stroke. *Brain* 1996; 119:1737–749.

26. Farmer S, James M. Contractures in orthopaedic and neurological conditions: A review of causes and treatment. *Disability and Rehabilitation* 2001; 23(13):549–558.

27. Mortenson P, Eng J. The use of casts in the management of joint mobility and hypertonia following brain injury in adults: A systematic review. *Physical Therapy* 2003; 83:648–658.

28. Bonutti P, Windau J, Ables B, Miller B. Static progressive stretch to reestablish elbow range of motion. *Clinical Orthopedics and Related Research* Jun 1994; 303:128–134.

29. Gelinas J, Faber K, Patterson S, King G. The effectiveness of turnbuckle splinting for elbow contractures. *Journal of Bone and Joint Surgery* Jan 2000; 82-B(1):74–78.

30. O'Driscoll S. Patient adjusted static elbow splints for elbow contractures: A preliminary report. *Journal of Shoulder and Elbow Surgery* 1996; 5:S73.

31. Bonutti P, Hotz M, Gray T, et al. Joint contracture rehabilitation: Static progressive stretch. Paper presented at: Meeting of the American Academy of Orthopedic Surgeons, March 19–22, 1998; New Orleans, LA.

32. Glasgow C, Wilton J, Tooth L. Optimal daily total end range time for contracture: Resolution in hand splinting. *Journal of Hand Therapy* Jul–Sep 2003; 16(3):207–218.

33. Farmer S, Woollam P, Patrick J, et al. Dynamic orthoses in the management of joint contracture. *Journal of Bone and Joint Surgery* 2005; 87-B(3):291–295.

34. Wong M, Carter D. Articular cartilage functional histomorphology and mechanobiology: A research perspective. *Bone* 2003; 33(1):1–13.

35. Williams P, Catanese T, Lucey E, Goldspink G. The importance of stretch and contractile activity in the prevention of connective tissue accumulation in muscle. *Journal of Anatomy* 1988; 158:109–114.

36. Farrell J. Splinting the neurologically impaired hand: It's time for a change. *Advance for Occupational Therapy Practitioners* 3 April 2006; 22(7):41–43.

37. Magee D. *Orthopedic Physical Assessment.* Philadelphia, PA: WB Saunders Company, 1987.

38. Norkin C, Levangie P. *Joint Structure and Function.* Second ed. Philadelphia: F.A. Davis, 1992.

39. Van Peppen R, Kwakkel G, Wood-Dauphinee S, et al. The impact of physical therapy on functional outcomes after stroke: What's the evidence? *Clinical Rehabilitation* 2004; 18(8):833–862.

40. Winstein C, Rose D, Tan S, et al. A randomized controlled comparison of upper-extremity rehabilitation strategies in acute stroke: A pilot study of immediate and long-term outcomes. *Archives of Physical Medicine and Rehabilitation* 2004; 85(4):620–628.

41. Cauraugh JH, Summers JJ. Neural plasticity and bilateral movements: A rehabilitation approach for chronic stroke. *Progress in Neurobiology* 2005; 75(5):309–320.

42. Nudo R. Adaptive plasticity in motor cortex: Implications for rehabilitation after brain injury. *Journal of Rehabilitation Medicine* 2003; 41:7–10.

43. Nudo R, Plautz E, Frost S. Role of adaptive plasticity in recovery of function after damage to motor cortex. *Muscle and Nerve* 2001; 24(8):1000–1019.

44. Butler A, Blanton S, Rowe V, Wolf S. Attempting to improve function and quality of life using the FTM Protocol: Case report. *Journal of Neurologic Physical Therapy* Sep 2006; 30(3):148–156.

45. Hanna D, Harvey R. Review of preorthotic biomechanical considerations. *Topics in Stroke Rehabilitation* 2001; 7(4):29–37.

46. Gard S, Fatone S. Biomechanics of lower limb function and gait. In: Condie E, Campbell J, Martina J, eds. *Report of a Consensus Conference on the Orthotic Management of Stroke Patients*. Copenhagen, Denmark: International Society for Prosthetics and Orthotics, 2004:55–63.

47. Scribner G, Dealy L. Principles of gait analysis. In: Aisen M, ed. *Orthotics in Neurological Rehabilitation*. New York: Demos Publications, 1992:25–45.

48. Platts M, Rafferty D, Paul L. Metabolic cost of over ground gait in younger stroke patients and healthy controls. *Medicine and Science in Sports and Exercise* 2006; 38(6):1041–1046.

49. Zamparo P, Francescato M, De Luca G, et al. The energy cost of level walking in patients with hemiplegia. *Scandinavian Journal of Medicine and Science in Sports* Dec 1995; 5(6):348–352.

50. Shamp J. Neurophysiologic orthotic designs in the treatment of central nervous system disorders. *Journal of Prosthetics and Orthotics* 1990; 2(1):14–32.

51. Morrison B, Creasy T, Polliack A, Fite R. A new fabrication technique utilizing a composite material applied to orthopedic bracing. *Polymer Composites* 2002; 23(1):10–20.

52. Fatone S, Hansen A, Gard S, Malas B. Effects on gait of ankle alignment and foot-plate length in ankle foot orthoses (AFOs). Paper presented at: Annual Meeting of the American Academy of Orthotists and Prosthetists, 16-19 March, 2005; Orlando, Florida.

53. Lehmann J, Condon S, Price R, deLateur B. Gait abnormalities in hemiplegia: Their correction by ankle-foot orthoses. *Archives of Physical Medicine and Rehabilitation* Nov 1987; 68(11):763–771.

54. Lehmann J, Ko M, deLateur B. Knee moments: Origin in normal ambulation and their modification by double-stopped ankle-foot orthoses. *Archives of Physical Medicine and Rehabilitation* Aug 1982; 63(8):345–351.

55. Lehmann J, Warren C, deLateur B. A biomechanical evaluation of knee stability in below knee braces. *Archives of Physical Medicine and Rehabilitation* Dec 1970; 51(12):688–695.

56. Kakurai S, Akai M. Clinical experiences with a convertible thermoplastic knee-ankle-foot orthosis for post-stroke hemiplegic patients. *Prosthetics and Orthotics International* December 1996; 20(3):191–194.

57. Cook T, Cozzens B. The effects of heel height and ankle-foot-orthosis configuration on weight line location: A demonstration of principles. *Orthotics and Prosthetics* 1976; 30(4):43–46.

58. Loke M. Triplanar control dynamic response orthoses based on new concepts in lower limb orthotics. *Physical Medicine and Rehabilitation Clinics of North America* 2006; 17:181–202.

59. Perry J. *Gait Analysis: Normal and Pathological Function*. New York: McGraw-Hill, 1992.

60. Michael J. KAFOs for ambulation: An orthotist's perspective. *Journal of Prosthetics and Orthotics* 2006; 18(3S):187–191.

61. Blaya J, Herr H. Adaptive control of a variable-impedance ankle-foot orthosis to assist drop-foot gait. *IEEE Transactions in Neural Systems and Rehabilitation Engineering* Mar 2004; 12(1):24–31.

62. Ferris D, Czerniecki J, Hannaford B. An ankle-foot orthosis powered by artificial pneumatic muscles. *Journal of Applied Biomechanics* May 2005; 21(2):189–197.

63. Duncan W. Tonic reflexes of the foot. *Journal of Bone and Joint Surgery.* 1960; 42-A (5):856.

32

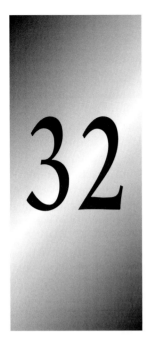

Alternative, Complementary, and Integrative Medicine

Samuel C. Shiflett

T he use of alternative or nonconventional therapies by patients to supplement or complement conventional medical treatments has been commonplace for many decades. These therapies have historically been used without the knowledge of the patients' health care providers, thus raising the risk of unknown interactions with standard medical treatments. The existence of this phenomenon was first brought to the attention of the medical community with the publication of a major national survey published in 1993, along with a follow-up survey confirming the findings seven years later (1, 2). These surveys revealed that the use of alternative therapies in the general population has grown from an estimated 34% in 1990 to 42% in 1997, and it is likely that this trend is continuing. These surveys not only demonstrated the widespread use of alternative therapies, but also indicated that more money was being spent on these therapies than on conventional medicine. These findings spurred a major move toward a better understanding of the nature of these alternative therapies along with the development of a major research agenda to study them initiated by the National Institutes of Health (NIH). The majority of this research is funded and monitored by the National Center for Complementary and Alternative Medicine (NCCAM), a division of the Office of the Director of NIH.

According to NCCAM, the expression *complementary and alternative medicine* (CAM) covers a broad range of interventions that can be categorized as follows:

1. Biologically based practices
2. Manipulative and body-based practices
3. Energy medicine
4. Mind-body medicine
5. Whole medical systems

The exact definitions of these categories can be found on their website at nccam.nih.gov. Although many therapies in the NCCAM lists are clearly alternative, many others may be considered either mainstream or alternative, depending on who is doing the categorizing. For example, many supplements and herbal extracts that are considered alternative in the United States have been used routinely for many years in European medical practice, and their use is taught in medical schools there.

The question of what is alternative becomes even more problematic when we move to the field of physical medicine and rehabilitation (PM&R). The modern medical field of PM&R basically began during World War II as an identifiable discipline utilizing a number of complementary treatments that addressed not only the broken body but also the mind, spirit, and soul, with the goal of uplifting and restoring the whole person into a meaningful and productive life, rather than simply focusing on physiological or anatomical healing (3). Over the years, many complementary treatments involved in PM&R have become accepted as standard of care, and the evidence base for these treatments is slowly growing. The whole-person nature of this field means that, more than is the case in most medical disciplines, PM&R has been willing to explore and utilize potential new therapies that appear to be beneficial even while those same therapies are being subjected to the time-consuming and costly process of evaluation based on randomized, controlled trials. In fact, many modern and alternative movement and manipulation techniques have actually emerged from the field of rehabilitation medicine, and many of these techniques were developed by physical therapists. Examples include such movement and manipulation techniques as Feldenkrais®, Rolfing® or Structural Integration, and Trager® psychophysical integration. Thus, the division between complementary/alternative medicine and conventional medical therapy is not always clear in rehabilitation. For example, most conventional category systems defining CAM, including that of the NCCAM of the NIH, include biofeedback as an example of a mind-body alternative therapy. And biofeedback is indeed typically offered at most New Age and alternative health clinics. Yet, various forms of biofeedback have been available at many rehabilitation centers for many years now. Thus, the status of biofeedback as alternative versus conventional medical therapy is unclear.

The Ottawa Evidence-Based Clinical Practice Guidelines (EBCPG) Development Group recently published an extensive and exhaustive review of therapies for post-stroke rehabilitation (4). They reviewed a broad range of interventions, both conventional and nontraditional, including biofeedback and constraint-induced therapy, along with other ostensibly alternative therapies such as massage, electrical stimulation, TENS, and acupuncture. At no time were any of the therapies that were reviewed—and for which EBCPGs were developed—referred to as alternative or complementary. They were included because there was research literature providing evidence for or against the effectiveness of the therapy. Their approach thus epitomizes the call for evidence-based medicine rather than alternative versus conventional medicine, issued by the JAMA editors in the first special issue on CAM ever published in that journal (5).

Many alternative therapies currently practiced in the West have their origins in the ancient medical traditions of Eastern cultures, such as Traditional Chinese Medicine (TCM) and the Ayurvedic tradition of India. These ancient approaches treat the body and its health as an integrated system, and illness is seen as an imbalance or disharmony of vital energy within the whole body. Treatment of illness is thus seldom focused on the symptoms of the illness but on the believed underlying imbalance of subtle energy. Restoring the body to equilibrium usually requires a set of integrated interventions that focus on the body, mind, and soul. As a result, TCM has an arsenal of treatments that include not only various forms of acupuncture, but also a vast pharmacopeia of herbs and supplements barely known in Western medicine; various physical movement and physical manipulation techniques such as tui na, a technique similar to chiropractic manipulation; and exercises designed to strengthen the body and to move and balance the subtle energy (chi or qi), including Tai Chi and Qi Gong. Many meditation and breathing techniques supplement these physical interventions. The same situation holds true for Indian medicine, where yoga postures, Ayurvedic herbs, meditation, sound, and breathing exercises may all be prescribed for a particular disease, all focusing on the restoration of the health of the overall system.

Even though these ancient models of the human organism often do not seem to have any relationship to modern (Western) concepts of physiology, anatomy, and the ontogeny of disease, many of the techniques that they have generated over the centuries continue to be practiced today and are often felt by their recipients to be of help. Interestingly, many of these ancient techniques have parallels in modern therapies, which sometimes are derived from these early traditions and, in other cases, were developed independently of them. Thus, stretching exercises, massage, and other techniques routinely used by physical therapists are surprisingly similar to the alternative techniques of tui na, yoga, and pranayama (breathing exercises), and so forth.

A major premise of this chapter is the idea that no unconventional therapies should be thought of as alternative, that is, unconventional therapies are not expected to replace conventional therapies and current standard of care. Rather, their use is expected to be complementary, being used in conjunction with regular care. Practitioners seeking to combine these two approaches together into a systematic and evidence-based set of protocols often refer to this combined approach as integrative medicine.

All of the therapies discussed below are presented with an explanation of their proposed mechanism(s) of action and evaluated in terms of the research evidence that supports their use. As will be seen, the evidence varies in quality, from moderately strong to very weak. The chapter is organized around the category system proposed by NCCAM, with the exception that the whole medical systems category is not used here; rather, certain specific therapies within those systems are discussed here and categorized in one of the more specific NCCAM categories. An expanded discussion of acupuncture is provided because it is the most extensively studied of all of the body-based techniques and because the studies of this technique illustrate several recurring methodological challenges present in research on CAM techniques for stroke recovery. These methodological issues include:

1. Variability in the severity and anatomy of stroke within a study population
2. Inadequate consideration of the impact of baseline level of functioning
3. Timing of the outcome measures

The chapter concludes with a discussion of strategies for managing therapies that appear promising and safe but for which empiric evidence of efficacy is not yet available.

MANIPULATIVE AND BODY-BASED THERAPIES

Manipulative and pressure-based therapies encompass any of a number of techniques that involve touching the body with an external object, such as massage therapy, or a penetrating needle, as in acupuncture. Manipulative therapies are used in the treatment of a number of medical and physical conditions and are also used as a general technique for relaxing the body and generating a feeling of well-being in otherwise healthy individuals. Many fundamental therapies, such as massage, myofascial adjustments, or osteopathic manipulation, have numerous variations, with different names based on the particular variations in the application of the fundamental technique.

Acupuncture

Acupuncture has been used for over 2,000 years to treat stroke in China and other parts of Asia. According to traditional Oriental medical theory, upon which acupuncture is based, the body contains a system of energy channels called *meridians*. These meridians are not physical vessels that can be identified by anatomical dissection; rather, they are hypothetical pathways through which energy flows. The energy that flows through these meridians is considered a life-force and is referred to as *qi* or *chi*. (Both spellings are pronounced "chee.") Illness is viewed as an imbalance in the flow of qi throughout the body. Acupuncture and related TCM therapies are all designed to alter the flow of qi and to return the body to a state of health and balanced qi. Numerous variations have evolved over the centuries, including the relatively recent use of electrical stimulation of needles at some acupuncture points during treatment sessions. Other (non-TCM) potential mechanisms by which acupuncture might be effective for certain conditions have been proposed as alternatives to TCM theories (6).

A modest amount of research on the effectiveness of acupuncture in stroke recovery has appeared in the Chinese research literature for several decades. Unfortunately, most of this early research does not meet current standards of clinical research methodology, so it is of limited utility in evaluating the effectiveness of acupuncture. Beginning in the early 1990s, research of much improved rigor began to appear, with variable findings regarding the efficacy of acupuncture to facilitate stroke recovery. The evidence in favor of therapeutic efficacy for stroke recovery was sufficiently strong to warrant a conclusion by the 1997 NIH Consensus Development Conference on acupuncture (7) that there was limited and encouraging evidence for the relationship between acupuncture and stroke recovery, although not yet enough to recommend its use as a medical procedure.

In the past 10 years, however, several controlled, randomized clinical trials examining the effects of acupuncture on stroke recovery have appeared that have failed to demonstrate a meaningful effect on recovery. Recently, several systematic reviews, including one meta-analysis, have concluded that the evidence for acupuncture is either weak or nonexistent (8–11). In the extensive meta-analysis by Sze et al. (12), however, the authors conclude that acupuncture is associated with a weak to moderate effect on motor recovery and activities of daily living, but they dismiss the relevance of these findings, attributing this effect to a true placebo effect rather than an effect specific to acupuncture. Conversely, this author conducted a review and reanalysis of these studies (13–15) and found that, after accounting for methodological flaws in several of the clinical trials, the evidence may, in fact, support the efficacy of this technique. Three of the more common methodological problems are briefly discussed here because of their relevance to other studies of stroke rehabilitation techniques.

Improvement Versus Absolute Level of Functioning as the Primary Outcome Measure. Many of the clinical trials of acupuncture do not statistically analyze the data as improvement (change) scores, but rather as absolute performance levels at follow-up. The use of change scores helps correct for baseline differences among subjects, an important issue given that baseline functional ability has been shown to be a key predictor of functional outcome after stroke.

Stroke Severity. There is some evidence that the anatomy and severity of a stroke play an important role in the responsiveness to acupuncture therapy and perhaps other treatment modalities as well. Many recent studies of therapies for stroke recovery, such as the EXCITE trial (16), exclude patients outside of a certain range of motor deficits, and some exclude subjects with brain stem strokes because of concerns that these individuals are less able to benefit from cortical plasticity. Naeser et al. (17) studied CT scan findings for 20 stroke survivors treated with acupuncture and found that efficacy correlated with stroke location and extent. Subjects who responded to acupuncture were found to have less than one-half of pyramidal tracts and periventricular white matter infarcted on the CT scan. Even though this finding has not yet been replicated, this preliminary study does suggest that stroke anatomy and severity need to be included when characterizing participants in acupuncture studies in stroke survivors. The possibility of both floor and ceiling effects for acupuncture therapy needs to be further explored as well to determine if patients with excessively severe or very mild strokes are unable to benefit from this treatment. Failure to consider this possibility poses a risk of diluting clinically meaningful effects in the moderately affected population.

Timing of Post-Treatment Assessment. Recovery from stroke commonly takes weeks to months, depending on severity. Because the biological mechanisms by which acupuncture might influence stroke recovery are not yet known, it is difficult to predict the time course of any beneficial effect acupuncture may provide. A number of studies of acupuncture for stroke recovery have chosen post-treatment assessment time frames that are quite short, such as assessing efficacy immediately at the completion of a two- to four-week treatment period. Given the uncertainty regarding the onset and duration of potential beneficial effects of acupuncture, it is important that studies provide adequate follow-up assessment (at least several months) to evaluate for the possibility of late improvement as a result of treatment. This pattern of continued improvement is evident in studies that have included a longer follow-up periods (18–20).

Systematic Reviews of Acupuncture and Stroke Rehabilitation. As mentioned above, several systematic reviews have appeared since the NIH consensus statement on acupuncture (7). All of which have concluded that there is no convincing evidence for the effectiveness of acupuncture in treating stroke (8–11). Although a potentially useful technique for aggregating the results of a number of clinical trials, systematic review and meta-analyses are inherently problematic as a means of determining efficacy of a therapy. Divergent results have often been found between meta-analyses and subsequent large, randomized, controlled clinical trials (21). Shiflett (15) has commented on a number of the flaws and limitations in these systematic reviews of acupuncture and stroke rehabilitation, including heterogeneous inclusion criteria. The efforts by the authors of these analyses to maintain a relatively homogenous population often leads to exclusion of important studies that do not fit their criteria, for example, exclusion of the study by Kjendahl et al (20) from the recently published reviews.

Other Outcomes. The systematic reviews of acupuncture have focused on motor recovery and global

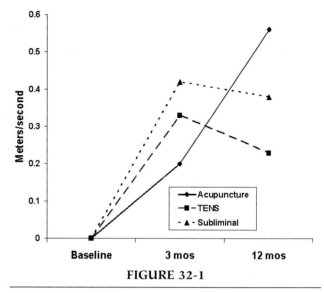

FIGURE 32-1

Walking speed as a function of acupuncture condition. (From Johansson et al. 2001)

measures of functional outcome, but several other aspects of recovery have been studied in specific studies. Even though the evidence base for these other applications is modest, these results do suggest that further study of these potential applications is warranted. The ability to maintain postural control in the presence of perturbation was found to be improved in acupuncture recipients compared with a control group of stroke survivors in one study (22). Similarly, walking speed was found to benefit from acupuncture in two studies (18, 19) (see Figure 32-1).

Two studies of acupuncture for treatment of dysphagia in stroke patients have recently been reported. Seki et al. (23), using video fluoroscopic swallowing study (VFSS) as an assessment tool, compared acupuncture to standard care in post-stroke patients with episodes of choking while eating or drinking. Thirty-two elderly subjects were randomly selected from elder care facilities and then randomly assigned to two groups: acupuncture plus usual care or usual care only. Acupuncture was administered three times a week for four weeks. A VFSS was performed at baseline and four weeks later at the end of the treatment period. Even though the control group showed no change or a slight increase in retention and aspiration, the acupuncture group showed major reductions in retention, from approximately 45% retention to 15–20% retention, and there was complete elimination of aspiration of water, fluid food, and solid food. Similar results for acupuncture on swallowing problems in stroke patients, also using VFSS, have been reported in a study performed several years earlier (24). In contrast, Park et al. (25) found that an acupuncture group had a higher percentage of unsafe swallows, as assessed by a bedside swallow screening test, than did the control group (p < 0.04). Unfortunately, no baseline assessment of swallowing was reported in this study, so that change in swallowing status cannot be determined.

Summary. The evidence for the efficacy of acupuncture after stroke is still best described as mixed, and definitive conclusions for or against the efficacy of this technique seem premature. In the absence of any specific medical contraindications, acupuncture generally seems safe and well-tolerated by stroke survivors, and patients and their families can thus be reassured that acupuncture is unlikely to interfere with the recovery process. The possibility of benefit combined with the favorable risk profile may lead some individuals to try this therapy even though data on efficacy remain indeterminate.

Massage and Pressure-based Techniques

Acupressure. Acupressure is a form of manual therapy that is based on the same TCM theory underlying acupuncture. Based on this meridian system, acupressure, like acupuncture, aims to balance the flow of qi and is used either preventatively or as a means of healing an illness. Even though acupuncture involves the insertion of needles in specific points along the meridians, acupressure uses the fingers to press these points. Because the same points are used in acupuncture as in acupressure, there is a general assumption that both techniques should have similar effects, although nonpenetrating acupressure might be expected to show milder effects. Practitioners suggest that acupressure might be appropriate for situations where acupuncture seems appropriate but the subject or patient is not willing to submit to needle insertion or acupuncture was unacceptably painful.

There are many different types of Oriental bodywork therapies that use acupressure. Among the most widely used in the United States are:

* Shiatsu (literally translated as "finger pressure" in Japanese)
* Jin shin jyutsu ("the art of circulation awakening")
* Jin shin do ("the way of the compassionate spirit")

What is common to all of the different acupressure systems is the use of sequenced applications of pressure to the meridian points (or *acupoints*) in order to tonify or sedate them (26, 27). Fundamental differences between the different forms of acupressure relate to the amount of pressure applied to the points, length of application, the intent of treatment (for example, overall relaxation or balance versus treating a specific condition), and philosophy (for example, the extent to which the treatment approach is integrated with other methods, such as Western manual manipulation techniques, dietary or herbal methods, or

psychology) (26). Only one study has examined the effectiveness of acupressure in stroke rehabilitation. In a small, poorly controlled study, Hogg (28) found that acupressure was more effective on several outcome measures than a control treatment consisting of lightly laying on of hands (therapeutic touch).

Marma Therapy. Marma therapy is a massage-based therapy originating in Indian Ayurvedic medicine. It involves stimulating Marma points with vigorous pressure to promote healing. In stroke, the pressure would typically be applied primarily to the affected side. There are 107 Marma points where flesh, veins, arteries, tendons, bones, and joints meet (29). The points are related to the yogic system of channels through which prana flows (nadis) rather than to the acupuncture meridian system. The effectiveness of Marma therapy is proposed to be related to the sensitivity of these points. Marma points are therefore selected on the basis of their sensitivity, which reduces as function returns (29).

What appears to be the first controlled study of Marma therapy for stroke is a small (N = 30), nonrandomized, controlled pilot trial on stroke patients with Barthel score <75 in an acute stroke unit (29). Outcomes for Marma therapy (three 45-minute sessions plus standard rehabilitation) were compared to outcomes for standard rehabilitation only. Although no statistically significant effect was detected on the Barthel at 12 weeks post-treatment, motoricity scores showed greater improvement for the Marma group at both 6 and 12 weeks after treatment. Despite its methodological limitations, this study demonstrates promise for this therapy and a larger, randomized, controlled trial seems appropriate. Similarly, further formal study of the related Ayurvedic and yoga-based interventions is needed.

MIND-BODY THERAPIES

The mind-body category of NCCAM contains a huge number of diverse interventions. Mind-body interventions, as the name implies, focus their therapeutic efforts on the interrelationship between mental and physical activities. In Eastern models, the two, mind and body, are inextricably intertwined, so physical and cognitive techniques are often discussed together in Western treatments of the subject. Techniques in this area can focus primarily on the mind (for example, hypnosis and meditation), on the body through physical movements (for example, exercise, Tai Chi, and yoga), or on a combination of both (for example, yoga exercises with meditation). For clarity and to more directly reflect the categories often used in PM&R, we divide these techniques into two sections: movement and mind-focused interventions.

Movement Therapies

A number of movement-based therapies, such as balance training and dance therapy, are utilized in physical rehabilitation, and a few can be thought of as alternative. Because of the limited mobility of many stroke patients, however, the application of these approaches is limited and often must be modified and simplified in order to safely accommodate their capabilities. Nevertheless, there is some evidence, often with non-stroke elderly patients, that suggests that these approaches should be considered and developed for future clinical use. Two therapies are briefly discussed here: Tai Chi and yoga.

Tai Chi and Qi Gong.   Tai Chi and the closely related Qi Gong are whole-body movement approaches based in TCM that use gentle, rhythmical, and ritualized movements of the arms and legs. Tai Chi is associated with and has emerged from the martial arts; Qi Gong, although using similar movements, generally refers to the use of breathing as well as stylized movements for healing purposes. Qi Gong can also refer to a form of subtle energy healing in which subtle energy or chi is emitted from a master into another person for healing purposes. In this chapter, Qi Gong refers to the stylized movements of a person with the purpose of moving the chi within his or her own bodies.

Tai Chi has been used with success in improving balance and reducing falls and fear of falling in fall-prone elderly subjects (30, 31), but research on stroke patients is limited. A small (N = 18) controlled study in Israel found that community-dwelling stroke survivors showed improvement in balance and speed of walking after a 12-week program of Tai Chi training twice per week. More research on this promising technique is warranted.

Yoga.   Yoga is a philosophical system that originated in India approximately 4,000 years ago and was primarily intended as a means toward increasing self-awareness. The term *yoga* means "union," referring to the universal self, and includes any practice designed to enhance this self-awareness. Thus, meditation, study of the Scriptures, pure devotion to God, repetition of a mantra, selfless service, physical, and many other practices are all forms of yoga. In the West, however, the term yoga usually refers to hatha yoga and encompasses a number of systems focusing on the physical body, using postures (asanas) along with other yogic practices. Yoga postures are designed to prepare the body for maximizing self-awareness. One advantage of yoga is that many poses can be performed in sitting or supine positions, so they thus may be safer and easier to perform for people with limited mobility.

Although there are numerous studies of the effect of yoga interventions on hypertension and cardiovascular physiology, which have some relevance to stroke prevention, a recent systematic review of the literature yielded no controlled trials of yoga for stroke rehabilitation (32). However, two small case series have been reported. One case series, involving four chronic (nine months to eight years post-CVA) stroke patients with hemiparesis, reported improvement in several outcome measures (Berg Balance Scale, Timed Movement Battery, and Stroke Impact Scale) after participation in an eight-week integrative yoga therapy program involving a number of classical seated, supine, and standing yoga postures, a short period of breathing exercises (pranayama), and a short meditation period (33). Lynton et al. (32) present the results of a small pilot study involving yoga in chronic stroke patients. The three participants in this study attended yoga classes twice a week for 12 weeks and underwent pre- and post-assessments using the O'Connor Tweezer Dexterity test, a timed test where the participant places pins in a peg board with tweezers, and the Boston Aphasia Exam for speech. All three participants showed improvement on both measures. The small sample size makes it impossible to draw definite conclusions, but the positive trends in these two small case series suggest that further research examining the usefulness of yoga in stroke recovery is warranted. In spite of the minimal published evidence on the utility of this treatment, a number of clinical rehabilitation programs do offer yoga as an option to patients, given its favorable safety profile and favorable anecdotal patient reports.

Mind-focused Therapies

This section includes interventions focused directly on cognitive processes that are intended to favorably affect the whole body.

Meditation.   With regard to stroke prevention, the most robust finding from the extensive research literature on meditation is the success of meditation for reducing hypertension (34–37) , and there is also evidence of reduction in cholesterol level in one study (38). Given the success of meditation for reducing hypertension and the fact that hypertension is a predisposing factor for stroke and recurrence of stroke, it seems reasonable to conclude that meditation may be effective in reduction of risk of recurrent stroke. In a well-controlled, randomized study comparing several relaxation techniques, regular practice of Transcendental Meditation by elderly nursing home residents was associated with significantly reduced systolic blood pressure and significantly increased three-year survival rate, when compared to the simple relaxation and no-treatment conditions (39), though the prevalence of stroke was not reported in this study population.

Biofeedback. Biofeedback is a therapeutic technique originally developed for muscle relaxation, but it has recently been used in a number of other ways as well. It is a good example of a family of techniques that remain on the boundary between alternative and mainstream, despite a substantial body of research evidence, including several meta-analyses (40–42).

Biofeedback for Physical Rehabilitation. The Ottawa Panel on EBCPGs reviewed and recommended several forms of EMG-based biofeedback therapy, finding the evidence supports its use for upper and lower extremities at all stages of stroke recovery. The Ottawa Panel also concluded that there is strong support for audio and video feedback training for unilateral neglect reduction in subacute stroke and general facilitation EMB-BFB training for upper and lower extremities, including rhythmic positional training in chronic stroke. They concluded that EMG-BFB should be included as an intervention for post-stroke patients who have a high level of motor return and where gait and standing are focuses of rehabilitation. More details on the specifics of the use of EMB-BFB in stroke rehabilitation can be found in the Ottawa Panel report (4). Positive, but less conclusive, research evidence for other uses of BFB in stroke recovery have been reported and should be considered when other interventions are not successful. For example, BFB may be helpful in controlling urinary incontinence (43–45). It appears to assist with some aspects of the rehabilitation of hemiparesis and mobility recovery, may be useful in the rehabilitation of swallowing in patients with dysphagia, and shows promise in the domain of controlling urinary incontinence.

Biofeedback for Cognitive Rehabilitation. A newer form of feedback is EEG-based feedback, or neurofeedback (43). In this approach, electrodes monitor the EEG activity at one or more scalp locations, and a computer displays information about the brain's activity to the patient. Then, operant conditioning combined with various cognitive strategies or functional tasks are used to train the patient to alter his or her own EEG activity in the desired direction. Given the relationship between EEG activity in particular frequency bands over specific cortical locations and metabolic rates of various cortical structures (46), this approach has been hypothesized to allow the therapist and patient to alter cortical metabolism and thereby influence neural activity and neuroplasticity in various regions of the brain (47, 48). Neurofeedback has been hypothesized to alter or accelerate the processes of functional reorganization of the cortex following stroke, thereby enhancing or accelerating functional recovery. Aside from two case reports in chronic stroke survivors suggesting improved cognitive functioning (49, 50), this technique remains untested in stroke patients, and its efficacy remains speculative at this time.

Interactive Metronome Therapy. Another novel technique for cognitive rehabilitation following stroke is Interactive Metronome Therapy (43). This technology uses operant conditioning of an individual's motor planning, sequencing, timing, and attention by having him or her engage in simple, repetitive motor tasks such as clapping the hands or tapping the feet in time with a set beat. The system provides both visual and auditory feedback to indicate how far off beat each repetition of the task is (in milliseconds) and whether the repetition was early (before the beat) or late (after the beat) to allow the individual to alter the rate of movement on a beat-by-beat basis. The tempo of the beat is adjustable. Thus, in the course of just over a second, the individual receives audio and visual feedback about his or her last response, tracks the next beat, adjusts his or her behavior accordingly, and makes the next response. The deceptively simple task is cognitively demanding, and many patients find it frustrating and confusing in the beginning of their treatment. The research on Interactive Metronome technology has focused largely on the remediation of attention deficit disorder in children (51), and, as yet, there is no published research evidence for its efficacy in stroke rehabilitation.

Mental Practice/motor Imagery. Mental practice (MP), or motor imagery, is a technique by which physical skills can be mentally rehearsed in a safe, repetitive manner. MP increases motor skill learning and performance in elderly individuals (52, 53), and the same neural and muscular structures are activated when movements are mentally practiced as during physical practice of the same skills (54–56). Other similarities between MP and physical practice include:

1. The time taken to mentally and physically perform movements is highly similar (57).
2. During MP, the speed/accuracy trade-off is maintained (58).
3. MP produces similar autonomic events as physical practice of the same skills (59).

Pilot data suggest that the addition of MP to motor therapy may actually yield greater motor improvement than conventional motor therapy in subacute (60, 61) and chronic stroke (62–67).

Optimizing Self-Healing Through Expectations and Beliefs. Virtually all alternative therapies acknowledge the inextricably intertwined nature of the mind and the body. Alternative systems of therapy seldom use only a single intervention, instead using multiple interventions that work on various aspects of both the mind and the body. Thus, a TCM practitioner might use acupuncture, herbs, massage (tui na), and energy healing (Qi Gong, and so forth) in a systematic and integrated treatment of the whole body, including the mind, rather than focusing on a single diagnosis or symptom. Similarly, in Ayurvedic medicine, herbs are a basic part of a treatment, but they are usually combined with physical manipulations (yoga and Marma therapy), breathing exercises, mantras or healing sounds, and meditation to quiet the mind and reduce stress. All of these systems of intervention work on both the mind and the body.

In Western medicine, the connection between the mind and the body is also well-known and acknowledged as a legitimate way of conceptualizing the way the body maintains a healthy state. Well-defined fields such as behavioral medicine, psychoneuroimmunology, psychiatry, and psychology all recognize and focus on the mind-body connection in health and healing. However, with the advent of powerful surgical and pharmacological interventions, conventional medicine has tended to push the mind part of the equation into the background, considering it to be a minor, if not irrelevant, component of the healing process. In fact, these belief-based processes have often been considered confounders in clinical research that is designed to look at the pure underlying mechanisms and healing ability of a medical intervention, free of any artifacts that might make the treatment look better or worse than it really was. The unwanted effects of these beliefs and expectations have come to be called *placebo*, from the Latin for "I please," in effect implying that patients are mindlessly following their doctor's suggestions. Rigorous, placebo-controlled, clinical research protocols have become the only true test of the underlying effectiveness of a treatment because they control, not only for the placebo effect, but also for placebo-like effects such as natural healing and other artifacts in the healing process.

Recently, some biomedical researchers have begun to look at the placebo effect more closely, not merely as a confounding phenomenon that occurs in research designs, but also as a possible source of healing per se (68–70). In an extensive review of the literature on the placebo effect, Walach and Jonas (70) have suggested that the placebo process should really be called something that reflects the fact that it is a "meaning attribution" process, and they provide suggestions, based on the literature, for enhancing the process whereby positive meaning is given to a clinical situation. From a therapeutic point of view, the placebo response can best be defined as the effect that is caused by the meaning of a therapeutic intervention for a particular patient and context (70). Notice that this "meaning response" definition acknowledges that humans are not deterministic machines mechanically reacting to external causes such as drugs, physical therapy, and so forth, but we respond in part as a result of our interpretation of what is happening to us, including the meaning

attached to a particular treatment and the manner in which the health-giver presents it. To the extent that a patient responds to the extracausal components of the intervention itself, it must be considered to be a real effect. If the environmental cues send a negative message about the therapy (technically referred to as a *nocebo*), we should expect to see a poorer result from the treatment. Similarly, if the cues are positive and supportive, the pure effects of the therapy can be expected to be enhanced. And the changes in treatment effectiveness are not simply because of willfulness or weak-mindedness on the part of the patient; they are real effects that emerge from the patient's attribution of meaning to the situation.

Health care providers who are developing integrative approaches to medicine, involving both conventional and nonconventional therapies, have begun to stress the importance of this mental component of the healing process. They are encouraging its use in the clinic and even conducting research designed specifically to assess the extent of and effectiveness of various placebo-inducing factors. It is also being argued that the term *placebo* should no longer be used to characterize this phenomenon because it has the negative connotation of weak-willed compliance to an authority figure (68). The suggestive component of this process not only includes the bedside manner of the caregivers, but it also includes the physical environment itself. More and more clinics are utilizing a healing environment approach to their space. Walls and equipment are in warm colors. Soothing music is available in the waiting room as well as the clinical suite. Invasive and complex-looking equipment is placed as unobtrusively as possible and so forth. Research on the effectiveness of these techniques is still in very early stages, but the importance of harnessing this meaning aspect of the placebo effect needs to be recognized (68, 70–72).

A useful list of ways to enhance the healing effects of a therapeutic intervention based on research literature on placebo has been presented by Walach and Jonas (70). Based on their literature review, they propose a number of ways to enhance the meaning attribution process in a clinical setting, which is presented here in Table 32-1.

Even though not all of these interventions may be easily applicable to a rehabilitation setting, they should suggest, by generalization, the types of things a clinician can do and say that will encourage the patient and facilitate the healing process. A whole body of research is emerging in which the effects of these interventions are being tested in rigorous research designs (68, 69). But, in the meantime, clinicians should take to heart the fact that the mind is a major component of healing and, over time, can facilitate or thwart the effects of even the most powerful physically focused intervention.

TABLE 32-1

Ways a Health Care Provider Can Optimize the Meaning Attribution Process in the Doctor-Patient Relationship (from Walach and Jonas 2004).

- Always work with—and not against—patient's expectations.
- If patients' expectations are unhealthy or harmful, work to change them first before jumping from intervention to intervention.
- Talking can induce a response toward cure. Rapport between doctor and patient is an important vehicle for suggesting therapeutic effects and enhancing expectations.
- One of the greatest skills of a doctor—and a topic often left out of the debate around evidence-based medicine—is individualization. It is in the subtle changes to therapy and how they are delivered by a skilled healer that the meaning response is harnessed to its fullest.
- Raising hope and alleviating anxiety in a credible way is one of the most therapeutic acts in general.
- It has been shown empirically that a simple act, such as giving a clear diagnosis and prognosis, improves outcome.
- A frequent assumption is that only specific causal effects count, like those produced by drugs or surgery. Other effects also count.
- Giving placebos is not identical to using the meaning response therapeutically. One need not give sugar pills. However, in some cases, the use of nonactive or minimally active drugs might be a better option than continuous medication of toxic, but effective, therapies.
- Therapeutic rituals might be helpful in eliciting the meaning response. It may be useful to help patients develop their own rituals, like taking a drug after a morning bath, in a special room, before or with prayer, or having it administered by a friend.

ENERGY MEDICINE

According to the NCCAM definition of energy medicine, this category includes any form of stimulation with external energy, such as electricity, as well as the more controversial forms of subtle energy, such as chi, Reiki, and so forth. The latter forms of energy are controversial because they cannot be detected with currently existing technology, hence the use by NCCAM of the term *putative* for these forms of energy. Because there is so little evidence for the subtle energy forms of therapy, except where observable interventions are used to influence this energy (as in yoga and Tai Chi), they will not be discussed further here.

Electrical Stimulation

Various forms of electrical stimulation have been used in treating specific medical problems associated with stroke. TENS is used to stimulate nerves in an effort to control pain, and therapeutic electrical stimulation is often used to stimulate paretic muscles in an effort to induce recovery of muscle function. The conventional applications of these techniques are covered in detail in Chapter 18. Electroacupuncture is another type of electrical stimulation used in stroke survivors. Unfortunately, the use of electricity with acupuncture in these studies is quite variable and inconsistent from study to study, so few conclusions can be drawn regarding the direct effects of the electrical stimulation independent of the effects caused by acupuncture per se. These studies are included in the general discussion of acupuncture above.

At least one study in which acupuncture is the primary focus used a form of TENS as the control condition (19). In this study, surface electrodes were applied to acupuncture points, and either a strong current (TENS) or an extremely low, undetectable current (sham TENS) was applied to acupuncture points, so the effectiveness of TENS relative to sham TENS, as well as (electro)acupuncture, could be estimated. No difference between acupuncture point TENS and sham TENS was seen for functional and motor recovery, though, on reanalysis, electroacupuncture appeared more effective than either in improving functional independence or walking speed (15). In a study by Wong (73), electrical acupuncture was defined as the application of electricity via surface electrodes over acupuncture points. In other words, it was a nonconventional form of TENS. Subjects with this form of treatment, combined with rehabilitation, did better on several neurologic and functional outcomes when compared to a rehabilitation-only control group. Based on these two studies, the evidence for what could be called *acupuncture-point TENS* appears mixed, but encouraging enough to warrant further research.

BIOLOGICALLY BASED INTERVENTIONS

Supplements, Herbs, and Homeopathic Remedies

A number of nutritional supplements and herbs have been suggested for the prevention of CVA and related diseases with varying degrees of research evidence. However, there is little evidence that these compounds can help in stroke recovery except perhaps in their ability to reduce the likelihood of a recurrence of a stroke (74). Natural agents, such as the antioxidant alpha lipoic acid, certain traditional Asian herbal mixtures, and some homeopathically prepared remedies, have been studied as a means of reducing infarct size. A number of nutrients and herbs have been proposed to assist in treatment of stroke-related complications such as pressure sores, urinary tract infections, and pneumonia (75). At this time, the evidence is insufficient to recommend nutritional supplements as well as herbal and homeopathic treatment options as adjuncts in stroke prevention, treatment, and rehabilitation. Moreover, some of these supplements may have interactions with conventional medications, such as warfarin, anticonvulsants, and so forth. Physicians should inform patients of these concerns, and they should review the appropriateness of any proposed herbal or nutritional supplement before patients initiate usage. The reader is referred to a more thorough review of these adjunctive treatments (74).

Ginkgo Biloba. The one herbal supplement for which there is a substantial amount of research in neurologic and vascular disorders is an extract of the ginkgo biloba leaf (76). The leaf of the ginkgo tree has been part of the traditional Chinese pharmacopoeia for 5,000 years. Standardized extracts of the ginkgo leaf are widely used in Asia, Germany, and France, and they are increasingly being used in the United States. Ginkgo shows promise in the treatment of some of the most salient and debilitating symptoms associated with stroke, cognitive functioning in particular, and other vascular and neurologic disorders. One example of this evidence reported that 50 subarachnoid hemorrhage patients who were administered ginkgo extract in a placebo-controlled, double-blind study showed significant improvements in attention and verbal short-term memory (77). Similarly, in another placebo-controlled study of patients with multi-infarct dementia or Alzheimer's disease showed modest, but significant, improvement in cognition on a geriatric assessment scale (78). The evidence for the use of ginkgo has been extensively reviewed by Diamond et al (76, 79), and their conclusions were that the evidence for ginkgo's effectiveness is mixed, but encouraging. More recently, however, a systematic review (80) concluded that gingko as a sole herb appears to have no consistent benefit in treatment of acute ischemic stroke; however, its role as part of more traditional herbal mixtures was not assessed (81). Discrepancies in the results of these reviews may be related to the strictness of the criteria for inclusion. The clinical applications and precautions for ginkgo use are discussed in detail by Diamond et al (76). One important caveat is that ginkgo has an anticoagulant effect and should be administered with caution in the presence of warfarin or aspirin and in individuals who have had a hemorrhagic stroke.

Hyperbaric Oxygen (HBO) Therapy. Hyperbaric oxygen (HBO) therapy is defined as the provision of oxygen at pressures above sea level (1 atmosphere absolute or ATA). This normally is accomplished by enclosing the patient within a pressurized (hyperbaric) chamber. Hyperbaric oxygen has been primarily used to treat decompression sickness and air embolism, but has been proposed as a treatment for stroke. Advocates note that stroke patients experience a deprivation of oxygen to areas of the brain and suggest that this treatment might enhance neuronal viability by its ability to increase the amount of dissolved oxygen in the blood without changing blood viscosity (82).

The evidence for hyperbaric oxygen therapy in chronic stroke is limited and controversial at best. Early, poorly controlled studies and surveys suggested that it might be helpful, but more recent studies come to the opposite conclusion. The treatment parameters remain uncertain, with a range of 1.5 ATM to 2.5 ATM proposed, and some suggest that treatment with pressures as high as 3.0 ATM for the initiation of therapy (83).

A recent, small clinical trial (84) randomized a small sample of chronic stroke patients to receive either 60 minutes of HBO in a chamber at 2.5 ATA versus a control treatment of 100% oxygen treatment in an HBO chamber at 1.14 ATA. The small amount of additional pressure in this condition was designed to facilitate blinding patients. Results indicated that a very low pressure of 100% oxygen (1.14 ATM) was more effective than a treatment at 2.5 ATM. Safety and toxicity have been concerns regarding HBO therapy (85–88). In the absence of convincing evidence of efficacy, this therapy cannot be recommended for clinical use at this time.

Chelation. Although EDTA-chelation therapy has long been FDA-approved for removing heavy metals from the blood, its use for other purposes is controversial. It has been advocated for the treatment and prevention of cardiovascular and cerebrovascular disorders, but there are no controlled trials to substantiate its use. In one uncontrolled trial, cerebral arterial occlusion was measured in 57 patients before and after treatment with 10 to 46 sessions of chelation therapy. Eighty-eight percent of the patients improved, with the criteria for improvement not stated, and cerebral arterial stenosis was reported to be reduced from a mean 28% to 10% (89). A retrospective analysis was conducted in Brazil of 2,870 patients who were treated with chelation therapy between 1983 and 1985 (90). These patients had a variety of vascular and degenerative diseases, with about 18% of the patients (504) diagnosed with cerebrovascular disease or degenerative CNS disease. The investigators reported "marked recovery" in 24% of the patients and "good recovery" in 60%. Animal studies with another chelating agent, deferoxamine, show that the hypoxic-ischemic injury is reduced if deferoxamine is administered soon after the injury (91–93). At present, the evidence of efficacy and safety is insufficient to recommend this treatment for stroke survivors.

CONCLUSION

The therapies presented above are by no means an exhaustive listing. The research-based evidence for the therapies discussed here varies from minimal to moderately positive. Many other CAM therapies have and will be proposed in the future, often with little empiric or theoretical basis for their use. Even though many of these therapies may be innocuous, ultimately, the criterion for incorporating any therapy into routine treatment (mainstream or nonconventional) must be researched, showing evidence of safety and efficacy. Some maintain that this fundamental requirement will eventually erase the distinction between conventional and alternative medicine (5). Unfortunately, this evidence base is likely to be long in coming.

In the meantime, however, clinicians need to treat patients while awaiting an adequate research evidence base. By way of comparison with allopathic (conventional) medicine, more than one-half of treatment recommendations in the area of antithrombotic therapy for cardiovascular disease lacked "Grade A" evidence in a recent consensus conference on this relatively well-researched area (94). Thus, even within conventional medicine, practitioners who aspire to provide evidence-based medicine often lack high-quality evidence to support this approach.

These facts should not be construed to justify the indiscriminant use of unproven therapies, but do highlight the fact that health care providers today utilize a more informal, but time-honored, method of selecting treatments. Even though the same evidence-basing procedures need to be applied to all therapies, whether conventional or nonconventional, it is important to recognize that many alternative therapies have a very low risk of adverse reactions. In the absence of clear evidence of efficacy, but with a low risk of harm, many patients and their caregivers are willing to accept CAM therapies to treat symptoms that are otherwise not yet amenable to proven therapies.

Most alternative therapies will be used in conjunction with other therapies, and the most judicious use of alternative or complementary therapies will generally be as an adjunct to well-established conventional therapies that are considered to be standard of care. In some cases, alternative therapies can be explored when other therapies appear to have run the course of their effectiveness. In many cases, the use of CAM therapies is initiated by patients, and clinicians need to determine how to deal with these therapies. Communication with patients, including an honest appraisal of the evidence base for both conventional and CAM treatments, is the best approach for safely and appropriately using these therapies in clinical practice.

References

1. Eisenberg DM, Kessler RC, Foster C, et al. Unconventional medicine in the United States: Prevalence, costs, and patterns of use. *N Engl J Med* 1993; 328:246–252.
2. Eisenberg DM, Davis RB, Ettner SL, et al. Trends in alternative medicine use in the United States, 1990–1997: Results of a follow-up national survey. *JAMA* 1998; 280:1569–1575.
3. Kessler HH. The knife is not enough. New York: WW Norton, 1968.
4. Ottawa Panel. Ottawa Panel evidence-based clinical practice guidelines for post-stroke rehabilitation. *Topics in Stroke Rehabilitation* 2006; 13(2):1–269.
5. Fontanarosa PB, Lundberg GD. Alternative medicine meets science. *JAMA* 1998; 280:1618–1619.
6. Andersson S, Lundeberg T. Acupuncture—from empiricism to science: Functional background to acupuncture effects in pain and disease. *Med Hypotheses* 1995; 45:271–281.
7. NIH Consensus Conference. Acupuncture. *JAMA* 1998; 280:1518–1524.
8. Park J, Hopwood V, White AR, Ernst E. Effectiveness of acupuncture for stroke: A systematic review. *J Neurol* 2001; 248:558–563.
9. Zhang SH, Liu M, Asplund K, Li L. Acupuncture for stroke. *Cochrane Database Syst Rev* 2005; 18(2):CD003317.
10. Sze FK-H, Wong E, Yi X, Woo J. Does acupuncture have additional value to standard poststroke motor rehabilitation? *Stroke* 2002; 33:186–194.
11. Wu HM, Tang JL, Lin XP, et al. Acupuncture for stroke rehabilitation. *Cochrane Database Syst Rev.* 2006; 19(3):CD004131.
12. Sze FK, et al. Does acupuncture improve motor recovery after stroke? A meta-analysis of randomized controlled trials. *Stroke* 2002; 33:2604–2619.
13. Shiflett SC. Commentary on Akupunktur bei Schlaganfall (Acupuncture with Stroke). *Forschende Komplementarmedizin/Research in Complementary Medicine* 1999; 6:274–276.
14. Shiflett SC. Acupuncture and stroke rehabilitation. *Stroke* 2001; 34:1934–1936.
15. Shiflett SC. Evidence for the effectiveness of acupuncture in stroke rehabilitation. *Topics in Stroke Rehabilitation* in press.
16. Wolf SL, Winstein CJ, Miller JP, et al. Effect of constraint-induced movement therapy on upper extremity function 3 to 9 months after stroke: The EXCITE randomized clinical trial. *JAMA* 2006.

17. Naeser MA, Alexander MP, Stiassny-Eder D, et al. Real versus sham acupuncture in the treatment of paralysis in acute stroke patients: A CT scan lesion site study. *J Neurol Rehabil* 1992; 6:163–173.
18. Johansson K, Lindgren I, Widner H, et al. Can sensory stimulation improve the functional outcome in stroke patients? *Neurology* 1993; 43:2189–2192.
19. Johansson BB, Haker E, von Arbin M, et al. Acupuncture and transcutaneous nerve stimulation in stroke rehabilitation: A randomized, controlled trial. *Stroke* 2001; 32:707–713.
20. Kjendahl A, Sallstrom S, Osten PE, Stanghelle JK. A one year follow-up study on the effects of acupuncture in the treatment of stroke patients in the subacute stage: A randomized, controlled study. *Clinical Rehabilitation* 1997; 11:192–200.
21. LeLorier J. Gregoire G. Benhaddad A. Lapierre J. Derderian F. Discrepancies between meta-analyses and subsequent large randomized, controlled trials. *New England Journal of Medicine* 1997; 337(8):536–542.
22. Magnusson M, Johansson K, Johansson BB. Sensory stimulation promotes normalization of postural control after stroke. *Stroke* 1994; 25:1176–1180.
23. Seki T, Iwasaki K, Arai H, et al. Acupuncture for dysphagia in post-stroke patients: A videofluoroscopic study. *JAGS* 2005: 53:1083–1084.
24. Nowicki NC, Averill A. Acupuncture for dysphagia following stroke. *Medical Acupuncture: A Journal for Physicians by Physicians* 2003; 14(3):17–19.
25. Park J, White AR, et al. Acupuncture for subacute stroke rehabilitation: A sham-controlled, subject- and assessor-blind, randomized trial. *Arach Intern Med* 2005; 165:2026–2031.
26. Rubik B, Pavek R. Manual healing methods. In: *Alternative Medicine: Expanding Medical Horizons, A Report to the National Institutes of Health on Alternative Medical Systems and Practices in the United States.* Chantilly, VA: 1992.
27. Vickers A. *Complementary Medicine and Disability: Alternatives for People with Disabling Conditions.* London: Chapman & Hall, 1993.
28. Hogg PK. The effects of acupressure on the psychological and physiological rehabilitation of the stroke patient. *Dissertations Abstract International* 1986; 47(2-B):841.
29. Fox M, Dickens A, Greaves C, et al. Marma therapy for stroke rehabilitation: A pilot study. *J Rehabil Med* 2006; 38:268–271.

30. Wolf SL, Barnhart HX, Kutner NG, et al. Reducing frailty and falls in older persons: An investigation of Tai Chi and computerized balance training. *J Am Geriatr Soc* 2003; 51:1794–1803.

31. Choi JH, Moon JS, Song R. Effects of sun-style Tai Chi exercise on physical fitness and fall prevention in fall-prone older adults. *J Adv Nurs* 2005; 51:150–157.

32. Lynton H, Kligler B, Shiflett SC. Yoga in stroke rehabilitation: A systematic review and results of a pilot study. *Topics in Stroke Rehabilitation* in press.

33. Bastille JV, Gill-Body KM. A yoga-based exercise program for people with chronic post-stroke hemiparesis. *Physical Therapy* 2004; 84(1):33–48.

34. Benson H. Systemic hypertension and the relaxation response. *New England Journal of Medicine* 1977; 296:1152–1156.

35. Hafner RJ. Psychological treatment of essential hypertension: A controlled comparison of meditation and meditation plus biofeedback. *Biofeedback and Self Regulation* 1982; 7:305–316.

36. Schneider RH, Alexander CN, Wallace RK. In search of an optimal behavioral treatment for hypertension: a review and focus on transcendental meditation. In: Gentry WD, Julius S, eds. *Personality, Elevated Blood Pressure, and Essential Hypertension.* Washington DC: Hemisphere, 1992.

37. Wallace RK, et al. Systolic blood pressure and long-term practice of the Transcendental Meditation and TM-Sidhi program: Effects of TM on systolic blood pressure. *Psychosomatic Medicine* 1983; 45:41–46.

38. Cooper MJ, Aygen MM. A relaxation technique in the management of hypercholesterolemia. *Journal of Human Stress* 1979; 5:24–27.

39. Alexander CN, et al. Transcendental meditation, mindfulness, and longevity: An experimental study with the elderly. *Journal of Personality and Social Psychology* 1989; 57(6):950–964.

40. Moreland JD, Thomson MA, Fuoco AR. Electromyographic biofeedback to improve lower extremity function after stroke: A meta-analysis. *Archives of Physical Medicine and Rehabilitation* 1998; 79(2):134–140.

41. Schleenbaker RE MA. Electromyographic biofeedback for neuromuscular reeducation in the hemiplegic stroke patient: A meta-analysis. *Archives of Physical Medicine and Rehabilitation* 1993; 74(12):1301–1304.

42. Glanz M, Klawansky S, Stason W, et al. Biofeedback therapy in post-stroke rehabilitation: A meta-analysis of the randomized controlled trials. *Arch Phys Med Rehabil* 1995; 76:508–515.

43. Nelson LA. The role of biofeedback in stroke rehabilitation: Past and future directions. *Topics in Stroke Rehabilitation* in press.

44. Thomas LH BJ, Cross S, French B, et al. Prevention and treatment of urinary incontinence after stroke in adults. *Cochrane Database of Systematic Reviews* 2005; (3):CD004462.

45. Capelini MV RC, Dambros M, Tamanini JT, et al. Pelvic floor exercises with biofeedback for stress urinary incontinence. *Int Braz J Urol* 2006; 32:462–469.

46. Alper KR, John ER, Brodie J, et al. Correlation of PET and qEEG in normal subjects. *Psychiatry Research: Neuroimaging* 2006; 146(3):271–282.

47. Lee JS, Lee DS, Oh SH, et al. PET Evidence of neuroplasticity in adult auditory cortex of postlingual deafness. *J Nucl Med* 2003 2003; 44(9):1435–1439.

48. Detre JA. Clinical applicability of functional MRI. *Journal of Magnetic Resonance Imaging* 2006; 23(6):808–815.

49. Rozelle GR BT. Neurotherapy for stroke rehabilitation: A single case study. *Biofeedback Self Regul* 1995; 20(3):211–228.

50. Bearden TS, Cassisi JE, Pineda M. Neurofeedback training for a patient with thalamic and cortical infarctions. *Applied Psychophysiology and Biofeedback* 2003; 28(3):241–253.

51. Shaffer RJ JL, Cassily JF, Greenspan SI, et al. Effect of interactive metronome training on children with ADHD. *Am J Occup Ther* 2001; 55(2):155–162.

52. Fansler CL, Poff CL, Shepard KF. Effects of mental practice on balance in elderly women. *Phys Ther* 1985; 65(9):1332–1337.

53. Linden CA, Uhley JE, Smith D, Bush MA. The effects of mental practice on walking balance in an elderly population. *Occ Ther J Res* 1989; 9:155–169.

54. Decety J, Ingvar DH. Brain structures participating in mental simulation of motor behavior: A neuropsychological interpretation. *Acta Psycholog.* 1990; 73(1):13–34.

55. Weiss T, Hansen E, Beyer L, et al. Activation processes during mental practice in stroke patients. *Int J Psychophysiol* 1994; 17(1):91–100.

56. Ito M. Movement and thought: Identical control mechanisms by the cerebellum. *Trends Neurosci* 1993; 16(11): 453–454.

57. Decety J, Jeannerod M, Prablanc C. The timing of mentally represented actions. *Behav Brain Res* 1989; 34(1–2):35–42.

58. Decety J, Jeannerod M. Mentally simulated movements in virtual reality: Does Fitts's law hold in motor imagery? *Behav Brain Res* 1995; 72(1–2):127–134.

59. Roure R, Collet C, Deschaumes-Molinaro C, et al. Autonomic nervous system responses correlate with mental rehearsal in volleyball training. *Eur J Appl Physiol Occup Physiol.* 1998 Jul; 78(2):99–108.

60. Page SJ, Levine P, Sisto S, Johnston M. A randomized, efficacy, and feasibility study of imagery in acute stroke. *Clin Rehabil* 2001; 15(3):233–240.

61. Page SJ, Levine P, Sisto S, Johnston M. Imagery combined with physical practice for upper limb motor deficit in sub-acute stroke: A case report. *Phys Ther* 2001; 81(8):1455–1462.

62. Page SJ. Imagery improves motor function in chronic stroke patients with hemiplegia: A pilot study. *Occ Ther J Res* 2000; 20(3):200–215.

63. Page SJ, Levine P, Leonard AC. Effects of mental practice on affected limb use and function in chronic stroke. *Arch Phys Med Rehabil* 2005; 86(3):399–402.

64. Crosbie JH, McDonough SM, Gilmore DH, Wiggam MI. The adjunctive role of mental practice in the rehabilitation of the upper limb after hemiplegic stroke: A pilot study. *Clin Rehabil* 2004; 18(1):60–68.

65. Dijkerman HC, Letswaart M, Johnston M, MacWalter RS. Does motor imagery training improve hand function in chronic stroke patients? A pilot study. *Clin Rehabil* 2004; 18(5):538–549.

66. Dunsky A, Dickstein R, Ariav et al. 2006. Motor imagery practice in gait rehabilitation of chronic post-stroke hemiparesis: Four case studies. *Int J Rehabil Res.* 2006 Dec; 29(4):351–356.

67. Sharma N, Pomeroy VM, Baron JC. Motor imagery: A back door to the motor system after stroke? *Stroke* 2006; 37:1941–1952.

68. Kaptchuk TJ, Goldman P, Stone DA, Stason WB. Do medical devices have enhanced placebo effects? *Journal of Clinical Epidemiology* 2000; 53:786–792.

69. Hammerschlag R. Methodological and ethical issues in clinical trials of acupuncture. *J Altern Complement Med* 1998; 4:159–171.

70. Walach H, Jonas WB. Placebo research: The evidence base for harnessing self-healing capacities. *Journal of Alternative and Complementary Medicine* 2004; 10(Suppl 1):S103–S112.

71. Birch S. A review and analysis of placebo treatments, placebo effects, and placebo controls in trials of medical procedures when sham is not inert. *J Altern Complement Med* 2006; 12:303–310.

72. Frenkel O. A phenomenology of the "placebo effect": Taking meaning from the mind to the body. *Journal of Medicine and Philosophy* 2008; 33:58–79.

73. Wong AMK, Su T, Tang F, et al. Clinical trial of electrical acupuncture on hemiplegic stroke patients. *American Journal of Physical Medicine and Rehabilitation* 1999; 78:117–122.

74. Bell IR. Adjunctive care with nutritional, herbal, and homeopathic complementary and alternative medicine modalities in stroke treatment and rehabilitation. *Topics in Stroke Rehabilitation* in press.

75. Loeb M, High, K. The effect of malnutrition on risk and outcome of community-acquired pneumonia. *Respir Care Clin N Am* 2005; 11(1):99–108.

76. Diamond BJ, Shiflett SC, Feiwel N, et al. Ginkgo biloba extract: mechanisms and clinical indications. *Archives of Physical Medicine and Rehabilitation* 2000; 81:668–678.

77. Weiss H, Kallischnigg G. Ginkgo-biloba-extrakt (EGb 761): Meta-analyse von Studien. *Munchner Medizinishe Wochenschrift* 1991; 133(Suppl 1):S34–S37.

78. Le Bars PL, Katz MM, Berman N, et al. A placebo-controlled, double-blind, randomized trial of an extract of Ginkgo biloba for dementia. *JAMA* 1997; 278:1327–1332.

79. Diamond BJ, Shiflett SC, Feiwel N, et al. Ginkgo biloba extract: Mechanisms, clinical indications and comments. In: B Vellas, JL Fitten, et al., eds. *Research and Practice in Alzheimer's Disease*, 2002.

80. Zeng X, Liu M, Yang Y, et al. Ginkgo biloba for acute ischaemic stroke. *Cochrane Database Syst Rev* 2005; 4:CD003691.

81. Liu J. The use of Ginkgo biloba extract in acute ischemic stroke. *Explore* 2006; 2(3):262–263.

82. Mink RB, Dutka AJ. Hyperbaric oxygen after global cerebra ischemia in rabbits reduces brain vascular permeability and blood flow. *Stroke* 1995; 26:2307–2312.

83. Hart GB, Strauss MB. Hyperbaric oxygen therapy. *Stroke* 2003; 34:e153–155.

84. Rusnyiak DE. Oxygen therapy in ischemic stroke. *Stroke* 2003; 34:e154–155.

85. Anderson DC, Bottini AG, et al. A pilot study of hyperbaric oxygen in the treatment of human stroke. *Stroke* 1991; 22:1137–1142.

86. Nighoghossian N, Trouillas P, Adeleine P, Salord F. Hyperbaric oxygen in the treatment of acute ischemic stroke. *Stroke* 1995; 26:1369–1372.

87. Blenkarn GD, Schanberg SM, Saltzman HA. Cerebral amines and acute hyperbaric oxygen toxicity. *J Pharmacol Exp Ther* 1969; 166:346–353.

88. Weinstein PR, Anderson GG, Telles DA. Results of hyperbaric oxygen therapy during temporary middle cerebral artery occlusion in unanaesthetized cats. *Neurosurgery* 1987; 20:518–524.

89. McDonagh EW, Rudolph CJ, Cheraskin E. An oculocerebrovasculometric analysis of the improvement in arterial stenosis following EDTA chelation therapy. In: Cranton EM, ed. *A Textbook on EDTA Chelation Therapy.* New York, Human Sciences Press, 1989:155–166.

90. Olszewer E, Carter JP. EDTA chelation therapy in chronic degenerative disease. *Medical Hypotheses* 1988; 27(1):41–49.

91. Palmer C, Roberts RL, Bero C. Deferoxamine post-treatment reduces ischemic brain injury in neonatal rats, *Stroke* 1994; 25(5):1039–1045.

92. Hurn PD, et al. Deferoxamine reduces early metabolic failure associated with severe cerebral ischemic acidosis in dogs. *Stroke* 1995; 26(4):688–695.

93. Babbs CF. Role of iron ions in the genesis of reperfusion injury following successful cardiopulmonary resuscitation: Preliminary data and a biochemical hypothesis. *Annals of Emergency Medicine* 1985; 14(8):777–783.

94. Dalen JE. "Conventional" and "unconventional" medicine: Can they be integrated? *Arch Int Med* 1998; 158:2179–2181.

33 Seating, Assistive Technology, and Equipment

Rory A. Cooper
Bambi Roberts Brewer
Rosemarie Cooper

Katya Hill
Patricia Karg
Amol Karmarkar

Amy Karas Lane
Roger Little
Tamara L. Pelleshi

Assistive technology (AT) plays a significant role in the lives of individuals with disabilities to help maintain, increase, or improve the functional activities of daily living (ADLs) within the home and community. Appropriate selection and application of technology has a great potential to not only contribute but also improve the quality of life of the individual.

This chapter will provide a brief insight into the range of AT applicable for individuals who have experienced physical impairments as a result of a severe stroke. An important step to ensure appropriate selection of AT is to start with an AT team that consists of qualified AT professionals who have a keen interest to include and encourage active participation of the end user in the AT evaluation and selection process as described in the AT service delivery model. Sections covered in this chapter include AT interventions in wheelchair seating and mobility, electronic aids for daily living, augmentative and alternative communication adaptive driving, wheelchair transportation safety, and robotic rehabilitation devices, as they may be applied and fit into the individual's stroke recovery and rehabilitation process.

AT SERVICE DELIVERY MODEL

A successful AT service delivery model requires specialized knowledge in the design and application of AT, as it has tremendous potential to have a positive impact on the community integration of people with disabilities.

The specialized knowledge starts out with the AT assessment team that consists of physiatrists, occupational and/or physical therapists, speech language therapists with specialty training/certification, rehabilitation engineering technologists, and qualified equipment suppliers. Other professionals may also be consulted depending on the needs and goals of the client. Rehabilitation counselors, nurses, personal care assistants, and other similar professionals can also make important contributions to the AT service delivery team.

To assure that specialized knowledge is present within the AT assessment team, the Rehabilitation Engineering and Assistive Technology Society of North America (RESNA) (www.resna.org) offers a credentialing program in AT to clinicians and suppliers. RESNA offers three levels of credentials, as outlined in the following paragraphs: Assistive Technology Supplier (ATS),

543

Assistive Technology Provider (ATP), and Rehabilitation Engineering Technologist (RET).

RESNA offers the Assistive Technology Supplier (ATS) credential. In order to attain the ATS credential, an individual must demonstrate compensated employment in the field of AT and pass an examination that consists of fundamental elements and case-based scenarios. Suppliers with the ATS credential have demonstrated a minimum level of knowledge and experience with AT. Clinics should give careful consideration to encouraging the suppliers who work with them to demonstrate that their employees hold the ATS credential.

In order to identify clinicians who are specialized in AT service provision, RESNA created the Assistive Technology Provider (ATP) credential. The ATP requires demonstrated experience in a mentored AT service environment and the passage of an examination. Many of the most highly regarded AT clinics have therapists with the ATP credential (1).

For engineers and technicians who have been supporting AT clinics, RESNA created the Rehabilitation Engineering Technologist (RET) credential. The RET credential first requires an individual to hold an engineering or technology degree. After a suitable period of clinical AT service delivery experience, individuals are eligible to sit for the ATP examination and the supplemental RET examination. Individuals earn the RET designation if they pass both of these examinations. These credentials help consumers to identify individuals who have acquired specialized knowledge of AT and are committed to providing high-quality services.

The design and application of the AT service delivery starts out with the introduction of the client to the AT assessment team and empowering the client to be an active decision-making member of that team.

A proper assessment begins with an initial interview that involves listening and paying attention to the client's needs, concerns, and goals for a device. It is important to understand the medical variables—assessed by the physiatrist and shared with the team on how underlying medical conditions may impact the prescription of a AT device—as well as the physical and functional variables assessed by the therapists on how physical capacities and limitations affect mobility and instrumental ADLs. It is important to know how the client performs tasks, where the deficits are, and how AT can compensate for deficits to augment task performance. The user is given an opportunity to try the equipment to determine how he or she best performs and assesses this. Transportation variables are also important to consider if transporting the wheelchair and seating system is an essential goal. The person who will be stowing the device should get an opportunity to try it prior to the final prescription being written.

The AT team members will explain the outcomes, reasons, and facts upon which they based the final recommendation of the device to the client; however, the final decision on the mobility device lies with the client, the family, and/or caregivers.

The assessment and service delivery process is completed during delivery of the new device with the client, and the therapist signs off on the correctness of the final fitting and operation of the new AT device.

SEATING/MOBILITY

Seating

AT for seating and positioning for a person after a stroke can vary according to the individual's needs. Several seating challenges can occur following a CVA. These challenges are secondary to but not limited to two main factors:

1. Poor trunk balance and muscle tone caused by hemiplegia
2. Increased extensor tone more notably evident following a left CVA with right-sided involvement

Several residuals from the stroke can affect the person's ability to complete many daily tasks that he or she was able to previously perform. These residuals include impairments with motor skills, cognition, and vision. It is important that the individual requiring the use of a mobility device become more functionally independent with his or her ADL needs while seated in the wheelchair. A key to functional seating involves stabilizing the pelvis. A rule of thumb to remember with seating is that pelvic stability leads to enhanced upper trunk stability.

As aforementioned, stabilizing the pelvis is the first step in improving upper trunk mobility, thus increasing ability to perform ADL skills. There are several seat cushions available on the market, which include solid and contoured bases (Figure 33-1; Figure 33-2). If pressure management is an issue, seat cushions can be comprised of air, gel, or simply just a soft foam. Knowing your patient's skin integrity is crucial to cushion selection.

A contoured seat base can be utilized for the individual with hemiplegia. The contour of the base will aid in maintaining the pelvis, hips, and lower extremities in neutral alignment. The degree of the contour will depend on the amount of support that the individual needs to maintain the position.

An anti-thrust cushion will prevent the individual with extensor tone from sliding forward on the seat (Figure 33-3). The anti-thrust cushion is higher in the front, thus providing a shelf that makes it difficult for the individual to overcome. Placing a seat dump, that is, the front of the seat frame is higher than the back, in the frame of the wheelchair can provide the same effect as the cushion.

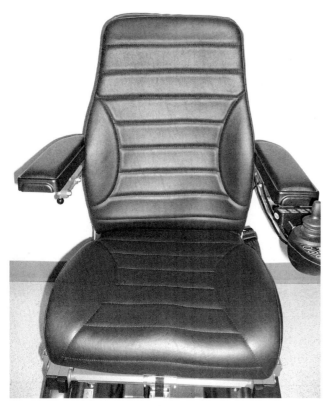

FIGURE 33-1

Example of an Ergo contoured seating system.

Thigh guides placed along the lateral aspect of the upper portion of the lower extremity will provide lower extremity support and alignment (Figure 33-4). The thigh guide will prevent external rotation and abduction of the hip joint.

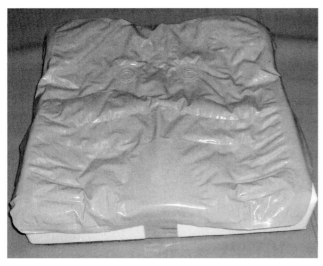

FIGURE 33-2

Example of a contour molded cushion with gel-filled inserts.

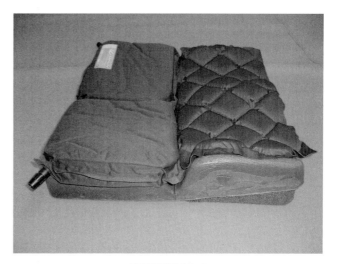

FIGURE 33-3

Example of anti-thrust cushion.

Adductor pads can be placed lateral to the knee joint to provide support and prevent adduction, thus improving neutral alignment. An abductor pad for lower extremity alignment will prevent abduction and internal rotation of the hip. The abductor is placed between the knees. This can be an external pad that is removable, or it can be incorporated into the contoured seat base.

A solid seat provides a static surface on which the cushion can be placed. This support prevents the cushion

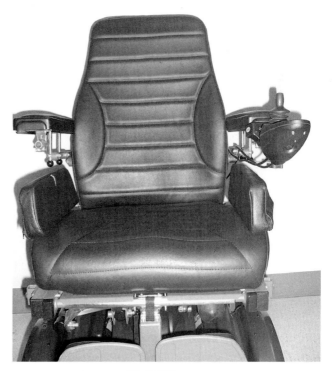

FIGURE 33-4

Example of thigh guide placement.

from contouring to the surface it is placed upon. A pelvic belt will also assist in maintaining the pelvis in position. The belt can be a standard two-point or four-point. The point value refers to numbers of attachment to the frame. Four points of attachment provides greater contact, thus controlling and supporting the pelvis.

Lower extremity alignment and support is critical in maintaining pelvic stability. It is necessary that the individual achieves full foot contact and placement on the footplates. Without foot support, the individual will slide and shift on the seat. The hanger angle of the wheelchair frame is an important part of achieving foot placement. A range of motion assessment will provide information needed to determine the appropriate leg rest hanger configuration. When using elevating legrests, the individual should maintain foot contact as well as knee extension throughout the elevation process. Angle adjustable footplates can be adjusted to assure foot contact in the event of decreased ankle range of motion or ankle instability at neutral posturing.

Stability of the upper trunk can be achieved by utilizing a variety of back supports. Back support can be provided through the use of a solid or flat surface, a contoured (mild, moderate, or deep) surface, or upholstery (Figure 33-5; Figure 33-6; Figure 33-7). The decision and type of back support to be utilized depends largely upon the individual's trunk balance. A large variety of back supports not mentioned is also available and is more specific for spinal deformities.

A solid back support provides static stability. The solid support allows for greater wheel strikes when

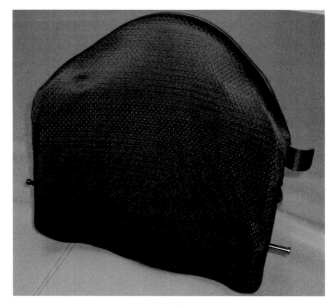

FIGURE 33-6

Moderate contoured back.

propelling as the upper extremities have full range of movement without contact of an external source. The use of a lateral support can be utilized with the solid back to prevent the individual from leaning sideways when sitting or traveling.

The contoured back support provides for lateral stability of the upper trunk. The amount of contour depends on the amount of support the individual requires to remain upright. Adjustable tension back upholstery can provide upper trunk stability without the need to utilize

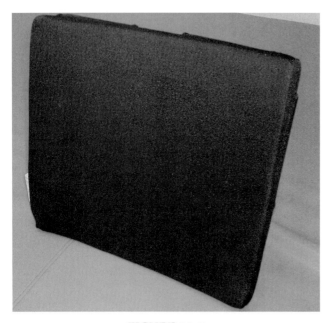

FIGURE 33-5

Flat solid back.

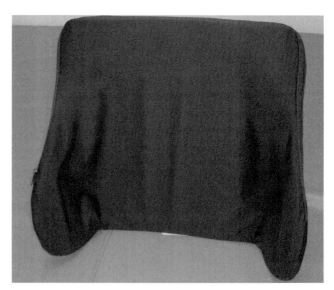

FIGURE 33-7

Deep contoured back.

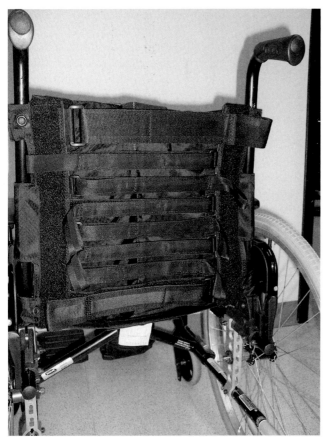

FIGURE 33-8

Example of adjustable tension back upholstery.

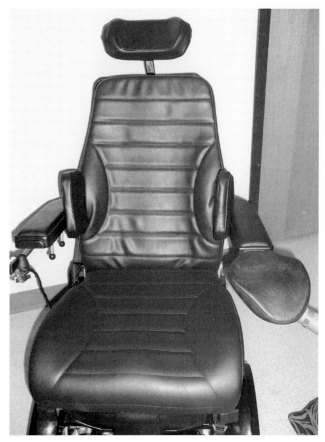

FIGURE 33-9

Example of seating system with arm trough with custom palmer support and lateral trunk supports.

a back support (Figure 33-8). This will aid in keeping the overall weight of the wheelchair down for the individual who is a self-propeller.

Lateral trunk supports attached to the side frame of the wheelchair provide stability and support of the upper trunk. The sizes of the supports vary and should be ordered according to the individual's size. Placement of the support is also crucial, as it should not be placed directly under the axilla because it may cause nerve impingement.

Support of the effected upper extremity for the individual with hemiplegia is also important. Assortments of arm troughs are available on the market. The arm trough will provide for full contact and support of the distal portion of the upper extremity, thus preventing it from falling from the armrest (Figure 33-9). The palmer portion of the arm trough can be provided in a variety of shapes, depending on the individual's hand positioning needs. The arm troughs are attached to the frame of the armrest. Height adjustable armrests are necessary, as they assure adequate shoulder placement and support. A subluxation is often evident with hemiparesis, so proper height adjustment is needed to assure the shoulder joint

is placed properly in the socket. A lap tray can also be utilized for upper extremity support. The tray can be a full- or half-design.

Other seating features that can be incorporated into the frame of the wheelchair are tilt-in-space and recline. Tilt-in-space can be utilized for the individual who is unable to sit upright against gravity. The tilt-in-space provides a gravity-decreased plane, thus improving sitting (Figure 33-10). Tilt-in-space can also provide pressure relief for the individual who is unable to independently change position and shift the weight for effective pressure relief maneuvers. When utilizing a tilt-in-space seating system, it is recommended to add a headrest for cervical support and stability. Headrests also come in a large variety of shapes and sizes, and selection is based on comfort and functional support.

The reclining back wheelchair can first be utilized in the event that the individual has systemic issues that may prevent him or her from sitting upright. Overall, the use of a reclining back wheelchair is typically not beneficial to the individual with hemplegia. Reclining the back opens the hip angle, thus decreasing the stability of the pelvis.

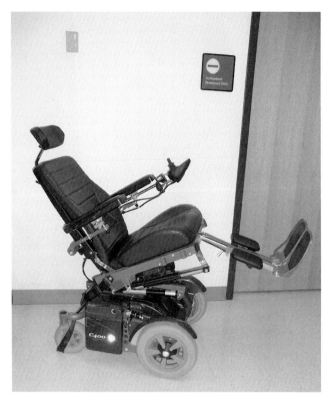

FIGURE 33-10

Example of tilt-in-space seating system.

The lack of control of the pelvis can lead to poor support and alignment of the upper and lower trunk. Tilt-in-space is the preferred alternative to meet individual's seating and positioning needs.

This section was completed as an attempt to provide a basic insight into the specific seating and positioning needs for persons after CVA. For more in-depth reading into this topic, please refer to the reference list at the end of this chapter.

Mobility

Use of wheelchairs, including both manual and electric power, could be a transient or long-term need for individuals after CVA. Therefore, like any other piece of AT device, wheelchair selection, customization, and delivery process after CVA has to be an individually tailored procedure. Also, utilization of wheelchairs could significantly alter limitations that could result after CVA, which could be based on changes in physical functioning and use of alternative mobility aids, especially during the first year after CVA (2). Periodic assessments before wheelchair prescription is a key factor, which should include physical, sensory, cognitive, perceptual, behavioral, and environmental assessment along with identification of other barriers for use of a wheeled mobility device. Recent

literature have indicated use of Wheelchair Skills Test (WST) and Wheelchair Collision Test (WCT) as screening measures specifically designed for individuals after CVA for identifying problems related to use of wheeled mobility devices, which could also serve as a guideline for customization of the prescribed device (3, 4).

Manual Wheelchairs

For individuals after CVA, manual wheelchair (MWC) propulsion could become very tiresome because of several factors such as primary use of one upper/lower extremity for propulsion, limited coordination between the available extremities, and problems with visual-perceptual abilities. Despite these difficulties, MWCs have been considered as a primary aid for independent mobility for this population (5).

Attendant-Propelled. This type of MWC is typically used as a dependent mobility option for individuals who are not able to functionally self-propel any type of MWC because of physical and/or cognitive limitations (Figure 33-11). An attendant-propelled MWC frame usually comes equipped with a tilt/recline combination seating system for gravity-assisted postural support. Also, in early stages of post-CVA, attendant-propelled wheelchairs could be a safer option as self-propulsion could result in dislocation of joints of extremities with flaccid muscle tone. The previous notion was that self-propulsion in early stages of post-stroke could result in increased abnormal muscle tone, resulting in further physical disability. However, recent studies have indicated no such detrimental effect of providing self-propulsion wheeled mobility on physical disability in early post-CVA stages (6).

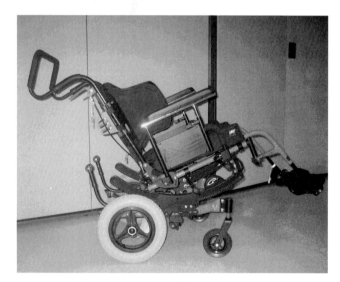

FIGURE 33-11

Attendant-propelled with tilt-in-space (Quickie IRIS).

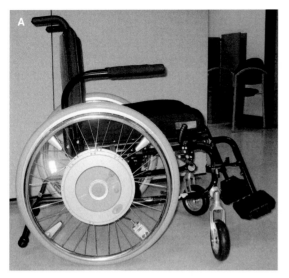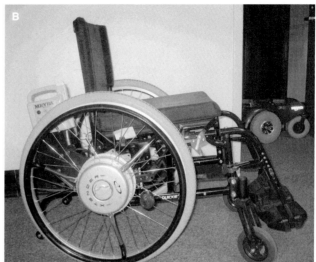

FIGURE 33-12

(A) PAPAW (e.motion); (B) PAPAW (Quickie Xtender).

Manual Self-Propelled. The traditional self-propelled MWC can be classified in five basic categories for medical justification purposes:

- Standard wheelchairs
- Standard hemi (low seat)
- Lightweight
- High-strength lightweight
- Ultralight weight wheelchairs

The hemi wheelchairs have characteristics of low seat to floor height with provisions for modifications that enable a person after CVA to be able to use a wheelchair with one side of his or her body (upper and/or lower extremity). Self-propelled MWCs can fall in the following three categories.

Pushrim-Activated Propelled. Even though this is the most commonly used interface, it could result in repetitive strain injuries (RSI), which, coupled with preexisting conditions of muscle weakness, reduced physical capacity, pain, and fatigue, could make MWC propulsion significantly inefficient. Pushrim-activated power-assisted wheelchairs (PAPAWs) have recently become an alternative option to MWCs to reduce the risk of RSI and maintain physical conditioning of the users (Figure 33-12). Studies investigating individuals with spinal cord injury reported effectiveness of PAPAWs in improving mechanical efficiency of propulsion by significantly reducing energy expenditure, stroke frequency, upper extremity range of motion, and power requirement for wheelchair propulsion (7). A PAPAW should be considered as a therapeutic intervention for addressing learned non-use as the individual wheels of

the PAPAW system may be programmed separately to enhance and encourage function of the affective side during self-propulsion.

Lever Drive. Lever drive mechanisms may be attached to the MWC on either one or both sides, which indirectly transfers push or pull forces that are applied to the rod/lever system to wheels (Figure 33-13). This mechanism facilitates use of the shoulder and elbow muscle group and reduces tiresome effects on wrist and hand muscles. Also, this form of propulsion method was reported to be energy-efficient, inducing less physical restraint as compared to unilateral/bilateral pushrim use (8).

Foot-Propelled. This form of propulsion method has been reported to be physiologically efficient, resulting in faster speed of propulsion as compared with the traditional mode of propulsion after CVA using one side of body (hand and foot) (9). However, assessment of the client is a prerequisite before prescribing the system, which includes seat to floor height to allow for heel strike and toe pulling, appropriate seat depth to allow for knee flexion, a stable back and seat support, and high friction surfaces for seat and shoe (10).

Power Wheelchairs

One concern and sometimes limiting factor for prescription of power wheelchairs (PWCs) after CVA is based on a visual-perception deficit known as unilateral neglect (UN), which can be defined as neglect of one side of the environment during any task performance, and hence raises safety concerns for individuals with right-side affected CVA to use power mobility safely and independently (11).

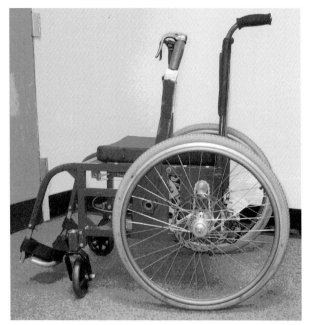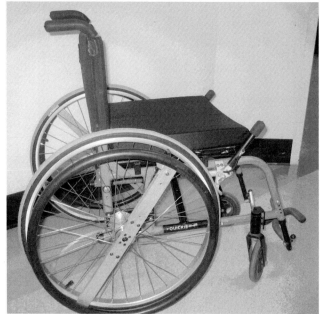

FIGURE 33-13

Lever drive system.

Computer-assisted training was reported to be effective in reducing unsafe driving behavior that may cause incidents and improving ability to complete a real-world wheelchair obstacle course for individuals with UN (12). Similarly, use of a virtual reality (VR) environment is suggested as one of the intervention techniques for improving safety with an application to provide wheeled mobility training for individuals with CVA and UN (13). PWCs can be classified in three major categories according to the Center for Medicare and Medicaid (CMS) Healthcare Common Procedure Coding System (HCPCS):

Standard Power Wheelchair.   Standard power wheelchairs do not have any option for customized programmability and/or customized seating and postural support (Figure 33-14). These low-cost and very basic PWCs are commonly prescribed and used by individuals diagnosed with CVA as their use is anticipated in low-active indoor environments. A study conducted by Pearlman et. al. (14) revealed that these chairs do not hold up to the American National Standards Institute (ANSI) and RESNA standard requirements testing as they are unstable and have a limited durability. Caution is advised when prescribing this type of power wheelchair.

Programmable Power Wheelchair.   These PWCs provide options for customization of control parameters for speed adjustment, tremors damping, acceleration control, and braking. This type of PWC can be equipped with customized power seat options and is therefore a preferred recommendation for individuals with CVA (Figure 33-15).

Lightweight, Portable Power Wheelchair.   Lightweight, portable PWCs are base-equipped with basic seating designed for ease of transportation (Figure 33-16). This type of PWC should only be considered for end users with very limited and specific mobility needs.

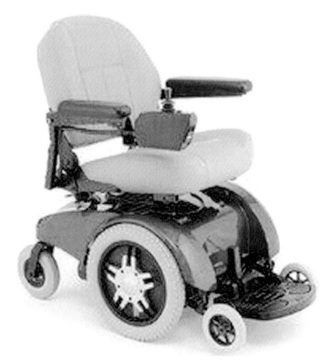

FIGURE 33-14

Example of a standard power wheelchair.

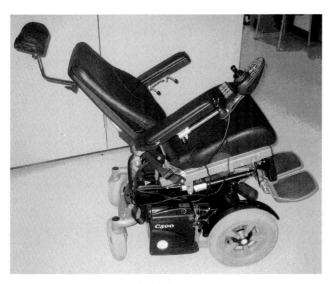

FIGURE 33-15

Example of a programmable power wheelchair.

Customized, Motorized Power Wheelchair. Customized, motorized PWCs are base-equipped along with a provision of other seating options like elevating seat and footrest, tilt and recline, lateral tilt, and standing frame. These PWCs are typically equipped with high-performance motors, batteries needed to support increased weight capacities, and higher-performance power seating systems. Precise and sound medical justification is needed when prescribing this type of PWC. Typically, it is not a PWC frequently recommended for an individual

diagnosed with a CVA of weight (less than 300 pounds) and average body structure.

Justification of an appropriate PWC that can meet all requirements of the end user and is a safe option in terms of durability and ability to withstand repeated use is a complicated process, in spite of previous research indicating higher durability and cost-effectiveness of customizable PWC as compared to standard PWC (14). Besides the CMS classification system, PWCs can be divided into three main categories based on the presence of drive wheels in relation to the seat of the user (Figure 33-17):

- Front-wheel drive (FWD)
- Mid-wheel drive (MWD)
- Rear-wheel drive (RWD)

For FWD, the drive wheels are located in the front of the seat, and it is effective over uneven grounds and rough terrains. The main disadvantage of FWD is the fish-tailing effect, where the PWC tends to sway in lateral directions while going up and down ramps. MWDs are the most efficient PWC for indoor use with availability of limited space because their turning radius is small. However, MWDs sometimes pose problems when traversing over uneven ground or rough terrains. RWDs are considered to be the fastest PWC, and they can provide good stability on most of the surfaces. However, they require a good amount of space for turning and could be unsafe while going up a ramp (15). Decisions regarding types of PWC are based on several factors, especially depending on frequency of usage and environment of use.

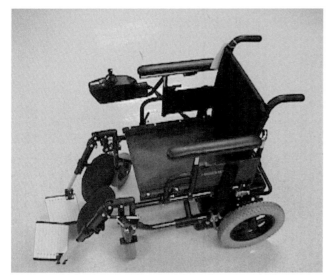
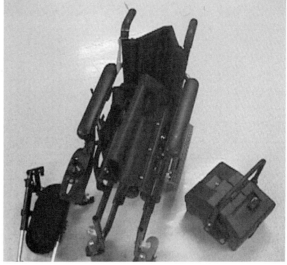

FIGURE 33-16

Example of a portable power wheelchair.

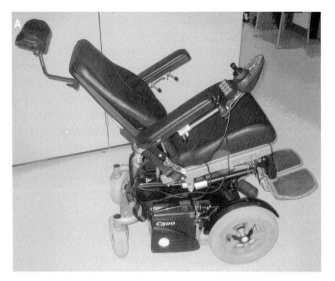
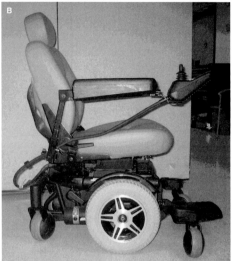
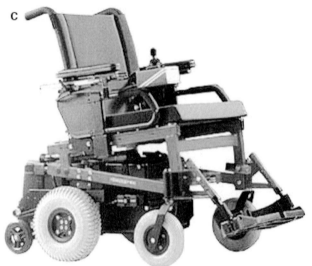

FIGURE 33-17

Three categories based on the presence of drive wheels in relation to seat of user: (A) front-wheel drive (FWD), (B) mid-wheel drive (MWD), and (C) rear-wheel drive (RWD).

ELECTRONIC AIDS FOR DAILY LIVING

Electronic aids for daily living (EADLs) are devices used to access, operate, and control electrical appliances. EADLs can be used in a home, school, or workplace. The primary purpose of an EADL is to enable a person to independently perform daily functions that he or she could not otherwise accomplish. Typical functions that an EADL enables people to perform include alerting caregivers of needs, using the telephone, changing bed positions, managing lights and room temperature, opening and securing doors, and operating TV/stereo equipment. Other names for EADLs are environmental control systems (ECSs) and environmental control units (ECUs) (16).

Persons who use and benefit most from such devices are those with severe physical limitations that affect one's mobility and upper extremities. Individuals with the diagnosis of quadriplegia, muscular atrophy, muscular dystrophy, cerebral palsy, multiple sclerosis, and amyotrophic lateral sclerosis (ALS) are often aided by the use of an EADL. A person who has had a CVA could benefit from such devices, but, oftentimes, he or she is not considered a candidate for the typical funding sources. In fact, this technology has been limited largely because of funding barriers (7, 17, 18). However, age-appropriateness for vocational potential, skill base, and technological savvy can increase the funding prospective.

TABLE 33-1
A Comparison Between Computer-Based and Stand-alone Systems

	COMPUTER-BASED	STAND-ALONE
Use of a computer	• Can be easier to program • Offers the most programming flexibility	• May still need a computer for programming the device • No computer is generally needed
Prompting	• More versatility • Larger displays	• Smaller visual displays • Limited prompting features
Feedback	• More customizable • Better graphics and auditory feedback	• limited words or beeps • Less customization
Cost	• Can be less expensive to add home automation to an existing system	• Initial expense can be higher • Technology advances slower than the computer industry and will not be outdated as quickly
Remote access	• Can be limited to use while in front of the computer • Functionality can be greatly decreased with remote operation	• Most are portable or offer remote access packages
Voice recognition	• Best available	• Sometimes available, but much lower recognition accuracy/reliability
Switch access	• Can limit the ability to operate the other computer functions • Often is a secondary consideration	• Built for use with switches

EADLs are controlled either through a switch, touchscreen, or voice recognition or integrated with other controls such as alternate computer access, wheelchair controls, and augmentative communication devices. Using integrated controls to operate an EADL is helpful and often necessary when a person has a limited number of switch/control sites available.

Categories

There are two broad categories of EADL: computer-based and stand-alone. A computer-based EADL is a combination of hardware and software that is added to a computer system to allow one to control his or her environment. A stand-alone EADL does not rely on a computer for its function. In general, a computer-based, voice-activated EADL can offer superior voice recognition, vast amounts of visual and auditory prompting and feedback, as well as more advanced programmability. Although a computer-based system can be used for other functions than controlling the environment, using the EADL will make the system more vulnerable to viruses, glitches, and crashes. Stand-alone EADLs offer a closed system that is not prone to vulnerabilities that can plague a computer system used for multiple applications. Stand-alone systems usually offer fewer options in terms of feedback, prompting, and

programmability. They are usually more compact and can be more portable (Table 33-1).

Device Feedback

The EADL feedback to the user may be visual or auditory. Visual feedback can be either static or dynamic. Static, visual feedback consists of a fixed label on each option. Usually, a light advances from one option label to the next. Dynamic, visual feedback allows the options to change in accordance with the user input or option being presented. Auditory feedback could be in the form of a beep or a word/phrase given. Depending on the EADL, a combination of visual/auditory feedback is possible.

Controlled Devices

Common types of electrical appliances controlled by EADL are telephones, lights, door openers, door locks, fans, drapes, blinds, beds, audiovisual equipment, home climate controls, call systems, and security cameras (19). These appliances are usually controlled through one of the following methods: infrared (IR), direct connection, or power line.

IR offers control of many different functions the same way a TV/VCR/DVD remote control does. IR transmission requires line of sight. As a result, the controlling signal cannot operate a device located in another room or even in the same room if the controller cannot see the device. If IR control is required and the device is located in a different room, then an IR extension cable or IR distribution box can be used to extend the signal to the remote area. Another way to control IR devices that are not in the line of sight is to transform the IR signal into a radio frequency (RF) signal. The main disadvantage of using RF is the possible interference of the signal. Direct connection of devices can include telephone lines, intercom systems, bed control, external speakers/microphones/switches, IR extenders, and external relays.

The power line control method has historically been accomplished through X-10, an industry standard for communication among devices used for home automation. It uses household wiring (power line) to carry short-wave RF signals to the devices to be controlled (20). This type of control is limited to turning devices on and off. Lights can also be dimmed or brightened. An advantage of this type of control is that, in many cases, the home electrical service does not need to be modified and no additional wires need to be run.

Insteon is a newer technology that sends dual signals, a power line communication (like X-10) and a RF signal, that travels through the air. Insteon has several reliability advantages over X-10:

- Two different types of signals are sent.
- Each sending module resends the signal if an error is detected by the receiving module.
- Each receiving device resends the signal once it is received. This allows the network to be stronger as more devices are added.
- Insteon is backwards-compatible with X-10, which implies that an Insteon controller can control X-10 modules.
- Insteon accepts multiple addresses. The ability to accept multiple addresses increases the flexibility of the system. For example, a door opener and hall light can be set up to operate independently. When using multiple addresses, in addition to independent operation, the same door and light can also be operated simultaneously on another address.

Telephones are something that most individuals want/need to control. Various EADL systems operate different types of telephones. The types of telephones can be hardwired (one or two lines), cordless, cell, IR, and phone access through the computer's modem.

EADL Evaluation Considerations

When considering an EADL for someone, many factors need to be considered (Figure 33-18). Personal factors include accessibility needs, preferences, cognitive and physical abilities, technology background, desire to use technology, degenerative conditions, voice quality, and voice changes. Factors when considering equipment include the places where the device will be used, the layout and size of each area, the devices to be controlled, the electrical condition of the controlled environment, mounting to bed/chair, switch type, required integration with existing AT equipment, and particular EADL limitations and benefits. Funding factors include cost and the goals/requirements of the funding agency.

Costs

The basic cost of full EADL systems can range from $3,500–$6,000. A completely installed system with door openers and other options can cost $8,000–$15,000. Typically the only funding available for EADL comes from vocational rehabilitation agencies, Veterans Administration, worker's compensation, civil and nonprofit organizations, and philanthropists. Medical insurance does not cover EADLs.

Lower-Cost Alternatives

Persons diagnosed with a CVA often have function on one side of their body. Such persons may find it helpful to consider lower-end home automation options. Specifically, a large button, universal remote can assist by decreasing needed hand dexterity and making it easier to see the buttons. A remote control that combines IR features with X-10 capabilities can lessen the need to get up to turn on lights as well as open or lock doors and provides a means to signal assistance from someone in another room. Switch-activated telephones and cell phones are also available. These devices can give a person more security and independence. If a person's speech is significantly affected, switch-activated telephones that play a prerecorded message can be considered.

AUGMENTATIVE AND ALTERNATIVE COMMUNICATION

The process of achieving communication success for individuals with complex communication needs that are the result of a stroke may be perceived as an insurmountable challenge to their families and those providing clinical services. Yet, the goal of augmentative and alternative communication (AAC) intervention is to optimize the communication of individuals with significant communication disorders (18). AAC AT provides a viable rehabilitation solution to assist individuals who cannot speak to achieve maximum potential.

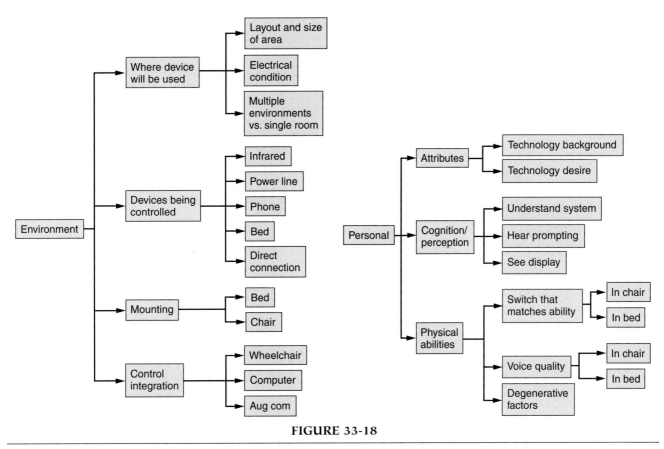

FIGURE 33-18

EADL evaluation considerations.

Individuals recovering from strokes who are candidates for AAC may have a motor speech disorder, language impairment, or a combination of both speech and cognitive-linguistic considerations that result in a complex communication disorder. These considerations present issues that influence the selection and design of AAC AT (21). In addition, candidates for AAC will have immediate short-term needs for technology as well as possible long-term use beyond rehabilitation. Regardless of the duration of use for an individual, the AAC AT must be considered based on how language is represented and generated using the system before specific technologies are considered. These language considerations include whether the AAC system provides for spontaneous novel utterance generation (SNUG), prestored messages, or both and how core and extended vocabulary is stored and accessed on the system. Several AAC systems may be considered, trialed, and recommended over the course of rehabilitation and a lifetime. How the systems handle these language considerations and transitions and maintain consistency when change occurs is important to achieving long-term effective communication.

Graphic symbols are used on AAC AT to construct messages. AAC language representation methods (LRMs) refer to the ways that symbols are used to generate communication. The three commonly used LRMs in AAC can be divided into three categories: single-meaning pictures, alphabet-based methods, and Semantic Compaction™ (22).Understanding the characteristics of each method is important when taking into consideration the specific characteristics and degree of a possible cognitive-linguistic impairment. In addition, people with aphasia may have impaired resource capacity and resource allocation abilities that will influence using AAC interventions (23). Therefore, language considerations (cognitive-linguistic functioning) should take priority in selecting AAC AT in order to match technology features to how language is best represented for an individual. Many AAC systems provide for multiple methods to access vocabulary and generate messages. Research has shown the communication performance for the different methods varies significantly (24). Consequently, selecting the LRMs based on the communication abilities, needs, and potential for improvement is critical for achieving the best possible performance.

A thorough appreciation of AAC LRMs is needed in order to evaluate how LRMs may be accessed using the range of aided AAC technology and types of AAC display technology recommended for individuals with acquired communication disabilities. High-performance

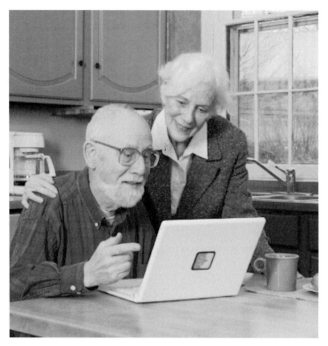

FIGURE 33-19

A laptop computer designed specifically for persons with aphasia.

technology solutions can then be identified as nondedicated or dedicated AAC systems. Nondedicated systems are computers, PDAs, and other mass-market hardware with software applications designed to support communication. For example, Lingraphica® is software running on a laptop computer that is designed specifically for persons with aphasia (Figure 33-19). The voice output used with computers is synthesized speech (text-to-speech).

Dedicated systems are designed specifically for the purpose of communication and can be classified into low, light, and high-performance technology. The range of aided technology increases as availability of power, voice output, electronics, and computer chips become part of the system. Table 33-2 shows the complex nature of decision-making for selecting AAC technology once a comprehensive assessment for communication abilities, needs, and expectations has been conducted by the team.

The display technology used to generate messages can be a static keyboard, touchscreen, or hybrid device (combination of a keyboard and touchscreen). The display configuration supports any of the chosen LRMs or multiple LRMs. The appearance of the display can vary in the number, arrangement, and organization of the keys. Display configurations used with individuals with acquired communication disorders include visual scenes, various grid organizational patterns, and a core and activity row pattern. Single-meaning picture or Semantic Compaction™ symbols/icons may be used on visual scenes and grids or page-based displays while alphabet-based methods are configured on a grid display (25). The core and activity row pattern is used exclusively with recursive semantic encoding for one-hit access as a single-meaning picture method or with sequencing. Most AAC manufactures provide a range of devices that offer one or more display configurations on a system. For example, visual scenes may be used for one communication activity such as retelling a story while a core/activity row would be used for another level of participation such as requesting, commenting, or questioning (26). A careful exploration of the features and components of systems is critical to understanding how the technology may support language/communication functioning and goals.

TABLE 33-2
Components of Dedicated AAC Technology (Hill©)

LANGUAGE REQUIREMENTS	CONTROL INTERFACE (HARDWARE)	HARDWARE COMPONENTS	SELECTION METHODS	ACCESSORIES	ADDITIONAL CONSIDERATIONS
Alphabet-based methods	**Touchscreen** Visual scenes	**Speech Outputs** Digitized	**Direct Selection** Keyboard	Mounting systems	Technical support
Single meaning pictures	Page or activity-based displays	Synthesized Combination	Headpointing Eye gaze	Carrying case	Training
Semantic compaction	Core/activity row display	**Auditory Outputs**	Neuro-controls	Peripherals (switches,	Repair services
		Visual Outputs	**Scanning** 1-switch	headsticks, and joystick)	Warranties
Multiple methods	**Static Display** Keyboard	**Electronic Outputs**	2-switch		Portability and weight
	Pictorial Overlay	**Data logging**	Joystick Neuro-controls		
	Hybrid System Static keyboard and touchscreen	**Memory capacity**	**Morse Code**		

An important aspect of successful AAC intervention is the considerable training and practice required to become efficient (27). Today's technology includes tools and features to monitor performance and outcomes for AAC intervention. Many AAC systems have built-in language activity monitoring (LAM) to collect data on the use of an AAC system (28). Any AAC system under consideration can be compared with other possible options for making the most informed choice. LAM data can be analyzed using the Performance Report Tool (PeRT) to generate a report of quantitative summary measures of communication (29). Clinical data on the number of symbols and/or words used, frequency of methods used to generate utterances, and frequency of vocabulary use provide insights for intervention. Outcome measures on the days, time, frequency, type of activity, and preferred use have been reported that indicate strong user satisfaction with AAC intervention (30).

Because communication performance is so important to the life experience of people who use AAC, significant clinical effort should be focused to optimize performance. Identifying the activities and type of participation important to a person with a disability can maximize the potential use of an AAC system (Table 33-2). AAC AT can function as a keyboard emulator to provide access to computers and enhance access to email and the Internet. AAC systems with IR technology can support environment controls and enhance independence. LAM tools can support telerehabilitation services for persons recovering in remote areas and with other transportation and health issues (31). Internet resources and support organizations specific to AAC provide the most current information to practitioners, family members, and consumers to support the complex questions about AAC AT.

ADAPTIVE DRIVING

One of the many important goals in the rehabilitation recovery process after a stroke is the ability to return to independent living in one's community. Community mobility, specifically driving, can contribute to a person's quality of life. Transportation into the community allows access to activities outside the confinement of one's home. Individuals who are no longer able to drive are more likely to report worsening depressive symptoms (32). Many stroke survivors express an interest in returning to driving during their rehabilitation process. It has been reported that 30% of stroke survivors who drove prior to their stroke are said to resume driving after their stroke (33).

Stroke can cause physical-motor, cognitive, visual, and psychological impairments that can impact a person's driving performance. A Certified Driving Rehabilitation Specialist (CDRS) can provide a comprehensive driving evaluation to assess the extent of the neurologic impairments and determine the ability of a person to operate a vehicle safely after a stroke (34). A typical comprehensive driving evaluation consists of a pre-driver's evaluation and on-road assessment. The pre-driver's evaluation assesses the basic skills necessary for driving, such as vision, perception, cognition, physical functioning, and knowledge of driving. This aspect of the process can help to identify strengths or deficit areas related to driving. Actual driving skills then can be assessed in a vehicle with the stroke survivor and the CDRS. The vehicle can be modified with adaptive equipment that the person may need to use for improved independent operation of the vehicle.

After completion of the driving evaluation, education and training may be indicated with or without the use of adaptive equipment. Adaptive equipment can be recommended by a CDRS to compensate for the loss of physical skills after a stroke. Adaptive equipment for the individual's vehicle is prescribed after completion of a comprehensive driving evaluation and training program and only after it is determined that the person will be able to develop competency to drive with the prescribed equipment.

A steering device, such as a spinner knob, can be attached to the steering wheel to allow a person to steer with one hand (Figure 33-20). A left-sided accelerator can be used if a person is unable to use his or her right foot to operate the gas or brake pedal (Figure 33-21). A turn signal crossover (Figure 33-22) shows the relocation of the turn signal indicator from the left side of the steering wheel to the right side. This allows a person without the use of his or her left hand to access the turn signal using only his or her right hand. Other secondary vehicle controls such as windshield wipers, lights, and horn can be relocated onto the steering wheel next to the steering device or at any other location within the vehicle. This can be done so that the driver is able to access all vehicle controls quickly and accurately with his or her dominant hand. If sitting balance is impaired and the person tends to lose his or her balance as the vehicle goes around a curve in the road, a chest harness may be indicated. This allows for additional trunk control beyond what a seat belt provides, but it does not replace the use of the seat belt. A strap or other modifications can be used for seat belt retrieval if the person is unable to grasp or reach his or her seat belt. A parking brake extension can be attached to a floor-mounted parking or emergency brake pedal (Figure 33-23). Using this type of device, the person without the use of his or her left foot then can apply the parking braking using his or her hand. Partial loss of visual fields or the presence of scotomas can sometimes be compensated for by the use of specially placed mirrors. As with all adaptive equipment, specialized education and training is required to assure correct placement and proper use of the additional mirrors (35).

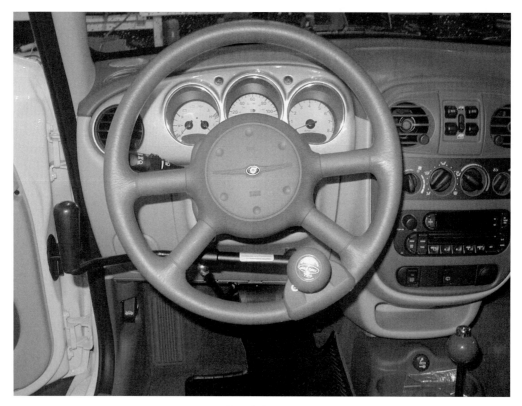

FIGURE 33-20

Spinner knob attached to the steering wheel. Courtesy of Howell Ventures Ltd.

The ability to drive uses a set of visual, perceptual, cognitive, and psychological skills. Impairment in any or all of these areas will affect the individual's driving performance. These deficit areas can be more challenging and difficult to compensate for, as compared to the physical impairment areas, especially when driving a vehicle in an ever-changing dynamic environment.

Common driving behaviors that may be observed in an individual after a stroke and would require additional training and education for remedial purposes include (36):

• Difficulty in maintaining a centered lane position or drifting across the lane lines into other lanes

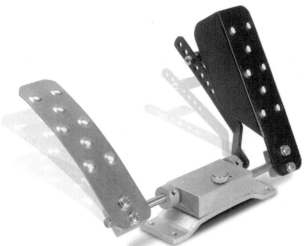

FIGURE 33-21

Left foot accelerator with gas pedal guard. Courtesy of Howell Ventures Ltd.

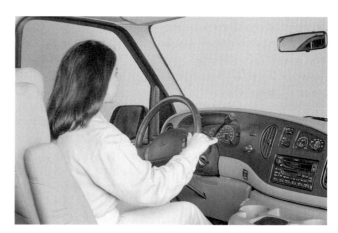

FIGURE 33-22

Right side turn signal. Courtesy of Mobility Products and Design.

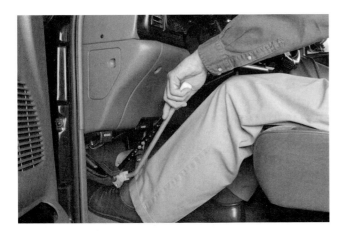

FIGURE 33-23

Parking brake extension. Courtesy of Mobility Products and Design.

- Poor speed modulation (driving either too fast or too slow)
- Poor judgment of distances (positioning too close to the other vehicles)
- Delayed response or reaction time
- Poor decision-making skills
- Difficulty in completing lane changes, merges, and blending with traffic
- Poor anticipation of other drivers or pedestrians

- Missing of traffic signs and signals
- Near misses, close calls, and frequent blowing of horns by other drivers directed at the driver

Unfortunately, not all functional deficits caused by a stroke can be easily compensated for by means of adaptive equipment or dedicated training. Severe cognitive impairments, uncontrolled spasticity, and significant visual field loss (for example, visual homonymous hemianopsia or unilateral visual attention deficits) are examples of problem areas that may prevent a person from permanently driving a vehicle after a stroke. When it is determined that an individual is no longer able to drive, suggestions and materials should be provided for alternative means of transportation. The individual's family and friends are encouraged to support the no-driving recommendation and assist the stroke survivor with ongoing access to the community (34).

A variety of adaptive equipment and vehicle modifications can be used for vehicle ingress and egress. Persons with impaired hand function can use automatic car door openers (also known as keyless entry), built-up key holders, or key turners. Power-based seats can be installed in the car seat to allow a driver or passenger to transfer from his or her wheelchair to the vehicle seat. These power-based seats have options that allow the car seat to swivel out, glide out of the vehicle, and then lower to a desired level for ease in transfers. Wheelchair lifts (Figure 33-24;

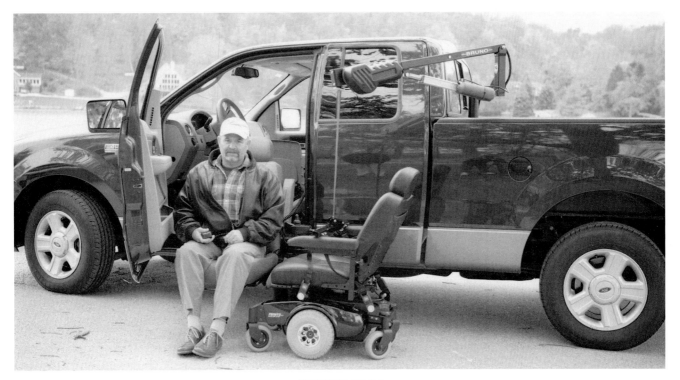

FIGURE 33-24

Turning automotive seat and wheelchair lift. Courtesy of Bruno Independent Living Aids, Inc.

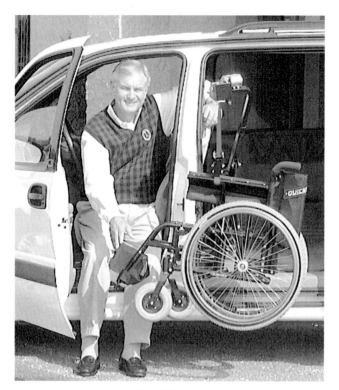

FIGURE 33-25

Wheelchair lift-side door application. Courtesy of Bruno Independent Living Aids, Inc.

Figure 33-25) are available to load and unload mobility equipment, such as MWCs, PWCs, or scooters, into the vehicle without significant vehicle modifications. Car toppers are another type of lift that attaches to the top of a sedan-type vehicle and can lift and store a MWC. Wheelchair or scooter users may require a vehicle ramp or lift to either get into their vehicle or lift their mobility device into the vehicle. These major vehicle modifications are typically prescribed by a CDRS and installed by a mobility equipment dealer. It is critical that, prior to prescribing and installing the adaptive equipment in the vehicle, compatibility between the individual, mechanical device, and vehicle is assured before the vehicle is modified.

WHEELCHAIR TRANSPORTATION SAFETY

Individuals recovering from a stroke may travel in a motor vehicle to seek medical care and continue to participate in family and community activities. It is safest to ride seated in a vehicle seat using the vehicle's seat belt system that complies with federal safety standards. However, an individual relying on a wheelchair for mobility may not be able to safely transfer to a vehicle seat. If transferring is not feasible, the person must ride while seated in the wheelchair. When this occurs, it is very important to ensure the safety of the wheelchair-seated occupant by using after-market safety systems that meet voluntary standards (37).

To ensure the safety of the wheelchair-seated occupant during vehicle transportation, the entire wheelchair transportation safety system must be considered. This system includes three main components: the wheelchair, the wheelchair securement, and the occupant restraint. This section will address selecting crashworthy wheelchairs and wheelchair securement equipment, securing the wheelchair, and properly restraining the occupant.

The Wheelchair

It is best to have a wheelchair that has been designed and tested for use as a seat in a motor vehicle. This means that the wheelchair has been designed to withstand forces generated in a crash, provides occupants with effective support during impact loading so that the occupant's restraint belts remain properly positioned, considers access and fit of the vehicle occupant restraints, and provides attachment points to secure the wheelchair to the vehicle. Such wheelchairs comply with voluntary standard ANSI/RESNA WC19 or ISO 7176-19 and are referred to as WC19, transit, or transit option wheelchairs (38, 39). These wheelchairs have four, crash-tested, and clearly labeled securement points for attachment of tiedown/securement straps or hooks (Figure 33-26). If a WC19 wheelchair is not an option, a

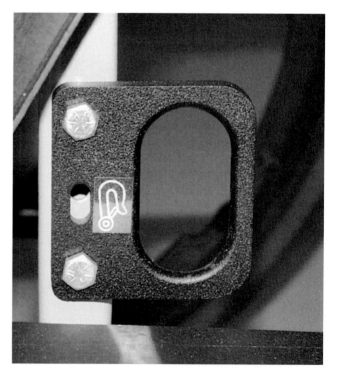

FIGURE 33-26

WC19-compliant wheelchair securement point with required label.

wheelchair with an accessible frame to allow securement straps to be attached to nonremovable, frame junctions is the next best choice. It is best to keep the wheelchair back at an angle of no more than 30 degrees to the vertical. Hard wheelchair trays should be removed and secured elsewhere during travel. Medical and other equipment should be secured to the wheelchair or vehicle to prevent it from breaking free and causing injury in an accident.

Wheelchair Securement

The wheelchair must not add to the forces on an occupant during emergency maneuvers or an accident. Therefore, the wheelchair must be secured using a means independent from restraining the occupant. For example, the same strap should not be used to restrain the occupant and secure the wheelchair. The securement system must be designed to attach to the wheelchair frame, prevent excessive movement or tipping during driving events, and withstand crash forces.

The wheelchair should be positioned facing forward in the vehicle and secured using a system that has been crash-tested and complies with the voluntary standard SAE J2249 or ISO 10542 (40, 41). The system should be installed according to the manufacturer's instructions by a reputable vehicle modifier. The most common type of securement is the four-point tiedown system (Figure 33-27) (42). This system consists of four

tiedown straps that anchor to the vehicle floor and four points on the wheelchair (two front and two rear). The end fittings that attach to the wheelchair can be hooks or loops that wrap around the wheelchair frame or designated securement attachment points. Although this system can be used with a wide variety of wheelchairs and does not require additional hardware be placed on the wheelchair, it does require an attendant or caregiver to secure and release the wheelchair.

If the wheelchair is not a WC19 wheelchair with four designated securement points to attach the four tiedown straps, the straps should be attached to the welded junctions of the wheelchair frame. The attachment points should be as close to the seat surface as possible to improve the stability of the wheelchair and result in rear tiedown strap angles preferably between 30 and 45 degrees to the horizontal. Tiedown straps should not be attached to removable or adjustable components of the wheelchair, such as armrests, footrests, or wheels. The four straps should be tightened to remove any slack.

Wheelchairs can also be secured using automatic docking systems. This type of securement utilizes a wheelchair adaptor (that is, special hardware mounted on the wheelchair), which engages with a docking station or receptacle mounted to the vehicle floor or sidewall. The advantages of wheelchair docking technology have been demonstrated by proprietary systems that have been used for independent securement of wheelchairs in private vehicles for many years (Figure 33-28). These systems offer increased independence by the wheelchair user and reduced attendant intervention (37). They also

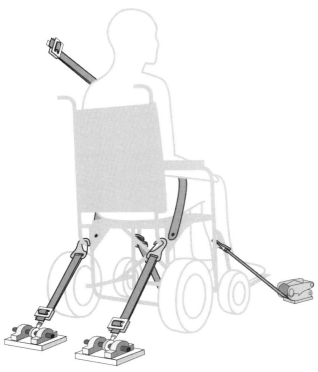

FIGURE 33-27

Example of a four-point tiedown system used to secure a wheelchair.

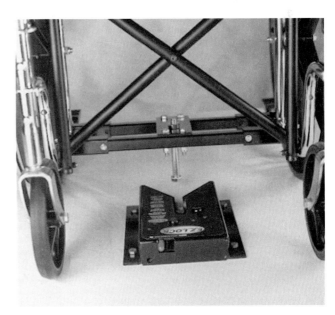

FIGURE 33-28

Example of a docking-type wheelchair securement system. Courtesy of EZ Lock Incorporated.

remove the need for human judgment, resulting in more consistent and proper use of the systems. However, they require a unique proprietary adaptor be retrofitted to the wheelchair and may add unwanted weight, impact ground clearance if mounted underneath, or add to the overall length if mounted in the rear. Docking systems also tend to cost more to purchase and maintain than the traditional four-point tiedown system. Docking systems should also have been crash-tested to meet voluntary safety standards and should have been successfully crash-tested with the specific wheelchair model being used.

Occupant Restraint

In addition to wheelchair securement, a crash-tested occupant restraint system is necessary to prevent occupant ejection from the vehicle or contact with the interior structure of the vehicle. Postural supports are not designed to withstand crash forces and are often not positioned correctly for effective restraint in a crash. Both pelvic and shoulder restraints are needed to safely limit the excursion of the head, chest, and pelvis (37, 41). The pelvic belt should be placed across the front of the pelvis near the upper thighs, not over the abdomen, at an angle between 45 and 75 degrees to the horizontal when viewed from the side. To allow proper placement on the pelvis, the pelvic belt should not be routed around armrests. This can often be avoided by inserting the lap belt under the armrest or between the armrest and the seatback. The shoulder belt should cross the middle of the shoulder and the center of the chest and connect to the lap belt near the hip. The shoulder belt should be anchored to the vehicle above and behind the occupant's shoulder in order to allow proper contact with the shoulder and chest. A WC19-compliant wheelchair has the option of a crash-tested pelvic belt that is anchored to the wheelchair, increasing the ease of achieving proper fit. This crash-tested pelvic belt will have labeling to indicate that it complies with ANSI/RESNA WC19. A vehicle-mounted shoulder belt should be attached to the pelvic belt to provide complete protection. A headrest positioned directly behind and in close proximity to the head can help protect the head and neck in rear impact. Space around the wheelchair rider should be as clear as possible to reduce the chance of injury from contact with items in the vehicle's interior during travel or a crash.

ROBOTIC REHABILITATION DEVICE

One focus of current research in stroke rehabilitation is the use of robotic devices in therapy. Such devices are not designed to replace human therapists. Rather, robotic therapy is a way to increase the amount of therapy available to individuals and enable therapists to administer new types of therapy (43). Robotic therapy allows the therapist to provide the user with a variety of feedback concerning his or her performance and has the potential to be customized to the individual, which is consistent with the values of traditional therapy (44). A variety of robotic devices exist with applications in the areas of upper extremity, lower extremity, and cognitive rehabilitation. A thorough overview can be found in "Health Care and Rehabilitation Robotics" (45). Here we will consider only one representative of each category.

The most widely tested robotic device targeted toward upper extremity rehabilitation is the MIT-MANUS, now commercially available under the name InMotion2 from Interactive Motion Technologies, Inc. (Figure 33-29). The MIT-MANUS is a robotic arm. The user grasps a handle on the robot and makes reaching movements in the horizontal plane (46). While the user reaches, he or she views a computer screen that displays feedback about performance in the form of a simple video game. The robot arm contains motors that can be used to assist or resist the user as he or she completes the target movements (47). Individuals with acute stroke who received extra therapy via the MIT-MANUS showed, relative to controls, greater gains in muscle control and muscle strength for the shoulder and elbow (48). Subjects with chronic stroke have also shown improvements after training with the device (47). Other systems addressing gross movements of the upper extremity include the ARM Guide (49) and the Mirror-Image Motion Enabler (MIME) (50) while systems for hand rehabilitation have also been proposed (51).

A representative example of the type of robotic devices available for lower extremity rehabilitation is the Lokomat from Hocoma (Figure 33-30). This device is designed as a therapeutic aid for body weight-supported treadmill training, which traditionally requires up to three therapists per individual. A harness supports the user's weight over the treadmill while a robotic exoskeleton placed on the user's legs moves him or her through a gaitlike pattern (52). Individuals with chronic partial spinal cord injury who received therapy using this device improved in gait speed, endurance, and performance on the timed "up & go" test (53). A variety of other devices exist as aids to body weight-supported treadmill training and weight-supported overground walking; these include the Gait Trainer GT (29) and the KineAssist device, among others (45).

The last category of robotic devices for therapy is robots designed to address cognitive of emotional issues. For instance, the PARO robot, developed by researchers in Japan, is a small robot that resembles a baby seal (Figure 33-31). Interacting with this robot has been shown to reduce stress in elderly residents of a care facility (54). Other researchers are investigating the use of toylike robots with children with disabilities, including autism and Down syndrome (45).

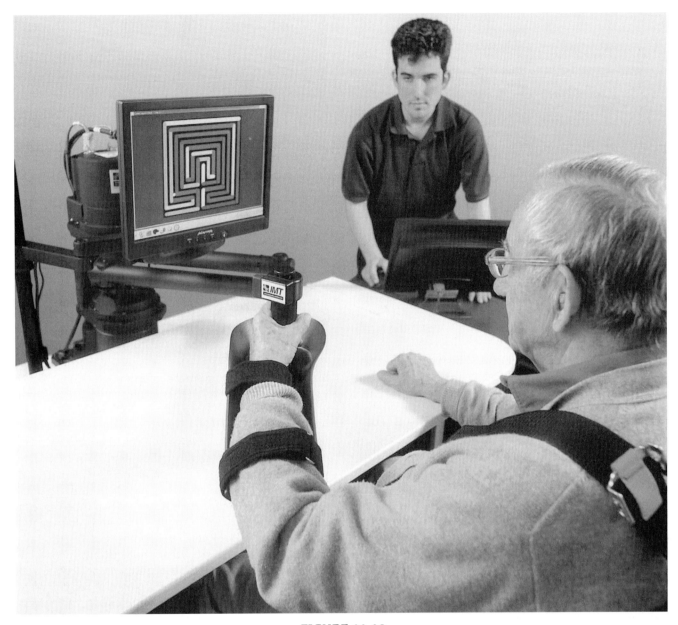

FIGURE 33-29

The InMotion2, a robot used for upper extremity rehabilitation of individuals with stroke. With permission from Interactive Motion Technologies, Inc.

This extremely brief overview of the field of rehabilitation robotics indicates the variety of applications being pursued by researchers. This field is relatively new, but has the potential to provide therapists with a wide range of technological tools to increase their ability to assist clients.

Research Frontiers—Future Technologies

There is a large and growing segment of our world population, people with reduced functional capabilities because of aging or disability. Recent advancements in technologies, including computation, robotics, machine learning, communication, and miniaturization of sensors, bring us closer to a futuristic vision of compassionate intelligent devices and technology-embedded environments. Even though many intelligent systems have been developed, most of them are for manufacturing, military, space exploration, and entertainment. Their use for improving health-related quality of life has been treated as a specialized and minor area. AT, for example, has fallen in the cracks between medical and intelligent-system technologies. The missing element is a basic understanding of how to relate human functions (physiological, physical,

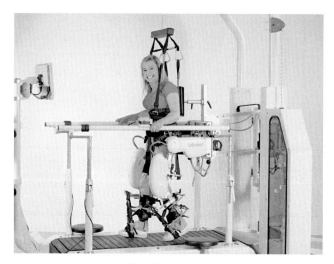

FIGURE 33-30

Lokomat, a robotic aid to body weight-supported treadmill training. With permission from Hocoma.

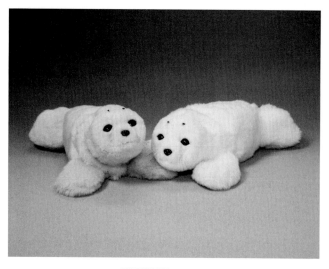

FIGURE 33-31

PARO, a robot developed by researchers in Japan as a companion to elderly residents of care facilities. With permission from AIST, Japan.

and cognitive) to the design of intelligent devices and systems that aid and interact with people.

A dilemma faced by clinicians is reconciling the fact that observations of patients only occur during (infrequent) face-to-face meetings in a clinic or laboratory, while what is really needed are assessments that reflect the patient's capabilities in the real world, where distractions are present and multitask performance is often required. As such, there is a need for ecologically valid tests that can provide information about a patient's ability to function in a real-life environment. One way to obtain ecologically valid measures is through the use of ubiquitous computing.

People with cognitive impairments often have difficulty with executive functions and prospective memory, including such tasks as organizing a schedule, initiating activities, and remembering to perform the appropriate task at the correct time. External cueing systems can assist people with cognitive disabilities by reminding them to perform a task at the appropriate time or providing guidance through a task. Such systems can range from low-tech, paper-and-pencil solutions, to mainstream voice recorders and PDAs, to specialized software designed for people with cognitive impairments.

Despite attempts at using simple reminders (timers, pressure monitors, and PDA reminders/surveys), user's guides (handouts and note cards), and consumer booklets developed to promote clinical practice guidelines,

users do not seem to follow clinician instructions. Novel approaches are emerging that use machine learning and artificial intelligence for real-time coaching of the person with disabilities for long-term monitoring of the person's use of the equipment and provide hard information for clinicians to use to augment their education of people with disabilities. This research is patient-centered and is likely to allow clinicians and people with disabilities to take more proactive roles in the ways technology can enhance their lives, for example, by avoiding detrimental health affects of prolonged seated postures.

A gap in current technology is to effectively combine manipulation and mobility assistance with perception and decision-making wherever a person goes. When end users were consulted, they reported they wanted a zero gap in mobility and manipulation between them and an unimpaired person. A primary challenge is to overcome the shortcomings and unmet needs with a device that provides coordinated mobility and manipulation. Some of the new functionalities required are to detect and/or predict user intent, provide coordinated movement between a power base and multiple manipulators, include natural and intuitive user interfaces and control modes, and incorporate real-world navigation and docking assistance. In order to make interaction easier, a wide range of natural and intuitive interfaces that reduce the time to complete tasks and produce fluid, human-like motions are needed.

Additional Readings

Angelo J. *Assistive Technology for Rehabilitation Therapists.* Lane S, ed. F. A. Davis Company, 1997.

Cook A, Hussey S. *Assistive Technologies: Principles and Practice.* 2nd ed. Mosby Publishing, 2001.

Trefler E, Hobson DA, Taylor SJ, et al. *Seating and Mobility for Persons with Physical Disabilities.* Communication Skill Builders/Therapy Skill Builders, 1993.

References

1. Cooper RA, Cooper RM. Powering On. *Paraplegia News* 2006; 60(9):13–20.
2. Garber SLB, Monga R. Wheelchair utilization and satisfaction following cerebral vascular accident. *Journal of Rehabilitation Research and Development* 2002; 39(4):521–533.
3. Kirby RL, Adams CD, MacPhee AH, et al. Wheelchair-skill performance: Controlled comparison between people with hemiplegia and able-bodied people simulating hemiplegia. *Archives of Physical Medicine and Rehabilitation* 2005; 86(3):387–439.
4. Qiang W, Sonoda S, Suzuki M, et al. Reliability and validity of a wheelchair collision test for screening behavioral assessment of unilateral neglect after stroke. *American Journal of Physical Medicine & Rehabilitation* 2005; 84(3):161–166.
5. Barker DJ, Reid D, Cott C. The experience of senior stroke survivors: Factors in community participation among wheelchair users. *Canadian Journal of Occupational Therapy—Revue Canadienne d Ergotherapie* 2006; 73(1):18–25.
6. Pomeroy VM, Mickelborough J, Hill E, et al. A hypothesis: Self-propulsion in a wheelchair early after stroke might not be harmful. *Clinical Rehabilitation* 2003; 17(2):174–180.
7. Algood SD, Cooper RA, Fitzgerald SG, et al. Impact of a pushrim-activated power-assisted wheelchair on the metabolic demands, stroke frequency, and range of motion among subjects with tetraplegia. *Archives of Physical Medicine & Rehabilitation* 2004; 85(11):1865–1871.
8. van der Woude LH, Dallmeijer AJ, Janssen TW, Veeger D. Alternative modes of manual wheelchair ambulation: an overview. *American Journal of Physical Medicine & Rehabilitation* 2001; 80(10):765–777.
9. Makino K, Wada F, Hachisuka K, et al. Speed and physiological cost index of hemiplegic patients pedaling a wheelchair with both legs. *Journal of Rehabilitation Medicine* 2005; 37(2):83–86.
10. Buck S. Wheelchair propulsion by foot: Assessment considerations. *Topics in Stroke Rehabilitation* 2004; 11(4):68–71C.
11. Dawson J, Thornton H. Can patients with unilateral neglect following stroke drive electrically powered wheelchairs? *British Journal of Occupational Therapy* 2003; 66(11):496–504.
12. Webster JS, McFarland PT, Rapport LJ, et al. Computer-assisted training for improving wheelchair mobility in unilateral neglect patients. *Archives of Physical Medicine & Rehabilitation* 2001; 82(6):769–775.
13. Katz N, Ring H, Naveh Y, et al. Interactive virtual environment training for safe street crossing of right hemisphere stroke patients with unilateral spatial neglect. *Disability and Rehabilitation* 2005; 27(20):1235–1243.
14. Pearlman JL, Cooper RA, Karnawat J, et al. Evaluation of the safety and durability of low-cost nonprogrammable electric powered wheelchairs. *Archives of Physical Medicine & Rehabilitation* 2005; 86(12):2361–2370.
15. Cooper RA. *Powered Mobility.* New York: Demos Medical Publishing, 1998
16. Tam C, et al. Development of a measuring tool using electronic aids to daily living, *Technology and Disability* 2003; 15:181–190.
17. Barnes MP. Environmental control systems: An audit and review. *Clinical Rehabilitation* 1994; 8(4):362–366.
18. American Speech-Language-Hearing Association (ASHA). *Preferred practice patterns for the profession of speech-language pathology.* Rockville, MD: Author, 2004.
19. Lang M. Electronic aids to daily living. *Rehab Report* 1997:24–27.
20. 55.www.insteon.net
21. Garrett KL, Kimelman MDZ. AAC and aphasia: Cognitive-linguistic considerations. In: Beukelman DR, Yorkston KM, Reichle J, eds. *Augmentative and Alternative Communication for Adults with Acquired Neurologic Disorders.* Baltimore, MD: Paul H. Brookes Publishing Co., 2000:339–374.
22. Romich B, Vanderheiden G, Hill K. Augmentative communication. In: Bronzino JD, ed. *The Biomedical Engineering Handbook.* 2nd ed. Boca Raton, FL: CRC Press, 2001:144-1–8.
23. McNeil MR, Odell K, Tseng CH. Toward the integration of resource allocation into a general model of aphasia. In: Prescott T, ed. *Clinical Aphasiology.* Austin, TX: PRO-ED, 1991:21–39.
24. Hill K. AAC evidence-based practice and language activity monitoring. *Topics in Language Disorders: Language and Augmented Communication* 2004; 24:18–30.
25. Baker B. Semantic compaction lets speech-impaired people quickly and effectively communicate in a variety of environments. *Byte* 1986; 11(3):160–168.
26. Stuart S, Kasker JP, Beukelman DR. AAC message management. In: Beukelman DR, Yorkston KM, Reichle J, eds. *Augmentative and Alternative Communication for Adults with Acquired Neurologic Disorders.* Baltimore, MD: Paul H. Brookes Publishing Co. 2000:330–374.
27. Koul R, Arvidson HH, Pennington GS. Intervention for persons with acquired disorders. In: Lloyd LL, Fuller DR, Arvidson HH, eds. *Augmentative and Alternative*

communication: A handbook of Principles and Practices.* Boston: Allyn And Bacon, 1997:340–366.
28. Hill K, Romich B. A language activity monitor for supporting AAC evidence-based clinical practice. *Assistive Technology* 2001; 13:12–22.
29. AAC Institute. *PeRT (Performance Report Tool): A computer program for generating the AAC Performance Report.* [Computer software]. Pittsburgh, PA: Author, 2003.
30. Steele R. *How do persons with aphasia use their Lingraphica SGDs?* Poster at the Annual American Speech-Language-Hearing Association (ASHA) Convention. Miami, FL. November 2006.
31. Cohn E, Hill K. *Telerehabilitation Clinical Practice & AAC: An interactive SWOT Analysis.* Seminar at the Annual American Speech-Language-Hearing Association (ASHA) Convention. Miami, FL. November 2006.
32. Fonda SJ, Wallace RB, Herzog AR. Changes in driving patterns and worsening depressive symptoms among older adults. *Journal of Gerontology: Social Sciences* 2001; 56(6):S343–S351.
33. Fisk GD, Owsley C, Pulley LV. Vision, attention, and self-reported driving behaviors in community-dwelling stroke survivors. *Archives of Physical Medicine and Rehabilitation* 2002; 83(4):496–477.
34. The physician's guide to assessing and counseling older drivers. Available at www.ama-assn.org/ama/pub/category/10791.html. Accessed March 1, 2007.
35. Transportation, adaptive driving equipment. Available at www.birf.info/home/library/transport/trans_adapt.html. Accessed March 1, 2007.
36. Driving after a stroke. Available at www.driver-ed.org. Accessed March 1, 2007.
37. Schneider LW, Manary MA. Wheelchairs, wheelchair tiedowns, and occupant restraints for improved safety and crash protection. In: Pellerito JM, ed. *Driver Rehabilitation and Community Mobility: Principles and Practices.* Elsevier Mosby, 2006:357–372.
38. ANSI/RESNA. Wheelchairs/Volume 1: Requirements and test methods for wheelchairs (including scooters); Section 19: Wheelchairs used as seats in motor vehicles. Arlington: American National Standards Institute (ANSI)/Rehabilitation Engineering Society of North America (RESNA), 2000.
39. ISO 7176-19. Wheelchairs: Wheeled mobility devices for use in motor vehicles. International Organization for Standardization, 2001.
40. ISO 10542. Technical systems and aids for disabled or handicapped persons: Wheelchair tiedown and occupant-restraint systems. Parts 1–5. International Organization for Standardization, 2001.
41. SAE. Recommended Practice J2249. Wheelchair tiedown and occupant restraint systems for use in motor vehicles. Warrendale, PA: Society of Automotive Engineers, 1999.
42. Hardin JA, Foreman C, Callejas L. Synthesis of securement device options and strategies (Technical report No. 416-07). Tampa: National Center for Transit Research (NCTR), 2002.
43. Patton JL, Mussa-Ivaldi FA. Robot-assisted adaptive training: Custom force fields for teaching movement patterns. *IEEE Trans Biomed Eng* 2004; 51:636–646.
44. Krebs HI, Palazzolo JJ, Dipietro L, et al. Rehabilitation robotics: Performance-based progressive robot-assisted therapy. *Autonomous Robots* 2003; 15:7–20.
45. Van der Loos HF, Reinkensmeyer DJ. Health care and rehabilitation robotics. In: Siciliano B, Khatib O, eds. *Springer Handbook of Robotics* in press.
46. Krebs HI, Hogan N, Aisen ML, Volpe BT. Robot-aided neurorehabilitation. *IEEE Trans Rehabil Eng* 1998; 6:75–87.
47. Stein J, Krebs HI, Frontera WR, et al. Comparison of two techniques of robot-aided upper limb exercise training after stroke. *Am J Phys Med Rehabil* 2004; 83:720–728.
48. Volpe BT, Krebs HI, Hogan N. Is robot-aided sensorimotor training in stroke rehabilitation a realistic option? *Curr Opin Neurol* 2001; 14:745–752.
49. Reinkensmeyer DJ, Kahn LE, Averbuch M, et al. Understanding and treating arm movement impairment after chronic brain injury: Progress with the ARM guide. *J Rehabil Res Dev* 2000; 37:653–662.
50. Lum PS, Burgar CG, Shor PC, et al. Robot-assisted movement training compared with conventional therapy techniques for the rehabilitation of upper limb motor function after stroke. *Arch Phys Med Rehabil* 2002; 83:952–959.
51. Boian R, Sharma A, Han C, et al. Virtual reality-based post-stroke hand rehabilitation. *Stud Health Technol Inform* 2002; 85:64–70.
52. Hesse S, Schmidt H, Werner C, Bardeleben A. Upper and lower extremity robotic devices for rehabilitation and for studying motor control. *Curr Opin Neurol* 2003; 16:705–710.
53. Wirz M, Zemon DH, Rupp R, et al. Effectiveness of automated locomotor training in patients with chronic incomplete spinal cord injury: A multicenter trial. *Arch Phys Med Rehabil* 2005; 86:672–680.
54. Wada K, Shibata T. Robot therapy in a care house: Its sociopsychological and physiological effects on the residents. Presented at IEEE International Conference on Robotics and Automation. Orlando, FL. 2006:3966–3971.

VII

STROKE CARE SYSTEMS AND OUTCOMES

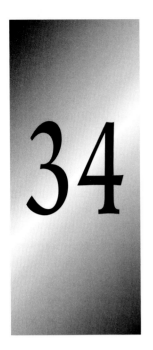

34 Stroke-specific Functional Assessment Instruments

Nancy K. Latham
Chiung-ju Liu
Alan M. Jette

The manifestations of stroke are heterogeneous and depend on many factors, including the size of the lesion, the affected brain region, and the patient's premorbid status. Although no two stroke patients are exactly the same, the ultimate goal of treatment for stroke survivors is to diminish sequelae of the disease and help patients return to community life. Functional assessments evaluate a patient's abilities beyond the primary affected cerebral functions related to movement, cognition, and language.

As evidence-based practice and initiatives to improve the quality of health care have grown around the world, recognition of the need to measure functional status in all health care settings has also increased (1). There are many instruments that have been used in clinical practice and research to assess functional outcomes in patients who have suffered a stroke. Some are designed for general use (usually called generic instruments), while others are designed for use specifically with patients with a stroke (called condition-specific functional instruments). The most commonly used generic instruments in stroke are the Functional Independence Measure (FIM) and the Barthel Index (BI) to assess basic daily activities and the SF-36 to assess health-related quality of life. The use of these generic measures in stroke has been extensively reviewed elsewhere (2–5). The focus in this chapter will be on reviewing condition-specific instruments that have been designed for use with patients who have suffered a stroke.

Functional status instruments vary widely in the scope of functional content included in the instrument. Some focus on the assessment of specific body movements or discrete functional tasks. Others assess a patient's ability to accomplish self-care activities; others address more broadly defined concepts of quality of life. The selection of an appropriate functional assessment measure is a complex process, and many factors need to be considered, including the scope of the instrument, the purpose for which it has been developed, the administration and scaling methods used, the psychometric properties of the instrument, as well as its feasibility in a particular context.

The aim of this chapter, therefore, is to provide readers with a conceptual framework for reviewing functional assessment instruments, introduce the range of condition-specific functional status instruments that are available to use with patients who have suffered a stroke, review some of the key criteria to guide one's selection among the variety of available instruments that might best meet a user's specific needs, and highlight some newer methodological techniques available to improve the assessment of function with patients who have suffered a stroke.

WHAT IS FUNCTIONAL ASSESSMENT?

Before selecting a functional assessment measure, it is necessary to have a clear understanding and definition of the concept being assessed and the range of functional content to be considered for a particular application. Currently, there is no clear and commonly accepted definition of functional status or a clear delineation between instruments that assess function and those that assess other health concepts. As work to define and quantify health concepts has taken place, many different types of instruments assessing overlapping health and functional concepts have been developed. These include instruments that purport to assess disability, function, activities of daily living, activity performance, advanced activities, physical performance, health, health status, quality of life, and health-related quality of life. To date, there is no consensus on how these terms should be used or measured (6).

The World Health Organization's (WHO) International Classification of Functioning, Disability, and Health (ICF) has tried to address this concern by providing the field with a useful conceptual framework for considering the definition and scope of functional assessment in stroke rehabilitation (7). In 2001, the WHO released the ICF to provide researchers and clinicians with a biopsychosocial view of health states from a biological, personal, and social perspective. The ICF organizes concepts in two parts. The first deals with function and disability, and the second deals with contextual factors. The function and disability domains of the ICF, expressed in either neutral or negative terms, are described from the perspective of body systems, the individual, and society. *Body functions and structures* are defined as physiological functions of body systems or anatomical elements such as organs, limbs, and their components. Hemiparesis is an example of a common impairment in a body function following the onset of a stroke. *Activity*, in contrast, is defined as the execution of specific tasks or actions by an individual. An example of the activity concept is a person's ability to walk independently or transfer from bed to chair. And finally, participation is described as encompassing involvement in life situations, such as the ability to return to one's former occupation following a stroke. Health-related quality of life includes aspects of all three ICF dimensions, but it is a distinct concept that usually includes domains that assess social functioning, emotional well-being, life satisfaction, as well as physical functioning.

The focus of this chapter is on stroke-specific measures of activity, participation, or health-related quality of life. The ICF organizes the areas of activity and participation into several domains, which include the following:

- Learning and applying knowledge
- General tasks and demands
- Communication
- Mobility
- Self-care
- Domestic life
- Interpersonal interactions and relationships
- Major life areas
- Community, social, and civic life

The two contextual elements of the ICF are environmental and personal factors. Environmental factors are all aspects of the external or extrinsic world that form the physical, social, and attitudinal circumstances in which people live and conduct their lives. Personal factors include gender, race, age, lifestyle, habits, social background, and other individual characteristics or experiences that are not classified elsewhere in the ICF. Even though these contextual factors may act as facilitators or barriers as they affect functioning and disability, they are not directly included within a functional assessment instrument.

Purpose of Functional Assessment

A patient's functional status can be assessed for several different purposes that have important bearing on the criteria that should be considered when choosing an assessment instrument. For this chapter, we focus on two distinct purposes to which functional assessment instruments are typically applied. The first can be characterized as discrimination. Discriminative functional instruments are designed to differentiate among patients at a point in time. At the level of a group of patients, a discriminative functional assessment can be done for the purpose of describing a patient population or for selection purposes in recruiting patients for a study, while, at an individual patient level, discriminative assessment can be done to set patient treatment goals or to gauge a patient's prognostic potential. Alternatively, a functional assessment can be used for evaluative purposes. In this situation, the assessment instrument has to be adequate to measure meaningful change in function over time. At the group level, this type of index can be used to evaluate hypotheses pertaining to the impact of therapeutic interventions on function when applied in clinical studies. At the individual patient level, evaluative instruments can be used to monitor change in a patient's functional status or to modify treatment approach during an episode of care.

Key Psychometric Properties

In addition to considering the scope of the functional content needed in a functional assessment, a user should consider the psychometric quality of the functional assessment instrument for the purpose to which it will be put, be it discrimination or evaluation. For discriminative instruments, standards of validity and reliability must be achieved. For the purpose of evaluation, the additional criterion of responsiveness much also be considered.

Validity. Validity concerns the degree to which the functional assessment instrument actually measures what it is intended to measure. There are several approaches to examining an instrument's validity. If the score represents the specific theoretical domain or universe of content, the assessment has content validity. For example, a questionnaire on quality of life should contain items that are related to the concept of quality of life but not gait control. If the score is in accordance with an established functional measurement administrated at the same time, the assessment has concurrent validity. For example, a new self-care measure should be highly correlated to the BI. If the functional score can predict a future criterion score, the assessment has predictive validity. For example, results of a patient's functional assessment at hospital admission may predict functional outcome at discharge.

Reliability. Reliability of an assessment is the extent to which repeated measurements yield the same outcome. The concepts of validity and reliability are related. An instrument with poor reliability will have diminished validity as well because it gives different outcomes at each measurement. However, it is possible that a highly reliable instrument still cannot measure the intended concept well and thus have poor validity.

Reliability assessment can include how consistent the result of an instrument is if readministered over time by the same person (test-retest) and/or if administrated by different people (inter-rater reliability). Similar results should be obtained regardless of who administers the assessment. For example, scores should be nearly the same when the assessment is administered by a therapist or a nurse. Internal consistency reliability reflects how consistent items are under the same category in an assessment. For example, items that measure self-care activities should have a higher correlation with each other than with items that measure instrument activities of living.

Responsiveness. Choosing a functional assessment with suitable responsiveness is a crucial criterion if the intended application is evaluative. A functional assessment with good responsiveness is sensitive to clinically meaningful change over time within a patient and the change is responsive to intervention effects (8). An assessment with good reliability and validity does not guarantee that it also has good responsiveness. Responsiveness can be seen as a form of longitudinal validity, meaning that a functional instrument should be able to detect changes in function in patients whose function actually changes and no or small changes in persons whose function remains stable over time (8).

Additional Factors to Consider

Validation in Stroke Population. When evaluating the psychometric properties of a stroke functional assessment instrument, it is important to consider the population in which the psychometric testing was performed. A generic instrument should be tested in a stroke population before it is used in research or clinical practice. For stroke-specific instruments, the similarity of the validation population to the target population needs to be considered. Ideally, the psychometric testing will have been performed in a representative sample of stroke patients that has a broad range of important characteristics. If a more restrictive sample of stroke patients was used, it is important to consider whether the type of stroke, severity of stroke, degree of functional limitation, and the timing of the assessment post-stroke are adequately similar between the two groups.

Feasibility. Many factors affect the feasibility of using a particular instrument. The setting of use and the subjects' severity of stroke will influence the amount of time that can be spent doing the assessment and the number of items that can be used. Even if a functional instrument is ideal in other ways, if an assessment requires special training, takes an excessive amount of time to administrate, or has complex scoring procedure, it increases the burden for health care professionals and may rarely be applied.

Mode of Assessment. Many functional assessments rely on self-reported functional abilities rather than observed direct performance by an assessor. Some instruments are designed to rely primarily on the patient's self-report, while others rely on caregivers or family members. The focus of self-report assessments is on the activities that people regularly perform in their own environment.

Use of Proxy Reports of Function. It is sometimes necessary to rely on proxy reports of function if a patient has a problem in communication because of affected cognition and language, and, as a result, an interview with the patient is not possible. Proxy reports might be more suitable when trying to obtain data from some populations, such as for people with severe functional problems. One study has found that a proxy was more likely to complete a mail survey if the patient had more functional limitations (9).

Because the source of information can influence reliability and validity of the functional assessment, it is important to clarify whether the score obtained from a proxy provides the same information as that obtained from the patient's own self-report, especially with patients who experience cognitive and communicative problems. When a proxy is used to provide a functional assessment, the agreement between the proxy and patient should have been assessed.

Self-Report Versus Direct Performance. An alternative approach to self-report functional assessments is to observe participants directly while performing a series of set functional tasks. Direct performance tests can be a useful alternative when patients have communication or cognitive problems that limit their ability to report their function. In addition, the direct performance tests can provide an accurate assessment of a person's capacity to do specific functional tasks, including tasks that he or she might not regularly undertake as part of his or her daily activities. Many studies have shown that direct performance measures provide similar but slightly different outcomes than self-report assessments (10). This is probably because direct performance tests are evaluating what a person is capable of doing under set conditions, while self-report assessments ask people what they actually do in their own environment.

Overview of Stroke-specific Functional Assessments

This section of the chapter describes the most commonly used stroke-specific measures of activity, participation, and health-related quality of life. For each measure, we summarize the instrument's background, scope, purpose, and psychometric properties. Table 34-1 summarizes the intended purpose, ICF conceptual domains covered, mode of administration, and psychometric properties of nine stroke-specific functional assessments reviewed.

American Heart Association Stroke Outcome Classification. The American Heart Association Stroke Outcome Classification (AHA.SOC) was developed by a multidisciplinary panel to measure the full range of deficits following stroke (11). The global classification identifies the severity and extent of neurologic impairments as well as the level of independence according to basic and instrumental activities of daily living (BADLs and IADLs). Therefore, the instrument covers all the three domains in the ICF: body structures and functions, activities, and participation. The primary purpose of the instrument is to serve as a standardized and comprehensive classification system to document the impairments and disability resulting from a stroke. A secondary aim is to gauge the effect of treatment.

The AHA.SOC contains three scales. The first scale, AHA.SOC-Domain, classifies the extent of neurologic impairments in six domains: motor, sensory, vision, affect, cognition, and language. The scale ranges from

0 (0 domains impaired) to 3 (more than two domains impaired). The second scale, AHA.SOC-Severity, classifies the severity of neurologic impairments into one of three levels: A (no/minimal neurologic deficit because of stroke in any domain), B (mild/moderate deficit because of stroke in >1 domain), and C (severe deficit due to stroke in >1 domain). The third scale, AHA.SOC-Function, classifies the dependency in BADLs and IADLs. The scale ranges from I (independent in BADLs and IADLs and tasks required of roles that patient had before the stroke) to V (completely dependent in of BADLs in more than five areas and IADLs). The classification score is meant to document

---

TABLE 34-1
Chedoke-McMaster Stroke Assessment Disability Inventory

Gross Motor Function Index
1. Supine to side lying on strong side
2. Supine to side lying on weak side
3. Side lying to long sitting through strong side
4. Side lying to sitting on side of the bed through strong side
5. Side lying to sitting on side of the bed through weak side
6. Standing
7. Transfer to and from bed toward strong side
8. Transfer to and from bed toward weak side
9. Transfer up and down from floor and chair
10. Transfer up and down from floor and standing

Walking Index
11. Walking indoors
12. Walking outdoors, over rough ground, ramps, and curbs
13. Walking outdoors several blocks
14. Stairs
15. Age- and sex-appropriate walking distance (in meters) for 2 minutes (2-point bonus)

Scoring key from the Functional Independence Measure, Uniform Data System For Medical Rehabilitation, State University of New York at Buffalo

Independence (no helper)
7. Complete independence (timely, safely)
6. Modified independence (device)

Modified dependence (helper)
5. Supervision
4. Minimal assist (subject = 75%)
3. Moderate assist (subject = 50%)

Complete dependence (helper)
2. Maximal assist (subject = 25%)
1. Total assist (subject = 0%)

the limitations resulting from the most recent episode of stroke. It is recommended that clinicians should use clinical examinations and standardized assessments to support their rating decisions for each scale (11). Time to complete the classification was not reported, but it may depend on the completion of standardized assessments.

Concurrent validity was assessed by correlations with the Modified Rankin Scale ($r = 0.70$), the BI ($r = -0.87$), Lawton Instrumental Activities of Daily Living (IADL) Scale ($r = -0.85$), and physical function in SF-36 ($r = -0.70$) (12). The inter-rater reliability is good for the number of impaired neurologic domains classification ($k = 0.56$) and excellent for the severity of impairment classification ($k = 0.76$) and for the functional disability classification ($k = 0.77$) (11). It can discriminate ADL-related disabilities after one, three, and six months after a stroke (12).

The AHA.SOC is a comprehensive clinical assessment of impairment, severity, and function after a stroke and a useful tool to classify stroke severity. Although the classification covers all the three conceptual domains in the ICF, the AHA.SOC-Function assesses basic ADLs and IADLs together and shows no clear division between activities and participation. Administration of AHA.SOC may require experienced health care professionals to obtain required information and to decide the rating. It is recommended that the classification should not be completed unless related standardized assessments are available.

Modified Rankin Scale and Oxford Handicap Scale. Rankin initially described functional recovery of a group of stroke patients on a five-level scale (13). The scale later was used as a global disability measure. To avoid ambiguity, the scale was revised with six levels and clearer wording to differentiate levels one and two (14). The scale was renamed as the Modified Rankin Scale and has become a popular outcome measure for stroke clinical trials (15, 16). The instrument was changed a third time by changing the word *disability* to *handicap*, and the term *lifestyle* was incorporated to expand the scale to measure handicap. This version is referred to as the Oxford Handicap Scale. Both scales are classification instruments to discriminate functional levels of patients. The Modified Rankin Scale covers the conceptual domain of activities whereas the Oxford Handicap Scale covers activities and participation.

Administration relies on professional judgment. Both scales have six grades ranging from 0 (no symptoms) to 5 (severe disability; bedridden, incontinent and requiring constant nursing care and attention in the Modified Rankin Scale; or severe handicap-totally dependent patient requiring constant attention night and day in the Oxford Handicap Scale) (14, 17). Time to complete the scale varies, depending on how familiar the clinician is with the patient. The structured interview takes approximately 15 minutes (18).

Concurrent validity of the Modified Rankin Scale was determined by comparing this scale with the BI (19). Concurrent validity of the Oxford Handicap Scale was assessed with a regression with multiple functional health indicators, including the BI and subscales of the Sickness Impact Profiles (20). The results showed that the Oxford Handicap Scale is a global functional health index but with a focus on physical disability (20). The inter-rater reliability of the Modified Rankin Scale is moderate for raters with similar professional background ($k = 0.56$) but low for raters with different background ($k = 0.25$) (14, 21). A structured interview was suggested to improve its inter-rater reliability. The inter-rater reliability was improved ($k = 0.74$) when the structured interview was followed (22). The inter-rater reliability of the Oxford Handicap Scale showed moderate agreement ($k = 0.42$) (17). The test-retest reliability was only available for the Modified Rankin Scale ($k = 0.81$) (22). The Modified Rankin Scale was less responsive to change when compared with the BI and the FIM in a group of stroke patients who received a rehabilitation service (23).

The Modified Rankin Scale and the Oxford Handicap Scale are simple outcome measures designed for use with patients post-stroke. The vague scale categories may be time-efficient and adequate to classify patients in a clinical setting but appear less psychometrically adequate for evaluating change. The Oxford Handicap Scale captures the domain of participation restrictions following a stroke, but is not designed for use with inpatients because it measures lifestyle issues that are not relevant while a patient is in the hospital. The lack of standardized criteria for administering both scales reduces the reliability of the scales. Training to improve the agreement of rating is needed if multiple testers will be used.

Chedoke-McMaster Stroke Assessment. The Chedoke-McMaster Stroke Assessment includes two outcome domains: a physical impairment inventory and an activity inventory (previously called a *disability inventory*) (24). The physical impairment inventory is a discriminative measure that is based on the body structures and functions conceptual domain in the ICF. The activity inventory is an evaluative measure that assesses change in mobility function, which is part of the activities conceptual domain in the ICF (Table 34-1).

The Chedoke-McMaster Stroke Assessment is a direct performance exam. Time to complete the assessment is approximately one hour. Administration and scoring rules are provided in a users' manual (25).

The physical impairment inventory has six dimensions: shoulder pain, postural control, the arm, the hand, the leg, and the foot. Each dimension is measured using a seven-point ordinal scale corresponding to the stage of motor recovery. The activity inventory has two subscales: gross motor function and walking. There are 10 items measuring rolling, sitting, transferring, and standing in the gross motor function subscale and 5 items measuring walking indoors, outdoors, stairs, and distance in the walking subscale. The activity inventory is suggested to be used with Uniform Data System for Medical Rehabilitation, which includes the FIM (24). Scoring for each item is on a seven-point Likert scale based on the assistance needed except for the last item, a two-minute walk test. A higher score indicates more independence. The maximum score of the activity inventory is 100.

Concurrent validity of the physical impairment inventory was assessed with correlation with Fugl-Meyer Test ($\gamma = 0.95$), and the activity inventory was with the FIM ($\gamma = 0.79$) (24). All the reliabilities were estimated with intraclass correlation coefficient (ICC) (24). The internal consistency of the six dimensions in the physical impairment inventory ranges from 0.93–0.98. The inter-rater reliability of the physical impairment inventory is 0.97, and the activity inventory is 0.99. The test-retest reliability of the activity inventory is 0.98. Variance ratio was used to assess the responsiveness between admission and discharge of a group of stroke patients (24). The Chedoke-McMaster Stroke Assessment was 1.92 times more responsive when compared with the FIM.

The Chedoke-McMaster Stroke Assessment is a stroke-specific instrument that has demonstrated high levels of validity and reliability. The two-inventory design can facilitate measuring treatment effects because it provides a way to classify stroke survivors into homogeneous subgroups based on motor recovery. However, the scope of the activity inventory may be too narrow if administered alone because it only measures mobility function. To fully assess functional domains commonly affected after a stroke—for example, self-care and communication—supplemental assessments are necessary.

Frenchay Activities Index. The Frenchay Activities Index (FAI) is a 15-item questionnaire that assesses activities performed inside and outside the home, including one mobility, seven IADL, and seven indoor or outdoor social/role activities (21, 26). The instrument covers activities and participation domains in the ICF. The FAI is designed as an evaluative instrument, which intends to obtain information on the premorbid lifestyle and up to three to six months after a stroke to help determine rehabilitation goals and record progress in activities (21, 26).

The FAI measures three domains: domestic (preparing main meals and washing clothes), leisure/work (reading books and gainful work), and outdoor activities (local shopping and outings/car rides). Administration can be done through self-report of patients and/or relatives (27). The questionnaire takes less than 10 minutes to complete, which makes it feasible to use in a clinic. Scoring is based on a four-point Likert frequency scale ranging from never (1) to the highest frequency (4). The use of a frequency scale is assumed to reduce the subjective judgment of quality of an activity (21).

Concurrent validity was assessed by examining correlations with the BI ($\gamma = 0.66$) and subscales of the Sickness Impact Profile Scale (γ is from -0.14 to -0.73) (21, 27). The FAI has excellent inter-rater reliability ($\gamma > 0.80$) (21, 28). The test-retest reliability is not reported. There is a high agreement between patients and their proxies on the FAI (ICC = 0.87 for the total FAI; ICC = 0.85 for the domestic domain; ICC = 0.63 for work/leisure domain; ICC = 0.87 for outdoor activities domain) (29). Although the FAI has been shown to detect change in the year following a stroke, data on the responsiveness of the FAI instrument is not available (21).

The FAI allows health care professionals to understand premorbid lifestyle of patients so rehabilitation goals can be set to fit individual needs. Although items in the three domains cover concepts of activity and participation in the ICF, the two concepts are merged in the three domains. The FAI has been validated in older patients; the coverage of activities may be not sufficient for younger age groups, who have different social roles and task demands (30). For example, a young female patient may have to fulfill a mother's role and carry out caring activities that are not covered by the FAI. Moreover, items of leisure activities lack diversity to capture the experiences of younger patients who may have different hobbies, which could further affect the responsiveness in this population.

Hamrin Activity Index. The Hamrin Activity Index (AI) was specifically designed for a study to measure an activity program for patients with stroke in nursing care in Sweden (31). The AI is an evaluative instrument. The instrument includes 16 items in three domains: mental capacity, motor activity, and ADL function. These items cover the conceptual domains of body structures and functions and activities in the ICF.

Administration involves a structured interview with the patients and relatives (31). It may take up to one hour to have the assessment done properly. The mental capacity domain includes four subscales: degree of consciousness, orientation in time, space and person, ability to communicate verbally, and psychological activities. The maximum score of this domain is

32 with a higher score indicating a better capacity. The motor activity domain measures functions of the four extremities with six subscales: right arm, right hand, right leg, left arm, left hand, and left leg. Scoring is from a functional point of view in relation to ADL performance, such as functional grip. The maximum score is 24 with a higher score indicating higher functioning. The ADL function domain includes six subscales: ambulation, personal hygiene, dressing, feeding, and continence with two items, emptying function of bladder and bowels. Scoring is based on the assistance needed to complete the activity. The maximum score is 36 with a higher score indicating more independence.

The concurrent validity was tested through a correlation with the Rankin disability scale, but the value of correlation was not reported (31). Similarly, the internal consistency was assessed but not reported (31). No inter-rater reliability was specifically assessed because mainly one researcher conducted the interviews in the activity intervention study (31). The instrument did not demonstrate responsiveness in patients three and twelve months after stroke (32).

One feature of AI is that it measures patient's ability to communicate verbally, which may be affected by the disease. However, the application of the scale to patients with communication or language deficits has not been tested. Moreover, motor activity only focuses on unilateral motor function whereas most daily activities require coordination between right and left extremities to complete. The application of this instrument can be limited given that AI was created within a research context to evaluate specific outcome domains of an intervention program. In addition, psychometric properties should be carefully assessed before applying this instrument.

Rivermead ADL Scale. The Rivermead ADL scale was designed to evaluate ADLs for stroke patients in the United Kingdom (33). Activities selected in the scale were considered important for people's daily life. It is an evaluative instrument that records the functional progress of stroke patients. The instrument measures a patient's ability to perform specific tasks, so it reflects the conceptual domain of activities in the ICF.

The Rivermead ADL scale is a task performance exam. The administrator follows a standardized procedure, and patients are required to demonstrate each task. The evaluation is terminated after three consecutive failed items. The instrument includes 16 ADLs and 15 IADLs and uses a hierarchical scaling. Namely, the order of the items reveals increasing difficulty. Scoring is based on three levels:

- 1 = Independent with or without aid
- 0v = Independent but verbal assistance is required
- 0 = Dependent

The administration time varies from 30 to 60 minutes.

The validity of the Rivermead ADL scale was established through Guttman scaling. The results showed the existence of a valid cumulative and unidimensional Guttman scale with acceptable reproducibility (coefficient > 0.89) and scalability (coefficient > 0.79) (34). The inter-rater reliability ($\gamma = 0.89$), and the test-retest reliability is excellent ($\gamma = 0.95$) (33). Whether the scale is responsive to clinically meaningful change is unknown.

The application of hierarchical scaling is one advantage of the Rivermead ADL scale. The total score not only reflects the functional limitation, but it also shows the actual items that the patient can do. Although the standardized procedure and direct physical performance increases the instrument's reliability, substantial time may be required for proper training and administration. Its responsiveness remains unknown. Some activities in the scale may be culturally sensitive, and a cross-culture comparison should be conducted before applying the instrument to the United States population.

Stroke-Specific Quality of Life Scale. Domains and items for the Stroke-Specific Quality of Life Scale (SS-QOL) were developed from interviews with patients with ischemic stroke (35). It is an evaluative instrument for stroke-specific, health-related quality of life (Table 34-2).

The SS-QOL is a self-report measure that is interview administered. Time to complete the interview is not reported. Twelve domains in the scale cover areas that may be affected by a stroke: energy, family roles, language, mobility, mood, personality, self-care, social roles, thinking, upper extremity function, vision, and work/productivity. All items are rated on a five-point Likert scale with a higher score indicating desirable outcomes.

The concurrent validity was assessed by comparing SS-QOL scores with established measures for each domain (35). Patients with language and cognitive deficits were excluded from the validation study, and, as a result, there was inadequate variation in the scores for the language, thinking, and social role domains to allow the assessment of their validity. Each domain in the SS-QOL was considered to have adequate internal consistency based on estimated Cronbach's α values; however, these values were not reported (35). No test-retest or inter-rater reliabilities are available. The responsiveness was evaluated on patients one and three months after an ischemic stroke. Most of the domains were shown moderate responsiveness (standardized effect sizes > 0.4) (35).

One advantage of SS-QOL is that it is a comprehensive measure of stroke. For example, it assesses language function, which has been ignored

TABLE 34-2
Stroke-Specific Quality of Life Scale

We would like to know how you're doing with activities or feelings that can sometimes be affected by stroke. Each question will ask about a specific activity or feeling. For each question, think about how that activity or that feeling has been in the past week.

The first group of questions asks about how much trouble you have with a specific activity. Each question deals with problems that some people have after their stroke. Circle the number in the box that best describes how much trouble you have had with that activity in the past week.

DURING THE PAST WEEK:

	COULDN'T DO IT AT ALL	A LOT OF TROUBLE	SOME TROUBLE	A LITTLE TROUBLE	NO TROUBLE AT ALL
SC1. Did you have trouble preparing food?	1	2	3	4	5
SC2. Did you have trouble eating, for example, cutting food or swallowing?	1	2	3	4	5
SC4. Did you have trouble getting dressed, for example, putting on socks or shoes, buttoning buttons, or zipping?	1	2	3	4	5
SC5. Did you have trouble taking a bath or shower?	1	2	3	4	5
SC8. Did you have trouble using the toilet?	1	2	3	4	5
V1. Did you have trouble seeing the television well enough to enjoy a show?	1	2	3	4	5
V2. Did you have trouble reaching for things because of poor eyesight?	1	2	3	4	5
V3. Did you have trouble seeing things off to one side?	1	2	3	4	5
L2. Did you have trouble speaking, for example, get stuck, stutter, stammer, or slur your words?	1	2	3	4	5
L3. Did you have trouble speaking clearly enough to use the telephone?	1	2	3	4	5

DURING THE PAST WEEK:

	COULDN'T DO IT AT ALL	A LOT OF TROUBLE	SOME TROUBLE	A LITTLE TROUBLE	NO TROUBLE AT ALL
L5. Did other people have trouble understanding what you said?	1	2	3	4	5
L6. Did you have trouble finding the word you wanted to say?	1	2	3	4	5
L7. Did you need to repeat yourself so others could understand you?	1	2	3	4	5
M1. Did you have trouble walking? (If you can't walk, circle 1 and go to question M7)	1	2	3	4	5
M4. Did you lose your balance when bending over or reaching for something?	1	2	3	4	5
M6. Did you have trouble climbing stairs?	1	2	3	4	5
M7. Did you have trouble with needing to stop and rest when walking or using a wheelchair?	1	2	3	4	5

TABLE 34-2
(Continued)

	COULDN'T DO IT AT ALL	A LOT OF TROUBLE	SOME TROUBLE	A LITTLE TROUBLE	NO TROUBLE AT ALL
M8. Did you have trouble with standing?	1	2	3	4	5
M9. Did you have trouble getting out of a chair?	1	2	3	4	5
W1. Did you have trouble doing daily work around the house?	1	2	3	4	5
W2. Did you have trouble finishing jobs that you started?	1	2	3	4	5
W3. Did you have trouble doing the work you used to do?	1	2	3	4	5

DURING THE PAST WEEK:

	COULDN'T DO IT AT ALL	A LOT OF TROUBLE	SOME TROUBLE	A LITTLE TROUBLE	NO TROUBLE AT ALL
UE1. Did you have trouble writing or typing?	1	2	3	4	5
UE2. Did you have trouble putting on socks?	1	2	3	4	5
UE3. Did you have trouble buttoning buttons?	1	2	3	4	5
UE5. Did you have trouble zipping a zipper?	1	2	3	4	5
UE6. Did you have trouble opening a jar?	1	2	3	4	5

The next set of questions asks about how much you agree or disagree with each statement. Each question deals with a problem or feeling that some people have after their stroke. Circle the number in the box that best says how you felt about each statement during the past week.

DURING THE PAST WEEK:

	STRONGLY AGREE	MODERATELY AGREE	NEITHER AGREE NOR DISAGREE	MODERATELY DISAGREE	STRONGLY DISAGREE
T2. It was hard for me to concentrate.	1	2	3	4	5
T3. I had trouble remembering things.	1	2	3	4	5
T4. I had to write things down to remember them.	1	2	3	4	5
P1. I was irritable.	1	2	3	4	5
P2. I was impatient with others.	1	2	3	4	5
P3. My personality has changed.	1	2	3	4	5
MD2. I was discouraged about my future.	1	2	3	4	5
MD3. I wasn't interested in other people or activities.	1	2	3	4	5
FR5. I didn't join in activities just for fun with my family.	1	2	3	4	5
FR7. I felt I was a burden to my family.	1	2	3	4	5
FR8. My physical condition interfered with my family life.	1	2	3	4	5
SR1. I didn't go out as often as I would like.	1	2	3	4	5
SR4. I did my hobbies and recreation for shorter periods of time than I would like.	1	2	3	4	5

TABLE 34-2
(Continued)

	STRONGLY AGREE	MODERATELY AGREE	NEITHER AGREE NOR DISAGREE	MODERATELY DISAGREE	STRONGLY DISAGREE
SR5. I didn't see as many of my friends as I would like.	1	2	3	4	5
SR6. I had sex less often than I would like.	1	2	3	4	5
SR7. My physical condition interfered with my social life.	1	2	3	4	5

DURING THE PAST WEEK:

	STRONGLY AGREE	MODERATELY AGREE	NEITHER AGREE NOR DISAGREE	MODERATELY DISAGREE	STRONGLY DISAGREE
MD6. I felt withdrawn from other people.	1	2	3	4	5
MD7. I had little confidence in myself.	1	2	3	4	5
MD8. I was not interested in food.	1	2	3	4	5
E2. I felt tired most of the time.	1	2	3	4	5
E3. I had to stop and rest often during the day.	1	2	3	4	5
E4. I was too tired to do what I wanted to do.	1	2	3	4	5

Now, we would like to ask how you feel you are doing today in some general areas compared to how you were before your stroke. Put an "X" in the box to show whether each area is a lot worse, a little worse, or the same as your before your stroke. Please remember to compare how you are doing today with how you were before your stroke happened.

	A LOT WORSE THAN BEFORE MY STROKE	SOMEWHAT WORSE THAN BEFORE MY STROKE	A LITTLE WORSE THAN BEFORE MY STROKE	THE SAME AS BEFORE MY STROKE
1. E. My energy level is …				
2. L. My speech is …				
3. M. My walking is …				
4. V. My vision is …				
5. UE. The use of my arms or hands is …				
6. T. My thinking is …				
7. MD. My mood is …				
8. P. My personality is …				
9. W. I do my jobs at home or at work.				
10. SC. I can take care of myself.				
11. FR. I do things for my family.				
12. SR. I do things for my friends.				
13. Overall, my quality of life is …				

by most functional assessments. Because SS-QOL is a condition-specific quality of life measure, it is more related to the overall quality of life in stroke patients than generic QOL measures (36). However, the scoring procedure can be confusing, as one domain may use two response set keys. The Likert response scale for each key is inconsistent with each other, that is, in one scale, 5 may indicate "no help needed" or may indicate "strongly disagree." Consequently, the domain sum score may be difficult to interpret. In addition, this is a lengthy questionnaire and, therefore, might be inefficient to use in some settings. SS-QOL was validated only using direct self-reports of patients with ischemic stroke. Caution is needed in applying it to different populations or if proxies are used.

Stroke Adapted Sickness Impact Profile. The Stroke Adapted Sickness Impact Profile (SA-SIP30) is adapted from the 136-item Sickness Impact Profile (SIP) to measure quality of life post-stroke (37). The scale eliminates the disadvantage of length in the SIP by excluding irrelevant and unreliable items. It is an evaluative instrument and covers body structures and functions, activities, and participation in the ICF.

Administration is via a structured interview with the patient. The SA-SIP30 includes 30 yes/no items in eight domains: body care and movement, ambulation, mobility, household management, social interaction, communication, emotional behavior, and alertness behavior (37). The first four domains assess a physical dimension, and the other four assess a psychosocial dimension. Items are weighted for scoring with a lower score indicating more desirable outcome. Time to complete the questionnaire is less than 30 minutes.

Validity was compared with the 136-item SIP ($\gamma_s = 0.96$) as well as with the BI ($\gamma_s = 0.50$) and the Rankin Scale ($\gamma_s = 0.68$) (37). The internal consistency was moderate to good ($\alpha > 0.68$) (38). No test-retest and inter-rater reliabilities were specifically reported for the SA-SIP30. Responsiveness was assessed on patients at six and twelve months and showed moderate effect sizes (effect size = 0.6) (38, 39).

SA-SIP30 is a time-efficient quality of life measure for stroke patients. However, the scale has few psychosocial items and has a tendency to measure physical functioning rather than health-related quality of life (40). The scale has not been validated in patients with cognitive or language impairments or with proxy reporting.

Stroke Impact Scale. The Stroke Impact Scale (SIS) was developed from the perspective and input of stroke patients, caregivers, and health professionals with stroke expertise (41). It is a comprehensive evaluative instrument that tries to capture the heterogeneous consequences after a stroke. It covers all three conceptual domains in the ICF (Table 34-3).

It is a self-report measure administered through a structured interview with a patient and includes 59 items in 8 domains: strength, hand function, ADLs/IADLs, mobility, communication, emotion, memory and thinking, and social participation. SIS scoring uses a five-point Likert scale with a higher score indicating higher function. Time to complete is approximately 15 to 20 minutes. If the patient has trouble following a three-step command because of cognitive impairment or aphasia, a proxy can be used to complete the interview (42). The instrument also can be administered via telephone interview and mail survey, which increases the feasibility to follow up functional recovery in a community setting (43).

Validity was assessed with correlations with established measures (41). The correlation coefficients are from 0.82–0.84 for items in the mobility and ADL/IADL. The correlation coefficients are from 0.44–0.58 for items in the memory and communication domains. The correlation coefficient is 0.70 for items in the participation domain. The internal consistency of the eight domains are from 0.7–0.92 (ICCs) (41). Rasch analysis also demonstrated that most items in each domain are unidimensional, and five misfit items identified by the analysis were dropped from the latest version of SIS (42). The sensitivity to change of the SIS depends on the patient's stage of stroke severity. Even though the scale has been shown to detect change from one to three months and one to six months for minor and moderate stroke ($t > 1.73$), from three to six months for people with moderate stroke with higher-functioning ($t > 2.14$) (41), the ability to be responsive to clinically meaningful change has yet to be established.

Recently, SIS has demonstrated good test-retest reliability through telephone interview (ICCs range from 0.75–0.95) and mail survey mode (ICCs range from 0.68–0.98) in a sample of veterans (43). SIS has demonstrated a moderate level of agreement between the proxy and patient (ICCs range from 0.50–0.83), especially in the domains that are related to physical function (strength, hand function, ADLs/IADLs, and mobility) (44). These four domains can be combined as one physical domain score. A short version (SIS-16), in which items are selected from these four domains, has demonstrated less ceiling effect for patients with mild stroke than the BI (45).

To our knowledge, SIS is the first stroke-specific instrument validated in a large and diverse group of stroke survivors, including ischemic and hemorrhagic stroke, from multiple clinical sites in the United States and Canada. Test content is comprehensive, and the scale can differentiate among patients with various functional states because of its broad range of item difficulty (42). The scale can be widely applied because it has been validated for use by mail or telephone and when a proxy respondent is required. Another advantage is that the short version of SIS-16 can be an alternative to traditional ADL scales.

Research Frontiers: Future Directions for Functional Assessment

The Precision vs. Feasibility Dilemma. As the above review of instruments demonstrates, we have greatly improved the breadth in functional status measurement used in the stroke field and broader health care arena (46, 47). However, even those functional outcome instruments with excellent breadth still have problems of inadequate depth of measurement (48). Thus, although

TABLE 34-3
Stroke Impact Scale (Version 3.0)

The purpose of this questionnaire is to evaluate how stroke has impacted your health and life. We want to know from your point of view how stroke has affected you. We will ask you questions about impairments and disabilities caused by your stroke, as well as how stroke has affected your quality of life. Finally, we will ask you to rate how much you think you have recovered from your stroke.

These questions are about the physical problems that may have occurred as a result of your stroke.

1. IN THE PAST WEEK, HOW WOULD YOU RATE THE STRENGTH OF YOUR …	A LOT OF STRENGTH	QUITE A BIT OF STRENGTH	SOME STRENGTH	A LITTLE STRENGTH	NO STRENGTH AT ALL
a. Arm that was most affected by your stroke?	5	4	3	2	1
b. Grip of your hand that was most affected by your stroke?	5	4	3	2	1
c. Leg that was most affected by your stroke?	5	4	3	2	1
d. Foot/ankle that was most affected by your stroke?	5	4	3	2	1

These questions are about your memory and thinking.

2. IN THE PAST WEEK, HOW DIFFICULT WAS IT FOR YOU TO …	NOT DIFFICULT AT ALL	A LITTLE DIFFICULT	SOMEWHAT DIFFICULT	VERY DIFFICULT	EXTREMELY DIFFICULT
a. Remember things that people just told you?	5	4	3	2	1
b. Remember things that happened the day before?	5	4	3	2	1
c. Remember to do things (keep scheduled appointments or take medication)?	5	4	3	2	1
d. Remember the day of the week?	5	4	3	2	1
e. Concentrate?	5	4	3	2	1
f. Think quickly?	5	4	3	2	1
g. Solve everyday problems?	5	4	3	2	1

These questions are about how you feel, about changes in your mood, and about your ability to control your emotions since your stroke.

3. IN THE PAST WEEK, HOW OFTEN DID YOU …	NONE OF THE TIME	A LITTLE OF THE TIME	SOME OF THE TIME	MOST OF THE TIME	ALL OF THE TIME
a. Feel sad?	5	4	3	2	1
b. Feel that there is nobody you are close to?	5	4	3	2	1
c. Feel that you are a burden to others?	5	4	3	2	1
d. Feel that you have nothing to look forward to?	5	4	3	2	1
e. Blame yourself for mistakes that you made?	5	4	3	2	1
f. Enjoy things as much as ever?	5	4	3	2	1
g. Feel quite nervous?	5	4	3	2	1
h. Feel that life is worth living?	5	4	3	2	1
i. Smile and laugh at least once a day?	5	4	3	2	1

TABLE 34-3
(Continued)

The following questions are about your ability to communicate with other people, as well as your ability to understand what you read and what you hear in a conversation.

4.	IN THE PAST WEEK, HOW DIFFICULT WAS IT TO …	NOT DIFFICULT AT ALL	A LITTLE DIFFICULT	SOMEWHAT DIFFICULT	VERY DIFFICULT	EXTREMELY DIFFICULT
a.	Say the name of someone who was in front of you?	5	4	3	2	1
b.	Understand what was being said to you in a conversation?	5	4	3	2	1
c.	Reply to questions?	5	4	3	2	1
d.	Correctly name objects?	5	4	3	2	1
e.	Participate in a conversation with a group of people?	5	4	3	2	1
f.	Have a conversation on the telephone?	5	4	3	2	1
g.	Call another person on the telephone, including selecting the correct phone number and dialing?	5	4	3	2	1

The following questions ask about activities you might do during a typical day.

5.	IN THE PAST TWO WEEKS, HOW DIFFICULT WAS IT TO …	NOT DIFFICULT AT ALL	A LITTLE DIFFICULT	SOMEWHAT DIFFICULT	VERY DIFFICULT	COULD NOT DO AT ALL
a.	Cut your food with a knife and fork?	5	4	3	2	1
b.	Dress the top part of your body?	5	4	3	2	1
c.	Bathe yourself?	5	4	3	2	1
d.	Clip your toenails?	5	4	3	2	1
e.	Get to the toilet on time?	5	4	3	2	1
f.	Control your bladder (not have an accident)?	5	4	3	2	1
g.	Control your bowels (not have an accident)?	5	4	3	2	1
h.	Do light household tasks/chores (dust, make a bed, take out garbage, and do the dishes)?	5	4	3	2	1
i.	Go shopping?	5	4	3	2	1
j.	Do heavy household chores (vacuum, laundry, or yard work)?	5	4	3	2	1

The following questions are about your ability to be mobile at home and in the community.

6.	IN THE PAST TWO WEEKS, HOW DIFFICULT WAS IT TO …	NOT DIFFICULT AT ALL	A LITTLE DIFFICULT	SOMEWHAT DIFFICULT	VERY DIFFICULT	COULD NOT DO AT ALL
a.	Stay sitting without losing your balance?	5	4	3	2	1
b.	Stay standing without losing your balance?	5	4	3	2	1
c.	Walk without losing your balance?	5	4	3	2	1
d.	Move from a bed to a chair?	5	4	3	2	1
e.	Walk one block?	5	4	3	2	1
f.	Walk fast?	5	4	3	2	1

TABLE 34-3
(Continued)

6. IN THE PAST TWO WEEKS, HOW DIFFICULT WAS IT TO ...	NOT DIFFICULT AT ALL	A LITTLE DIFFICULT	SOMEWHAT DIFFICULT	VERY DIFFICULT	COULD NOT DO AT ALL
g. Climb one flight of stairs?	5	4	3	2	1
h. Climb several flights of stairs?	5	4	3	2	1
i. Get in and out of a car?	5	4	3	2	1

The following questions are about your ability to use your hand that was MOST AFFECTED by your stroke.

7. IN THE PAST TWO WEEKS, HOW DIFFICULT WAS IT TO USE YOUR HAND THAT WAS MOST AFFECTED BY YOUR STROKE TO ...	NOT DIFFICULT AT ALL	A LITTLE DIFFICULT	SOMEWHAT DIFFICULT	VERY DIFFICULT	COULD NOT DO AT ALL
a. Carry heavy objects (a bag of groceries)?	5	4	3	2	1
b. Turn a doorknob?	5	4	3	2	1
c. Open a can or jar?	5	4	3	2	1
d. Tie a shoelace?	5	4	3	2	1
e. Pick up a dime?	5	4	3	2	1

The following questions are about how stroke has affected your ability to participate in the activities that you usually do, things that are meaningful to you and help you to find purpose in life.

8. DURING THE PAST FOUR WEEKS, HOW MUCH OF THE TIME HAVE YOU BEEN LIMITED IN ...	NONE OF THE TIME	A LITTLE OF THE TIME	SOME OF THE TIME	MOST OF THE TIME	ALL OF THE TIME
a. Your work (paid, voluntary, or other)?	5	4	3	2	1
b. Your social activities?	5	4	3	2	1
c. Quiet recreation (crafts, reading)?	5	4	3	2	1
d. Active recreation (sports, outings, travel)?	5	4	3	2	1
e. Your role as a family member and/or friend?	5	4	3	2	1
f. Your participation in spiritual or religious activities?	5	4	3	2	1
g. Your ability to control your life as you wish?	5	4	3	2	1
h. Your ability to help others?	5	4	3	2	1

9.   STROKE RECOVERY

On a scale of 0 to 100, with 100 representing full recovery and 0 representing no recovery, how much have you recovered from your stroke?

_____ 100 Full Recovery
_____ 90
_____ 80
_____ 70
_____ 60
_____ 50
_____ 40
_____ 30
_____ 20
_____ 10
_____ .

we now have the capability to quantify many different functional dimensions, most instruments are relatively crude and imprecise, which particularly restricts their utility as evaluative instruments designed to monitor clinical relevant change in function for clinical use, quality improvement, and/or research. Those instruments that do provide more depth of measurement along with breadth are quite lengthy and are thus impractical to use in most settings and for most applications.

Contemporary test development techniques, relatively new to the health care arena, may provide the field with innovative means of solving this measurement dilemma and open the way to more responsive instruments to monitor change in function. Although these newer measurement techniques have yet to be applied to the development of a stroke-specific functional status instrument, this is an active area of research.

Contemporary Methods to Improve Functional Assessment. We believe two contemporary measurement techniques—item response theory (IRT) and computer-adaptive testing (CAT)—have the ability to overcome many limitations in traditional functional status instruments and have the potential to transform how functional assessment is done within rehabilitation. Although these advances have been used in educational testing for decades, they have only just recently begun to be applied to functional outcome assessment in rehabilitation and other arenas of health care.

Item Response Theory Techniques. IRT methods examine the associations between individuals' response to a series of items designed to measure a specific concept such as functional status (49). Data collected from samples of rehabilitation patients are fit statistically to an underlying IRT model that best explains the covariance among item responses (50, 51). IRT measurement models are a class of statistical procedures used to develop measurement scales. The measurement scales are comprised of items with a known relationship between item responses and positions on an underlying functional domain, called an *item characteristic curve.* The form of the relationships is typically nonlinear. Using this approach, probabilities of patients scoring a particular response on an item at various functional ability levels can be modeled. Persons with more functional ability have higher probabilities of responding positively to functional items than persons with lower functional abilities. These probability estimates are used to determine the individual's most likely position along the functional dimension. When assumptions of a particular IRT model are met, estimates of a person's functional ability do not strictly depend on a particular fixed set of items. This scaling feature allows one to compare persons along a functional outcome dimension even if they have not completed the identical set of functional items.

Because items and functional outcome scores are defined on the same scale, items can be optimally selected to provide good estimates of each domain of function at any level of the scale. This feature of IRT creates important flexibility in administering tests in a dynamic and tailored approach for each individual. See Hambleton (1989) for a more detailed explanation of IRT methods (52).

IRT is currently being applied in rehabilitation to develop new measures, improve existing measures, investigate group differences in item and scale functioning, equate different instruments, and, as we highlight, develop efficient test applications, such as CATs.

To apply IRT to functional outcome assessment, an appropriate item pool of functional tasks or activities needs to be assembled. An item pool is a collection of outcome items that represent a range of levels of a particular outcome domain. Item pools used in IRT analyses are developed by equating outcome items from different sources so they can be meaningfully compared together on a common underlying scale. IRT methods open the door to understanding the linkages among items used to assess a common functional outcome domain and, in this way, serve as the psychometric foundation underlying CAT (53–55).

CAT Methodology. CAT programs use a simple form of artificial intelligence that selects questions tailored to the test-taker and thereby shortens or lengthens the test to achieve the level of precision desired by a user. Functional status CAT applications rely on extensive item pools constructed for each outcome area. It contains items that consistently scale along each functional domain from low to high proficiency and includes rules guiding starting, stopping, and scoring procedures. CAT methodology uses a computer interface for the patient/clinician report that is tailored to a patient's unique functional ability level. The basic notion of a CAT test is to mimic what an experienced clinician does. A clinician learns most when he or she directs questions at the patient's approximate level of proficiency. Administering functional items that represent tasks that are either too easy or too hard for the patient provides little information. In contrast to traditional, fixed form functional tests that ask the same questions of everyone, regardless of how the respondent answers, CAT instruments, like a skilled clinician, tailor their assessment by asking only the most informative questions based on a person's response to previous questions.

A CAT is programmed to first present an item from the midrange of an IRT-defined item pool and then directs subsequent functional items to the level based on the patient's (or clinician's) previous responses without asking unnecessary questions. The selection of an item in the midrange is arbitrary, and the CAT can be set to select an initial item based on other information entered about the patient such as age, diagnosis, or severity of his or her

TABLE 34-4

Stroke-specific Functional Assessment Instruments

	Name	American Heart Assoc.	Modified Rankin Scale	Chedoke-McMaster Scale	Frenchay Activities Index	Hamrin Activity Index	Rivermead ADL scale	Stroke-Specific QOL	Stroke-Adapted SIP	Stroke Impact Scale
Intended purpose	Classification	√	√	√						
	Evaluation of change	√	√	√	√	√	√	√	√	√
ICF domains	Body structures and functions	√		√		√		√	√	√
	Activities	√	√	√	√	√	√	√	√	√
	Participation	√			√			√	√	√
Mode of administration	Patient interview				√			√	√	√
	Professional judgment	√	√							
	Physical performance			√			√			
Psychometric properties	Validity	*	*	*	*	*	*	*	*	*
	Test-retest reliability		*	*			*			*
	Inter-rater reliability	*	*	*	*		*			
	Responsive-ness		*	*	*	*		*	*	*

Note. * = Related psychometric property was assessed and reported. Please see text for detailed review.

condition. By having comprehensive item banks available in each functional outcome domain of interest, the selection of additional items after the initial one is based on responses to the previous items. This allows for fewer items to be administered while gaining precise information regarding an individual's placement along an outcome continuum.

We will illustrate how the CAT works using a functional activity scale developed in our research group (56). In this functional activity scale, we assume that the midpoint of the scale is 50, and this serves as the initial (default) score estimate prior to the CAT administration. For this example, we used data collected in a prospective rehabilitation outcome study (57). We set the CAT precision stopping rule as a 95% CI < 3.0. The case is an individual who suffered a stroke and is now receiving rehabilitation therapy in a community-based outpatient center.

The initial item administered is, "How much difficulty do you have coming to sit at side of a bed?" A response of "a little difficulty" yields a score estimate of 38.2 with a large confidence interval (49).

A second question is administered, based on the estimate from the first response, "How much difficulty do you have carrying a suitcase?" The person responds, "No difficulty." A new score estimate is then calculated (44.4 ± 9.2), and the CAT program checks to see if the stop rule has been satisfied. Because the stop rule in this case is a confidence interval of <5, a third item is administered.

To the third item, "How much difficulty do you have running to catch a bus?" the person responds, "A little difficulty." A new score estimate is calculated (44 ± 6). The stop rule has not yet been satisfied, so a fourth item is administered.

The item "How much difficulty do you have doing heavy housework?" is given to the person, and the answer is "a little difficulty," with a new score estimate of 44.2 ± 3. Because this meets the stop rule, no additional items are administered, and a final score estimate based on four items is 44.2 with a confidence interval of ±3. In this case, the four items administered were able to reproduce closely the score of 43.8, which was obtained by the administration of all 101 items in the full item pool. The number of items administered can be increased to achieve the desired level of precision.

Though intuitively appealing on its surface, to be truly innovative and useful in rehabilitation, functional status CATs must be shown to meet several standards for acceptance for clinical and research applications. These include:

1. Acceptable score accuracy in comparison to the entire item pool
2. Adequate score precision for group and individual assessments
3. Sufficient content breadth for application across a wide array of care settings
4. Adequate responsiveness for monitoring clinically relevant change
5. Feasibility with respect to user burden and administration cost for widespread use. This is an active area of research investigation within rehabilitation.

SUMMARY

Functional assessment is now an essential part of stroke research and clinical practice. The selection of the most appropriate instrument is a complex process that requires careful consideration. Health professionals, researchers, and others who utilize functional assessments need to carefully evaluate the existing instruments to determine which one is most appropriate to meet their needs. The field of functional assessment has progressed so that there are now many stroke-specific functional assessments to choose from (Table 34-4). Potential users should consider the scope of the instrument, the purpose for which it has been developed, the administration and scaling methods used, the psychometric properties of the instrument, as well as its feasibility in a particular context.

Even though the breadth of content in functional status instruments used in the stroke field and broader health care arena has improved in recent decades, existing instruments still have problems with the balance between feasibility and breadth as well as depth of coverage. Fortunately, new methodologies such as item response theory (IRT) and computer-adaptive testing (CAT) provide a way to overcome these problems. It is anticipated that these methods will be applied to stroke-specific measures in the future and allow further improvements in our ability to accurately and efficiently measure functional status in a wide range of people following a stroke.

References

1. Iezzoni LI, Greenberg MS. Capturing and classifying functional status information in administrative databases. *Health Care Financ Rev* 2003; 24:61–76.
2. Barak S, Duncan PW. Issues in selecting outcome measures to assess functional recovery after stroke. *NeuroPx* 2006; 3:505–524.
3. Jette AM. Disability assessment for patients with stroke. *Top Stroke Rehabil* 1997; 3:21–37.
4. Kelly-Hayes M. Stroke outcome measures. *J Cardiovasc Nurs* 2004; 19:301–307.
5. Salter K, Jutai JW, Teasell R, et al. Issues for selection of outcome measures in stroke rehabilitation: ICF participation. *Disabil Rehabil* 2005; 27:507–528.
6. Johnston M, Steinman M, Velozo CA. Assessing medical rehabilitation practices: The promise of outcomes research. In: Fuhrer M, ed. *Outcomes Research in Medical Rehabilitation: Foundations from the Past and Directions to the Future.* Baltimore, MD: Paul H. Brookes Publishing Company, 1997:1–41.
7. World Health Organization. *International Classification of Functioning, Disability and Health.* Geneva, Switzerland: World Health Organization, 2001.
8. Guyatt G, Walter S, Norman G. Measuring change over time: Assessing the usefulness of evaluative instruments. *J Chronic Dis* 1987; 40:171–178.

9. Duncan PW, Reker DM, Horner RD, et al. Performance of a mail-administered version of a stroke-specific outcome measure, the Stroke Impact Scale. *Clin Rehabil* 2002; 16:493–505.

10. Stretton C, Latham N, Carter K, et al. Determinants of physical health in frail older people: The importance of self-efficacy. *Clin Rehabil* 2006; 20:357–366.

11. Kelly-Hayes M, Robertson JT, Broderick JP, et al. The American Heart Association Stroke Outcome Classification. *Stroke* 1998; 29:1274–1280.

12. Lai S-M, Duncan PW. Evaluation of the American Heart Association Stroke Outcome Classification. *Stroke* 1999; 30:1840–1843.

13. Rankin J. Cerebral vascular accidents in patients over the age of 60: II. Prognosis. *Scot Med J* 1957; 2:200–215.

14. van Swieten JC, Koudstaal PJ, Visser MC, et al. Interobserver agreement for the assessment of handicap in stroke patients. *Stroke* 1988; 19:604–607.

15. Duncan PW, Jorgensen HS, Wade DT. Outcome measures in acute stroke trials: A systematic review and some recommendations to improve practice. *Stroke* 2000:1429-1438.

16. New PW, Buchbinder R. Critical appraisal and review of the Rankin scale and its derivatives. *Neuroepidemiology* 2006; 26:4–15.

17. Bamford JM, Sandercock PA, Warlow CP, Slattery J. Interobserver agreement for the assessment of handicap in stroke patients (letter). *Stroke* 1989; 20:828.

18. Salter K, Jutai JW, Teasell R, Foley NC, Bitensky J, Bayley M. Issues for selection of outcome measures in stroke rehabilitation: ICF activity. *Disabil Rehabil.* 2005; 27:315-340.

19. Wolfe CD, Taub NA, Woodrow EJ, Burney PG. Assessment of scales of disability and handicap for stroke patients.[see comment]. *Stroke* 1991; 22:1242–1244.

20. de Haan R, Limburg M, Bossuyt P, et al. The clinical meaning of Rankin 'handicap' grades after stroke. *Stroke* 1995; 26:2027–2030.

21. Wade DT, Legh-Smith J, Hewer RL. Social activities after stroke: Measurement and natural history using Frechay Activities Index. *Int Rehabil Med* 1985; 7:176–181.

22. Wilson JT, Hareendran A, Hendry A, et al. Reliability of the modified Rankin Scale across multiple raters: Benefits of a structured interview. *Stroke* 2005; 36:777–781.

23. Dromerick A, Edwards D, Diringer M. Sensitivity to changes in disability after stroke: A comparison of four scales useful in clinical trials. *J Rehabil Research Dev* 2003; 40:1–8.

24. Gowland C, Stratford P, Ward M, et al. Measuring physical impairment and disability with the Chedoke-McMaster stroke assessment. *Stroke* 1993; 24:58–63.

25. Gowland C, Van Hullenaar S, Torresin W, et al. *Chedoke-Mcmaster Stroke Assessment: Development, Validation, and Administration Manual.* Hamilton, Ontario, Canada: School of Occupational Therapy and Physiotherapy, McMaster University; 1995.

26. Holbrook M, Skilbeck CE. An activities index for use with stroke patients. *Age Ageing* 1983; 12:166–170.

27. Schuling J, de Haan R, Limburg M, Groenier KH. The Frenchay Activities Index: Assessment of functional status in stroke patients. *Stroke* 1993; 24:1173–1177.

28. Post MWM, de Witte LP. Good inter-rater reliability of the Frenchay Activities Index in stroke. *Clin Rehabil* 2003; 17:548–552.

29. Tooth LR, McKenna KT, Smith M, O'Rourke P. Further evidence for the agreement between patients with stroke and their proxies on the Frenchay Activities Index. *Clin Rehabil* 2003; 17:656–665.

30. Turnbull JC, Kersten P, Habib M, et al. Validation of the Frenchay Activities Index in a general population aged 16 years and older. *Arch Phys Med Rehabil* 2000; 81:1034–1038.

31. Hamrin E, Wohlin AI. Evaluation of the functional capacity of stroke patients through an activity index. *Scand J Rehabil Med* 1982; 14:93–100.

32. Lindmark B, Hamrin E. Instrumental activities of daily living in two patient populations, three months, and one year after a stroke. *Scand J Caring Sci* 1989; 3:161–168.

33. Whiting S, Lincoln N. An ADL assessment for stroke patients. *British Journal of Occupational Therapy* 1980; 43:44–46.

34. Lincoln NB, Edmans JA. A revalidation of the Rivermead ADL scale for elderly patients with stroke. *Age Ageing* 1990; 19:19–24.

35. Williams LS, Weinberger M, Harris LE, et al. Development of a stroke-specific quality of life scale. *Stroke* 1999; 30:1362–1369.

36. Williams LS, Weinberger M, Harris LE, Biller J. Measuring quality of life in a way that is meaningful to stroke patients. *Neurology* 1999; 53:1839–1843.

37. van Straten A, de Haan RJ, Limburg M, et al. A stroke-adapted 30-item version of the Sickness Impact Profile to assess quality of life (SA-SIP30). *Stroke* 1997; 28:2155–2161.

38. van de Port IGL, Ketelaar M, Schepers VPM, van den Bos GAM. Monitoring the functional health status of stroke patients: The value of the Stroke-Adapted Sickness Impact Profile-30. *Disabil Rehabil* 2004; 26:635–640.

39. Schepers VP, Ketelaar M, Visser-Meily JM, et al. Responsiveness of functional health status measures frequently used in stroke research. *Disabil Rehabil* 2006; 28:1035–1040.

40. van Straten A, de Haan RJ, Limburg M, van den Bos GA. Clinical meaning of the Stroke-Adapted Sickness Impact Profile-30 and the Sickness Impact Profile-136. *Stroke* 2000; 31:2610–2615.

41. Duncan PW, Wallace D, Lai SM, et al. The Stroke Impact Scale Version 2.0: Evaluation of reliability, validity, and sensitivity to change. *Stroke* 1999; 30:2131–2140.

42. Duncan PW, Bode RK, Min Lai S, Perera S. Glycine antagonist in neuroprotection Americans I. Rasch analysis of a new stroke-specific outcome scale: the Stroke Impact Scale. *Arch Phys Med Rehabil* 2003; 84:950–963.

43. Duncan P, Reker D, Kwon S, et al. Measuring stroke impact with the stroke impact scale: Telephone versus mail administration in veterans with stroke. *Med Care* 2005; 43:507–515.

44. Duncan PW, Lai SM, Tyler D, et al. Evaluation of proxy responses to the Stroke Impact Scale. *Stroke* 2002; 33:2593–2599.

45. Duncan PW, Lai SM, Bode RK, et al. Stroke Impact Scale-16: A brief assessment of physical function. *Neurology* 2003; 60:291–296.

46. McHorney C. Generic health measurement: Past accomplishments and a measurement paradigm for the 21st century. *Ann of Intern Med* 1997; 127:743–750.

47. Patrick DL, Chiang YP. Measurement of health outcomes in treatment effectiveness evaluations: Conceptual and methodological challenges. *Med Care* 2000; 38:II-14–II-25.

48. Liang M, Lew R, Stucki G, et al. Measuring clinically important changes with patient-oriented questionnaires. *Med Care* 2002; 40:II-45–II-51.

49. Embretson SE, Reise SP. *Item Response Theory for Psychologists.* Mahwah, NJ: Lawrence Earlbaum Associates, 2000.

50. Hambleton RK. Emergence of item response modeling in instrument development and data analysis. *Med Care* 2000; 38:II-60–II-65.

51. Thissen D, Steinberg L. Data analysis using item response theory. *Psychol Bull* 1988; 104:385–395.

52. Hambleton R. Principles and selected applications of item response theory. In: Linn R, ed. *Educational Measurement.* 3rd ed. New York: MacMillian, 1989:147–200.

53. Revicki DA, Cella DF. Health status assessment for the twenty-first century: Item response theory, item banking, and computer-adaptive testing. *Qual Life Res* 1997; 6:595–600.

54. van der Linden W, Glas C. *Computerized-adaptive Testing: Theory and Practice.* Dordrecht, Netherlands: Kluwer Academic Publishers, 2000.

55. Wainer H. *Computerized-adaptive Testing: A Primer.* Mahwah, NJ: Lawrence Erlbaum Associates, 2000.

56. Haley S, Coster WJ, Andres PL, et al. Score compatibility of short forms and computerized adaptive testing: Simulation study with the activity measure for post-acute care. *Arch Phys Med Rehabil* 2004; 85:661–666.

57. Jette A, Keysor J, Coster W, Ni PS. Beyond function: Predicting participation outcomes in a rehabilitation cohort. *Arch Phys Med Rehabil* 2005; 86:2087–2094.

35 Predictive Factors for Recovery

Robert W. Teasell
Norine Foley
Katherine Salter

FACTORS CONTRIBUTING TO STROKE RECOVERY

Stroke often results in significant neurologic deficits leading to loss of function or independence, which can be devastating to both patients and families. Fortunately, many patients demonstrate significant recovery following stroke, although the degree to which individuals recover is highly variable. Even though a number of processes have been identified as contributing to neurologic recovery following a stroke, the role of each is not completely understood. Recovery from stroke has long been attributed to the resolution of edema and return of circulation within the ischemic penumbra, prompting skeptics to speculate that rehabilitation does not influence stroke recovery (1). However, it is now well-recognized that recovery can be a prolonged process, extending well past the resolution period of acute structural changes caused by the stroke. Results from animal and clinical studies have shown that the cerebral cortex undergoes functional and structural reorganization for weeks and months following a stroke, with compensatory changes extending up to six months in more severe strokes (2). Physiological factors that account for stroke recovery include resolution of post-stroke edema, reperfusion of the ischemic penumbra, resolution of diaschisis, and cortical reorganization in response to learning and rehabilitation training.

Post-stroke Edema

Edema surrounding the ischemic or infarcted area may disrupt neuronal functioning locally, at least in the early period following stroke. A portion of the early recovery following a stroke may be caused by the resolution of edema (3). As the edema subsides, neurons begin to function again. This process takes place relatively early in the course of recovery; however, it can extend for as long as eight weeks (4). Greater edema is associated with cerebral hemorrhages, which, in turn, may take longer to subside and may partially explain why patients with hemorrhagic stroke tend to enter rehabilitation after a delay and yet achieve similar outcomes once discharged (5).

Reperfusion of the Ischemic Penumbra

A focal ischemic lesion of the brain consists of a core area of infarcted tissue, caused by low blood flow, which is surrounded by a region of moderate, but reduced, blood flow, known as the ischemic penumbra (6, 7). The penumbra is known to be at risk for infarction, but is still salvageable. Reperfusion of this area early following a stroke permits ischemic and nonfunctioning, but still viable, neurons to regain function with subsequent clinical recovery.

Diaschisis

Diaschisis is a reversible state of low reactivity or depressed function as a consequence of a sudden interruption or loss of excitation in regions of the brain remote from, but neuronally connected to, the site of tissue damage. Nudo et al. noted that diaschisis occurs early after injury and is an inhibition or suppression of the surrounding cortex or distant areas of cortex with a connection to the damaged area (8). The reversibility may be partially caused by the resolution of edema, which may account for a portion of spontaneous recovery. Neuronal function may return following the resolution of diaschisis, particularly if the affected area of the brain recovers itself.

Cortical Reorganization

Rehabilitation helps to facilitate cortical reorganization, an important contributor to the recovery process and one that responds to rehabilitation. Neuroplasticity post-stroke, following damage to the motor cortex, is based on three main concepts:

1. In normal (non-stroke) brains, acquisition of skilled movements is associated with predictable functional changes within the motor cortex.
2. Injury to the motor cortex post-stroke results in functional changes in the remaining cortical tissue.
3. After a cortical stroke, these two observations interact so that reacquiring motor skills is associated with functional neurologic reorganization occurring in the undamaged cortex (9).

Neuroplasticity, or cortical reorganization, is an important underlying rationale for post-stroke rehabilitation.

Size of the Stroke

The cerebral cortex undergoes functional and structural reorganization for weeks and months following injury, with compensatory changes extending up to six months in more severe strokes (10). There is considerable evidence that both humans and laboratory animals are capable of some spontaneous (independent of rehabilitation therapies) return of lost function after cortical injury, particularly if the lesion is small (11, 12).

Animal Studies.   It has been demonstrated that animals with induced, small strokes may experience functional and structural recovery occurring spontaneously (without rehabilitation therapy) for weeks to months post-stroke (13, 14). Underlying neural changes appear to be related to surrounding intact brain regions taking over the lost function. Animals with larger lesions show much less return of function, and what function that does return may take weeks or months to stabilize (15, 16). Compensatory movements may play an important role here with activation and reorganization occurring in more distant cortical areas (15).

Kolb suggested that the differences between recovery from small and larger strokes is related to the mechanisms of neural recovery (15). For smaller strokes, the mode of recovery is most likely related to changes in the remaining intact motor cortex, while, for larger lesions, changes in related, but more distant, cortical regions facilitate compensatory behavior, which improves with practice.

Initial Severity

As a general rule, the severity of the initial deficit following stroke is inversely proportional to the prognosis for recovery. Most recovery occurs during the first three to six months following the stroke. The course of recovery decelerates as a function of time and is generally a predictable phenomenon (17).

The majority of patients with less-severe strokes demonstrate no or only mild disabilities, while many patients suffering from very severe strokes will remain dependent in activities of daily living (ADLs), even after the completion of rehabilitation. The results from several studies highlight the association between stroke recovery and initial severity. In the Copenhagen Stroke Study, 95% of patients with mild strokes reached their maximal neurologic recovery within six weeks. For patients with moderate, severe, and very severe strokes, 95% of the group had achieved their maximal recovery within 10, 13, and 15 weeks respectively (18, 19). Maximal neurologic recovery occurred, on average, two weeks earlier than marginal functional recovery. The specific timeline for neurologic and functional disability recovery is presented in Tables 35-1 and 35-2. Among the surviving patients, the best neurologic recovery occurred within four-and-a-half weeks in 80% of the patients, while best ADL function was achieved by six weeks. For 95% of the patients, best neurologic recovery was reached by eleven weeks and best ADL function within twelve-and-a-half weeks. Similarly, Jorgensen et al. reported that the best walking function was reached within four weeks for patients with mild paresis of the affected lower extremity, six weeks for those with moderate paresis, and eleven weeks for those with severe paralysis (20). Consequently, the time course of both neurologic and functional recovery was strongly related to both initial stroke severity and functional disability. Two-thirds of all stroke survivors with mild to moderate strokes achieve independence in ADLs (18–20).

TABLE 35-1

Impairment and Neurologic Recovery of Stroke Patients in the Copenhagen Stroke Study

Category (SSS)	Admission[1]	Discharge[2]	Survival (%)	Weeks to 80% Best Recovery[3]	Weeks to 95% Best Recovery[3]
Very severe (0–14)	19%	4%	38	10	13 (11.6–14.4)
Severe (15–29)	14%	7%	67	9	15 (13–17)
Moderate (30–44)	26%	11%	89	5.5	10.5 (9.5–11.5)
Mild/No (45–58)	41%	78%	97	2.5	6.5 (5.4–7.6)

[1] Percentage patient distribution on admission, grouped by stroke severity subgroups, as measured by SSS (scores range from 0–58 points)
[2] Percentage distribution of survivors (79% of initial group) after completion of stroke rehabilitation
[3] Neurologic recovery as measured by Scandanavian Stroke Scale

Age

Animal Studies. The impact of age on stroke and recovery in animals is not entirely clear. Shapira et al., examining the effects of age on the development of ischemic injury in rats, discovered that young rats were affected more by the stroke than old rats were, as exhibited by more pronounced neurologic impairments and poorer performance in a water maze task. However, the duration of motor impairment post-brain lesion appears to increase with age (21, 22). The regenerative response of neurons and glial cells, although largely preserved with age, appears to be delayed or occurs at a diminished rate the older the animal (23, 24). Reactive neuronal synaptogenesis declines (25), sprouting responses are less robust (24, 26), and synaptic replacement rates diminish (27).

Clinical Studies. In humans, age has long been thought to limit post-stroke neurologic recovery. Evidence suggests that, compared with older patients, younger patients recover at a faster rate and more completely (28, 29).

When compared with older patients, younger patients—defined as persons less than 65 years old—may have a better chance of regaining independence in ADLs and returning home at discharge (30). Herman et al. reported that, when compared to those patients over 85 years of age, odds of successful discharge home were 18 times greater if the stroke patient was under 65 (31). The effect of age on recovery was demonstrated even within a cohort of younger patients. Bogousslavsky and Pierre (32) reported that, following first-ever ischemic stroke, the prognosis of patients between the ages of 16 to 30 was better than that of patients aged 31 to 45 years. Nakayama et al. (33) reported that, although older stroke patients achieved the same degree of neurologic recovery as younger patients, the functional gains were lower. It was suggested that elderly patients had less compensatory abilities than younger stroke patients with comparable neurologic impairments.

Even though younger age has been associated with improved recovery, the results from several studies contest the concept that age limits recovery. Kugler et al. studied the effect of patient age on early stroke

TABLE 35-2

Disability and Outcome of Stroke Patients in the Copenhagen Stroke Study

Category (BI)	Discharge[1]	Survival (%)	Weeks to 80% Best Recovery[2]	Weeks to 95% Best Recovery[2]
Very Severe (0–20)	14%	50	11	17 (15–19)
Severe (25–45)	6%	92	15	16 (13.5–18.5)
Moderate (50–70)	8%	97	6	9 (7.5–10.5)
Mild (75–95)	26%	98	2.5	5 (4–6)
No (100)	46%			

[1] Percentage patient distribution on discharge, grouped by stroke severity subgroups, as measured by BI
[2] Functional recovery as measured by BI

recovery and found that relative improvement decreased significantly with increasing age. Patients younger than 55 years achieved 67% of the maximum possible improvement, compared with only 50% for patients above 55 years (34). They also found that age had a significant, but relatively small, impact on the speed of recovery; younger patients demonstrated slightly faster functional recovery. The authors concluded that, although age had a significant impact, it was a poor predictor of individual functional recovery and could not be regarded as a limiting factor in the rehabilitation of stroke patients. However, younger patients did demonstrate more complete recovery. Bagg et al. found that, even though age was a significant predictor of motor and total functional improvement measure (FIMTM) scores at discharge, age alone accounted for only 3% of the variance in a multivariable model (35).

Stroke Type

Approximately 10% of all strokes are the result of intracerebral hemorrhage (ICH) (36, 37). Although primary ICH has been associated with more severe neurologic impairment and higher mortality in the acute phase (up to one-half of patients with primary ICH die within the first month), it is generally believed that patients with ICH have better recovery compared to patients with ischemic strokes. After controlling for potential confounders, Jørgensen et al. found that stroke type (ischemic vs. hemorrhagic) did not influence mortality, the time course of neurologic recovery, neurologic outcome, or the time course of recovery from disability (38). The apparent effect of poorer outcome among patients with hemorrhagic stroke was because of initial greater stroke severity. Paolucci et al. matched patients on the basis of initial stroke severity, age, sex, and onset to admission time and reported that ICH patients had superior rehabilitation outcomes and demonstrated a higher therapeutic response on ADLs (37). ICH patients had higher Canadian Neurological Scale and Rivermead Mobility scores as well as greater efficiencies in gains. Lengths of hospital stays were similar between the groups. The authors attribute the greater gains, relative to patients with ischemic strokes, to improved neurologic recovery associated with resolving brain compression. Kelly et al. reported similar results (36). In this study, although patients with ICH admitted to a rehabilitation hospital had significantly lower FIMTM scores compared to patients with ischemic stroke, there were no differences in discharge FIMTM scores between the groups. Patients with ICH had higher FIM change scores. Although initial disability did not significantly predict the amount of recovery during rehabilitation, initial stroke severity was a strong predictor of functional status at discharge.

Depression

In general, depression, identified acutely or within the first three months following stroke, has an adverse effect on both functional status and physical recovery in both the short (39–44) and long-term (41, 42, 44–48). However, the presence of depression does not preclude recovery, and, over the course of rehabilitation, patients with post-stroke depression may experience significant improvements, although functional ability may remain at a lower level despite rehabilitation interventions (49, 50). Physical impairment and post-stroke depression appear to act upon each other, and each influences the recovery of the other. Reports on the contribution of physical functioning impairments to the development of post-stroke depression vary from a low of 5–15% (51) to a high of 48% (52).

Van de Port et al. recently published the results of a prospective cohort study (n = 205), which demonstrated that mobility decline was experienced by 21% of participants between one and three years post-stroke (53). Significant predictors of this decline in mobility status were level of activity, cognitive problems, fatigue, and depression. Given that the relationship between depression and physical impairment may be reciprocal, depression may contribute to deteriorations in mobility, which may, in turn, contribute to increased feelings of depression.

Because depression is a treatable condition, which impacts both function and functional recovery, it should be taken into account in the evaluation and treatment of all stroke patients (43). As Ramasubbu et al. pointed out, early recognition and treatment of depression may "optimize rehabilitation potential" and reduce "significant human and financial costs associated with post-stroke functional impairment" (43).

Cognitive Impairment

It has been suggested that higher order cognitive abilities such as abstract thinking, judgment, short-term verbal memory, comprehension, and orientation are important in predicting the stroke survivor's functional status at discharge (54–56). Reduced cognition has been associated with a decreased ability to perform ADLs, with poorer physical functioning at discharge and a greater likelihood of mortality within one year of discharge (56–62). Zinn et al. reported fewer discharges home among patients with cognitive impairment than among cognitively intact patients (85.9% vs. 93.4%, p = 0.07) (63).

Although the presence of cognitive impairment may be associated with decreased ADL function, it has been demonstrated that it is not a significant predictor of ADL function at six months post-stroke (63). Instrumental function may be more severely impacted by the presence of cognitive ability. At six months post-stroke, the presence of cognitive impairment was associated with and predictive of decreased instrumental activities of daily living (IADL function) (63). Similarly, Mok et al. determined that higher levels of cognitive impairment post-stroke were associated with greater deficits in IADL function and greater levels of pre-stroke cognitive decline (64). Identified predictors of IADL performance were stroke severity, executive dysfunction, age, and pre-stroke cognitive decline (64). Patients with cognitive impairments may require more therapy over a longer period of time (63). This is, of course, associated with greater expenditure of health care resources (60).

Comorbid Burden

Greater medical complexity contributes to the severity of functional impairment following stroke and may impede recovery. In general, the presence of multiple comorbid diagnoses or increased comorbid burden is associated with decreased functional status, both at admission to and discharge from rehabilitation (65–67). Individuals with more than one comorbid diagnosis may experience less functional gain and a more incomplete recovery than individuals with no comorbid burden. In a study of 1,020 adult rehabilitation patients, Stineman and colleagues determined that the odds of full functional recovery decreased as the number of comorbid medical conditions increased (68). Similarly, within populations of individuals with stroke, increasing comorbid burden has been associated with reduced gain in functional ability over the course of rehabilitation as well as decreased rehabilitation efficiency (67, 69). Furthermore, among community-dwelling stroke survivors, comorbid burden has been identified as a significant predictor of functional outcome (70) and was associated with an increased risk for physical decline and new problems in basic activities of daily living (71).

There is an association between age and comorbid burden such that elderly individuals tend to experience an increasing number of comorbidities (66, 67). Hence, the presence of multiple comorbidities is not uncommon in the stroke population (70, 71). Rigler et al. reported that, in a sample of community-dwelling stroke survivors, only 6% were free from comorbid conditions while more than 40% had three or more (71). Even though comorbid burden may be an important modifier in the prediction of future functional status, it may not be as important as either age or initial/baseline functional status (70, 71).

Even though increasing age and number of comorbidities may have a negative impact on functional status and recovery, this does not necessarily prevent the individual with stroke from making significant gains in function. Giaquinto et al. demonstrated that, even though comorbid burden was associated with functional status, it was not associated with functional gain in rehabilitation (66). Similarly, Lew et al. reported that all participants with stroke made significant gains in function over the course of rehabilitation and that comorbid burden was not associated with change in function or status (72).

THE EFFECT OF TIMING ON REHABILITATION

Animal Research

Recent evidence suggests that the brain is not only able to reorganize, but it is, in fact, primed to do so early on after the stroke (15, 73, 74). The results from animal studies have demonstrated that, if therapy is delayed for several weeks post-stroke, dendritic arborisation is markedly reduced. The concept of a detrimental effect with rehabilitation delay was best shown through the animal work of Biernaskie et al. (75). After small strokes were induced in rats, they were subjected to five weeks of rehabilitation beginning at days 5, 14, and 30 post-stroke. A group of control rats received no rehabilitation and were placed in social housing. Rats receiving early (day 5) rehabilitation showed marked improvement in neurologic recovery. Rats beginning rehabilitation at day 14 showed moderate improvement, while rats at day 30 showed no greater improvement than the control animals. The same authors examined dendritic morphology in the undamaged animal cortex contralateral to the stroke lesion. Enriched rehabilitation provided very early post-stroke (at day 5) resulted in an increased number of dendritic branches and greater complexity of layer V neurons when compared to those rats receiving rehabilitation at day 30 and to those exposed to social housing only. The authors concluded that the post-stroke brain was more responsive to rehabilitation early in the post-stroke period and that responsiveness declined linearly with time, such that rehabilitation, when delayed (beginning at day 30 in rats), is no longer effective. The clinical implications of this finding are apparent; rehabilitation will have the greatest impact during the window when the brain is primed for behavior-dependent changes or cortical reorganization.

Clinical Studies

Several studies have supported the association between early admission to rehabilitation and improved functional outcomes and/or decreased length of rehab hospital stay (76–79). Paolucci et al. suggested that early initiation of rehabilitation post-stroke may be a "relevant prognostic factor of functional outcome" (78). Certainly, this viewpoint is supported by recent reports based on both American (80, 81) and Canadian (76) data, which suggest that early admission to rehabilitation, regardless of initial severity of disability, is associated with greater functional gain and shorter lengths of stay. Horn et al. reported a strong, consistent, inverse association between the time from stroke onset to rehabilitation admission and functional outcome, even when controlling for overall severity or complexity of illness, and suggested that "the sooner a patient with stroke starts rehabilitation after his/her stroke, no matter how severe, the better the outcome" (81). The authors recognized that this could mean transferring patients to rehabilitation before they are medically stable. Within many institutions, altering the time of stroke rehabilitation would require a more flexible and responsive approach, but would result in a decreased acute care stay and better outcomes.

Maulden et al. reported on the findings of the Post-Stroke Rehabilitation Outcomes Project (PSROP), an observational, prospective study that enrolled 1,161 patients from six inpatient rehabilitation facilities in the United States (Table 35-3) (80). Increases in the length of time from stroke onset to admission to rehabilitation were associated with lower discharge FIM scores and increased rehabilitation length of stay (LOS) for patients with both moderate and severe strokes. Time (days) from stroke onset to admission was also a significant predictor of discharge total FIMTM score, discharge motor FIMTM

score, discharge mobility FIMTM score, and rehabilitation LOS, after controlling for medical comorbidity and complications. The subgroup that demonstrated the strongest relationship between early admission to rehabilitation and improved functional outcome was the most severely impaired patients. The authors concluded that:

> For moderately and severely impaired patients with stroke, fewer days between onset of stroke symptoms and admission to inpatient rehabilitation are associated with better functional outcomes at discharge. For moderately impaired patients with stroke, fewer days between onset of stroke symptoms and admission to acute inpatient rehabilitation also is associated with shorter rehabilitation LOS. Providers should strive to transfer patients with stroke as soon as possible from an acute care hospital into acute rehabilitation to improve functional outcomes. (80)

Horn et al., also using data from the PROSP, noted that, in the United States:

> Rehabilitation providers often wonder if the acute care hospital payment system encourages acute care providers to discharge patient to rehabilitation when

---

TABLE 35-3
The PSROP (2005) Data on Early Interventions

STUDY AUTHOR(S), YEAR, LOCATION	DESCRIPTION	RESULTS
Maulden et al. (2005) Post Stroke Rehabilitation Outcomes Project USA (80)	969 patients with moderate or severe stroke for whom the time from stroke onset to rehabilitation admission was recorded. Records were obtained from six rehabilitation facilities. Outcomes included FIM total and subscores as well as length of stay. Patients were stratified by severity as per case-mix group (used for Medicare payment purposes).	In both the moderate and severe case-mix groups, more time from stroke onset to rehabilitation admission was associated with lower total FIM scores at discharge as well as lower motor FIM, mobility FIM, and ADL FIM subscale scores. In the group of moderately disabled patients only, greater delays in admission to rehabilitation were associated with significantly longer lengths of stay ($p < 0.001$). Even when taking severity of illness (comprehensive severity index score) into account, days from stroke to rehabilitation admission was a significant independent predictor of functional status as assessed by the FIM.
Horn et al. (2005) Post Stroke Rehabilitation Outcomes Project USA (81)	830 patients with moderate or severe stroke included in the PSROP database. Regression models were created for discharge FIM (total, cognitive & motor FIM scores) as well as discharge destination (home or assisted living)	Time from onset of stroke symptoms to rehabilitation admission was a significant predictor of total FIM and motor FIM scores at discharge in patients with both moderate and severe stroke.

they are not yet medically stable. The findings here suggest that 'sicker and quicker' may in some cases be better . . . A longer time between onset of stroke symptoms and admission to inpatient rehabilitation was associated with reduced discharge FIMTM score, after controlling for overall severity of illness or its components. This suggests that earlier admission to rehabilitation, even if a patient's severity of illness is increased according to a higher CSI score or its components, is associated with better outcomes. In any event, the findings should encourage more timely coordination in the handoff from acute care to rehabilitation for patients with stroke and more willingness of rehabilitation facilities to admit medically challenging, sicker patients. (81)

The authors concluded that

the sooner a patient with stroke starts inpatient rehabilitation after his/her stroke, no matter how severe, the better the outcome. Moreover, . . . earlier gait activities . . . have a significant association with outcome, regardless of how much additional therapy a patient receives or what his/her admission functioning level (FIMTM score) is. (81)

Although the practice of including early mobilization in acute stroke care has been incorporated into many best practice guidelines, insufficient evidence exists to suggest that early mobilization is associated with safety, improved outcomes, or cost-effectiveness. Therefore, in Australia, A Very Early Rehabilitation Trial (AVERT) has been initiated with the goal of establishing the efficacy and cost-effectiveness of early intervention. If the results support the hypothesis, the study will provide level-1 evidence that early mobilization is effective. The AVERT phase III trial commenced in 10 centers in Australia in July 2006 (82).

Even though stroke results in premature death and disability, its major burden is chronic disability. Provision of very early mobilization (VEM) in a stroke care unit has been associated with a 64% reduction in death or disability. Indredavik et al. demonstrated that, together, blood pressure and VEM were the strongest predictors of improved outcomes and were the factors that distinguished stroke unit care from general medical ward care (83). VEM accounted for 78% of the benefit associated with stroke unit care.

INTENSITY OF REHABILITATION

Best Evidence for Intensity of Stroke Rehabilitation Therapies

Both animal and clinical studies demonstrated that training or inpatient rehabilitation increases cortical representation with subsequent functional recovery, whereas a lack of rehabilitation or training decreases cortical representation and delays recovery. Animals exposed to enriched environments post-stroke have improved functional outcomes when compared with animals exposed to nonenriched environments. Socialization alone can improve stroke recovery in animals with the mediating factor appearing to be increased activity. In animal studies, the key factors promoting neurologic recovery include increased activity and a complex and stimulating environment. Therefore, it follows that, if training and stimulation lead to increased cortical reorganization, neurologic recovery, and functional improvements, then more intensive therapy is likely to result in a greater degree of recovery and improved functional outcomes. However, the relationship may not be linear.

The intensity of rehabilitation therapies is often cited as an important factor associated with both specialized stroke rehabilitation and improved functional outcome. Do patients who receive therapy for longer periods of time or at a higher level of intensity realize greater benefits compared to patients who receive conventional care? Although many studies have been designed and conducted to answer this question, the intensity of therapy was often only weakly correlated with improved functional outcome. Even though a universally accepted definition of the term *intensity* does not exist, it is usually defined as the number of minutes per day of therapy or the number of hours of consecutive therapy. Studies evaluating the effects of increased intensity of therapy usually provide more therapy over a given course of total treatment time compared to the alternative, which receives a lesser amount. This weak association may be explained by differences in the time, duration, and composition of therapies provided and/or the characteristics of the stroke patients under study. Page argues that intensity of therapy has been overemphasized and that:

[L]ess intense (30–45 min/day) task-specific training regimens with the more affected limb can produce cortical reorganization and correlative, meaningful functional improvements. (84)

Turton and Pomeroy acknowledge the widely held clinical belief that too much of or the wrong type of activity early on in the rehabilitation of the upper extremity may produce a worse outcome, increasing spasticity in particular (85).

The intensity of the package of rehabilitation therapies offered also needs to be considered. The total amount of time that a patient spends engaged in rehabilitation activities can vary considerably between units, institutions, and countries. De Weerdt et al. used behavioral mapping to quantify the amount of time that patients spent in therapeutic activities on two rehabilitation units, one in Belgium and one in Switzerland (86). Patients in the rehab unit in Belgium were engaged in rehabilitation for a longer percentage of the day than those from Switzerland (45% vs. 27%). De Wit et al. also observed significant differences in the amount of time patients spent in rehabilitation activities among four European countries (Belgium, UK, Switzerland, and Germany) (87). Patients from Germany spent a larger percentage of the day in therapy time (23.4%), while those from the UK spent the least (10.1%). Therapy time ranged from one hour per day in the UK to about three hours per day in Switzerland. In all of the centers, patients spent 72% of the time in nontherapeutic activities. A number of studies have reported that the majority of a patient's time on a stroke rehabilitation unit is spent idle and alone (88–91). In one study, patients on a stroke rehabilitation unit were engaged in interactive behaviors for only 25% of their time (90).

There is conflicting evidence that intensity of therapy is associated with improved functional outcome. A review authored by Teasell et al. found evidence that greater intensity of physiotherapy and occupational therapy resulted in improved functional outcomes, although the overall beneficial effect was modest and not maintained over time (92). Wodchis et al. found that, for patients with an uncertain prognosis on admission, the intensity of rehabilitation therapies was positively associated with an increased likelihood of going home (93). Evidence from four meta-analyses also suggests that increased intensity of therapy is beneficial. Langhorne et al., examining the effects of differing intensities of physical therapy, showed significant improvements in ADLs, function, and reduction of impairments with higher intensities of treatment (94). However, Cifu and Stewart identified only three moderate quality studies and one meta-analysis that examined the intensity of rehabilitation services and functional outcomes and reported that the intensity of rehabilitation services was only weakly associated with improved functional outcomes after stroke (95). Kwakkel et al. found a small, but statistically significant, intensity effect on ADLs and functional outcome parameters (96). In an extension of their previous meta-analysis, the same authors evaluated the benefit of augmented physical therapy, including 20 studies that had assessed many interventions: occupational (upper extremity), physiotherapy (lower extremity), leisure therapy, home care, and sensorimotor training (97). After adjusting for differences in treatment intensity contrasts, augmented therapy was associated with statistically significant treatment effects for the outcomes of ADLs and walking speed, although not for upper extremity therapy assessed using the Action Research Arm test. A 16-hour increase in therapy time during the first six months following stroke was associated with a favorable outcome.

However, Duncan et al. recently reviewed all randomized trials and meta-analyses examining the effect of intensity on improved functional outcome and concluded that there was weak evidence of a dose-response relationship. The authors suggest that all subsets of patients may not benefit equally and could not recommend specific guidelines about the intensity or duration of rehabilitation therapies (98). Chen et al. also examined the relationship between intensity of therapy and functional gains and found that, even though admission function, LOS, and therapy intensity collectively contributed to greater functional gains, LOS and therapy intensity did not always predict those gains (99).

Interdisciplinary specialized stroke rehabilitation units are also associated with better outcomes when compared to conventional multidisciplinary care. The benefit has been attributed, in part, to the provision of higher intensities of stroke rehabilitation therapies. Despite baseline similarities between groups, Kalra et al. demonstrated that patients who received care on a stroke unit two weeks following an acute stroke had higher median Barthel Index discharge scores, which were achieved in a shorter length of time, compared with patients who were rehabilitated on a general ward (100). Although patients treated on the general ward received more hours of physical therapy compared with patients on the stroke unit (21.5 vs. 16.6 hrs, p < 0.05), their length of hospital stay was significantly longer. The rate of change of median Barthel score was higher among stroke unit patients (gain of 2.2 points/week compared with 0.9 points/week). The hospital costs of those patients admitted to the general ward were higher, even though their outcomes were not nearly so favorable.

SUMMARY

A stroke can be a devastating event in patients' lives, leaving them with impairments and disabilities that can threaten their independence. Stroke patients do recover to varying degrees, although the extent of recovery is dependent upon a number of factors. There is irrefutable evidence that, even though cortical reorganization is an important component of recovery, stroke rehabilitation is necessary for it to occur. Our increasing understanding of factors that contribute to cortical reorganization, gleaned through the animal model, including complex stimulating environments and high activity levels, have corollaries in the clinical realm, such as early admission to rehabilitation, intensity of therapies, and task-specific therapies. Depression, comorbid medical conditions, and cognitive deficits may negatively influence recovery by interfering with learning and through disruption of the rehabilitative process. Clearly, rehabilitation, which is both focused and intensive, is essential to ensure maximal recovery achieved post-stroke.

References

1. Dombovy ML. Stroke: Clinical course and neurophsyiologic mechanisms of recovery. *Physical and Rehabilitation Medicine* 1991; 2(3):171–188.

2. Green JB. Brain reorganization after stroke. *Top Stroke Rehabil* 2003; 10(3):1–20.

3. Lo RC. Recovery and rehabilitation after stroke. *Can Fam Physician* 1986; 32: 1851–1853.

4. Inoue Y, Takemoto K, Miyamoto T, et al. Sequential computed tomography scans in acute cerebral infarction. *Radiology* 1980; 135(3):655–662.

5. Lipson DM, Sangha H, Foley NC, et al. Recovery from stroke: Differences between subtypes. *Int J Rehabil Res* 2005; 28(4):303–308.

6. Astrup J, Siesjo BK, Symon L. Thresholds in cerebral ischemia: The ischemic penumbra. *Stroke* 1981; 12(6):723–725.

7. Lyden PD, Livin JA. Cytoprotective therapies in ischemic stroke. In: Cohen SN, ed. *Management of Ischemic Stroke.* New York: McGraw-Hill, Health Professions Division, 2000:225–240.

8. Nudo RJ, Plautz EJ, Frost SB. Role of adaptive plasticity in recovery of function after damage to motor cortex. *Muscle Nerve* 2001; 24(8):1000–1019.

9. Nudo RJ. Adaptive plasticity in motor cortex: Implications for rehabilitation after brain injury. *J Rehabil Med* 2003; (41 Suppl):7–10.

10. Green JB. Brain reorganization after stroke. *Top Stroke Rehabil* 2003; 10(3):1–20.

11. Duncan PW, Lai SM, Keighley J. Defining post-stroke recovery: Implications for design and interpretation of drug trials. *Neuropharmacology* 2000; 39(5):835–841.

12. Kolb B. Overview of cortical plasticity and recovery from brain injury. *Phys Med Rehabil Clin N Am* 2003; 14(1 Suppl):S7–25, viii.

13. Whishaw IQ. Loss of the innate cortical engram for action patterns used in skilled reaching and the development of behavioral compensation following motor cortex lesions in the rat. *Neuropharmacology* 2000; 39(5):788–805.

14. Nudo RJ, Milliken GW. Reorganization of movement representations in primary motor cortex following focal ischemic infarcts in adult squirrel monkeys. *J Neurophysiol* 1996; 75(5):2144–2149.

15. Kolb B. *Brain Plasticity and Behavior.* New Jersey: Erlbaum Mahwah, 1995.

16. Frost SB, Barbay S, Friel KM, et al. Reorganization of remote cortical regions after ischemic brain injury: a potential substrate for stroke recovery. *J Neurophysiol* 2003; 89(6):3205–3214.

17. Skilbeck CE, Wade DT, Hewer RL, Wood VA. Recovery after stroke. *J Neurol Neurosurg Psychiatry* 1983; 46(1):5–8.

18. Jorgensen HS, Nakayama H, Raaschou HO, Olsen TS. Recovery of walking function in stroke patients: The Copenhagen Stroke Study. *Arch Phys Med Rehabil* 1995; 76(1):27–32.

19. Jorgensen HS, Nakayama H, Raaschou HO, et al. Outcome and time course of recovery in stroke. Part I: Outcome. The Copenhagen Stroke Study. *Arch Phys Med Rehabil* 1995; 76(5):399–405.

20. Jorgensen HS, Nakayama H, Raaschou HO, et al. Outcome and time course of recovery in stroke. Part II: Time course of recovery. The Copenhagen Stroke Study. *Arch Phys Med Rehabil* 1995; 76(5):406–412.

21. Shapira S, Sapir M, Wengier A, et al. Aging has a complex effect on a rat model of ischemic stroke. *Brain Res* 2002; 925(2):148–158.

22. Brown AW, Marlowe KJ, Bjelke B. Age effect on motor recovery in a post-acute animal stroke model. *Neurobiol Aging* 2003; 24(4):607–614.

23. Popa-Wagner A, Schroder E, Schmoll H, et al. Upregulation of MAP1B and MAP2 in the rat brain after middle cerebral artery occlusion: Effect of age. *J Cereb Blood Flow Metab* 1999; 19(4):425–434.

24. Whittemore SR, Nieto-Sampedro M, Needels DL, Cotman CW. Neuronotrophic factors for mammalian brain neurons: Injury induction in neonatal, adult and aged rat brain. *Brain Res* 1985; 352(2):169–178.

25. Scheff SW, Bernardo LS, Cotman CW. Decrease in adrenergic axon sprouting in the senescent rat. *Science* 1978; 202(4369):775–778.

26. Schauwecker PE, Cheng HW, Serquinia RM, et al. Lesion-induced sprouting of commissural/associational axons and induction of GAP-43 mRNA in hilar and CA3 pyramidal neurons in the hippocampus are diminished in aged rats. *J Neurosci* 1995; 15(3 Pt 2):2462–2470.

27. Cotman CW, Anderson KJ. Synaptic plasticity and functional stabilization in the hippocampal formation: Possible role in Alzheimer's disease. *Adv Neurol* 1988; 47:313–335.

28. Kalra L. Does age affect benefits of stroke unit rehabilitation? *Stroke* 1994; 25(2): 346–351.

29. Alexander MP. Stroke rehabilitation outcome: A potential use of predictive variables to establish levels of care. *Stroke* 1994; 25(1):128–134.

30. Kotila M, Waltimo O, Niemi ML, et al. The profile of recovery from stroke and factors influencing outcome. *Stroke* 1984; 15(6):1039–1044.

31. Herman JM, Culpepper L, Franks P. Patterns of utilization, disposition, and length of stay among stroke patients in a community hospital setting. *J Am Geriatr Soc* 1984; 32(6):421–426.

32. Bogousslavsky J, Pierre P. Ischemic stroke in patients under age 45. *Neurol Clin* 1992; 10(1):113–124.

33. Nakayama H, Jorgensen HS, Raaschou HO, Olsen TS. The influence of age on stroke outcome. The Copenhagen Stroke Study. *Stroke* 1994; 25(4):808–813.

34. Kugler C, Altenhoner T, Lochner P, Ferbert A. Does age influence early recovery from ischemic stroke? A study from the Hessian Stroke Data Bank. *J Neurol* 2003; 250(6):676–681.

35. Bagg S, Pombo AP, Hopman W. Effect of age on functional outcomes after stroke rehabilitation. *Stroke* 2002; 33(1):179–185.

36. Kelly PJ, Furie KL, Shafqat S, et al. Functional recovery following rehabilitation after hemorrhagic and ischemic stroke. *Arch Phys Med Rehabil* 2003; 84(7):968–972.

37. Paolucci S, Antonucci G, Grasso MG, et al. Functional outcome of ischemic and hemorrhagic stroke patients after inpatient rehabilitation: A matched comparison. *Stroke* 2003; 34(12):2861–2865.

38. Jorgensen HS, Nakayama H, Raaschou HO, Olsen TS. Intracerebral hemorrhage versus infarction: stroke severity, risk factors, and prognosis. *Ann Neurol* 1995; 38(1):45-50.

39. Sinyor D, Amato P, Kaloupek DG, et al. Post-stroke depression: Relationships to functional impairment, coping strategies, and rehabilitation outcome. *Stroke* 1986; 17(6):1102–1107.

40. Ebrahim S, Barer D, Nouri F. Affective illness after stroke. *Br J Psychiatry* 1987; 151:52–56.

41. Parikh RM, Robinson RG, Lipsey JR, et al. The impact of post-stroke depression on recovery in activities of daily living over a 2-year follow-up. *Arch Neurol* 1990; 47(7):785–789.

42. Pohjasvaara T, Vataja R, Leppavuori A, et al. Depression is an independent predictor of poor long-term functional outcome post-stroke. *Eur J Neurol* 2001; 8(4):315–319.

43. Ramasubbu R, Robinson RG, Flint AJ, et al. Functional impairment associated with acute post-stroke depression: The Stroke Data Bank Study. *J Neuropsychiatry Clin Neurosci* 1998; 10(1):26–33.

44. Herrmann N, Black SE, Lawrence J, et al. The Sunnybrook Stroke Study: A prospective study of depressive symptoms and functional outcome. *Stroke* 1998; 29(3):618–624.

45. Robinson RG, Bolduc PL, Price TR. Two-year longitudinal study of post-stroke mood disorders: Diagnosis and outcome at one and two years. *Stroke* 1987; 18(5):837–843.

46. Bacher Y, Korner-Bitensky N, Mayo N, et al. A longitudinal study of depression among stroke patients participating in a rehabilitation program. *Canadian Journal of Rehabilitation* 1990; 4(1):27–37.

47. Morris PL, Raphael B, Robinson RG. Clinical depression is associated with impaired recovery from stroke. *Med J Aust* 1992; 157(4):239–242.

48. Kotila M, Numminen H, Waltimo O, Kaste M. Post-stroke depression and functional recovery in a population-based stroke register. The Finnstroke study. *Eur J Neurol* 1999; 6(3):309–312.

49. van de Weg FB, Kuik DJ, Lankhorst GJ. Post-stroke depression and functional outcome: A cohort study investigating the influence of depression on functional recovery from stroke. *Clin Rehabil* 1999; 13(3):268–272.

50. Nannetti L, Paci M, Pasquini J, et al. Motor and functional recovery in patients with post-stroke depression. *Disabil Rehabil* 2005; 27(4):170–175.

51. Robinson R. Post-stroke mood disorders. *Hospital Practice* 1986:83–89.

52. Loong CK, Kenneth NK, Paulin ST. Post-stroke depression: Outcome following rehabilitation. *Aust N Z J Psychiatry* 1995; 29(4):609–614.

53. van dP, I, Kwakkel G, van W, I, Lindeman E. Susceptibility to deterioration of mobility long-term after stroke: A prospective cohort study. *Stroke* 2006; 37(1):167–171.

54. Jongbloed L. Prediction of function after stroke: A critical review. *Stroke* 1986; 17(4):765–776.

55. Mysiw WJ, Beegan JG, Gatens PF. Prospective cognitive assessment of stroke patients before inpatient rehabilitation: The relationship of the Neurobehavioral Cognitive Status Examination to functional improvement. *Am J Phys Med Rehabil* 1989; 68(4):168–171.

56. Tatemichi TK, Desmond DW, Stern Y, et al. Cognitive impairment after stroke: Frequency, patterns, and relationship to functional abilities. *J Neurol Neurosurg Psychiatry* 1994; 57(2):202–207.

57. Prencipe M, Ferretti C, Casini AR, et al. Stroke, disability, and dementia: Results of a population survey. *Stroke* 1997; 28(3):531–536.

58. Desmond DW, Moroney JT, Paik MC, et al. Frequency and clinical determinants of dementia after ischemic stroke. *Neurology* 2000; 54(5):1124–1131.

59. Ruchinskas R, Curyto K. Cognitive screening in geriatric rehabilitation. *Rehabilitation Psychology* 2003; 48(1):14–22.

60. Claesson L, Linden T, Skoog I, Blomstrand C. Cognitive impairment after stroke: Impact on activities of daily living and costs of care for elderly people. The Goteborg 70+ Stroke Study. *Cerebrovasc Dis* 2005; 19(2):102–109.

61. Leys D, Henon H, Mackowiak-Cordoliani MA, Pasquier F. Post-stroke dementia. *Lancet Neurol* 2005; 4(11):752–759.

62. Hinkle JL. Variables explaining functional recovery following motor stroke. *J Neurosci Nurs* 2006; 38(1):6–12.

63. Zinn S, Dudley TK, Bosworth HB, et al. The effect of post-stroke cognitive impairment on rehabilitation process and functional outcome. *Archives of Physical Medicine and Rehabilitation* 2004; 85:1084–1090.

64. Mok VC, Wong A, Lam WW, et al. Cognitive impairment and functional outcome after stroke associated with small vessel disease. *J Neurol Neurosurg Psychiatry* 2004; 75(4):560–566.

65. Patrick L, Knoefel F, Gaskowski P, Rexroth D. Medical comorbidity and rehabilitation efficiency in geriatric inpatients. *J Am Geriatr Soc* 2001; 49(11):1471–1477.

66. Giaquinto S. Comorbidity in post-stroke rehabilitation. *Eur J Neurol* 2003; 10(3):235–238.

67. Ferriero G, Franchignoni F, Benevolo E, et al. The influence of comorbidities and complications on discharge function in stroke rehabilitation inpatients. *Eura Medicophys* 2006; 42(2):91–96.

68. Stineman MG, Maislin G, Williams SV. Applying quantitative methods to the prediction of full functional recovery in adult rehabilitation patients. *Arch Phys Med Rehabil* 1993; 74(8):787–795.

69. Ween JE, Alexander MP, D'Esposito M, Roberts M. Factors predictive of stroke outcome in a rehabilitation setting. *Neurology* 1996; 47(2):388–392.

70. Studenski SA, Lai SM, Duncan PW, Rigler SK. The impact of self-reported cumulative comorbidity on stroke recovery. *Age Ageing* 2004; 33(2):195–198.

71. Rigler SK, Studenski S, Wallace D, et al. Comorbidity adjustment for functional outcomes in community-dwelling older adults. *Clin Rehabil* 2002; 16(4):420–428.

72. Lew HL, Lee E, Date ES, Zeiner H. Influence of medical comorbidities and complications on FIM change and length of stay during inpatient rehabilitation. *Am J Phys Med Rehabil* 2002; 81(11):830–837.

73. Schallert T, Fleming SM, Woodlee MT. Should the injured and intact hemispheres be treated differently during the early phases of physical restorative therapy in experimental stroke or Parkinsonism? *Phys Med Rehabil Clin N Am* 2003; 14(1 Suppl):S27–S46.

74. Johansson BB. Brain plasticity and stroke rehabilitation. The Willis Lecture. *Stroke* 2000; 31(1):223–230.

75. Biernaskie J, Chernenko G, Corbett D. Efficacy of rehabilitative experience declines with time after focal ischemic brain injury. *J Neurosci* 2004; 24(5):1245–1254.

76. Salter K, Jutai J, Hartley M, et al. Impact of early vs. delayed admission to rehabilitation on functional outcomes in persons with stroke. *J Rehabil Med* 2006; 38(2):113–117.

77. Shah S, Vanclay F, Cooper B. Predicting discharge status at commencement of stroke rehabilitation. *Stroke* 1989; 20(6):766–769.

78. Paolucci S, Antonucci G, Grasso MG, et al. Early versus delayed inpatient stroke rehabilitation: A matched comparison conducted in Italy. *Arch Phys Med Rehabil* 2000; 81(6):695–700.

79. Ancheta J, Husband M, Law D, Reding M. Initial functional independence measure score and interval post stroke help assess outcome, length of hospitalization, and quality of care. *Neurorehabil Neural Repair* 2000; 14:127–134.

80. Maulden SA, Gassaway J, Horn SD, et al. Timing of initiation of rehabilitation after stroke. *Arch Phys Med Rehabil* 2005; 86(12 Suppl 2):S34–S40.

81. Horn SD, DeJong G, Smout RJ, et al. Stroke rehabilitation patients, practice, and outcomes: Is earlier and more aggressive therapy better? *Arch Phys Med Rehabil* 2005; 86(12 Suppl 2):S101–S114.

82. Bernhardt J, Dewey H, Collier J, et al. A very early rehabilitation trial (AVERT). *International Journal of Stroke* 2006; 1(August):169–171.

83. Indredavik B, Bakke F, Solberg R, et al. Benefit of a stroke unit: A randomized controlled trial. *Stroke* 1991; 22(8):1026–1031.

84. Page SJ. Intensity versus task-specificity after stroke: How important is intensity? *Am J Phys Med Rehabil* 2003; 82(9):730–732.

85. Turton A, Pomeroy V. When should upper limb function be trained after stroke? Evidence for and against early intervention. *NeuroRehabilitation* 2002; 17(3):215–224.

86. De Weerdt W, Selz B, Nuyens G, et al. Time use of stroke patients in an intensive rehabilitation unit: a comparison between a Belgian and a Swiss setting. *Disabil Rehabil* 2000; 22(4):181–186.

87. De Wit L, Putman K, Dejaeger E, et al. Use of time by stroke patients: A comparison of four European rehabilitation centers. *Stroke* 2005; 36(9):1977–1983.

88. Bernhardt J, Dewey H, Thrift A, Donnan G. Inactive and alone: Physical activity within the first 14 days of acute stroke unit care. *Stroke* 2004; 35(4):1005–1009.

89. Wade DT, Skilbeck CE, Wood VA, Langton HR. Long-term survival after stroke. *Age Ageing* 1984; 13(2):76–82.

90. Lincoln NB, Willis D, Philips SA, et al. Comparison of rehabilitation practice on hospital wards for stroke patients. *Stroke* 1996; 27(1):18–23.

91. Keith RA, Cowell KS. Time use of stroke patients in three rehabilitation hospitals. *Soc Sci Med* 1987; 24(6):529–533.

92. Teasell R, Bitensky J, Salter K, Bayona NA. The role of timing and intensity of rehabilitation therapies. *Top Stroke Rehabil* 2005; 12(3):46–57.

93. Wodchis WP, Teare GF, Naglie G, et al. Skilled nursing facility rehabilitation and discharge to home after stroke. *Arch Phys Med Rehabil* 2005; 86(3):442–448.

94. Langhorne P, Wagenaar R, Partridge C. Physiotherapy after stroke: More is better? *Physiother Res Int* 1996; 1(2):75–88.

95. Cifu DX, Stewart DG. Factors affecting functional outcome after stroke: A critical review of rehabilitation interventions. *Arch Phys Med Rehabil* 1999; 80(5 Suppl 1):S35–S39.

96. Kwakkel G, Wagenaar RC, Koelman TW, et al. Effects of intensity of rehabilitation after stroke: A research synthesis. *Stroke* 1997; 28(8):1550–1556.

97. Kwakkel G, van Peppen R, Wagenaar RC, et al. Effects of augmented exercise therapy time after stroke: A meta-analysis. *Stroke* 2004; 35(11):2529–2539.

98. Duncan PW, Zorowitz R, Bates B, et al. Management of adult stroke rehabilitation care: A clinical practice guideline. *Stroke* 2005; 36(9):e100–e143.

99. Chen CC, Heinemann AW, Granger CV, Linn RT. Functional gains and therapy intensity during subacute rehabilitation: A study of 20 facilities. *Arch Phys Med Rehabil* 2002; 83(11):1514–1523.

100. Kalra L. The influence of stroke unit rehabilitation on functional recovery from stroke [see comments]. *Stroke* 1994; 25(4):821–825.

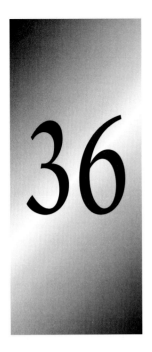

36 Stroke Services: A Global Perspective

Peter Langhorne
Anthony George Rudd

GLOBAL BURDEN OF STROKE

Stroke is now recognized as being a global problem. In developed countries, it is the third most common cause of death after coronary heart disease and cancer (1). Stroke is also one of the most important causes of severe disability (1, 2). A broader estimate of the global burden of disease (3) suggests that the top three causes of death globally are ischemic heart disease (7.2 million deaths), stroke (5.5 million), and lower respiratory diseases (3.9 million) out of a total of 56 million deaths. The leading causes of disability-adjusted life years (DALY) are those that affect predominantly younger patients such as perinatal conditions (7.1% of global DALY), lower respiratory infections (6.7%), and diarrheal diseases (4.7%). Ischemic heart disease and stroke rank sixth and seventh, respectively, as causes of global disease burden (3). It is therefore a common misperception that stroke is predominantly a disease of developed countries.

Despite a prolonged investment in efforts to identify effective drug therapies, we still lack a medical therapy that significantly impacts the burden of stroke in a population. Acute treatment with aspirin can reduce death and disability to a modest extent (one extra independent survivor per 100 patients treated) (4). Thrombolysis with tissue plasminogen activator is more potent, but

it is applicable to only a small minority of patients (5). Therefore, for the foreseeable future, the greatest hope for reducing the burden of stroke will depend upon prevention measures and effective systems for managing stroke patients (5).

Governments, and in particular those responsible for providing health care, are increasingly aware of the impact that stroke has on the health of the population and the cost to the community. Stroke patients account for about 5% of all Health Service costs in the UK (6). Studies from other countries (e.g., Sweden, the United States, Canada, the Netherlands, and Japan) suggest that the financial burden may be even greater than in the UK, possibly because of greater health service expenditure (7–14). Furthermore, demographic changes are likely to cause increasing mortality and morbidity in the developing world (15, 16).

This chapter will focus on the organization of services for people who have had a stroke. We will focus on care in hospital, but we will also mention the early post-discharge period. The discussion will emphasize models of care targeted at a broad range of stroke patients rather than at those with specific problems (e.g., aphasia). The discussion will largely reflect models of care in the UK and other European countries, but we will also mention other areas—particularly Australia and Canada.

FACTORS INFLUENCING STROKE SERVICES

The overall aim of stroke services should be to deliver the care required by stroke patients and their families in the most efficient, effective, equitable, and humane manner possible. These services may not always be exclusively stroke-specific; parts may be embedded in general (internal) medicine, geriatric medicine, neurology, or rehabilitation medicine services.

In an ideal world our decisions about the delivery of stroke services would always be informed by robust evidence from randomized trials, and priority given to those aspects of care that have been proven to be effective. However, we must recognize that carrying out randomized trials of complex interventions such as stroke services is challenging (17). At present there are relatively few clinical trials available, and these trials can be difficult to interpret and generalize.

Several factors other than evidence of effectiveness or cost-effectiveness may shape stroke-service delivery and constrain the options available to clinicians and service planners. These include the following:

a) Local healthcare culture and economy. The existing approach to providing healthcare, and the way it is funded or reimbursed, will influence the way services are delivered. Developing a stroke service in the United States or Germany will present different challenges from doing so in Scandinavia or the United Kingdom.

b) Needs of different patient groups. Stroke presents a complex challenge to service planners, in that most patients require a common basic service, although a small number (for instance, those eligible for hyperacute interventions) may require more specialized services.

c) Views of patients and families. One of the common complaints from patients and caregivers is the discontinuity of services they receive (18, 19), resulting in fragmentation of care and dissatisfaction with services.

d) Resources available. It is relatively easier to organize or reorganize a stroke service if the basic levels of staffing and investigation services are already available. For this reason, much of our discussion will be relevant mainly to well-resourced services in developed countries.

EVIDENCE-BASE FOR STROKE SERVICES

Before describing the pattern of stroke services in different regions, and the evidence-base underpinning them, we should outline some service terms and descriptions.

Comprehensive Stroke Service

We have used the term "comprehensive stroke service" to mean a stroke service that covers most of the needs of patients with stroke, and which is integrated in a way that provides a continuous patient journey—a "seamless service" (Table 36-1).

Organized Inpatient (Stroke-unit) Care

Throughout most European countries (and, indeed, further afield), there is now widespread acceptance that stroke services in hospitals should be organized within

---

TABLE 36-1
Objectives and Common Service Solutions for Managing Patients With Stroke

OBJECTIVES	PROPOSED SERVICE OPTIONS
Specific acute medical and surgical treatment	Acute or comprehensive stroke units; stroke centers
Identification and assessment of patient problems	Acute or comprehensive stroke units
Secondary prevention of further vascular events	Acute or comprehensive stroke units
General care, including interventions to resolve problems (includes many aspects of rehabilitation)	Comprehensive or rehabilitation stroke units
Terminal care for patients who are unlikely to survive	Stroke units
Hospital discharge and reintegration into the community	Early supported discharge services; discharge planning
Continuing or long-term care for severely disabled patients	Therapy-based rehabilitation services; stroke liaison worker services; day hospital services
Follow-up to detect and manage late-onset problems	Chronic disease management; outpatient clinics

See Table 4 for some definitions of terms.

TABLE 36-2
Summary of Patient Outcomes in the Stroke Unit Trials

	STROKE UNIT	CONVENTIONAL CARE	ODDS RATIO (95% CI)	APPROXIMATE NUMBER OF OUTCOMES PER 100 ADMITTED
Home (independent)	45%	40%	1.25 (1.12, 1.40)	5
Home (dependent)	17%	15%	1.16 (0.88, 1.53)	1
Institutional care	14%	16%	0.84 (0.72, 0.98)	−2
Dead	23%	28%	0.80 (0.70, 0.91)	−4

This table shows the proportion (%) of patients with various outcomes at the end of scheduled follow-up (median 1 year) in the randomized trials of stroke-unit care vs. conventional care. The absolute risk difference is the proportion of outcomes achieved (+) or avoided (−) with stroke-unit care. The next column is the number of outcomes achieved (+) or avoided (−) for every 1000 patients cared for in a stroke unit, assuming the absolute risk of an outcome in the population is similar to that in the trials. These figures are based on data from 24 trials (4900 patients). Stroke Unit Trialists Collaboration 2001 (51).

stroke units (20, 21). Much of the evidence comes from a systematic review of clinical trials that compared the outcomes for stroke patients cared for in a specialist stroke unit with the outcomes of those cared for in general wards. Patients managed in stroke units are more likely to survive, return home, and regain independence (Table 36-2). The units included in the systematic review were run by geriatricians, neurologists, general (internal) physicians, and rehabilitationists. Patients with mild, moderate, and severe strokes, of all age groups, appear likely to benefit from stroke-unit care (20, 21).

Although comprehensive stroke-unit care is a complex and multifaceted intervention, the key components are reasonably well described (22) and include all of the following (Table 36-3):

- Ward base—effective stroke units have usually been based in a distinct ward with dedicated nursing staff.
- Specialist staffing—they have been staffed with medical, nursing, and therapy staff with a specialist interest and expertise in stroke and/or rehabilitation.
- Multidisciplinary teamwork—they have always included good multidisciplinary communication (defined as a formal meeting of all staff once per week to plan the management of individual patients).
- Education and training—they have included programs of education and training for staff and provision of information for patients and caregivers.

Several consistent features of the process of care in stroke units have also been described (20, 22). These typically did not depend on high-technology facilities but include a systematic approach to care (Table 36-3) that incorporated the following:

- Careful assessment and monitoring of medical, nursing, and therapy needs.
- Early active management, incorporating management of food and fluids, control of pyrexia, hypoxia, hyperglycemia, early mobilization, careful positioning and handling, and avoidance of urinary catheterization.
- Ongoing multidisciplinary rehabilitation, with early goal-setting, early involvement of caregivers in rehabilitation, and provision of information to patients and caregivers. This also includes early planning of discharge needs.

Many of these processes of care will come as no surprise to those experienced in stroke care, but recent audits raise concerns that many are not routinely provided (23).

Beyond describing the basic components of stroke-unit care, it is difficult to determine whether the effectiveness of the stroke units is a result of the total package of care, or of particular components. Although the basic principles of stroke-unit care are reasonably well described, they have been delivered in a variety of ways, and the term "stroke unit" means different things to different people. So it is important to define our terms (see Table 36-4).

Acute Stroke Unit. "Acute" refers to the policy of rapid admission of the stroke patient to the stroke unit. In some regions, particularly in North America and Germany, there has been a pattern of admitting stroke patients to ward areas with facilities for intensive monitoring of physiological functions (cardiac, respiratory, and neurologic). Interventions are introduced to correct these abnormalities (e.g., raised intracranial pressure, systemic hypertension). Broadly speaking, two approaches have been described:

- Intensive-care units, which can offer all monitoring (including intracranial monitoring) and life-support options (e.g., respiratory support).

TABLE 36-3
Characteristics of Comprehensive Stroke-unit Care

Structure
- Geographically discrete ward
- Multidisciplinary staffing (nursing, medical, physiotherapy, occupational therapy, speech therapy, social work)
- Medical staff with specialist interest in stroke and rehabilitation
- Nursing staff with specialist interest in stroke and rehabilitation

Coordination of care
- Regular multidisciplinary team meetings (formal meeting of all staff once weekly, informal meetings 2–3 times per week)
- Close linking of nursing and multidisciplinary team care
- Educational programs for staff

Assessment and monitoring
- Rapid admission to stroke unit
- Medical history and examination
- Standard routine investigations (biochemistry, hematology, ECG, CT scanning)
- Further selective investigations (carotid Doppler US, echocardiogram, MRI scanning)
- Nursing assessments (vital signs, general care needs, swallow test, fluid balance, pressure areas, neurologic monitoring)
- Therapy assessments of impairments and disability

Early management
- Careful management of fluids/food
- Pyrexia management, paracetamol for pyrexia, antibiotic for suspected infection
- Hypoxia management; oxygen if hypoxia, drowsiness, or cardiorespiratory disease
- Glycemic management, insulin for hyperglycemia
- Careful positioning and handling
- Pressure-area care
- Avoid urinary catheterization if possible
- Early mobilization: up to sit, stand, and walk as soon as possible

Ongoing multidisciplinary rehabilitation
- Early goal-setting
- Early involvement of caregivers in rehabilitation
- Provision of information to patients and caregivers

Discharge planning
- Early assessment of discharge needs
- Discharge plan involving patient and caregivers

- "Semi-intensive" units are similar to coronary-care units, where monitoring and intervention focus on physiological variables but not life-support.

There have been three small clinical trials of semi-intensive units that have reported rather inconclusive findings.

Comprehensive Stroke Units. Perhaps the most successfully implemented model has been the comprehensive stroke unit, which admits patients acutely and then provides at least a few weeks of rehabilitation. This approach, which is widespread in Norway and Sweden, is supported by several clinical trials included in the systematic review and results from a national stroke register in Sweden (24). A major advantage of this approach is that rehabilitation can start on the day of the stroke. In practice, although these units provide most care for most patients, it is common to refer some patients with ongoing, complex rehabilitation needs to other rehabilitation services.

Rehabilitation Stroke Units. Several trials have indicated benefit from rehabilitation units that admit patients a few days after stroke onset and continue rehabilitation for several weeks. These trials have inevitably examined a more select patient group, who are stable enough for that environment and have ongoing rehabilitation needs (21).

Some trials also explored the impact of organizing stroke care within generic rehabilitation services (e.g., geriatric medicine or neurologic rehabilitation services); patients achieve better outcomes in mixed rehabilitation units than in general wards (21). Comparisons with stroke-specific units indicate a trend toward better outcomes in stroke-specific units, but the data are limited.

Mobile Stroke Teams. Overall the trials in the meta-analysis indicated that a stroke team working across several general wards may improve aspects of the processes of care (e.g., access to specialist assessments) but cannot achieve patient outcomes as good as those of a team based in a stroke unit (25, 26).

Transfer from Hospital to Community

One of the main areas of concern to patients, and perhaps still more so to caregivers, is the organization (or rather the lack of organization) of hospital discharge (18, 19). A number of approaches have been attempted to reduce the stress of the transition from hospital to home:

- Providing adequate information and training to the caregivers while the patient is in the hospital—for example, inviting the caregivers to therapy sessions and involving them in the patient's care on the unit. However, trials of information provision and patient education do not provide clear evidence to guide practice.
- A program of training caregivers to manage their new role has been tested in one moderately large randomized trial (27). This involved stroke-unit staff training caregivers about stroke and in practical caring skills. This approach was surprisingly

TABLE 36-4

Classification of Different Forms of Organized Inpatient (Stroke-unit) Care

TYPE	PHILOSOPHY OF CARE	PATIENT GROUP	MDT BASE	TIMING OF ADMISSION	TIMING OF DISCHARGE	TYPE OF CARE
Acute (intensive) stroke unit	Acute	Stroke	Ward	Acute (hours)	Early (3–7 days)	Acute medical and nursing care (with high staffing levels)
Acute (semi-intensive) stroke unit	Acute	Stroke	Ward	Acute (hours)	Early (3–7 days)	Acute medical and nursing care. Monitoring and management of physiological variables
Comprehensive stroke unit	Acute care and multidisciplinary rehabilitation	Stroke	Ward	Acute (hours)	Later (days–weeks); some referral to specialist rehabilitation	Acute medical and nursing care. Non-intensive management of physiological variables. Early active multidisciplinary rehabilitation.
Rehabilitation stroke unit	Multidisciplinary rehabilitation	Stroke	Ward	Delayed (days)	Later (weeks)	Multidisciplinary rehabilitation
Mixed rehabilitation unit	Multidisciplinary rehabilitation	Stroke and other disabling illness	Ward	Early (hours–days)	Later (weeks)	Multidisciplinary rehabilitation
Mobile stroke team	Acute care and/or multidisciplinary rehabilitation	Stroke	Mobile (no ward) base	Early (hours–days)	Later (weeks)	Acute medical care and/or multidisciplinary rehabilitation. No specialist nursing input

This table summarizes, in broad terms, the characteristics of different types of stroke unit. MDT = Multidisciplinary team effective and cost-effective, reducing the overall cost of caring (28), and it is the subject of further research.

- Pre-discharge home visits with the patient and one or more members of the team, to ensure that the home environment is tailored to the patient's needs. Although this is a well-established procedure in many centers, we could not identify any clinical trials of such policies.
- Pre-discharge case conferences to allow the patient and caregiver to meet with the hospital-based team and any professionals who are to be involved in their care in the community, including clear guidelines of who to contact in the event of problems. Once again, this is a well-established approach for which we could not identify any clinical trials.

Early Supported Discharge Services

Early supported discharge services aim to accelerate discharge home from the hospital but provide more continuity of rehabilitation in the home setting. To date, twelve randomized trials have tested this approach to care in a variety of settings around the world (29, 30). Most were centered around a small, multidisciplinary team of physiotherapy, occupational therapy, nursing, and assistant staff—with input from medical, speech and language therapy, and social work staff. These teams were either hospital-based (and went out to the patient's home) or community-based (and came into the hospital to recruit patients). All incorporated regular multidisciplinary team meetings to plan patient care. A typical pathway of care (30) is shown in Table 36-5. Typically these services

---

TABLE 36-5

Typical Care Pathway in an Early Supported Discharge (ESD) Service

- Early identification of eligible patients in hospital.
- Early assessment by a "key worker" from the early supported discharge team (one individual who supervised the care of the patient).
- Assessment of home needs through a home visit (with or without the patient present).
- Identification of recovery goals with the patient and caregivers.
- Discharge home with very early input (within 24 hours) by members of the early supported discharge team.
- Continuing rehabilitation in the home setting (up to five days per week if necessary).
- Negotiated withdrawal of the team as recovery goals are achieved.
- Multidisciplinary review of the patient's progress.
- Planned discharge from the service with later follow-up and review.

---

can input for up to three months, but this has been shorter with hand-over to other community services (30).

Even when compared with high-quality care from a hospital-based stroke unit, an early supported discharge team could not only accelerate discharge home (with an average reduction in length of stay of eight days), but could also result in the patient having a greater chance of remaining at home and regaining independence. Overall, for every 100 patients randomized to early supported discharge services, an extra 5 remained at home and/or were independent at 6 to 12 months after the stroke. Good results were most likely with a well-resourced, coordinated multidisciplinary supported discharge team, and if patients were recruited with mild to moderate stroke severity. There is a suggestion that such services may not work as well in more dispersed rural populations (31), but this requires confirmation. Overall early supported discharge services may be relevant to about half the stroke patients admitted to hospitals (30).

Economic analyses (29) indicate that the additional costs of community rehabilitation are more than outweighed by the savings in hospital bed days. In addition to the "harder" outcomes above, it is also noteworthy that patients and caregivers allocated to early supported discharge services were more likely to report satisfaction with their services. Early supported discharge services appear to be an important component of a truly comprehensive stroke service and should particularly target patients with mild to moderately severe strokes.

Continuing Rehabilitation and Reintegration Back to Normal Life. Even when stroke patients have received good care in hospital and around the discharge period, they may still have difficulty maintaining independence and reintegrating to normal life. At this stage of the patient journey, services are often quite variable and may be completely nonexistent (32). This probably reflects the diversity of approaches in different countries but also a limited evidence base to suggest that effective interventions really can improve recovery. In general two broad approaches have been tested in clinical trials:

- Therapy-based rehabilitation services (provided by physiotherapy, occupational therapy, or multidisciplinary staff and primarily aiming to increase activities in daily living). In practice this might include a range of task-related interventions aiming to improve mobility, activities of daily living, or specific tasks such as dressing. In a systematic review (33) of therapy-based rehabilitation services, therapy-based rehabilitation (when compared with no routine intervention) helped prevent stroke patients from deteriorating in their ability to carry out activities of daily living (ADL), and improved ADL scores. Therefore, even relatively late after stroke onset (several months), patients may gain from input from a therapist. What is less clear is the absolute benefit likely to be achieved and the cost-effectiveness of these services.

- Stroke liaison-worker services provided by stroke nurses, family support workers, or specialist social workers primarily aim to improve participation in normal living and quality of life (34). In practice these have included a mix of interventions, which could deliver a programme of rehabilitation or respond to identified problems. These services often involve approaching patients and families during hospital admission, when staff can provide information and education about stroke. Assistance is also available for input after discharge home, particularly to identify problems or unmet needs and to develop customized solutions. At least fifteen randomized trials have tested this type of service in the UK, Australia, the United States, and the Netherlands. Their impact on patient outcomes is unclear (35), but they do appear to be valued by patients and caregivers.

STROKE SERVICES IN DIFFERENT REGIONS

Having outlined some general principles, background research, and different approaches to providing stroke care, we can discuss in more detail the delivery of stroke services in various parts of the world, particularly in Europe.

The subsequent discussion will, of course, be very general, and there will inevitably be many local exceptions. However, we aim to indicate the different approaches that have been adopted in different parts of the world (Table 36-6). For each section, we will try to briefly mention the local health care economy, those medical specialties largely providing stroke-unit care, the types of stroke-unit care and coverage available (including issues of equity of access), and access to other services. Finally, we will try to mention evidence of successful implementation of service components.

Scandinavia (Norway, Sweden, Denmark, Finland)

This group of countries have mature social democratic economies with largely publicly funded health services (24, 36). The main medical specialties managing stroke in Norway, Sweden, and Denmark tend to have been general (internal) medicine and geriatric medicine, although neurologists also play an important role, particularly in Finland. The most common stroke-unit model is the comprehensive stroke unit, which was developed and pioneered in Norway and Sweden, and some of the most important clinical trials come from these countries.

Recent surveys suggest that most hospitals (over 90%) have stroke units, and the majority of patients (70–80%) obtain access to stroke units during their hospital stay.

Evidence of successful service implementation comes from studies of the Swedish Stroke Register (24), which has studied all 85 Swedish hospitals, registering all admitted stroke patients and following them up after discharge from hospital. These publications (24) indicate that admission to a hospital with a stroke unit is an independent predictor of good outcome. For every 100 patients admitted to a stroke unit, there were six fewer deaths and three more surviving to return home.

Scandinavian countries have also pioneered the development and evaluation of early supported-discharge services (29). Such services are becoming more widespread, but current figures are unclear.

United Kingdom (England, Scotland, Wales, Northern Ireland)

The UK also has a largely publicly funded health service (23, 37–39). Traditionally, stroke care has been provided in departments of geriatric medicine and general (internal) medicine (40), and stroke units have tended to evolve from rehabilitation services. Some specialist rehabilitation services (e.g., for younger adults) are provided by rehabilitation medicine physicians.

Relatively little attention was paid to stroke in the UK until the publication of the King's Fund Consensus Conference (1988). This highlighted the many deficiencies in the services provided for stroke patients, concluding that "services were often haphazard and poorly tailored to the patient's needs (19)." Since then, stroke has moved up in the political agenda. These changes have led to a substantial interest in stroke in general, and in stroke services in particular. Over the last few years, an increasing amount of research has been done to determine the best and most cost-effective ways of providing care for stroke patients.

In the most recent audits of services in England and Wales (23), 92% of hospitals reported having a stroke unit, and approximately 60% of patients gained access to a unit during their admission. In a recent study of the National Sentinel Audit (23), admission to a stroke unit was an independent predictor of better survival, with an odds ratio of death of 0.75 among those admitted to a stroke unit. Recent data from Scotland show similar patterns (41).

Supported discharge services provided by community teams are relatively uncommon (32%) but have increased in recent years (23).

TABLE 36-6

Summary of Predominant Service Patterns in Different Regions

	SCANDINAVIA	UNITED KINGDOM	CONTINENTAL EUROPE	MEDITERRANEAN	AUSTRALIA AND NEW ZEALAND	CANADA	DEVELOPING WORLD
Healthcare economy	Public health services	Public health services	Mixed health economies	Mixed health economies	Mixed	Mixed	Variety
Specialties providing stroke-unit care	General medicine, geriatric medicine	Geriatric medicine, general medicine	Neurology, rehabilitation medicine	Neurology, general (internal) medicine	Neurology, rehab medicine	Neurology, rehab medicine	Variety
Type of stroke-unit care and coverage	Comprehensive stroke-unit model	Rehabilitation (and comprehensive) units	Acute and rehabilitation units	Acute and rehabilitation units	Acute and rehab units	Acute and rehab units	Very limited access
Equity of access to stroke units	Most hospitals (>90%) have stroke units, and most patients get access (70–80%)	80%–90% of hospitals have stroke unit (60% of patients gain access)	Less than 50% access at last surveys	Variable access (10–20%) in PROSIT register in Italy	23% of patients treated in SU in Australia	31% of patients treated in SU in Canada	Very few stroke units established (usually in private hospitals)
Evidence of successful implementation of stroke units	Swedish RIKS-Stroke register shows effective implementation	National sentinel audit showed improved outcome with admission to stroke unit	Registries show some effective implementation (but also inequities of access)	PROSIT register (Italy) suggests effective implementation is possible	Report indicates improved outcomes with stroke-unit care	Limited information available	Limited information available
Services after hospital discharge	Some early supported discharge services	Some community rehabilitation services	Variable	Limited	Variable	Variable	Very limited access

NB Most survey data were published in 2003.

West Continental Europe (France, Germany, Austria, Switzerland, the Netherlands)

This group of countries tend to have mixed healthcare economies with a mixture of public funding and private insurance (42–45). Traditionally, the acute phase of stroke care tends to be provided in neurology services (and sometimes geriatric medicine services for older stroke patients), with rehabilitation medicine providing the main rehabilitation services. In neurology departments, acute units (intensive care or semi-intensive care units) appear to predominate. After the acute illness, rehabilitation services tend to be provided in rehabilitation stroke units. Some publications (46) have suggested less than 50% access for stroke patients in Germany, but this appears to vary from region to region.

Studies of stroke-unit registries (45) suggest effective implementation but also some reduction in access for older patients.

Mediterranean Europe (Spain, Portugal, Italy, Greece)

This group of countries also have mixed healthcare economies, with a mixture of public funding and insurance (47, 48). Once again, the acute management of stroke frequently occurs in departments of neurology and sometimes general (internal) medicine. In many neurology departments, acute semi-intensive units have been adopted, as well as rehabilitation services based in rehabilitation units. Studies from Italy (48) suggest very variable access to stroke-unit care, frequently less than 20%. Unpublished data from the Italian register suggests that effective implementation of stroke-unit care is possible in Italy.

Eastern Europe (Poland, the Czech Republic, Hungary, Russia, Baltic States)

Many of these countries have undergone a rapid economic transition, with health services moving from a publicly funded model to a more mixed economy (49, 50). Traditionally stroke services have often been provided in departments of neurology. Organized (stroke-unit) care has been developed in Poland and Hungary (49, 50) but appear less well-established in other areas. Post-discharge services appear to be very variable.

Australia and New Zealand

The structures of health care in Australia and New Zealand originally developed from a UK model of service. However, in recent years both countries have developed a more mixed health care economy.

Much of acute stroke care in Australia is carried out in departments of neurology, with more of a mixed picture in New Zealand. There have been considerable concerns about the limited provision of stroke-unit care, and several promising initiatives have been implemented in Australia to try to develop stroke units in both acute settings and rehabilitation units (51). Rehabilitation is frequently provided by rehabilitation medicine specialists or in departments of geriatric medicine.

A recent report from Australia, comparing services in different hospitals, indicated that stroke-unit care was associated with improved outcomes in Australian settings (51). Post-discharge services appear variable.

Canada

The Canadian health care economy is based on a national health insurance system. Traditional stroke care has been provided by a range of specialties, predominantly neurology, rehabilitation medicine, and general (internal) medicine. Stroke-unit care has been available in a minority of hospitals (52), but steps are being taken to expand coverage. A variety of post-discharge services exist, which appear variable in nature.

Developing countries (esp. Africa, Asia, South America)

It is recognized that developing countries have some of the highest stroke mortality rates, accounting for two-thirds of stroke deaths worldwide (36). A recent review (49) has demonstrated a lack of organized stroke-unit care and rehabilitation services in these nations. Some excellent services do exist, but frequently with poor access for the majority of the population. The authors concluded that there is a need to develop basic organized stroke-unit care in developing countries.

CONCLUSIONS AND CHALLENGES

The challenges facing developed countries clearly differ from those of developing regions. Scandinavian countries appear to be facing the challenge of maintaining established standards through clinical guidelines and possibly the accreditation of stroke units. In the UK there has been an underdevelopment of acute care, and we may see strategic investment to improve acute services. In western continental Europe, issues have been raised around the cost and the equity of access to services, and we may see an expansion of stroke-unit care or the adoption of a less intensive model of acute stroke care. In the Mediterranean region, there has been underdevelopment of specialist stroke services, and it is expected that strategic investment may be required. In the developing world, the major challenge is how to provide stroke services that are effective, affordable, tailored to local needs, and available to the majority of people who need such services.

Research Frontiers

The value of the stroke-unit model of care is clearly demonstrated. Future studies should explore the impact of different components of the stroke-unit "package" (e.g., early mobilization). In particular, we need to identify simple, widely applicable inventions that could be applied in low-resource settings in developing countries. Effective ways of improving discharge home, reintegrating to normal life, and relieving caregiver burden also require identification.

*R*eferences

1. Murray CJL, Lopez AD. Mortality by cause for eight regions of the world: Global Burden of Disease Study. *Lancet* 1997; 349:1269–1276.
2. Warlow C, Sudlow C, Dennis M, et al. Stroke. *Lancet* 2003; 362:1211–1224.
3. Lopez AD, Mathers CD. Measuring the global burden of disease and epidemiological transitions 2002–2030. *Ann Trop Med Parasitol* 2006; 100:481–499.
4. Chen ZM, Sandercock P, Pan HC, et al. Indications for early aspirin use in ischemic stroke: A combined analysis of 40,000 randomized patients from the Chinese Acute Stroke Trial and International Stroke Trial. *Stroke* 2000; 31:1240–1249.
5. Gilligan AK, Thrift AG, Sturm JW, et al. Stroke units, tissue plasminogen activator, aspirin and neuroprotection: Which stroke intervention could provide the greatest community benefit? *Cerebrovascular Dis* 2005; 20:239–244.
6. Isard PA, Forbes JF. The cost of stroke to the National Health Service in Scotland. Cerebrovascular Diseases 1992; 2:47–50.
7. Caro JJ, Huybrechts KF, Duchesne I. for the Stroke Economic Analysis Group. Management patterns and costs of acute ischaemic stroke. An international study. *Stroke* 2000; 31:582–590.
8. Dewey HM, Thrift AG, Mihalopoulos C, et al. Lifetime cost of stroke subtypes in Australia. Findings from the North East Melbourne Stroke Incidence Study (NEMESIS). *Stroke* 2003; 34:2502–2507.
9. Evers SMAA, Engel GL, Ament AJHA. Cost of stroke in the Netherlands from a societal perspective. *Stroke* 1997; 28:1375–1381.
10. Grieve R, Hutton J, Bhalla A, et al. On behalf of the Biomed II European Study of Stroke Care. *Stroke* 2001; 32:1684–1691.
11. Persson U, Silverberg R, Lindgren B, et al. Direct costs of stroke for a Swedish population. *International Journal of Technology Assessment in Health Care* 1990; 6:125–137.
12. Smurawska LT, Alexandrov AV, Bladin CF, Norris JW. Cost of acute stroke care in Toronto, Canada. *Stroke* 1994; 25:1628–1631.
13. Taylor TN, Davis PH, Torner JC, et al. Lifetime cost of stroke in the United States. *Stroke* 1996; 27:1459–1466.
14. Yoneda Y, Uehara T, Yamasaki H, et al. Hospital-based study of the care and cost of acute ischemic stroke in Japan. *Stroke* 2003; 34:718–724.
15. Bonita R, Solomon N, Broad JB. Prevalence of stroke and stroke-related disability: Estimates from the Auckland Stroke Studies. *Stroke* 1997; 28:1898–1902.
16. Feigin VL. Stroke epidemiology in the developing world. *Lancet* 2005; 365: 2160–2161.
17. Campbell M, Fitzpatrick R, Haines A, et al. Framework for design and evaluation of complex interventions to improve health. *BMJ* 2000; 321:694–696.
18. Chest, Heart, and Stroke Scotland Report. Improving stroke services: Patients and carers' views. 2001. (http://www.chss.org.uk/pdf/research/Improving_services_patients_and_carers_views.pdf).
19. Healthcare Commission. *Stroke: survey of patients.* London, 2005 (http://www.healthcarecommission.org.uk/_db/_documents/04018503.pdf).
20. Stroke Unit Trialists' Collaboration. Collaborative systematic review of the randomised trials of organised inpatient (stroke unit) care after stroke. *British Medical Journal* 1997; 314:1151–1159.
21. Stroke Unit Trialists' Collaboration. Organised inpatient (stroke unit) care for stroke. In the Cochrane Library. Oxford: Update Software, 2001.
22. Langhorne P, Dennis MS. Stroke units: the next 10 years. *Lancet* 2004; 363:834–835.
23. Rudd AG, Hoffman A, Irwin P, et al. Stroke Unit Care and Outcome. Results from the 2001 National Sentinel Audit of Stroke (England, Wales, and Northern Ireland). *Stroke* 2005; 36:103–106.
24. Stegmayr B, Asplund K, Hulter-Asberg K, et al. Stroke units in their natural habitat: Can results of randomized trials be reproduced in routine clinical practice? *Stroke* 1999; 30: 709–714.
25. Kalra L, Evans A, Perez I, et al. Alternative strategies for stroke care: a prospective randomised controlled trial. *Lancet* 2000; 356:894–899.
26. Langhorne P, Dey P, Woodman M, et al. Is stroke unit care portable? A systematic review of the clinical trials. *Age Ageing* 2005; 34:324–330.
27. Kalra L, Evans A, Perez I, et al. Training carers of stroke patients: randomised controlled trial. *British Medical Journal* 2004; 328:1099.
28. Patel A, Knapp M, Evans A, et al. Training care givers of stroke patients: Economic evaluation. *BMJ* 2004; 328:1102.
29. Early Supported Discharge Trialists. Services for reducing duration of hospital care for acute stroke patients. The Cochrane Database of Systematic Reviews 2005; 2:article number CD000443.pub2. DOI: 10.1002/14651858.CD000443.pub2.
30. Langhorne P, Taylor G, Murray G, et al. Early supported discharge services for stroke patients: An individual patient data meta-analysis. *Lancet* 2005; 365:501–506.
31. Askim T, Rohweder G, Lydersen S, Inderdavik B. Evaluation of an extended stroke unit service with early supported discharge for patients living in a rural community. A randomized controlled trial. *Clin Rehab* 2004; 18:238–248.
32. Wolfe CDA, Tilling K, Beech R, Rudd AG for the European BIOMED Study of Stroke Care Group. Variations in case fatality and dependency from stroke in Western and Central Europe. *Stroke* 1999; 30:350–356.
33. Outpatient Service Trialists. Therapy-based rehabilitation services for stroke patients at home. *Lancet* 2004; 363:352–356.
34. Ellis G, Mant J, Langhorne P, Dennis M, Winner S. Stroke liaison workers for stroke patients and carers (Cochrane Protocol). The Cochrane Database of Systematic Reviews 2005; 2.
35. Ellis G on behalf of the Stroke Liaison Workers Collaboration. Meta-analysis of Stroke Liaison Workers for Patients and Carers. *Cerebrovascular Dis* 2006; 21 suppl 4:120.
36. Indredavik, B. Stroke Units—The Norwegian experience. *Cerebrovascular Diseases* 2003; 15, suppl 1:19–20.
37. Dennis M. Stroke services in Scotland. *Cerebrovascular Diseases* 2003; 15, suppl 1:26–28.
38. Rudd AG, Irwin P, Rutledge Z, et al. The National Sentinel Audit for stroke: A tool for raising standards of care. *Journal of the Royal College of Physicians of London* 1999; 33:460–464.
39. Scottish Stroke Services Audit. Report on an Audit of the Organisation of Services for Stroke Patients, 1997–98. Royal College of Physicians and Surgeons of Glasgow, 1999.
40. Ebrahim S, Redfern J. Stroke care: A matter of chance—A national survey of stroke services. The Stroke Association: London, 1999.
41. Scottish Stroke Care Audit. National Report on Stroke Services in Scottish Hospitals 2005/2006. 2006 (http://www.strokeaudit.scot.nhs.uk/Downloads/files/SSCA).
42. Brainin M, Steiner M, Gugging M, for the participants in the Austrian Stroke Registry for Acute Stroke Units. *Cerebrovascular Diseases* 2003; 15, suppl 1; 29–32.
43. Busse O. Stroke units and stroke services in Germany. *Cerebrovascular Diseases* 2003; 15, suppl 1:8–10.
44. Hommel M, Deblasi A, Garambois K, Jaillard A. The French Stroke Program. *Cerebrovascular Diseases* 2003; 15, suppl 1:11–13.
45. Walter A, Seidel G, Thie A, Raspe HH, for the SSSH Study Group. German stroke units versus conventional care in acute ischemic stroke and TIA—A prospective study. Abstract. *Cerebrovasc Dis* 2005; 19, suppl 2: 30.
46. Habscheid W, Felenstein M, Pullwitt A. Characterization of medical and neurological care of stroke patients. An analysis of the data from the project "Safeguarding Quality in Stroke Care" of the Regional Medical Council of Baden-Wurttemberg. *Deutsche Medizinische Wochenschrift* 2004; 129(37):1911–1915.
47. Melo TP, Ferro JM. Stroke units and stroke services in Portugal. *Cerebrovascular Diseases* 2003; 15, suppl 1:21–22.
48. Sterzi R, Micieli G, Candelise L, on behalf of the PROSIT collaborators. Assessment of regional acute stroke unit care in Italy: The PROSIT Study. *Cerebrovascular Diseases* 2003; 15, suppl 1:16–18.
49. Bereczki D, Csiba L, Fulesdi B, Fekete I. Stroke units in Hungary—The Debrecen experience. *Cerebrovascular Diseases* 2003; 15, suppl. 1:23–25.
50. Czlonskowska A, Milewska D, Ryglewics D. The Polish experience in early stroke care. *Cerebrovascular Diseases* 2003; 15, suppl 1:14-15.
51. Cadhillac D. Evaluation of the New South Wales Greater Metropolitan Transition Taskforce. Stroke Unit Initiative, 2003/2004 Final Report. National Stroke Research Institute Report, Melbourne, Australia. May 2004.
52. Hill, MD. Stroke units in Canada *CMAJ* 2002; 167:649–650.

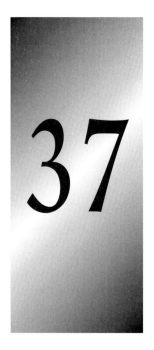

37 Levels of Rehabilitative Care and Patient Triage

Anne Epstein
Andrew M. Kramer

When stroke patients are ready to leave the hospital, they have several options to continue and expand their rehabilitation. These include inpatient rehabilitation facilities, skilled nursing facilities, home health agencies, outpatient facilities, and long-term acute care hospitals. This chapter compares and contrasts the settings available for stroke patients who require additional rehabilitation and support once out of the hospital. First, the various rehabilitation settings are described. Second, the factors that influence utilization of these settings, including patient characteristics, geographic variation, payment, and trends in utilization are discussed. Third, evidence about the relative costs and outcomes of the settings is presented. Finally, setting selection for stroke patients is discussed, including the indications for placing patients in each setting.

REHABILITATION SETTINGS

Five provider types are used for rehabilitation following an acute stroke:

1. Inpatient rehabilitation facilities (hospital-based units or freestanding hospitals)
2. Skilled nursing facilities (hospital-based units or freestanding)
3. Home health agencies
4. Outpatient facilities
5. Long-term acute care hospitals.

Inpatient Rehabilitation Facilities

Inpatient Rehabilitation Facilities (IRFs) are designed to provide multidisciplinary rehabilitation to patients who can tolerate up to three hours of physical, occupational, and/or speech therapy a day. IRFs provide comprehensive rehabilitation programs under physician supervision and access to a full range of therapists. The close medical supervision allows IRFs to care for patients with complicated medical conditions, provided they are capable of undergoing intense rehabilitation therapy. About 80% of the United States' 1,235 IRFs are hospital-based units, and the remainder are freestanding hospitals (1).

The number of IRFs has grown nearly 20% over the last ten years. The U.S. Medicare insurance system requires IRF patients to receive a minimum of three hours of rehabilitation therapy a day, and to demonstrate consistent functional improvement. Further, in order to qualify as an IRF rather than an acute inpatient hospital under the Medicare system, Medicare requires 60% of patients in the IRF over a 12-month period meet a list of thirteen medical conditions, including stroke. Stroke patients currently make up the second largest diagnostic group of IRF admissions, 16.5% in 2004 (1).

Skilled Nursing Facilities

Skilled Nursing Facilities (SNFs) are nursing homes that are certified by the U.S. Centers for Medicare and Medicaid Services (CMS) to provide skilled nursing and therapy services. Under the Medicare program, 78% of SNF patients receive rehabilitation services ranging from at least 45 minutes per week over three days (low intensity) to at least 720 minutes per week over five days, involving two different types of therapy (ultra-high intensity) (2). In 2005, there were 15,625 SNFs certified by CMS, a 7.4% increase from 1996 (1). SNFs may be freestanding nursing homes (over 90%) or distinct part units (sometimes called transitional care or sub-acute units) within an acute care or rehabilitation hospital. Freestanding SNFs usually also provide long-term nursing facility care. SNFs vary in terms of therapist availability and the scope of their rehabilitative services. Some use therapy management companies that provide all of the rehabilitation services under contract.

SNFs admit post-stroke patients who require daily skilled nursing care and/or skilled therapy services. These patients are not able to function in the community, nor are they strong enough to take part in the intensive therapy of an IRF. Both physician supervision and medical director availability are substantially less in SNFs than in IRFs. SNFs are often used for patients that demonstrate the potential for improvement in function, but who previously resided in a long-term nursing home or are unlikely to return to the community. These patients may move from the skilled portion of the nursing facility into residential care when recovery plateaus. Over 30% of SNF admissions were discharged back to the community in 2005 (3).

Long-Term Acute Care Hospitals

Long-term acute care hospitals (LTACs) care for medically complex patients with significant potential for improvement. These patients may have underlying chronic conditions, or acute conditions that require substantial monitoring or ongoing medical care. Examples include organ failure, respiratory problems requiring ventilator support, and multiple comorbidities. Only about 10% of LTACs have been classified as specializing in rehabilitation based upon the Major Diagnostic Categories of their patient population (4). LTACs meet the certification requirements for acute hospitals, but must also have a length of stay greater than 25 days to meet Medicare requirements for payment.

Many of the long-established LTACs were originally freestanding tuberculosis or chronic condition hospitals. The number of LTACs rose from 90 in 1990 to 357 in 2004, and the rapid growth in facilities has continued over the past few years (5). Many of the newer LTACs are physically located within an acute care hospital. While studies suggest that LTACs may be substituting for longer acute care stays or for SNF care (4, 6), relative to other rehabilitation settings, LTACs have higher average nurse staffing hours per patient day, have respiratory therapists available 24 hours a day, and have daily physician involvement with patients (6).

Outpatient Rehabilitation

Outpatient therapy may be provided in various settings, including facilities that also provide inpatient rehabilitation services. The vast majority (94%) of acute care hospitals also have outpatient centers (1). In 2002, 30% of Medicare outpatient payments were made to SNFs, and 24% to hospital-based outpatient departments. Outpatient rehabilitation facilities (ORFs) and comprehensive outpatient rehabilitation facilities (CORFs) combine for another 19 percent. The remainder was divided between physician offices, therapists in private practice, and other settings (7). Outpatient facilities may be able to provide tests and procedures to monitor a stroke patient's medical condition as well as provide therapy services.

Outpatient care is designed for patients who are capable of self-care in a residential setting, or who have caregivers available and are able to leave their homes on a regular basis. Outpatient treatment can be multidisciplinary. Facilities can offer rehabilitation programs that are as intense as inpatient rehabilitation programs, or may provide less-demanding regimens, depending on the needs of the patient.

Home Health Agencies

Home health agencies (HHA) provide nursing, therapy, and caregiver services to patients through home visits. A physician works with the HHA to develop a plan of care, and the HHA staff communicates with the physician on a regular basis; however, direct physician supervision in the home is rarely available. HHAs may be associated with an acute hospital, an IRF, a SNF, or an outpatient facility, or may operate independently. Medicare recognized 8,082 HHAs in 2005, a drop of nearly 18% from 1996, but with steadily increasing numbers over the past four years.

Home health care is suited to patients who are medically stable and who have caregivers in the home capable of managing the patient's daily needs. Many insurers, including Medicare, require that patients meet strict criteria for a "homebound" designation. Medicare requires that patients are able to leave home only with great difficulty and for absences which are infrequent and of short duration.

UTILIZATION OF REHABILITATION SETTINGS

All of the five settings described in the previous section can serve as the primary rehabilitation setting following a stroke, that is, the setting where the patient first receives rehabilitation services following discharge from the acute hospital. They can also be a subsequent rehabilitation provider in a multiple provider episode of care. Patterns of rehabilitation use vary from patient to patient. A stroke patient may be discharged to an IRF and then transferred to an SNF as their rehabilitation needs decline, or they may go home from the IRF, utilizing either home health services or outpatient services.

Primary Rehabilitation Settings and Factors Influencing Use

The primary rehabilitation setting has been studied most thoroughly in the Medicare population; however, a recent study within a large teaching hospital of 1,012 patients examined patients of all ages presenting with ischemic stroke (8). Fifty-eight percent (58%) were discharged home, 10% were discharged home with home care services, 15% were discharged to a rehabilitation hospital, 11% were discharged to a skilled or intermediate care facility, and 6% died. In older patients, around two-thirds of stroke patients alive at discharge go on to a rehabilitation provider, excluding outpatient care. Nearly one-half of these enter an inpatient setting, IRF, SNF, or LTAC (8).

Patient Characteristics. Multiple studies have noted that SNF patients tend to be older, on average, than patients in other rehabilitation settings (9–12). The age relationship can be seen in Figure 37-1A–D, which breaks down the initial discharge destination for stroke patients from the 2003 Nationwide Inpatient Sample (NIS) data set from the Agency for Healthcare Research and Quality (AHRQ) (13). This data set includes over 8 million discharges nationwide. Discharge to IRF gets less common as the age group increases, while discharge to SNF increases as age group increases.

Kramer and colleagues (1997) found a number of overall differences between stroke patients treated in IRFs and in SNFs. On average, IRF patients were more functionally independent upon admission, had better cognitive function, and were more likely to have an able and willing caregiver than SNF patients (12). Stroke patients who had no caregivers and lower cognitive function were found only in SNFs, whereas stroke patients who had caregivers and higher cognitive function were prevalent in both settings, although moreso in IRFs. Stroke patients in IRFs were more likely to participate in social and recreational activities than patients in SNFs.

Other research comparing only IRF and SNF patients found similar differences between SNF and IRF stroke patients (10). SNF patients were more likely to have lived alone prior to stroke, have a longer period of time between stroke onset and rehabilitation admission, and have lower FIM (functional independence measure) motor scores upon admission. FIM cognition scores were also lower for SNF patients.

Not only are SNF patients likely to be less functionally independent upon admission than IRF, HHA, or outpatient admissions, they are also likely to have been less functionally independent prior to their stroke. Recent data suggest that SNF patients had worse premorbid function in ambulation, activities of daily living (ADLs), instrumental activities of daily living (IADLs), and social role function than IRF patients, as well as worse premorbid function in ADLs and IADLs than HHA patients (14).

HHA patients tended to have shorter acute hospital lengths of stay, suggesting lower severity of the acute stroke and related conditions, and the shortest total rehabilitation stays relative to either of the other provider types. Other conditions that may determine rehabilitation setting include findings that patients with a history of Alzheimer's disease were more likely to use SNFs than HHAs, and that patients with emphysema were more likely to use HHAs than SNFs (15).

Geographic Variation and Bed Availability. Geographic variation includes variation in the use of any rehabilitation services, and in the distribution of primary rehabilitation settings. The supply of one setting relative to another setting and the distance from the patient to each type of care influence which setting is chosen. One study found the use of any rehabilitation services (IRF, SNF, or HHA care) among Medicare stroke patients varied from 82.1% in the state of Washington to 59.1% in the state of Oklahoma in 1997 (11). The distribution of the use of any inpatient rehabilitation also varies widely across states. Recent Medicare data showed inpatient rehabilitation use ranged from highs of 57% in Massachusetts and 56% in Connecticut, to lows of 34%, 39%, and 39% in Alaska, Mississippi, and Maryland, respectively. States that have high IRF usage tended to have low SNF usage. Conversely, only some states with low IRF usage tended to have high SNF usage. This leads to broad differences in the ratio of IRF to all inpatient care received across states, from a low of 22% in Connecticut to a high of 59% in Nevada (8).

Other work has noted differences in census regions in the use of IRF and HHAs: the West South Central states are high IRF users, and both East and West South Central states are high HHA users (16). Research by Neu, Harrison, and Heilbrunn explored utilization rates across different health service market areas to determine whether market areas with unusually high utilization

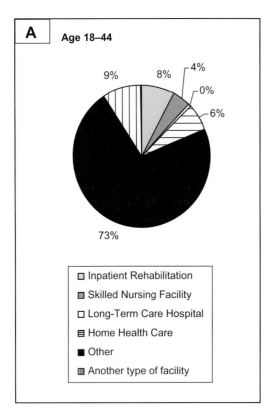

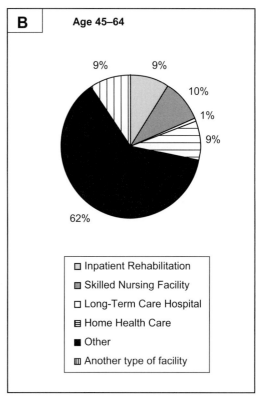

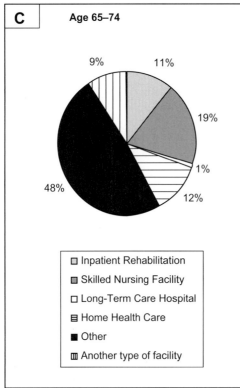

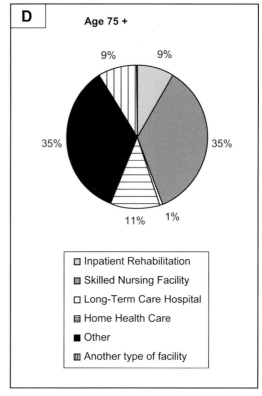

FIGURE 37-1

Primary rehabilitation setting by age group.

of one type of rehabilitation setting demonstrate relatively low utilization of other types of rehabilitation settings (17). These authors found some evidence for substitution between SNF and HHA care. Similarly, Lee, Huber, and Stason found wide geographic variation in the use of different rehabilitation settings for stroke rehabilitation, indicating substantial variation in treatment practices and substitution between different rehabilitation settings across different geographic regions (18).

Other work has looked more directly at the relationship between availability and use. One study found that use of SNF care increased as SNF bed availability increased (19). Due to the number of SNFs compared to the number of IRFs, the average distance to the nearest SNF is much smaller than the average distance to the nearest IRF. The distance to the nearest IRF has an inverse relationship to the likelihood of primary rehabilitation in an IRF, and the distance to the nearest SNF has an inverse relationship to the likelihood of primary rehabilitation in SNF. Further, the number of IRFs in the patient's locality is positively related to the likelihood of discharge to IRF and negatively related to the likelihood of SNF use. Similar findings for the number of SNFs were reported. The same study included the presence of distinct-part units in the discharging acute hospitals. Over 50% of stroke patients received care in an acute hospital with a SNF distinct-part unit, and nearly 38% received care in one with an IRF distinct-part unit. Having an IRF distinct-part unit greatly increased the likelihood of discharge to IRF, while decreasing the likelihood of discharge to SNF. Having a SNF distinct-part unit had the inverse effects on these likelihoods (9).

Payer and Payment Design.   Payer and payment design also influences discharge destination. Studies have noted that HMOs are much less likely to discharge stroke patients to IRFs (20). Payment design in post-acute care has undergone radical changes over the last decade. Medicare has switched from cost-based payment to separate prospective payment systems for each of the major rehabilitation settings. These systems differ both in the overall organization of payment units, and in the financial incentives for treating certain kinds of patients. IRFs and LTACs are paid on a per episode basis, regardless of length of stay. SNFs are paid on a per diem basis with an upper limit on the number of days of care (100 days). HHA care is paid on an episode basis where the episode is a 60-day time period, but the number of visits can vary.

The patient payment burden for care also varies. Using Medicare as an example, patients discharged to IRFs and LTACs pay no additional deductible, but the IRF days count against their hospital day limits per illness. Beneficiaries do not have any copayment for home health services, either. They do, however, have a 20% coinsurance payment for SNF care. Additionally, outpatient therapy requires a 20% coinsurance payment from patients, and outpatient care is also subject to an illness cap, currently set at $1,740. While the effect of out-of-pocket payments on rehabilitation setting choice is relatively unstudied, one study found that patients with a second source of health insurance (Medicaid or supplemental insurance) were more likely to use SNFs than HHAs (19). Payer differences in primary rehabilitation setting can be found in the NIS distribution for stroke patients aged 15 and older.

As shown in Figure 37-2, privately insured patients are nearly equally likely to go to SNF or IRF (10% and 9%, respectively). Medicare and Medicaid patients are far more likely to go to SNF than to an IRF. While the Medicare distribution is driven, at least in part, by age disparities with privately insured individuals, the Medicaid distribution is less so.

Other Sources of Variation.   One study found the discharge destination of stroke patients was related to the specialty of the attending physician. Neurologists were more likely to discharge patients to IRFs (21.9%), as compared to internists (16.0%) or family practice physicians (13.0%). Neurologists were less likely to discharge patients to a SNF or nursing home (22.2%) compared to internists (33.1%) or family practice physicians (39.6%) (21).

Much of the distribution of stroke patients across rehabilitation settings remains unexplained. One study found that one-half to two-thirds of practice variation in the utilization of rehabilitation services could not be explained by the differences in patient characteristics and market conditions (18). Of six diagnoses that commonly use post-acute care, stroke had the lowest percentage of patients correctly classified (52%) by using patient and market characteristics (22).

Multiple-Provider Rehabilitation Episodes.   Stroke patients commonly use multiple care settings for rehabilitation following the acute hospitalization. Patients with stroke are more likely than other common rehabilitation diagnoses to use two or more rehabilitation services (15). At 60 days, 22% of Medicare patients will have used a combination of rehabilitation setting when these settings were limited to IRF, SNF, and HHAs (11). A more recent study (14) found that nearly 90% of a sample of IRF patients continued to use at least one additional rehabilitation setting (SNF, HHA, and/or outpatient) within 90 days following a primary rehabilitation admission. Almost 40% of IRF patients also used outpatient services within 90 days, 49% used home health services, and 21% used SNF services. The majority of stroke patients (over 62%) admitted to SNF as

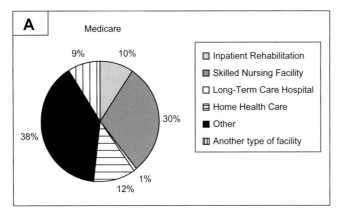

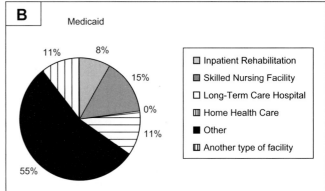

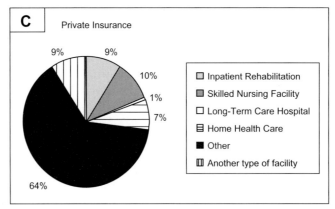

FIGURE 37-2

Primary rehabilitation setting by primary payer.

primary rehabilitation location also used a subsequent rehabilitation provider.

Changing Utilization Patterns

A recent study by Direct Research LLC, which compared episodes of rehabilitation use in 1996 (prior to implementation of any prospective payment system (PPS)) and 2001 (after PPS implementation in SNFs and HHAs) across medical conditions, found that the number of episodes involving only HHAs decreased by 46%; whereas episodes involving only SNF care increased by 28%, and those involving care by LTACs, IRFs, or psychiatric hospitals increased by 33% (7). Episodes consisting of SNF care followed by HHA care decreased by 13%, and those involving other combinations of providers increased by 17% (7).

Another study by McCall, et al. examined patterns of rehabilitation utilization for Medicare beneficiaries with stroke, COPD, heart failure, hip fracture, and diabetes during the period when the HHA PPS was in effect and the SNF PPS was being instituted (23). They found substantial changes in patterns of rehabilitation, with use of IRFs increasing and use of HHA services falling, as both an initial rehabilitation setting and a subsequent setting following initial treatment in an institutional setting.

Earlier research by Liu, et al. in 1999 revealed that prior to implementation of PPS, 51% of post-acute patients used HHA care only, 26% used SNF care only, 4% used IRF care only, and 19% used more than one rehabilitation setting (24).

A study looking at the trend in primary discharge destination for inpatient rehabilitation from 1998 to 2004 revealed change in the distribution of stroke discharges. The overall percentage of stroke patients receiving inpatient rehabilitation remained fairly steady across the time period, at close to 50%. The distribution of destinations changed over time as IRF and LTAC use increased while SNF use decreased. The drop in SNF use and increase in IRF use appeared more dramatic in 2004. Although LTAC discharges remained a small percentage of inpatient care over time, they increased by nearly 90% (from 0.82% to 1.53%). This study also examined the trend of using SNF after an initial discharge to IRF over this time period. While the use of this combination did increase over the time period, it appeared to be associated with the overall increase in IRF use. Between 1998 and 2004, the percentage of Medicare patients discharged to an IRF that also used a SNF within 90 days of hospital discharge fluctuated around 25%. In another sample, 30% of IRF stroke patients used three or more rehabilitation providers in the 90 days following rehabilitation admission (14).

COSTS OF REHABILITATION BY SETTING

The cost of stroke rehabilitation varies widely by setting. Several studies over the past decade have compared the Medicare cost of rehabilitation for stroke across settings, including both the primary setting and the full episode of rehabilitation. In the first six weeks following stroke, the total Medicare cost for patients admitted to an IRF as the primary setting was found to be about $17,000, in contrast to about $6,000 for a patient admitted to SNF, and $4,000 for a patient admitted to HHA in the late 1990s (25). However, most of the higher cost for patients admitted first to IRF occurred in the first six weeks. That is, while the total rehabilitation cost remained larger for IRF patients over six and twelve months, the cost gap between patients discharged to IRF and those discharged to SNF was reduced as the time frame lengthened. At one year, total Medicare costs in the late 1990s were about $26,000 for patients admitted to IRFs, $24,000 for patients admitted to SNFs, and $13,000 for patients admitted to HHAs.

In a more recent study in 2003 to 2005, Kramer, et al found that in the first 90 days of rehabilitation, Medicare rehabilitation costs were $26,000, $14,500, and $3,000, respectively, for patients discharged to IRF, SNF and HHA. However, total Medicare costs in the first 90 days were substantially higher ($32,000, $23,000, and $6,000) respectively. Outpatient therapy is a lower cost alternative, with Medicare outpatient spending on stroke patients averaging about $1,700 per patient (7, 26).

LTACs are even more expensive than IRFs. For patients with the next to lowest severity score, the average total LTAC payment in 2001 for stroke patients was $31,164, compared to $15,191 for patients who used other forms of rehabilitation care. Even in the highest severity patients, the cost difference was significant: $36,053 in LTACs, in contrast to $21,161 for other types of rehabilitation (7).

OUTCOMES OF REHABILITATION BY SETTING

Multiple studies have attempted to compare outcomes of rehabilitation across settings. No randomized trials exist, so these are all quasi-experimental designs that attempt to control for case mix differences across settings. Representing stroke patients from 17 states and up to 92 IRFs and SNFs, Kramer (1997) found IRFs to produce better outcomes than SNFs in three areas: recovery scores

in five ADLs, overall functional losses from pre-stroke levels, and discharge to community (12). Recovery scores were dichotomies representing the return to a pre-morbid state. Overall functional losses were the sum of all ADLs in which the patient did not return to their pre-morbid level, and ranged from a score of zero to five. Assessment of recovery was made at six months after admission to the rehabilitation setting.

Case-mix adjustments were made using two separate methods: propensity scores and multivariate regression. After adjustment for case mix using multiple regression, the difference in the number of ADLs recovered was significantly better in IRFs as compared to SNFs. Propensity scores mirrored these findings; SNF stroke patients in every strata had significantly more ADL difficulties than IRF stroke patients at six months.

This study also separated SNFs into subacute and traditional SNFs, where subacute SNFs were identified as nursing homes with high volumes of Medicare skilled nursing patients, as opposed to traditional nursing homes that had a larger ratio of custodial care patients. While no significant differences were found between the two types of SNFs in functional recovery, subacute SNFs did a better job returning patients to the community at six months than traditional SNFs.

Another study of recovery included stroke patients discharged home with home health care and those discharged home without formal care (although they could have received outpatient therapy) (27). The study utilized patients in three cities from multiple providers. Functional recovery was defined as an improvement in a dependency score that combined ADLs together. Other outcomes included residence in a nursing home, rehospitalization, and mortality. Each was measured at six weeks, six months, and one year. Case mix adjustment was made using instrumental variables.

Among stroke patients, those discharged to a nursing home had consistently significantly higher adjusted mortality rates and were significantly more likely to be in a nursing home at each follow-up point. Adjusted rehospitalization rates were similar among settings until the one year end point, at which time IRF patients and patients that went home without formal care were most likely to be rehospitalized, while those who went home with HHA care were the least likely to be rehospitalized. At six weeks, stroke patients discharged to IRFs showed statistically significantly higher functional recovery than those discharged to SNF or home without formal care. Stroke patients discharged to HHAs also had significantly greater functional recovery than those discharged to SNF or home without formal care. The difference between IRF and HHA care was not significant. At six months and one year, home with HHA care had significantly greater improvement in dependency scores than all other modalities.

More recent data supports the earlier outcome relationship between IRF and SNF care. Categorizing patients by motor disabilities and cognitive ratings, Deutsch (2006) compared IRF and SNF patients, using all Medicare beneficiaries in 1996 and 1997 that had reported FIM scores in the Uniform Data System for Medical Rehabilitation (10). This sample included approximately 60% of IRFs, but only about 11% of SNFs; the SNFs included are likely to be more specialized in rehabilitation than other SNFs. However, this sample mirrored earlier findings. Patients treated in IRFs had better outcomes than SNF patients, in most of the subcategories of disability and cognition. IRFs did not result in a higher FIM motor rating at discharge for patients with minimal motor disabilities or for patients with mild motor disabilities and significant cognitive disabilities. These two categories of patients also failed to achieve higher rate of community discharge from IRF compared to SNF. IRFs also did not increase the likelihood of discharge to the community for older patients with severe motor disabilities.

The most recent data looked at stroke patients in the era after Medicare instituted payment reforms in the form of prospective payment systems for all rehabilitation settings (28). This study found very little substitution or overlap between SNF, IRF, and HHA patients, and thus the authors did not believe comparisons between these primary settings were warranted. However, the study also looked at the next step for IRF patients. Out of 522 IRF patients, 419 received further rehabilitation care in SNF, HHA, or outpatient facilities. Overall, relative to direct discharges to SNF, discharges to IRF followed by SNF care (a subgroup of the IRF group with similar characteristics) had apparently comparable outcomes. Relative to patients admitted to outpatient therapy from IRFs, patients receiving HHA following their IRF stay had greater functional losses and lower rates of recovery in ADLs, IADLS, and ambulation. Not only does the IRF-outpatient therapy option appear to lead to enhanced outcomes, but costs were significantly lower during the rehabilitation episode and over 90 days.

One study attempted to quantify the cost-outcome relationship between rehabilitation settings. With an instrumental variables specification to account for the differences in patient characteristics related to setting choice, Chen (2000) modeled both cost and outcomes in five conditions, including stroke (25). The models were fitted to a Medicare patient sample from 51 hospitals in three cities (Minneapolis-Saint Paul, Pittsburgh, and Houston), and coefficients from the second stages allowed selection-adjusted functional outcomes and costs to be calculated for each patient from the four rehabilitation settings: IRF, SNF, HHA, and home without formal rehabilitation.

Rehabilitation setting could then be compared using a cost-effectiveness ratio. If a more expensive setting produced higher functional outcomes, the cost difference with the next most expensive setting could be divided by the additional outcome improvement for a cost-effectiveness ratio. Any rehabilitation setting associated with higher cost and lower functional improvement is an inferior alternative. The cost-effectiveness ratio for the average percentage of ADL improvement in patients treated within that setting was calculated. SNFs were found to be an inferior option for stroke patients as compared to all other settings. Discharge home with home care was found to have greater functional improvement with no or little cost difference as compared discharge home without formal rehabilitation care (outpatient care would not be formal care). Relative to SNFs, IRF patients experienced a $460 incremental cost in total rehabilitation costs for a 1% improvement in ADL score at six months post-discharge. This was nearly one-fifth of the incremental cost for hip fracture patients, suggesting that stroke patients had more benefit for the additional cost than hip fracture patients. The incremental cost of IRF care (total rehabilitation costs) for stroke patients as compared to home without formal rehabilitation was $14,906 at one year.

The available literature, although limited, suggests that IRFs provide better outcomes than SNFs in post-stroke rehabilitation, at least for patients with functional disabilities but not significant cognitive disabilities. Home health services may be more cost effective for rehabilitation goals, if patients are ready and capable of discharge home. In the next section we delve into the decision-making process for selecting the best rehabilitation alternative for stroke patients.

SELECTING A REHABILITATION SETTING

The decision about the appropriate rehabilitation setting requires two steps. First, the clinicians, patient, and family must decide whether to use inpatient rehabilitation care or to provide rehabilitation in the home. Second, if further inpatient care is indicated, the most appropriate inpatient setting for which the patient is eligible must be determined. If the patient is to return to the community, eligibility for home health care or appropriateness of outpatient rehabilitation services must be determined.

Published clinical guidelines for stroke treatment suggest that the decision for or against inpatient rehabilitation should be made after a comprehensive assessment for rehabilitation services, including the nature and extent of rehabilitation services needed, medical stability, the functional status of the patient, and his or her social supports. Further information is necessary for the decision among inpatient settings.

Patients that would benefit most from inpatient rehabilitation services include both those requiring 24-hour nursing services, and those whose functional deficits would most benefit from intensive daily rehabilitation services. Some selected reasons for continued inpatient rehabilitation include

- the need for continuous observation and treatment of medical conditions
- the inability of the patient and/or caregiver to adequately care for the patient at home
- disabilities that would benefit from intensive, daily therapy services
- the presence of unstable complex medical conditions
- the need for multidisciplinary rehabilitation routinely updated and adapted

Once the decision to use inpatient rehabilitation has been made, a choice must be made among the inpatient options. The three inpatient rehabilitation settings vary with respect to the intensity of physician and skilled nurse monitoring/observation available, the intensity of therapy services required, the staff expertise and experience in rehabilitation, and the availability of technology and equipment.

IRFs provide a comprehensive rehabilitation program that is physician directed and a range of ability to clinically monitor co-existing conditions or perform medical interventions. Advantages to a patient who is capable of sustaining an intensive rehabilitation schedule include the design of a goal-directed treatment plan that is aggressive and responsive to change in the patient status in a timely manner. IRF care is delivered by a highly trained, experienced, and licensed team of specialists in rehabilitation. Patients that are suitable for IRF care include

- those who can tolerate at least three hours of therapy a day
- patients needing multidisciplinary rehabilitation such as motor, speech, and occupational therapy
- patients capable of learning
- patients who are able to follow instructions with either verbal or non-verbal communication
- patients with moderate levels of disability
- medically stable patients with co-existing conditions that benefit from monitoring

Selecting SNF as the discharge location should be based on a need for inpatient care, need for personal care services, and the patient's inability to tolerate very intense rehabilitation. It may be designed as a short stay—just until the patient has recovered enough strength to endure an active three-hour-a-day program, at which time admission to IRF would occur. SNFs are the best setting for patients with functional impairments, and cognitive impairments that limit either learning or comprehension. Finally, patients who need only limited rehabilitation,

but are unable to care for themselves at home and are without a caregiver at home, may benefit most from a SNF stay. Patient characteristics suggesting a SNF stay are therefore

- cognitive disability related to comprehension
- cognitive disability related to learning
- lack of caregiver/ inability to care for self
- co-existing conditions that need skilled nursing care
- rehabilitation needs that can be met in one to two hours per day

Indications that an LTAC may be the best setting for the stroke patient are medical co-morbidities or complications of the primary stroke. Some selected medical conditions that suggest the consideration of an LTAC include multiple co-morbidities such as

- unstable diabetes
- renal failure with dialysis
- respiratory insufficiency requiring respiratory therapy
- infectious disease monitoring and management
- a need for blood or blood products

LTACs may be the best place for medically unstable patients who require a high degree of monitoring, including frequent laboratory tests and/or repeated nursing observation, or interventions around the clock.

If it is instead decided that the patient is to be discharged to the community, the use of home health services versus outpatient rehabilitation services must be considered. Home health care may be appropriate if the patient is homebound (i.e., has difficulty leaving the home), or if the person requires personal care services in the home or even regular transportation to and from outpatient facilities. The patient may be more likely to adhere to treatment regimens in the home, and the copayment is less than for outpatient therapy. Patients that are suitable for HHA care include patients

- with difficulty leaving their home or finding regular transportation
- who require intermittent skilled nursing services (less than daily) for medical monitoring
- who do not require physician-directed rehabilitation services
- who are unlikely to be compliant with outpatient visits
- who need some outside assistance with bathing, meal preparation, or medication management

Ultimately, the choice may come down to the criteria for insurance coverage. Home health care usually requires that the patient meet 'homebound' criteria.

These criteria force the patient to leave home only for limited periods that are infrequent, of short duration, or in order to receive medical treatment. Leaving home must require a considerable and taxing effort, some examples of which may be shown by the need of personal assistance or the help of a wheelchair or crutches to leave the house.

Patient and caregiver preferences should be taken into account. Even though a caregiver may be available, he or she may be unable or unwilling to provide transportation services or in-home support services. For patients that have mobility and adequate social supports, outpatient services are preferable. Outpatient facilities give patients access to equipment and services not available in home care. Rehabilitation services in an outpatient setting can vary from physician-directed team care to individual therapist visits. Indications for outpatient therapy include

- ability to travel to an outpatient clinic at least daily
- need for multiple therapy disciplines
- complex rehabilitation needs requiring oversight of a physiatrist
- if Medicare, ability to afford copayment

A comprehensive rehabilitation plan frequently starts with some type of inpatient rehabilitation followed by a step down to a home or outpatient setting.

CONCLUSION

Settings for rehabilitation following hospitalization for stroke can vary, and the same setting is not appropriate for all patients. Rehabilitation settings differ in terms of the types of patients they are most equipped to serve. Setting utilization is also dependent upon availability of the different options and payment design. Evidence exists of differences in outcomes and costs across rehabilitation options. Indications for the most appropriate initial rehabilitation setting can be derived from all of this information. In some cases, a stroke patient's recovery may be further aided by using a combination of settings, often moving from a setting that provides more intensive rehabilitation and support to one that provides less. Familiarity with the patient's resources, clinical status, functional status, and the services offered at each level aid the clinician in selecting the most appropriate setting at any point in a patient's recovery.

References

1. Medicare Payment Advisory Commission. Health care spending and the Medicare program: A data book. Section 9: Post-acute care. Washington, D.C.: MedPAC, 2006.
2. Donelan-McCall N, Eilertsen T, Fish R, Kramer A. Small patient populations and low frequency event effects on the stability of SNF quality measures. University of Colorado, 2006. www.medpac.gov/publications/contractor_reports/Sep06_SNF_CONTRACTOR.pdf. 2006.
3. Kramer A, Min S, Goodrich G, Fish R. Trends between 2000 and 2005 in SNF rates of community discharge and rehospitalization. University of Colorado, 2008. Available March 2008 at www.medpac.gov.
4. Liu K, Baseggio C, Wissoker D, Maxwell S, et al. Long-term care hospitals under Medicare: Facility-level characteristics. Health Care Fin Rev 2001; 23(2):1–18.
5. Medicare Payment Advisory Commission. Report to the Congress: Medicare payment policy. Chapter 4: Long-term care hospital services: Assessing payment adequacy and updating payments. Washington, D.C.: MedPAC, 2006:205–221.
6. Medicare Payment Advisory Commission. Report to the Congress: New Approaches in Medical Care. Chapter 5: Monitoring post-acute care. Washington, D.C.: MedPAC, 2004: 119–135.
7. Medicare Payment Advisory Commission. Report to Congress: Variation and innovation in Medicare. Chapter 5: Monitoring post-acute care. Washington, D.C: MedPAC, 2003:69–88.
8. Epstein A, Kramer A. Trends in inpatient post-acute care for stroke. In: Kramer A, Holthaus D, eds. Study of Stroke Post-Acute Care and Outcomes: Final Report. Aurora, CO: Division of Health Care Policy and Research, University of Colorado at Denver and Health Sciences Center, 2006:99–114.
9. Beeuwkes Buntin M, Garten AD, Paddock S, et al. How Much Is Post-Acute Care Use Affected by Its Availability? Santa Monica, CA: RAND Health, 2004.
10. Deutsch A, Granger CV, Heinemann AW, et al. Poststroke rehabilitation: Outcomes and reimbursement of inpatient rehabilitation facilities and subacute rehabilitation programs. Stroke 2006; 37:1477–1482.
11. Kane RL, Wen-Chieh L, Blewett LA. Geographic variation in the use of post-acute care. Health Serv Res 2002; 37(3):667–682.
12. Kramer AM, Steiner JF, Schlenker RE, et al. Outcomes and costs after hip fracture and stroke: A comparison of rehabilitation settings. JAMA 1997; 277(5):396–404.
13. HCUP NIS Database Documentation. Healthcare Cost and Utilization Project (HCUP). http://www.ahrq.gov/data/hcup. 2007.

14. Kramer AM, Goodrich G, Holthaus D, Epstein A. Patterns of post-acute care following implementation of PPS. In: Kramer A, Holthaus D, eds. Study of Stroke Post-Acute Care and Outcomes: Final Report. Aurora, CO: Division of Health Care Policy and Research, University of Colorado at Denver and Health Sciences Center, 2006: 58–80.
15. Liu K, Gage B, Harvell J, et al. "Medicare's Post-Acute Care Benefit: Background, Trends, and Issues to Be Faced." 1999 Urban Institute. U.S. Department of Health and Human Services, Office of the Assistant Secretary for Planning and Evaluation, January 1999.
16. Gage B. Impact of the BBA on post-acute utilization. Health Care Fin Rev 1999; 20(4):103.
17. Neu CR, Harrison SC, Heilbrunn JZ. Medicare patients and postacute care: Who goes where? Santa Monica, CA: The RAND Corporation, 1989.
18. Lee AJ, Huber JH, Stason WB. Factors contributing to practice variation in post-stroke rehabilitation. Health Serv Res 1997; 32(2):197–221.
19. Liu K, Wissoker D, Rimes C. Determinants and costs of Medicare post-acute care provided by SNFs and HHAs. Inquiry 1998; 35:49–61.
20. Smith MA, Frytak J, Liou JI, Finch MD. Rehospitalization and survival for stroke patients in managed care and traditional Medicare plans. Med Care 2005; 43(9):902–910.
21. Mitchell JB, Ballard DJ, Whisnant JP, et al. What role do neurologists play in determining the costs and outcomes of stroke patients? Stroke 1996; 27:1937–1943.
22. Kane RL, Finch M, Blewett LA. Use of post-hospital care by Medicare patients. J Am Geriatr Soc 1996; 44(3):242–250.
23. McCall N, Korb J, Petersons A, Moore S. Reforming Medicare payment: Early effects of the 1997 balanced budget act on postacute care. Milbank Q 2003; 81(2):277–303.
24. Liu K, Gage B, Harvell J, et al. Medicare's post-acute care benefit: Background, trends, and issues to be faced. For contract 3# HHS-100-97-0010. 1999. The Urban Institute.
25. Chen Q, Kane RL, Finch MD. The cost-effectiveness of post-acute care for elderly Medicare beneficiaries. Inquiry 2000; 37:359–375.
26. Ciolek DE, Hwang D. Utilization Analysis: Characteristics of High Expenditures of Outpatient Therapy Services, CY 2002 Final Report. Columbia, MD: AdvanceMed, 2004.
27. Kane RL, Chen Q, Finch M, et al. Functional outcomes of posthospital care for stroke and hip fracture patients under Medicare. J Am Geriatr Soc 1998; 46:1525–1533.
28. Holthaus D, Kramer A. Post-acute care policy issues. In: Kramer A, Holthaus D, eds. Study of Stroke Post-Acute Care and Outcomes: Final Report. Aurora, CO: Division of Health Care Policy and Research, University of Colorado at Denver and Health Sciences Center, 2006:8–21.

38 Rehabilitation of Children After Stroke

Donna L. Nimec
Robin M. Jones
Eric F. Grabowski

The last ten years have brought about a growing appreciation of the incidence, prevalence, and rehabilitation needs of childhood stroke survivors. Historically, the incidence of stroke in the pediatric population was thought to be two to three per 100,000 children (1–5). More recently, studies indicate that this number is low and more accurate data is now being collected, with some studies identifying more than double this number (3, 6, 7). As noninvasive imaging techniques have improved, diagnoses are being made earlier (8–11). There is also significant mortality associated with stroke in the pediatric population. Six to ten percent of children who have a stroke will die (12–14). Hence, stroke is now a more recognized cause of chronic morbidity and mortality in children that interferes with the development of gross motor, fine motor, communication, and psychosocial skills. As a result, services need to be provided over an extended period of time to address the deficits caused by stroke in this young population.

In pediatrics, there are different classifications of stroke, depending upon when the event occurs. *Perinatal stroke* is defined as a cerebrovascular event that occurs between 28 weeks of gestation and 28 days of postnatal age. *Childhood stroke* is defined as a cerebrovascular event that occurs between 29 days and 18 years of age. This chapter reviews etiology, diagnostic techniques, and acute management for all classifications of stroke in children, though the primary focus will be on the post acute rehabilitation program.

Stroke recovery and rehabilitation in the perinatal/childhood population differ from recovery and rehabilitation in the adult population due to ongoing maturation of the central nervous system (CNS). While the CNS lesion from the stroke is not progressive, the associated neurophysiologic symptoms may affect growth and development. Residual neurologic dysfunction is seen in more than 50% of pediatric stroke survivors.

For example, cognitive development describes an ongoing learning process for children as they acquire information and build on new experiences. Neurologic injury can interfere with this process from many perspectives, including auditory processing, visual perceptual skills, and motor coordination. It is important for families to understand and have information regarding potential problems, depending on the site and extent of the injury. While a number of studies in adults demonstrate that the most significant recovery occurs during the first three months after stroke, there is no such data available in the pediatric population (15, 16).

Once the stroke has been diagnosed and the child is stable in the acute hospital setting, a decision must be made about moving forward with rehabilitation. A family centered care approach is essential. For infants and children who have sustained a stroke, using a pediatric rehabilitation framework model may enable families to better embrace the multidisciplinary approach to the recovery process. The framework encourages planning for needs beyond medical and direct therapy services, and encourages consideration of how the child and family are coping with community reintegration and involvement in activities outside the home.

INCIDENCE, PREVALENCE, AND ETIOLOGY

Statistics from the National Institute of Neurologic Disorders and Stroke (NINDS) show that newborn strokes occur at a rate of one in 4,000 births (14). The stroke rate in newborns is similar to that of individuals 75 years of age and older. There are age-related differences in susceptibility of the mature brain to oxidative stress and inflammation, as well as in the rate and degree of apoptotic neuronal death (17). Fullerton et al. have determined that while there is a peak in pediatric stroke incidence at the time of birth and in the first year of life, there is a second peak in the teenage years (5).

The Canadian Pediatric Ischemic Stroke Registry has compiled one of the largest cohorts of pediatric patients diagnosed with arterial ischemic stroke and sinovenous thrombosis. This registry collects data from all 16 children's hospitals in Canada as part of a national collaborative study. The results have provided the first population-based data on incidence, risk factors, treatment, and outcomes (13). This is part of the International Pediatric Stroke Study (IPSS) group that has enrolled more than 1,500 children with stroke in 31 countries (18).

Three types of stroke are described in the pediatric age group. About one in 3,000–4,000 pediatric strokes result from blood clots that cause arterial ischemic strokes (AIS). The incidence of hemorrhagic stroke is similar if you include perinatal stroke. Sinovenous thrombosis is less common and occurs more frequently in infants. In adults, arterial ischemic strokes are four times more common than hemorrhagic strokes.

Arterial Ischemic Stroke

In the Canadian Ischemic Stroke Registry, the incidence of arterial ischemic stroke (AIS) (Figure 38-1) in newborns has been expressed as 93 per 100,000 live births. In the long term, the effects can be devastating (7). The most common cause of AIS in children is congenital or acquired heart disease, accounting for 30% of strokes (12). This is related to the development of intracardiac thrombi that may embolize to the brain. Most of these children have congenital heart lesions identified well before an infarction occurs. During cardiac surgery, the risk of stroke is higher.

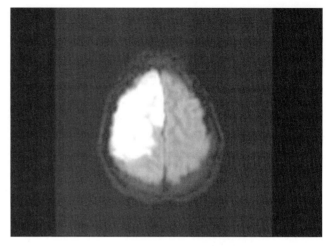

FIGURE 38-1

Large MCA arterial ischemic stroke; diffusion weighted image.

Blood disorders are the second most common cause of AIS in children, with sickle cell disease being the most common hematologic etiology. Children with sickle cell anemia are 200 times more likely to develop a stroke than other children. An estimated 5% of individuals with sickle cell disease have clinical features of cerebrovascular dysfunction. A much larger number are found to have asymptomatic ischemic lesions on imaging studies, up to 15–20% by MR imaging. Other inherited or acquired defects of coagulation are receiving increasing attention, as these defects can shift the balance between coagulation and anticoagulation and lead to thrombosis.

Perinatal AIS is the most common known cause of spastic diplegia and quadriplegia in term and near-term infants (19). The greater deformability of newborn RBCs compensates for the greater Hct. Arterial ischemia occurring during the three days surrounding birth is reported to be responsible for 50 to 70% of congenital hemiplegic cerebral palsy (20). Ischemic strokes during the newborn period are also related to maternal or placental infections that contribute to the prothrombotic state in the fetus and newborn. These infections cause inflammation of the brain's blood vessels and can alter clotting mechanisms in the blood.

Hemorrhagic Stroke

Over one-third of pediatric strokes are hemorrhagic (Figure 38-2) if you include the perinatal population (5). They can be characterized by intraparenchymal hemorrhages and subarachnoid hemorrhages from non-traumatic etiologies. Structural anomalies of the cerebral vasculature also produce intracranial hemorrhage. Strokes that occur during the newborn period are often hemorrhagic in nature, and are associated with premature birth. These hem-

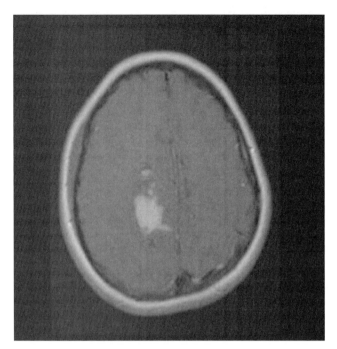

FIGURE 38-2

T1 weighted MRI of a hemorrhagic stroke.

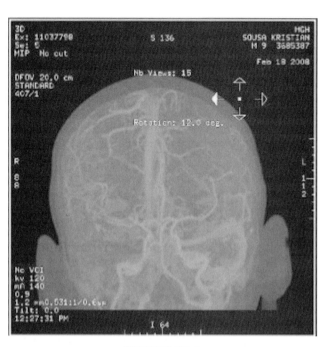

FIGURE 38-3

Computerized Tomographic Angiography (CTA) showing a sinus venous occlusion of the transverse sinus on the right.

orrhages are usually due to the immaturity and fragility of the germinal matrix, with the most common presentation being an intraparenchymal hemorrhage. The lower the birth weight, the greater the risk of an intraventricular hemorrhage.

In the older child, arteriovenous malformations (AVM), intracranial aneurysms, and hematologic disorders are responsible for most intracranial hemorrhages. Mortality is approximately 25% in children, higher than mortality with AIS. Of those who survive, 42% have significant disability (21). Idiopathic thrombocytopenic purpura, hemophilia, and sickle cell disease are known risk factors.

Sinovenous Thrombosis

Venous occlusion was previously difficult to identify, and the reported number of children known to have sinovenous thrombosis (SVT) was underreported. MRI/MRA have now made this easier to diagnose. The factors that contribute to SVT are variable. Many children have more than one risk factor (22). Even with a thorough work-up, the reason for the venous thrombosis cannot always be identified (23).

The clinical features of sinovenous thrombosis (Figure 38-3) are age related and may be subtle. They usually develop gradually over many hours. Neonates and infants constitute half the pediatric patients with cerebral sinovenous thrombosis (9, 12), and usually present with seizures or lethargy (24). Seizures occur in three-fourths of neonates compared to one-half of older infants and chil-

dren. Symptoms at presentation in older children include seizures, fever, and vomiting.

Etiology

The conditions that lead to stroke in adults such as diabetes, high blood pressure, or atherosclerosis are uncommon in children (25, 26). For the pediatric patient, the variety of risk factors is much broader (see Table 38-1) (27). Congenital conditions such as heart disease and blood disorders predispose children to stroke. Infectious disorders and vascular anomalies may be contributing factors. Some children have more than one risk factor present. However, approximately one-half of children presenting with stroke have no previous medical history. The cause of one-third of stroke cases in children remains unknown despite investigation. The difficulty in determining the etiology of a stroke has implications for efforts to prevent recurrence.

In sickle cell disease, cerebral ischemia can develop as a result of multiple factors as well. Multiple microstenoses are induced by vessel wall injury from abnormal red blood cells, and by the adhesion to vascular endothelium in the microcirculation of poorly deformable but "sticky" discocytes. This leads to increased red blood cell residence times and the formation of irreversibly sickled red blood cells and plugging of microvessels.

The possible etiologies for arterial ischemic strokes during the perinatal period are unique and include maternal factors, fetal/neonatal factors, and other miscellaneous

TABLE 38-1
Risk Factors for Pediatric Stroke

CONGENITAL HEART DISEASE
Ventricular septal defect
Atrial septal defect
Patent ductus arteriosus
Aortic stenosis
Mitral stenosis
Coarctation
Cardiac rhabdomyoma
Complex congenital heart defects

ACQUIRED HEART DISEASE
Rheumatic heart disease
Prosthetic heart valve
Libman-Sacks endocarditis
Bacterial endocarditis
Cardiomyopathy
Myocarditis
Atrial myxoma
Arrhythmia

SYSTEMIC VASCULAR DISEASE
Systemic hypertension
Systemic hypotension
Hypernatremia
Superior vena cava syndrome
Diabetes
Vasculitis
Meningitis
Systemic infection
Systemic lupus erythematosus
Polyarteritis nodosa
Granulomatous angiitis
Takayasu's arteritis
Rheumatoid arthritis
Dermatomyositis
Inflammatory bowel disease
Drug abuse (cocaine, amphetamines)
Hemolytic-uremic syndrome

VASCULOPATHIES
Ehlers-Danlos syndrome
Homocystinuria
Moyamoya syndrome
Fabry disease
Malignant atrophic papulosis
Pseudoxanthoma elasticum
NADH-CoQ reductase deficiency
Williams syndrome

VASOSPASTIC DISORDERS
Migraine
Ergot poisoning
Vasospasm & subarachnoid bleed

HEMATOLOGIC DISORDERS/COAGULOPATHIES
Hemoglobinopathies (sickle cell anemia, sickle
    cell-hemoglobin C)
Immune thrombocytopenic purpura
Thrombotic thrombocytopenic purpura
Thrombocytosis
Polycythemia
Disseminated intravascular coagulation
Leukemia or other neoplasm
Congenital coagulation defects
Oral contraceptive use
Pregnancy/postpartum period
Antithrombin III deficiency
Factor V Leiden
Protein S deficiency
Protein C deficiency
Congenital serum C2 deficiency
Liver dysfunction-coagulopathy
Vitamin K–deficiency
Lupus anticoagulant
Anticardiolipin antibodies

STRUCTURAL ANOMALIES
Arterial fibromuscular dysplasia
Agenesis or hypoplasia of the internal carotid or
    vertebral artery
Arteriovenous malformation
Hereditary hemorrhagic telangiectasia
Sturge-Weber syndrome
Intracranial aneurysm

TRAUMA
Child abuse
Fat or air embolism
Foreign body embolism
Carotid ligation (eg, ECMO)
Vertebral occlusion after abrupt cervical rotation
Post-traumatic arterial dissection
Blunt cervical arterial trauma
Arteriography
Carotid cavernous fistula
Coagulation defect with minor trauma
Amniotic fluid/placental embolism
Penetrating intracranial trauma

Reprinted with permission from Elsevier.

factors (28). Figure 38-4 shows the complex, multifactorial relationship of risk factors identified in cases of perinatal AIS. On the maternal side, pregnancy is a naturally prothrombotic state due to various hemostatic factors. In the fetus, thrombotic episodes on the fetal side of the placenta can lead to embolic phenomenon secondary to the patent foramen ovale. Because neonatal blood is denser, dehydration increases the risk of stroke in neonates. Despite these associations, the causal pathways and the nature of their interactions are not well understood.

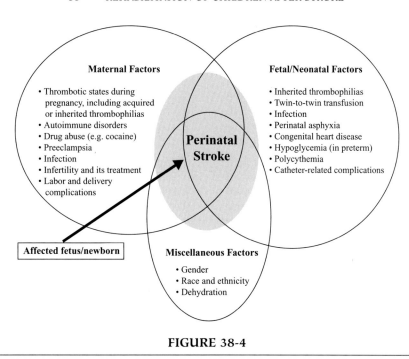

FIGURE 38-4

Conceptualization of risk Factors for perinatal AIS. *(Reprinted with permission from The American Academy of Pediatrics.)*

In older children, thromboembolism is a more frequent cause of ischemia, similar to adult patients, but with a greater input from plasma-phase risk factors.

In the Canadian Registry, the recurrence rate of children with neonatal stroke was 3 to 5%. In survivors, outcome was normal in 33% of cases (6). This is much less than the recurrence rate of childhood stroke (6). Brankovic-Sreckovic followed 36 children over time to evaluate recurrence risk of ischemic stroke in childhood. Results showed that congenital and acquired heart disease was the most common cause of repeated stroke in the study patients.

For hemorrhagic stroke, vascular malformations including arteriovenous malformations, aneurysms, and cavernous malformations are the most common causes. Fewer hemorrhagic strokes remain cryptogenic when compared to ischemic strokes. Leukemia, coagulopathies, and intracranial tumors are important causes of hemorrhagic stroke.

Fullerton et al. evaluated the recurrence risk of hemorrhagic stroke in 16 hospitals in northern California (29). The initial incidence was 1.18 per 100,000 person years. In this study, etiology was 54% structural, 21% trauma related, and 17% idiopathic. Initial events were higher in boys secondary to trauma related etiologies. Recurrence rate was higher in girls during this time period. Recurrence rate over a six year period was 17.4% in structural etiologies.

In sinovenous thrombosis, risk factors are age-related. Dehydration is a risk factor in neonates. In older children, chronic systemic diseases are an underlying risk factor. The mechanism for sinovenous thrombosis in most chronic diseases is an acquired prothrombotic state.

Thrombophilia and AIS. A number of plasma-phase risk factors have been considered in the pathophysiology of AIS. The following section focuses on the current state of knowledge and understanding of the hypercoagulability factors important to consider in evaluating acute AIS in childhood (30). It is important to note that many of these factors are thought to contribute to venous thromboembolism in all age groups.

Factor V Leiden. Factor V Leiden (FVL) is a recently identified mutant factor V that produces the subsequent resistance in the degradation of the factor by activated protein C. It is the most common cause of activated protein C resistance (APC-R). Case reports and case series have demonstrated an association between FVL and ischemic stroke in neonates, children, and young adults (31–33). In contrast, FVL was not found to be a risk factor for pediatric or neonatal stroke in another study (34).

Lipoprotein (a). Elevated lipoprotein a [Lp (a)] has also been identified as a genetically determined risk factor for ischemic stroke in neonates and children (31, 33, 35). In vitro studies show that Lp (a) competes with plasminogen binding sites and may interfere with endogenous endothelial cell-mediated fibrinolysis.

Antithrombin III, Protein C, Protein S, and PAI-1. The role of the hereditary deficiencies of the naturally occurring coagulation inhibitors, specifically antithrombin III (AT), protein C (PC), and protein S (PS), in the development of ischemic pediatric stroke remains debatable. AT inhibits serine esterase activity, and this inhibition accounts for its effects not only on thrombin but also on activated forms of factors XII, XI, IX and X. PC, a glycoprotein, is activated by the thrombomodulin-thrombin complex on the endothelial cell surface, thereby becoming a serine protease with both anticoagulant and profibrinolytic activities. In the presence of protein S, activated protein C degrades the thrombin-activated forms of factors V and VII and neutralizes a circulating inhibitor of tissue-plasminogen activator. Tissue-plasminogen activator, in turn, converts plasminogen into the enzyme plasmin. Case reports and case-control studies (31, 36–38) showed a positive correlation between AT, PS, and PC deficiency and stroke, whereas other studies failed to confirm this correlation (32, 34, 39, 40).

Acquired deficiencies of anti-clotting factors. Neonatal and childhood stroke have also been reported in the context of acquired deficiencies of PC or PS due to the presence of antibodies in patients with sepsis and viral infections such as varicella, and acquired deficiency of ATIII (41). In a study by de Veber et al., acquired deficiencies of PC, PS, and/or AT were present in children following thromboembolic stroke, but their causative role could not be determined (42).

Hyperhomocysteinemia. Classic homocystinuria, a rare inborn error due to cystathionine beta-synthase deficiency, predisposes to cardiovascular and cerebrovascular disease. An association between mild hyperhomocysteinemia and stroke in children has been found (43).

Antiphospholipid antibodies. Antiphospholipid antibodies (APLA) constitute a heterogeneous group of antibodies directed against cell surface phospholipids. The two APLA most commonly tested for are lupus anticoagulant (LA) and anticardiolipin antibodies (ACLA). Kenet et al. reported that anticardiolipin antibody (ACLA) was associated with a six-fold risk of pediatric stroke (32). The presence of ACLA in children has also been reported by de Veber et al. (42). Transplacentally derived maternal APLA (LA, ACLA) are considered a risk factor for neonatal stroke (35, 44).

Compound Heterozygous Conditions. A significant proportion of children have multiple prothrombotic disorders. These children are heterozygous for two of the prothrombotic conditions mentioned above. The combination of thrombophilia markers increases the risk of stroke. There is evidence for interaction between FVL and hyperhomocysteinemia, and FVL and PC deficiency. If one marker is identified, a thorough search for others should be undertaken (32, 45). Furthermore, many studies suggest an interaction

between underlying non-hematologic diseases or conditions (e.g. patent foramen ovale) and prothrombotic risk factors as important triggering mechanisms in the etiology of childhood stroke (32).

In a study looking at deaths from stroke in children in United States between 1979 to 1998, Fullerton et al. (2) found that mortality from childhood stroke declined by 58% overall with reductions in all major subtypes. They analyzed death certificate data for ischemic and hemorrhagic stroke and intracerebral hemorrhage in children under 20 years of age in the United States. Black ethnicity was a risk factor for mortality from all stroke types. Male sex was a risk factor for mortality from SVT and ICH, but not from ischemic stroke. They concluded that African American children were at greater risk of death from all stroke types compared to white children.

DIAGNOSIS

Unless a child has a known predisposing factor for stroke such as congenital heart disease, sickle cell disease, or protein deficiencies in the blood, an immediate diagnosis based on presenting symptoms may be delayed. The differential diagnosis for the presentation of neurologic symptoms is broad (Table 38-2).

Past studies have shown that delay in diagnosis has been problematic (8, 46) (Figure 38-5). In a prospective study covering a 12 month period by Shellhass et al., charts on 143 patients with acute presentations suspicious for cerebrovascular disease were reviewed for mimics of childhood stroke. Results showed that history and clinical presentation often do not distinguish one-third of patients with benign disorders from the two-thirds with more serious conditions (27). Recent advances in the detection of childhood stroke have enabled more timely diagnoses, due in part to the development of noninvasive low risk neuroimaging techniques, especially MRI (10, 47).

TABLE 38-2
Differential Diagnosis of Neurologic Symptoms

Stroke	Cerrebellitis
Seizures	Syncope
Migraine	Metabolic Disorder
Trauma	Hydrocephalus
Abscess	ADEM
Toxin Ingestion	Tumor
Drug Reaction	Psychogenic
Meningitis	

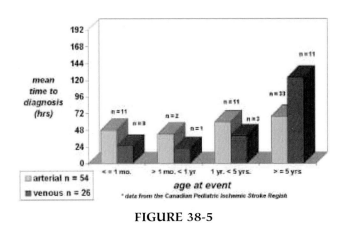

FIGURE 38-5

Effect of age at event on mean diagnosis time* (0–18 years; N = 80) (17).

Braun et al. (9) published the results of a study that reviewed the case histories of 45 children with ischemic stroke. The initial clinical diagnosis, based on the interpretation of presenting symptoms, was compared with the etiologic stroke diagnosis after completion and review of diagnostic workup. The type of diagnostic change, subsequent time delay until correct diagnosis, reasons for change of diagnosis, and alterations to management were evaluated. Out of the 45 children, 25 diagnostic changes were identified. Nineteen changes were in the primary stroke diagnosis. Five were in the etiological diagnosis. The median interval between the initial and final diagnosis was seven days. The change in diagnosis led to therapeutic alterations in 17 patients.

Clinical Presentation and History-Taking

The clinical presentation varies according to age, cause, and location of the stroke, and can therefore be difficult to diagnose (Table 38-3). Neonates often have perinatal events that are silent. A premature infant or newborn has limited gross and fine motor activity. Patterns of movement reflect the presence of primitive reflexes. Problems with movement become more evident when the reflexes either fail to emerge or, if present, do not become integrated at the appropriate time. As more advanced skills fail to develop, functional deficits become more apparent. Imaging may then demonstrate that such hemiparesis is associated with a remote, even in-utero, vascular event.

In ischemic stroke, hemiplegia and headache associated with seizures are the most common presentations (17, 48–50). For children experiencing hemorrhagic stroke, headache and vomiting are often the presenting symptoms. In sinovenousvenous thrombosis, decreased level of consciousness and headache are seen.

Another type of an event that may present as a stroke is a transient ischemic attack (TIAs). A TIA is a

TABLE 38-3
Stroke Type and Presenting Symptoms

STROKE TYPE	PRESENTING SYMPTOMS
Acute Ischemic Stroke	Hemiplegia
	Headache
	Speech Difficulties
	Numbness
	Facial Droop
	Salivary Drool
Hemorrhagic Stroke	Headache
	Vomiting
Sinovenous Thrombosis	Gradual Progression
	Seizures
	Fever
	Vomiting
	Decreased Level of Consciousness

transient neurologic deficit referable to a cerebral arterial territory in which a MRI shows no acute ischemia. However, the child's history and other workup may suggest cerebrovascular disease. With a TIA, the child may show signs of rapid recovery.

Initial screening should include enough history to identify congenital thrombophilic states, as well as risk factors such as cardiac disease, infections, dehydration, trauma and possible dissection, sickle cell anemia, and malignancy. Family history should be recorded for thrombotic events (deep venous thromboses, pulmonary emboli, myocardial infarction, stroke) occurring in the patient or any first-degree relatives under age 55.

Diagnostic Imaging

The purpose of the imaging work-up is to

1) confirm that an acute ischemic event has occurred
2) determine the extent and location of acute cerebral injury
3) determine the patency of major neck and intracranial arteries
4) determine the relative cerebral perfusion

For newborns and infants, the imaging modality is magnetic resonance imaging (MRI), as computerized tomography (CT) can be insensitive to the detection of acute ischemic events in this age group. In older children, CT with computerized tomographic angiography (CTA) may precede MRI if intravascular thrombolysis is being considered. These studies can be obtained more rapidly than MRI in most centers. CTA is very sensitive at detecting intralumenal thrombus, and may be more sensitive at

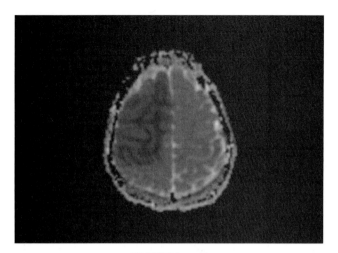

FIGURE 38-6

Large right MCA acute infarction. The diffusion weighted image is bright and the dark ADC confirm acute ischemia and diagnosis of stroke.

detecting vertebral artery dissections than MRI or magnetic resonance arteriogram (MRA) in older children. Otherwise MRI is the modality of choice.

Standard imaging for suspected ischemic events would include CT scan and MRI with diffusion weighted imaging (Figure 38-6). It may also be helpful to obtain vascular imaging, to include an MRA and CTA as indicated to diagnose a dissection. CTA is more sensitive.

MRA will identify vascular pathology (e.g., Moya-Moya disease; multiple stenotic cerebral vessels as in sickle cell anemia; dissections; vascular malformations). Infarction in a non-vascular distribution, however, might suggest the presence of a metabolic defect or a mitochondrial disorder. Hemorrhage might suggest tumor, or trauma in the setting of a bleeding disorder.

Echocardiogram and bubble studies should be considered for all patients. In patients under age 7, transesophageal echocardiograms will increase test sensitivity to detect a patent foramen ovale or other cardiac malformations, allowing for significant right-to-left shunting. This predisposes the child to thrombi reaching the arterial circulation from the heart itself, sites of deep venous thrombosis, or, in a newborn, a diseased placenta. In the latter case, it is reasonable to request, where and when available, the pathology results of the placenta and umbilical cord.

Studies for Thrombophilia

Blood work for thrombophilia should include evaluation for the risk factors cited earlier. Sometimes multiple risk factors can be found, especially in the absence of major underlying illness or other medical conditions.

When family history suggests, and when blood volumes are limited, as in the newborn, studies performed on both parents can be useful and should include anticardiolipin antibodies in the mother, as these can cross the placenta.

TREATMENT AND MANAGEMENT

Clinical management of pediatric stroke varies dependent on the category of stroke and age of the child. Medical stabilization should address adequate oxygenation, rehydration, seizure control, and management of infection. In the case of an evolving and rapidly progressing stroke, consideration should be given to early use of thrombolytic therapy. In the case of sickle cell disease, however, prompt red cell pheresis is indicated. Ongoing management after the initial event involves helping the child and family achieve the greatest level of independence possible.

In the hematologic management, we consider the three most common stroke populations: the newborn, the child with sickle cell disease, and the older child. This section reviews the current state of knowledge and understanding of the hypercoagulability factors important to consider in evaluating acute AIS in childhood, and current recommendations for diagnostic assessment and management of AIS in these populations.

The Newborn

The role of plasma-phase risk factors in the management of newborn stroke is controversial, since more than 90% of newborns suffering stroke appear to do well clinically and have no recurrence. The neurologic examination may be subtle or even non-apparent, despite the occurrence of a major in-utero or perinatal ischemic event. Seizures and lethargy are the most common findings.

In the neonate, sequential brain imaging is paramount to assess stroke progression, especially in the setting of an underlying plasma-phase risk factor. This, combined with prospective outcome studies, demonstrates more clearly the role or non-role of anticoagulant prophylaxis. There is early data on diffusion tensor imaging that can be predictive of outcome in neonatal stroke (51). In the presence of plasma-phase risk factors, the use of anticoagulants or antiplatelet therapy in newborns should be considered only in cases demonstrating clear progression and/or recurrence, and should include consultation with members of the local stroke team.

Sickle Cell Disease

Prothrombotic risk factors are controversial in stroke of sickle cell disease. Although an underlying prothrombotic state has long been acknowledged in this condition, no studies have yet demonstrated a clear role for plasma-phase risk factors in stroke pathogenesis. This is possibly because of the dominant effects of sickle erythrocyte adhesion to microvascular endothelium with subsequent irreversible sickling of later-arriving red blood cells and frank flow obstruction. The standard of care is to use transcranial Doppler to measure the flow velocity of blood. If the rate exceeds 200 cm/sec, there is justification for red cell pheresis (52).

Prevention for recurrent strokes has been most effective in children with sickle cell disease. In 1998, the STOP trial identified that transfusion to HgbS less than 30% was beneficial in sickle cell patients with carotid transcranial Doppler (TCD) velocities greater than 200 cm/sec (47). Population-based data from Fullerton in 2004 noted a significant decrease in the incidence of stroke in California, from 10% to 1%, due to a vigilant transfusion protocol (53). STOP II, published in 2005, identified that discontinuation of transfusion in patients with TCDs less than 200 cm/sec due to increased iron overload was not safe, and resulted in increased incidence of large vessel infarction. Alternatives to managing iron overload were recommended (52). It has been found that ischemic stroke is associated with small asymptomatic subcortical infarcts to large territorial lesions causing major disability. To prevent recurrent or progressive CNS damage, the institution of regular red blood cell transfusions is the standard of care.

Older Children and Adolescents

In older children with AIS but no plasma-phase risk factors, therapy with intravenous standard unfractionated heparin is indicated for three to five days, followed by warfarin for a period of 6 to 12 weeks. In the case of dissection of a vessel, treatment should continue until evidence of healing and restreamlining of the affected vessel is apparent on reimaging. Strokes marked by recurrent symptoms may be an indication for the addition of antiplatelet therapy, usually aspirin.

Children with severe hemiparesis are at risk of deep venous thromboses (DVTs) in the immobilized limb, and may benefit from prophylaxis with subcutaneous (SC) low molecular weight heparin. One simple regimen is to offer 0.5 mg/kg SC enoxaparin bid, or, with somewhat less efficacy, 1.0 mg/kg SC enoxaparin qd. An alternative that is rapidly gaining favor among younger patients is the use of fondaparinux, which offers true once-daily dosing insofar as its half-life is approximately 18 hours, versus 5–6 hours for the low molecular weight heparins. Dosing of this agent for prophylactic intent is 2.5 mg SC qd, or, 0.08 mg/kg SC for children under 45 kilograms.

In the presence of an underlying plasma-phase risk factor, duration of therapy should be extended or even made indefinite and/or until the underlying condition is corrected. For example, hyperhomocysteinemia responds to folate and vitamin B12; lipoprotein (a) can be lowered by oral niacin therapy.

THE COURSE OF REHABILITATION

The impact of pediatric stroke is substantial. Childhood stroke often results in significant impairments, including movement disorders, seizures, speech and language delay, visual impairments, orthopedic deficits, and cognitive and behavioral difficulties. Depending on the extent and the location of the stroke, the presentation of symptoms will vary. The acute rehabilitation program usually begins as soon as the child is stabilized in the acute hospital setting and medical treatment is underway. The earlier therapy is initiated, the greater the opportunity for preventing contractures and maximizing functional gains. There is no guarantee that symptoms or neurologic deficits will completely resolve. However, children can make substantial gains with the proper therapeutic interventions.

The initial assessment is best carried out in a playful, interesting, and non-threatening manner. Observation of the child's quality of movement and interactions should precede hands on examination. Use of familiar toys to initiate interest may help the child's willingness to participate. Sessions should be time limited to enable a child to concentrate on activities without getting fatigued. The assessment can take more than one session to complete, depending on the child's mood, endurance, and ability to cooperate.

After the acute stroke, children can receive rehabilitation services in a hospital-based inpatient setting, an outpatient setting, or at home. Much of this depends upon the severity of medical issues that need to be monitored (i.e. respiratory, nutrition, neurologic, hematologic). Children admitted to an inpatient rehabilitation program often have the most severe motor and cognitive deficits. Therapy can be customized based upon clinical status and endurance. There are other aspects of care that move beyond the purely medical issues, primarily involving the role of the family in all aspects of recovery.

The decision around level of rehabilitation must address both the child's and family's needs. The inpatient setting often provides more support as the family learns to cope with the child's needs to transition into the community. The central principle of family-centered care in pediatric rehabilitation is that the child's family is a constant presence, available to provide comfort and reassurance during times of stress. In the rehabilitation setting, family members need to be involved in the process of their child's recovery, as they are expected to participate in the therapy programs.

A pediatric rehabilitation framework (Table 38-4) can be utilized to help parents understand the multidisciplinary process, and enables a case manager or family member to keep track of progress being made in each area of the child's recovery. After an initial evaluation by the physician, nurses, and therapists on the team, an individualized program is put in place based on the child's areas of strengths and needs. For example, a child with multiple medical problems, such as impaired feeding, respiratory compromise, and seizures, will require more focused medical care and an oral motor program.

Discharge planning includes the goals identified by the family for a safe return home. Outpatient or home services are then scheduled to continue program goals initiated in the inpatient setting. Follow-up should be scheduled with a multidisciplinary stroke team including a physiatrist and neurologist, and when indicated, a hematologist, cardiologist, or metabolic specialist. Children with specific plasma-phase disorders predisposing to thrombosis require longer follow-up for their strokes, given the likely longer period of anticoagulant therapy (except most newborns and all children with sickle cell disease) and more significant risk of recurrence (except newborns). Those with hypercoagulable states will require follow-up also, to ensure proper care for planned and emergency surgery, and for trauma.

In children who have hemiplegia, arm and leg lengths and the alignment of the spine need to be evaluated regularly for development of worsening asymmetry (Figure 38-7). Active and passive ranges of motion at the shoulders, elbows, wrists, fingers, hips, knees, and ankles need to be assessed, as well as the quality of movement. Radiographic studies of the spine and hips may be needed on a yearly basis during periods of rapid growth. The child may require referral to an orthopedic surgeon to discuss the surgical management of these complications. Surgical interventions can take many forms including tendon lengthening/transfer, osteotomy, release of the covering around the muscle followed by serial casting, or epiphydesis. For children with evolving scoliosis, further evaluation and spine stabilization surgery may be needed for rapidly progressive curves beyond 60 degrees.

The role of the physiatrist is to help prioritize goals and make recommendations for treatment strategies with therapists at school that enable the child to gain functional independence. Physiatrists often manage prescriptions for spasticity treatment, orthoses, equipment for school, home adaptations, and therapy outside the school. In addition, the physiatrist maintains contact with school and community therapists to monitor progress and changes in motor and cognitive domains, and communicates essential information to the primary care physician.

Tone management is key as the child is growing. Spasticity and dystonia are common sequelae after an injury to the motor areas of the brain. With the

---

TABLE 38-4
Pediatric Rehabilitation Framework

1. Medical Issues
   a. nutrition
   b. respiratory
   c. neurologic
   d. cardiovascular
   e. orthopaedic
   f. skin
   g. bowel
   h. bladder
   i. social and emotional skill development
   j. sleep
   k. hematologic
   l. vision and hearing

2. Mobility
   a. quality of movement in different positions
   b. equipment needs
   c. home environment/accessibility
   d. community mobility

3. Functional Skills (54)

   Performance Areas
   a. activities of daily living (grooming, hygiene, dressing, feeding, etc.)
   b. work and productive activities (educational and work activities, etc.)
   c. sensorimotor (sensory, neuromusculoskeletal, and motor)
   d. psychosocial and psychologic components (psychological, social, self-management, and self-control)

   Performance Contexts
   a. temporal aspects (chronologic, developmental, disability status, etc.)
   b. environmental (physical, social, and cultural)
   c. adaptation and coping

4. Speech/Language/Cognition
   a. oral motor skills
   b. articulation
   c. receptive language skills
   d. expressive language skills
   e. auditory/language processing
   f. reading/reading comprehension
   g. education and neuropsychological evaluation
   h. cognitive integration and cognitive components (attention span, memory, etc.)

5. Community Integration and Family Teaching
   a. resources/supports
   b. advocacy
   c. school
   d. play and leisure skills
   e. community activities

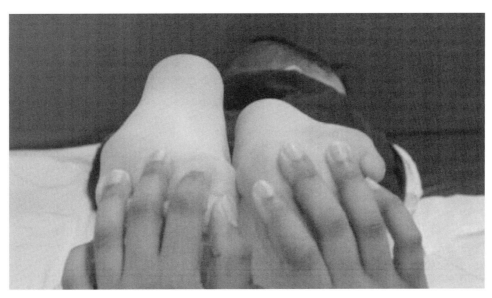

FIGURE 38-7

A 2 cm leg length discrepancy, decreased growth of the tibia on the right in a child with right hemiplegia.

combination of tone management, therapy, and bracing, a child can gain maximal functional mobility and minimize the risk of joint deformity. The physiatrist, neurologist, or orthopedic surgeon may treat these conditions with a variety of medications including baclofen, valium, tizanidine, and botulinum toxin for relaxation of overactive agonist muscles. A dilute solution of phenol may be used for motor branch blocks in the lower extremity. The goal is to improve coordination of the muscles around a joint to allow for more effective movement patterns. The prescription for therapy should focus on stretching the muscles that were treated, strengthening the antagonists, and improving selective motor control around each joint.

Therapy programs for children who experience a stroke early in life take place over the course of the developmental period beginning with Early Intervention and continuing through the preschool, elementary, middle, and high school years. A therapist identifies impairments and emerging functional abilities relevant to each child's developmental level. Motor and language learning principles need to be incorporated into the treatment plan integrating emotional, cultural, and social aspects of the child and family. The initial injury can have different long-term effects on acquisition of skills and psychosocial development for each child.

The pediatric rehabilitation framework further encourages planning for needs beyond direct therapy services. The goal of therapy in the schools is to keep the child safe within the school environment, as well as to facilitate the acquisition of grade-appropriate skills and information. A child's qualification for therapy at school is based on whether or not it will help the child access the academic curriculum. Medical goals are different in that they focus more directly on treatment of the neurologic and musculoskeletal systems. Therefore, a combination of school and outpatient therapy is appropriate.

Other Therapeutic Options

In addition to the more traditional therapy programs, a variety of different treatment approaches have been used to help children who have had a stroke improve the quality of their patterns of movement and communication skills throughout the developmental process. Examples include conductive education, constraint-induced movement therapy (CIMT), hippotherapy, and aquatic therapy. New therapeutic techniques are also becoming available, such as robotic therapy for improving gait and upper extremity function.

Conductive Education. Conductive Education was introduced in Hungary 60 years ago. It was developed to help children with motor disorders learn to overcome problems of movement resulting from damage to the central nervous system. It approaches motor disorders as a problem of learning or relearning—a problem that will respond to the appropriate patterned teaching. If the children can move and they can learn, they can learn to move differently. By repeating tasks and integrating intentional movement with learning, the theory is that the brain creates alternate pathways to send messages to muscle groups creating the desired movements. Most of the students have underlying weakness in the trunk and hyper- or hypotonic extremities.

Constraint-Induced Movement Therapy. CIMT has been utilized for improving upper limb function in adults after stroke. It involves three main elements: restraint of the noninvolved limb, an extensive movement program for the involved limb, and use of strategies to continue the use of two hands in activities of daily living. More recently, children have participated in studies utilizing a variety of CIMT techniques (55, 56). Treatment groups have demonstrated improved movement and efficacy as well as dexterity of the involved upper extremity. This has been sustained through six-month evaluation as measured by the Jebson-Taylor Test of Hand Function and fine motor subtests of the Bruininks-Oseretsky Test of Motor Proficiency (55, 57).

In a study by Taub et al., children ages two through six years were diagnosed with hemiparesis secondary to prenatal, perinatal, or early antenatal stroke. The control group, after receiving usual and customary care for six months, was crossed over to receive CIMT and exhibited results that were as good as those for children receiving CIMT first. Retention of treatment gains was approximately 70% at six months after the end of the initial program. One of the important factors contributing to good retention was the compliance of parents with the recommended post-treatment regimen. The children followed the recommended protocol during the treatment time five days per week (58).

Willis et al. evaluated twelve children ages one through eight years who received a plaster cast on the unimpaired arm for one month. When compared to a control group, the children in the treatment group showed significant improvement on the Peabody Developmental Motor Scales test. Again, gains were appreciated in this group six months after follow-up (59).

The amount of time in the restraint can vary, enabling the child to continue to explore and learn from the environment using the more functional hand. For some children, frustration may also be a major issue, especially if the cast is removed intermittently. Psychological concerns regarding restraining movement in a child is an issue that has been discussed. Of note, children who have fractured a bone and require casting for the purpose of allowing a bone to heal have not shown significant psychological problems. Decisions regarding the structure of this therapeutic program may require modification, depending on the child's needs. CIMT can be modified to be child-friendly and well tolerated (60).

Hippotherapy. In hippotherapy, the horse is used as a dynamic treatment tool that influences the child's postural reactions, as the base of support provided by the horse is constantly in motion (Figure 38-8). Therapy sessions are conducted by an occupational, speech, or physical therapist with a horse handler, side walker, and a trained horse. The therapist guides the child through a series of positions on horseback, thereby challenging different aspects of the child's balance responses. These positions progress through forward sitting, backward sitting, forward quadruped, backward quadruped, lying

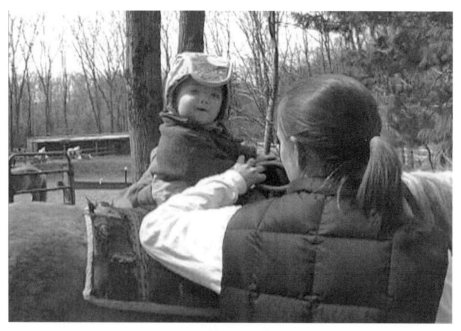

FIGURE 38-8

Hippotherapy with a therapist and a side-walker.

prone or supine, forward tall kneeling, backward tall kneeling, forward standing, and backward standing. The therapist can also ask the child to perform tasks with eyes closed. The child can toss a ball or manipulate objects from the moving base of support. These positions can be done with the horse moving in straight lines, circles, or other patterns accompanied by changes in speed and stride length.

It is believed that the rhythmic walking motion of the horse stimulates the child's vestibular system and improves his or her automatic balance responses. A rider sitting passively on a horse experiences pelvic displacement and trunk movement similar to that in human walking. This was confirmed by Fleck, using preadolescent riders on a horse walking on an equine treadmill moving in speed of 1.3 meters per second. With the use of adhesive surface markers placed on the anatomical reference points, Fleck evaluated the vertical displacement of center of gravity and lateral pelvic shift (61). The study demonstrated similarity between the mechanics of human walking and horseback riding in terms of lateral pelvic tilt, direction of displacement, and temporal sequences. It is believed that facilitating pelvic and trunk stability may contribute to the development of a stable base of support for the walking motion.

Hippotherapy has been identified as one therapeutic technique that can help improve balance, posture, mobility, and function in children with underlying weakness, including those with stroke (62–64). It may also affect psychological, cognitive, behavioral, and communication functions. The duration of treatment will vary, depending on the goals of the program and level of skill acquisition by the child.

Aquatic Therapy. Aquatic therapy or pool therapy consists of an exercise program that is performed in the water. It uses the physical properties of water to assist in healing and exercise performance. In children who have had a stroke, there may be significant underlying weakness that makes it difficult for them to move through space. While submerged in water, the buoyancy provided by the water helps support the weight of the child, thereby making it easier for him or her to move against gravity. The goals of therapy are to increase functional mobility, range of motion, balance and coordination, trunk stability and postural alignment, motivation and arousal, and muscle strength and endurance. In a therapeutic pool, the warmth of the water can also help relax muscles. Children with muscle spasms and increased tone find this aspect of aquatic therapy especially beneficial.

The viscosity of water also provides an excellent source of resistance that can be easily incorporated into an aquatic therapy exercise program. This resistance allows for muscle strengthening without the need of weights. Using resistance coupled with the water's buoyancy allows a child to strengthen muscle groups. Aquatic therapy also utilizes hydrostatic pressure to improve joint position awareness. The hydrostatic pressure produces forces perpendicular to the body's surface. This pressure provides increased joint position awareness that can help a child coordinate movement in a more effective manner.

Robotic Therapy. As robotic technology enables us to modify the size of a robotic device, more treatment options for children are becoming available for both fine motor and gross motor programs (Figure 38-9). In a study conducted at Spaulding Rehabilitation Hospital in Boston, twelve children ages 5 to 12 years participated in sixteen 1-hour robotic therapy sessions, two times per week for eight weeks (65). During each session, children used the paretic arm to perform 640 repetitive, goal-directed planar reaching movements, with robot assist as needed. Initially, the robot guided the movement. As time progressed, the child was able to direct more of the movement patterns without the assistance of the robot.

Primary outcome measures were the Quality of Upper Extremity Skills Test (QUEST) and the Fugl-Meyer Assessment (FMA) upper limb subtest. Secondary outcomes included the Modified Ashworth Scale, peak isometric strength of shoulder and elbow muscles, and parent questionnaire scores. Single group repeated-measures analyses of variance revealed significant gains beyond measurement error in total QUEST and FMA scores at discharge and follow up, and in isometric strength of elbow extensors at discharge. In addition, the parent questionnaire showed significant improvements in "how much" and "how well" children used the paretic arm during daily functional tasks at home.

Recent studies have demonstrated beneficial effects of intensive, task specific gait training on motor recovery in children with injury to the motor areas of the brain and adults with paraparasis and hemiparesis. Developments in the neurorehabilitation field have been stimulated by information on neuronal recovery processes and their modulation by various physical and pharmacological interventions. Robotic devices that control gait are being developed to help a child develop a greater appreciation of a heel to toe gait pattern (Figure 38-10). There is a growing body of evidence demonstrating that the human brain is capable of significant recovery, providing that the volume and frequency of treatments are adequate. The quality of intervention is equally important, with task-specific interventions enhancing neural reorganization and recovery.

Meyer-Heim et al. presented the preliminary results of a study in which six children and six adolescents with

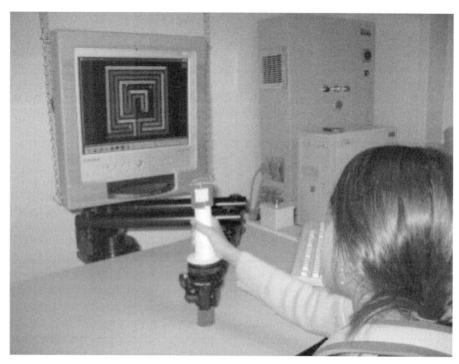

FIGURE 38-9

A child with right hemiplegia works to improve shoulder and elbow movement using the maze pattern on the robot.

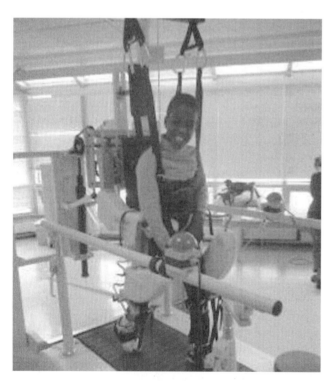

FIGURE 38-10

The Lokomat is a robotic device that controls the movement of the hips and the knees to facilitate a more symmetric efficient gait pattern.

acquired or congenital central gait impairment utilized a driven gait orthosis (DGO) to improve the quality of their ambulation. Results of the clinical experience of this series of children and adolescents were promising. Walking speed, the Gross Motor Functional Mobility (GMFM) score, and the distance in the six minute walk test improved in all children. Results of the walking section in the GMFM were superior to findings in the standing section, reflecting the task-oriented specificity in the DGO training. A positive relation was found between increasing numbers of sessions and walking distance during the training sessions. Preliminary findings in the outcome measurements suggest an improvement of locomotor performance (66).

FUNCTIONAL OUTCOME

Functional outcomes for children with stroke are being studied more aggressively. In the setting of the acute rehabilitation program, the Wee-Functional Independence Measure (Wee-FIM) (67) or the Pediatric Evaluation of Disability Inventory (PEDI) (68) are used to track progress over time (Table 38-5). Different programs use different tools. Use of these tools enables a program to compare recovery with the national average for similar conditions. The selection of outcome variables may differ between facilities as well.

TABLE 38-5
Comparison of Outcome Measures

OUTCOME MEASURE	AGE RANGE	DESCRIPTION
Wee-Functional Independence Measure (Wee-FIM)	6 months–7 years	Administered by observation or structured questions. Item clusters include self-care, sphincter control, mobility, locomotion, communication, social, and cognition. Ratings of child on 7-point scale of burden of care.
Pediatric Evaluation of Disability Inventory	6 months–7 years	Rated by informant or by interview. Includes three major content domains: self-care, mobility, social function. Assesses separate measurement dimensions of functional skills, caregiver assistance, and modifications.

There has been speculation that recovery from stroke in children has a better outcome compared to recovery in adults. Mosch and colleagues studied pairs of children and adults with similar lesions to determine if the children had different functional outcomes. The results showed that children with right hemisphere lesions had significantly better social outcomes than adults with matched lesions. This may suggest a process of plasticity buffering the children from more severe social outcome impairment (69).

Over the last few years, there have been more research projects involving cognitive recovery after stroke during childhood. By considering some of the many variables that may affect intellectual outcome (i.e., hemisphere damaged, child's age at injury, site and extent of damage, and presence or absence of seizures) it is hoped that a better understanding of the prognosis for intellectual functioning after childhood can be determined (70).

In 1995, de Veber initiated a two center longitudinal comprehensive outcome study involving collaborations with neuropsychologists and occupational therapists. No adequate outcome measures existed for children with focal, non-progressive cerebral disorders including stroke, and standard adult measures do not apply (13). The Pediatric Stroke Outcome Measure (PSOM) was developed to quantify recovery following the diagnosis of a stroke in a child. The results showed that 57% of pediatric patients with ischemic infarction recover fully or with only mild dysfunction. Twenty-six percent had moderate dysfunction, and 16% had severe dysfunction.

Gordon et al. described functional consequences of childhood stroke that were described in terms of activity limitation, extent of brain damage, impairment, and functional sequelae (60). Seventeen children and adolescents with cerebral infarction in the territory of the middle cerebral artery were assessed with a 4-point Likert scale (the Pediatric Stroke Activity Limitation Measure) to examine the degree of difficulty experienced by the children in daily activities. Activity limitation was evident in the domains of education, self-care, and motor skills. In comparison with population norms, the subjects scored below average in both physical and psychologic health. Parental health also rated generally lower than expected.

Ganesan et al. used a parent survey to better define deficits in 90 children diagnosed with ischemic strokes. Sixty percent of the children needed help in the areas of activities of daily living. Seventy-four percent had motor deficits. Forty-three percent had speech and language deficits (71).

In 1999, Hogan et al. published results of a literature review that looked at intelligence in children after stroke. Hogan found that after stroke, mean IQ falls significantly below the population mean but remains within the average range. There was no significant difference between hemispheric side of injury. The Verbal and Performance IQ lateralization profile widely recognized in adults with unilateral injury is not apparent in younger children. Older children who sustained a stroke only trended toward this profile (70, 72).

Academic skill impairments were more likely to be seen in children than their adult counterparts. This finding was consistent with those studies that suggested that lesions acquired in childhood before literacy acquisition detrimentally affected the development of reading skills, both in children who suffer general declines in verbal processing and in children who merely showed a deficit in basic phonics skills without poor verbal IQ (73).

Verbal learning and memory (VLM) following pediatric stroke was characterized in a cross-sectional neuropsychologic and neuroimaging study of 26 subjects, aged 5 to 17, with a history of pediatric stroke and gender matched orthopedic controls. Further comparisons were made between the VLM profiles of stroke subjects with right versus left hemisphere lesions and early (<12 months) versus late (12 months) strokes.

Overall, stroke subjects scored significantly lower than control subjects on several VLM indices (California Verbal Learning Test-Children; CVLT-C), as well as on measures of intellectual functioning (IQ), and auditory attention/working memory (Digit Span). Subgroup analyses of the stroke population found no significant differences in VLM, Digit Span, Verbal IQ, or Performance IQ when left-hemisphere lesion subjects were compared to right-hemisphere lesion subjects. In contrast, early strokes were associated with significantly fewer words recalled after delay, reduced discriminability (fewer correct hits relative to false positive errors on recognition testing), and relatively worse auditory attention/working memory scores (Digit Span). These findings indicate that pediatric stroke subjects demonstrated more VLM impairment than control subjects, and early strokes were associated with greater recall and recognition deficits (72).

Hurwitz et al. found that children and adolescents with a history of stroke demonstrated fairly good outcomes in terms of transition to adulthood, including high rates of high school graduation and higher education. Thirty-two patients were followed over the course of about ten years. Study results found that in early adulthood, most individuals were employed (90%) and could drive (76%). As far as general functional status, mobility outcomes were excellent, although assistive devices and orthotic use was common. Daily living skills, communication, and socialization fell in the moderately low range and were influenced by medical status (74).

CONCLUSION

Stroke in children is an important cause of morbidity and mortality in the pediatric population. The risks and benefits of stroke treatments in children may differ significantly from those in adults, attributed to developmental differences in the cerebrovascular, neurologic, and coagulation systems. The variety of etiologies of pediatric stroke makes it difficult to develop stroke

prevention strategies based on adult studies. Despite the fact that the incidence of pediatric stroke is lower than stoke in adults, the consequences of stroke in children can have a lifelong impact on function, families, and use of resources. Lo et al. determined the median cost for pediatric post-stroke care during the first year after diagnosis was $42,338. The cost for stroke care was higher for hemorrhagic stroke than for ischemic stroke. Cost had a significant positive correlation with neurologic impairment (68).

There is a growing consensus among those who study pediatric stroke that a common terminology is needed to enhance research and multicenter trials (21, 75, 76). Increased awareness of unique pediatric stroke subtypes, their clinical presentations, and findings on imaging studies can improve early identification and development of optimal treatment strategies. Furthermore, improved recognition of subtypes may lead to more effective secondary stroke prevention measures (18).

No single type of therapy has been identified as being superior, and a collaborative approach must be utilized in helping children maximize their functional gains. The goals should focus on improving postural stability and symmetry of movement, minimizing joint deformities, and facilitating communication, cognitive, and social skill acquisition to improve function with everyday life skills.

A pediatric rehabilitation framework model can be utilized to help parents and the treatment team embrace the multidisciplinary process for recovery. Encouraging family members to become active participants in the rehabilitation process may help with advocacy that may be needed in the educational setting. Preconceived notions of what a child may or may not be able to accomplish may interfere with his or her ability to participate fully in athletic and social activities. As is true with all children, it is incumbent on the caregiver to help maximize each child's functional potential. The pediatric rehabilitation team is a resource for families to help accomplish this goal.

References

1. Giroud M, Lemesle M, Madinier G, Manceau E, Osseby GV, Dumas R. Stroke in children under 16 years of age. Clinical and etiological difference with adults. *Acta Neurol Scand* Dec 1997; 96(6):401–406.
2. Fullerton HJ, Chetkovich DM, Wu YW, Smith WS, Johnston SC. Deaths from stroke in US children, 1979 to 1998. *Neurology* Jul 9 2002; 59(1):34–39.
3. Schoenberg BS, Mellinger JF, Schoenberg DG. Cerebrovascular disease in infants and children: A study of incidence, clinical features, and survival. *Neurology* Aug 1978; 28(8):763–768.
4. Broderick J, Talbot GT, Prenger E, Leach A, Brott T. Stroke in children within a major metropolitan area: The surprising importance of intracerebral hemorrhage. *J Child Neurol* Jul 1993; 8(3):250–255.
5. Fullerton HJ, Wu YW, Zhao S, Johnston SC. Risk of stroke in children: Ethnic and gender disparities. *Neurology* Jul 22 2003; 61(2):189–194.
6. de Veber G, Roach ES, Riela AR, Wiznitzer M. Stroke in children: Recognition, treatment, and future directions. *Semin Pediatr Neurol* Dec 2000; 7(4):309–317.

7. de Veber GA, MacGregor D, Curtis R, Mayank S. Neurologic outcome in survivors of childhood arterial ischemic stroke and sinovenous thrombosis. *J Child Neurol* May 2000; 15(5):316–324.
8. Gabis LV, Yangala R, Lenn NJ. Time lag to diagnosis of stroke in children. *Pediatrics* Nov 2002; 110(5):924–928.
9. Braun KP, Kappelle LJ, Kirkham FJ, Deveber G. Diagnostic pitfalls in paediatric ischaemic stroke. *Dev Med Child Neurol* Dec 2006; 48(12):985–990.
10. Wiznitzer M, Masaryk TJ. Cerebrovascular abnormalities in pediatric stroke: Assessment using parenchymal and angiographic magnetic resonance imaging. *Ann Neurol* Jun 1991; 29(6):585–589.
11. Warach S, Baron JC. Neuroimaging. *Stroke* Feb 2004; 35(2):351–353.
12. Carvalho KS, Garg BP. Arterial strokes in children. *Neurol Clin* Nov 2002; 20(4):1079–1100, vii.
13. de Veber G, Adams M, Andrew M. Canadian pediatric stroke registry (abstract). *Can J Neurol Sci* 1995; 22:S24.

14. Lynch JK, Hirtz DG, de Veber G, Nelson KB. Report of the National Institute of Neurological Disorders and Stroke workshop on perinatal and childhood stroke. *Pediatrics* Jan 2002; 109(1):116–123.

15. Wade DT, Wood VA, Hewer RL. Recovery after stroke—the first 3 months. *J Neurol Neurosurg Psychiatry* Jan 1985; 48(1):7–13.

16. Skilbeck CE, Wade DT, Hewer RL, Wood VA. Recovery after stroke. *J Neurol Neurosurg Psychiatry* Jan 1983; 46(1):5–8.

17. Vexler ZS, Sharp FR, Feuerstein GZ, et al. Translational stroke research in the developing brain. *Pediatr Neurol* Jun 2006; 34(6):459–463.

18. Fullerton H, Lynch JK, de Veber G. The call for multicenter studies of pediatric stroke. *Stroke* Feb 2006; 37(2):330–331.

19. Nelson KB. Thrombophilias, perinatal stroke, and cerebral palsy. *Clin Obstet Gynecol* Dec 2006; 49(4):875–884.

20. Kirton A, de Veber G. Cerebral palsy secondary to perinatal ischemic stroke. *Clin Perinatol* Jun 2006; 33(2):367–386.

21. Lynch JK, Han CJ. Pediatric stroke: What do we know and what do we need to know? *Semin Neurol* Dec 2005; 25(4):410–423.

22. Lanthier S, Carmant L, David M, Larbrisseau A, de Veber G. Stroke in children: The coexistence of multiple risk factors predicts poor outcome. *Neurology* Jan 25 2000; 54(2):371–378.

23. Scotti LN, Goldman RL, Hardman DR, Heinz ER. Venous thrombosis in infants and children. *Radiology* Aug 1974; 112(2):393–399.

24. Rivkin MJ, Volpe JJ. Strokes in children. *Pediatr Rev* Aug 1996; 17(8):265–278.

25. Roach ES. Etiology of stroke in children. *Semin Pediatr Neurol* Dec 2000; 7(4):244–260.

26. Riela AR, Roach ES. Etiology of stroke in children. *J Child Neurol* Jul 1993; 8(3):201–220.

27. Shellhass RA, et al. Mimics of childhood stroke: Characterisitics of a prospective cohort. *Pediatrics* 2006; 118(2):704–709.

28. Raju TN, Nelson KB, Ferriero D, Lynch JK. Ischemic perinatal stroke: Summary of a workshop sponsored by the National Institute of Child Health and Human Development and the National Institute of Neurological Disorders and Stroke. *Pediatrics* Sep 2007; 120(3):609–616.

29. Fullerton HJ, Wu YW, Sidney S, Johnston SC. Risk of recurrent childhood arterial ischemic stroke in a population-based cohort: The importance of cerebrovascular imaging. *Pediatrics* Mar 2007; 119(3):495–501.

30. Nestoridi E, Buonanno FS, Jones RM, et al. Arterial ischemic stroke in childhood: The role of plasma-phase risk factors. *Curr Opin Neurol* Apr 2002; 15(2):139–144.

31. Nowak-Gottl U, Strater R, Heinecke A, et al. Lipoprotein (a) and genetic polymorphisms of clotting factor V, prothrombin, and methylenetetrahydrofolate reductase are risk factors of spontaneous ischemic stroke in childhood. *Blood* Dec 1 1999; 94(11):3678–3682.

32. Kenet G, Sadetzki S, Murad H, et al. Factor V Leiden and antiphospholipid antibodies are significant risk factors for ischemic stroke in children. *Stroke* Jun 2000; 31(6):1283–1288.

33. Gunther G, Junker R, Strater R, et al. Symptomatic ischemic stroke in full-term neonates: Role of acquired and genetic prothrombotic risk factors. *Stroke* Oct 2000; 31(10):2437–2441.

34. McColl MD, Chalmers EA, Thomas A, et al. Factor V Leiden, prothrombin 20210G--JA and the MTHFR C677T mutations in childhood stroke. *Thromb Haemost* May 1999; 81(5):690–694.

35. Andrew ME, Monagle P, de Veber G, Chan AK. Thromboembolic disease and antithrombotic therapy in newborns. *Hematology Am Soc Hematol Educ Program* 2001:358–374.

36. Israels SJ, Seshia SS. Childhood stroke associated with protein C or S deficiency. *J Pediatr* Oct 1987; 111(4):562–564.

37. Simioni P, Battistella PA, Drigo P, Carollo C, Girolami A. Childhood stroke associated with familial protein S deficiency. *Brain Dev* May–Jun 1994; 16(3):241–245.

38. Brenner B, Fishman A, Goldsher D, Schreibman D, Tavory S. Cerebral thrombosis in a newborn with a congenital deficiency of antithrombin III. *Am J Hematol* Mar 1988; 27(3):209–211.

39. Mayer SA, Sacco RL, Hurlet-Jensen A, Shi T, Mohr JP. Free protein S deficiency in acute ischemic stroke. A case-control study. *Stroke* Feb 1993; 24(2):224–227.

40. Zenz W, Bodo Z, Plotho J, et al. Factor V Leiden and prothrombin gene G 20210 A variant in children with ischemic stroke. *Thromb Haemost* Nov 1998; 80(5):763–766.

41. Ganesan V, McShane MA, Liesner R, Cookson J, Hann I, Kirkham FJ. Inherited prothrombotic states and ischaemic stroke in childhood. *J Neurol Neurosurg Psychiatry* Oct 1998; 65(4):508–511.

42. de Veber G, Monagle P, Chan A, et al. Prothrombotic disorders in infants and children with cerebral thromboembolism. *Arch Neurol* Dec 1998; 55(12):1539–1543.

43. Cardo E, Vilaseca MA, Campistol J, Artuch R, Colome C, Pineda M. Evaluation of hyperhomocysteinaemia in children with stroke. *Eur J Paediatr Neurol* 1999; 3(3):113–117.

44. Golomb MR, Garg BP, Williams LS. Outcomes of children with infantile spasms after perinatal stroke. *Pediatr Neurol* Apr 2006; 34(4):291–295.

45. Heller C, Becker S, Scharrer I, Kreuz W. Prothrombotic risk factors in childhood stroke and venous thrombosis. *Eur J Pediatr* Dec 1999; 158 Suppl 3:S117–121.

46. Carlin TM, Chanmugam A. Stroke in children. *Emerg Med Clin North Am* Aug 2002; 20(3):671–685.

47. Adams RJ. Lessons from the Stroke Prevention Trial in Sickle Cell Anemia (STOP) study. *J Child Neurol* May 2000; 15(5):344–349.

48. Brankovic-Sreckovic V, Milic-Rasic V, Jovic N, Milic N, Todorovic S. The recurrence risk of ischemic stroke in childhood. *Med Princ Pract* May–Jun 2004; 13(3):153–158.

49. Fullerton HJ. The emerging quandary of childhood stoke: Better aim but no magic bullet. *Stroke* Jan 2006; 37(1):3.

50. de Veber G. Cerebrovascular disease. In: Swaiman K, Ashwal S, Ferriero DM, eds. *Pediatric Neurology*. 4th ed. Oxford: Elsevier, 2006:1759–1801.

51. Kirton A, Shroff M, Visvanathan T, de Veber G. Quantified corticospinal tract diffusion restriction predicts neonatal stroke outcome. *Stroke* 2007; 38(3):974 - 980.

52. Adams RJ, Brambilla D. Discontinuing prophylactic transfusions used to prevent stroke in sickle cell disease. *N Engl J Med* Dec 29 2005; 353(26):2769–2778.

53. Fullerton HJ. Declining Stroke Rates in Californian Children with Sickle Cell Disease. *Blood* 2004; 15(1104) 2:336–339.

54. American Occupational Therapy Association. Uniform terminology for occupational therapy (third edition). *Am J Occup Ther* Nov–Dec 1994; 48(11):1047–1054.

55. Karman N, Maryles J, Baker RW, Simpser E, Berger-Gross P. Constraint-induced movement therapy for hemiplegic children with acquired brain injuries. *J Head Trauma Rehabil* May–Jun 2003; 18(3):259–267.

56. Dickerson AE, Brown LE. Pediatric constraint-induced movement therapy in a young child with minimal active arm movement. *Am J Occup Ther* Sep–Oct 2007; 61(5):563–573.

57. Charles JR, Wolf SL, Schneider JA, Gordon AM. Efficacy of a child-friendly form of constraint-induced movement therapy in hemiplegic cerebral palsy: A randomized control trial. *Dev Med Child Neurol* Aug 2006; 48(8):635–642.

58. Taub E, Ramey SL, DeLuca S, Echols K. Efficacy of constraint-induced movement therapy for children with cerebral palsy with asymmetric motor impairment. *Pediatrics* Feb 2004; 113(2):305–312.

59. Willis JK, Morello A, Davie A, Rice JC, Bennett JT. Forced use treatment of childhood hemiparesis. *Pediatrics* Jul 2002; 110(1 Pt 1):94–96.

60. Gordon AM, Charles J, Wolf SL. Methods of constraint-induced movement therapy for children with hemiplegic cerebral palsy: Development of a child-friendly intervention for improving upper-extremity function. *Arch Phys Med Rehabil* Apr 2005; 86(4):837–844.

61. Fleck, CA. Hippotherapy: Mechanics of human walking and horseback riding. In Engel BT, ed. *Rehabilitation with the Aid of the Horse: A Collection of Studies*. Durango, CO, Barbara Engel Therapy Services, 1997.

62. Bertoti DB. Effect of therapeutic horseback riding on posture in children with cerebral palsy. *Phys Ther* Oct 1988; 68(10):1505–1512.

63. McGibbon NH, Andrade CK, Widener G, Cintas HL. Effect of an equine-movement therapy program on gait, energy expenditure, and motor function in children with spastic cerebral palsy: A pilot study. *Dev Med Child Neurol* Nov 1998; 40(11):754–762.

64. McPhail AHE, Edwards J, Golding J, Miller K, Mosier C, Zwiers T. Trunk postural reactions in children with and without cerebral palsy during therapeutic horseback riding. *Pediatr Phys Ther* 1998; 10:143–147.

65. Fasoli SE, Krebs HI, Stein J, Frontera WR, Hogan N. Effects of robotic therapy on motor impairment and recovery in chronic stroke. *Arch Phys Med Rehabil* Apr 2003; 84(4):477–482.

66. Meyer-Heim A, Reiffer C, Sennhauser FH, Colombo G, Knecht B. First steps with the pediatric lokomat: Feasibility of robotic assisted locomotor training in children with central gait impairment. *Dev Med Child Neurol* 2006; 48(Suppl 107):15.

67. Ottenbacher KJ, Msall ME, Lyon N, et al. The WeeFIM instrument: Its utility in detecting change in children with developmental disabilities. *Arch Phys Med Rehabil* Oct 2000; 81(10):1317–1326.

68. Lo W, Zamel K, Ponnappa K, et al. The cost of pediatric stroke care and rehabilitation. *Stroke* Jan 2008; 39(1):161–165.

69. Mosch SC, Max JE, Tranel D. A matched lesion analysis of childhood versus adult-onset brain injury due to unilateral stroke: Another perspective on neural plasticity and recovery of social functioning. *Cogn Behav Neurol* Mar 2005; 18(1):5–17.

70. Hogan AM, Kirkham FJ, Isaacs EB. Intelligence after stroke in childhood: Review of the literature and suggestions for future research. *J Child Neurol* May 2000; 15(5):325–332.

71. Ganesan V, Hogan A, Shack N, Gordon A, Isaacs E, Kirkham FJ. Outcome after ischaemic stroke in childhood. *Dev Med Child Neurol* Jul 2000; 42(7):455–461.

72. Lansing AE, Max JE, Delis DC, et al. Verbal learning and memory after childhood stroke. *J Int Neuropsychol Soc* Sep 2004; 10(5):742–752.

73. Pitchford NJ. Spoken language correlates of reading impairments acquired in childhood. *Brain Lang* Apr 2000; 72(2):129–149.

74. Hurvitz E, Warschausky S, Berg M, Tsai S. Long-term functional outcome of pediatric stroke survivors. *Top Stroke Rehabil* Spring 2004; 11(2):51–59.

75. Sofronas M, Ichord RN, Fullerton HJ, et al. Pediatric stroke initiatives and preliminary studies: What is known and what is needed? *Pediatr Neurol* Jun 2006; 34(6):439–445.

76. Zahuranec DB, Brown DL, Lisabeth LD, Morgenstern LB. Is it time for a large, collaborative study of pediatric stroke? *Stroke* Sep 2005; 36(9):1825–1829.

39

Stroke in Young Adults

Randie M. Black-Schaffer

pproximately 4% of strokes in the United States occur in adults younger than 45 years old (1). While the 28,000 strokes in this age group are a small fraction of the 700,000 total events in the United States each year, they are a significant source of neurologic impairment in this group. The fact that stroke occurs in those under 45 years old over twice as frequently as both spinal cord injury (11,000/year for all ages) and multiple sclerosis (11,000/year for all ages) in the United States has been underappreciated (2, 3), perhaps due to the tendency to consider young adult stroke in the context of all strokes rather than in the context of all causes of neurologic impairment in the young. In contrast to the United States, in developing countries with younger populations, stroke in adults under the age of 40 accounts for as many as 19% of all strokes, leaving no doubt about its significance as a source of neurologic impairment in these societies (4). Numerous investigations over the past 25 years have established important differences in the incidence, epidemiology, etiology, treatment, and outcomes of stroke in young adults compared to older populations. These will be discussed in this chapter.

EPIDEMIOLOGY

Incidence

The incidence of stroke in adults under 45–50 years of age has been found to range from 8.8 to 23 per 100,000 in European and American populations (Table 39-1) (5–12). Notably higher rates are reported in two studies of African populations (4, 13). These numbers contrast with the much higher incidence of stroke in older adults, which, in the United States, ranges between 230 per 100,000 in white females to 660 per 100,000 in black males for those 45–84 years old (14).

Not only is the frequency of stroke different in young adults compared to adults of all ages, but the distribution of stroke types differs as well. Among people in the United States of all ages, 87% of strokes are ischemic infarctions, and 13% are intracerebral (ICH) or subarachnoid (SAH) hemorrhages (14). In most studies of young adults, there is a higher frequency of hemorrhagic events. The population-based study of young Italians by Marini et al. found 57% infarction and 42% hemorrhages (ICH and SAH) (15). Moreover, Leno et al. in Spain and Nencini et al. in Florence found fewer than 50% infarctions in their young adult

TABLE 39-1

Incidence of Stroke in Young Adults (Population-based Studies)

STUDY	POPULATION	AGE RANGE	TYPE OF ARTERIAL STROKE	INCIDENCE /100,000
Nencini, 1988 (5)	Florence, Italy	15–44	All	8.8
Guidetti, 1993 (12)	Northern Italy	15–44	All	13.6
Kristensen, 1997 (6)	Northern Sweden	18–44	Infarction	11.3
Lidegaard, 1986 (7)	Denmark	15–44	Infarction, TIA	15
Jacobs, 2002 (8)	Northern Manhattan	20–44	All	23
Leno, 1993 (9)	Cantabria, Spain	16–45	All	12.0
Naess, 2002 (10)	Western Norway	15–49	Infarction	11.4
Rosenthul-Sorokin, 1996 (11)	Israel	17–49	All	10.4
Radhakrishnan, 1986 (4)	Benghazi, Libya	15–40	All	47
Rosman, 1986 (13)	Pretoria, South Africa	20–54	Infarction, ICH	33
Gross, 1984 (15)	Alabama	20–54	All All	Whites: 42 Blacks: 50
Ghandehari, 2006 (16)	Southern Khorasan, Iran	15–45	Infarction	8
Corbin, 2004 (17)	Barbados	25–34 35–44	All All	11 30

stroke populations (5, 9). On the other hand, studies in Israel and Libya have chronicled rates of 78% and 81% infarction among young adults with stroke (Table 39-2). The reasons for this variation from one population to another are unclear, but may relate to differences in genetic susceptibility, acquired risk factors, or temporal bias. Location of infarct, however, appears similar in young and older populations, though comparative data is limited. Anterior circulation infarcts comprise 70% of infarcts in older populations and 59–64% in two Scandinavian young adult populations (6, 10, 19).

Gender

Women, as a group, experience an increase in stroke risk during their childbearing years because of the hazards of pregnancy and the puerperium as well as the use of oral contraceptive medications, particularly in combination with smoking. In many studied populations, young women's incidence of stroke exceeds that of young men. This was the case for all strokes in Rochester, Minnesota, during most of the period from 1955–1989 (20); in Denmark from 1977–1982, where Lidegard et al. found an increased incidence of

TABLE 39-2

Distribution of Stroke Subtypes in Population-based Studies of Young Adults with Stroke

STUDY	POPULATION	INFARCT %	ICH %	SAH %
Marini, 2001 (15)	L'Aquila, Italy	57	20	23
Leno, 1993 (9)	Cantabria, Spain	47	27	25
Nencini, 1988 (5)	Florence, Italy	38	21	36
Rozenthul-Sorokin, 1996 (11)	Israel	81	10	8
Radhakrishnan, 1986 (4)	Benghazi, Libya	78	13	10

cerebral infarction in women aged 15–34 compared to men; in Western Norway for those under age 30 (10); in Cantabria, Spain, where strokes were more frequent in women in the 31–35 age cohort (9); and in Florence, Italy, where women aged 15–34 suffered more strokes than men (5). In southern Alabama, black women in the 20–54 age cohort were found to have twice as many strokes as black men and white women. In Barbados, women aged 25–44 also exceeded men in the number of strokes (15, 17).

This trend was not found in the Northern Manhattan study, where men aged 20–44 had 1.2 times the risk of stroke and a high proportion of ICH (8). In the African population of Ibadan, Nigeria, the incidence of stroke in those ages from 20–29 was equal in men and women and higher in men in all other decades (21). Population differences in prevalence of different risk factors in men could account for these differences.

Race and Ethnicity

Population-based studies in American cities have documented a higher incidence of stroke in young blacks compared to whites. In the Greater Cincinnati/ Northern Kentucky area, the incidence of stroke was higher for blacks at all ages, but the greatest increase in risk (fivefold) was in young and middle-aged blacks. The risk of first-ever stroke was twice as high for blacks in the <35 age group, rising to fivefold higher in those aged 35–44 and then declining in succeeding age groups to a 1.3-fold increase in those older than 85. The authors hypothesized that the higher incidence in blacks was related to a higher burden of hypertension and diabetes and to socioeconomic factors (22). A similar trend was seen in Northern Manhattan study, where the increase in risk of stroke in blacks compared to whites, present in all age cohorts, peaked at ninefold in those aged 35–44 years (23). In southern Alabama, the increase in stroke risk for blacks compared to whites peaked at 2.5-fold in the 55–64 age range. In the Baltimore/Washington area, blacks had a 2.1-fold higher risk of ischemic stroke and a 3.1-fold higher risk of intracerebral hemorrhage compared to whites (15, 24). In addition, in 1984, Gross et al. found a higher risk of stroke in black females but not males, compared to their white counterparts aged 20–54 in southern Alabama. The actual numbers of strokes in each age and race category in this study were small, and confidence intervals were not given (15).

These findings corroborate those of the pre-CT era literature (25). Eckstrom et al. in 1965 in Missouri and Heyman et al. in 1971 in Evans County, Georgia, found a higher incidence of stroke in young blacks compared to whites, with young black women showing the highest risk in the latter study (25, 26).

The question of black and white racial differences outside of the United States has been less explored. Stewart et al., studying a mixed population in South London, found a higher incidence of stroke in blacks under the age of 45 compared to whites (44 per 100,000 in blacks age 25–34, compared to 5 per 100,000 in whites and 42 per 100,000 in blacks age 35–44 compared to 28 per 100,000 in whites) (27). Whether there are regional differences throughout the world, the susceptibility of different, young black populations to stroke has yet to be investigated.

The Northern Manhattan Stroke Study examined relative risk of stroke in Hispanics aged 20–44 and found a 2.5-fold higher risk compared with whites while blacks showed a relative risk of 2.4 (8). A population-based study of stroke rates over a twenty-year period among New Zealand women found an increasing incidence in Pacific women, a decline in European women, and no change of rate in Maori women. These two studies illustrate the need for further exploration of ethnic and racial differences in stroke incidence around the globe.

ETIOLOGY

An Evolving Spectrum of Causes

Over 60 different disorders causing stroke in young adults were identified in a comprehensive list published in 1983 (28). A few of these, particularly valvular disease caused by rheumatic fever and infectious arteropathies, have diminished in importance in developed nations since that time. On the other hand, a number of new potential causes of stroke in young adults have appeared. Prothrombotic states caused by antiphospholipid antibodies (first described in 1978), deficiency of proteins C (1981) and S (1984), Factor V Leiden (1993), and the prothrombin 20210A mutation (1996) can increase the risk of arterial stroke as well as venous thrombosis in young adults. Venous thrombosis in young adults has also been characterized (29). Drugs of abuse, including cocaine, heroin, and the ephedra alkaloids, have been recognized as significant causes of stroke at the same time that the risk of stroke from oral contraceptives has declined with the advent of lower dosing. The risk of stroke in young adults with HIV/AIDS, cerebral autosomal dominant arteriopathy with subcortical infarcts and leukoencephalopathy (CADASIL), and reversible vasospastic disorders, including Call-Fleming syndrome, has been discovered (30). Finally, there is dawning acknowledgement of the role played by our increasing array of medical and surgical interventions that promote the incidence of stroke in young adults. For example, cervical radiation, transplant surgery, artificial valves, carotid stenting, and chiropractic maneuvers all have an associated risk of stroke, and all tend to be offered to younger patients. The failure of stroke incidence rates in the US to decline since the 1980s may, to some extent, reflect an increase in the iatrogenic opportunities for stroke (31–37).

Advances in craniocervical imaging in the past two decades have improved detection of several important causes of stroke in young adults. Magnetic resonance and computed tomography imaging and angiography, have greatly enhanced our ability to diagnose large vessel dissection, intracranial vasospasm, vasculitis, and cerebral venous thrombosis.

Distribution of Causes by Age Subgroup

While an extensive literature on aspects of stroke in young adults has developed over the past 30 years, the definition of *young* has not been standardized. Case series variably use 30, 40, 45, or 50 as their upper age limit for young adult patients. This fact—and the small sample size of most reported series—have made it difficult to discern natural age subgroups within the broader category of young adult stroke. Nonetheless, it is clear that the distribution of causes of stroke in adults 15–35 years of age differs from that in adults 35–50 years of age. In the younger group, cardiogenic embolism, drugs (both therapeutic and illicit), migraine, traumatic dissection, prothrombotic states, and premature atherosclerosis caused by inherited conditions such as homocystinuria are prominent factors, whereas, in the older subgroup dissection, antiphospholipid antibodies and atherosclerosis caused by hypertension and other traditional risk factors are prominent (38–41). Neto et al., using the TOAST criteria (42), examined the distribution of stroke mechanisms of a series of 106 patients admitted to a university hospital in Sao Paulo with cerebral infarction and found that those 15–29 years old had a higher proportion of strokes due to "other determined causes" and the group ages 30–40 had more "cardioembolism"-related events (43). The study of larger populations and series will enable further definition of etiology patterns in different decades of adulthood.

Many case series have considered the causes of stroke in young adults. These studies frequently come from tertiary care hospitals, with their attendant bias toward cases of unusual/complex etiology. For this reason, true frequencies of the specific etiologies of stroke in young adults have been difficult to determine. There is fair agreement on broad categories of causation, however, and Hart and Miller's 1983 categories have proven durable, with the addition of drug use, which is an increasing cause of stroke in urban settings in the developed world (44). Hart and Miller attributed stroke in young adults to atherosclerotic disease in 20%;

cardiac emboli in 20%; arteropathies, particularly large vessel dissection, in 10%; coagulopathy in 10%; and peripartum cerebrovascular events in 5%. Another 20% was related to mitral valve prolapse, migraine, and oral contraceptive use, and 15% remained unexplained after full evaluation (28, 41).

Specific etiologies of stroke in young adults described in the literature are listed in Table 39-3. Even though it is beyond the scope of this chapter to discuss all of these in detail, we will review several of the important and controversial causes of stroke in this age group.

Etiologies

Cervicocranial Dissection. After cardioembolic stroke, dissection is the second-leading cause of stroke in patients younger than 45 (46). This mechanism accounts for 10–25% of strokes in young and middle-aged adults (47). Large vessel dissection is a disorder of midlife; its incidence peaks in the fifth decade. A population-based study from Rochester, Minnesota, found a mean age of 45.8 for dissection cases (48). Both internal carotid and vertebral arteries have segments vulnerable to the effects of head and neck movement. In the internal carotid artery (ICA), the distal half of the extracranial segment is most often affected, whereas in the vertebral artery, the V3 segment from C2 to the artery's entrance into the skull and the V1 segment in the neck are commonly involved. The external and common carotid arteries are rarely affected. The mechanism usually involves an intimal tear with dissection of arterial blood between the intimal and medial layers of the arterial wall. This can cause bulging of the inner arterial wall and stenosis or occlusion of the lumen. The intimal tear can become a nidus for formation and embolization of platelet and/or fibrin thrombi. In some cases, trauma to the artery may instead cause intramural hematoma formation with secondary rupture from the intima into the lumen, or there may be primary intramural hematoma dissecting between arterial layers and causing luminal stenosis or occlusion without rupture into the lumen. Cerebral infarctions resulting from a carotid dissection can thus be small, cortical insults caused by emboli, watershed territory lesions caused by low flow from a sudden carotid stenosis, or major anterior circulation infarction from rapid development of carotid occlusion. The current belief is that approximately 80% of dissection-related strokes are due to embolization and 20% to carotid thrombosis.

Carotid dissection has historically been difficult to diagnose. Patients present with pain, often above or behind the eye or along the side of the neck, jaw, and face. They may describe pulsatile tinnitus and transient monocular blindness. They may see scintillating scotomata and have transient cranial nerve dysfunctions,

TABLE 39-3
Causes of Stroke in Young Adults (27, 29, 37, 38, 43)

Cardiac	Congenital anomalies	
	Rheumatic valvular disease	
	Calcific aortic stenosis	
	Mitral valve prolapse	
	Patent foramen ovale/atrial septal defect with venous thrombosis	
	Endocarditis	
	Atrial myxoma	
	Cardiomyopathy	
	Arrhythmias	
	Ventricular thrombus	
Vascular	Premature atherosclerosis	
	Craniocervical dissection	
	Infectious vasculitis	Syphilis, tuberculosis, Lyme disease, AIDS
	Moya Moya disease	
	Takayasu's disease	
	Intracranial aneurysm	
	Cerebral arteriovenous malformation	
	Susac's syndrome (microangiopathy of brain, ear, retina)	
	Call-Fleming syndrome	
	Buerger's disease	
Collagen vascular disease	Systemic lupus erythematosus	
	Rheumatoid arthritis	
	Sjogren's syndrome	
	Polyarteritis nodosa	
	Behcet's disease	
	Scleroderma	
Hematologic	Sickle cell disease	
	Hemoglobin SC disease	
	Hypercoagulable states	Antiphospholipid syndrome, Factor V Leiden, PT 20210A, protein C or S deficiency, antithrombin III deficiency, elevated factor VIII
	Disseminated intravascular coagulation	
	Polycythemia vera	
	Idiopathic thrombocytopenic purpura (ITP)	
	Thrombotic thrombocytopenic purpura	
	Hemophilia	
	Leukemia	
Other acquired conditions	Wegener's granulomatosis	
	Lymphomatoid granulomatosis	
	Cryoglobulinemia	
	Sarcoidosis	
	Churg-Strauss syndrome	
	Inflammatory bowel disease	
	Migraine	

TABLE 39-3
Causes of Stroke in Young Adults (Continued)

Inherited conditions	Ehlers Danlos Homocystinuria Fabry's disease Fibromuscular dysplasia Pseudoxanthoma elasticum CADASIL (cerebral autosomal dominant arteriopathy with subcortical infarcts and leukoencephalopathy	
Pregnancy/Puerperium	ITP Eclampsia Post-partum CNS angiopathy Cerebral venous thrombosis Peripartum cardiomyopathy	
Drugs	Therapeutic	Oral contraceptives, sympathomimetics, MAO inhibitors, L-asparaginase, cytosine arabinoside
	Drugs of Abuse	Cocaine, heroin, amphetamine, alcohol, phenylcyclidine LSD
Medical interventions	Craniocervical vascular procedures Prosthetic valves Surgery Radiation-induced arterial injury Chiropractic maneuvers	Stents, angioplasty, CEA

especially of XII, which may be irritated by an expanding ICA in the neck. An important clue in nearly half of patients is a partial Horner's syndrome with miosis and mild ptosis on the side of the pain. This is caused by irritation of the sympathetic plexus carrying oculomotor fibers, which runs along the internal carotid artery. Sympathetic fibers supplying the ipsilateral facial sweat glands run along the external carotid artery and are not affected in ICA dissection, hence sweating function remains intact.

The symptoms of vertebral dissection include pain in the posterior neck and face, which typically precedes vertigo, nausea, staggering, and/or dysarthria. Embolization is most often to the PICA territory. Signs of lateral medullary dysfunction, including nystagmus, skew deviation, and first division trigeminal sensory loss, may occur (49–52).

Dissection of a major artery may be related to a variety of diseases and types of trauma, many of them seemingly trivial. The spectrum of these is illustrated in Table 39-4. Symptoms of dissection frequently evolve from migraine-like headache to neurologic deficit over days to weeks, making recognition of the inciting event difficult for the patient and clinician. The diagnosis of dissection can be made by MRI/MRA, ultrasound, or catheter angiography. Axial cuts on MRI can be helpful in demonstrating a contracted arterial lumen surrounded by clot, and MRA can demonstrate segmental narrowing or rapid tapering of the arterial lumen in sagittal views. Treatment commonly is with six months of full-dose Coumadin or aspirin to prevent further embolization, though these treatments have not yet been subjected to randomized trials to establish efficacy (46).

Pregnancy and Childbirth (53). Pregnancy and the puerperium are a time of increased risk of stroke for young women. The overall incidence of stroke during this period in the United States in 2000–2001 has been calculated at 34.2 per 100,000 deliveries (54). Recent studies suggest that the risk of stroke is less during the first two trimesters and surges in the peri- and postpartum period. In the Baltimore/Washington area, the relative risk was 5.4 [95% Confidence Interval (CI) 2.9–10] for cerebral infarction and 18.2 (95% CI 8.7–38.1) for intracerebral hemorrhage during the peripartum weeks (51). A Swedish population-based cohort study found a markedly elevated relative risk of SAH of 46.9 (95% CI 19.3–98.4), of ICH 95.0 (95% CI 42.1–194.8), and cerebral infarction 33.8 (95% CI 10.5–84.0) from two days before to one day after delivery, compared to the non-pregnant state (55). Figure 39-1 shows the distribution of stroke risk during

TABLE 39-4
Associated Factors in Cervicocranial Dissection

Diseases	Ehlers-Danlos syndrome type IV
	Marfan syndrome
	Fibromuscular dysplasia
	Cystic medial necrosis
	Pseudoxanthoma elasticum
	Polycystic kidney disease
	Osteogenesis imperfecta type I
	Alpha-1 antitrypsin deficiency
	Coarctation of the aorta
	Syphilitic arteritis
	Pharyngeal infection
	Sympathomimetic drug use
Trauma	Attempted strangulation
	Blunt trauma to neck (cow's tail, car door, car shoulder seatbelt)
	Sharp trauma to neck (gun, knife injuries)
	Hyperextension of neck (dental chair, beauty parlor stroke, bottoms-up dissection, painting a ceiling, CPR)
	Head rotation (chiropractic manipulation, shoveling snow, backing up car, yoga, tennis, bow hunter's stroke)
	Forceful head and body rotation (golfer's stroke)
	Vigorous aerobic exercise (treadmill, rowing machine)

pregnancy in this study. The most frequent cause of both ischemic and hemorrhagic stroke in the puerperium is eclampsia, found in 24–47% of infarctions and 14–44% of intracerebral hemorrhages (53, 56). Rapid and severe elevation of blood pressure is a likely mechanism, and women with underlying aneurysm, arteriovenous malformation (AVM), or other vasculopathy are particularly vulnerable. Other less common associations with pregnancy-related stroke include amniotic fluid embolism, choriocarcinoma, postpartum cerebral angiopathy, infection, cardiomyopathy, and use of ergot derivatives (54, 57). A Nationwide Inpatient Sample analysis from the United States using 2000–2001 data found a number of factors associated with increased risk with an odds ratio (OR) of six or higher:

- Age older than 35 years
- Migraine
- Thrombophilia
- Preexisting heart disease or hypertension
- Systemic lupus erythematosus
- Sickle cell disease
- Thrombocytopenia

Regarding race and ethnicity, black women had a higher risk of stroke than Hispanic or white women

in this study. Of those who suffer a pregnancy-related stroke, 4–15% die, and 10–22% of survivors are too impaired to be discharged home from the acute hospital (54).

Cerebral Venous Thrombosis (CVT).   Cerebral venous thrombosis (CVT) also occurs in late pregnancy and the postpartum period, as well as in hypercoagulable states of other causes. It may cause ischemic and/or hemorrhagic stroke. Its incidence in a recent United States population-based study of pregnancy-related stroke was calculated at 11.6 cases per 100,000 deliveries, nearly as high as the incidence of arterial stroke (13.1 per 100,000). The risk of CVT increases in the presence of an underlying coagulopathy or malignancy, and it is associated with Cesarean delivery, infection, and hypertension (58). The initial symptom is most often headache, which may progress after days or weeks to seizures and/or focal neurologic deficits. Sinus thrombosis causes increased intracranial pressure caused by impaired venous drainage. This may progress to venous infarction, usually of superficial cortical veins, often bihemispheric. The superior sagittal, transverse, and straight sinuses are most often involved. MRI, which clearly delineates the venous sinuses, has greatly improved diagnostic accuracy. Treatment in cases without intracerebral hemorrhage is evolving from anticoagulation with heparin toward targeted thrombolysis, both followed by warfarin for several months.

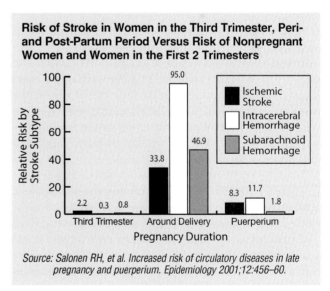

Risk of Stroke in Women in the Third Trimester, Peri- and Post-Partum Period Versus Risk of Nonpregnant Women and Women in the First 2 Trimesters

Source: Salonen RH, et al. Increased risk of circulatory diseases in late pregnancy and puerperium. Epidemiology 2001;12:456–60.

FIGURE 39-1

Risk of stroke in women in the third trimester, peri- and postpartum period versus risk of nonpregnant women and women in the first two trimesters.
Rosamond W, Flegal K, Friday G, et al. Heart Disease and Stroke Statistics: 2007 Update. American Heart Association (14)

Functional outcomes of cerebral venous thromboses are usually good, with 75–85% achieving full, functional recovery (59).

Migraine. Migrainous infarction is a fixed, focal neurologic deficit following an attack of migraine. In population studies, it accounts for 0.5–1.5% of all ischemic strokes and 10–14% of ischemic strokes in young patients (60). Infarction occurs more often in migraine with aura. The mechanism is thought to involve unusually severe cortical spreading depression with hypoperfusion during the aura and/or the head-ache. One-third of these infarcts involve the occipital lobe. Common deficits include visual field cuts, visual-perceptual disturbances, and dysphasias. Migraine is a disease of younger adults and is three times more common in women than men. Consistent with this, a recent meta-analysis found the risk of ischemic stroke to be increased 2.7-fold in women younger than 45 years who suffer from migraine headaches (61). That risk rises further in those with migraines who smoke and/or use oral contraceptives (60, 62). Despite this data, the relationship between migraine and cerebral infarction, and its true incidence has been difficult to clarify because it is difficult to obtain a detailed and precise headache history from patients during an acute neurologic episode. In addition, the definition of migraine has changed over time in the literature. Finally, some large vessel dissections cause unilateral headache with migraine-like features, but they are not true migraine episodes.

Drugs. A number of drugs of abuse and medications have been linked to stroke in young adults. This section will review the major drugs of both classes and their relationship to ischemic and hemorrhagic stroke. Illicit drug use is an important risk factor for stroke in urban young adults. It was associated with 12% of strokes in the Baltimore/Washington young adult population and with 2–39% of strokes in other published case series (63).

Cocaine. Cocaine is responsible for the majority of strokes caused by illicit drug use and has been most studied. It is a local anesthetic and sympathomimetic alkaloid first extracted from the leaf of Erythroxylon coca, a tree native to Peru and Bolivia, in the mid-nineteenth century. For thousands of years in that region, the leaves have been chewed (mixed with lime) or drunk as tea for their stimulant effects. In the early 1900s, cocaine was a frequent component of medicinal tonics for a variety of ailments in the United States, and it was an ingredient in early cola formulations. Growing recognition of its abuse potential led to its inclusion as a Category II drug in the Controlled Substances Act of 1970. The two chemical forms for illicit use are the hydrochloride salt and the freebase. The hydrochloride salt, or powdered form of cocaine, is water-soluble and can be taken intravenously or intranasally. Crack cocaine is a freebase formulation, and, although it is short-acting, it is the most concentrated form of cocaine. The smoke of the freebase is inhaled. Cocaine is sold on the street as a fine, white, crystalline powder, known as coke, C, snow, flake, or blow. It is often diluted with cornstarch, talcum powder, sugar, or the active drugs procaine and amphetamine (64). The incidence of new cocaine users in the United States peaked in 1983 at 1.5 million and then declined to 0.5 million in 1992. In 2000, the number of new users had risen again to 0.9 million (65).

Cocaine use is associated with an increased risk of both hemorrhagic and ischemic stroke. In an HMO population in California, young women reporting cocaine or amphetamine use had an OR for stroke of 6.5 (95% CI = 2.5–16.6) compared to those reporting no drug use, with the OR for hemorrhagic stroke 9.6 (95% CI = 2.7–33.5) and for ischemic stroke 4.5 (95% CI = 0.9–21.6). Case series have reported 2–39% of young stroke patients having associated illicit drug use, predominantly cocaine (66), and the population-based Baltimore/Washington Young Stroke Study found 9.7% of young stroke patients to have a history of recent cocaine use. A number of mechanisms that may lead to hemorrhage have been suggested, such as drug-induced acute hypertension, particularly in individuals with AVM or aneurysm. Other mechanisms include increased platelet aggregation, vasospasm, vasculitis, and apoptosis of cerebral vascular smooth muscle. Complications of cocaine use that can cause stroke include cardiomyopathy leading to arrhythmia or ventricular clot, endocarditis with embolization of septic material, and contaminants in intravenous preparations that embolize to the brain through a preexisting patent foramen ovale (PFO) or atrial septal defect (ASD).

The plasma half-life of cocaine is 60–80 minutes. Smoking provides the fastest route of entry into the cerebral circulation (6–8 seconds), with the intravenous route taking 12–16 seconds. The majority of strokes occur within one hour of ingestion. In one series, a positive urine toxicology screen at the time of presentation was associated with more severe stroke (64, 67).

Amphetamines have similar sympathomimetic effects and spectrum of potential mechanisms in causing hemorrhagic and ischemic stroke (68). Methamphetamine is most often implicated in stroke cases.

Heroin. Heroin, a derivative of morphine, is usually taken intravenously but can be used by oral, nasal, subcutaneous, or inhalational routes. It has been associated with ischemic stroke, with deficits appearing from immediately to more than 24 hours after use. Hypoxia caused by hypotension or respiratory depression, vasculitis, positional vascular compression, and septic embolization caused by endocarditis have been proposed as mechanisms (64, 69).

Clinical studies of the cerebrovascular effects of individual illicit drugs have been hampered by patients' reluctance to admit to use, inconsistent toxicology screening, frequent concomitant ingestion of multiple drugs of unknown purity and potency, and patient populations who have, in addition, a substantial burden of traditional risk factors for stroke.

Sympathomimetics. A number of sympathomimetic agents available in the United States without prescription have been associated with stroke. Dietary supplements containing ephedrine and related alkaloids (also known as ma huang) are taken by young women and others to promote weight loss and boost energy. Pseudoephedrine, phenylephrine, phentermine, oxymetazoline, and fenoxazoline are decongestants included in cough and cold preparations. Phenylpropanolamine has both appetite suppressant and decongestant effects and has been used in both types of preparations. These drugs have all been implicated in cases of stroke, primarily hemorrhagic. In a prospective tertiary center series of 2,500 strokes, 2.5% were associated with use of decongestant preparations, and all but one of these were hemorrhagic. A series of 702 hemorrhagic stroke cases in patients 18–49 years of age found a significant association between stroke and phenylpropanolamine use (70–72). The mechanism of a causal relationship may include drug-induced hypertension, vasoconstriction and secondary hemorrhage, and/or vasculitis (70, 72, 73). In 2004, the Food and Drug Administration (FDA) prohibited the use of ephedra in dietary supplements because of health risks (74). Additionally, since March 2006, the FDA has limited the availability of medications containing pseudoephedrine, phenylpropanolamine, and ephedrine to behind-the-counter rather than over-the-counter sales, with quantity limits and purchaser identification required. The Combat Methamphetamine Epidemic Act of 2005 mandated these restrictions, not because of adverse health effects of the agents, but because of their frequent use in the illicit production of methamphetamine (75). Manufacturers of cough and cold preparations have responded by removing them from most formulations.

Alcohol. In many societies, alcohol consumption begins in adolescence, increases during the young adult period, plateaus during midlife, and decreases in the eighth and ninth decades. The relationship of alcohol consumption to stroke is thus germaine to young adults. While few studies have looked for an association between alcohol and stroke in young adults specifically, many studies of subjects of all adult ages have found that alcohol use increases the risk of ICH and SAH in a linear manner as dose increases. Heavy drinkers, usually defined as persons imbibing more than 40 grams of alcohol per day (three cans of beer or 15 ounces of wine) have a two- to elevenfold increase in their risk of hemorrhagic stroke (76, 77). The relationship between alcohol consumption and ischemic stroke, on the other hand, follows a U- or J-shaped curve, where moderate drinkers have fewer events than either nondrinkers or heavy drinkers. This finding was confirmed specifically in young women in the Baltimore/Washington area (78). However, the definition of *moderate drinking* in this literature has varied from less than once per day to amounts up to two drinks per day, and concern has been expressed that the comparison groups of nondrinkers in some studies may have been self-selected for greater burden of comorbidity (79). The mechanism of the protective effect of moderate alcohol vis-à-vis ischemic stroke is unclear, but may involve raising HDL cholesterol levels, thereby slowing plaque formation (64). A prospective community study of 826 subjects in northern Italy found a slower progression of carotid atherosclerosis over a five-year period among drinkers of 1–50 grams of alcohol per day than among those who drank less or more (79, 80). Alcohol also decreases platelet aggregation and fibrinolytic activity, which may play a role both in increasing risk of hemorrhagic stroke and in protecting moderate drinkers from ischemic events (64). The association of alcohol abuse with cardiomyopathy and atrial arrhythmias provides another possible mechanism for ischemic stroke (77). No specific vascular territory or brain structure has been associated with stroke related to alcohol use. Clinical features and treatment are the same as for other strokes, with the caveat that the presence of an overt coagulopathy caused by alcoholism may complicate therapeutic anticoagulation. Chronic heavy drinkers may experience slower and/or less complete recovery because of prior alcohol-induced brain damage.

Oral Contraceptives. Oral contraceptive (OC) medications came into use in the United States in the 1960s. It was first suggested that they might increase the risk of cerebrovascular events in 1962. The mechanism of thrombosis from OC medication may involve the elevation of plasma levels of Factors VIIc and XIIc, which occurs in a dose-related fashion in OC users and may promote generation of thrombin (81).

There is convincing evidence that current low-dose OCs (less than 50 mcg estrogen) do not increase the risk of arterial stroke in women without vascular risk factors. Hypertensive users, however, as well as smokers and women with migraine headaches have an increased risk of arterial infarction, and the risk of cerebral venous thrombosis is increased. In the WHO international study, relative risk (RR) was 10–14 for hypertensive OC users and 4.7 for OC users who smoke (82).

Low-dose OCs should be used with caution in women with migraine headaches, who smoke, who are hypertensive, or who have genetic thrombophilic defects due to variably increased, though still low, risk of stroke (83).

Thrombophilic States

A number of acquired and inherited thrombophilic states related to stroke in young adults have been described in recent decades. Even though all of them [deficiency of proteins C, S, and antithrombin III (AT3), Factor V Leiden, Prothrombin gene 20210A, and the antiphospholipid antibody syndrome] are strongly associated with venous thrombosis, only the antiphospholipid antibody syndrome has a strong correlation with arterial stroke. The latter is also the only one of these conditions with distinctive clinical features. First described in 1983, the antiphospholipid antibody syndrome (APS) is diagnosed when a patient has had one or more episodes of arterial or venous thrombosis in any organ leading to tissue infarction or fetal loss and when the patient is demonstrated to have antiphospholipid antibodies (lupus anticoagulant [LA] and/or cardiolipin) in plasma on at least two occasions six weeks apart (84). Other frequently associated findings in APS are thrombocytopenia (40–50%); livedo reticularis, a lacey pattern of microvascular occlusion occurring in the skin of the back and extremities (11–22%); and hemolytic anemia (14–23%) (85). The brain is the most common site of arterial thromboembolism, and neurologic manifestations may include TIA, cerebral infarction, cerebral venous thrombosis, multi-infarct dementia, seizures, encephalopathy, migraines, transverse myelitis, chorea, and mononeuritis multiplex. In situ arterial thrombosis of vessels of all sizes and embolism from cardiac valvular vegetations that occur in approximately 4% of patients are the mechanisms underlying these diverse phenomena. A wide variety of effects involving other organs has been described as well (85).

Primary APS occurs in patients without an autoimmune disease; secondary APS occurs in patients with autoimmune or other disease, most often systemic lupus erythematosus. Treatment recommendations continue to evolve with accumulating evidence. Anticoagulation with warfarin, but not antiplatelet agents, is beneficial in preventing recurrent thrombosis, and the benefit of antiplatelet therapy for asymptomatic individuals with LA or anticardiolipin antibodies is unclear (84–86).

Factor V Leiden, Prothrombin 20210A, and deficiencies of protein C, S, and antithrombin III cause thrombosis by impairing the normal modulation of thrombin generation and inactivation. They are strongly associated with venous thrombotic events and variably with arterial stroke. Their frequent clinical expression in the early adult years, with the majority of patients experiencing their first thrombotic event before the age of 45, makes them relevant to our discussion (29).

Resistance to activated protein C is caused by base substitution (adenine for guanine) at position 1691 on the Factor V gene. The resulting mutation is called Factor V Leiden (FVL). This mutation occurs in about 5% of the Caucasian population, but is rare in Africans and Asians. Even though its association with increased risk of venous thrombotic disease is clear, its relationship to arterial stroke is less certain. A recent meta-analysis found a modest increase in risk of ischemic stroke primarily among patients <55 years of age carrying FVL (29, 86, 87).

Another substitution of adenine for guanine, at nucleotide 20210 of the Prothrombin gene (G20210A), has similarly been associated with increased risk of venous thrombosis at all ages and modest risk of arterial stroke in younger adults. The greater effect of these two mutations on producing venous rather than arterial thrombosis may relate to the difference in the thrombotic process, with stasis an important predisposing factor on the venous side and endothelial damage with platelet activation driving arterial clot formation.

In large blood vessels, proteins C, S, and antithrombin III all act by different mechanisms to control thrombin generation (29). Several case series of stroke in young adults have found approximately 5% of patients with protein C deficiency, though others have seen no increase over the control rate (88). Case reports and series describing stroke associated with deficiency of protein S, which may be inherited or acquired in sepsis or pregnancy or caused by hormonal therapy, are more extensive. Arterial stroke and cerebral venous thrombosis may occur in the same individual, and the frequency of protein S deficiency appears to be higher in young adult stroke patients than in older groups (86). Evidence linking deficiency of antithrombin III to arterial stroke is weak, and it appears that this deficiency, which slows thrombin inactivation, is nearly exclusively involved in venous thromboses.

The above conditions of modest effect in promoting stroke may be potentiated by the addition of acquired thrombophilic factors, including pregnancy, oral contraceptives, smoking, migraine, hypertension, diabetes mellitus, and dyslipidemia. Most experts currently believe that population screening for inherited thrombophilic states is not warranted because of the low incidence of major vascular events. Clinicians treating individual patients must exercise judgment on this point based on the patient's composite of medical and family history as well as acquired risk factors.

Patent Foramen Ovale

Patent foramen ovale (PFO) is a persistent fetal communication between the right and left atria of the heart. It is present in >25% of adults and is associated with ischemic stroke in adults <55 years old and less clearly with stroke in older adults. PFOs are thought to cause stroke by allowing paradoxical embolization across the opening from venous to arterial sites, although the possibility of in situ thrombus formation in a tunnel-like PFO or an increased risk of atrial arrhythmia and thrombus because of the presence of the defect has not been excluded. First described in 1877, PFO was difficult to diagnose in vivo until the advent of contrast echocardiography.

The presence of an atrial septal aneurysm with a PFO significantly increases the risk of ischemic stroke. Additionally, atrial anatomic variants, including a prominent Eustachian valve or Chiari's network, and lower extremity or pelvic venous thrombi or a predisposition to these—caused by presence of the Factor V Leiden mutation, G20210A, an elevated factor VIII level, the antiphospholipid antibody syndrome, or May-Thurner syndrome—can increase the chance of a PFO leading to a stroke. An intriguing association between PFO and migraine with aura has been found in case control studies, and others have noted a decrease in migraine attacks after PFO closure. The mechanism of this association remains speculative, but may involve the presence of a gene modulating both cardiac and vascular development, left to right shunting of an endogenous substance normally metabolized in the lung (such as serotonin) into the systemic arterial circulation, or left to right shunting of microemboli (60, 89).

Strokes of Undetermined Cause

An important feature of the literature on stroke in young adults is the high percentage of strokes of undetermined cause in most series. A number of these are summarized in Table 39-5. Additionally, Bevan et al., reviewing the literature in 1990, noted that a cause is found 55–93% of the time in young adults (90). Even though it is reassuring in clinical practice to be able to say to a young stroke patient after an exhaustive workup that no serious disease or defect has been found to explain the stroke, it is at the same time frustrating and worrisome when no cause can been identified. Without a cause, no estimate of risk of recurrence can be made, and no focused plan developed to minimize that risk.

Several definitional issues contribute to the high rate of strokes of unknown etiology. First, the TOAST criteria, a five-category classification of stroke mechanism developed for the Trial of ORG 10172 in Acute Stroke Therapy (TOAST), have been used in a number of young stroke series and also have the advantage of widespread use and familiarity (42). However, the five categories—large artery atherosclerosis, small vessel occlusion, cardioembolism, other determined etiology, and unknown etiology—were designed for an older population with a predominance of atherosclerotic disease. Other than the 10–20% caused by large artery atherosclerosis and the 20% of young adult strokes caused by cardioembolism, most strokes in young adults fall into the "other determined etiology" and "undetermined etiology" categories of this classification. Further, these categories are broad and refer to the vascular mechanism rather than the specific etiology of the stroke. Other than TOAST, however, there are no widely recognized classification systems for stroke etiology, and young stroke studies have used a variety of ad hoc instruments, with variable definitions of *unknown* or *cryptogenic, probable cause*, and *possible cause*. Conditions of disputed or unclear etiologic importance—migraine, mitral valve prolapse, PFO, alcohol, and oral contraceptives—are classified differently by different authors. An etiologic classification scheme specifically for young adult stroke has been proposed, taking into account our recently acquired ability

---

TABLE 39-5
Stroke of Undetermined Cause in Young Adults

AUTHOR	STUDY TYPE	LOCATION	UNDETERMINED CAUSE (%)
Kittner, 1998 (44)	Population-based	Baltimore, Maryland	31.8
Adams, 1995 (91)	Population-based	Iowa	34.3
Camerlingo, 2000 (92)	Hospital series	Bergamo, Italy	21.5
Naess, 2004 (93)	Population-based	Western Norway	47.8
Quereshi, 1995 (66)	Hospital series	Atlanta, Georgia	26
Lee, 2002 (94)	Hospital series	Taiwan	23.5

to diagnose large vessel dissection and CVT reliably via MR. Hoffman et al. propose the following categories for stroke in young adults:

- Large vessel
- Small vessel
- Cardiogenic
- Dissection
- Prothrombotic states
- Migraine-induced
- Cerebral venous thrombosis
- Vasculitides
- Vasculopathy other
- Miscellaneous
- Unknown (95)

Use of classification schemes such as this one designed for this population segment may help to reduce the number of strokes reported as "unknown cause."

The historical emphasis in American and European medical culture on finding the one unifying cause for an illness or group of symptoms is beginning to yield to the recognition that a constellation of factors—some genetic and some environmental or behavioral—often come together to cause a medical event (96). Many strokes in young adults are likely multifactorial, the result of several mild genetic predispositions or the intersection of genetic predisposition and acquired risk factors. A case control study by Martinelli et al. found women taking oral contraceptives to have 13 times the risk of stroke if they also have the Factor V Leiden and 9 times the risk if they have the prothrombin 20210A mutation, compared to women on oral contraceptives without either mutation (97). Smoking and hypertension also appear to increase the risk created by genetic predispositions. Pezzini et al. found that patients with two of four predisposing polymorphisms [Prothrombin 20210A, Factor V Leiden, the TT677 genotype of the methylenetetrahydrofolate reductase (MTHFR) gene, and epsilon-4 carriership of the apolipoprotein gene] had OR for stroke of 3.5 (CI 1.40–9.98), but, if they also smoked, the OR rose to 15.99 (CI 4.01–63.3). If they had two polymorphisms and were hypertensive, the OR for stroke rose to 10.79 (95% CI 1.01–115.4) (96). It may turn out that many of the strokes categorized as "cryptogenic" occur because of alignment of several genetic and acquired risk factors in the individual.

Population Differences

Population-based studies, though superior to case series in gauging the spectrum and distribution of causes of stroke, are subject to the variations among populations studied. In United States urban populations, for example, stroke caused by illicit drug use accounts for as many as 12% of young adult cases, whereas, in a Saudi university hospital series, it accounted for 2% and, in the Bern and Zurich stroke registries, just 0.5% of cases (98, 99). In Khorasan province in Iran, 54% percent of infarctions in young adults are of cardio-embolic origin, twice the frequency found in American and European populations. Chagas disease, rare or absent as a cause of stroke in most studies, accounted for 4 of 106 young adult stroke cases in a Brazilian series (16, 43). As knowledge of stroke in young adults accumulates, our appreciation of its variability over time and from place to place increases.

DIFFERENTIAL DIAGNOSIS OF STROKE IN YOUNG ADULTS

A number of other illnesses can confuse the diagnosis of stroke in young adults. A list of these is provided in Table 39-6. The relative rarity of stroke in young adults predisposes providers to consider first and sometimes exclusively the more routine etiologies of headache, neck pain, ear pain, and dizziness. Reliance on noncontrast head CT as the sole imaging screen for CNS disease will allow some strokes in young adults to be missed because of CT's limited sensitivity to acute infarction and ischemic territory at risk. In a recent series of 15 misdiagnosed cases of cerebellar infarction, half of the patients were younger than 50 years. A normal head CT and a poorly

---

TABLE 39-6

Differential Diagnosis of Stroke in Young Adults

Brain infection
Brain neoplasm
Cranial nerve palsy
Peripheral nerve palsy
Hemiplegic migraine
Demyelinating diseases
Benign positional vertigo
Vestibulitis
Unrecognized seizure with postictal neurologic deficit
Toxic metabolic encephalopathy (hypoglycemia, hepatic encephalopathy)
Brown-Sequard syndrome (hemiplegia and contralateral hemisensory loss)
Conversion disorder
Progressive multifocal leukoencephalopathy (PML)
Subcortical leukoencephalopathy (Binswanger's disease)
Mitochondrial Encephalopathy, Lactic Acidosis and Stroke-like episodes (MELAS)

documented neurologic exam were frequent findings in this series, and incorrect diagnoses included migraine, toxic encephalopathy, gastritis, meningitis, myocardial infarction, and polyneuropathy (100). Younger adults may be more prone to misdiagnosis because of both their lesser frequency of stroke and their higher prevalence of certain, easily confused conditions, such as multiple sclerosis and conversion disorder. Increased recognition of the importance of stroke in the younger population and routine availability of more definitive imaging techniques will improve our ability to identify stroke rapidly in this group.

On the other hand, patients may be diagnosed with stroke in the emergency room and later be found to have other illnesses. Postictal weakness and confusion, for example, may persist for days to weeks after an unwitnessed seizure, and serial scans, EEG, and further history may be needed to clarify the diagnosis. Brain tumors, multiple sclerosis, and PML may present with neurologic findings, and scan appearances consistent with stroke and the diagnosis may not become clear until deficits progress and/or scans evolve. In an emergency department study of 463 patients given diagnoses of stroke or TIA, 19 were later discharged from the hospital with different diagnoses, including seizure, migraine, peripheral neuropathy, cranial nerve neuropathy, and psychogenic paralysis. The mean age of those misdiagnosed was 55, whereas it was 65 for those correctly diagnosed (101). Conversion disorder with motor symptoms occurs on average at age 39. Symptoms include paralysis, ataxia, tremor, sensory loss, pain, blindness, and dysphonia in patterns consistent with stroke (102). This disorder may be suspected, but is infrequently diagnosed early in the patient's hospital course, particularly during the first episode of psychogenic symptoms. Conversion symptoms typically respond well to rehabilitative therapies, though relapse is common.

TREATMENT

Young patients are offered the most advanced and aggressive treatments available for all illnesses more readily than elderly patients. In acute stroke treatment, this tendency is reflected in use of hemicraniectomy for malignant middle cerebral territory infarction. This procedure is offered to appropriate patients under 50–60 years of age because of accumulating evidence that younger patients have better survival and functional outcome (103, 104). Younger patients are also offered the most aggressive and technologically advanced rehabilitation treatments because of their lesser burden of comorbidity and prior disability and, therefore, their greater tolerance and lower risk of complications.

OUTCOMES

Survival

The case fatality rate (death within 30 days of the ictus-CFR) for stroke in young adults ranges between 10–34% in published series. As in the older population, CFRs are higher in ICH and SAH than infarction. In an epidemiological study evaluating racial differences in CFR in the 1990s, no significant difference between white and black young stroke patients in Cincinnati was found (8, 105). Mortality is highest in the first year after stroke, declining in subsequent years (106). Mortality was 1.7% per year among ischemic stroke patients under the age of 45 in the Iowa Registry of Stroke in Young Adults (107), and 86% of these patients were alive at follow-up, a mean of six years after the stroke. This last finding was consistent with that of Marini et al., who found an 86.5% 10-year survival for ischemic stroke in patients ages 15–44 in a multisite series (107, 108). As would be expected given these survival rates, the prevalence of young stroke survivors has increased over time. In the United States, there were 590,000 ages 25–59 in 1973, growing to 965,000 in 1991 (109). Individual survival, of course, depends on the cause and severity of the stroke and the burden of comorbid conditions.

Function

Global functional outcomes for young adults are generally good. In Western Norway, 80% of young infarction patients achieved a Modified Rankin Scale (mRS) ≤ 2 at three months post-stroke and 78% at long-term follow-up (mean 5.7 years) (10, 93). Case series have consistently corroborated this finding, with 96% of the 272 cases studied by Varona et al. achieving mRS ≤ 2 at three years post-stroke (101). Camerlingo et al. found that 91% of their 135 cases evaluated at one year had achieved mRS scores ≤ 3 (92), and Neau et al. found that 86% of their 65 cases at follow-up (mean 32 months) had RS ≤ 3 (110). In the series of Musolino et al., 89% of 54 young patients evaluated a mean of 6.12 years after stroke had mRS ≤ 3 (111).

In population-based studies as well as case series, the great majority of young stroke survivors achieve good functional outcome in self-care and mobility. Marini et al. in northern Italy recorded 84% achieving a Barthel Index of ≥ 90 at the end of follow-up (108). Varona et al. found that 90% of their 272 cases were independent in ADLs and 95% could walk without assistance at follow-up (mean 12 years) (106), and Kappelle et al. noted 92% with Barthel Index scores >90 (107). Poor outcome after stroke in young adults has been associated with a history of diabetes mellitus, severe deficit at presentation, stroke involving the total anterior circulation, and large artery atherosclerosis (93, 99, 106). There is evidence that functional recovery occurs more quickly in younger than elderly patients in an inpatient rehabilitation setting. In analyzing a large consecutive series of stroke patients stratified into five age subgroups, Black-Schaffer and Winston found that younger patients had significantly higher FIM efficiencies (FIM points gained per day) during inpatient rehabilitation (112). Older patients often enter rehabilitation at a lower level because of pre-stroke functional limitations and progress more slowly related to a greater burden of comorbid conditions (112–115). Because treating staff feel that young patients have greater functional potential and more complex goals than their elderly counterparts, young adult stroke patients tend to remain in rehabilitation facilities longer than the elderly (112) and are offered the newest and most aggressive rehabilitation regimens.

Community Discharge

In keeping with their higher functional level at discharge, young adult stroke patients are discharged back to the community more often than the elderly. Black-Schaffer and Winston found that, in a cohort of 979 stroke rehabilitation inpatients, 84% of those under age 55 were discharged home, in contrast to 54% of those older than 85 years. Alexander, Granger, et al. found the same trend in separate American cohorts of inpatient rehabilitation patients examined a decade earlier (112, 116, 117). In the United States, skilled nursing facilities are often reluctant to accept young patients because of lack of appropriate programming, further reinforcing this trend.

Return to Work

The ability to perform valued work is central to self-esteem and an important goal for most young stroke patients (118). Between 3–84% of patients achieve this goal, with the wide range reported in this literature caused by differing age ranges of patients reported, variable definitions of work, and disability compensation systems with different incentive structures (119). Numerous series have examined the percentage of patients returning to work after the stroke. Those that evaluate patients less than 45 years of age find notably higher percentages of patients returning to work than those that evaluate patients up to the age of 65. These studies are summarized in Table 39-7.

Many case series have been analyzed for factors associated with success in returning to work. Variables cited have included:

- Pure motor or no hemiparesis (126, 131)
- Good self-care and mobility function (93, 119, 132–134)
- No aphasia or apraxia (110, 119, 120)

- Advanced education (93, 110, 135, 136)
- Preserved cognition (118, 126)
- White-collar job (133–136)
- Married status (93)
- Younger age (93, 132, 130, 134)

Variables identified as barriers to successful vocational rehabilitation include, in addition to the reverse of these factors:

- Visual/perceptual impairment (126)
- Depression (110, 126)
- Economic disincentives related to disability and retirement benefits (133, 137)

Of those returning to work after a stroke, about two-thirds reduce hours and/or duties (118, 138). The rehabilitation physician is often asked to certify that the young stroke patient is "medically cleared" to return to work. This may mean certifying only that the patient has sufficient cardiovascular capacity to perform the job, but, more often, it is a request for a detailed evaluation of the patient's cognitive, physical, and psychological capacity as they relate to specific job requirements. This assessment is complex and is ideally accomplished with the assistance of a coordinated multidisciplinary team, including physical, occupational, speech therapist, neuropsychologist, and vocational rehabilitation counselor (137).

Patients who are able to resume work after a stroke on average do so within the first six months. In the United States, the 1990 Americans with Disabilities Act had a positive impact on employers' responsiveness to the requests of stroke survivors for accommodations on their pre-stroke job, not only regarding physical access and equipment, but also for personal assistance, schedule flexibility, and task modification (137). On the other hand, employers' concerns regarding possible costs associated with stroke survivors as new hires may, in some cases, make it hard for survivors to change to a different job.

Driving

Throughout the developed world, a return to driving has become a necessary step to resuming a normal lifestyle and avoiding social isolation. In many locations, it is a prerequisite for returning to gainful employment. It has been estimated that half of stroke survivors in the United States return to driving without advice or reevaluation of their fitness to drive (139). Of those who do seek reevaluation, approximately half are successful in passing driving evaluations (140, 141). In the United States, many rehabilitation clinics offer written tests of driving ability. These can be useful for screening out patients with significant perceptual or cognitive problems who would be unsafe in a road test setting. In one study, two

TABLE 39-7
Return to Work after Stroke

Studies of patients under the age of 46

Author	Year	N	RTW	Ages	Work
Adunsky et al. (153)	1992	30	81%	20–45	FT, other
Bogousslavsky & Regli (120)	1987	41	81%	<30	FT
Camerlingo et al. (92)	2000	135	62%	16–45	unspecified
Ferro & Crespo (121)	1994	140	73%	<46	FT, PT, HM, S
Hindfelt & Nilsson (122)	1977	52	84%	16–40	FT, PT
Kappelle et al. (107)	1994	274	42%	15–44	unspecified
Leys et al. (123)	2002	265	60%	15–45	unspecified
Marini et al. (108)	1999	330	56%	15–44	unspecified
Musolino et al. (111)	2003	60	69%	17–45	FT, PT
Naess et al. (93)	2004	134	68%	15–44	unspecified
Neau et al. (110)	1998	63	73%	15–45	FT, PT, HM, S
Varona et al. (106)	2004	240	53%	15–44	unspecified

Studies of patients under the age of 65

Authors	Year	N	RTW	Ages	Work
Black-Schaffer&Osberg (119)	1990	79	49%	21–65	FT, PT, HM, S
Coughlan & Humphrey (124)	1982	170	33%	<65	FT, PT
Fugl-Meyer et al. (125)	1975	83	41%	<65	FT, PT, HM
Kotila et al. (126)	1984	58	55%	<65	CE, HM, S
Mackay & Nias (127)	1979	45	38%	<65	unspecified
Saeki et al. (128)	1993	230	58%	<65	FT, PT, HM, S
Weisbroth et al. (129)	1971	62	37%	<65	CE
Wozniak et al. (130)	1999	109	53%	mean 55	FT, PT

FT = full-time, PT = part-time, HM = homemaking, S = student, CE = competitive employment

commonly used tests, the Motor Free Visual Perception Test and the Trail Making B test, were found to correlate closely with on-the-road driving performance (142). Computerized driving simulators also hold promise both as screening tools and training devices (143, 144), though their adoption in clinical rehabilitation settings has been slow. In the published case series on this topic, a number of factors have been associated with driving performance after stroke:

- Right hemisphere location of stroke (141, 145, 146)
- Visual perceptual deficits (142, 147)
- Reduced sustained and selective attention (148, 149)
- Impulsivity or poor judgment (141, 147)
- Lack of organizational skills (149)

All correlate with poor performance behind the wheel. Aphasia, though it may negatively impact performance on written and road tests because of compromised processing of verbal or written instructions, does not always interfere with self-directed driving (139, 147, 150). And physical impairment alone does not increase the risk of accidents or traffic violations (141). Physicians are often consulted about a patient's readiness to resume driving, and, though visual perception can be readily screened, the evaluation of attention, judgment, and organizational ability is more complex and benefits from involvement of a neurologic rehabilitation team (151). An on-the-road test performed either by a driving instructor or by a state licensing agency remains the gold standard for assessing driving ability.

Parenting

The young adult stroke survivor who needs to return to parenting faces physical as well as cognitive and perceptual challenges in the performance of child bathing, dressing, feeding, and transporting tasks. Fortunately, many helpful items of equipment are readily available. Disposable diapers with adhesive tabs require less dexterity than cloth diapers with pin closures. Microwaves make heating bottles of formula easier and safer than warming them in a pan of boiling water. Baby tub inserts help to stabilize an infant for bathing and so on. Other adult family members, home care occupational therapists, and/or hired childcare assistants can provide valuable assistance to the stroke survivor in problem-solving performance of these tasks. When the survivor requires physical assistance to accomplish a childcare activity, he or she should be encouraged to assume the supervisory role whenever possible.

Even more challenging, potentially, is the establishment and maintenance of a loving and effective relationship between a disabled parent and a growing child because children's needs and perceptions of their parents evolve as psychosocial development proceeds. The child's second parent, or another adult important to the child, can play an important role in helping both parties negotiate this relationship over time.

RECURRENCE

The likelihood of a second stroke increases as young patients' vascular disease risk factors multiply. In Hordaland County, Norway, risk of recurrence ranged from 2.1% during the mean six-year follow-up period for those young adult stroke survivors without hypertension, diabetes, hypercholesterolemia, smoking, angina, myocardial infarction, or intermittent claudication to 67% recurrence for those with five of these risk factors (152). Recurrence rates are highest in the first year after ischemic stroke, ranging from 1–3% (106, 108, 123). For certain nonatherosclerotic stroke etiologies, recurrence risk is well-defined. After carotid dissection, recurrences occur in approximately 10% at the rate of 1% per year, and they are usually in a different artery. Recurrences are more common in those with first dissection under age 45 (47). Cerebral venous thrombosis carries an overall recurrence rate of 11%, which may reflect comorbid conditions such as cancer with continuing thrombophilia (59). Risk of recurrence after a drug- or pregnancy-induced stroke depends on whether intake of the drug is resumed or pregnancy is again undertaken.

It is important for the young stroke survivor and his or her physician to review the etiology of the patient's stroke, identify modifiable risk factors for recurrence, and jointly develop a plan to minimize these. The patient's motivation to comply with treatment for hypertension and diabetes, develop a habit of compliance with newly prescribed anticoagulation therapy, quit smoking, avoid excessive alcohol intake, and turn away from the use of street drugs will be maximal in the months following the stroke. Close medical follow-up to reinforce the risk reduction plan and monitor its effects will improve the likelihood of success. Young adult survivors with stroke of unknown etiology face unavoidable uncertainty regarding the risk of recurrence. It is not clear that empiric prescribing of preventive medications for these individuals in the absence of corresponding risk factors, though sometimes an attractive way to deal with the natural desire to do something, is beneficial (152). Significant progress has been made in elucidating components of the stroke of unknown etiology category in recent years, and we can anticipate that future research will shed further light on this area.

References

1. Weinfeld FD. National survey of stroke. *Stroke* 1981; 12(No. 2 Suppl 1):11–90.
2. National Institute on Disability and Rehabilitation Research. Multiple sclerosis: Hope through research. 1996:75.
3. The National SCI Statistical Center. Spinal cord injury: Facts and figures at a glance. 2006.
4. Radhakrishnan K, Ashok PP, Sridharan R, Mousa ME. Stroke in the young: Incidence and pattern in Benghazi, Libya. *Acta Neurol Scand* 1986; 73:434–438.
5. Nencini P, Inzitari D, Baruffi MC, et al. Incidence of stroke in young adults in Florence, Italy. *Stroke* 1988; 19:977–981.
6. Kristensen B, Malm J, Carlberg B, et al. Epidemiology and etiology of ischemic stroke in young adults aged 18 to 44 years in Northern Sweden. *Stroke* 1997; 28:1702–1709.
7. Lidegaard O, Soe M, Andersen MVN. Cerebral thromboembolism among young women and men in Denmark 1977–82. *Stroke* 1986; 17:670–675.
8. Jacobs BS, Boden-Albala BB, Lin IF, Sacco RL. Stroke in the young in the Northern Manhattan Stroke Study. *Stroke* 2002; 33:2789–2793.
9. Leno C, Berciano J, Combarros O, et al. A prospective study of stroke in young adults in Cantabria, Spain. *Stroke* 1993; 24:792–795.
10. Naess H, Nyland HI, Thomassen L, et al. Incidence and short-term outcome of cerebral infarction in young adults in Western Norway. *Stroke* 2002; 33:2105–2108.
11. Rozenthul-Sorokin N, Ronen R, Tamir A, et al. Stroke in the young in Israel. *Stroke* 1996; 27:838–841.
12. Guidetti D, Baratti M, Zucco RG, et al. Incidence of stroke in young adults in the Reggio Emilia area, northern Italy. *Neuroepidemiology* 1993; 12:82–87.
13. Rosman KD. The epidemiology of stroke in an urban black population. *Stroke* 1986; 17(4):667–669.
14. Rosamond W, Flegal K, Friday G, et al. Heart disease and stroke statistics—2007 update: A report from the American Heart Association Statistics Committee and Stroke Statistics Subcommittee. *Circulation* 2007; 115(5):169–171.
15. Gross CR, S KC, Mohr JP, et al. Stroke in South Alabama: Incidence and diagnostic features—a population-based study. *Stroke* 1984; 15:249–255.
16. Ghandehari K, Moud ZI. Incidence and etiology of ischemic stroke in Persian young adults. *Acta Neurol Scand* 2006; 113(2):121–124.
17. Corbin DOC, Poddar V, Hennis A, et al. Incidence and case fatality rates of first-ever stroke in a black Caribbean population: The Barbados Register of strokes. *Stroke* 2004; 35:1254–1258.
18. Marini C, Totaro R, De Santis F, et al. Stroke in young adults in the community-based L-Aquila registry. *Stroke* 2001; 32:52–56.
19. Baird A. Anterior Circulation Stroke. *emedicine/webMD*.
20. Brown RD, Whisnant JP, Sicks JD, et al. Stroke incidence, prevalence, and survival: Secular trends in Rochester, Minnesota, through 1989. *Stroke* 1996; 27:373–380.
21. Osuntokun BO, Bademosi O, Akinkugbe OO, et al. Incidence of stroke in an African city: Results from the Stroke Registry at Ibadan, Nigeria, 1973–75. *Stroke.* 1979; 19:205–207.
22. Kissela B, Schneider A, Kleindorfer D, et al. Stroke in a biracial population. *Stroke* 2004; 35:426–431.
23. Sacco RL, Boden-Albala B, Gan R, et al. Stroke incidence among white, black, and Hispanic residents of an urban community: The Northern Manhattan Stroke Study. *American Journal of Epidemiology* 1998; 147:259–268.
24. Kittner SJ, McCarter RJ, Sherwin RW, et al. Black-white differences in stroke risk among young adults. *Stroke* 1993; 24 (Suppl I):I13–I15.

25. Eckstrom PT BF, Ediavitch SA, Parrish HM. Epidemiology of stroke in a rural area. *Public Health Reports* 1969; 84:878–882.

26. Heyman A, Karp HR, Heyden S, et al. Cerebrovascular disease in the biracial population of Evans Country, Georgia. *Arch Intern Med* 1971; 128:949–955.

27. Stewart JA, Dundas R, Howard RS, et al. Ethnic differences in incidence of stroke: Prospective study with stroke register. *British Medical Journal* 1999; 318:967–971.

28. Hart RG, Miller VT. Cerebral infarction in young adults: A practical approach. *Stroke* 1983; 14(1):110–114.

29. Seligsohn U, Lubetsky A. Genetic susceptibility to venous thrombosis. *N Engl J Med* 2001; 344(16):1222–1231.

30. Singhal AB. Cerebral vasoconstriction syndromes. *Top Stroke Rehabil* 2004; 11(2):1–6.

31. Rothwell DM, Bondy SJ, Williams JI. Chiropractic manipulation and stroke: A population-based case-control study. *Stroke* 2001; 32:1054–1060.

32. Schultz-Hector S, Trott KR. Radiation-induced cardiovascular diseases: Is the epidemiologic evidence compatible with the radiobiologic data? *Int J Radiat Oncol Biol Phys* Jan 1 2007; 67(1):10-18.

33. Friedlander AH, August M. The role of panoramic radiography in determining an increased risk of cervical atheromas in patients treated with therapeutic irradiation. *Oral Surg Oral Med Oral Pathol Oral Radiol Endod* 1998; 85(3):339–344.

34. Loftus ML, Schumacher HC, Meyers PM. Interventional therapy for carotid artery disease using angioplasty and stenting with embolic protection. *Minerva Cardioangiol* 2006; 54(5):679–685.

35. Kevorkian CG. Stroke rehabilitation and the cardiac transplantation patient. *Am J Phys Med Rehabil* 2000; 79:558–564.

36. Ponticelli C, Campise MR. Neurological complications in kidney transplant recipients. *J Nephrol* 2005; 18(5):521–528.

37. Meeske KAN, Marvin D, Lavey RS, et al. Premature carotid artery disease in long-term survivors of childhood cancer treated with neck irradiation: A series of 5 cases. *J Pediatr Hematol Oncol* 2007; 29(7):480.

38. Wiebers DO, Feigin VL, Brown RD. Cerebrovascular disease in children and young adults. *Handbook of Stroke*. 2nd ed. Lippincott Williams & Wilkins, 2006:273–276.

39. Bendixen BH, Posner J, Lango R. Stroke in young adults and children. *Current Neurology and Neuroscience Reports* 2001; 1:54–66.

40. Williams LS, Garg BP, Cohen M, et al. Subtypes of ischemic stroke in children and young adults. *Neurology* 1997; 49(6):1541–1545.

41. Blecic S, Bogousslavsky J. Stroke in young adults. In: Barnett HJM, Mohr JP, Stein BM, Yatsu FM, eds. *Stroke: Pathophysiology and Management*. 3rd ed. New York: Churchill Livingstone, 1998:1001–1012.

42. Adams H. Stroke mechanism categories from the Trial of ORG 10172 in Acute Stroke Study 1)small vessel occlusion, 2) large artery atherosclerosis, 3) cardioembolism, 4) other determined etiology, 5) undetermined etiology. *JAMA* 1998; 279:1265–1272.

43. Neto JIS, Santos AC, Fabio SRC, Sakamoto AC. Cerebral infarction in patients aged 15 to 40 years. *Stroke* 1996; 27:2016–2019.

44. Kittner RJ, Stern BJ, Wozniak M, et al. Cerebral infarction in young adults: The Baltimore-Washington Cooperative Young Stroke Study. *Neurology* 1998; 50:890–894.

45. Stern BJ, Wityk RJ. Stroke in the young. *Current Diagnosis in Neurology* 1994:34–40.

46. Lyrer P, Engelter S. Antithrombotic drugs for carotid artery dissection. *Cochrane Database of Systematic Reviews* 2005; 2005(4).

47. Biller J. Strokes in the young. In: JF T, ed. *Cerebrovascular Disorders*. 5th ed. 1999:283–316.

48. Lee VH, Brown RD, Mandrekar JN, Mokri B. Incidence and outcome of cervical artery dissection: A population-based study. *Neurology* 2006; 67:1809-1812.

49. Brandt T, Orberk E, Werner H. Cervical artery dissection syndromes. *Stroke Syndromes*. 2nd ed. Bogousslavsky J, Caplan L. eds. Edinburgh, Cambridge University Press, 2001:660–666.

50. Caplan LR, Biousse V. Cervicocranial arterial dissections. *J Neuro-Opthalmol* 2004; 24(4):299–305.

51. Schievink WI. Spontaneous dissection of the carotid and vertebral arteries. *NEJM* 2001; 344(12):898–906.

52. Wityk RJ. Stroke in a healthy 46-year-old man. *JAMA* 2001; 285:2757–2762.

53. Kittner SJ, Stern BJ, Feeser BR, et al. Pregnancy and the risk of stroke. *N Engl J Med* 1996; 335(11):768–774.

54. James AH, Bushnell CD, Jamison MG, Myers ER. Incidence and risk factors for stroke in pregnancy and the puerperium. *Obstetrics and Gynecology* 2005; 106(3):509–516.

55. Salonen Ros H, Lichtenstein P, Bellocco R, et al. Increased risks of circulatory diseases in late pregnancy and puerperium. *Epidemiology* 2001; 12(4):456–460.

56. Sharshar T, C L, Mas JL. Incidence and causes of strokes associated with pregnancy and puerperium: A study in public hospitals of Ile de France. *Stroke* 1995; 26:930–936.

57. Bousser MG. Stroke in women. *Circulation* 1999; 99:463–467.

58. Lanska DJ, Kryscio RJ. Risk factors for peripartum and postpartum stroke and intracranial venous thrombosis. *Stroke* 2000; 31(6):1274–1282.

59. Dzialo AF, Black-Schaffer RM. Cerebral venous thrombosis in young adults: Two case reports. *Arch Phys Med Rehabil* 2001; 82(5):683–688.

60. Bousser MG, Welch K, Michael A. Relation between migraine and stroke. *Lancet Neurol* 2005; 4:533–542.

61. Etminan M, Takkouche B, Isorna FC, Samii A. Risk of ischaemic stroke in people with migraine: Systematic review and meta-analysis of observational studies. *BMJ* 2005; 330:63–65.

62. Lampl C, Marecek S. Migraine and stroke: Why do we talk about it? *European Journal of Neurology* 2006; 13:215–219.

63. Sloan MA, Kittner SJ, Feeser BR, et al. Illicit drug-associated ischemic stroke in the Baltimore-Washington Young Stroke Study. *Neurology* 1998; 50(6):1688–1693.

64. Kelly MA, Gorelick PB, Mirza D. The role of drugs in the etiology of stroke. *Clin Neuropharmacol* 1992; 15(4):249–275.

65. National Institute on Drug Abuse. NIDA Research Report: Cocaine Abuse and Addiction. 2002.

66. Qureshi AI, Safdar K, Patel M, et al. Stroke in young black patients. *Stroke* 1995; 26:1995–1998.

67. Nanda A, Vannemreddy P, Willis B, Kelley R. Stroke in the young: Relationship of active cocaine use with stroke mechanism and outcome. *Acta Neurochurgica* 2006; 96S:91–96.

68. Perez JA, Jr., Arsura EL, Strategos S. Methamphetamine-related stroke: Four cases. *J Emerg Med* 1999; 17(3):469–471.

69. Buttner A, Mall G, Penning R, Weis S. The neuropathology of heroin abuse. *Forensic Science International* 2000; 113:435–442.

70. Kernan WN, Viscoli CM, Brass LM, et al. Phenylpropanolamine and the risk of hemorrhagic stroke. *N Eng J Med* 2000; 343:1826–1832.

71. Cantu C, Arauz A, Murillo-Bonilla LM, et al. Stroke associated with sympathomimetics contained in over-the-counter cough and cold drugs. *Stroke* 2003; 34:1667–1672.

72. Haller CA, Benowitz NL. Adverse cardiovascular and central nervous system events associated with dietary supplements containing ephedra alkaloids. *N Engl J Med* 2000; 343:1833–1838.

73. Morgenstern LB, Viscoli CM, Kernan WN, et al. Use of ephedra-containing products and risk for hemorrhagic stroke. *Neurology* 2003; 60:132–135.

74. Food and Drug Administration US. Sales of supplements containing ephedrine alkaloids (ephedra) prohibited. February 11, 2004.

75. Food and Drug Administration US. Legal Requirements for the legal sale and purchase of drug products containing pseudoephedrine, ephedrine, and phenylpropanolamine. May 8, 2006.

76. O'Connor AD, Rusyniak DE, Bruno A. Cerebrovascular and cardiovascular complications of alcohol and sympathomimetic drug abuse. *Med Clin N Am* 2005; 89:1343–1358.

77. Reynolds K, Lewis LB, Nolen JDL, et al. Alcohol consumption and risk of stroke: A meta-analysis. *JAMA* 2003; 289(5):579–588.

78. Malarcher AM, Giles WH, Croft JB, et al. Alcohol intake, type of beverage, and the risk of cerebral infarction in young women. *Stroke* 2001; 32(1):77–83.

79. Berger K, Ajani UA, Kase CS, et al. Light-to-moderate alcohol consumption and risk of stroke among U.S. male physicians. *N Engl J Med* 1999; 341(21):1557–1564.

80. Kiechl S, Willeit J, Rungger G, et al. Alcohol consumption and atherosclerosis: What is the relation? Prospective results from the Bruneck Study. *Stroke* 1998; 29(5):900–907.

81. Kelleher CC. Clinical aspects of the relationship between oral contraceptives and abnormalities of the hemostatic system: Relation to the development of cardiovascular disease. *Am J Obstet Gynecol* 1990; 163(1 Pt 2):392–395.

82. Bousser MG, Kittner SJ. Oral contraceptives and stroke. *Cephalalgia* 2000; 20(3):183–189.

83. American College of Obstetrics and Gynecology PBN. Use of hormonal contraception in women with coexisting medical conditions. *Obstetrics & Gynecology* 2006; 107:1453–1466.

84. Brey RL. Antiphospholipid antibodies in young adults with stroke. *Journal of Thrombosis and Thrombolysis* 2005; 20(2):105–112.

85. Levine JS, Branch W, Rauch J. The antiphospholipid syndrome. *N Eng J Med* 2002; 346(10):752–763.

86. Green D. Thrombophilia and stroke. *Top Stroke Rehabil* 2003; 10(3):21–33.

87. Kim RJ, Becker RC. Association between factor V Leiden, prothrombin G20210A, and methylenetetrahydrofolate reductase C677T mutations and events of the arterial circulatory system: A meta-analysis of published studies. *Am Heart J* 2003; 146:948–957.

88. Moster ML. Coagulopathies and arterial stroke. *J Neuro-Ophthalmol* 2003; 23(1):63–71.

89. Schwedt TJ, Dodick DW. Patent foramen ovale and migraine: Bringing closure to the subject. *Headache* 2006; 46:663–671.

90. Bevan H, Sharma K, Bradley W. Stroke in young adults. *Stroke* 1990; 21:382–386.

91. Adams HP, Kappelle LJ, Biller J, et al. Ischemic stroke in young adults: Experience in 329 patients enrolled in the Iowa Registry of Stroke in young adults. *Arch Neurol* 1995; 52:491–495.

92. Camerlingo M, Casto L, Censori B, et al. Recurrence after first cerebral infarction in young adults. *Acta Neurologica Scandinavica* 2000; 102(2):87–93.

93. Naess H, Nyland HI, Thomassen L, et al. Long-term outcome of cerebral infarction in young adults. *Acta Neurol Scand* 2004; 110(2):107–112.

94. Lee T-HH, Wen-Chuin C, Chi-Jen C, Sien-Tsong. Etiologic study of young ischemic stroke in Taiwan. *Stroke* 2002; 33:1950–1955.

95. Hoffman M, Chichkova R, Ziyad M, Malek A. Too much lumping in ischemic stroke: A new classification. *Med Sci Monit* 2004; 10:CR285–287.

96. Pezzini A, Grassi M, Del Zotto E, et al. Cumulative effect of predisposing genotypes and their interaction with modifiable factors on the risk of ischemic stroke in young adults. *Stroke* 2005; 36:533–539.

97. Martinelli I, Battaglioli T, Burgo I, et al. Oral contraceptive use, thrombophilia, and their interaction in young women with ischemic stroke. *Haematologica* 2006; 91:844–847.

98. Awada A. Stroke in Saudi Arabian young adults: A study of 120 cases. *Acta Neurol Scand* 1994; 89:323–328.

99. Nedeltchev K, der Maur TA, Georgiadis D, et al. Ischaemic stroke in young adults: Predictors of outcome and recurrence. *J Neurol Neurosurg Psychiatry* 2005; 76:191–195.

100. Savitz SI, Caplan LR, Edlow JA. Pitfalls in the diagnosis of cerebellar infarction. *Academic Emergency Medicine* 2007; 14:63–68.

101. Kothari RU, Brott T, Broderick JP, Hamilton CA. Emergency physicians: Accuracy in the diagnosis of stroke. *Stroke* 1995; 26:2238–2241.

102. Krem MM. Motor conversion disorders reviewed from a neuropsychiatric perspective. *J Clin Psychiatry* 2004; 65:783–790.

103. Chen CC, Cho DY, Tsai SC. Outcome and prognostic factors of decompressive hemicraniectomy in malignant middle cerebral artery infarction. *J Chin Med Assoc* 2007; 70(2).

104. Rabinstein AA, Mueller-Kronast N, Maramattom BV, et al. Factors predicting prognosis after decompressive hemicraniectomy for hemispheric infarction. *J Neurosurg* 2007; 106(1):59–65.

105. Kleindorfer D, Broderick J, Khoury J, et al. The unchanging incidence and case-fatality of stroke in the 1990s: A population-based study. *Stroke* 2006; 37:2473–2478.

106. Varona JF, Guerra JM, Bermejo F. Stroke in young adults. *Med Clin (Barc)* 2004; 122(2):70–74.

107. Kappelle LJ, Adams HP, Jr., Heffner ML, et al. Prognosis of young adults with ischemic stroke: A long-term follow-up study assessing recurrent vascular events and functional outcome in the Iowa Registry of Stroke in Young Adults. *Stroke* 1994; 25(7):1360–1365.

108. Marini C, Totaro R, Carolei A. Long-term prognosis of cerebral ischemia in young adults. *Stroke* 1999; 30:2320–2325.

109. Muntner P, Garrett E, Klag MJ, Coresh J. Trends in stroke prevalence between 1973 and 1991 in the US population 25–74 years of age. *Stroke* 2002; 33:1209–1213.

110. Neau J-P, Ingrand P, Mouille-Brachet C, et al. Functional recovery and social outcome after cerebral infarction in young adults. *Cerebrovascular Disease* 1998; 8:296–302.

111. Musolino R, La Spina P, Granata A, et al. Ischaemic stroke in young people: a prospective and long-term follow-up study. *Cerebrovasc Dis* 2003; 15(1–2):121–128.

112. Black-Schaffer RM, Winston C. Age and functional outcome after stroke. *Top Stroke Rehabil* 2004; 11:23–32.

113. Colantonio A, Kasi SV, Ostfeld AM, Berkman LF. Pre-stroke physical function predicts stroke outcomes in the elderly. *Arch Phys Med Rehabil* 1996; 77:562–566.

114. Sze K-H, Wong E, Or KH, et al. Factors predicting stroke disability at discharge: A study of 793 Chinese. *Arch Phys Med Rehabil* 2000; 81:876–880.

115. Ergeletzis D, Kevorkain CG, Rintala, D. Rehabilitation of the older stroke patient. *AJPMR* 2002; 81(12):881–889.

116. Alexander MP. Stroke rehabilitation outcome: A potential use of predictive variables to establish levels of care. *Stroke* 1994; 25:128–134.

117. Granger CH, Fiedler RC. Discharge outcome after stroke rehabilitation. *Stroke* 1992; 23:978–982.

118. Vestling M, Tufvesson B, Iwarsson S. Indicators for return to work after stroke and the importance of work for subjective well-being and life satisfaction. *J Rehabil Med* 2003; 35:127–131.

119. Black-Schaffer RM, Osberg JS. Return to work after stroke: Development of a predictive model. *Arch Phys Med Rehabil* 1990; 71(5):285–290.

120. Bogousslavsky J, Regli F. Ischemic stroke in adults younger than 30 years of age: Cause and prognosis. *Arch Neurol* 1987; 44(5):479–482.

121. Ferro JM, Crespo M. Prognosis after transient ischemic attack and ischemic stroke in young adults. *Stroke* 1994; 25(8):1611–1616.

122. Hindfelt B, Nilsson O. The prognosis of ischemic stroke in young adults. *Acta Neurol Scand* 1977; 55(2):123–130.

123. Leys D. Clinical outcome in 287 consecutive young adults (15–45 years) with ischemic stroke. *Neurology* 2002; 59:26–33.

124. Coughlan AK, Humphrey M. Presenile stroke: Long-term outcome for patients and their families. *Rheumatology and Rehabilitation* 1982; 21:115–122.

125. Fugl-Meyer AR, Jaasko L, Norlin V. The post-stroke hemiplegic patient: Incidence, mortality, and vocational return in Goteborg, Sweden. *Scandanavian Journal of Rehabilitation* 1975; 7:73–83.

126. Kotila M, Waltimo O, Neimi J, et al. The profile of recovery from stroke and factors influencing outcome. *Stroke* 1984; 15:1039–1044.

127. Mackay A, Nias BC. Strokes in the young and middle-aged: Consequences to the family and to society. *Journal of the Royal College of Physicians of London* 1979; 13:106–112.

128. Saeki S, Ogata H, Toshiteru O, et al. Factors influencing return to work after stroke in japan. *Stroke* 1993; 24:1182–1185.

129. Weisbroth S, Esibill, Zuger RR. Factors in the vocational success of hemiplegic patients. *Arch Phys Med Rehabil* 1971; 52(10):441–446 passim.

130. Wozniak MA, Kittner SJ, Price TR, et al. Stroke location is not associated with return to work after first ischemic stroke. *Stroke* 1999; 30:2568–2573.

131. Saeki S, Ogata H, Okubo T, et al. Return to work after stroke: A follow-up study. *Stroke* 1995; 26:399–401.

132. Heinemann AW, Roth EJ, Cichowski K, Betts HB. Multivariate analysis of improvement and outcome following stroke rehabilitation. *Arch Neurol* 1987; 44:1167–1172.

133. Saeki S. Disability management after stroke: Its medical aspects for workplace accommodation. *Disability and Rehabilitation* 2000; 22:578–582.

134. Howard G, Till S, Toole JF, et al. Factors influencing return to work following cerebral infarction. *JAMA* 1985; 253:226–232.

135. Smolkin C, Cohen S. Socioeconomic factors affecting the vocational success of stroke patients. *Arch Phys Med Rehabil* 1974; 55:269–271.

136. Bergmann J, Kuthmann M, von-Ungern-Sternberg A, Weimann V. Medical, educational and functional determinants of employment after stroke. *Journal of Neuronal Transmission* 1991; 33(Supplement):157–161.

137. Black-Schaffer RM, Lemieux L. Vocational outcome after stroke. *Top Stroke Rehabil* 1994; 1:74–86.

138. Gresham GF, Fitzpatrick TE, Wolf PA, et al. Residual disability in survivors of stroke: The Framingham study. *NEJM* 1975; 293:954–956.

139. Golper LAC, Rau MT, Marshall RC. Aphasic adults and their decisions on driving: An evaluation. *Arch Phys Med Rehabil* 1980; 61:34–40.

140. Nouri FM, Tinson DJ, Lincoln NB. Cognitive ability and driving after stroke. *Int Disabil Studies* 1987; 9:110–115.

141. Van Zomeran AH, Brouwer WH, Minderhoud JM. Acquired brain damage and driving: A review. *Arch Phys Med Rehabil* 1987; 68:697–705.

142. Mazer BL, Korner-Bitensky NA, Sofer S. Predicting ability to drive after stroke. *Arch Phys Med Rehabil* 1998; 79:743–749.

143. Klavora P, Gaskovski P, Martin K, et al. The effects of Dynavision rehabilitation on behind-the-wheel driving ability and selected psychomotor abilities of persons after stroke. *Am J Occup Ther* 1995; 49:534–542.

144. Akinwuntan AK, De Weerdt W, Feys H, et al. Effect of simulator training in driving after stroke: A randomized controlled trial. *Neurology* 2005; 65:843–850.

145. Akinwuntan AE, Feys H, De Weerdt W, Pauwels J, Baten G, Strypstein E. Determinants of driving after stroke: A retrospective study. *Arch Phys Med Rehabil* 2002; 83:334–341.

146. Quigley FL, DeLisa JA. Assessing the driving potential of cerebral vascular accident patients. *American Journal of Occupational Therapy* 1983; 37:474–478.

147. Bardach JL. Psychological factors in the handicapped driver. *Arch Phys Med Rehabil* 1971; 60:328–332.

148. Galski T, Ehle HT, Bruno RL. An assessment of measures to predict the outcome of driving evaluations in patients with cerebral damage. *Am J Occup Ther* 1989; 44:709–713.

149. Galski T, Bruno RL, Ehle HT. Driving after cerebral damage: A model with implications for evaluation. *Am J Occup Ther* 1992; 46:324–332.

150. Hartje W, Willmes K, Pach R, et al. Driving ability of aphasic and non-aphasic brain-damaged patients. 1991.

151. Heikkila VM, Korpelainen J, Turkka J, et al. Clinical evaluation of the driving ability in stroke patients. *Acta Neurol Scand* 1999; 99:349–355.

152. Naess H, Wage-Andreassen U, Thomassen L, et al. Do all young ischemic stroke patients need long-term secondary preventive medication? *Neurology* 2005; 65:609–666.

153. Adunsky A, Hershkowitz M, Rabbi R, et al. Functional recovery in young stroke patients. *Arch Phys Med Rehabil* 1992; 73(9):859–862.

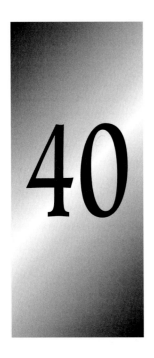

40 Stroke in Older Adults

Marianne Shaughnessy
Kathleen Michael

S troke is the third-leading cause of death and a foremost cause of serious, long-term disability in the United States (1). As cardiovascular and metabolic disease incidence rises with age, so does the risk of stroke, and clinical and functional consequences may be compounded by other conditions associated with aging. But stroke is not an inevitable consequence of aging. By identifying and modifying risk factors in older people, there are opportunities to reduce the incidence and mortality of this condition (2) and improve function, independence, and quality of life after stroke. Recent advances in emergency medical care have reduced mortality and stroke severity, resulting in greater numbers of older adults who survive strokes (3). Even though stroke incidence in America appears stable and stroke mortality is slowly declining, the absolute magnitude of stroke is likely to grow over the next 30 years. With aging of the population, the number of older stroke survivors is likely to increase substantially (1). The very old are expected to become a growing part of the stroke survivor population (4).

This chapter presents a discussion of special considerations in the management of stroke recovery and rehabilitation for older adults. We describe the incidence, prevalence, and economic impact of stroke in the aging population. We discuss the management of

common risk factors for recurrent stroke. We address challenges to successful rehabilitation in older adults with stroke and suggest strategies to overcome barriers and optimize outcomes.

INCIDENCE, PREVALENCE, AND ECONOMIC IMPACT

Age is the single most important risk factor for stroke. For each successive 10 years after age 55, the stroke rate more than doubles in both men and women (5). Nearly three-quarters of all strokes occur in people over the age of 65. Stroke incidence rates are 1.25 times greater in men, but, because women tend to live longer than men, more women than men die of stroke each year (1).

Not only are they more likely to have strokes, but the physical, psychological, and social consequences may be more severe for older adults. The burden of stroke is heterogeneous and is greatest among the elderly, men, and African Americans (1). Furthermore, age is an independent predictor of outcome after ischemic stroke. Older patients, especially those over 80 years old, are more likely to die in the hospital after stroke and less likely to make a favorable long-term recovery (4). Other factors, such as onset stroke severity, preexisting disability, and atrial fibrillation, are also significant age-related, independent predictors of prognosis after stroke (4).

Many stroke survivors (50–70%) regain functional independence, but 15–30% are permanently disabled, and 20% require institutional care at three months after onset (1). Effective rehabilitation interventions initiated early after stroke can enhance the recovery process and minimize functional disability (6). Stroke rehabilitation begins during the acute hospitalization as soon as the diagnosis of stroke is established and life-threatening problems arc under control. The highest priorities during this early phase are to prevent recurrent stroke and complications, manage health issues, promote mobility and self-care activities, and provide emotional support to the patient and family (6). Post-stroke guidelines recommend transfer to a stroke-specific rehabilitation unit as soon as possible to ensure early mobilization, availability of speech, physical and occupational therapy, rehabilitation psychology, and the social support derived from interaction with other stroke survivors (6). There is a body of evidence indicating that patients have better outcomes with an organized, multidisciplinary approach to post-acute rehabilitation after a stroke (7, 8).

The economic impact of stroke is substantial. The direct and indirect cost of stroke for 2007 is estimated to total approximately $62.7 billion (1). This cost is derived from the anticipated number of strokes, combined with average lifetime costs for ischemic and hemorrhagic strokes. Ischemic strokes account for 87% of all strokes in the United States (9), and the mean lifetime cost of ischemic stroke is estimated at $140,048, including inpatient care, rehabilitation, and follow-up care for residual deficits. This estimate was converted to 1999 dollars using the medical component of the Consumer Price Index (1). Demographic variables, including age, sex, and insurance status, are not associated with stroke cost. Severe strokes, that is, National Institute of Health Stroke Scale scores greater than 20, are estimated to cost twice as much as mild strokes, despite similar diagnostic testing profiles (10). Death within seven days, subarachnoid hemorrhage, and stroke while hospitalized for another condition are associated with higher costs in the first year. Conversely, lower costs are associated with mild cerebral infarctions or residence in a nursing home before the stroke (11).

Comorbidities, such as ischemic heart disease and atrial fibrillation, predict higher costs (12). Other uncontrolled risk factors dramatically increase costs associated with stroke. An analysis of data from the National Health and Nutrition Examination Survey (NHANES) II study examining cost data from short-term hospitalization and estimated first-year loss of productivity or premature death concluded that the annual costs of one undermanaged cardiovascular risk factor for subjects who had already suffered an Myocardial Infarction (MI) or stroke are estimated

between $3.2 and $11.1 billion (13). Among persons with previous MI or stroke, two or more inadequately controlled risk factors accounted for incurred cost ranging between $4.1 to 12.2 billion (13). Estimates using the same data for years of life lost because of uncontrolled risk factors range from 7.5 years for one uncontrolled risk factor to 8.9 years for two or more (13).

Yet stroke risk factors remain suboptimally managed in the post-stroke population at large. In a group of 364 community-dwelling chronic stroke survivors who were assessed by history, physical examination, and laboratory analysis of a fasting sample:

- 99% had at least one suboptimally controlled stroke risk factor.
- 91% had two or more risk factors inadequately treated.
- 80% of the participants had pre-hypertension or hypertension.
- 67% were overweight or obese.
- 60% had suboptimal LDL.
- 45% had impaired fasting glucose.
- 34% had low HDL.
- 14% were current smokers.

All were reportedly receiving routine medical care (14).

Clearly, in addition to public health efforts to educate all Americans about stroke risk and recognition of signs and symptoms, risk factors that persist must be managed as aggressively as possible.

MANAGING COMMON RISK FACTORS FOR RECURRENT STROKE IN THE OLDER ADULT

Risk factors and the incidence of stroke peak in individuals 75 years or older. Patients with the highest risk benefit the most from effective risk reduction therapy (15). For this reason, all strategies of demonstrated value in stroke prevention are pertinent in the care of older adults. Control of hypertension, resolution of dyslipidemia, management of diabetes mellitus, anticoagulation for atrial fibrillation, promotion of exercise and healthy diet, and cessation of cigarette smoking are obligatory at all ages, but they are of particular importance in older adults (15).

Management of Hypertension

High blood pressure, once believed to represent a normal and progressive component of the aging process, is now recognized as a sign of structural and physiologic abnormalities of vascular function (16). Elevated blood pressure is a significant determinant of the long-term risk of stroke (17). Casual systolic hypertension is a prevalent finding in older adults. 50% of women over the age of 80 have casual systolic blood pressures >160 mm Hg (18). Isolated systolic hypertension, defined as a systolic blood pressure ≥140 mm Hg with a diastolic blood pressure <90 mm Hg, affects most individuals aged 60 years and older (16).

Antihypertensive treatment has established efficacy in primary prevention of fatal or nonfatal stroke in hypertensive and high-risk patients >60 years of age, particularly through treatment of systolic hypertension (19). In a summary of 17 treatment trials of hypertension throughout the world involving nearly 50,000 patients, investigators found a 38% reduction in all stroke and a 40% reduction in fatal stroke resulting from systematic treatment of hypertension (20). Treatment was also highly effective in preventing stroke in individuals >65 years with systolic hypertension (20). Importantly, there was no less impact on stroke prevention above age 80, with incidence reduced by 40% (1). To prevent stroke, it is necessary to treat older adults with hypertension aggressively to the same target blood pressures as those identified for younger patients (16). Thiazide diuretics and ACE inhibitors are the drug classes of choice from which therapy may be initiated in this population (21).

There appears to be no age threshold beyond which treatment of hypertension would not be beneficial (22). In older adults up to the age of 80 who have systolic blood pressures over 160 mm Hg, antihypertensive treatment is associated with significant reductions in stroke and cardiovascular events (18). Optimal clinical management accounts for specific aspects of pathophysiology and metabolic characteristics of older adults. Treatment should be initiated with lower doses of antihypertensive agents, bringing pressure down slowly while monitoring for orthostatic hypotension, impaired cognition, and electrolyte abnormalities (16). Although goal blood pressure is <140/90 mm Hg, a decrease of 20–30 mm Hg in systolic blood pressure, even if the overall treatment goal is not achieved, is still associated with reduced cardiovascular risk (22). For every 5 mm Hg reduction in systolic blood pressure, stroke mortality may decrease by as much as 14% (21).

Management of Dyslipidemia

Elevated cholesterol levels are common in older adults. Sixty-one percent of women between the ages of 65 and 74 are reported to have total cholesterol levels over 240 mg/dL (23). Elevated total cholesterol and decreased high-density lipoprotein (HDL) levels predispose older adults to ischemic stroke (23).

Possible benefits from lipid-lowering therapy are particularly relevant for the older population at high risk for stroke (23). Though associations are relatively weak, epidemiological evidence indicates that elevated total cholesterol and subfractions increase stroke risk (23). Lowering high serum cholesterol with HMG-CoA

reductase inhibitors (statins) has been beneficial in the primary and secondary prevention of myocardial infarction, but further research is needed to determine the effect of lipid lowering on stroke occurrence (23). Few large-scale studies have investigated the specific effect of statins on stroke prevention in older individuals. To date, the largest trials suggest a beneficial effect for stroke prevention with statins in high-risk elderly subjects ≤ 82 years of age (19).

Indirect evidence suggests that the reduction in the stroke risk with statins is larger than would be expected with reduction of serum cholesterol level alone. Antioxidant and endothelium-stabilizing properties of statins may contribute to reducing the risk of stroke by protecting vascular walls (23). Although the relative risk of stroke associated with elevated lipids is only moderate, its population-attributable risk is high, given the increase in the elderly population worldwide (23). It is important to note that elevated serum cholesterol seldom occurs in isolation from other cardiovascular risk factors.

Original Adult Treatment Panel III (ATP III) guidelines recommended that the low-density lipoprotein (LDL) level be targeted for intervention, with the goal below 100 mg/dl in this population. However, an update released in 2005 suggests a more ambitious goal of less than 70 mg/dl for very high-risk patients, defined as those with a recent MI, cardiovascular disease with diabetes, severe/poorly controlled risk factors, or metabolic syndrome (24). After lifestyle modifications of diet and exercise, statin agents are recommended as first-line choice of treatment, followed by the addition of bile acid sequestrants as needed (25).

Management of Diabetes

There is an age-related increase in total body fat and visceral adiposity that often is accompanied by diabetes or impaired glucose tolerance. The prevalence of type 2 diabetes increases progressively with age, peaking at 16.5% in men and 12.8% in women at 75–84 years old. Over age 65, glucose intolerance or diabetes was present in 30–40% of Framingham Study subjects (26). In a recent report, 80 chronic hemiparetic stroke patients were evaluated by fasting plasma glucose and oral glucose tolerance test to assess the utility of screening for abnormalities using fasting plasma glucose alone. Seventy-five of the 216 (35%) had type 2 diabetes by medical history. Another 70 were either diabetic (n = 11) or had impaired fasting glucose (n = 59) based on a single blood draw at the time of screening. Fasting plasma glucose among nondiabetic stroke patients had a sensitivity of 49% for predicting abnormalities in the two-hour glucose level during oral glucose tolerance test. Cumulative results identify 77% as abnormal (impaired or diabetic) on the basis of medical history, fasting plasma glucose, and/or two-hour glucose level, reflecting a very high prevalence of diabetic states in these chronic stroke survivors (27).

Type 2 diabetes and obesity are both associated with a clustering of atherogenic risk factors. Diabetes, often associated with high blood pressure, contributes to increased frequency and severity of cerebral vascular events (28). The risk of macrovascular disease is actually increased before glucose levels reach the diagnostic threshold for diabetes, and 25% of newly diagnosed diabetics already have overt cardiovascular disease (26). Diabetes and related complications, including untreated or poorly treated hypertension, may lead to premature arterial stiffening. The resulting stiffening and hypertrophy of the left ventricle yield a predisposition to coronary heart disease, heart failure, stroke, and other conditions (29). Other aspects of glucose metabolism may play a role in stroke risk, specifically hyperinsulinemia and increased insulin resistance. Both were shown to be risk factors for ischemic stroke, even among subjects with normal glucose status by laboratory values (1).

The risk of cardiovascular sequelae in diabetics is variable. The majority of events occur in those with two or more additional risk factors. Comprehensive stroke risk reduction in older adults should include not only normalization of the blood sugar, but also weight reduction, dietary fat restriction, strict blood pressure and lipid control, exercise, and avoidance of tobacco (26).

Atrial Fibrillation Management

Atrial fibrillation (AF) is the most common clinically relevant arrhythmia in persons aged >75 years and is strongly associated with ischemic stroke and other adverse outcomes. AF is also the most treatable cardiac precursor of stroke (30). AF describes quivering of the upper chambers of the heart, leading to pooling of blood where clots may develop. The incidence and prevalence of AF increase with age. With each successive decade of life above age 55, incidence of AF doubles (1). Data from the Framingham Study and hospital discharges suggest that the prevalence of AF in the United States population is increasing (17). More than 2.2 million Americans currently have AF, and this number is expected to increase by at least 2.5-fold over the next 50 years (30).

Stroke is the most feared complication of AF. Multiple clinical trials have shown that warfarin sodium anticoagulation is effective in reducing the risk of stroke in older adults (31). However, the complex pharmacokinetics and narrow therapeutic window of warfarin make its use challenging. An adjusted dose of warfarin with a target International Normalized Ratio (INR) of between 2 to 3 prevents ischemic stroke in elderly patients with an acceptable hemorrhagic risk, but is still largely underprescribed (19). Novel approaches to anticoagulation, including more potent antiplatelet agents and direct thrombin inhibitors, are currently undergoing clinical trials (31).

Carotid Stenosis Treatment

Carotid stenosis refers to the buildup of atherosclerotic materials within the carotid arteries, leading to occlusion of vital circulation to the brain. Carotid endarterectomy is indicated in carotid artery stenosis >70%, and outcomes are even better in elderly than in younger patients. However, medical treatment is preferred in asymptomatic elderly patients with <70% stenosis (19). Elderly patients with severely symptomatic stenotic carotid artery disease should undergo endarterectomy. Evidence for benefit from endarterectomy in asymptomatic subjects at any age is weak and cannot be recommended as a preventive strategy (15, 32). Carotid stenting, recently approved by the FDA for stroke risk reduction, has had mixed results in clinical trials and is currently being evaluated in more rigorous studies (32).

Antiplatelet Therapy in Stroke Prevention

Finally, for most patients with noncardioembolic stroke, daily treatment with an antiplatelet agent is recommended by the American Association of Chest Physicians. Aspirin (50–325 mg daily) is the least expensive option. Other antiplatelet agents, such as clopidogrel or extended-release dipyridamole with aspirin, may also be used in the absence of contraindications (32). Because of increased risks of bleeding, clinicians are advised to avoid combining clopidogrel and aspirin unless there is a specific cardiac indication (32).

CHALLENGES TO SUCCESSFUL REHABILITATION

Even with identical stroke severity, increasing age was associated with greater disability in activities of daily living (ADLs) and mobility. Patients >85 years were nearly ten times as likely to show a low response to rehabilitation in ADLs and nearly six times as likely to show low response in mobility as younger patients (33). Nevertheless, rehabilitation treatment is still valuable in patients older than 85 years because even small changes in function can improve independence and quality of life. Possibly less effective than for younger patients, inpatient rehabilitation is still substantially helpful for older patients (33).

Rehabilitation and gerontology care professionals share a function-based assessment and management paradigm. Clinical challenges post-stroke, therefore, should be considered within the context of age and any preexisting disability.

Biological Changes with Aging

Visual Changes. Visual loss is usually defined as <20/40 in the better eye and is associated with functional consequences. Blindness is traditionally defined as vision <20/200 in the better eye. Blindness or low vision affects 3.3 million Americans age 40 and over, or 1 in 28, and this figure is projected to reach 5.5 million by the year 2020. Low vision and blindness increase significantly with age, particularly in people over age 65 (34). Presbyopia, or the loss of accommodative ability, is the major age-associated ocular change leading to low vision. It begins at approximately age 40 and progresses so that, by the seventh decade, little ability to accommodate remains. Other changes with senescence include increased light absorption by the lens, cornea, and vitreous, leaving less to reach the retina and resulting in decrease in sharpness of vision and the need for more light for certain activities, such as reading and driving. The prevalence of common ophthalmologic diseases also dramatically rises with advancing age, with those older than 80 years of age suffering an increase in cataracts (68%), age-related macular degeneration (35%), and open-angle glaucoma (7.7%) (34).

Consequences of stroke may also manifest in visual disturbances, such as homonymous hemianopsia, visual field defects, visual neglect, disturbances in color vision, or paralysis of conjugate gaze. Ocular motility disturbances may produce diplopia, vertigo, oscillopsia, or visual distortions. All of these visual disturbances have potential to complicate or hinder the progress of rehabilitation. For example, visual deficits may make it difficult for an older adult to orient to new surroundings, follow directions, or receive feedback and cues for mobility and self-care activities. Visual deficits may contribute to fear of falling and impede progress in ambulatory activities. All stroke survivors should be screened for visual impairment as soon as they are medically stable, conscious, and communicative enough to participate in the examination and an individualized plan has been formulated by the rehabilitation team to compensate for losses.

Auditory Changes. Hearing loss is one of the most prevalent chronic conditions in the elderly population, affecting 31% of people over the age of 65 and 40–50% of persons over the age of 75 and is defined as the inability to hear a pure tone softer than 40 dB at more than one frequency in one or both ears (35). The most common cause of hearing loss in the elderly is presbycusis, which is sensorineural loss marked by difficulty hearing high frequency tones, and impaired speech comprehension. Other common causes of hearing loss in the elderly include cerumen plugs, otosclerosis, ototoxicity, tinnitus, Meniere's disease, and acoustic neuromas.

Again, stroke may impose comprehension or communication deficits that may compound hearing loss and negatively impact rehabilitation, such as aphasia, dysarthria, and apraxia of speech. Individuals with stroke are usually assessed for these problems, but all stroke survivors, especially the elderly, should also be screened for hearing loss and referred for treatment or adaptive strategies as needed. Adequate auditory acuity is critical for stroke survivors to understand the rehabilitation team's instructions, participate in problem assessment and decision-making, and communicate effectively with family and members of the rehabilitation team, thereby improving chances for successful rehabilitation.

Body Composition. A potential confounder to reaching physical therapy goals for older stroke patients may be sarcopenia (age-related loss of muscle mass), commonly seen in older adults (36, 37). By the seventh and eighth decade of life, maximal voluntary contractile strength is decreased on average by 20–40% for both men and women in proximal and distal muscles and caused in large part to decreased muscle mass (38). Loss of skeletal muscle fibers is a major contributing factor to sarcopenia, but other factors, including decreased physical activity, altered hormonal status, decreased total caloric and protein intake, inflammatory mediators, and factors contributing to protein synthesis are also involved. Together, they may contribute to functional decline (38). Interventions targeted at combating sarcopenia of aging have included testosterone replacement, growth hormone replacement, and resistive strength training. Of these, only strength training has been demonstrated as an effective means of increasing muscle mass and strength in healthy older adults (39).

The additional loss of muscle in the hemeparetic limb(s) creates further difficulties for stroke survivors as they attempt to mobilize again following stroke. A recent study examining 30 chronic stroke survivors showed lean mass of the paretic leg and thigh were 4% and 3% lower than the nonaffected leg; arm lean mass of the paretic side was 7% lower than the nonaffected side. Midthigh muscle area was 20% lower in the paretic limb than in the nonaffected leg (40). The mechanism of muscle atrophy following stroke is not well understood at this time, nor is the timeframe over which the atrophy occurs. However, it appears that the sarcopenia associated with aging—combined with the disability of stroke—may conspire to place the survivor at a disadvantage from a rehabilitation perspective. Most stroke patients are carefully assessed for muscle strength throughout the rehabilitation course, and more research is needed to identify specific strength training recommendations for these patients.

Comorbidities

Early exercise rehabilitation is critical to maximizing functional outcomes following stroke (41); however, sedentary older adults with stroke often suffer from comorbidities that may limit their ability to fully participate or maximize physical therapy in the subacute and chronic phases of stroke recovery.

Disorders of the cardiovascular system can potentially impact rehabilitation therapy by limiting exercise tolerance. Such disorders are very common in older adults. Preexisting coronary artery disease (often seen coincident with cerebrovascular disease), congestive heart failure, valvular dysfunction, and arrhythmias all increase in prevalence with age. Chronic obstructive pulmonary disease, emphysema, and chronic bronchitis are also more prevalent in older adults. Stroke survivors with these and similar comorbid illnesses are likely to face additional challenges with rehabilitation and life beyond. For example, these individuals may experience severe limitations in activity tolerance and progress more slowly toward their rehabilitation goals. It is likely that comorbid cardiovascular or pulmonary problems played a role dictating a previously sedentary lifestyle that precipitated the stroke.

Rehabilitation may also be challenged by musculoskeletal disorders (osteoarthritis, rheumatoid arthritis, and history of muscle or bone injury). Careful evaluations of preexisting disability, the extent of neurologic deficit, and motor control are critical to developing a realistic exercise prescription. Identifying and addressing barriers to mobilization (premedication prior to physical therapy appointments, braces/orthotics for support, appropriate assistive devices, and environmental modifications) will maximize chances for success in reaching therapeutic goals.

Cognitive impairment is another potential barrier to successful rehabilitation. Stroke survivors are likely to have long-standing hypertension and other cardiovascular risk factors, which can lead to vascular-related cognition impairments or dementia, and cognition may be further impaired by the stroke event. In a study comparing stroke survivors to match controls, cognitive impairment was seen in 35.2% of patients with stroke and 3.8% of controls (42). Cognitive domains most likely to be defective in stroke compared with control subjects were memory, orientation, language, and attention, and functional impairment was greater with cognitive impairment (42). These problems are very likely to impact the course of rehabilitation therapy and are discussed more comprehensively elsewhere in this text, but all older stroke survivors should be carefully screened in these domains of cognition to maximize therapeutic intervention.

Access to Care

In general, older adults face more barriers in accessing health care services than their younger counterparts. Older disabled stroke survivors face even more hurdles in their quest for both restorative and preventive health care services. Many older adults are dependent

on Medicare benefits to pay for health care services and may or may not carry an additional group or private gap coverage policy. The Medicare insurance system was developed to ensure that the older workers had insurance for health care expenses, and many have used it for incidental care only (43), as coverage for preventive services has been added incrementally over time. In a recent study of 46,659 respondents aged 65 years and older, 93% reported having a regular care provider, 98% had a regular place of care, and 98% were able to obtain needed medical care (44). Those with a regular care provider or a regular place of care were more likely to receive clinical preventive services than those without either of these. Reasons given for not obtaining needed medical care were cost (27%), too long a wait for an appointment (20%), no transportation or distance (9%), office not open when the individual could get there (8%), and other reasons (32%) (44). Another large study of older adults revealed that a perceived lack of responsiveness to patient concerns, cost, transportation, and street safety were substantial barriers for many older adults (45). Some older adults in the United States have no health care coverage at all and therefore experience significant cost barriers to care and do not regularly receive annual checkups or preventive health screenings (46).

Access to care may be further compromised because of shrinking reimbursement for physicians caring for those insured by Medicare. A recent survey by the American Medical Association revealed that 45% of respondents surveyed reported a threatened Medicare cut will force them to either decrease or stop seeing new Medicare patients (47).

For stroke survivors, economic barriers are only the beginning of the battle. As listed above, transportation becomes problematic as driving ability is frequently lost because of disabilities resulting from the stroke. Previously independent older adults are forced to rely on family, neighbors, or public transportation to access health care services. Those who provide transportation for the stroke survivors must adjust schedules to accommodate appointments to primary and subspecialty physician's appointments and multiple weekly physical occupational and/or speech therapy appointments throughout the subacute rehabilitation period. These barriers have potential to significantly impact the ability of stroke survivors to access the care necessary to optimize recovery. Health care providers should remember to query stroke survivors regarding these potential barriers and be sensitive to the multiple demands placed on survivors and caregivers.

Behavioral Barriers

Lack of physical activity is an important contributor to many of the most important chronic diseases for older Americans, including heart disease, diabetes, colon cancer, and high blood pressure. Few older adults achieve the minimum recommended 30 or more minutes of moderate physical activity on five or more days per week. Data from the Centers for Disease Control and Prevention (CDC) indicate 35–44% of adults ages 75 or older are inactive, meaning they engage in no leisure time physical activity. National data indicate that few older persons engage in regular physical activity. Only 31% of individuals aged 65 to 74 report participating in 20 minutes of moderate physical activity three or more days per week, and even fewer (16%) report 30 minutes of moderate activity five or more days per week (48). For those aged 75 and older, levels of activity are even lower. 23% engage in moderate activity for 20 minutes three or more days per week, and only 12% participate in such activity for 30 minutes five or more days per week (48).

The tendency for older adults to be sedentary places them at risk in multiple ways. Inactive lifestyles alone or in combination with other inadequately controlled risk factors like hypertension, hyperlipidemia, diabetes, smoking, and imprudent diet creates a scenario that makes a stroke likely to happen. Post-stroke, an inactive lifestyle not only inhibits optimal recovery, but accelerates the muscle atrophy and resultant cellular changes that raise the risk of recurrent stroke (27). Further, older adults who have been sedentary may be reluctant to adopt active lifestyles because of affective disorders, fear, or fatigue.

A substantial proportion of individuals with stroke (ranging from 39–76%) report significant and persistent fatigue affecting their daily lives (49–52). The frequency of self-reported fatigue is about twice as high in individuals with stroke as in age-matched controls and is not related to time post-stroke, stroke severity, or lesion location (50). Self-reported fatigue has been identified as an independent predictor for having to move into an institutional setting after stroke (49). Fatigue also predicts dependency in primary ADLs. In older adults with stroke, fatigue may be a sentinel for decline in general health status, accompanied by reductions in functional independence. For further discussion of fatigue after stroke, refer to Chapter 28.

OVERCOMING BARRIERS

Common post-stroke problems include cardiovascular deconditioning, impairments in gait and balance, diminished muscle tone and weakness, alterations in glucose metabolism, and persistent cardiovascular disease risk factors. When it is more difficult to get around and requires more energy to do so, survivors of stroke often become sedentary. Without regular physical activity, cardiovascular fitness may be lost, further compounding the imbalance of energy resources and expenditure. If you add fatigue, loss of confidence, and social isolation to the mix, a cyclical pattern emerges that negatively affects function, independence and quality of life.

With effective interventions, many of these problems are remediable, if not reversible. The potential for recovery is not time-limited, and relatively simple task-oriented activity programs can induce meaningful physiologic changes in function, fitness, metabolism, and brain activity.

The Role of Exercise

Conventional rehabilitation care typically provides little or no structured therapeutic exercise beyond the subacute stroke recovery period. Emerging evidence indicates that task-oriented exercise has the potential to improve upper and lower extremity motor function regardless of time since stroke (53–57). Low-intensity treadmill training three times per week can significantly improve motor and gait function in 12 weeks, even in distant chronic stroke survivors (55–57). Motor function can also be improved in the paretic upper extremity. In a recent study, 14 chronic hemiparetic stroke survivors who trained on a custom arm extension machine gained significant strength in elbow and wrist flexion and extension on the paretic side after six weeks of training three times per week (54, 58). The task-oriented exercises referenced in these studies were conducted under close medical supervision, and new studies are underway to specifically identify appropriate training protocols for use in community settings.

Following stroke, regular exercise can facilitate motor recovery and help control the common comorbidities that influence recurrent stroke risk. Exercise can reduce hypertension, enhance glucose regulation, improve blood lipid profiles, and reduce body fat. Many older adults with stroke have never been advised by a health care professional to engage in a regular exercise or walking program (59), yet generalized recommendations have been formalized to promote physical activity following stroke (41). Even though the field of post-stroke exercise rehabilitation is still developing, stroke survivors can work with their health care providers to fight back against disability and limit risk profiles. All stroke survivors should be questioned regularly about physical activity and exercise patterns, habits, and beliefs. If a stroke survivor reports little to no physical activity and he or she is capable of performing physical activity safely, each office visit is an opportunity to educate and prescribe daily exercise activity.

Role of Self-efficacy in Behavior Change

Many of the cardiovascular risk factors associated with stroke require changes in health behaviors, such as choosing a healthier diet, losing weight, beginning an exercise program, stopping smoking, or adhering to a medication regimen (60). Social cognitive theory indicates that specific efficacy expectations affect behavior, motivational level, thought patterns, and emotional reactions to any situation (61). Perceptions and beliefs affecting behavior include self-efficacy (an individual's judgment of his or her capabilities to perform a specific action) and outcome expectations (beliefs that there will be a specific outcome or benefit if a certain behavior is performed). These beliefs are essential to the adoption and maintenance of self-care ADL after stroke (62) and exercise following stroke (59). Bolstering self-efficacy to make significant lifestyle modifications is accomplished through the following four steps:

1. Educate and encourage
2. Provide specific tasks to accomplish as well as directions to completion of task
3. Identify and address barriers to compliance
4. Cuing with role-modeling or self-modeling

Finally, education regarding expected benefits may provide further incentive and motivation to change behaviors (63, 64). Helping an older adult to begin an exercise program, choose a healthier diet, or adhere to a medication regimen requires time, care, and encouragement, and discussing these and other behavior modification goals should be a part of routine assessment and surveillance. An example of a self-efficacy based intervention to encourage exercise in older stroke survivors is given in Table 40-1.

Evaluation and Activation of Support Systems

For many older adults, particularly those affected by stroke, support systems can make the difference between returning to home in the community and life in an assisted living or skilled nursing facility. The support system of older adults is comprised of three components: the informal network, the formal support system, and semiformal supports (65). Informal supports are provided by family and friends, are based on long-standing relationships, and form the basis for the older adult's social network. Neighbors who see the older adult on a daily basis perform chores or errands or offer to shop are another example of informal support. Formal supports are those paid for and provided by Social Security, Medicare, Medicaid, other service providers, and social welfare agencies. Home-based therapists, home health nurses, and personal care aides are examples of formal supports. Semiformal supports refer to the support provided by local or neighborhood organizations, churches, or senior centers. A local stroke support group may be another example of a semiformal support.

It is critically important to identify and mobilize social supports and resources as quickly as possible in order to smooth the transition to home and begin community reintegration. Identification of the informal and semiformal resources allows for an inventory of persons or services that can be called upon while waiting for formal supports to become available, such as applying for transportation service for the disabled. Similarly, home-based therapies and nursing/personal care assistance may be prescribed immediately upon discharge to home to allow the stroke survivor the additional time necessary to become independent with ADLs or allow for identification of an informal or semiformal support to take up care provision when formal services end.

Care providers should routinely inquire about support systems and changes in available supports for stroke survivors over time. In particular, providers should inquire about the well-being of the primary caregiver for the stroke survivor. Multiple studies have indicated that primary caregivers experience strain that is described as mild to severe in the first year following a stroke (66, 67), and the chronic strain on caregivers over the long term takes a toll on health in higher levels of emotional and physical distress (68). Respite resources should be identified and used as needed to preserve the health and well-being of the primary caregiver.

Continuing Patient/Family Education: Recognizing Signs and Symptoms

Of the more than 700,000 strokes that occur each year, 200,000 are recurrent (1). About 25% of people who recover from their first stroke will have another stroke within five years. Unless specific interventions are directed toward modifying stroke risk factors, the potential for recurrence persists. Stroke survivors should be monitored regularly for recurrent stroke risk, and they and their families should be educated to self-monitor as well.

To minimize impact from stroke, early recognition of signs and symptoms as well as immediate initiation of evaluation and treatment is imperative. Quantitative estimates of the rate of neural circuitry loss in ischemic stroke emphasize the urgency of timely and definitive care. The adage that "time lost is brain lost" takes on added significance when one realizes that the typical patient loses 1.9 million neurons each minute during which acute stroke goes untreated (69).

Older adults often do not associate new onset symptoms with acute stroke, but rather attribute them to other illnesses (arthritis, weakness, headaches, or fatigue) and fail to take immediate action. The American Stroke Association has launched an educational campaign to educate the general public about the signs and symptoms of stroke. The campaign has been somewhat effective. 70% of respondents in a recent random telephone survey of 2,173 correctly named one stroke warning sign, up from only 57% in 1995 (70), but

TABLE 40-1
Self-efficacy-based Intervention to Encourage Exercise in Older Stroke Survivors

ASSESSMENT/PLAN	EXAMPLE
Analyze risk factor profile for primary prevention	Comorbidities (diabetes, high blood pressure, hyperlipidemia) Medication regimen Lifestyle influences (smoking, poor diet, physical inactivity)
Consider deficit profile for stroke survivor	Hemiparesis, cognitive, language deficits, and depression are common in survivors of stroke.

INTERVENTION	EXAMPLE
Educate and encourage	Provide education on influences of comorbidities on risk for first or second stroke Encourage patient to make changes in behavior to minimize risk
Provide explicit direction and verify ability to perform activity	Give patient (and family, if available) clear instructions on self-monitoring, prescribed medication regimen and symptom management In conjunction with primary health care provider, provide detailed, customized activity program and calendar to mark off days as activity is accomplished. If an exercise program is warranted, a physical therapist or exercise physiologist may be consulted
Identify barriers and physiological feedback	Pain, fatigue, and anxiety are some examples of physiological barriers. Depression may influence perceived ability to carry out activities. Age-related sensory changes may influence ability to perform tasks. Transportation and finances may be also identified as barriers to adherence to prescribed regimens.
Cuing and role-modeling/self-modeling	Patient derives confidence in his or her own ability to perform any activity by watching others who are similar to himself or herself performing the same activity or seeing himself or herself successfully performing the activity. A photograph may be helpful as cue.

EVALUATION	EXAMPLE
Provide routine surveillance of risk factors/profile	Review risk factor profile at every visit
Revise prescribed regimens as needed	Medications and physical activity programs should be modified as needed in collaboration with primary provider.
Routinely provide encouragement to reach patient goals	Continue positive reinforcement for work accomplished. Behavior change is hard. Continue gentle reminders for healthy behaviors yet to be adopted.
Continue education as needed	Routine review of comorbidities, symptoms, and new diagnoses as needed

there is ongoing need for education and reinforcement. A recent report of the Reasons for Geographic and Racial Differences in Stroke Study (REGARDS) indicated that 18% of more than 18,000 participants with no history of diagnosed stroke or TIA reported having had at least one stroke symptom, most reporting unilateral numbness, weakness, or sudden visual disturbance. Symptoms were more prevalent among African Americans compared with white participants and among those with lower income, lower educational level, and fair to poor perceived health status, indicating that continued educational efforts are required (71).

CONCLUSION

There are nearly 5 million persons in the United States aging with the chronic disability of stroke, and, with advancing age, the risk for first-time stroke increases (1). Older adults often have age-associated factors that compound the risk for stroke and can potentially affect recovery trajectories. Rehabilitation therapies are effective at any age if comorbidities and functional changes associated with aging are taken into account. Careful, comprehensive assessment of the older stroke survivor, along with the family and support network is necessary to design a customized, progressive exercise program to maximize recovery.

References

1. Writing Group M, Rosamond W, Flegal K, et al. Heart Disease and Stroke Statistics: 2007 Update. Report from the American Heart Association Statistics Committee and Stroke Statistics Subcommittee. *Circulation* 2006; 2006:CIRCULATIONAHA.106.179918.
2. Rodgers H, Greenaway J, Davies T, et al. Risk factors for first-ever stroke in older people in the northeast of England: A population-based study. *Stroke* 2004 2004; 35(1):7–11.
3. Barker WH, Mullooly JP. Stroke in a defined elderly population, 1967–1985: A less lethal and disabling but no less common disease. *Stroke* 1997; 28(2):284–290.
4. Kammersgaard L, Jorgenson HS, Reith J, et al. Short- and long-term prognosis for very old stroke patients. The Copenhagen Stroke Study. *Age and Aging* 2004; 33:149–154.
5. Centers for Disease Control. Stroke facts and statistics. *Heart Disease and Stroke Prevention* 2006.
6. Duncan PW, Zorowitz R, Bates B, et al. Management of adult stroke rehabilitation care: A clinical practice guideline. *Stroke* 2005 2005; 36(9):e100–143.
7. Cifu D, Stewart DG. Factors affecting functional outcome after stroke: A critical review of rehabilitation interventions. *Archives of Physical Medicine and Rehabilitation* 1999; 80(5 Suppl 1):S35–S39.
8. Stroke Unit Trialists' Collaboration. Organized inpatient (stroke unit) care for stroke. *Cochrane Database System Review* 2002; 1(CD000197).
9. NHLBI. *Incidence and Prevalence: 2006 Chart Book on Cardiovascular and Lung Diseases* Bethesda, MD: National Heart Lung and Blood Institute, 2006.
10. Taylor TN, Davis PH, Torner JC, et al. Lifetime cost of stroke in the United States. *Stroke* 1996; 27(9):1459–1466.
11. Leibson C, Hu T, Brown RD, et al. Utilization of acute care services in the year before and after first stroke: A population-based study. *Neurology* 1996; 46:861–869.
12. Diringer MN, Edwards DF, Mattson DT, et al. Predictors of acute hospital costs for treatment of ischemic stroke in an academic center. *Stroke* 1999 1999; 30(4):724–728.
13. Qureshi AI, Suri MFK, Kirmani JF, Divani AA. The relative impact of inadequate primary and secondary prevention on cardiovascular mortality in the United States. *Stroke* 2004; 35(10):2346–2350.
14. Kopunek S, Michael KM, Shaughnessy M, et al. Cardiovascular risk in survivors of stroke. *American Journal of Preventive Medicine* in press.
15. Barnett H. Stroke prevention in the elderly. *Clinical & Experimental Hypertension* 2002; 24(7–8):563–571.
16. Sander G. Hypertension in the elderly. *Current Hypertension Reports* 2004; 6(6):469–476.
17. Seshadri S, Beiser A, Kelly-Hayes M, et al. The lifetime risk of stroke: Estimates from the Framingham Study. *Stroke* 2006; 37(2):345–350.
18. Beckett N, Nunes M, Bulpitt C. Is it advantageous to lower cholesterol in the elderly hypertensive? *Cardiovascular Drugs & Therapy* 2000; 14(4):397–405.
19. Andrawes W, Bussy C, Belmin J. Prevention of cardiovascular events in elderly people. *Drugs & Aging* 2005; 22(10):859–876.
20. Waeber B. Trials in isolated systolic hypertension: An update. *Current Cardiology Reports* 2003; 5(6):427–434.
21. Chobanian A, Bakris GL, Black HR, et al. National High Blood Pressure Education Program Coordinating Committee. The Seventh Report of the Joint National Committee on Prevention, Detection, Evaluation, and Treatment of High Blood Pressure: The JNC 7 report. *JAMA* 2003; 289(19):2560–2572.
22. Asmar R. Benefits of blood pressure reduction in elderly patients. *Journal of Hypertension Supplement* 2003; 21:S25–30.
23. Sarti C, Kaarisalo M, Tuomilehto J. The relationship between cholesterol and stroke: Implications for antihyperlipidaemic therapy in older persons. *Drugs and Aging* 2000; 17:33–51.
24. Stone N, Bilek S, Rosenbaum S. Recent National Cholesterol Education Program Adult Treatment Panel III update: Adjustments and options. *American Journal of Cardiology* 2005; 96:53E–59E.
25. Expert Panel on Detection EaToHBCiA. Executive Summary of the Third Report of the National Cholesterol Education Program (NCEP) Expert Panel on Detection, Evaluation, and Treatment of High Blood Cholesterol in Adults (Adult Treatment Panel III). *JAMA* 2001; 285(19):2486–2497.
26. Wilson P, Kannel WB. Obesity, diabetes, and risk of cardiovascular disease in the elderly. *American Journal of Geriatric Cardiology* 2002; 11:119–123, 125.
27. Ivey F, Ryan AS, Hafer-Macko CE, et al. High prevalence of abnormal glucose metabolism and poor sensitivity of fasting plasma glucose in the chronic phase of stroke. *Cerebrovascular Diseases* 2006; 22(5–6):368–371.
28. Bauduceau B, Bourdel-Marchasson I, Brocker P, Taillia H. The brain of the elderly diabetic patient. *Diabetes Metabolism* 2005; 31 Spec(2):5S92–95S97.
29. Franklin S. Hypertension in older people: Part 1. *Journal of Clinical Hypertension (Greenwich)* 2006; 8:444–449.
30. Go A. The epidemiology of atrial fibrillation in elderly persons: The tip of the iceberg. *American Journal of Geriatric Cardiology* 2005; 14:56–61.
31. Cooper H. Trials of newer approaches to anticoagulation in atrial fibrillation. *Journal of Interventional Cardiac Electrophysiology: An International Journal of Arrhythmias and Pacing* 2004; 10 Suppl(1):27–31.
32. Sacco RL, Adams R, Albers G, et al. Guidelines for prevention of stroke in patients with ischemic stroke or transient ischemic attack: A statement for healthcare professionals from the American Heart Association/American Stroke Association council on stroke: Co-sponsored by the Council on Cardiovascular Radiology and Intervention: The American Academy of Neurology affirms the value of this guideline. *Stroke* 2006; 37(2):577–617.
33. Paolucci S, Antonucci G, Troisi E, et al. Aging and stroke rehabilitation: A case-comparison study. *Cerebrovascular Diseases* 2003; 15(12):98–105.
34. The Eye Diseases Prevalence Research G. Causes and prevalence of visual impairment among adults in the United States. *Arch Ophthalmol* 2004; 122(4):477–485.
35. National Institute on Deafness and Other Communication Disorders. Statistics about hearing disorders, ear infections, and deafness. www.nidcd.nih.gov/health/statistics/hearing.asp#1.
36. Nair K. Age-related changes in muscle. *Mayo Clinic Proceedings* 2000; 75(Suppl):S14–18.
37. American College of Sports Medicine. Exercise and physical activity for older adults. *Medicine and Science in Sports and Exercise* 1998; 30(6):992–1008.
38. Doherty T. Invited review: Aging and sarcopenia. *Journal of Applied Physiology* 2003; 95(4):1717–1727.
39. Borst S. Interventions for sarcopenia and muscle weakness in older people. *Age and Ageing* 2004; 33(6):548–555.
40. Ryan A, Dobrovolny CL, Smith GV, et al. Hemiparetic muscle atrophy and increased intramuscular fat in stroke patients. *Archives of Physical Medicine & Rehabilitation* 2002; 83(12):1703–1707.
41. Gordon NF, Gulanick M, Costa F, et al. Physical activity and exercise recommendations for stroke survivors: An American Heart Association scientific statement from the Council on Clinical Cardiology, Subcommittee on Exercise, Cardiac Rehabilitation, and Prevention; the Council on Cardiovascular Nursing; the Council on Nutrition, Physical Activity, and Metabolism; and the Stroke Council. *Circulation* 2004; 109(16):2031–2041.
42. Tatemichi TK, Desmond DW, Stern Y, et al. Cognitive impairment after stroke: Frequency, patterns, and relationship to functional abilities. *J Neurol Neurosurg Psychiatry* 1994 1994; 57(2):202–207.
43. Janes GRB, Bolen DK, Kamimoto JC, et al. Surveillance for use of preventive health-care services by older adults, 1995–1997. *Morbidity & Mortality Weekly Report CDC Surveillance Summaries* 1999; 48(8):51–88.
44. Okoro C, Strine TW, Young SL, et al. Access to health care among older adults and receipt of preventive services. Results from the Behavioral Risk Factor Surveillance System, 2002. *Preventive Medicine* 2005; 40(3):337–343.
45. Fitzpatrick AL, Powe NR, Cooper LS, et al. Barriers to health care access among the elderly and who perceives them. *Am J Public Health* 2004; 94(10):1788–1794.
46. Okoro C, Young SL, Strine TW, et al. Uninsured adults aged 65 years and older: Is their health at risk? *Journal of Health Care for the Poor & Underserved* 2005; 16(3):453–463.
47. American Medical Association. New AMA survey shows Medicare cuts will harm seniors' access to physician care. Press release, March 16, 2006.
48. Agency for Healthcare Research and Quality and the Centers for Disease Control. Physical activity and older Americans: Benefits and strategies. www.ahrq.gov/ppip/activity.htm. Accessed February 5, 2007.
49. Glader E, Stegmayr B, Asplund K. Post-stroke fatigue: A two-year follow-up study of stroke patients in Sweden. *Stroke* 2002; 33(5):1327–1333.
50. Ingles J, Eskes GA, Phillips SJ. Fatigue after stroke. *Archives of Physical Medicine and Rehabilitation* 1999; 80(2):173–178.
51. Michael K. Fatigue and stroke. *Rehabil Nurs* 2002; 27(3):89–94, 103.
52. Staub F, Bousslavsky J. Fatgue after stroke: A major but neglected issue. *Cerebrovascular Diseases* 2001; 12(2):75–81.
53. Duncan P, Richards L, Wallace D, et al. A randomized, controlled pilot study of a home-based exercise program for individuals with mild and moderate stroke. *Stroke* 1998; 29(10):2055–2060.

54. Harris-Love M, mcCombe Waller S, Whiall J. Exploiting interlimb coupling to improve paretic arm reaching performance in people with chronic stroke. *Archives of Physical Medicine and Rehabilitatation* 2005; 86(11):2131–2137.

55. Harris-Love ML, Macko RF, Whitall J, Forrester LW. Improved hemiparetic muscle activation in treadmill versus overground walking. *Neurorehabilitation & Neural Repair* 2004; 18(3):154–160.

56. Silver KH, Macko RF, Forrester LW, et al. Effects of aerobic treadmill training on gait velocity, cadence, and gait symmetry in chronic hemiparetic stroke: A preliminary report. *Neurorehabil Neural Repair* 2000; 14(1):65–71.

57. Smith GV, Silver KH, Goldberg AP, Macko RF. "Task-oriented" exercise improves hamstring strength and spastic reflexes in chronic stroke patients. *Stroke* 1999; 30(10):2112–2118.

58. Luft A, McCombe Waller S, Whitall J, et al. Repetitive bilateral arm training and motor cortex activation in chronic stroke: A randomized, controlled trial. *JAMA* 2004; 292(15):1853–1861.

59. Shaughnessy M, Resnick B, Macko RF. Testing a model of exercise behavior following stroke. *Rehabilitation Nursing* 2006; 31(1):15–21.

60. Shaughnessy M, Michael, K, Normandt P. When stroke strikes: Minimizing impact and maximizing recovery. *Advance for Nurse Practitioners* 2006; 14(9).

61. Bandura A. Self-efficacy: Toward a unifying theory of behavioral change. *Psychological Review* 1977; 84:191–215.

62. Robinson-Smith G, Pizzi E. Maximizing stroke recovery using patient self-care self-efficacy. *Rehabilitation Nursing* 2003; 28(2):48–51.

63. Resnick B, Zimmerman SI, Orwig D, et al. Outcome expectations for exercise scale: Utility and psychometrics. *J Gerontol B Psychol Sci Soc Sci* 2000; 55(6):S352–356.

64. Resnick B. Testing a model of exercise behavior in older adults. *Research in Nursing & Health* 2001; 24(2):83–92.

65. Gallo J, Fulmer T, Paveza GJ, Reichel W, eds. *Handbook of Geriatric Assessment.* Gaithersburg, MD: Aspen Publishers, Inc., 2000.

66. Bugge C, Alexander H, Hagen S. Stroke patients' informal caregivers: Patient, caregiver and service factors that affect caregiver strain. *Stroke* 1999; 30:1517–1523.

67. Low J, Payne S, Roderick P. The impact of stroke on informal careers: A literature review. *Social Science & Medicine* 1999; 49:711–725.

68. Scholte op Reimer W, de Haan RJ, Rijnders PT, et al. The burden of caregiving in partners of long-term stroke survivors. *Stroke* 1998; 29:1605–1611.

69. Saver JL. Time is brain-quantified. *Stroke* 2006 2006; 37(1):263–266.

70. Schneider A, Pancioli AM, Khoury JC, et al. Trends in community knowledge of the warning signs and risk factors for stroke. *JAMA* 2003; 289:343–346.

71. Howard VJ, McClure LA, Meschia JF, et al. High prevalence of stroke symptoms among persons without a diagnosis of stroke or transient ischemic attack in a general population: the Reasons for Geographic and Racial Differences in Stroke (REGARDS) Study. *Arch Intern Med* 2006; 166(18):1952–1958.

VIII

PSYCHOSOCIAL AND COMMUNITY REINTEGRATION

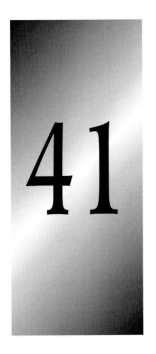

41 Ethical Issues in the Care of Stroke Survivors

Lynne C. Brady Wagner
Kristi L. Kirschner

I wanted to communicate: Yelling louder does not help me understand you any better! . . . Speak more slowly. Enunciate more clearly. Again! Please try again! S-l-o-w down . . . See that I am a wounded animal, not a stupid animal. I am vulnerable and confused. (1)

Suddenly and without warning, 37-year-old neuroanatomist Jill Bolte Taylor sustained a large, left hemispheric intracranial hemorrhage from an arteriovenous malformation. After several years of rehabilitation, she wrote an account of her stroke experience and recovery, *My Stroke of Insight: A Brain Scientist's Personal Journey* (1). Embedded in her recollections and fragmented memories are examples of the moral dilemmas that are familiar to health care professionals who work with people after strokes. Questions that commonly confront the clinician working with stroke patients and the families of stroke survivors include:

- Does the stroke survivor have decision-making capacity (DMC)?
- How does one evaluate DMC when there is an obvious language disorder?
- Is the patient the "same person" with the same values as before, or is he or she forever altered? Should this matter?
- Should life-sustaining medical treatments be initiated or continued in the face of sometimes devastating neurologic impairment?

These questions are just a few of the common ethical issues that are frequently encountered after stroke. This chapter is intended to provide some guidance for health care professionals navigating these uncertain waters. There are no easy answers. There are only some ethical principles and guidelines that can help clarify the range of acceptable choices. The rapid pace of change in this field compounds the complexity of these ethical dilemmas. As new research is produced, new stroke treatments become clinically available, and the equations related to the potential benefits and burdens of existing treatment choices change. Individual outcomes are often uncertain, not only in terms of level of impairment, but in disability, handicap, and life satisfaction as well. Patients and families frequently feel overwhelmed and daunted by the decisions that must be made—often within a constrained time frame—about the most routine to the more complicated interventions and procedures. The lack of societal and financial resources to support people who need care after stroke can add a layer of complexity, with ripple effects on family members, friends, and others in the environment. Stroke, though an individual medical event, affects a community of people.

This chapter addresses a range of potential ethical issues faced by patients, family members, and various individuals who are part of the health care team. One of the most common ethical issues encountered in the care of stroke survivors are questions regarding decision-making ability. Because stroke can result in a host of neuropsychologic impairments that may affect a person's cognitive-communication skills, questions regarding the stroke survivor's ability to participate in decision-making after stroke are familiar to all clinicians caring for this population. Other common dilemmas include issues related to personhood, social justice, and restrictions people face in choices of where and how to live, the role of the family and surrogate decision-makers (2, 3), as well as controversies that arise when patients need alternative nutrition and hydration caused by dysphagia (4–6).

We will use excerpts from patient narratives about the lived experience of stroke to illustrate how the ethical problems may present to clinicians. Rehabilitation clinicians have stated that they face a number of clinical ethical issues in their daily practice (7); these are often recognizable as situations when values are in conflict and the right course of action is not clear. Teasing apart the clinical questions or options from the ethical questions or duties can often be accomplished by considering how the question should be phrased. Clinical questions begin with the phrase "Can we?" Can we achieve the medical goals for this patient by applying this treatment approach? For example, "Can we technically place a feeding tube in Mr. Jones? Is it medically feasible and reasonable?" Ethical questions begin with the phrase "Should we?" Should this particular outcome be a goal for this person at this time? For example, "Given that Mr. Jones values the pleasure of eating above his nutritional status, should we insert a gastrostomy tube for this purpose?"

INFORMED CONSENT

> Later in the morning, it was time for me to have an angiogram that would outline the blood vessels in my brain . . . Although, I thought it absolutely absurd that anyone would ask me to sign a form of consent while in this condition, I realized that policy is policy! How do we define "of sound mind and body" anyway? (1)

The first and most pressing issue that commonly arises after a stroke is whether the patient is able to understand and make important medical decisions or not. From the time the person enters the emergency room through the course of rehabilitation, the medical team will need to engage in an evaluative process to decide if the person has the requisite capacity to make decisions (8). The ethical principle of respect for autonomy demands that medical decisions be a result of a shared communication process between the health care professional(s) and the patient whenever possible (9, 10). As a conceptual framework, the terminology of informed consent is fairly recent and

did not become fully integrated into medical care in the United States until the 1970s (9).

Though the initial emphasis for obtaining informed consent focused on the obligations of the health care professional or researcher to disclose the appropriate information, the process of assessing the patient's or subject's comprehension and ability to make an uncoerced choice quickly became of paramount interest. For this reason, some bioethicists began to use the terminology *valid consent* rather than *informed consent* to emphasize the interactional nature of the process. In his classic textbook, *Ethical Issues in Neurology*, neurologist and bioethicist James L. Bernat identifies three critical elements for valid consent:

> (1) physicians must convey adequate information to their patients; (2) consent must be obtained without coercion (or be "voluntary"); and (3) patients must be competent to consent or refuse. (11)

"Adequate information" is further clarified to include the basic facts about the available medical therapies, including their risks and benefits, the risk of no treatment at all, the course of treatment recommended by the health care professional, and the rationale thereof (11).

Assessment of Decision-making Capacity

As one of the three criteria required for valid consent, assessing competence, or decision-making capacity (DMC), is a critical skill for all health care professionals. In the hospital setting, people who were previously competent may become temporarily or permanently compromised in their ability to make decisions on their own behalf. Sometimes, as with stroke, a direct injury to the brain may be involved. Other times, it may involve secondary factors such as medications, metabolic abnormalities, hypoxia, or psychiatric conditions (12–14).

In the health care setting, competency is more accurately referred to as decision-making capacity (DMC). The distinction is not merely a matter of semantics. In our society, adults greater than age 18 are presumed to be competent and able to make their own decisions. Only a court of law can declare someone "incompetent," and the specific areas of incompetence must be delineated in the court decision. For example a person may be declared incompetent to manage his financial affairs, but be deemed competent to participate in medical decisions (15, 16). Usually, a guardian is appointed by the court to oversee the areas in which the person has been judged incompetent.

It is important to note that the assessment of DMC is not a global concept, but is assessed in the context of the question at hand. In other words, it is a situation- or question-specific assessment. In the classic model for assessing decision-making, as articulated by Appelbaum and Grisso (15, 16), the person must in some way—either verbally or behaviorally—be able to communicate a choice. Thus, adequate consciousness and a method of reliable communication are essential. The person must also be able to understand relevant information, such as the nature and rationale of the treatment and its risks and benefits as well as alternatives to the proposed treatment. Applying this information to his or her particular circumstances, which requires insight and appreciation of one's own medical condition, is the next critical capacity. Finally, the person should be able to demonstrate a logical process of reasoning.

Various tools have been developed to assist clinicians in assessing DMC in the health care setting, including the Aid to Capacity Exam (ACE) developed by the University of Toronto Joint Centre of Bioethics. (See www.utoronto.ca/jcb/disclaimers/ace.htm) (14, 17). In addition to providing training and a framework for the assessment of DMC, a series of suggested questions and a scoring system allow the evaluator to tabulate a total score. The determination of capacity thus falls along a continuum, acknowledging that capacity is not an all-or-none phenomenon. Depending on the score, at that specific point in time, the person may be considered:

- Definitely capable
- Probably capable
- Probably incapable
- Definitely incapable

The circumstances of the assessment are noted, as are any factors that might be interfering with DMC so that these issues can be addressed medically, if possible. Ideally, a final determination of DMC will be deferred until such confounders are corrected (17).

It is important to note that it is possible for patients to have DMC for some medical decisions and not others. For example, a patient may not be able to decide if the benefits of a carotid endarterectomy are worth the risks, but the same person may be able to tell clinicians who he or she wants to speak for him or her if there are important medical questions to be addressed. The issue here is the congruence between the complexity of the information involved in the decision and the person's capabilities. It is also possible that, for decisions that involve greater risks, for example, a patient's refusal of life-sustaining treatment, a higher level of evidence may be required than for decisions with less consequence, such as whether to wear a splint or what to eat (9, 14, 16–18). It is not the outcome that is at issue here, that is, whether the health care team agrees with the decision or not. It is the evidence that the process the person used to arrive at a decision is sound. This concept is also known as the sliding scale for standards of evidence in the assessment of DMC (9).

The Effects of Stroke on Decision-making Capacity

To someone looking on, I may have been judged as less than what I had been before because I could not process information like a normal person. I was saddened by the inability of the medical community to know how to communicate with someone in my condition . . . I wanted my doctors to focus on how my brain was working rather than on whether it worked according to their criteria or timetable. I still knew volumes of information and I was simply going to have to figure out how to access it again. (1)

When patients make choices that are compatible with the team's recommendations, there is typically little concern about DMC. It is when decisions are contrary to the team's recommendations or when certain medical conditions occur, such as brain diseases or injuries, that clinicians raise the question of DMC. Decisional processes, after all, involve a complex integration of neurologic systems and processes (12). A neurologic condition such as a stroke is one such brain disease that has the potential to affect the patient's ability to understand, contemplate, and communicate—all critical skills for decision-making—a choice (19–21).

The process of shared decision-making requires the patient to possess basic comprehension and expression skills, verbal or nonverbal (19, 21). Persons with impaired communication skills are at risk for unnecessary exclusion from this process (21, 22). A stroke can result in a myriad of problems, including dysarthria, aphasia, dyslexia, agraphia, dysphonia, abulia, and other cognitive-communication impairments. Patients with these impairments may be especially vulnerable to judgments that their participation in the informed consent process would be invalid because they may not be able to communicate without accommodation or facilitation from a trained assistant (either a clinician, family member, or volunteer) (19, 21, 23). In general, post-stroke deficits that can affect DMC fall into four general categories: disorders of consciousness, communication, insight and awareness of one's condition, and mood. Freedman et al. have further classified that the cognitive processes fundamental to decision-making include attention, language, memory, and frontal lobe function (12).

DMC and Disorders of Attention

Attention can be considered the sine qua non for all other cognitive neurologic processes (24). Without which, encoding, problem-solving, and essentially all other cognitive functions cannot optimally operate. It is also highly distributed in the brain, from the brain stem/reticular activating system to the thalamus and bilateral frontal and nondominant parietal lobes. Another way of thinking about the neural network for attentional processing is that the reticular activating structures are critical for arousal, whereas the cingulate cortex provides the motivational components, the posterior parietal lobe provides the sensory representation, and the frontal lobe the motor representation (24).

In the context of such a neurologic model, it is easy to see how attentional mechanisms may be disrupted when a stroke occurs. Patients who have had strokes may have attentional problems from both the brain lesions as well as from seizures or toxic-metabolic factors such as medications, hypoxia, infectious processes, or electrolyte abnormalities that can result in acute confusional states (24). Patients who are unconscious are de facto unable to participate in decision-making until they regain consciousness. If attention is fluctuating or drifting, capacities may be emerging, but they are often not adequate for in-depth discussions and assessments about medical decisions (12). Patients need to be able to attend to information long enough to decode information, apply the information to their circumstances, and reason.

Another interesting attentional problem occurs with lesions in the nondominant hemisphere, resulting in neglect syndromes. For example, there are well-described syndromes that result in disruptions of the internal template of the body (24), such as anosoagnosia, as well as syndromes that disrupt the exploratory motor components. Such lesions can result in disconnection syndromes in which patients can verbally comprehend information, but have difficulty applying this information to their particular circumstances. Such verbal-behavioral disconnections pose particular difficulties for clinicians when assessing DMC (12, 25), as the assessments tend to be heavily weighted to the verbal realm. It is possible for patients to demonstrate verbally an accurate understanding of information, but be unable to apply this information to their own particular circumstances. Such defects in intrapersonal awareness or perception can pose serious challenges to DMC.

DMC and Aphasia

"Answer this, squeeze that, sign here!" they demanded of my semi-consciousness, and I thought, How absurd! Can't you see I've got a problem here? What's the matter with you people? Slow down! I can't understand you! Be patient! Hold still! That hurts! What is this chaos? . . . They couldn't hear me because they couldn't read my mind. (1)

Aphasia is an acquired disorder of the language system that can result from a stroke or other damage to the language centers of the brain (26, 27). Linguistic or verbal (language) ability is critical to decision-making. As noted above by Appelbaum and Grisso, among the requisite skills for DMC is that the person must in some way—either vocally or behaviorally—be able to communicate a choice. Furthermore, the person must also be able to understand relevant information, such as the nature and rationale of the treatment and its risks and benefits as well as alternatives to the proposed treatment. The complexity of the decision will thus determine the level of detail required for accurate communication.

Under the diagnosis of aphasia, many taxonomies exist (27). Relative to the area and size of the neurologic lesion, diastasis, and an individual's premorbid linguistic capabilities, aphasia can present a number of challenges for a stroke survivor. The most recognizable form of this impairment presents as problems with word-finding that can range from the very mild (minimally affecting a person's word choice and fluency) to the very profound (resulting in the absence of the ability to produce or communicate words). The situation may be further complicated by the fact that the person with an aphasia affecting verbal expression and others who interact with him or her may not be be fully aware of extent of any accompanying impairment of comprehension, raising the risk of incorrectly assuming accurate communication (21, 28).

Unfortunately, health care professionals receive little or no formal training in working with patients who have communication impairments, specifically in methods to facilitate and accommodate communication with persons who are aphasic (29, 30). Kagan (31) demonstrated that, even without objective improvement in the linguistic abilities of a person with aphasia, training medical professionals and other caregivers who work with persons with aphasia can lead to more successful communication outcomes. The presence of aphasia should not preclude attempts to involve the patient in making decisions with appropriate accommodations as needed. Indeed, it would be an injustice to the patient to exclude him a priori (12, 23, 31). When a patient has a way to demonstrate that he or she can comprehend the information provided and make a choice regarding treatment, a very significant measure of respect for individual self-determination is fulfilled.

When patients with communication impairments have the ability to participate in decision-making but are denied the opportunity because of lack of either awareness or of training on the part of their health care providers, their autonomy is usurped. The opposite can also occur. Linguistic representation in the brain is complex, and one's ability to recognize and convey nonverbal communication can be preserved while the ability to encode specific words and concepts may be severely limited. Because of this, persons with some language impairments may communicate by responding to head nods, tone of voice, or gestures and might therefore be assumed to understand information that they do not. In this example, DMC may be assumed when it is not present, and the stroke survivor is denied the protection and involvement of a surrogate (19, 21). When possible, a detailed assessment of language abilities by a speech-language pathologist (SLP) is critical if questions of DMC arise in the context of aphasia. Not only can the SLP clarify the type and extent of aphasia, but he or she can also provide guidance for compensatory strategies in many cases. For example, communication with a patient with comprehension impairments may be more successful if information is presented visually, in shortened segments, or accompanied by diagrams, rather than through lengthy auditory presentations (30).

DMC and Disorders of Speech

So I usually have the skimpiest arsenal of facial expressions, winks, and nods to ask people to shut the door, loosen a faucet, lower the volume on the TV, or fluff up a pillow. I do not succeed every time. As the weeks go by, this forced solitude has allowed me to acquire a certain stoicism and to realize that the hospital staff are of two kinds: the majority, who would not dream of leaving the room without first attempting to decipher my SOS messages; and the less conscientious minority, who make their getaway pretending not to notice my distress signals. (32)

In his book, *The Diving Bell and the Butterfly* (32), Jean-Dominique Bauby described the devastating loss of his communication abilities following a stroke at the age of 43. He became "locked in" as a result of a massive stroke affecting his brain stem. Though his cognition was intact, he was paralyzed and unable to phonate or articulate (anarthria). His only preserved movement was blinking his left eye. It was through this movement that Bauby communicated, meticulously and tediously blinking in response to the presentation of letters from the alphabet to spell out his thoughts, needs, wishes, and feelings. Indeed, his book is a remarkable product of such efforts. It provides a distressing perspective on the health care system, in which a man with a rich inner life is considered by some as a vegetable or treated as an object with his only interaction with staff through the provision of tube feedings, baths, and repositioning. This is in striking contrast with the many care providers and friends who invested the time to learn the laborious communications strategies and facilitate Bauby's connection with humanity.

Though a number of authors have addressed the various ethical issues that are a consequence of aphasia (19, 21, 29, 31), less has been written about the issues involved in the face of speech disabilities (23, 33, 34). Yet, the impact of motor impairments of speech on DMC can be devastating. A person like Bauby, who clearly has the ability to make decisions when give the opportunity to do so with appropriate facilitation, can easily be discounted or prevented from doing so. Even health care professionals may have limited understanding of the association between cognitive abilities and one's ability to speak, often presuming that a person who is unable to articulate well has related difficulty with the ability to

understand and think. The importance of a careful neurologic evaluation and frequent reevaluations by trained professionals cannot be overstated; furthermore, once the appropriate methods and techniques for facilitated communication are identified, all staff and contacts with the person need to be trained in their use (23, 33).

Augmentative and alternative communication (AAC) techniques have been used successfully to assist in the decision-making process for persons with neurologic disease or disorders that have severely affected motor control of speech (23). The aid of a knowledgeable facilitator and the necessary high-tech (for example, electronic or computerized equipment) or low-tech (for example, alphabet boards and picture books) device(s) can reveal the decisional abilities of persons whose profound communication difficulties may lead clinicians and families to believe that the patient could not possibly participate. SLPs and occupational therapists with experience in the use of these strategies are invaluable resources for the physician, nurses, family, and all other team members (23) and should be involved early after the stroke.

AAC solutions are frequently not easy to implement. Their use often requires a great deal of time on the part of both the patient and facilitator. (See Table 41-1 for suggestions to maximize communication.) Allowing patients to participate fully in discussions contributes to respect for individual autonomy and fosters clinician understanding of the patient's authentic wishes. An additional challenge to allowing patients with severe motor output impairment to participate in medical choices is the lack of trained personnel as well as the availability and funding for AAC devices (35). Even though some individuals who need this kind of equipment are able to obtain insurance coverage of higher-tech and expensive systems, other insurers fail to accept the medical necessity of this equipment. The onus is often on the clinician to advocate and appeal such adverse funding decisions, arguing that accurate and timely communication is essential to good, safe, medical care.

DMC and Mood Disorders

My own mood seesawed wildly—at times I felt almost euphoric with relief and at the satisfaction of being alive, and other times almost suicidally depressed. (36)

In his book *My Year Off: Recovering Life after a Stroke*, British editor Robert McCrum, 42 years old and newly married at the time of his cerebral hemorrhage, describes his experience of emotional turmoil after his stroke. Neuropsychologic processes involved in mood regulation can be both caused and affected by the presence of stroke (37–40). Even though an affective disorder may be transitory and fluctuating, depression and anxiety can limit a stroke survivor's ability to engage fully in the process of deliberating about daily problems and considering future events and issues.

TABLE 41-1
Strategies for Maximizing Communication When a Patient Requires Increased Time to Interact

1. Partner with the patient to develop strategies together so he or she knows you are purposefully attempting to optimize communication.
2. Be thoughtful about scheduling. For non-urgent discussions, try to schedule meetings when you are not rushed to get to another appointment.
3. Encourage the patient to record questions or statements ahead of time. If the patient has computer access, he or she can email the questions before the appointment or may be able to work with an assistant who can write down the questions ahead of time. These can either be sent to you or read at the appointment.
4. Physicians and other team members may call on the SLP or other trained individuals to assist by asking the patient specific questions. The physician can then schedule time to be there at the end of the appointment, and the information gathered can be shared. The trained facilitator can then assist in facilitating a discussion about the particular issue.
5. If you cannot understand the message and do not have more time to stay with the patient, make a specific promise to return to this question at a later time or use one of the above strategies.

Depression and anxiety can impede two critical elements of DMC. First, a person may be unable to fully appreciate or remember the perspective conveyed by others and therefore may be unable to comprehend various treatment choices presented. Additionally, the patient who is depressed or anxious may experience interference in the cognitive processes typically referred to as executive functioning (38), that is, the ability to identify problems, generate possible solutions, remember factors of these solutions, and weigh them against one another and select a reasonable approach to the challenge. In this situation, a patient may be unable to fully deliberate on the options presented in making a medical choice. Treatment for the underlying depression and/or anxiety may not only alleviate the patient's suffering, but it may help the patient imagine possibilities and process information in a more balanced fashion.

When a Patient Lacks DMC: The Role of a Surrogate

Honestly, I didn't really understand all of the details about what they were proposing to do—partly because the cells in my brain that understood language were swimming in a pool of blood and partly because of the sheer speed of their conversation . . . In my condition, I thought I understood that they were planning on passing a suction instrument up through my femoral artery into my brain to suck out the excess blood and threatening tangle of vessels. I was aghast when I realized it was their plan to cut my head open! . . . I made it perfectly clear to everyone that under no circumstances would I ever agree to permit them to open my head . . . The meeting ended with the craniotomy option temporarily tabled, and though it was clear to everyone (except me) that it was G.G.'s job to convince me to have the surgery. (1)

When a determination is made that a person lacks the capacity to make a particular decision—even with

the proper supports, compensatory strategies, and facilitation—then a proxy or surrogate decision-maker is required (Figure 41-1). The least common, but most straightforward, situation for naming the surrogate is when the patient had previously executed an advance directive naming the individual he or she would want to act on his or her behalf in the event of incapacity. At the present, it is estimated that only about 20% of the population have completed advance directives, though this percentage varies widely by geographic region, socioeconomic background, ethnicity, and other factors (41–44).

The Patient Self-Determination Act of 1990 requires that all hospitals and health care facilities query patients upon admission about whether they have an advance directive and, if not, if they wish to complete one (45).

There are two general types of advance directives: instructional documents such as the living will and proxy directives such as the durable power of attorney for health care (DPAHC) (9). There are also a growing number of hybrid documents, such as the physicians' orders for life-sustaining treatment paradigm (POLST) (www.ohsu.edu/ethics/polst/) and Five Wishes (www.agingwithdignity.org/5wishes.html). The level of legal recognition each state gives to these documents varies, and it is therefore imperative to know the law in the state in which you reside.

The living will is the earliest form of an advance directive and became prominent in the 1970s after the case of Karen Ann Quinlan (46) as a tool for allowing a person to exercise autonomy into states of future incompetence (47). The early living will was typically effective only when a person became terminally ill and unable to make his or her own decisions and included instructions that allowed the physician to withhold death-delaying treatments. Unfortunately, these documents do not provide guidance for situations in which

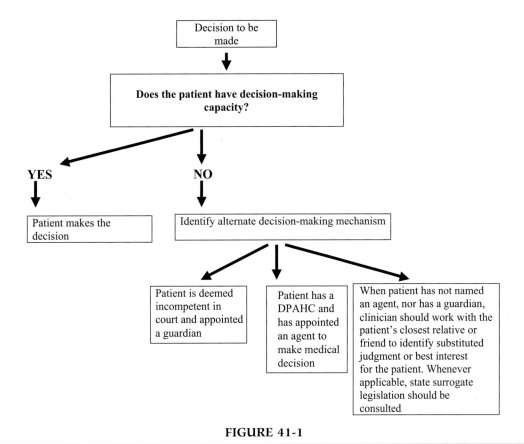

FIGURE 41-1

Who is the decision-maker? Adapted from Kothari and Kirschner (17)

a person may become temporarily or permanently incapable of making health care decisions, but are not terminally ill, such as in the case of a stroke or brain injury. In general, living wills also do not include provisions for withholding artificial nutrition and hydration. After the case of Nancy Cruzan (48), a woman with a traumatic brain injury in a state of persistent unconsciousness whose father petitioned the courts to allow her feeding tube to be removed, the DPAHC became of greater interest. With a DPAHC, a person can name an individual to speak on his or her behalf (a proxy) if he or she becomes temporarily or permanently unable to participate in medical decision-making. It is thus a more powerful and flexible document than a living will. Both the living will and DPAHC must be executed while an individual is considered to be competent in order to be legally recognized.

If a person has not completed an advance directive and is not able to make health care decisions, then the health care team must identify a surrogate. As of 2007, 38 states and the District of Columbia have formal state surrogate statutes that provide guidance on naming the appropriate surrogate decision-maker (49). Usually, this follows a next of kin hierarchy, and the person highest on the list who is available and willing to serve in this

capacity is the default legal surrogate. As opposed to the DPAHC, in which proxies can make any health care decision that the patient could (unless the patient restricted the proxy's authority in some way), the state surrogate laws typically provide some limits and restrictions on the types of decisions the surrogate can make, particularly when it comes to withdrawing or withholding life-sustaining treatments. Again, it is best to know the specific standards for the state in which one practices, as these laws vary from state to state (49). In the absence of a formal state surrogate law, health care providers will usually ask the next of kin to serve in this capacity. As with any situation, if there is concern about the appropriateness of the surrogate, conflict within the family, or the magnitude and extent of the decisions, the courts can be asked to appoint a guardian.

Some organizations, such as the Gunderson Lutheran Respecting Choices Program (www.gundluth.org), have attempted to assist patients and families in beginning the difficult conversations involved in making choices for medical treatment. The concept of advance care planning focuses on helping people identify aspects of life that they value most in order to guide a surrogate decision-maker in selecting the most respectful choice for their loved one (50).

Whether the surrogate is named by the DPAHC or via a state surrogate law, the surrogate is first and foremost asked to make the same decision that he or she believes the patient would have if he or she were capable. This principle is known as substituted judgment (9). Written directions are one source of information that can be referenced. Conversations and, in some instances, even lifestyle decisions have also been considered (16). In the absence of knowledge of a person's wishes, the surrogate is counseled to make a decision based upon what he or she believes to be in the best interest of the patient (9). This involves weighing the benefits and burdens of a treatment decision in the context of the person's condition. Though, in theory, both substituted judgment and best interest standards have great appeal, they can be difficult to implement in practice. In particular, there is growing literature that questions whether it is ever really possible to put one's beliefs and values aside to make decisions on behalf of another (47, 51).

Adjustment to Disability and the Concept of Personhood

[Stroke] is an event that goes to the core of who and what you are, the You-ness of you. First of all, the event happens in your brain which is, without becoming unduly philosophical the command centre of the self. Your brain is you: your moods, your skills, your character, your intelligence, your emotions, your self-expression, your self. (36)

One of the thorniest problems with substituted judgment as a heuristic is the issue of personhood. Simply put, who is the person for whom the decision is being made (16)? The name, social security number, birth date, and even genealogy and personal history as defining characteristics of personhood are clear and unchanging. What is not clear, however, is whether somehow the survivor is literally a changed person after the stroke, with different personality characteristics, values, interests, and capacities. Grieving the loss of the old self is commonplace after stroke, but it is not only for the person who experiences the stroke. It is also his or her network of close family and friends. How then does a proxy take these issues into consideration when making decisions?

A rich and layered debate on this topic exists without clear a consensus (52–54). That being said, there are some general guidelines that can be offered (47). Patients who have very strong feelings about personhood are more likely to have made an advance directive and put their future care wishes in writing. Indeed, the advance directive is the best way for a person to maintain control of his or her treatment into states of future incompetence and should therefore be taken very seriously. It is also possible that the person may be temporally incapacitated and, with time, may recover to the point where he or she

can resume making personal health care decisions. People who are not fully capacitant may still be able to indicate wishes and preferences in such a way that their proxies and health care team can use this information to guide decisions. In the end, knowledge that people frequently change their minds when their circumstances change is relevant to decision-making and needs to be a part of an informed consent discussion about future treatment decisions (47, 55).

Balancing the Patient's "Best Interests" in the Context of a Family

But today we spend the whole of the symbolic day together, affirming that even a rough sketch, a shadow, a tiny fragment of a dad is still a dad. I am torn between joy at seeing them living, moving, laughing, or crying for a few hours, and fear that the sight of all these sufferings—beginning with mine—is not the ideal entertainment for a boy of ten and his eight-year-old sister. (32)

Though substituted judgment and best interest standards have been extensively discussed in the ethics literature and are widely accepted, these standards are not without controversy. Some ethicists advocate considering the interests of the family, not just the patient, when decisions must be made, particularly when those decisions will have a substantial impact on others. A decision to place a feeding tube in a person with a severe brain injury may have financial repercussions, for example, or create an unspoken expectation that the family will take the person home and provide substantial care, usually without compensation (2, 3, 56, 57). Some studies have found that, even if it is theoretically desirable, it is probably not truly possible to stand in another's shoes and put one's perspectives and wishes aside in making a decision on behalf of another (47, 55). Interestingly, despite this observation, studies have also shown that many patients, even when told that their identified surrogate does not understand and make decisions as he or she would want, would still want a family member, rather than a stranger, to make these decisions.

In general, despite the limitations of surrogate decision-making, the health care team should respect the choices made by a proxy unless there is evidence that the proxy is not acting in the best interest of his or her loved one. Disagreement among members of the patient's family or between the family and the patient's care team can lead to unresolved conflicts and has occasionally lead to the need for legal adjudication of these matters (58, 59). When reviewing questions regarding a surrogate's ability to authorize removal of life-sustaining treatments, the courts have affirmed that the state can stipulate the level of evidence required to support such decisions as being reflective of the patient's desires/wishes. Many states require the criterion of clear and convincing evidence based on a reasonable person standard. That is, would the evidence convince a reasonable person that the allegation is so? This standard is used in Missouri and other states. However, there has been some movement to accept a less stringent standard; for example, after the Wendland case in California (60).

When Conflicts Occur

Conflicts often arise because of fractured or incomplete communication (61). Ethics services in health care institutions promote education related to ethical distress and dilemmas in addition to providing ethics consultation when requested. This education gives team members a process and framework for understanding the ethical principles involved, such as autonomy, beneficence, nonmaleficence, justice, and virtue. One important goal for ethics consultation is to assist the team in prioritizing and balancing these principles and values in conflict and, ultimately, to achieve an ethically acceptable outcome in an individual case. Varied methods can be found in the literature (9, 10, 62, 63) (Table 41-2) as well as in approaches developed by individual institutions. The Joint Commission mandates that all accredited hospitals provide a mechanism for resolving ethics conflicts in the medical setting (64).

Caregiver Burdens and Lack of Resources: When Patient and Family Interests Conflict

Very often, when a conflict regarding a medical decision occurs, the parties involved hope to identify the course of action that is ethically correct. Unfortunately, in most ethics cases, there is no single right answer. More often, a range of ethically acceptable options can be identified as well as those that might be impermissible. Because the stroke survivor may have temporary or permanent disability that requires the care of another person, the interests of the patient are frequently intertwined with those of his or her involved family members.

In many ethics cases, clinicians are taught that the interests and wishes of the patient supersede those of family members. Several authors caution, however, that dealing with the family issues and interests should not be an afterthought (2, 3). Instead, clinicians should partner with families to optimize the choices for the patient. Indeed, when patients need care and/or supervision following a stroke, the patient's ability to recover may be directly related with the health of the family system. Family caregivers give assistance to loved ones who are ill or have disabilities. This care would otherwise cost tens to hundreds of thousands of dollars annually if the patient hired a third party to provide it. Some families may not be physically or psychologically equipped to participate in the care of their loved one. Others may lack the financial resources or flexibility to

---

TABLE 41-2
Selected Paradigms for Case-based, Ethical Decision-making

Jonsen, Siegler, and Winslade (2006) = The Four-box Model (10)
Consideration of four coexisting factors (medical indications, patient preferences, quality of life, and contextual features) present in the shared decision-making process. Primary focus is on the patient-clinician relationship acknowledging potential conflict between "Medical Recommendations" [beneficence] with "Patient Preferences" [autonomy]

McCormick-Gendzel and Jurchak (2006) = FESOR (62)
Facts: Collect the facts of the case
Ethics: Identify and apply the appropriate ethical principles
Stakeholders: Ensure that all stakeholders are involved in the process
Options: Identifying and implementing the ethically acceptable options
Results: Evaluating the outcome of the ethical analysis and decision for all stakeholders

Miller, Fletcher, and Fins (1997) = Clinical Pragmatism (65)
Detailed ethical decision-making model in outline/checklist format that gathers information for a moral diagnosis.
 Reflective analysis is used to develop approaches for managing similar situations in the future.

Purtilo (2005) = Six-Step Process of Ethical Decision-Making (63)
1. Getting the story straight: gather relevant information
2. Identify type of ethical problem (e.g., ethical distress, ethical dilemma, question of locus of authority)
3. Use ethics theories or approaches to analyze the problem(s)
4. Explore the practical alternatives
5. Complete the action
6. Evaluate the process and outcome

TABLE 41.3
Family-focused Team Approach

Dealing with family conflict and competing interests in
the care of a stroke survivor by addressing the following:
1. Recognize all family members with standing
2. Identify family-focused goals
3. Communicate a commitment to the whole family
4. Address competing interests
5. Identify and protect vulnerable family members
6. Construct family discharge plans

Adapted from Brashler (2)

---

reduce work hours or leave a job to care for a relative/
close friend.

Brashler (2) recommends a family-focused team
approach to identifying, recognizing, and addressing
conflicts between the interests of patients and those of
their family members. Central to this approach is the
understanding that the recovery and success of a person following stroke may be substantially dependent on
the involvement of family members willing to assist the
patient, so their interests are inseparable. The key considerations in Brashler's model include bringing all family
stakeholders into the discussion, dealing directly and
openly with competing interests, and developing shared
goals to create a family discharge plan (Table 41-3).

Management of Dysphagia: A Predictable Ethical Challenge after Stroke

In the last eight months I have swallowed nothing
save a few drops of lemon-flavored water and a half-
teaspoon of yogurt, which gurgled noisily down my
windpipe. The feeding test—as they grandly called this
banquet—was not a success. But no call for alarm;
I haven't starved. By means of a tube threaded into
my stomach, two or three bags of a brownish fluid
provide my daily caloric needs. For pleasure, I have
to turn to the vivid memory of tastes and smells, an
inexhaustible reservoir of sensations. Once, I was a
master at recycling leftovers. Now I cultivate the art
of simmering memories . . . (32)

Stroke can be a life-threatening event, and over 20%
of strokes are fatal (www.americanheart.org). There are
many medical sequelae of stroke that may result in death.
One commonly occurring condition is dysphagia with
subsequent aspiration pneumonia. Recent standardization of acute stroke care has highlighted the importance
of dysphagia screening as a means of mitigating this risk.
(See www.jointcommission.org/CertificationPrograms/
Disease-SpecificCare/DCSPM.)

Dysphagia is the impairment of one's ability to
chew and swallow food and liquid safely and efficiently
(taking in enough calories in a given time frame) to sustain life. It is estimated that anywhere from 64 to 78%
of all persons surviving stroke develop at least some
degree of dysphagia (68, 69). The severity of problems
following dysphagia can range from a mild condition
in which the person requires extra time to complete a
meal to very severe when an individual cannot manage
his or her secretions safely and requires a tracheostomy
tube to protect the airway. In cases of severe dysphagia,
an alternative method of nutrition and hydration may
be recommended and initiated in the acute phase of
the illness (68).

Clinicians and patients may disagree over treatment when severe dysphagia is diagnosed. Clinicians
may recommend alternative nutrition and hydration
with the goal of avoiding aspiration and its complications while maintaining sustenance. The issue of food
and nutrition often raises strong emotions for patients
and families. Food has high symbolic value and is not
simply a medical question. It is an issue rooted in social
habits and cultural values. Even though various ethical issues arise in the treatment of dysphagia, including
questioning the continuation of a life-sustaining treatment, perhaps the most challenging for many clinicians
is balancing a patient's desire to eat, regardless of the
hazard posed when the an alternative feeding approach
is believed to be lower risk by the clinical team. The
conflict between a clinicians' sense of beneficence and
the patients' preferences or desires frequently causes
considerable ethical distress for the clinician.

Beneficence and autonomy are two of the corner-
stones of Western bioethics principles. Beauchamp and
Childress (9) state that beneficence is the obligation of the
health care provider to do good for their patient, based on
what he or she believes to be in the patient's best interest.
The principle of autonomy is the duty of the health professional to respect, support, and facilitate the patient's
ability to make an authentic medical choice without coer-
cion. When clinicians find themselves in a situation where
these two principles directly conflict, the ethical distress
can be high. Further complicating this issue is the active
role that the health care team plays in assisting stroke
patients with dysphagia. Thus, a patient who is deemed
unsafe to take oral nutrition, but insists on receiving this
feeding nonetheless, may require assistance by the nurse
or SLP in eating. Health care professionals are trained
to make recommendations that promote health. When
a patient or a proxy makes a decision that appears to
place a person at risk for a poor health outcome, and the
health care team's participation is required, some clinicians are inclined to view such a decision as unethical
based upon the principle of nonmaleficence—that is, "Do
no harm."

Sharp and Genesen (69) describe how a case-based model of clinical ethical analysis can be useful in managing the ethical challenges inherent in such conflicts. Use of this model, based on Jonsen, Siegler, and Winslade (10) (Table 41-2), can assist clinicians and others in identifying ethically acceptable options. The primary challenge is balancing respect for a patient's autonomous wishes related to use of feeding tubes and oral intake after carefully weighing the risks and benefits of eating and drinking when one has dysphagia. As with all other medical decisions, recommendations related to dysphagia should occur in the context of an informed consent and shared decision-making process.

When such values conflicts arise in the clinical care of a patient post-stroke, some health care providers wonder if they should continue to be involved in the care of that patient, even if they fundamentally agree with the principle that patients have the right to reject medical recommendations. We believe this consideration is based on two concerns:

1. The treating clinician will be complicit in a "bad decision" that may result in harm to the patient.
2. The clinician may be liable from a legal perspective if the patient experiences a bad outcome.

Clinicians are highly immersed in a medical culture that promotes improving health, and find participation in a treatment plan that may result in "avoidable" medical complications uncomfortable at best. These situations can be very difficult to negotiate. Even though in most scenarios professionals have the right to withdraw from a clinical case where they feel that care is in conflict with their own ethical values (a conscientious objection clause

of sorts), it is critical to avoid abandoning the patient in the process. Because we recognize that people have the right to accept our recommendations, they also have the correlate right to refuse them. If a clinical recommendation is rejected, patients still may benefit from clinical interventions to mitigate potential harms. Additionally, patients may refuse recommendations for many reasons (Table 41-4). Without coercing or usurping a patient's right to make his or her own choices, clinicians should investigate the reasons behind a patient's refusal to accept treatment recommendations and to aid him or her in attaining as complete an understanding of the issues as feasible to ensure that this is an informed choice.

The degree of uncertainty regarding the outcome of a particular medical treatment (or foregoing that treatment) may guide the options and decisions made by patients, proxies, and health care providers. When the benefits of a certain treatment outweigh the risks, for example, an otherwise healthy person taking antibiotics for pneumonia, clinicians may try to assure or persuade patients through further education and discussion to accept the recommended treatment. In other cases, such as the treatment of dysphagia, the degree of uncertainty of the likelihood of a poor outcome (for example, development of aspiration pneumonia) can be quite high (70). The clinical consequences of aspiration or risk of aspiration are not fully understood. In a medical record review of nursing home residents, Langmore et al. (70) concluded that, even though dysphagia was a risk factor for the development of aspiration pneumonia, it was not a leading determinant. The fact that an individual was dependent upon another person for feeding or had poor dental and oral hygiene were stronger predictors of the development of aspiration pneumonia.

TABLE 41-4
Reasons for Patient/Surrogate Refusal of Medical Recommendations

1. Personal values and preferences (may include religious beliefs)
2. Desire to continue current behaviors (e.g., refusal to stop smoking, refusal to change diet). Patient values the behavior above the health-related concern (quality of life judgment).
3. Concern that the intervention will be painful or uncomfortable
4. Fear of the potential for negative outcome from the procedure (e.g., mortality risk in some surgeries)
5. Lack of full understanding of the recommendations (e.g., language barrier, belief that the treatment is something other than described, not yet realized lack of DMC)
6. Conflicting recommendations from various health care professionals
7. Cultural differences (e.g., family members helping persons with disabilities instead of facilitating independence in ADL)
8. Negative personal experience (self, family member, or friend) with the recommended treatment plan
9. Lack of understanding of the potential for recovery or possibility of a positive quality of life given the patient's current condition
10. Family conflict
11. Lack of insurance benefit (e.g., personal payment for the treatment would drain personal and family resources)
12. Lack of trust in the clinician or in medical personnel in general
13. Depression or thought disorder

Time-limited Trials

Clinical ethicists have promoted the use of a time-limited trial of treatment in order to assist decision-making and cooperation in cases of disagreement or uncertainty about the best course of action (71, 72). For example, the use of an alternative method of nutrition and hydration is often recommended when a patient experiences moderate or severe dysphagia. The goal of using enteral or parenteral feeding is to reduce the risk of prandial aspiration by bypassing the oral route altogether. It is also to ensure adequate caloric and nutritional intake and hydration to foster recovery and avoid malnourishment. There is growing literature that questions these assumptions for certain patient populations, in particular persons with advanced dementia (73, 74). Some studies (75) have found that the risk of aspiration of gastric reflux actually increases when feeding tubes are placed.

In a time-limited trial of treatment, the patient agrees to try a treatment for a limited period of time, followed by a period of reassessment and renegotiation. The patient will then either continue the trial treatment or change course (76). The following clinical vignette illustrates this concept:

> Mrs. E was admitted to a rehabilitation hospital after a pontine stroke. She presented with moderate to severe dyphagia and had a PEG placed in the acute care hospital. Several days after Mrs. E arrived, she told her SLP that she no longer wished to use the feeding tube and she wanted to eat and drink, despite her treatment team's strong recommendation that she continue to rely on tube feedings for the present time. After much discussion, Mrs. E and her team agreed to a time-limited trial of continuation of the PEG feedings and intensive swallowing therapy to target and remediate her difficulties. At the agreed reevaluation point two weeks later, the patient's swallowing was much improved. She was able to begin eating pureed solids at that time, consistent with the SLP's recommendations.

Another version of this time-limited trial scenario is as follows:

> Mrs. E was admitted to a rehabilitation hospital after a pontine stroke. She communicated to the staff via a letterboard that she would like to discontinue use of her PEG tube. Despite discussion and further education, the patient was not dissuaded from this decision, even though she was aspirating. Mrs. E agreed to begin eating a diet that had been deemed to be the safest and to use swallowing techniques taught her by her SLP for a period of two weeks. After this trial period, the patient had not developed any respiratory complications, and, indeed, her swallowing function had improved. The SLP upgraded her diet further.

Use of time-limited trials can be extremely valuable in many cases by clarifying what the goals and measurable risks are for a particular patient.

Combination Treatment

Another strategy for balancing conflicting values is to combine a therapy that has been recommended by the clinician with a high priority desire of the patient that also has some risk (76). This vignette provides an example:

> Mr. B was a 46-year-old gentleman who sustained a right hemisphere stroke and now had left-sided paralysis, visual neglect, and severe dysphagia. Although he demonstrated mild cognitive-communication impairments, he was felt to have adequate DMC regarding his feeding choices. Because of aspiration on all consistencies, Mr. B's physician recommended a feeding tube. After a thorough discussion about the risks, benefits, and alternatives, Mr. B refused. Though he wanted to get better, he placed higher value on eating and drinking orally and accepted the risk of aspiration pneumonia. The SLP considered removing herself from his case because of her discomfort with his decision. After discussing her concerns with the patient's physician and a clinical ethicist in the hospital, she was able to accept his decision as informed and authentic. She chose to stay involved and attempt to mitigate potential harms by educating Mr. B on a diet and techniques that were safest while carefully documenting all discussions and the process of decision making in the case (Table 41-5).

Using combination therapy allows clinicians to engage in providing patients with needed expertise and care while acknowledging and supporting the person's informed choice to refuse a particular medical treatment.

The use of feeding tubes is perhaps one of the most widely discussed life-sustaining treatments in the field of medical ethics, as evidenced by the recent controversies surrounding Terry Schiavo (59). Differing conceptual frameworks for the meaning of a feeding tube seem to underlie at least some of the debate (77). A traditional medical ethics perspective is that a feeding tube is a form of medical treatment, similar to a ventilator, and can be withheld or withdrawn as such. A second perspective is that a feeding tube provides basic humane care of food and fluids. Without which, a person cannot survive, so they should always be continued. A third perspective would be that a feeding tube is a disability accommodation. Just as a person uses a wheelchair for a mobility impairment, a person uses a feeding tube for a swallowing impairment. Understanding the perspective of the various parties involved when a discussion arises about withdrawing or withholding food and fluid can

---

TABLE 41-5
Critical Documentation of the Shared Decision-making Process

1. The clinical situation and recommendation(s)
2. Whether or not the patient has DMC to participate in the decision
3. If the patient is not the decision-maker, indicate who is
4. Report information shared with patient and/or the surrogate
5. The response of the patient or proxy
6. If the response was a rejection of the clinical recommendations, state the reasons given
7. Further information provided to the patient and/or surrogate to address questions or concerns that may have been raised
8. The agreed-upon plan
9. Plan for monitoring the intervention

* In general and importantly, documentation should consistently reflect who the decision-maker is and that questions about care are appropriately directed to that person.

---

help in negotiating difficult conversations (77). Decisions to withhold or withdraw a life-sustaining treatment are very emotionally charged because they are in most cases, by definition, final decisions.

Withdrawal or Withholding of Life-Sustaining Treatment

We make a distinction here between withholding and withdrawal of treatment and withholding and withdrawing care. Medical and basic care is/should always be provided to a patient, but, in all but the most exceptional of circumstances, the withholding and withdrawal of medical treatment is the personal preference of an autonomous patient or her surrogate. Withholding life-sustaining treatment is a term applied to a situation in which a medical treatment is not initiated. Withdrawal of life-sustaining treatment is the discontinuation of a medical treatment after it has been started (9).

Withholding and withdrawing life-sustaining treatment are often within the purview of a proxy decision-maker, just as they are for a patient (47, 78), though the circumstances may be limited by a patient's advance directive or state law. Based on the presumed right to privacy, that is, to be free of unwanted medical treatment, case law in the United States recognizes this personal choice as a defensible construct (46). Ethical study also supports this as a correlate for the respect for patient autonomy. Both legal and ethical frameworks hold that there is no moral difference between withdrawing or withholding life-sustaining treatments (79, 80), though clinicians do not always agree. Within the context of a clinical case, some clinicians feel that withdrawing life-sustaining medical treatment feels psychologically as if they have a direct responsibility for the patient's death (79, 81).

Team Conflicts: Goals of Rehabilitation

The biggest lesson I learned that morning was that when it came to my rehabilitation, I was ultimately the one in control of the success or failure of those caring for me. It was my decision to show up or not. I chose to show up for those professionals who brought me energy by connecting with me, touching me gently and appropriately, making direct eye contact with me, and speaking to me calmly. I responded positively to positive treatment. The professionals who did not connect with me sapped my energy, so I protected myself by ignoring their requests. (1)

The literature has suggested that team-based care, as is the model for rehabilitation, may inherently predispose individuals to conflict (82). As previously stated, conflicts often arise when a clinician's professional recommendation is at odds with a patient's choice. Sharp (82) delineates an often-experienced process of individuals coming together to form a team. She indicates that the way people come together and begin to make joint decisions may not be smooth. Often, groups test each other before they trust the judgment and recommendations of other group members. Teams then ideally reach a place where they can challenge one another safely and reach consensus for the best approach to a particular patient. Dowdy and his colleagues (83) demonstrated that challenging issues are predictable in certain clinical contexts and that use of a preemptive ethical consultation aided team members in feeling that they were each involved in the process of decision-making. Bringing clinical teams, patients, and families together to discuss problems and issues is often a very effective means of navigating and resolving conflict (61, 84).

The patient and family (2) are part of this team as well. They are prone to similar adjustment challenges to team interaction and communication as those faced by clinicians. However, at the end of the day, the patient and, in many cases, the family have the most at stake in any scenario. Having direct conversations with patients to learn and focus on their specific goals can aid interdisciplinary teams in avoiding unnecessary discord and in allowing patients' wishes to direct the plan of care to the greatest degree possible.

SUMMARY

> I think that one of the problems with stroke is that, as a condition, it offers a moving target. Compared to, say, cancer, stroke is not a degenerative condition. If you survive the initial crisis you are—with luck— constantly and imperceptibly getting better. I had to learn to adjust, and also to wait. (36)

Ethical issues are common in the clinical care of persons who survive a stroke, in part, because different individuals in an interdisciplinary team, including patients and families, can experience conflicting values and, in part, because the experience and sequelae of stroke may change a person's abilities and concept of himself or herself. This shift in perspective that stroke survivors commonly experience may require a period of reflection and redefinition for the stroke survivor to clarify his or her new vantage point. Stroke can result in cognitive and communication impairments that affect a survivor's ability to participate in both the routine and the complex decisions about medical care faced in the first hours, days, and even years following the event. Additionally, some potentially life-threatening medical conditions, such as dysphagia, require balanced consideration of the risks and benefits of common and sometimes invasive interventions.

This chapter has presented an overview of the kinds of ethical issues faced by health care providers, patients, and families in the care of stroke survivors. Understanding and use of ethical paradigms and principles will guide clinicians and clinical teams in identifying ethically acceptable options in difficult circumstances. Keeping the wishes of the patient paramount and supporting participation of patients who demonstrate significant communication impairment are critical in reaching optimal outcomes.

Illness can create defining moments in one's life. Clinicians have a role in fostering and facilitating self-actualized choices for the stroke survivor. In the face of great change (either temporary or lasting), patients can still maintain dignity and self-fulfillment with a considered and ethical approach to patient interaction and care.

As Marc Black Sings in "When You Get Back," "... you never get back to where you've been, always get back to where you're going on down the line" (85).

ACKNOWLEDGMENTS

The authors would like to gratefully acknowledge the diligent research and legal memorandum on state surrogacy legislation contributed by Priya Sazawal Koul, J.D. Candidate 2008, Chicago-Kent College of Law.

References

1. Taylor J. *My Stroke of Insight: A Brain Scientist's Personal Journey*. Lulu.com, 2006.
2. Brashler R. Ethics, Family Caregivers, and Stroke. *Top Stroke Rehabil* 2006; 13(4):11–17.
3. Levine C, Zuckerman C. The trouble with families: Toward an ethic of accommodation. *Ann Intern Med* 1999; 130(2):148–152.
4. Rabeneck L, McCullough L, Wray N. Ethically justified, clinically comprehensive guidelines for percutaneous endoscopic gastrostomy tube placement. *Lancet* 1997; 349(9050): 496–498.
5. Sharp H. Ethical issues in the management of dysphagia after stroke. *Top Stroke Rehabil* 2006; 13(4):18–25.
6. Sharp H, Bryant K. Ethical issues in dysphagia: When patients refuse assessment or treatment. *Seminars in Speech and Language* 2003; 24(4): 285–300.
7. Kirschner K, Stocking C, Wagner LB, et al. Ethical issues identified by rehabilitation clinicians. *Arch Phys Med Rehabil* 2001; 82(12 Suppl 2):S2–8.
8. Demarquay G, Derex L, Nighoghossian N, et al. Ethical issues of informed consent in acute stroke: Analysis of the modalities of consent in 56 patients enrolled in urgent therapeutic trials. *Cerebrovascular Diseases* 2005; 19:65–68.
9. Beauchamp T, Childress J. *Principles of Biomedical Ethics*. 5th ed. New York: Oxford, 2001.
10. Jonsen A, Siegler M, Winslade W. *Clinical Ethics: A Practical Approach to Ethical Decisions in Clinical Medicine*. 6th ed. New York: McGraw-Hill, 2006.
11. Bernat J. *Ethical Issues in Neurology*. 2nd ed. Boston: Butterworth Heinemann, 2002.
12. Freedman M, Stuss D, Gordon M. Assessment of competency: The role of neurobehavioral deficits. *Ann Intern Med* 1991; 115: 203–208.
13. Lo B. Assessing decision-making capacity. *Law Med Health Care* 1990; 18(3):193–201.
14. Tunzi M. Can the patient decide? Evaluating patient capacity in practice. *American Family Physician* 2001; 64(2).
15. Appelbaum P, Grisso T. Assessing patients' capacities to consent to treatment. *NEJM* 1988; 319:1635–1638.
16. Kothari S, Kirschner K. Decision-making capacity after TBI: Clinical assessment and ethical implications. In Zasler ND, Katz DI, Zafonte RD, eds. *Brain Injury Medicine*. New York: Demos Medical Publishing, 2007:1205–1222.
17. Etchells E, Darzins P, Silberfeld M, et al. Assessment of patient capacity to consent to treatment. *J Gen Intern Med* 1999; 14: 27–34.
18. Drane J. *Clinical Bioethics: Theory and Practice in Medical-Ethical Decision Making*. Kansas City, MO: Sheed & Ward, 1994.
19. Stein J, Wagner LB. Is informed consent at "yes or no" response? Enhancing the shared decision-making process for persons with aphasia. *Top Stroke Rehabil* 2006; 13(4):42–46.
20. Tippett D, Sugarman J. Discussing advance directives under the patient self-determination act: A unique opportunity for speech-language pathologists to help persons with aphasia. *Am J Speech-Lang Path* 1996; 5:31–34.
21. Wagner LB. Clinical ethics in the context of language and cognitive impairments: Rights and protections. *Seminars in Speech and Language* 2003; 24(3): 275–284.
22. Alexander M. Clinical determination of mental competence: A theory and a retrospective study. *Archives of Neurology* 1988; 45:23–26.
23. Diener B, Bischof-Rosarioz J. Determining DMC in individuals with severe communication impairments with the use of augmentative-alternative communication (AAC). *Top Stroke Rehabil* 2004; 11(1):84–88.
24. *Principles of Behavioral and Cognitive Neurology, Second Edition*. Edited by M.–Marsel Mesulam, M.D. Oxford, UK: Oxford University Press, 2000.
25. Kirschner K. Ethics in practice: Assessing decision-making capacity in a patient with nondominant hemisphere stroke. *Top Stroke Rehabil* 1994; 1:104–105.
26. Benson F, Geschwind N. Aphasia and related disorders: A clinical approach. In: Mesulam M, ed. *Principles of Behavioral Neurology*. Philadelphia: F.A. Davis, 1985.
27. Goodglass H. *Understanding Aphasia*. New York Academic Press, 1993.
28. Brady L, Kirschner K. Ethical issues for persons with aphasia and their families. *Top Stroke Rehabil* 1995; 2:84–87.
29. Holland A, Halper A. Talking to individuals with aphasia: A challenge to the rehabilitation team. *Top Stroke Rehabil* 1996; 2:27–37.
30. Kagan A. Supported conversation for adults with aphasia: Methods and resources for training conversation partners. *Aphasiology* 1998; 12(9):816–830.

31. Kagan A. Revealing the competence of aphasic adults through conversation: A challenge to health professionals. *Top Stroke Rehabil* 1995; 2:15–28.

32. Bauby J. *The Diving Bell and the Butterfly: A Memoir of Life in Death*. Paris: Alfred A Knopf, 1997.

33. Fried-Oken M, Bersani H, eds. *Speaking Up and Spelling It Out*. Baltimore: Paul H. Brookes, 2000.

34. Strand E. Clinical and professional ethics in the management of motor speech disorders. *Seminars in Speech and Language* 2003; 24(4):301–311.

35. Stinneford K, Kirschner K. Concepts of medical necessity in rehabilitation. *Top Stroke Rehabil* 2004; 11(2):69–76.

36. McCrum R. *My Year Off: Recovering Life After a Stroke*. New York: Horton, 1998.

37. Lezak M, Howieson D, Loring D, et al. *Neuropsychological Assessment*. 4th ed. New York: Oxford University Press, 2004.

38. Mukherjee E, Levin R, Heller W. The cognitive, emotional, and social sequelae of stroke: Psychological and ethical concerns in post-stroke adaption. *Top Stroke Rehabil* 2006; 13(4):26–35.

39. Nitschke J, Heller W. Distinguishing neural substrates of heterogeneity among anxiety disorders. *Int Rev Neurobiol* 2005; 67:1–42.

40. Ouimet M, Primeau F, Cole M. Psychological risk factors in post-stroke depression: A systematic review. *Can J Psychiatry* 2001; 46: 819–828.

41. Salmond S, David E. Attitudes toward advance directives and advance directive completion rates. *Orthopedic Nursing* 2005; 24(2):117–129.

42. Gordon N, Shade S. Advance directives are more likely among seniors asked about end-of-life care preferences. *Arch Intern Med* 1999; 159:701–704.

43. Mezey M, Leitman R, Mitty E, et al. Why hospital patients do and do not execute an advance directive. *Nursing Outlook* 2000; 48:165–171.

44. Morrison R, Zayas L, Mulvihill M, et al. Barriers to completion of health care proxies: An examination of ethnic differences. *Arch Intern Med* 1998; 158:2493–2497.

45. 1990 OBRAo. *Pub Law 101–508, 4206, 4751*. 1990.

46. *In Re Quinlan*. 70 N.J. 10, 355 A.2d 647 1976.

47. Kirschner K. When written advance directives are not enough. *Clin Geriatr Med* 2005; 21:193–209.

48. *Cruzan v. Director*. Department of Health, 58 U.S. L. W. 4916. 1990.

49. Koul P. *Research on Health Care Surrogate Acts*. Kirschner K, Wagner LB, eds. Chicago, 2007.

50. Prendergast T. Advance care planning: Pitfalls, progress, promise. *Crit Care Med* 2001; 29(suppl.): N34–N39.

51. Kothari S, Kirschner K. Abandoning the golden rule: The problem with "putting ourselves in the patient's place." *Top Stroke Rehabil* 2006; 13(4):68–73.

52. Dworkin R. *Life's Dominion*. New York: Alfred A. Knopf Publishers, 1993.

53. Parfit D. *Reasons and Persons*. Oxford: Oxford University Press, 1984.

54. Dresser R. Dworkin on dementia: Elegant theory, questionable policy. *Hastings Cent Rep* 1995; 25:32–38.

55. Stein J. The ethics of advance directives: A rehabilitation perspective. *Am J Phys Med Rehabil* 2003; 82:152–157.

56. Hardwig J. What about the family? *Hastings Cent Rep* 1990; 20:5–10.

57. Kuczewski M, Kirschner K. Special issue: Bioethics & disability. *Theor Med Bioeth* 2003; 24(6):455–458.

58. *In re Michael Martin* (Nos. 99699, 99700) Supreme Court of Michigan, 1995.

59. *In re: guardianship of Theresa Marie Schaivo*, Case No. 2D02-5394, 2003.

60. Lo B, Dornbrand L, Wolf L, Groman M. The Wendland case: Withdrawing life support from incompetent patients who are not terminally ill. *N Engl J Med* 2002; 346: 1489–1493.

61. Spielman B. Conflict in medical ethics cases: Seeking patterns of resolution. *J Clin Ethics* 1993; 4(3):212–218.

62. McCormick-Gendzel M, Jurchak M. A pathway for moral reasoning. *Home Healthcare Nurse* 2006; 24(10):654–661.

63. Purtilo R. *Ethical Dimensions in the Health Professions*. Philadelphia: Elsevier Saunders, 2005.

64. JCAHO. *Comprehensive Accreditation Manual for Hospitals*. Oakbrook Terrace, IL: Author, 2004.

65. Miller F, Fletcher J, Fins J. Clinical pragmatism: a case method of moral problem solving. In Fletcher LP, Marshall FM, Miller FG, eds. *Introduction to Clinical Ethics*. Hagerstown: University Publishing Group, 1997:21–38.

66. Mann G, Hankey G, Cameron D. Swallowing disorders following acute stroke: Prevalence and diagnostic accuracy. *Cerebrovascular Diseases* 2000; 10(5): 380–386.

67. Martino R, Foley N, Bhogal S, et al. Dysphagia after stroke: Incidence, diagnosis and pulmonary complications. *Stroke* 2005; 36:2756–2763.

68. Logemann J. *Evaluation and Treatment of Swallowing Disorders*. 2nd. ed. Austin: ProEd, 1998.

69. Sharp H, Genesen L. Ethical decision-making in dysphagia management. *Am J Speech-Lang Path* 1996; 5:15–22.

70. Langmore S, Terpenning M, Schork, et al. Predictors of aspiration pneumonia: How important is dysphagia? *Dysphagia* 1998; 13:69–81.

71. Lo B. *Resolving Ethical Dilemmas: A Guide for Clinicians*. 2nd. ed. Philadelphia: Lippincott, Williams, Wilkins, 2000.

72. Ruark J, Raffin T, Ethics SUMCCo. Initiating and withdrawing life support. *N Engl J Med* 1988; 318:25–30.

73. Callahan C, Haag K, Weinberger M, et al. Outcomes of percutaneous endoscopic gastrostomy among older adults in a community setting. *J Am Geriatric Soc* 2000; 48(9):1048–1054.

74. Post S. Tube feeding and advanced progressive dementia. *Hastings Cent Rep* 2001; 31(1):36–42.

75. Finucane T, Christmas C, Travis K. Tube feeding in patients with advanced dementia: A review of the evidence. *JAMA* 1999; 282(14):1365–1370.

76. Sharp H, Wagner LB. Ethics, informed consent, and decisions about non-oral feeding for patients with dysphagia. *Topics in Geriatric Rehabilitation* July/September 2007; 23(3):240–248.

77. Brashler R, Savage T, Mukherjee D, Kirschner K. Feeding tubes: Three perspectives. *Top Stroke Rehabil* 2007; 14(6):74–77.

78. Lang F, Quill T. Making decisions with families at the end of life. *American Family Physician* 2004; 70(4):719–723.

79. Edwards M, Tolle S. Disconnecting a ventilator at the request of a patient who knows he will then die: The doctor's anguish. *Ann Intern Med* 1992; 117(3):254–256.

80. Ethics AMACoM. *E-2.20 Withholding or Withdrawing Life-Sustaining Medical Treatment*. 2005.

81. Levin P, Sprung C. Withdrawing and withholding life-sustaining therapies are not the same. *Critical Care* 2005; 9:230–232.

82. Sharp H. Ethical decision-making in interdisciplinary team care. *Cleft Palate Craniofac J* 1995; 32(6):495–499.

83. Dowdy M, Robertson C, Bander J. A study of proactive ethics consultation for critically and terminally ill patients with extended lengths of stay. *Crit Care Med* 1998; 26(2):252–259.

84. Orr R, deLeon D. The role of the clinical ethicist in conflict resolution. *J Clin Ethics* 2000; 11(1):21–30.

85. Black M. *A Stroke of Genius*. Marc Black, 2006.

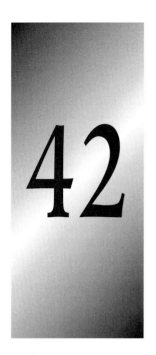

42 Stroke and the Family

Tamilyn Bakas

amilies are an integral part of stroke recovery and rehabilitation. A family caregiver can be a relative, partner, personal friend, or neighbor who provides assistance to an older person or adult with a chronic or disabling condition (1). Roughly 68–74% of stroke survivors are discharged home under the care of family members (2, 3). Stroke is different from other chronic conditions in that stroke caregivers must suddenly assume the caregiving role after a stroke event, whereas, for example, dementia caregivers typically assume the caregiving role gradually over time (4). Family caregivers must quickly learn how to help stroke survivors live with a variety of stroke-related impairments (for example, motor, sensory, visual, language, cognitive, and affective impairments) (5, 6) while also trying to adapt to the changes in their own lives that have resulted from providing care (7–11). Studies have shown that family caregivers are at risk for depression, psychosocial impairments, and mortality as a result of providing care (12–14). To make matters worse, family caregivers of stroke survivors are commonly neglected by health care providers in the practice setting (7, 13). In a study of 116 stroke caregivers, 11.7% reported that communication with health professionals was very or extremely difficult (15). Stroke affects the entire family, not just the stroke survivor and his or her caregiver. The survivor's children, siblings, parents,

extended family, and friends are also affected. The purpose of this chapter is to provide a general overview of the impact of stroke on the family and to explore existing literature regarding stroke caregiver interventions, which are designed to support families of stroke survivors through recovery and rehabilitation.

IMPACT OF STROKE ON FAMILY MEMBERS

Family caregivers have a variety of needs and concerns related to stroke care and also experience negative outcomes such as depression, declining health, and other life changes such as social and financial problems. Other family members may experience conflict, psychological distress, and other negative outcomes. The literature regarding these topics is reviewed in the following sections.

Caregiver Needs and Concerns

The assessment of caregiver needs and concerns from the caregivers' perspective and culture is important across inpatient, outpatient, and community-based settings (1, 7, 16). The Caregiver Needs and Concerns Checklist (CNCC) is one instrument with which health care providers can assess caregivers in the context of stroke care (Figure 42-1) (7) The CNCC, originally developed based on qualitative comments from stroke caregivers, addresses five main areas of needs and concerns:

1. Information
2. Emotions and behaviors
3. Physical care
4. Instrumental care
5. Personal responses to caregiving

Information.   Finding information about stroke is especially important for families because spouses and other family members are commonly the initiators of emergency care for stroke survivors (17). Of the estimated 700,000 strokes that occur each year in the United States, 200,000 are recurrent strokes (5). Moreover, 14% of persons experiencing a stroke or a transient ischemic attack (TIA) for the first time will have a reoccurrence within one year (5). Family caregivers of stroke survivors have expressed concerns about whether they would be able to recognize a second stroke, and they want more information from health professionals about stroke warning signs (7, 18). For example, one caregiver reported that she thought her father was drinking when he was actually suffering a stroke. She was concerned that she might not be able to recognize signs of another stroke (7). Stroke warning signs can be difficult to distinguish from other conditions, particularly when a stroke survivor already has some residual deficits from the initial stroke. It is imperative that health professionals assess and reinforce knowledge of stroke warning signs in both patients and caregivers during follow-up visits.

Stroke caregivers also have needs and concerns about recommended lifestyle changes and risk factors for recurrent stroke. One caregiver reported that she had only received information about her husband's diet and speech therapy and commented that, if he had had a heart attack, she would have received more information on smoking, exercise, and other lifestyle changes (7). Another study reported that only 40% of stroke caregivers remembered receiving any information about stroke prevention (16). Providing information for stroke survivors and families regarding lifestyle changes and risk factors for recurrent stroke is critical for secondary stroke prevention. Current guidelines recommend management of hypertension, diabetes, and cholesterol in stroke survivors, along with counseling to avoid smoking, heavy alcohol consumption, and obesity (19). Stroke survivors should also undergo a supervised therapeutic exercise regimen that includes a pre-exercise evaluation (19, 20). Family caregivers need information about these recommendations so they can encourage and reinforce prescribed healthy behaviors and lifestyle changes throughout stroke recovery and rehabilitation.

Additional areas of stroke caregiver informational needs and concerns relate to:

- Medication management
- The survivor's condition and treatment plans
- Management of specific symptoms or problems that the survivor may have (for example, constipation, bowel or bladder incontinence, dizziness, fatigue, and pain)
- Which health professionals to call for advice
- Where to find books or written materials, support groups, or organizations that can help (7)

Stroke organizations, such as the American Stroke Association (www.strokeassociation.org; 1-888-478-7653) and the National Stroke Association (www.stroke.org; 1-800-787-6537), can be valuable resources for stroke survivors and their families. They offer written information on a variety of stroke-related topics, monthly magazine subscriptions addressing the latest issues in stroke care, websites for stroke survivors and caregivers, and lists of stroke support groups for specific geographical areas. Informational needs may not be the same for each caregiver, so individualization is often indicated. This can be challenging given the limited time that health professionals usually have with family members. In fact, caregivers often report that health professionals ignore them (7, 13). Nevertheless, caregivers recommend trying to get as much information as they can before the survivor is discharged home, asking for names of health professionals they can call for advice, attending therapy sessions, talking with other stroke survivors and caregivers, and looking for books or written materials, stroke support groups, home health care, financial counseling, and other resources that may assist them in providing care (7, 16).

Emotions and Behaviors.   Managing emotional and behavioral reactions of the stroke survivor are among the most stressful aspects of providing care for family caregivers (5, 10, 15, 16, 21–25). Some studies have also described how caregivers were unaware that difficult behaviors might be stroke-related and therefore responded with either anger or excessive sympathy (26, 27). Emotional and behavioral problems experienced by stroke survivors that caregivers typically face include depressive symptoms and other emotional reactions to stroke, changed personality or cognitive impairment resulting in disruptive behaviors, and communication deficits, including dealing with aphasia.

Studies have documented that approximately one-third of ischemic stroke survivors suffer from post-stroke depression, a condition that is often misdiagnosed, undertreated, and associated with poor outcomes and

Information: At this time, I would like more information about...

(Check all that apply.)

❑ the warning signs of another stroke.

❑ recommended lifestyle changes after stroke (e.g., eating a healthy diet, being physically active, stopping smoking, getting regular checkups).

❑ risk factors for stroke (e.g., controlling high blood pressure, diabetes).

❑ the stroke survivor's medications (e.g., drug name, what it's for, dosage, possible side effects).

❑ the stroke survivor's condition or what to expect before going home.

❑ how to manage specific problems the stroke survivor may have (e.g., constipation, bowel or bladder incontinence, dizziness, fatigue, pain).

❑ which health professionals to call for advice (e.g., doctor, nurse, physical therapist, occupational therapist, speech therapist, social worker).

❑ where to find books or written materials, support groups, or organizations that can help.

❑ where I can go for my healthcare needs.

Emotions and behaviors: At this time, I need help...

(Check all that apply.)

❑ dealing with the stroke survivor's emotions (e.g., mood fluctuations, anxiety, nervousness, anger, depression, poor future outlook).

❑ dealing with the stroke survivor's feelings about himself or herself (e.g., feelings of dependency, feelings of being a burden on others, worthlessness).

❑ keeping the stroke survivor socially active (e.g., keeping in touch with friends, holding an interest in others, finding someone to talk to who's had a stroke).

❑ communicating with the stroke survivor (e.g., trying to understand him or her, getting him or her to understand me, using the telephone, dealing with the frustration of communication).

❑ dealing with the stroke survivor's changed personality from the stroke.

❑ dealing with the stroke survivor's problems with thinking (e.g., loses or forgets things, has poor judgment, can't make decisions, confusion).

❑ dealing with the stroke survivor's difficult behaviors (e.g., cries easily, acts childlike, loses temper, uses foul language, waits for others to do things, doesn't appreciate caregiver).

Physical care: At this time, I need help...

(Check all that apply.)

❑ getting the stroke survivor to take medications on time.

❑ getting the stroke survivor to do prescribed exercises.

❑ learning how to help the stroke survivor walk, transfer to a wheelchair, move about, or avoid falls.

❑ getting the stroke survivor to eat (e.g., forgets to eat, refuses to eat, or has trouble swallowing).

❑ assisting the stroke survivor with bathing, dressing, or going to the bathroom.

Instrumental care: At this time, I need help ...

(Check all that apply.)

❑ learning how to manage checkbooks, bills, forms, or finances related to the stroke survivor's health care.

❑ trying to cover the cost of the stroke survivor's health care (e.g., medications, glasses, adult day care, therapy, services).

❑ transporting the stroke survivor places, going public with the wheelchair, or driving.

❑ finding care for the stroke survivor while I am away.

Personal responses to caregiving: At this time, I need help...

(Check all that apply.)

❑ dealing with my own emotions while providing care (e.g., mood fluctuations, anxiety, nervousness, anger, depression, poor future outlook, feelings of loss).

❑ with new responsibilities that I am not used to (e.g., taking on unfamiliar household tasks or things the stroke survivor used to do).

❑ finding the best way to ask family and friends for help with the stroke survivor's care.

❑ dealing with other things in my life (e.g., balancing work with caregiving, caring for other family members).

❑ taking care of my own health.

❑ keeping my energy level up.

❑ keeping my own social life going (e.g., getting out with friends and family, attending church, having free time for myself).

FIGURE 42-1

Caregiver Needs and Concerns Checklist. From "Needs, Concerns, Strategies, and Advice of Stroke Caregivers the First 6 months After Discharge," by T. Bakas, J. K. Austin, K. F. Okonkwo, R. R. Lewis, and L. Chadwick, 2002, *Journal of Neuroscience Nursing, 34(5)*, p. 245. Copyright 2002 by American Association of Neuroscience Nurses. Reprinted with permission.

increased mortality (28–31). Dealing with post-stroke depression is a primary concern for family caregivers, particularly because, although physical deficits are usually recognized in the hospital environment, cognitive-behavioral deficits may not become apparent until after discharge (4). Clark and colleagues (22) reported that 74% of their sample of 130 stroke caregivers indicated that their survivor appeared sad or depressed, and this was the most frequent memory or behavior change found in their study. Pierce and Steiner (32) reported in their qualitative study that male caregivers were most concerned about how to deal with their wife's depression and irritability. Although screening for depressive symptoms in stroke survivors using the PHQ-9 Depression Severity Scale is gaining attention in the literature (33), information provided to stroke caregivers on how to screen and seek treatment for post-stroke depressive symptoms is lacking. Caregiver communication with health care providers regarding survivor depressive symptoms can be challenging at times. For example, one caregiver reported that during a clinic visit she tried to inform the physician about her spouse's feelings of worthlessness and negative attitudes, but the survivor displayed a more positive attitude in the presence of doctors, making assessment and treatment for the depression difficult (7).

Additional survivor emotions and behaviors that are troublesome for stroke caregivers to manage include:

- Feelings of worthlessness and being a burden on others
- Moodiness
- Irritability
- Anger
- Loss of temper
- Frustration
- Indifference
- Negative interpersonal exchanges
- Emotional dependency
- Confusion
- Cognitive difficulty
- Memory loss
- Personality changes
- Inertia
- Waiting for others to do things the survivor can do
- Lack of participation in social activities
- Communication difficulties (7, 10, 15, 22, 24, 25, 27, 32, 34, 35)

Providing care to a stroke survivor who has aphasia has been associated with more negative caregiver outcomes and difficulties with tasks compared with caregivers of nonaphasic stroke survivors (10). In a sample of 42 family caregivers of aphasic stroke survivors, communication with the survivor, closely followed by managing behaviors,

were rated as the most difficult tasks caregivers faced (10). The challenges that caregivers have in communicating with aphasic survivors have been found in other studies as well (36, 37).

Unfortunately, no reported stroke caregiver intervention studies have specifically addressed how to help caregivers manage the emotional and behavioral reactions displayed by stroke survivors. Not all caregivers must deal with the same types of survivor emotions and behaviors; therefore, there is no one-size-fits-all solution to this problem. Nevertheless, supporting caregivers in their role of managing these difficult emotions and behaviors is paramount. Including the family caregiver in the assessment of stroke survivor depressive symptoms and other emotions and behaviors is a starting point where health professionals may begin to quickly identify areas for treatment or referral. Simply asking family caregivers about the emotions and behaviors they are dealing with and how they are communicating with the survivor may uncover serious barriers to stroke recovery and rehabilitation that may be amenable to treatment or psychological counseling for the survivor and his or her caregiver.

Physical Care.   Physical care provided by stroke caregivers may include such things as assisting the survivor with bathing, toileting, getting dressed, walking, mobility, exercises, meals, managing symptoms and deficits, and medication management. Studies have shown that caregivers do have concerns about managing stroke-related symptoms and deficits as well as providing basic stroke care (7, 15, 25). Although the provision of personal care (for example, bathing, toileting, getting dressed, and feeding) and assisting with mobility and exercises were not among the most difficult tasks on average in a sample of 116 stroke caregivers, 9.1% found personal care to be very or extremely difficult, and 14.3% found assisting with mobility to be very or extremely difficult (15). In a qualitative study of 14 stroke caregivers within six months after discharge, getting survivors to take their medications and exercise were major concerns, as were getting survivors to eat; assisting with bathing, dressing, or toileting; and avoiding falls (7). Caregivers suggested such things as using pill boxes for medications, taking the survivor to the mall for exercise, avoiding clutter to prevent falls, taking advantage of resources like Meals on Wheels, following a bladder and bowel regimen, and encouraging the survivor to do as much self-care as possible (7). Health professionals are encouraged to assist caregivers in providing personal care by encouraging them to attend therapy sessions with the survivor to learn transfer techniques and how to assist with activities of daily living. Medication instruction for stroke survivors should also include the family caregiver, especially if the stroke survivor has trouble reading or has poor sensory perception or cognitive deficits (38). Health professionals should encourage caregivers to ask questions about the survivor's medications, symptoms, and other stroke-related care issues (38).

Instrumental Care.   Instrumental care provided by stroke caregivers include such things as dealing with financial issues, providing transportation, assisting with household tasks (for example, laundry, cooking, cleaning, yard work, and home repairs), shopping, running errands, managing services and resources, as well as finding someone to care for the survivor while away. In one study of 116 stroke caregivers, household tasks and managing finances were among the top four most difficult tasks, with approximately 17–18% finding these activities to be very or extremely difficult (15). Providing transportation (14.2%), finding respite care while away (15.3%), and finding resources (9.1%) were rated as very or extremely difficult as well (15). In another study, six caregivers shared their concerns regarding finances, with one caregiver fearing she would run out of money, which would result in institutionalization of the stroke survivor. Financial management was also a concern for caregivers in another study across all time periods up to two years after stroke (16). These are only a few examples of the needs and concerns that family caregivers have in providing instrumental care. Referral of stroke caregivers to a social worker to assist them in dealing with financial problems and finding appropriate community resources are clearly areas where health professionals may better serve families of stroke survivors.

Personal Responses to Caregiving.   Caregivers will often share their needs and concerns about their stroke survivors before they will share their own personal needs and concerns (7). However, in one qualitative study, caregivers reported needs and concerns about their own emotions while providing care, shouldering new responsibilities, balancing caregiving with existing responsibilities (for example, employment and care of other family members), asking friends and family members for help, keeping their own social life going, as well as keeping their energy level up and taking care of their own health (7). It was evident from the findings of this study that caregivers experienced great stress while providing care (7). One caregiver stated she would cry late at night at home, but try to hold up for her sister. Another caregiver mentioned how she and the survivor used to have frequent gatherings and cookouts, but that had stopped since the stroke. Another caregiver was assertive enough to ask the doctor why everyone always asked how her husband was doing, but never asked her how she was doing. This caregiver felt neglected by the health professionals involved in her husband's care and was reaching out for help. In a similar study (16), a wife indicated she wanted more attention from health professionals and they did not have anything for caregivers. The most

difficult times for caregivers have been reported to occur during hospitalization and the first few months after the patient is discharged home (16), which underscores the need for early caregiver assessment followed by individualized caregiver interventions during these critical time periods following stroke. The next section provides a review of literature about negative caregiver outcomes, including depression, poor health, decreased social functioning, and other negative outcomes of providing care.

Caregiver Outcomes

Caregiver Depression.   Studies have explored caregiver psychological distress and depression as well as the many factors associated with these outcomes. Estimates of the prevalence of depression in stroke caregivers have ranged between 30–52% (12, 34, 39), with poorest mental health when the stroke survivors were discharged home early (40). In fact, some studies have reported higher depression rates in caregivers than in the stroke survivors that they provided care for (39, 41). The treatment of stroke caregiver depression is important because caregiver stress has been found to be a leading cause of long-term institutionalization of stroke survivors (12). In one landmark prospective study, family caregivers experiencing strain had a 63% higher risk of mortality compared with noncaregiving controls (14).

Factors directly associated with caregiver psychological distress and depression have included:

- Difficulty with caregiving tasks (15, 42)
- Burden (43)
- Lack of social support (41, 43, 44)
- Poorer family functioning (41)
- Concern for future care (45, 46)
- Negative caregiver appraisal of the situation (42, 47)
- Lower life satisfaction (44)
- Self-losses (44)

Positive factors that tend to be associated with lower caregiver depression and psychological distress include:

- Hope and meaningfulness (48)
- Optimism (45, 46)
- Self-esteem (42, 49)
- Resiliency (47)

Survivor characteristics such as stroke severity, physical impairment, depression, and negative personality characteristics have also been associated with caregiver depression (39, 44, 45, 48, 50, 51). Other studies, interestingly, have found that physical disability of the stroke survivor is often unrelated to caregiver depression (12, 13). Some studies have shown that Caucasian caregivers, as opposed to African American caregivers, and those providing care for older stroke survivors were at greater risk for developing depression (39, 43). Pinquart and Sorensen (52) conducted a meta-analysis of 228 caregiver studies involving informal caregivers of older adults. They found that care recipient behaviors were more strongly associated with caregiver burden and depression than care recipient physical limitations or cognitive status. Perceived benefits of caregiving, such as feeling useful or feeling closeness with the care recipient were associated with decreased burden and depression in caregivers. Pinquart and Sorensen (52) recommended that caregiver interventions be focused on reducing care recipient problem behaviors, improving caregiver skills in the management of problem behaviors, and promoting positive perceptions of providing care. Screening for depressive symptoms in stroke survivors using the PHQ-9 Depression Severity Scale has been recommended (33); however, the use of the PHQ-9 to screen for depression in stroke caregivers might also help to identify caregivers in need of antidepressant therapy or counseling (10).

Caregiver Health.   The research agenda for stroke caregiving must move beyond psychological distress and depression to explore the general health of family caregivers (12, 13). Researchers have noted that attention to the health status and health promotion activities of family caregivers is lacking in both descriptive and intervention studies (53, 54). More studies are needed to determine predictors of health outcomes. For example, Bakas and Burgener (42) found that low household income and appraisals of threat were significant predictors of self-perceptions of poorer general health in stroke caregivers. Tooth and colleagues (55) found that only patient characteristics, such as cognitive function and mental health and caregiver employment, were predictive of caregiver SF-36 mental and physical component scores. Many studies have used global health measures in stroke caregivers, such as the SF-36 Health Survey. Some reported scores close to published general population norms (40, 56, 57), while others reported lower scores (55, 58, 59). Bakas and Champion (8) found that, although stroke caregiver SF-36 general health scores were close to published norms, caregivers perceived that their physical health had changed for the worse as a result of providing care. Other studies have also found that stroke caregiver perceptions of their own health worsen as a result of providing care (49, 60). Although more research is needed to identify key indicators of stroke caregiver health, clinicians are urged to ask caregivers about their health, encourage them to seek regular checkups, and practice health promotion activities while providing care.

Other Caregiver Outcomes.   Quality of life issues associated with providing care other than depression, psychological distress, and health deserve more attention

in research studies (13, 61). White and colleagues (61) described the lack of clarity regarding the term *quality of life* in a review of stroke caregiver literature and asserted that quality of life involved not only health, but such things as participation in social and recreational activities, leisure, social relationships, family life, sexual life, ability to manage self-care, vocation, finances, and satisfaction with life as a whole. In an earlier review of the stroke caregiver literature, Low and colleagues (13) found that only 2 out of 31 studies had focused on the social health of stroke caregivers (34, 62), noting that, although social measures were most often used as variables associated with depression or psychological distress, they were rarely explored as outcomes (13).

Bakas and colleagues (8, 9) noted that, although there were a number of generic quality of life measures used in stroke caregivers, there was a need for an instrument that measured changes in caregivers' lives, specifically as a result of providing care. Based on Lazarus and colleagues' (63–65) definition of adaptational outcomes, the Bakas Caregiving Outcomes Scale (BCOS) was developed to measure changes in social functioning, subjective well-being, and health, specifically as a result of providing care (Figure 42-2) (8, 9). Extensive psychometric testing of the BCOS has found acceptable evidence for its reliability and validity in stroke caregivers (8, 9). Two comprehensive reviews of caregiver measures have recommended the BCOS because of its extensive psychometric testing compared with other measures (66) and because it had the highest rate of agreement among the authors for seven different factors considered to be important for stroke caregivers (67). The most current 15-item BCOS (9) consists of a comprehensive list of caregiver life changes rated on a scale from -3 (changed for the worst) to +3 (changed for the best), with 0 meaning no change. Life changes relate to such things as time for social and family activities, relationships with family and friends, relationship with the stroke survivor, roles in life, financial well-being, emotional well-being, ability to cope with stress, self-esteem, future outlook, level of energy, physical functioning, and general health. Unlike many other measures, an added benefit for the BCOS is the fact that it allows caregivers to rate these life changes as either negative or positive or having no change at all. Stroke caregiver studies using the BCOS have shown that the worst life changes were caregivers' time for family and social activities, relationship with friends, financial well-being, emotional well-being, level of energy, and physical health. Areas that changed for the better on average were relationship with the stroke survivor and self-esteem (8, 9). Factors found to be associated with total BCOS scores have included threat appraisal (8, 9, 42), difficulty with tasks (8, 9, 15), emotional distress (8, 42), or depressive symptoms (9, 10) The BCOS has been shown to be a valuable measure in stroke caregiver research (8–10, 66, 67)

BAKAS CAREGIVING OUTCOMES SCALE

This group of questions is about the possible changes in your life from providing care for the stroke survivor. For each possible change listed, circle one number indicating the degree of change. The numbers indicating the degree of change range from **–3 "Changed for the Worst"** to **+3 "Changed for the Best."** The number **0 means "Did Not Change."**

	Changed for the Worst			Did Not Change		Changed for the Best	
As a result of providing care for the stroke survivor:							
1. My self esteem	-3	-2	-1	0	+1	+2	+3
2. My physical health	-3	-2	-1	0	+1	+2	+3
3. My time for family activities	-3	-2	-1	0	+1	+2	+3
4. My ability to cope with stress	-3	-2	-1	0	+1	+2	+3
5. My relationship with friends	-3	-2	-1	0	+1	+2	+3
6. My future outlook	-3	-2	-1	0	+1	+2	+3
7. My level of energy	-3	-2	-1	0	+1	+2	+3
8. My emotional well-being	-3	-2	-1	0	+1	+2	+3
9. My roles in life	-3	-2	-1	0	+1	+2	+3
10. My time for social activities with friends	-3	-2	-1	0	+1	+2	+3
11. My relationship with my family	-3	-2	-1	0	+1	+2	+3
12. My financial well-being	-3	-2	-1	0	+1	+2	+3
13. My relationship with the stroke survivor	-3	-2	-1	0	+1	+2	+3
14. My physical functioning	-3	-2	-1	0	+1	+2	+3
15. My general health	-3	-2	-1	0	+1	+2	+3
16. In general, how has your life changed as a result of taking care of the stroke survivor?	-3	-2	-1	0	+1	+2	+3
If there any other changes in your life as a result of providing care for the stroke survivor, please write them below and rate them accordingly.							
17.	-3	-2	-1	0	+1	+2	+3
18.	-3	-2	-1	0	+1	+2	+3
19.	-3	-2	-1	0	+1	+2	+3

FIGURE 42-2

and might also serve as an assessment tool to determine deteriorating aspects of caregivers' lives so that individualized interventions or referrals can be made (8–10).

Impact of Stroke on Other Family Members

Although literature regarding the effect of stroke on family caregivers has grown substantially in recent years, very little research has focused on the effects of stroke on other family members such as minor children, spouses of adult child caregivers, siblings, and other relatives who may be involved in the care of stroke survivors (68). Even rarer are studies that document the effect of stroke on parents, most likely because pediatric stroke is an infrequent occurrence (69). Two recent studies have focused on the effect of a parent's stroke on minor children (70, 71). Visser-Meiley and colleagues (71) interviewed 82 children (ages 4–18; average of 13 years) of 55 parents who had suffered a stroke and were admitted to a rehabilitation center in The Netherlands. Shortly after admission, 54% of the children showed at least one behavioral problem or depression; 21% of those scored in the clinical range. Although these behavior problems and depression significantly improved by two months after discharge (p < 0.001), trends for increasing internalizing behavior problems and decreasing health status in the children were noted between two months and one year after their parent's discharge. Significant predictors of child depression scores at one year were the child's baseline depression scores, child's gender, and physical functioning of the parent at admission. Significant predictors of child's health status at one year were baseline health status, spouse depression, and spouse perception of marital relationship at the time of admission. These findings underscore the need to screen for children's functioning, spouse depression, and the quality of the marital relationship during rehabilitation for a more family-centered approach to care (71). Lackey and Gates (70) conducted a retrospective study of 51 adults who had been 3–19 years old at the time of their parent's stroke or diagnosis of other types of chronic conditions such as cancer, cardiovascular disease, amyotrophic lateral sclerosis, respiratory disease, diabetes, or arthritis. Providing personal care was most difficult. Household tasks were most time-consuming, and family life, school, and time with friends were most negatively affected by the caregiving situation.

Palmer and Glass (68) urged researchers and clinicians to consider the entire family system, not just stroke survivor-caregiver dyads, in trying to understand the ripple effect of stroke on families. Family roles, responsibilities, and patterns of emotional support and communication must be reconfigured to accommodate the recovery process for stroke survivors. This reconfiguration can pose challenges to preexisting family relationships as well as family functioning in general (68). Current research is

limited in studying family systems in the context of stroke, largely because of inadequate measures and the complexity of developing and studying family intervention methods. The limited research that exists provides some evidence that family functioning is associated with discharge disposition, treatment adherence, re-hospitalization, and post-stroke depression (68). Although stroke caregiver intervention research is on the rise, very few studies have focused on psychosocial interventions on whole family systems (68). The next section provides a review of existing stroke caregiver intervention research, followed by a section on recommendations for future research and practice that urges researchers and clinicians to consider a family systems approach to care.

STROKE CAREGIVER INTERVENTION RESEARCH

According to current stroke rehabilitation clinical practice guidelines (72), health care providers should involve family caregivers in decision-making and treatment planning for survivors, be alert to the stress and support needs of caregivers, provide information on community resources and services, as well as provide patient and family caregiver education about stroke and potential complications. Despite these recommendations, research has not produced sufficient evidence regarding the effectiveness of stroke caregiver interventions that can be easily incorporated into practice, although several recommendations have been provided (12, 13, 73–75).

Stroke Caregiver Clinical Trials

Visser-Meiley and colleagues (75) identified 22 studies from January 1966 to March 2003 (14 from Europe, 5 from the United States, 1 from Australia, 1 from New Zealand, and 1 from Canada). From March 2003 to August 2006, an additional three European studies were found (76–78). There was a broad range of outcomes and measures, making comparison of findings difficult, and many other limitations were identified. Only 10 of the 22 studies reviewed improved on one or more outcomes, meaning that 12 (54.5%) studies found no significant intervention effects (75). Potential reasons for the nonsignificant findings included insufficient interventions, incorrect timing of interventions, the use of measures that lacked sensitivity to detect relevant changes, and samples that included different mixtures of spouse and adult child caregivers (75). Of the 10 studies that reported positive outcomes on one or more measures:

- Two reported reduced depression.
- One reduced burden.
- Five improved knowledge.

- One improved satisfaction with care.
- One improved family functioning.
- Three improved quality of life.
- Two enhanced problem-solving skills.
- Three improved social activities and support (75)

A more recent study with 300 stroke caregivers randomized to caregiver training or conventional care during inpatient rehabilitation found lower costs, reduced caregiver burden, lower anxiety and depression scores, and improved quality of life for caregivers in the intervention group one year after the intervention (76). Patients of caregivers in the intervention group also reported less depression and anxiety and improved quality of life (76). The caregiver training in this study consisted of three to five sessions of hands-on caregiver training on:

- How to handle stroke problems and complications
- How to prevent future strokes
- Information about local benefits and services
- Training in lifting and mobility techniques, assistance with activities of daily living, and communication tailored to the needs of the stroke patients (76)

However, no interventions were tailored to the needs of caregivers. Caregiver intervention studies that better target the needs and concerns of family caregivers, rather than only the needs of stroke patients, have been strongly recommended (1, 7, 16, 75). Also evident in Visser-Meiley and colleagues' (75) review was the need for studies that document the effects of caregiver interventions on patient outcomes. A total of 17 out of 22 studies reviewed used combined patient and caregiver interventions, making it difficult to determine the effects of caregiver interventions by themselves on patient outcomes. Determining the effect of caregiver interventions on stroke survivor outcomes is recommended and would provide a stronger rationale for implementing caregiver programs in practice (75).

Forester et al. (73) concluded from their review of stroke caregiver intervention studies that the provision of information alone had no effect on mood, perceived health status, or quality of life for stroke patients or caregivers. A more recent study found similar results (78). Other studies that combined education with problem-solving strategies were much more effective at improving caregiver knowledge, family functioning, problem-solving strategies, and even patient adjustment than using education alone (26, 79). For example, Grant and colleagues (80) found that theoretically based telephone problem-solving sessions with family caregivers of stroke survivors significantly enhanced caregiver problem-solving skills, improved preparedness, reduced depression, and improved several SF-36 Health Survey scores. These sessions consisted of an initial face-to-face visit, followed by seven telephone calls over a twelve-week period to teach and reinforce caregiver problem-solving skills (80, 81). The advantage of these sessions was that they empowered family caregivers to identify, solve, and evaluate their own problems in providing care (80, 81).

Dennis and colleagues (82) found that stroke caregivers randomized to a treatment group receiving home visits by a family care worker had very few significant differences in outcomes compared to a control group; however, training and measurement problems may have biased the findings (83). A similar study by Mant and colleagues (84) found that the use of a trained family support organizer who made one hospital visit, one home visit, and three telephone calls significantly improved several SF-36 Health Survey scores, suggesting the importance of adequate training and adherence to a treatment protocol for interveners. Follow-up data from this study showed that the effect of the family support intervention persisted for up to one year after the intervention (77).

Caregiver Clinical Trials in Other Contexts

Most caregiver intervention research has been conducted in the areas of dementia and older persons. The most widely known intervention program, the Resources for Enhancing Alzheimer's Caregiver Health (REACH), evaluated the effectiveness of multiple caregiver interventions implemented across six sites to provide a comprehensive evidence base for caregiver intervention research (85). Meta-analytic findings from these interventions with 1,222 family caregivers showed active interventions to be superior to control interventions (86) and multicomponent interventions targeting multiple domains (knowledge, cognitive skills, behaviors, and affect) to be relatively more effective (87). Meta-analysis has also revealed that tailoring interventions to the individual needs of family caregivers is generally more effective than group interventions (88, 89). Other comprehensive reviews of caregiver intervention studies in dementia (90, 91) and old age (88, 89, 92, 93) exist. Two reviews emphasized the need to look beyond outcomes to methodological design factors such as intervention integrity and theoretical rationale (91, 92). Treatment fidelity, defined as strategies to improve the reliability and validity of behavioral interventions and address intervention integrity and theoretical rationale, is being increasingly emphasized in intervention research (91, 92, 94). Treatment fidelity consists of five components: treatment design, training, delivery of treatment, receipt of treatment, and enactment. Treatment design includes the theoretical model or clinical guidelines for the intervention, provider credentials, and information about the dosage (length, number, content, and duration of contacts) for both intervention and comparison conditions. Training includes detailed descriptions of how providers are trained, standardized, and maintained over time, for example, use of training manuals, role-playing, and audiotaping. Delivery of treatment involves ensuring that treatments are delivered as intended, for example, use of evaluation checklists to track adherence to protocol and need for retraining. Receipt of treatment refers to evidence that the study participants understood the intervention, for example, ability to verbalize what they have been taught, pretest/posttest, and ability to demonstrate skills. Enactment of treatment skills refers to evidence that study participants have incorporated treatment strategies into their everyday lives or that the strategies are used by the study participants in a variety of settings (94). Although implementation of these five components of treatment fidelity into clinical trials can be costly, time-consuming, and difficult to implement in clinical practice (95), rigorous attention to these components is likely to enhance scientific reporting, provide more plausible conclusions as to why interventions did or did not work, and improve treatment replication, making treatments more applicable to a wider variety of clinical practice settings (94).

RESEARCH FRONTIERS

The aging of the population, along with the current shortage of health care professionals to assist with the transition to home care, underscore the urgent need for public policies and programs to support family caregivers (96, 97). This is especially true for family caregivers of stroke survivors because the incidence of stroke is likely to increase as the population ages (5). As detailed earlier in this chapter, caregivers have a variety of needs and concerns about providing care, for example, information, managing the survivor's emotions and behaviors, providing physical care, providing instrumental care, and personal responses to caregiving. Caregiver depression, deteriorating health, and other negative caregiver outcomes such as decreased social functioning and financial well-being are common. Family caregivers often feel neglected by health professionals in practice settings. Although there are a few stroke caregiver intervention studies with positive results, this body of research as a whole has not produced sufficient evidence for the effectiveness of stroke caregiver interventions. Clinically tested interventions for family caregivers of stroke survivors are prerequisite to the development of effective public policies and programs that can be implemented into practice settings for family caregivers. Stroke also affects the entire family system (for example, minor children, spouses of adult child caregivers, siblings, and other relatives), although research is severely limited in this area. Interventions based on a family systems perspective have been recommended; however, further research is required to develop and clinically test interventions at the family systems level. The following sections summarize recommendations for future research

and practice implications pertinent to stroke recovery and rehabilitation for families.

Recommendations for Future Research

1. More research is needed that includes assessment tools to identify problem areas experienced by family caregivers so that individualized caregiver interventions can be delivered (1, 7, 16). For example, further studies using the CNCC (7) to assess caregiver needs and concerns, the Oberst Caregiving Burden Scale (OCBS) (15) to assess difficulty with caregiver tasks, and the BCOS (8, 9) to assess negative changes in caregiver lives as a result of providing care are needed (7–10, 15). The use of the PHQ-9 (33) to screen for caregiver depressive symptoms also warrants further testing (10).

2. Quality outcome measures relevant to stroke caregivers that have documented evidence of reliability, validity, and sensitivity to change are needed to evaluate stroke caregiver intervention programs (75).

3. Caregiver intervention research should include interventions that are tailored or individualized to specific caregiver needs and concerns (7, 10, 12, 15, 75, 89).

4. Stroke caregiver interventions that specifically address how to help caregivers manage the emotional and behavioral reactions displayed by stroke survivors are especially needed because managing survivor emotions and behaviors is among the most stressful aspects of providing care (5, 10, 15, 16, 21–25).

5. Multicomponent caregiver interventions covering multiple domains (knowledge, cognitive skills, behaviors, and affect) (87) and offering more than just information provision (73) should be the focus of future stroke caregiver intervention research.

6. Correct timing for interventions should receive attention when designing stroke caregiver intervention studies (75).

7. Studies that separate spouse data from adult child caregivers during analyses are needed to identify interventions appropriate for each group (75).

8. Studies that document the effects of caregiver interventions on stroke survivor outcomes are needed to provide a stronger rationale for caregiver interventions in practice (75).

9. Studies that look beyond outcomes to methodological design issues including treatment fidelity are recommended (91, 92, 94).

10. Studies that incorporate a theoretical rationale for interventions are also recommended (91, 92, 94).

11. More research from a family systems perspective is needed to document the impact of stroke on entire families as well as to develop and evaluate interventions at the family systems level (68).

Practice Implications

1. Because of the wide variety of needs, concerns, and negative outcomes experienced by family caregivers of stroke survivors, detailed assessment from the caregivers' perspective using tools such as the CNCC (7) are recommended so that individualized caregiver interventions or referrals can be provided (1, 7, 16, 75).

2. Health professionals should assess and reinforce both patient and caregiver knowledge of stroke warning signs, lifestyle changes (for example, diet, exercise, smoking, heavy alcohol consumption, and obesity), and risk factors for secondary stroke prevention (for example, management of hypertension, diabetes, and cholesterol) throughout stroke recovery and rehabilitation (7, 16, 19, 20, 72).

3. Family caregivers should be asked about the stroke survivor's depressive symptoms, emotions, and how they are communicating with the survivor to identify possible barriers to stroke recovery and rehabilitation that may be amenable to treatment, therapy, or psychological counseling (7, 10, 22, 36, 37, 72).

4. Family caregivers should be encouraged to attend therapy sessions and ask questions about the survivor's medications, symptoms, and other stroke-related care issues (7, 38, 72).

5. Family caregivers should be referred to a social worker as needed to assist them in dealing with financial problems and finding appropriate community resources (7, 15, 16, 72).

6. Stroke organizations, such as the American Stroke Association (www.strokeassociation.org; 1-888-478-7653) and the National Stroke Association (www.stroke.org; 1-800-787-6537), can be valuable resources for stroke survivors and their families (72).

7. Family caregivers should be asked how they are doing (7, 10, 16, 72), particularly about their depressive symptoms and health. Refer them for treatment and/or psychological counseling as needed. Encourage them to seek regular checkups and to practice health promotion activities while providing care.

8. The entire family system should be considered during recovery and rehabilitation, not just the stroke survivor-caregiver dyad (68). Ask the stroke survivor and his or her family caregiver how other family members are dealing with the stroke, including any minor children, and refer them for treatment and/or counseling when appropriate.

CONCLUSION

Providing care for a family member with stroke can be difficult and can lead to negative consequences not only for the family caregiver, but also for the entire family. Researchers and clinicians are urged to explore ways to better support families in providing care for stroke survivors during stroke recovery and rehabilitation. Research regarding the needs and concerns, depressive symptoms, poor health, and other negative outcomes experienced by family caregivers has been reviewed, along with stroke caregiver intervention research and the need for a family systems perspective in helping families adjust after stroke. Perhaps with attention to the several recommendations for future research and practice outlined in this chapter, families may receive better care and support from health professionals in the future.

Acknowledgment

Supported by the National Institute of Nursing Research, National Institutes of Health, Grant K01 NR0008712.

References

1. Family Caregiver Alliance. *Caregiver Assessment: Principles, Guidelines, and Strategies for Change.* Report from a National Consensus Development Conference. Vol. I. San Francisco: Author, 2006.

2. Dewey HM, Thrift AG, Mihalopoulos C, et al. Informal care for stroke survivors: Results from the North East Melbourne Stroke Incidence Study (NEMESIS). *Stroke* 2002; 33:1028–1033.

3. Dorsey MK. Vaca KJ. The stroke patient and assessment of caregiver needs. *Journal of Vascular Nursing* 1998; 16:62–67.

4. Wright LK, Hickey JV, Buckwalter KC, Clipp EC. Human development in the context of aging and chronic illness: The role of attachment in Alzheimer's disease and stroke. *International Journal of Aging and Human Development* 1995; 41:133–150.

5. American Heart Association. Heart disease and stroke statistics: 2006 update. A report from the American Heart Association Statistics Committee and Stroke Statistics Subcommittee. *Circulation* 2006; 113,e85:1–67.

6. Kelly-Hayes M, Robertson JT, Broderick JP, et al. The American Heart Association Stroke Outcome Classification. *Stroke* 1998; 29:1274–1280.

7. Bakas T, Austin JK, Okonkwo KF, et al. Needs, concerns, strategies, and advice of stroke caregivers the first six months after discharge. *Journal of Neuroscience Nursing* 2002; 34:242–251.

8. Bakas T, Champion V. Development and psychometric testing of the Bakas Caregiving Outcomes Scale. *Nursing Research* 1999; 48:250–259.

9. Bakas T, Champion V, Perkins SM, et al. Psychometric testing of the Revised 15-item Bakas Caregiving Outcomes Scale. *Nursing Research* 2006; 55:346–355.

10. Bakas T, Kroenke K, Plue LD, et al. Outcomes among family caregivers of aphasic versus non-aphasic stroke survivors. *Rehabilitation Nursing* 2006; 31:33–42.

11. Bakas T, Williams LS, Chadwick L, Jessup S. Task difficulty, depression, and life changes in family caregivers of stroke survivors. Oral abstracts of the 26th International Stroke Conference, Ft. Lauderdale, FL. *Stroke* 2001; 32:318.

12. Han B, Haley WE. Family caregiving for patients with stroke: Review and analysis. *Stroke* 1999; 30:1478–1485.

13. Low JTS, Payne S, Roderick P. The impact of stroke on informal caregivers: A literature review. *Social Science & Medicine* 1999; 49:711–725.

14. Schulz R, Beach, SR. Caregiving as a risk factor for mortality: The caregiver health effects study. *JAMA* 1999; 282:2215–2219.

15. Bakas T, Austin JK, Jessup SL, et al. Time and difficulty of tasks provided by family caregivers of stroke survivors. *Journal of Neuroscience Nursing* 2004; 36:95–106.

16. King RB, Semik PE. Stroke caregiving: Difficult times, resource use, and needs during the first two years. *Journal of Gerontological Nursing* 2006; 32:37–44.

17. Maze LM, Bakas T. Factors associated with hospital arrival time for stroke patients. *Journal of Neuroscience Nursing* 2004; 36:136–141, 151.

18. Hanger HC, Walker G, Paterson LA, et al. What do patients and their caregivers want to know about stroke? A two-year follow-up study. *Clinical Rehabilitation* 1998; 12:45–52.

19. Sacco RL, Adams R, Albers G, et al. Guidelines for prevention of stroke in patients with ischemic stroke or transient ischemic attack: A statement for healthcare professionals from the American Heart Association/American Stroke Association Council on Stroke. *Stroke* 2006; 37:577.
20. Gordon NF, Gulanick M, Costa F, et al. Physical activity and exercise recommendations for stroke survivors: An American Heart Association Scientific Statement. *Circulation* 2004; 109:2031–2041.
21. Cameron JI, Cheung AM, Streiner DL, et al. Stroke survivors' behavioral and psychological symptoms are associated with informal caregivers' experiences of depression. *Archives of Physical Medicine and Rehabilitation* 2006; 87:177–183.
22. Clark PC, Dunbar SB, Aycock DM, et al. Caregiver perspectives of memory and behavior changes in stroke survivors. *Rehabilitation Nursing* 2006; 31:26–32.
23. Clark PC, Dunbar SB, Shields CG, et al. Influence of stroke survivor characteristics and family conflict surrounding recovery on caregivers' mental and physical health. *Nursing Research* 2004; 53:406–413.
24. Davis LL, Grant JS. Constructing the reality of recovery: Family home care management strategies. *Advances in Nursing Science.* 1994; 17:66–76.
25. Stewart MJ, Doble S, Hart G, et al. Peer visitor support for family caregivers of seniors with stroke. *Canadian Journal of Nursing Research* 1998; 30:87–117.
26. Evans RL, Matlock AL, Bishop DS, et al. Family intervention after stroke: Does counseling or education help? *Stroke* 1988; 19:1243–1249.
27. Williams AM. What bothers caregivers of stroke victims? *Journal of Neuroscience Nursing* 1994; 26:155–161.
28. Burvill PW, Johnson GA, Jamrozik KD, et al. Prevalence of depression after stroke: The Perth Community Stroke Study. *Br J Psychiatry* 1995; 166:320–327.
29. Herrman N, Black SE, Lawrence J, et al. The Sunnybrook Stroke Study: A prospective study of depressive symptoms and functional outcomes. *Stroke* 1998; 29:618–624.
30. Kotila M, Numminen H, Waltimo O, Kaste M. Depression after stroke: Results of the FINNSTROKE study. *Stroke* 1998; 29:368–372.
31. Robinson RF, Starr LB, Kubos KL, Price RT. A two-year longitudinal study of post-stroke mood disorders: Findings during the initial evaluation. *Stroke* 1983; 14:736–741.
32. Pierce LL, Steiner V. What are male caregivers talking about? *Topics in Stroke Rehabilitation* 2004; 11:77–83.
33. Williams LS, Brizendine EJ, Plue L, et al. Performance of the PHQ-9 as a screening tool for post-stroke depression. *Stroke* 2005; 36:635–638.
34. Anderson CS, Linto J, Stewart-Wynne EG. A population-based assessment of the impact and burden of caregiving for long-term stroke survivors. *Stroke* 1995; 26:843–849.
35. Williams AM, Dahl CW. Patient and caregiver perceptions of stroke survivor behavior: A comparison. *Rehabilitation Nursing* 2002; 27:19–24.
36. Booth S, Swabey D. Group training in communication skills for careers of adults with aphasia. *International Journal of Language and Communication Disorders* 1999; 34:291–309.
37. Kagan A, Winckel J, Black S, et al. A set of observational measures for rating support and participation in conversation between adults with aphasia and their conversation partners. *Topics in Stroke Rehabilitation* 2004; 11:67–83.
38. Ostwald SK, Wasserman J, Davis S. Medications, comorbidities, and medical complications in stroke survivors: The CAReS Study. *Rehabilitation Nursing* 2006; 31:10–14.
39. Berg A, Psych L, Palomaki H, et al. Depression among caregivers of stroke survivors. *Stroke* 2005; 36:639–643.
40. Anderson C, Rubenach S, Mhurchu CN, et al. Home or hospital for stroke rehabilitation? Results of a randomized, controlled trial. *Stroke* 2000; 31:1024–1031.
41. King RB, Shade-Zeldow Y, Carlson CE, et al. Early adaptation to stroke: Patient and primary support person. *Rehabilitation Nursing Research* 1995; 4:82–89.
42. Bakas T, Burgener SC. Predictors of emotional distress, general health, and caregiving outcomes in family caregivers of stroke survivors. *Topics in Stroke Rehabilitation* 2002; 9:34–45.
43. Grant JS, Weaver M, Elliott TR, et al. Sociodemographic, physical, and psychosocial factors associated with depressive behavior in family caregivers of stroke survivors in the acute care phase. *Brain Injury* 2004; 18:797–809.
44. Grant JS, Bartolucci AA, Elliot TR, Giger JN. Sociodemographic, physical, and psychosocial characteristics of depressed and non-depressed family caregivers of stroke survivors. *Brain Injury* 2000; 14:1089–1100.
45. Schulz R, Tompkins CA, Rau MT. A longitudinal study of the psychosocial impact of stroke on primary support persons. *Psychology and Aging* 1988; 3:131–141.
46. Tompkins CA, Schulz R, Rau MT. Post-stroke depression in primary support persons: Predicting those at risk. *Journal of Consulting Clinical Psychology* 1988; 56:502–508.
47. Braithwaite V. Contextual or general stress outcomes: Making choices through caregiving appraisals. *Gerontologist* 2000; 40:706–717.
48. Thompson SC, Bundek M, Sobolew-Schubin A. The caregivers of stroke patients: An investigation of factors associated with depression. *Journal of Applied Social Psychology* 1990; 20:115–129.
49. Silliman RA, Fletcher RH, Earp JL, Wagner EH. Families of elderly stroke patients: Effects of home care. *J American Geriatric Society* 1986; 34:643–648.
50. Carnwath TC, Johnson DA. Psychiatric morbidity among spouses of patients with stroke. *British Medical Journal* 1987; 294:409–411.
51. Dennis M, O'Rourke S, Lewis S, et al. A quantitative study of the emotional outcome of people caring for stroke survivors. *Stroke* 1998; 29:1867–1872.
52. Pinquart M, Sorensen S. Associations of stressors and uplifts of caregiving with caregiver burden and depressive mood: A meta-analysis. *Journal of Gerontology: Psychological Sciences* 2003; 58B:P112–128.
53. Farran CJ, Loukissa D, Hauser PM, et al. Psychoneuroimmunological outcomes in dementia caregiver intervention studies: An idea whose time has come? *The Online Journal of Knowledge Synthesis for Nursing* 2001; 8:6.
54. Given BA, Given CW. Health promotion for family caregivers of chronically ill elders. *Annual Review of Nursing Research* 1998; 16:197–217.
55. Tooth L, McKenna K, Barnett A, et al. Caregiver burden, time spent caring, and health status in the first 12 months following stroke. *Brain Injury* 2005; 19:963–974.
56. Mant J, Carter J, Wade DT. The impact of an information pack on patients with stroke and their caregivers: A randomized, controlled trial. *Clinical Rehabilitation* 1998; 12: 465–476.
57. Rogers H, Atkinson C, Bond S, et al. Randomized, controlled trial of a comprehensive stroke education program for patients and caregivers. *Stroke* 1999; 30:2585–2591.
58. Bugge C, Alexander H, Hagen S. Stroke patient's informal caregivers: Patient, caregiver, and service factors that affect caregiver strain. *Stroke* 1999; 30:1517–1523.
59. White CL, Poissant L, Cote-LeBlanc G, Wood-Dauphinee S. Long-term caregiving after stroke: The impact on caregivers' quality of life. *Journal of Neuroscience Nursing* 2006; 38:354–360.
60. Williams AM. Caregivers of persons with stroke: Their physical and emotional well-being. *Quality of Life Research* 1993; 2:213–220.
61. White CL, Lauzon S, Yafe MJ, Wood-Dauphinee S. Toward a model of quality of life for family caregivers of stroke survivors. *Quality of Life Research* 2004; 13:625–638.
62. Periard ME, Ames BD. Lifestyle changes and coping patterns among caregivers of stroke survivors. *Public Health Nursing* 1993; 10:252–256.
63. Lazarus RS. *Psychological stress and the Coping Process.* New York: McGraw Hill, 1966.
64. Lazarus RS. *Emotion and Adaptation.* New York: Oxford University Press, 1991.
65. Lazarus RS, Folkman S. *Stress, Appraisal, and Coping.* New York: Springer, 1984.
66. Deeken JF, Taylor KL, Mangan P, et al. Care for the caregivers: A review of self-report instruments developed to measure the burden, needs, and quality of life of informal caregivers. *Journal of Pain and Symptom Management* 2003; 26:922–953.
67. Visser-Meily JMA, Post MWM, Riphagen I I, Lindeman E. Measures used to assess burden among caregivers of stroke patients: A review. *Clinical Rehabilitation* 2004; 18:601–623.
68. Palmer S, Glass TA. Family function and stroke recovery: A review. *Rehabilitation Psychology* 2003; 48:255–265.
69. Carlin TM, Chanmugam A. Stroke in children. *Emergency Medicine Clinics of North America* 2002; 20:671–685.
70. Lackey NR, Gates MF. Adults' recollections of their experiences as young caregivers of family members with chronic physical illnesses. *Journal of Advanced Nursing* 2001; 34:320–328.
71. Visser-Meiley A, Post M, Meijer AM, et al. When a parent has a stroke: Clinical course and prediction of mood, behavior problems, and health status of their young children. *Stroke* 2005; 36:2436–2440.
72. Duncan PW, Zorowitz R, Bates B, et al. Management of adult stroke rehabilitation care. *Stroke* 2005; 36:e100–e143.
73. Forster A, Smith J, Young J, et al. Information provision for stroke patients and their caregivers. *The Cochrane Library* 2004; 3.
74. Knapp P, Young J, House A, Forster A. Non-drug strategies to resolve psychosocial difficulties after stroke. *Age and Ageing* 2000; 29:23–30.
75. Visser-Meily A, van Heugten C, Post M, et al. Intervention studies for caregivers of stroke survivors: A critical review. *Patient Education and Counseling* 2005; 56:257–267.
76. Kalra L, Evans A, Perez I, et al. Training caregivers of stroke patients: Randomized, controlled trial. *British Medical Journal* 2004; 328:1099–1103.
77. Mant J, Winner S, Roche J, Wade DT. Family support for stroke: One year follow-up of a randomized, controlled trial. *J Neurol Neurosurg Psychiatry* 2005; 76:1006–1008.
78. Smith J, Forster A, Young J. A randomized trial to evaluate an education programme for patients and carers after stroke. *Clinical Rehabilitation* 2004; 18:726–736.
79. ven den Heuvel ETP, de Witte LP, Nooyen-Haazen I, et al. Short-term effects of a group support program and an individual support program for caregivers of stroke patients. *Patient Education and Counseling* 2000; 40:109–120.
80. Grant JS, Elliott TR, Weaver M, et al. Telephone intervention with family caregivers of stroke survivors after rehabilitation. *Stroke* 2002; 33:2060–2065.
81. Grant JS, Elliott TR, Giger JN, Bartolucci AA. Social problem-solving telephone partnerships with family caregivers of persons with stroke. *International Journal of Rehabilitation Research* 2001; 24:181–189.
82. Dennis M, O'Rourke S, Slattery J, et al. Evaluation of a stroke family care worker: Results of a randomized, controlled trial. *British Medical Journal* 1997; 314:1071–1076.
83. Chamberlain MA, Geddes JML, Wasti A. Stroke family care workers: Value of a support worker should not be dismissed on basis of only one trial. *British Medical Journal* 1997; 315:607.
84. Mant J, Carter J, Wade DT, Winner S. Family support for stroke: A randomized, controlled trial. *The Lancet* 2000; 356:808–813.
85. Schulz R, Belle SH, Czaja SJ, et al. Introduction to the special session on Resources for Enhancing Alzheimer's Caregiver Health (REACH). *Psychology and Aging* 2003; 18:357–360.
86. Gitlin LN, Belle SH, Burgio LD, et al. Effect of multicomponent interventions on caregiver burden and depression: The REACH multisite initiative at six-month follow-up. *Psychology and Aging* 2003; 18:361–374.
87. Burgio L, Corcoran M, Lichstein KL, et al. Judging outcomes in psychosocial interventions for dementia caregivers: The problem of treatment implementation. *Gerontologist* 2001; 41:481–489.
88. Knight BG, Lutzky SM, Macofsky-Urban F. A meta-analytic review of interventions for caregiver distress: Recommendations for future research. *Gerontologist* 1993; 33:240–248.
89. Yin T, Zhou Q, Bashford C. Burden on family members. *Nursing Research* 2002; 51: 199–208.
90. Acton GJ, Kang J. Interventions to reduce the burden of caregiving for an adult with dementia: A meta-analysis. *Research in Nursing and Health* 2001; 24: 349–360.

91. Bourgeois MS, Schulz R, Burgio L. Interventions for caregivers of patients with Alzheimer's disease: A review and analysis of content, process, and outcomes. *International Journal of Aging and Human Development* 1996; 43:35–92.

92. Kennet J, Burgio L, Schulz R. Interventions for in-home caregivers: A review of research (1990–present). In Schulz R, ed. *Handbook on Dementia Caregiving: Evidence-Based Interventions for Family Caregivers*. New York: Springer Publishing Co., 2000:61–125.

93. Sorensen S, Pinquart M, Dr habil, Duberstein P. How effective are interventions with caregivers? An updated meta-analysis. *Gerontologist* 2002; 42:356–372.

94. Borrelli B, Sepinwall D, Ernst D, et al. A new tool to assess treatment fidelity and evaluation of treatment fidelity across 10 years of health behavior research. *Journal of Consulting and Clinical Psychology* 2005; 73:852–860.

95. Leventhal H, Friedman MA. Does establishing fidelity of treatment help in understanding treatment efficacy? Comment on Bellg et al. (2004). *Health Psychology* 2004; 23: 452–456.

96. Healthy People. *Healthy People 2010*. www.health.gov/healthypeople. 2001; 7/13/02.

97. McLeod BW, ed. *And Thou Shalt Honor: The Caregiver's Companion*. Rodale, 2002.

43 Driving After Stroke

Arthur M. Gershkoff
Hillel M. Finestone

Returning to driving after stroke is a sensitive issue. Many stroke survivors relied on driving before their illness and consider it an essential component of independent living as well as a pleasure and privilege that they deserve. Stroke may cause physical, cognitive, and/or visuospatial impairments, which may or may not affect the ability to safely drive a vehicle. Health care providers who draw attention to these deficits may thus threaten stroke survivors' image of themselves. However, attention to driving safety is a necessary part of the overall rehabilitation plan for virtually all stroke survivors. The issue must be addressed from several points of view:

- *Societal:* While many stroke survivors safely return to driving, society must be protected from unsafe drivers, who expose themselves and others to the risk of bodily harm and property damage. Some stroke survivors may deny the severity of their deficits because of true anosognosia or severe impairment of judgment. The need to drive may be so strong that they purposely fail to report to their physicians symptoms such as seizures or episodic loss of consciousness that would lead to mandatory loss of driving privileges (1). Society therefore has an obligation to create and administer careful and thorough driving evaluations that assess the safety of the stroke survivor. In addition, safe and effective transportation is needed for those who are no longer able to drive.

- *Ethical:* Driving is a right, not a privilege. While the public must be protected from unsafe drivers, there is also an obligation to treat stroke patients fairly. It should *not* be assumed from the outset that residual neurologic deficits preclude safe driving (2). However, various jurisdictions have different regulations governing when and how a stroke survivor may return to driving.

- *Medicolegal:* The physician's potential liability for damages to others caused by an unsafe driver always lurks in the background. Several states and provinces have clarified physicians' responsibility by legislating mandatory reporting of potentially unsafe drivers. The jurisdiction may then either revoke the license of someone judged unsafe to drive or require the patient to undergo standard or specialized driving assessments.

While we are now more aware of driver safety following stroke, rehabilitation programs may not always address this issue. Of the approximately 78% of people who survive an acute stroke, 50%–70% regain functional independence. A substantial proportion

UQ1

of these have the potential to return to safe driving but often must overcome or adapt to residual deficits. Some deficits, especially those that impair judgment or awareness of deficits, preclude safe driving, while others do not. A 1997 survey of 290 stroke survivors three months to six years post-stroke showed that only 30% of subjects who drove before their illness resumed driving after the stroke. A total of 48% had not received advice about driving, and 87% had not received any type of evaluation of driver fitness before returning to driving (3).

CONCEPTUAL DRIVING MODELS

Driving requires multiple skills, and models have been developed to conceptualize the types of skill interactions that occur. Michon described three levels of driving-related decision-making: strategic, tactical, and operational (4). Strategic decision-making, the highest level, refers to trip planning, such as the route that will be taken and whether the weather or time of day or night is appropriate. Tactical decision-making refers to the driver's vehicle-handling decisions, such as how fast or slow to drive, whether to tailgate, and when to pass appropriately. Finally, operational decision-making refers to basic driving actions, such as braking, steering, and reaction to a sudden possibly dangerous event. Galski et al. developed a more dynamic model that incorporated sensory input, information processing, driving experience, and motor output skills (5). Marshall et al. combined the two models, as shown in Figure 43-1 (6).

The figure amply demonstrates the complexity of driving performance and how the physical, perceptual, and cognitive deficits that result from stroke may impede this performance at many levels.

NEUROLOGIC DISORDERS AND CRASH RISK

Diller et al. examined crash risk for Utah drivers based on medical conditions identified through a mandatory medical questionnaire at the time of licensure, followed by more extensive health screening (7). For each condition, the authors compared drivers whose licenses were restricted with drivers who were unrestricted. Neurologic conditions included a wide variety of diseases, but stroke was not separated out. Subjects with epilepsy in the absence of other neurologic disease were excluded. The data were linked to Utah Department of Transportation crash files. Among unrestricted drivers, those with neurologic conditions had 1.62 times the overall crash risk compared with a comparison group of 1,773 unrestricted drivers without medical conditions matched for age, sex, and county of residence; the relative risk for at-fault crashes was 2.20. Subjects with neurologic conditions and restricted licenses had an increased relative risk of crashes, but this did not reach statistical significance. Separate analysis of drivers with epilepsy and episodic disorders of consciousness showed a significantly increased overall and at-fault crash risk for both restricted and unrestricted drivers (7).

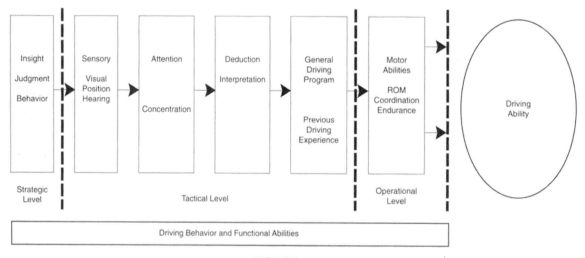

FIGURE 43-1

Model demonstrating the complexity of driving performance and how the physical, perceptual, and cognitive deficits that result from stroke may impede this performance at many levels. (Reprinted with permission from Marshall et al. 2007 (6).)

A retrospective study of 1,910 stroke patients indicated that the crash risk per person-year of driving for stroke survivors who return to driving is not higher than that for presumably healthy control subjects matched for age, sex, and zip code (8). The authors did not consider licensed drivers who voluntarily ceased driving or changed their driving exposure (9, 10). Reduction of driving exposure has been noted with increased age (11). The crash risk per mile driven rises substantially for drivers over age 65 (11); as the incidence of stroke increases substantially with aging, the crash risk per mile driven is therefore likely to be higher for stroke survivors as a group, regardless of neurologic deficits.

Nevertheless, specific neurologic deficits likely to be present following stroke play a role in driver performance and crash risk. In a study of visual impairments and their relationship to crash risk in 294 drivers aged 55–87 years, the most important deficit was restriction in useful field of view (UFOV), the visual field area over which a person can use rapidly presented visual information without moving the head or eyes (12). UFOV testing is different from visual field testing, which assesses visual sensitivity only. After adjustment for age, sex, race, chronic medical conditions, mental status, and number of days driven per week, impairment of UFOV of 40% or greater was associated with a 2.2-fold increased crash risk during three years of follow-up. Subcomponents of UFOV include processing speed, divided attention, and selective attention. Divided attention, which is frequently impaired following stroke, was associated with a 2.3-fold increased crash risk, while the other subcomponents were not significantly associated with increased risk. Other vision parameters (visual acuity, contrast sensitivity, stereo-acuity, visual field sensitivity [central and peripheral], and disability glare) were not significantly associated with increased crash risk (12). In another study, elderly drivers with substantial UFOV deficits had 15.6 times the crash rate at intersections compared with elderly drivers with normal UFOV (13). A meta-analysis by Clay et al. confirmed the significant relationship in older adults between UFOV and driving performance (14). In contrast to studies on UFOV, studies that examine the effect of visual field loss on driving have generally not shown a relationship between the loss and crash risk (9); however, stroke patients were not examined separately in these studies.

STROKE-RELATED DEFICITS AND DRIVING

Fisk et al. studied UFOV, visual acuity, peripheral vision, contrast sensitivity, and behavioral attention in 50 community-dwelling stroke survivors and a control group of 105 older adults without neurologic or visual impairment (10). They compared performance on these measures with a questionnaire of driving habits. Stroke survivors as a group demonstrated more impairment in UFOV, contrast sensitivity, and peripheral vision than controls, while stroke survivors who were drivers had less impairment of attention than those who were nondrivers. Stroke survivors who drove reported difficulty with challenging driving conditions and drove less than controls (10).

In general, the greater the severity of deficits, whether physical or cognitive, the lower the likelihood that the patient will return to driving. It has been estimated that every one-point increase in composite Functional Independence Measure score at discharge raises the likelihood that a stroke patient will return to driving by 5% (3). Smith-Arena et al. studied retrospectively the neurologic status at the time of admission to the rehabilitation hospital of 45 stroke patients referred to Occupational Therapy for driver prescreening (15). The 29 patients who passed the prescreening—23 of whom eventually passed an on-road assessment (ORA)—were significantly more likely than those who failed the prescreening to have intact visual fields and higher Mini Mental Status Examination (MMSE) and Motricity scores.

Aphasia presents a challenge to driving. In a 1980 study, 20 aphasic subjects (10 who had chosen to return to driving and 10 who had not) were evaluated as functional or nonfunctional to drive by a team including a physiatrist, driving instructor (off-road screening tests), occupational therapist, and speech therapist (16). The team's assessments of driving-related sensorimotor and cognitive domains were strongly predictive of the subject's decision whether or not to continue driving. Performance in spatial relationships was the most important variable that discriminated between those who chose to drive and those who did not, and that discriminated between subjects who were judged as functional and those who were judged as nonfunctional to drive. The severity of aphasia had a significant effect on the subject's decision to drive but not on the team's rating. All aphasic patients who chose to drive were judged as functional by the team (16).

Few studies have explored anatomic factors in driver performance following stroke. Using a driving simulator, Kotterba et al. studied 32 stroke survivors and found that patients with middle cerebral artery strokes performed more poorly than those with vertebral artery territory damage (17). This makes sense, given that middle cerebral artery strokes are likely to be larger in volume than vertebral artery strokes and are more likely to involve structures that affect cognition, vision, and perception. Patients with right-brain lesions are more likely than those with left-brain lesions to score poorly on visual and perceptual tests that are predictive of driver outcome (18). Akinwuntan et al. analyzed specific deficit areas in the ORA of 68 stroke survivors and found that subjects with attributes of visual neglect consistently drifted toward one side of the road and lacked adequate vision and perception during complex driving conditions (19).

DETERMINING FITNESS TO DRIVE

The majority of stroke survivors interested in return to driving will require an ORA, which is the gold standard for determining driver safety. However, it must be emphasized that the physician's interview, examination, and assessment is a vital component of the evaluation process. For the patient with apparent complete neurologic recovery, the physician may feel comfortable clearing the patient to return to driving, in which case neuropsychological tests, closed-course driving tests, and driving simulator performance described below can provide helpful corroboration of the validity of this decision. If the patient has residual deficits, these screening tools can assist the clinician in determining if the ORA is necessary and when it should take place.

The On-Road Assessment

The ORA can take place in the patient's own vehicle, with a trained driving instructor sitting in the front passenger seat assessing performance. More often, and especially in cases in which safety is unknown or a true concern, the instructor will require a dual-control vehicle in which both driver and instructor have control over the brakes. Most dual-control vehicles have automatic transmission. For standard transmission vehicles with a manual clutch, the instructor may have control over a second clutch; however, such vehicles are rarely, if ever, used or recommended for stroke patients.

Ideally, the instructor will be a driver rehabilitation specialist (DRS—see below) or at least have experience with stroke patients. In the province of Ontario, Canada, provincial law mandates that, for a specialized ORA for a disabled individual, an occupational therapist must ride in the vehicle and evaluate performance as well. However, many areas of North America lack driving instructors with such expertise, and the physician may have to (or be required to) send the patient for an ORA by the state or provincial license certifying agency. The experience of the agency's instructors working with stroke survivors and other disabilities may vary considerably.

The overall failure rate on the ORA by stroke survivors is 26%–83% (9). Such a wide variability in failure rate attests to the wide variation in testing methods for the ORA. The method of assessing on-the-road driving performance may be highly structured but often differs between centers. In addition, different instructors may score a structured assessment differently. For example, the validity and reliability of particular

structured 10-mile ORA were evaluated in a Belgian study involving 39 stroke survivors (20). The results of this study demonstrated a significant variability in the pass rate between driving instructors. The state-registered evaluator failed seven of nine patients who had been passed by a driving instructor who had had more experience working with patients with strokes and other disabling conditions (20). The findings indicate a need for stroke survivors to work with instructors who are skilled in evaluating disabled people.

The ORA can be costly, and failure can lead to the serious consequences of loss or inability to re-obtain a license to drive. Regaining the license may entail overcoming considerable bureaucratic hurdles (even to obtain a training or learner's permit) and substantial expense in driving lessons. When the ORA is necessary, the physician can play a key role in determining when it should be scheduled to insure the maximum likelihood that the patient will pass.

Predriving Cognitive and Neuropsychological Testing

A variety of studies have involved batteries of neuropsychological tests and correlated the results with on-road assessments (6, 9). These studies show significant relationships between a number of psychometric tests and fitness to drive as measured by the ORA. They suffer from tremendous variability in the kinds of tests administered and the timing of testing following stroke. In most cases small numbers of patients were studied. The exact locations and extent of cerebral damage are generally not identified (9).

Engum et al. developed the Cognitive Behavioral Driver's Inventory (CBDI), which consists of brief neuropsychological tests with 27 individual scoring items. These tests evaluate the following domains of driver-related cognitive functioning: attention, concentration, rapid decision-making, stimulus discrimination/response differentiation, visual scanning and acuity, and attention shifting (21). A summary score is average of the 27 items and is classified as pass, fail, or borderline. The CBDI has high internal consistency and validity based on correlations with the ORA. In a double-blind study of 81 patients, clearly passing the CBDI was 94% predictive of passing the ORA, and clearly failing the CBDI was 100% predictive of failing the ORA (22). The CBDI was further validated and shown to be sensitive in discriminating among 109 brain-injured subjects who passed the ORA, 54 brain-injured subjects who failed the ORA, and 41 non-brain-injured control subjects (23). In a recent retrospective study of 172 patients, including 28 with left-brain stroke, 20 with right-brain stroke, and 58 with traumatic brain injury, the CBDI was found to be a significant predictor of pass or fail on the ORA for patients with right-brain stroke and traumatic brain injury but not for those with left-brain stroke (24).

Klavora et al. found the CBDI alone to be only 66% accurate in predicting success or failure on the ORA in 56 stroke survivors (25). These authors also evaluated the accuracy of the Dynavision Performance Assessment Battery, which uses a computerized apparatus to test and train visual scanning, peripheral visual awareness, visual attention, and visuomotor reaction time, and found the accuracy of the battery and subtests to be 66%–77%. Some of the subtests of the Dynavision battery that take 5–10 minutes or less matched the predictive accuracy of the CBDI, which takes 60–90 minutes. Combining the CBDI and Dynavision battery yielded 100% accuracy (25).

In a study involving 23 subjects with stroke and 14 subjects with traumatic brain injury, Galski, et al compared 21 neuropsychological tests of attention, concentration, reaction time, memory, visual acuity, and visuospatial skills against a structured ORA consisting of 26 tasks (26). A driver evaluator converted the neuropsychological tests into a pass or fail score. Neither the pass/fail score nor any of the individual neuropsychological tests predicted the ORA outcome. The authors concluded that predriving evaluations should focus on screening out patients who are unsafe drivers rather than trying to predict reliably which patients are safe to drive (26).

In a study in Great Britain, 39 subjects who had had a stroke more than six weeks earlier were given a cognitive assessment by a psychologist and an ORA by the British School of Motoring (27). Significant relationships were noted for cube copy (spatial ability), dot cancellations time and misses (visual inattention, spatial ability, and memory), rey figure recall (visual inattention), "what else is in the square?" (a children's game that tests reasoning ability), pursuit rotor (eye-hand coordination), road sign recognition (visual comprehension), and hazard recognition (visual recognition from videotape of an open-road drive). Using these, the authors developed a model for predicting driving competency from the ORA; the model predicted pass or fail accurately for 95% of subjects. Complex reasoning skills seemed especially important (27).

A follow-up study, however, failed to validate the model in 40 stroke survivors (20 with left and 20 with right hemiparesis) (28), possibly because of a change in the ORA and driving evaluator used. A new model was developed using dot cancellation, square matrices (based on "what else is in the square?"), and road sign recognition; this model predicted performance on the ORA with 79%–82% accuracy and was eventually developed into the Stroke Drivers Screening Assessment. Two later studies involving a total of 66 patients showed this tool to be 80%–81% accurate in predicting performance on the ORA (20, 29). The instrument has

shown excellent concurrent validity with more extensive neuropsychological measures of attention and executive functioning (30).

Other studies using multivariate statistical analysis have shown a significant correlation between various tests, including the Motor Free Visual Perception Test (MVPT) (18, 31), single-letter cancellation test (18), trail-making test part B (18), and figure of rey complex drawing task (32), and subsequent performance on the ORA. In a multicenter trial of 269 patients, lower scores on the MVPT, increased age, and right-brain lesions were significantly associated with failure on the ORA, but the MVPT alone was insufficient to serve as the sole screening instrument for determining readiness for the ORA (31).

In a systematic review, Marshall et al. examined predictors of driving ability following stroke. They noted useful screening tests, such as trail-making parts A and B. Cognitive tests that assessed "multiple cognitive domains relevant to driving" were deemed to have the best reproducibility in predicting fitness to drive (6).

Thus, cognitive testing in a variety of domains can be helpful in identifying potentially unsafe drivers. However, no single test or battery of tests predicts this absolutely. If the physician believes the patient to be unsafe, that too has some validity; there is a significant correlation between the objective driving score derived from standardized ORA and the global subjective evaluation of fitness to drive (33). In general, regardless of the predriving screening method used, the threshold for requesting (or insisting) that the patient undergo an ORA should, in the opinion of the authors, remain low.

Driving Simulators and Closed-Course Driving Tests

Traditionally, driving simulation involved watching films or videos of a car driving through traffic and watching or tabulating the patient's reactions on mock driving controls, often adapted from an actual vehicle. Such simulation is noninteractive. Advances in computer simulation, video technology, and gaming have enabled development of highly realistic, interactive scenarios in which the video monitors wrap almost around the patient and the computer routine can change in response to the patient's actions. The computer can also monitor and record reaction time, errors, and appropriate or inappropriate use of steering and other controls (4).

Off-road, closed-course driving tests are recommended to evaluate vehicle operation skills and readiness for an in-traffic ORA (33). However one small study showed no significant correlation between measures of driving on a closed course and performance on an ORA (34). A closed course thus may require a different set of skills than those required on an open-road ORA, and some stroke survivors may perform better in open-road driving—which may be an over-learned skill—than in a novel, off-road closed-circuit test.

Szlyk et al. found decreased performance on a driving simulator in patients with hemianopsia associated with primarily occipital lobe damage from stroke compared with a control group of similar age (35). In a Belgian study, 83 stroke survivors were assigned to simulator-based driver training (experimental group) or driving-related cognitive tasks (control group) (36). The subjects trained for one hour three times weekly for five weeks. The simulator consisted of the controls from an actual vehicle, with adaptive equipment as needed and with large-screen video and audio that simulated a 13.5-kilometer (8.4-mile) course under varied driving conditions. Visual and neuropsychological performance improved in both groups. The experimental group improved significantly more than the control group only in a road sign recognition test. Before training, only 27% of either group was judged fit to drive based on an ORA. After training, improvements in the classification of fitness to drive favored the experimental group. Ultimately, 73% of the experimental group and 42% of the control group were legally permitted to resume driving.

Galski et al. found that neuropsychological test results explained only 64% of the variance in ORA performance, while performance on the Doron simulator (a realistic but noninteractive driving simulator) predicted 63% (37). Together, the neuropsychological testing and the simulator test explained 69% of the variance. The subjects' driving skills in a parking lot were also examined. The ability to follow directions, the presence of slow response, inattention and distractibility, and an index of overall behavior observed added 23% to the predictability, for a total of 92% of the variance. A factor analysis of the testing protocol identified five independent factors that predict performance on the Doron simulator: higher order visuospatial abilities, basic visual recognition and responding, anticipatory braking, defensive steering, and behavioral manifestations of complex attention (37).

In a study of 30 stroke survivors and 30 matched controls, a regression model was developed that included performance characteristics on a driving simulator and three psychological domains: attentional processing, executive capacity, and cognitive processing (38). A model based on performance variables on the simulator correctly predicted pass or fail on the ORA with 85% accuracy, while a model based on the psychological variables was 83% accurate.

A driving simulator may therefore provide a safer alternative to the ORA for evaluating the driving potential of a stroke survivor who is likely unsafe. The simulation of driving can also be used for educational purposes: poor performance may be more persuasive than paper and pencil neuropsychological test results to convince a patently unsafe patient to postpone an ORA and avoid driving.

However, to prove the patient is a safe driver, there is no adequate substitute for an ORA administered by competent and experienced personnel.

Other Screening Instruments Not Specifically Tested in Stroke Survivors

Clock drawing, which evaluates memory, visuoconstructional ability, and executive functioning, can be a quick, useful, and simple screening tool. Failure on the clock-drawing test was found to be 90% accurate in predicting failure on an ORA in 100 adults aged 65 years or more (39). Clock drawing also correlated highly with performance on a driving simulator in 119 community-dwelling, active older Virginia drivers (40).

General screening tools for dementia, such as the Clinical Dementia Rating Scale and Folstein Mini-Mental Status Examination (MMSE), have been studied in older adult drivers. Dubinsky et al. reviewed controlled studies of Alzheimer's disease and driving (41). Driving was found to be mildly impaired in drivers with probable Alzheimer's disease (Clinical Dementia Rating of 0.5, roughly equivalent to an MMSE score of 25, indicating only slight limitation in functional areas). The driving impairment was no different from that tolerated legally by other segments of the population (drivers aged 16–21 or drivers under the influence of alcohol with legal blood levels of less than 0.08%). Drivers with a Clinical Dementia Rating of 1 (roughly equivalent to an MMSE score of 19–24, indicating moderate limitation in memory and cognition that interferes with daily activities) had a significantly increased crash risk and performed more poorly on driving performance measurements. Stroke patients with cognitive deficits that correspond globally to these impairment levels probably share the respective levels of driving disability and crash risk.

The Assessment of Driving-Related Skills. The Assessment of Driving-Related Skills (ADReS) is the formal assessment tool developed by a consensus panel for the American Medical Association (AMA) (11). It was designed for assessing older drivers but is applicable to a wide variety of conditions, including stroke. For several of the subtests, there is evidence linking poor performance with increased risk of adverse driving events (11). The ADReS consists of the following subtests:

- Visual field testing by confrontation
- Visual acuity using a Snellen chart
- Rapid pace walk
- Manual test of range of motion, including neck rotation, finger curl, shoulder and elbow flexion, and ankle plantarflexion and dorsiflexion
- Motor strength (standard manual muscle test scored from 0 to 5) of shoulder abduction, adduction and

flexion, wrist flexion and extension, hand grip, hip flexion and extension, and ankle dorsiflexion and plantarflexion

- Trail-making test, part B
- Clock-drawing test (Freund method of scoring) (40)

If the patient fails any element of the ADReS, an ORA is recommended. Note that for stroke patients, significant hemiparesis will make it difficult for the patient to pass the motor strength screening (all muscles 4/5 or better in both upper extremities and the right lower extremity) and rapid pace walk test (10 feet and back in 9.0 seconds or less). Dominant upper extremity involvement will affect handwriting and may affect performance on the trail-making and clock-drawing tests.

The ADReS has good inter-rater reliability among nursing, medical, and occupational therapy professionals (42). In a study of 50 licensed adults aged 65 or older, McCarthy and Mann found the instrument to be 100% sensitive in identifying subjects who subsequently failed an ORA (43). However, it was only 38% specific, meaning that many safe drivers (those who passed the ORA) failed the ADReS. A major reason for the high false prediction of failure on the ORA was failure of the clock-drawing test. To pass this test, the patient must draw the clock without error by the Freund scoring method. The authors noted that lowering the cut-off scores for passing the clock-drawing test from 8/8 to 6/8 would not reduce the sensitivity but would improve the specificity to 62% (43).

In McCarthy and Mann's sample, which did not include any stroke survivors, only 16% of patients failed the ORA. The high sensitivity and specificity of the ADReS may be different in a stroke population, in which the likelihood of failing the ORA is much higher (26%–83%) (9). However, the battery of tests is useful because it is a quick screening tool (15–20 minutes) that incorporates elements of the functional examination that the rehabilitation clinician will likely perform.

RETURN TO DRIVING (OR OTHER SAFE COMMUNITY TRANSPORTATION)

AUQ4

Adaptive Equipment to Aid in Safe Driving

For stroke survivors with significant weakness of the hemiparetic side, a spinner knob attached to the steering wheel is required (Figure 43-2); this enables adequate control of the steering wheel and must be used at all times during operation of the vehicle. Spinner knobs are also now available with switches to make it possible for the driver to control the turn signals, windshield wipers, horn, and high beams without removing his or her hand from the knob (Figure 43-3). If the person cannot control his or her

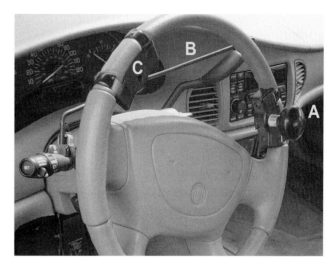

FIGURE 43-2

Adaptive equipment for hemiparetic drivers. A: Spinner knob to be used at all times with the right hand for driver with left hemiparesis. B: Left-to-right turn signal control. C: Note that spinner knob can be placed on the left side for a driver with right hemiparesis. (Equipment available from Mobility Products & Design, PO Box 306, 144 South 100 West, Winamac, IN 46996).

right ankle, a right-to-left accelerator pedal converter may be needed (Figure 43-4) (44). Similarly, for a stroke patient with left hemiparesis, controls on the left, such as a turn signal, will require left-to-right conversion (Figure 43-2). For all of these, the control is usually designed to be easily removed, so that the vehicle can be used by an able-bodied person as well (44).

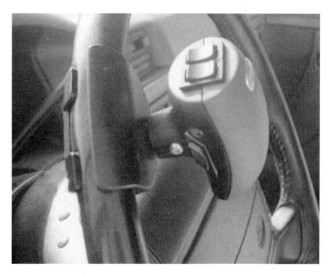

FIGURE 43-3

Spinner knob with controls (switches) for turn signals, windshield wipers, horn, and high beam. (Image courtesy of Driving Systems Incorporated, Van Nuys, CA.)

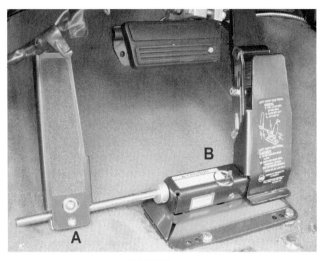

FIGURE 43-4

A: Right-to-left foot control for accelerator pedal for a driver with right hemiparesis. B: Note the pin for easy removal, so that the vehicle can also be used by an able-bodied driver. (Equipment available from Mobility Products & Design, PO Box 306, 144 South 100 West, Winamac, IN 46996.)

The Driver Rehabilitation Specialist

A Driver Rehabilitation Specialist (DRS) is a driving instructor who "plans, develops, coordinates, and implements driver rehabilitation services for individuals with disabilities" (45). A DRS generally undergoes a certification process through the Association for Driver Rehabilitation Specialists (formerly the Association for Driver Educators for the Disabled). Certification requirements include education, work experience, and passing a written examination. However, in most states and provinces there is no absolute requirement for certification to work as a DRS in adaptive driving instruction or administration of ORAs for people with disabilities. A DRS usually has certification or training in another discipline, most often occupational therapy but also physical therapy, kinesiotherapy, speech therapy, or recreational therapy. A driving instructor without training in another discipline (for example, a driving school instructor or state driver licensing bureau examiner) can gain certification with five years of full-time work experience in the field of driver rehabilitation (45).

The Association for Driver Rehabilitation Specialists has several categories of membership in addition to individual members: mobility equipment dealers, businesses involved in manufacturing and distributing products used by a DRS and by individuals with disabilities, and facilities and businesses that implement or administrate driver rehabilitation services. The association organizes and officiates the examination for certification, has developed best practice standards for delivery of driver rehabilitation

services, and has established ethical standards of practice. Thus, it serves as a major resource for all professionals involved in driver rehabilitation (45).

Adaptive driving programs are available in a variety of settings. Many comprehensive rehabilitation hospitals and programs offer driving schools for the disabled. A few programs are located within universities and are often connected to research facilities that are federally funded. Some are sponsored by local affiliates of national nonprofit organizations that serve the disabled, such as United Cerebral Palsy. Some private commercial driving schools have developed the expertise to advise on adaptive equipment and provide evaluation and training of stroke survivors. A few state vocational rehabilitation programs also offer such training, but most provide funding for patients to participate in adaptive driving programs in other settings (44).

The DRS performs a clinical evaluation of the patient, including medical and driving history, vision examination, assessment of selected physical aspects, cognitive assessment, and ORA. The medical history includes determining current medical status and stability to undergo further testing, reviewing medications for their potential deleterious effect on driving, assessing the patient's current communication status, reviewing the driving history, determining the license status (to determine whether an ORA can be performed legally), and assessing the availability of a suitable vehicle for the ORA. The DRS must also establish that the patient is actually medically cleared for an ORA and that performance of the ORA, given the medical condition, does not violate state or provincial regulations (46).

If the stroke survivor has had a seizure within the state-mandated period during which driving is not permitted, the DRS cannot perform an ORA, even if requested by a physician. In several states the mandated period of driving abstention can be overruled by the medical board of the state licensing agency if appropriate medical documentation is provided.

If a patient lacks a legal license but is cleared medically for the ORA, the DRS can facilitate the patient's obtaining a temporary license from the state authorizing the evaluation in a dual-control vehicle. This is required of the patient whose license is revoked because of a stroke and its sequelae but who recovers sufficiently to be evaluated.

For driving prescreening, the DRS performs an extensive functional and driving-oriented vision examination using assessment tools and clinical observation. Physical capacities required to control a motor vehicle are evaluated: strength, range of motion, grip strength, sensation, proprioception, coordination, and muscle tone. The level of cognitive impairment and self-awareness is also scrutinized, often with neuropsychological tests. Reaction time is usually measured objectively, especially movement of the foot from the accelerator to the brake pedal; this can now be tested with portable equipment in the patient's own vehicle. The DRS also evaluates the patient's assistive devices and orthotics needed for ambulation and must determine whether these will interfere with driving (46). Spastic talipes equinovarus, foot drop, and the use of an ankle-foot orthotic to block right ankle motion will usually impair control of the accelerator or brake pedal; the DRS can establish whether modification of the vehicle with adaptive equipment is indicated.

In a 2003 survey of driving evaluation practices of DRSs, more than 70% used a brake reaction timer, 70% the trail-making test part A or B, and 65% the motor-free visual perceptual test. In addition, 30% used the MMSE, and about 25% the letter cancellation test. Other measures of vision, perception, and cognition were used by 15% or less (47).

At the start of the ORA, the DRS assesses the patient's ability to enter and exit the vehicle and determines whether specialized equipment is needed (46). Rarely, stroke patients require a specialized wheelchair lift to access the vehicle independently. The patient's sitting posture and position with respect to the steering wheel and controls are evaluated. A major component of the evaluation is the patient's ability to operate controls while the vehicle is stationery or moving. If the vehicle already has adaptive equipment, the DRS evaluates its condition and appropriateness for the patient (46).

Out on the road, the DRS assesses the patient's driving performance in increasingly complex traffic conditions. The purpose of the examination is to observe the patient in road settings, traffic density, and weather conditions that approximate as closely as possible those likely to be encountered normally (46). For patients with suspected deficits that might interfere with safe driving, the DRS should design the ORA to emphasize driver actions that stress those deficit areas, for example, frequent left turns and performance at intersections with moderate to high degrees of traffic flow for patients with suspected left hemineglect (44). Some patients may be cleared for limited licenses, for example, to drive only during daylight hours. For most patients it is necessary to demonstrate satisfactory performance of all usual driving maneuvers required of able-bodied drivers seeking licensure.

At the end of the evaluation the DRS indicates to the patient—and the referring clinician—whether the patient is safe or unsafe to drive. If the patient is deemed unsafe to drive, the DRS recommends whether further training would help achieve safe driving or whether the patient should retire from driving. If adaptive equipment is required, the DRS trains and tests the patient to assure competence in its use while driving. If further training is likely to benefit the patient, the DRS can develop a program of goal-oriented driving lessons, with the ultimate purpose of passing a second ORA (46).

Stroke survivors who possess a valid license, require no special adaptive equipment, and are judged safe to drive by the DRS can generally return to driving. If new adaptive equipment is required, usually the patient must also be retested and certified by the state using that equipment. In most cases drivers seeking commercial certification must also be retested by the state to resume commercial occupations legally.

Evaluation and training by a DRS is expensive, generally costing $80–120 or more per hour. Some insurance companies may pay for this, but most do not. Federal and state vocational rehabilitation offices often pay for an ORA if it can be shown that return to driving will facilitate return to work.

The Physician's Approach to the Patient

Stroke patients vary considerably in their potential to be unsafe drivers, and physicians need to individualize their approach for each individual patient, depending on the severity of the stroke, the specific impairments involved, and associated comorbidities. Patients with moderate to severe deficits will be clearly unable to drive, either temporarily or permanently. Objective tests that characterize cerebral damage (computed tomography or magnetic resonance imaging) and quantify the impairments can help in developing a prognosis, but post-stroke functional ability and driving performance will ultimately determine the potential to resume driving.

Patients with severe impairments and disabilities may need counseling to avoid driving and to seek alternative forms of transportation. Patients who deny or are unaware of their neurologic deficits (including many with right-brain infarcts and anosognosia) and those with cognitive deficits who may impulsively decide to drive present a particular problem. In many, but not all, states and provinces the physician is legally obligated to report all potentially unsafe drivers to driver licensing agencies. Family members may need to be counseled to take measures to prevent the unsafe driver from driving (e.g., lock the car, hide the keys). Family members may also have the right to report the likelihood of unsafe driving practices to the driver licensing agency, and the threat of this may add weight to the physician's insistence that the patient cease driving. Patients who insist on an ORA may need counseling to postpone the assessment until further recovery has taken place.

Those with milder deficits and those who have recovered should be assessed using the ADReS or another objective, quantifiable test. Cognitive testing with the MMSE or other instrument is also useful. Patients who recover full motor, sensory, perceptual, and visual function, who lack cognitive deficits by testing, and who pass the ADReS are probably safe to drive. However, reaction time may still be affected and should be measured if possible. If there is *any* question that residual (or premorbid) visual, sensorimotor, or cognitive deficits exist, the patient should be referred for an ORA. Patients with hemiparesis severe enough to prevent bimanual grip of a steering wheel or regular use of brake and gas pedals need referral to a certified DRS for adaptive equipment or modification of the vehicle before the ORA.

Aphasic patients may recover in other neurologic domains to the point at which safe operation of a motor vehicle is feasible, but may have difficulty with written or oral examinations. The physician or therapist should anticipate such problems during testing and urge the testing or licensing agency to make accommodations for the patient's needs. This may include waiving the written test. If a written test cannot be avoided, patients with aphasia may benefit from extra time and the use of multiple-choice questions rather than prose or essay responses. Those with alexia or anomia may require someone to read the questions and choices for answers. Multiple-choice tests designed using pictures instead of words will also help the aphasic patient. Some with severe deficits may fail because they are untestable or because the agency cannot provide the necessary accommodations.

Physicians often encounter patients who have recovered from stroke but who present with new weakness. If the patient recovers fully, as with a transient ischemic attack, driving should be avoided until a full medical evaluation has been completed. Persistent (for more than 24 hours) new weakness warrants cessation of driving until completion of not only a medical reevaluation but also the ADReS, cognitive tests, and if appropriate, another ORA. A patient previously judged competent to use adaptive equipment—whether related to deficits from a prior stroke or from another disabling disease—may need reevaluation and training to use the equipment safely again. Repeated unpredictable transient ischemic attacks, syncope, or seizures require definitive medical treatment before driving can be resumed. If the medical condition can be controlled perfectly or is always preceded by adequate warning symptoms, return to safe driving may be possible. The physician should adhere to state or provincial regulations for reporting such transient neurologic changes. Most jurisdictions support the decision that the patient stop driving and require a period of freedom from episodes of altered consciousness before a license can be restored.

Patients who have undergone cerebrovascular or intracranial surgery should not drive until they are judged fully stable, free of post-surgical symptoms, and cleared by a neurosurgeon. Residual neurologic deficits should be addressed in the same way as persistent deficits following a stroke. Arteriovenous malformations and subarachnoid hemorrhage should be treated similarly; the risk of future bleeding/re-bleeding of arteriovenous malformations and aneurysms must be assessed. If the risk is low and residual neurologic deficits are stable and mild, return to driving can be considered. However, driving is contraindicated if the medical condition remains unstable or at high risk of recurrence (11).

Preexisting comorbidities may influence driver safety in stroke patients who may have previously been safe drivers. The presence of arthritis, mild Parkinsonism, visual acuity problems, deafness, mild dementia, or other disorders of aging may not in themselves preclude safe driving, yet when combined with even mild neurologic deficits after stroke, they may adversely affect driver safety. Thus, driver rehabilitation may require the physician to evaluate and treat such secondary comorbidities.

Regardless of state or provincial reporting requirements, it remains of paramount importance that the physician tell the patient who is potentially unsafe not to drive, until further recovery takes place, or until the patient undergoes a definitive ORA. The physician may be found negligent if the patient is not counseled in this way and subsequently drives or has an accident. To protect the physician, it is important to document that this counseling took place in the medical record.

It is important to offer support and counseling to patients who are unsafe to drive or who resist giving up driving or being tested. A list of tips to reinforce driving cessation is given in Table 43-1 (11). Referral to social services will help the patient to identify, apply for, and ultimately qualify for alternative community-based or subsidized transportation. The stroke survivor

---

TABLE 43-1

Tips to Reinforce Driving Cessation for Stroke Survivors Likely to be Unsafe Drivers

- Write on a prescription pad, "Do not drive." This emphasizes the strength of the message and can serve as a visual reminder to the patient.
- Ask whether the patient wishes to risk an accident in which injury could occur. The patient, his/her family, or an innocent party could be injured. How would the patient feel if someone else were injured as a result of causing an accident?
- Point out that an accident will very likely raise insurance premiums.
- Owning, insuring, fueling, and maintaining an automobile can be very expensive. If the patient retires from driving and sells the vehicle, how much money could be saved?
- Ask how much lower would the cost be to take taxis or public conveyances?
- Develop a plan for alternative transportation with family members. Present that plan to the patient.
- If the patient lacks a valid license or is not qualified to drive because of the medical condition, point out the legal risks of driving without a license.

Adapted from Wang et al. 2003 (11).

may require door-to-door public van service, which may require medical justification; the physician should expect requests for documentation when patients apply for such services.

AMA Physician's Guide to Assessing and Counseling Older Drivers

A useful resource to assist physicians and other rehabilitation personnel in addressing driver safety is the *Physician's Guide to Assessing and Counseling Older Drivers* (11). This was a cooperative effort between the AMA and the U.S. National Highway Traffic Safety Administration. It was developed by consensus of an advisory panel of clinicians, researchers, and representatives of medical specialty societies and organizations that serve the elderly. The primary goal of the guide was to educate physicians and provide them with assessment and management tools to address driving in elderly populations, but overall, it is also of value to physicians and therapists who work with stroke survivors of any legal driving age. The AMA guide is divided into chapters, many of which include specialized resources for evaluating and managing driver safety issues (Table 43-2).

TABLE 43-2

Specialized Resources in the American Medical Association's Physician's Guide to Assessing and Counseling Older Drivers

CHAPTER	SPECIAL RESOURCE
1. Safety and the Older Driver: an Overview	• Physician's plan for older drivers' safety
2. Is the Patient at Increased Risk for Unsafe Driving?	• Red flags for medically impaired driving
3. Formally Assess Function (Tools to Assess)	• Discussion of "What if your patient refuses assessment?" • Description of all parts of the Assessment of Driver-Related Skills (ADReS) • ADReS score sheet (can be copied) • Test sheet for Trail-making test, part B (can be copied)
4. Physician Interventions	• Discussion of evidence for driving restrictions based on visual acuity, visual fields, cognition, and motor ability
5. The Driver Rehabilitation Specialist	• Discussion of "What if driver assessment is not an option?"
6. Counseling the Patient Who is Longer Safe to Drive	• Tips to reinforce driving cessation • Sample letter to send to patient with recommendation to retire from driving
7. Legal and Ethical Responsibilities of the Physician	• Delineation of the conflicting responsibilities faced by physicians trying to assess and help patients who are patently unsafe to drive • Clinical approach to the patient: "Putting it all together"
8. State Licensing Requirements and Reporting Laws	• For each state: contact information, medical requirements for driver licensing, license renewal procedures, reporting procedures, and information about the medical advisory board
9. Medical Conditions and Medications that May Impair Driving	• A wide variety of medical conditions and diseases are discussed. Separate sections are devoted to cerebrovascular diseases, seizures, and medications
10. Moving Beyond This Guide: Research and Planning for Safe Transportation for the Older Population	• Goals for the AMA and other interested advocacy groups and researchers, to promote safe driving for our patients and alternative transportation
Appendices	Patient and caregiver educational materials: • Patient self-report questionnaire: "Am I a safe driver?" • Successful aging tips • Tips for driving • How to help the older driver (for family members/friends) • Getting by without driving

The AMA guide lists a series of "red flags" for medically impaired driving that should alert the physician to potential driver safety issues. Those particularly applicable to stroke include concerns about the patient's driving expressed by family members, the presence of multiple chronic medical conditions, polypharmacy use (especially medications with potential sedative effects), and a history of episodic or unpredictable events, such as hypoglycemia, cataplexy, angina, or syncope. Family members should be queried about recent crashes, near-misses, traffic tickets, unexpected or unexplained episodes of becoming lost, and forgetfulness. The presence of any of these should trigger a formal evaluation of driver safety as outlined above.

COMMON PROBLEMS AND MEDICAL DECISION-MAKING

Your patient has sustained a stroke. The following is a series of questions and answers concerning reporting, testing and medical responsibility.

1. Do Physicians have to Report to "The Authorities" that their Patient Sustained a Stroke?

The answer to this varies according to the patient's residence, the type of stroke sustained, and the sequelae of the stroke itself. States and provinces have different responsibilities. Most provinces and a few states have mandatory reporting, which means that the physician must report the patient to their state or provincial motor vehicle licensing authority if the stroke has caused any type of physical, cognitive, psychological, or other abnormality that could affect ability to drive. It does *not* mean that every patient with the diagnosis of stroke must be reported, as is the case in Belgium, where it is mandatory for physicians to report all acute stroke patients, who must then refrain from driving for six months.

There are stroke survivors without residual neurologic deficits who do not need to be reported; but it is the physician's responsibility to establish that fact with objective tests and examination. If the physician is uncertain about the apparent full recovery, reporting the patient may relieve the physician of potential liability for negligence or damages, if the patient is subsequently involved in an accident (see below). Not reporting the patient in a state with mandatory reporting may leave the physician in violation of civil law and may make defending a lawsuit for damages more difficult.

In some states and provinces, reporting potentially unsafe drivers is encouraged but not required. In that case, before the physician sends any driving-related information to the state or provincial authority, he or she should obtain the patient's consent to do so. Liability for reporting confidential information without patient permission (technically a breach of confidentiality) and immunity from prosecution or lawsuits arising out of such reporting vary from state to state.

For example, the state of Illinois, which has no mandatory reporting for physicians, legally obligates *drivers* to declare at the time of license application or renewal whether they have "any mental or physical condition that might interfere with driving," among other topics. The driver is thereafter obligated to produce a "physician's statement, a medical agreement, and/or the appropriate court documentation." The physician, however, is neither legally obligated to submit information regarding the medical condition of a patient nor can be held liable for providing this information. A specific form that provides medical documentation related to the patient's ability to drive safely has a corresponding patient section that must be completed as well. The physician can request that any or all of three components of a driving test (written, vision, and road) be performed. The state Medical Review Board may also compel the patient to take any or all of these tests (1).

In contrast, in Pennsylvania "all physicians and other persons authorized to diagnose or treat disorders and disabilities must report to The Pennsylvania Department of Transportation any patient 15 years of age or older, who has been diagnosed as having a condition that could impair his ability to safely operate a motor vehicle." Reporting is confidential, physicians are granted immunity from breach of confidentiality, and physicians are immune from civil or criminal liability related to a patient driving and becoming involved in an accident. Failure to report leaves the physician open to possible conviction of a summary criminal offense (for not reporting) and to possible liability in case the patient has a motor vehicle accident (48).

While the patient-physician relationship is usually built on trust, noncompliance with physician recommendations and treatment occurs frequently. The incidence of noncompliance with medical recommendations not to drive has not been studied in stroke survivors, but it has been studied in people with seizures. Salinsky et al. gave an anonymous questionnaire to 158 outpatients in an epilepsy clinic and found that if the patients were required by law to report seizures to the department of motor vehicles (but the physicians were not so required), 96% would tell their physicians if they had breakthrough seizures, but only 56% would report this to their department of motor vehicles. Under mandatory physician reporting, only 84% would inform their physician. A total of 17% endorsed that they would inform the physician but continue to drive, despite advice from the physician not to drive and despite the automatic license suspension from the state after being reported (49). Extrapolating to stroke patients, it cannot be assumed that just because the physician tells the stroke survivor not to drive, the patient will automatically comply.

2. Does my Patient with a Stroke have to Stop Driving? To Return to Driving is it Necessary to Undergo an On-Road Assessment?

According to the Canadian Medical Association (50), patients who have had a stroke "should not drive for at least one month. During this time they require assessment by their regular physician. They may resume driving if functionally able and if a neurologic assessment discloses no obvious risk of sudden recurrences and any underlying causes have been addressed with appropriate treatment. Where there is a residual loss of motor power, a road test may be required." While there is no absolute, evidenced-based foundation to the one-month restriction, many provincial legislative bodies agree with this decision. Delaying return to driving to give the patient time to recover more fully, assure stability, or undergo testing makes sense medically.

3. What is the Liability of the Physician if a Reported Patient is Involved in a Motor Vehicle Accident?

Most, but not all, states and provinces protect the physician from at least some liability (damages or breach of confidentiality) if a patient is reported for medical reasons to driving authorities. If a stroke patient who is not reported is personally involved in an accident (whether at fault or not), the physician could be sued for negligence and for damages resulting from the accident (11). The case against the physician would likely be strengthened if the plaintiffs can prove the physician was legally obligated to report the patient to state or provincial authorities or if the physician failed to counsel the patient not to drive. For example, if a post-stroke seizure is not reported and the patient is not instructed to stop driving, the physician could be held liable if the patient is involved in an accident.

4. Do Certain Strokes Require Different Types of Reporting or Attention by the Physician?

In general, there is no specific type of stroke that absolutely requires a report to a driving authority. However, the Canadian Medical Association guide indicates that "untreated cerebral aneurysms" are an absolute barrier to driving any class of vehicle, and a waiting period of three months for a private driver and six months for a commercial driver is required (50). These recommendations have face value but are wholly empirical and are not based on any specific research data that are currently available.

5. Can I Restrict the Type of Driving that my Patient Performs?

A restricted driving license—meaning a license that indicates that the person cannot drive at night, at certain speeds, or on certain roads—is available in only a few states and provinces in North America. In Utah, for example, the Utah Driver License Division indicates that a restricted license with speed and/or area restrictions may be issued if there are moderate impairments. The province of Saskatchewan has a restricted license as well. Marshall et al. studied whether people with restricted licenses were involved in more vehicle infractions or accidents than those without restricted licensing. The available data did not indicate a significant difference, but because of the use of provincial records, the driving patterns of the study subjects could not be ascertained (51). As a group, stroke patients appear to self-restrict when, where, and how much they drive (52).

6. Can my Patient with Isolated Homonymous Hemianopsia Return to Safe Driving?

Homonymous hemianopsia can affect safe operation of a motor vehicle, especially if the patient has associated perceptual deficits. In many, but not all, states patients with homonymous hemianopsia fail to meet visual field licensing criteria (usually >110°) (11). In Canada, however, hemianopsia alone is not an absolute contraindication for driving. A person with congenital homonymous hemianopsia took his case to the Supreme Court of Canada, where it was basically decided that if hemianopsia did not affect driving performance, it was not an absolute criterion preventing an individual from driving (53). Blindness of one eye also does not, by itself, make driving unsafe.

7. When Should the Physician Inform the Patient About the Decision to Report to Driving Authorities?

This issue should preferably be discussed as soon as the decision is made. In a state or province with mandatory reporting, the situation is made much easier. The physician emphasizes the legal obligations and necessity to report a person who may have impairments that could affect driving safety.

In jurisdictions without mandatory reporting laws, the physician risks liability for breach of confidentiality when reporting a patient without first obtaining consent. However, even when reporting is mandatory and anonymous, it is ethically appropriate to share with the patient the physician's legal obligation to report. The physician should limit information in the report to the minimum needed for the state to process the report appropriately. Being open with the patient is important to maintaining the patient-doctor relationship. It may also help the patient accept the reality that driving may not be safe. If at all possible, the physician should also obtain the permission of the patient before speaking to family members and caregivers (11).

8. What Therapy is Available to Improve my Patient's Potential to Drive Safely?

In general, there are no specific therapies that have been shown to speed up the recovery process to enable earlier return to safe driving. The physician should address stroke-related disabilities with appropriate therapies, including strengthening, conditioning, and coordination and visuoperceptual training. The study by Akinwuntan et al. suggests that training with a computerized driving simulator may be helpful in preparing some patients to be safe drivers (36). Training in UFOV may also be of benefit for patients with right brain lesions (54).

CONCLUSION

Driving after a stroke is possible. However, evaluation of the patient who has sustained a stroke must take into account any possible residual physical, cognitive, and perceptual impairments that may impede safe driving. The authors have identified the imperfect but relevant research on driving post-stroke as well as the physician responsibilities that may be required to report unsafe drivers. In general, if there is uncertainty about the stroke survivor's ability to drive, a formal driving evaluation including an on road assessment should occur. This may not always happen, but the authors believe that this is a principle that society should mandate. Future research will need to focus on the effects of specific neurologic deficits on driving, the consequences of driving cessation post-stroke, better screening tools to identify unsafe drivers, and alternate systems of community transportation to support stroke survivors.

References

1. Brandman JF. Cancer patients, opioids, and driving. *J Support Oncol.* 2005; 3(4):317–320.
2. Galski T, Ehle HT, McDonald MA, Mackevich J. Evaluating fitness to drive after cerebral injury: basic issues and recommendations for medical and legal communities. *J Head Trauma Rehabil.* 2000; 15:895–908.
3. Fisk GD, Owsley C, Pulley LV. Driving after stroke: driving exposure, advice, and evaluations. *Arch Phys Med Rehabil.* 1997; 78:1338–1345.
4. Beatson C, Gianutos R. Driver rehabilitation and personal transportation: the vital link to independence. In: Grabois M, Garrison SJ, Lehmkuhl LD, eds. *Physical Medicine and Rehabilitation: The Complete Approach.* Cambridge, MA: Blackwell Science, 2000; 777–802.
5. Galski T, Bruno RL, Ehle HT. Driving after cerebral damage: a model with implications for evaluation. *Am J Occup Ther.* 1992; 46:324–332.
6. Marshall SC, Molnar F, Man-Son-Hing M, et al. Predictors of driving ability following stroke: a systematic review. *Top Stroke Rehabil.* 2007; 14(1):98–114.
7. Diller E, Cook L, Leonard D, Reading J, et al. *Evaluating Drivers Licensed With Medical Conditions in Utah, 1992–1996.* Washington, DC: National Highway Traffic Safety Administration, 1999. US Department of Transportation, National Highway Traffic Safety Administration Publication No. DOT HS 809 023.
8. Haselkorn JK, Mueller BA, Rivara FA. Characteristics of drivers and driving record after traumatic and nontraumatic brain injury. *Arch Phys Med Rehabil.* 1998; 79:738–742.
9. Dobbs BM. *Medical Conditions and Driving: Current Knowledge.* Washington, DC: National Highway Traffic Safety Administration, 2002. US Department of Transportation, National Highway Traffic Safety Administration Project DTNH22-94-05297.
10. Fisk GD, Owsley C, Mennemeier M. Vision, attention, and self-reported driving behaviors in community-dwelling stroke survivors. *Arch Phys Med Rehabil.* 2002; 83:469–477.
11. Wang CC, Kosinski CJ, Schwartzberg JG, Shanklin AV. *Physician's Guide to Assessing and Counseling Older Drivers.* Washington, DC: National Highway Traffic Safety Administration, 2003.
12. Owsley C, Ball K, McGwin G, et al. Visual processing impairment and risk of motor vehicle crash among older adults. *JAMA.* 1998; 279:1083–1088.
13. Ball K, Owsley C. Identifying correlates of accident involvement for the older driver. *Hum Factors* 1991; 33:583–595.
14. Clay OJ, Wadley V, Edwards JD, et al. Cumulative meta-analysis of the relationship between useful field of view and driving performance in older adults: current and future implications. *Optom Vis Sci.* 2005; 82:724–731.
15. Smith-Arena L, Edelstein L, Rabadi MH. Predictors of a successful driver evaluation in stroke patients after discharge based on an acute rehabilitation hospital evaluation. *Am J Phys Med Rehabil.* 2006; 85:44–52.
16. Golper LAC, Rau MT, Marshall RC. Aphasic adults and their decisions on driving: an evaluation. *Arch Phys Med Rehabil.* 1980; 61:34–40.
17. Kotterba S, Widdig W, Brylak S, Orth M. Driving after cerebral ischemia—a driving simulator investigation. *Wien Med Wochenschr.* 2005; 155:348–353.
18. Mazer BL, Korner-Bitensky NA, Sofer S. Predicting ability to drive after stroke. *Arch Phys Med Rehabil.* 1998; 79:743–750.
19. Akinwuntan AE, Feys H, De Weerdt W, et al. Prediction of driving after stroke: a prospective study. *Neurorehabil Neural Repair.* 2006; 20:417–423.

20. Akinwuntan AE, De Weerdt W, Feys H, et al. The validity of a road test after stroke. *Arch Phys Med Rehabil.* 2005; 86(3):421–426.
21. Engum ES, Pendergrass TM, Cron L, et al. The cognitive behavioral driver's inventory. *Cogn Rehabil.* 1988; 6(5):34–50.
22. Engum ES, Lambert EW, Scott K, et al. Criterion-related validity of the cognitive behavioral driver's inventory. *Cogn Rehabil.* 1989; 7(4):22–31.
23. Engum ES, Lambert EW, Scott K. Criterion-related validity of the cognitive behavioral driver's inventory: brain-injured patients versus normal controls. *Cogn Rehabil.* 1990; 8(2):20–26.
24. Bouillon L, Mazer B, Gelinas I. Validity of the Cognitive Behavioral Driver's Inventory in predicting driving outcome. *Am J Occup Ther.* 2006; 60(4):420–427.
25. Klavora P, Heslegrave RJ, Young M. Driving skills in elderly persons with stroke: comparisons of two new assessment options. *Arch Phys Med Rehabil.* 2000; 81:701–705.
26. Galski T, Ehle HT, Bruno RL. An assessment of measures to predict the outcome of driving evaluations in patients with cerebral damage. *Am J Occup Ther.* 1990; 44:709–713.
27. Nouri FM, Tinson DJ, Lincoln NB. Cognitive ability and driving after stroke. *Int Disabil Stud.* 1987; 9(3):110–115.
28. Nouri FM, Lincoln NB. Validation of a cognitive assessment: predicting driving performance after stroke. *Clin Rehabil.* 1992; 6:275–281.
29. Nouri FM, Lincoln NB. Predicting driving performance after stroke. *BMJ.* 1993; 307:482–483.
30. Radford KA, Lincoln NB. Concurrent validity of the Stroke Drivers Screening Assessment. *Arch Phys Med Rehabil.* 2004; 85:324–328.
31. Korner-Bitensky NA, Mazer BL, Sofer S, et al. Visual testing for readiness to drive after stroke: a multicenter study. *Am J Phys Med Rehabil.* 2000; 79:253–259.
32. Akinwuntan AE, Feys H, De Weerdt W, et al. Determinants of driving after stroke. *Arch Phys Med Rehabil.* 2002; 83:334–341.
33. Fox GK, Bowden SC, Smith DS. On-road assessment of driving competence after brain impairment: review of current practice and recommendations for a standardized examination. *Arch Phys Med Rehabil.* 1998; 79(10):1288–1296.
34. Sivak M, Kewman DG, Henson DL. Driving and perceptual/cognitive skills: behavioral consequences of brain damage. *Arch Phys Med Rehabil.* 1981; 62:476–483.
35. Szlyk JP, Brigell M, Seiple W. Effects of age and hemianopic visual field loss on driving. *Optom Vis Sci.* 1993; 70(12):1031–1037.
36. Akinwuntan AE, De Weerdt W, Feys H, et al. Effect of simulator training on driving after stroke: a randomized controlled trial. *Neurology.* 2005; 65(6):843–850.
37. Galski T, Ehle HT, Williams JB. Off-road evaluations for persons with cerebral injury: a factor analytic study of predriver and simulator testing. *Am J Occup Ther.* 1997; 51:352–359.
38. Lundqvist A, Gerdle B, Rönnberg J. Neuropsychological aspects of driving after a stroke—in the simulator and on the road. *Appl Cogn Psychol.* 2000; 14(2):135–150.
39. Freund B, Gravenstein S, Dobbs A, Ferris R. Clock Drawing Test (CDT) may predict on-road driving performance [abstract]. *J Am Geriatr Soc.* 2001; 49(4):S113.
40. Freund B, Gravenstein S, Ferris R, et al. Drawing clocks and driving cars: use of brief tests of cognition to screen driving competency in older adults. *J Gen Intern Med.* 2005; 20:240–244.

41. Dubinsky RM, Stein AC, Lyons K. Practice parameter: risk of driving and Alzheimer's disease (an evidence-based review): report of the quality standards subcommittee of the American Academy of Neurology. *Neurology*. 2000; 54(12):2205–2211.

42. Posse C, McCarthy D, Mann WC. A pilot study of interrater reliability of the Assessment of Driver-related Skills: older driver screening tool. *Top Geriatr Rehabil*. 2006; 22(2):113–120.

43. McCarthy DP, Mann WC. Sensitivity and specificity of the assessment of driving related skills older driver screening tool. *Top Geriatr Rehabil*. 2006; 22(2):139–152.

44. Babirad J. Driver evaluation and vehicle modification. In: Olson DA, DeRuyter F, eds. *Clinician's Guide to Assistive Technology*. Philadelphia, PA: Mosby, 2002.

45. Association for Driver Rehabilitation Specialists. Certification. Available at: http://www.driver-ed.org/i4a/pages/index.cfm?pageid=120. Accessed May 6, 2007.

46. Association for Driver Rehabilitation Specialists Best Practices Committee. Best practices for the delivery of driver rehabilitation services, 2004. Available at: http://www.driver-ed.org/i4a/pages/index.cfm?pageid=279. Accessed May 6, 2007.

47. Korner-Bitensky N, Bitensky J, Sofer S, et al. Driving evaluation practices of clinicians working in the United States and Canada. *Am J Occup Ther*. 2006; 60(4):428–434.

48. Pennsylvania Department of Transportation. Physician reporting fact sheet, October, 2005. Available at: https://www.dotdev3.state.pa.us/pdotforms/fact_sheets/fs-pub7212.pdf. Accessed May 6, 2007.

49. Salinsky MC, Wegener K, Sinnema F. Epilepsy, driving laws, and patient disclosure to physicians. *Epilepsia* 1992; 33(3):469–472.

50. Canadian Medical Association. *Determining Medical Fitness to Operate Motor Vehicles: CMA Driver's Guide*. 7th ed. Ottawa, Ont: Canadian Medical Association, 2006; 65.

51. Marshall SC, Spasoff R, Nair R, van Walraven G. Restricted driver licensing for medical impairments: Does it work? *CMAJ*. 2002; 167(7):747–751.

52. Finestone HM, Rozenberg D, Moussa R, et al. Differences between post stroke drivers and non-drivers; medical factors, social attributes and driving consequences [poster]. Canadian Association of Physical Medicine & Rehabilitation Annual Meeting, Vancouver, June 7–10, 2006.

53. *British Columbia (Superintendent of Motor Vehicles) v. British Columbia (Council of Human Rights)*, [1999] 3 S.C.R. 868.

54. Mazer BL, Sofer S, Korner-Bitensky N, et al. Effectiveness of a visual attention retraining program on the driving performance of clients with stroke. *Arch Phys Med Rehabil*. 2003; 84:541–550.

44 Sports and Recreation

David Martin Crandell

There is more to life than putting on your pants.

Mary Vining Radomski (1)

Sports and recreation can play an important general role in stroke recovery and rehabilitation. The World Health Organization (WHO) defines recreation and leisure as engaging in programs of physical fitness, organized play, and sports (2). The WHO further defines sports as engaging in games or athletic events, performed individually or in a group. Sports need not be formally organized or competitive in nature to be enjoyed. Sports participation can also be rooted in the context of specific rehabilitation goals of increased flexibility, strength, endurance, balance, and coordination. With the recent adoption of the Convention on the Rights of Persons with a Disability, the United Nations has acknowledged sport, among other areas, as a human right for persons with a disability (3). This includes the encouragement and promotion of participation, to the fullest extent possible, of persons with disabilities into sporting activities.

Sport is a fundamental part of the lives of many people around the world and has significant benefits for persons with a disability.

Linda Mastrandrea (4)

Participation in sport improves physical and mental health outcomes (5, 6). Following enrollment in an individualized recreation program, disabled college students had the opportunity to participate in swimming, horseback riding, racquetball, fitness, bowling, tennis, Tai Chi, walking, fitness, and/or weightlifting. Participants engaged in the activity for 5–24 weeks and later reported their perceptions of their social self were expanded by their experiences and they initiated more social activities. Participants indicated that the program got them out of the house, gave them opportunities to meet new people, and offered opportunities for increased interaction with persons without disability. Greater control over social life was also noted as a social outcome of participation in this recreation program.

Social participation is positively associated with improving quality of life (QOL) after stroke (7–9). The participation in interpersonal relationships, responsibilities, fitness, and recreation are directly related to QOL (8). The failure of stroke survivors to resume pre-stroke leisure activities can interfere with post-stroke functioning (7). Bhogal et al. found that, when there was a reduction in social and leisure activities, both in and outside the home, there was increased depression, ineffective coping, and difficulties in social integration (7). This deterioration was more common in younger stroke survivors. Labe et al. (9) noticed that, even if stroke survivors regained their physical independence, they didn't return to their typical social activities. Stroke survivors who stayed at home became more isolated, lonely, and depressed. Kwok et al. (10) found that depression had a more generalized adverse effect on QOL than basic functional disabilities, but group exercises could promote socialization and community reintegration and thus lessen the negative effects of depression.

Therapeutic exercise is a mainstay to stroke rehabilitation efforts to improve physical function as well as increase flexibility, range of motion, muscle tone and strength, and coordination. Regular exercise can also help establish and maintain restorative sleep, maintain bone density, improve weight control, and help prevent secondary disabling conditions (11). A decline in aerobic fitness resulting from physical inactivity of stroke survivors may further increase the risk of cardiovascular disease in these individuals above than associated with stroke itself (12). Mackay-Lyons et al. (13) showed that the cardiovascular stress of a contemporary stroke rehabilitation program is much too low to induce a positive aerobic training effect. The safety and feasibility of a more vigorous exercise in stroke survivors is a concern, but the risks do not seem to be prohibitive (14–16). Duncan et al. (16) reported no major adverse events, that is, no deaths or cardiac events, during aerobic exercise sessions with stroke survivors. There were three recurrent strokes, with two occurring within the first two weeks of randomization and one after seven weeks, but no strokes occurred during an exercise treatment session. A meta-analysis of aerobic exercise training in individuals with stroke found very few adverse events, and the researchers concluded that it was unlikely that exercise training itself contributes to recurrent strokes (12). At this time, there is evidence to support the use of aerobic exercise to improve the aerobic capacity in stroke survivors, and the results seem generalizable to those who are mildly and moderately impaired, with low risk of cardiac complications with exercise.

A key feature of stroke rehabilitation research is the finding that earlier and more aggressive therapy may be better. Starting therapy soon after a stroke and initiating higher-order or more challenging activities earlier may lead to improved outcomes, even with lower-level functioning patients (17, 18). Horn et al. (19) reported results that indicate a strong and consistent association of rehabilitation activities that challenge patients and stress them well beyond their current level with better outcomes. An example would be moving quickly to practicing upper extremity functional activities rather than focusing on trunk strengthening. Their theory is that the trunk will strengthen secondarily out of necessity. They concluded that there would be positive benefits for patients who forge ahead into activities that might seem excessively challenging for them according to common clinical practice. So, beyond the pure sense of enjoyment, sports and recreation for stroke survivors should be viewed as an

increasingly important component of a comprehensive stroke rehabilitation program with the goals to improve QOL and recovery (20).

HISTORY

Through sports, every individual, with or without a disability, has the opportunity and ability to reach his or her potential. Sports can be a powerful tool to accentuate the ability and not the impairment or functional loss caused by stroke or other disabling conditions. The origins of the sports and recreation for the disabled can be traced to informal games at veterans' hospitals in the United States in the early 1940s. By playing wheelchair basketball in the gymnasium, veterans with spinal cord injuries rediscovered the joy of sports participation after injury. By the late 1940s, intra-hospital games led to eventual state and national competitions. During this period in England, Sir Ludwig Guttman, a neurosurgeon working on the spinal injuries unit at Stoke Mandeville Hospital, introduced sport and recreation as part of the standard rehabilitation program for the patients. Dr. Guttmann believed that

> [B]y restoring activity of mind and body, by instilling self-respect, self-discipline, a competitive spirit and comradeship, sport develops mental attitudes that are essential for social reintegration (21).

Even with these early successes, physicians were slow to express support for sports for the disabled, and some, including Dr. Guttmann himself, had concerns about patients with spinal cord injuries overexerting themselves. Despite these concerns, recreational and competitive sports continued to develop with additional disability groups beginning to participate at national and international events. In Toronto in 1976, amputee and blind athletes competed in the Summer Paralympic Games. In 1980, athletes with cerebral palsy competed with the other disabled groups in Arnhem, The Netherlands. This competition included athletes with stroke and brain injury for the first time.

Recognizing the growth of opportunities for individuals with cerebral palsy, traumatic brain injuries, and stroke, the National Association of Sports for Cerebral Palsy (NASCP) was formed in 1978 in the United States to meet the challenges of providing increased competitive experiences. In 1987, the NASCP became the United States Cerebral Palsy Athletic Association (USCPAA) and continued providing sports training and competition opportunities for its members. In 2001, the association changed its name again to the National Disability Sports Alliance (NDSA) (22). The new name reflected the growing number of sports with annual national championships offered in boccia, bowling, cross-country, cycling, equestrian, power lifting, soccer, swimming, track and field, and wheelchair team handball. Ambulatory basketball and sailing are in the planning stages for introduction.

In addition to national championships, the NDSA sanctions local and regional events annually throughout the United States. Athletes reside in over 40 states, and the membership exceeds 4,000. All athletes are classified on a medically approved system based on functional abilities, assuring equitable competition. There are four classes for wheelchair users and four classes for ambulatory individuals. Through training and competition, the athletes promote the NDSA motto: "Sports by ability . . . not disability" (22).

Over 60 years ago, Dr. Guttmann introduced sport and recreation as a tool in the spinal cord injury rehabilitation process. Recently, sport and training have been introduced into recommended guidelines of stroke rehabilitation (20). Merholz et al. (18) found that even jumping exercises are feasible for selected subacute stroke patients with hemiparesis. They recommended that further investigations should examine whether the introduction and combination of sport principles in rehabilitation programs could translate into quicker or better recovery of patients after stroke. Drawing on the principle of task-specific training, sports could be a new and engaging tool for post-stroke rehabilitation.

> Participation in disability sports rebuilds lives. When your life has been turned upside down by a disability, you need successes and you need accomplishments and you need them immediately. Participating in sports rebuilds. It's both a rehab tool and a lifestyle tool available to everyone (23).
>
> Kirk Bauer

CASE HISTORIES

To understand sports and recreation as a rehabilitation tool for stroke survivors, it is important to appreciate the individual's own concept of sports and recreation before and subsequently after his or her stroke. I characterize two major pre-stroke categories as the "dids" and the "did nots." The "dids" are those individuals who participated actively in either recreational or competitive sports prior to their stroke. The "did nots" are those individuals who, like many sedentary adults, did not participate actively in any sports or recreation program. It is useful to examine the stroke survivor's sports and recreation mind-set.

Case One

The first example is that of a 37-year-old engineer who had a cardioembolic stroke as a consequence of aortic valve replacement surgery. Sequelae included a mild left-sided hemiparesis and some mild visuospatial neglect.

Prior to his stroke, he was physically active, working in construction and playing regularly in an adult hockey program. He played college hockey at a competitive Division I program and was now the coach of his young son's hockey team. One of his rehabilitation goals was to return to skating and be able to continue to coach his son's team. He did well in acute rehabilitation, went home, and attended outpatient therapy. During his initial follow-up appointment, he reported that he was happy to be back at the hockey rink and able to coach his young son. During his next follow-up, he reported that he was back skating with his son. He continued to do well and, after several months, was back playing hockey himself. His comment was that he had "lost a step" and had some difficulty up against the boards, but was able to play competitively and safely as well as have fun. He reported that had always been better than his younger brother at hockey and the situation was now reversed. He stated that his new goal was to continue to improve and "get back" and be able to beat his brother. I felt that this was a healthy drive to compete that he didn't lose because of the stroke. This motivated him to push his rehabilitation efforts further.

Case Two

A 34-year-old psychologist had a brain stem hemorrhage stroke caused by an arteriovenous malformation at 38 weeks of her first pregnancy. She remained hospitalized and delivered her child via a C-section. She and her new son did well. She had mild residual left-sided weakness, intermittent double vision, and hemisensory deficit on the right side of her face.

Six months after her stroke, she expressed frustration with her ongoing standard outpatient PT and OT therapy program, especially with the rate and level of her functional recovery. Prior to her stroke, she was an accomplished athlete, competing at a Division I university as a singles tennis player. She was also the age-class winner in the previous years' triathlon in her region. Even well into her pregnancy, she was running and biking up to 30 miles per week. During her rehabilitation program, she had developed left patellar tendonitis and exacerbated back and shoulder problems from prior sports injuries.

During her outpatient follow-up, her rehabilitation program was refocused on her goals of wanting to be walk at typical speeds without asymmetry and be able to run again. She was referred to a local sports therapy program that was experienced in working with elite athletes and utilized aquatic therapy. It was a good fit for her because of the match between the treatment approach and her identification as an athlete, not as a stroke survivor. She was used to pushing herself, and her therapist was able to raise the effort to a level and intensity that she could relate to. She was not willing to settle for any goals that did not include running again.

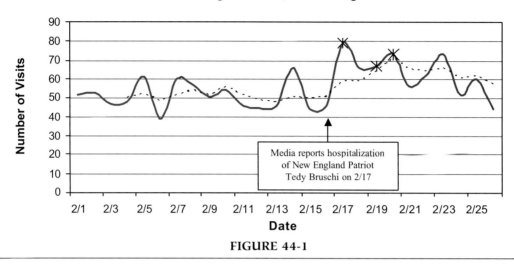

FIGURE 44-1

"Bruschi Effect." Reprinted with permission from Boston Public Health Commission.

These two examples of "dids" show the importance of sport in their lives, which did not change with their stroke. Setting the sport-specific goals became no different than establishing other short-term goals. I was convinced that returning to sports helped them reach the highest functional level possible, continuing to be a positive driving force in their rehabilitation.

Case Three

"You want me to go windsurfing?" This was the reaction of a 64-year old male patient who had had a hypertensive stroke, when he was asked to participate in the adaptive sports program where he was receiving inpatient acute rehabilitation. Despite his initial reluctance, he was medically cleared and did go down the waterfront dock adjacent to the hospital. He successfully sailed with the sports staff. This had a positive effect on his performance in the other non-sports-related therapy and had a big impact on his family. If he could windsurf after his stroke, both he and his family came to realize that he would be able to overcome many of the hurdles that remained as sequelae of his stroke.

He and the other "did nots" need to clearly understand the general benefits of sports participation for their recovery, and this education and opportunity should be expanded. Sports and recreation could help the advance the resumption of social, leisure, and productive activities that make life worth living (6).

QUALITY OF LIFE

Participation in sport represents the desire of individuals to have typical athletic experiences and to reach their optimum level of physical fitness, skill, enjoyment, and satisfaction. The goal of comprehensive rehabilitation for stroke survivors is the attainment of an optimal level of independent living and QOL. Combining the two components into a game plan can promote healthy lifestyles and reduce the effects of impairment and disability through sports and recreation.

Leisure satisfaction has been found to correlate highly with overall life satisfaction (24). Participation in physical activity and sport is an important key to familiar and many new experiences. Stroke survivors need to believe and experience that. Even after life-changing events, they can pursue and enjoy recreational activities.

The need for recreational experience has been incorporated into the post-stroke rehabilitation planning and treatment for stroke survivors in various settings. One example is the partnership of Spaulding Rehabilitation Hospital and AccessSportAmerica, which has created an innovative and exciting therapeutic sports and recreation program. Spaulding's Adaptive Sports and Recreation Program has taken advantage of its location on the banks of the Charles River in Boston to offer a variety of water- and land-based sports and recreational activities. Participants represent a wide spectrum of rehabilitation diagnoses and include both inpatient and outpatient stroke survivors.

The program staff includes members of the therapeutic recreation, physical therapy, and occupational therapy departments and is coordinated by outpatient services at the hospital. Recruitment is done internally on all the inpatient programs by team members and marketed to the outpatients attending therapy at the network of Spaulding facilities and to the community. Seasonal sporting activities currently include windsurfing, outrigger canoeing, kayaking, rowing, paddle boating, biking, wall climbing, weight

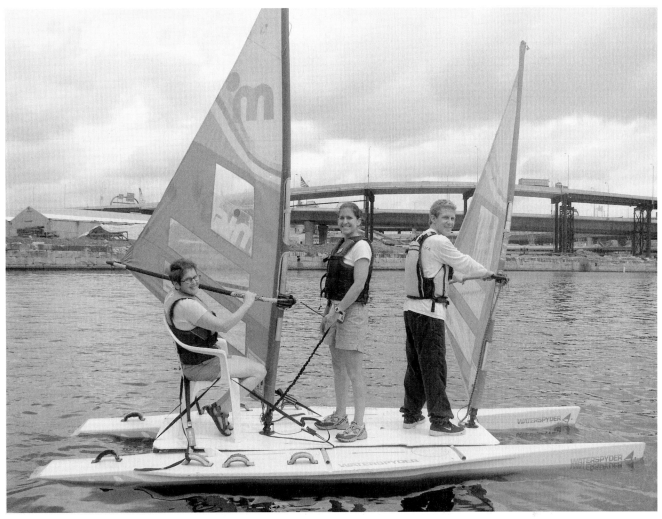

FIGURE 44-2

Adapted windsurfing.

training, and skiing. The staff has developed specially modified equipment that will allow stroke survivors with hemiparesis to row and windsurf (Figures 44-2 and 44-3).

Do sports and recreation improve the quality of life in stroke survivors? Some early research is being completed to show that it does. A pilot study on the impact of adaptive sports participation has been initiated, which included a participant survey (25). Questions of the participants included:

- Did the sport activity affect your emotional/mental outlook?
- What aspects of your emotional/mental outlook do you feel the sports helped?

76% of respondents said that the program helped significantly with increasing confidence, motivation, mood, and mental outlook. Stroke survivors need to believe and demonstrate for themselves that they can move beyond their physical limitations and participate in sports and recreation. For both the "dids" and "did nots," being an "I do" is an important part of stroke recovery, increasing their use of leisure time, enjoyment and pleasure, confidence, sense of achievement, as well as community access and social integration.

SPORT STRATEGY FOR STROKE RECOVERY

"Training is new brain." Recent studies on stroke recovery point to task repetition as a way to enhance recovery and for long-term maintenance of function (26). Utilizing this concept:

- Could sports and recreation be used as a strategy for stroke recovery?

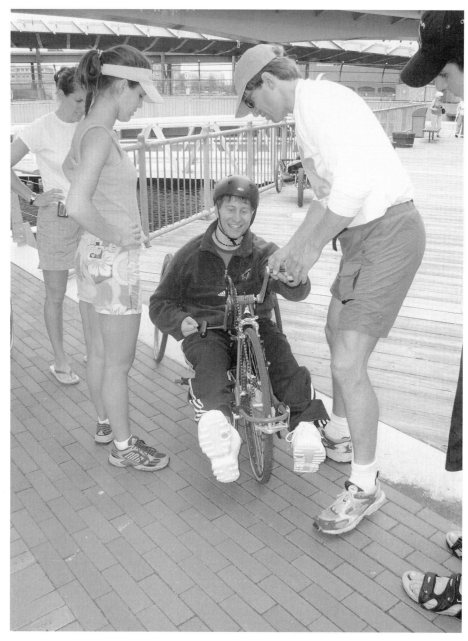

FIGURE 44-3

Adapted cycling.

- Could progress with task-specific training incorporating intensive practice of real-world activities improve motor control?
- Could the steps for motor learning after stroke including repetitive practice under varying conditions?
- Are tasks that are motivating and fun more apt to be repeated?

I believe that all of these concepts will be found to play a role with future research. Strategies for motor learning after stroke include progressively training components of goal-oriented, skilled movement tasks (27). Reinforcing the sensorimotor components of movement can provide kinematic, force, acceleration, directional, and temporal feedback for the patient's sensorimotor network. This repetition translates into "Practice, practice, practice." Forms of practice characterize all rehabilitation efforts to regain motor control, and sports experience and training may induce physiological plasticity. The more skilled the movement, the stronger the connections. Challenging posture and movement, using appropriate sensory inputs, along with specificity of the task, can represent a sports and recreation model of stroke recovery (28).

Yang et al. (29) reported in a single-blind, randomized, controlled trial that task-oriented, progressive resistance strength training programs improved lower extremity strength and resulted in reduction in functional limitations. This research shows the link between increases in muscle strength and improved functional performance. They theorized that the physiological mechanisms underlying their results related to improved motor unit recruitment and motor learning. The development of neuromotor patterns of coordination between agonist and antagonist muscles through the practice of a skill may be a lasting effect.

FUTURE IMPLICATIONS

On February 18, 2005, public health officials in Boston, Massachusetts, reported a significant increase in neurologic and stroke-like complaints in emergency departments around the city. An unusually large number of young men came in complaining of nontrauma related headache, blurred vision, and one-sided weakness (30). There was a 78% increase in stroke visits citywide, with no significant increase in any particular hospital. The greatest increase (59%) in these visits was found among young men ages 20–49. There was no geographical clustering and no known toxicological or unusual illness. They termed this phenomenon as the Bruschi Effect (Figure 44-3) after media coverage of New England Patriots professional football player Tedy Bruschi had suffered a mild stroke and was hospitalized at the Massachusetts General Hospital. Even though there was a significant increase in complaints, public health officials did not detect any corresponding increase in actual strokes in the city. "When there is heightened media coverage of a particular illness—in this case, stroke—it is not unusual for the public to react," said Dr. John Rich,

medical director of the Boston Public Health Department. A compensatory decrease in visit numbers was observed the following week.

Tedy Bruschi, age 31, a Pro Bowl defensive linebacker and nine-year veteran, was at the top of his game in the Patriots' 2005 Super Bowl victory, including a fourth-quarter interception. It was just 10 days later that he was taken urgently via ambulance to the hospital after complaining of left arm and leg numbness, blurred vision, and headache. He had a small right-sided stroke, and an echocardiogram revealed a patent foramen ovale (PFO). He did well with his rehabilitation and subsequently had his PFO closed. After only eight months, Bruschi returned to playing football professionally after being cleared medically.

His return to play has resulted in a secondary and more lasting Bruschi Effect, one in which there continues to be an overwhelming emotional response to his unprecedented comeback. Bruschi received thousands of letters from stroke survivors, letting him know he was an inspiration to them.

> I don't think America knows very much about strokes, that you can get back to your life after you have a stroke. There can be a full recovery. If your normal life after a stroke is just getting back to work, maybe your normal life is playing professional football. That was my normal life. That's what I wanted to get back to. I was fortunate enough that I was able to rehabilitate myself 100% and get back to playing football again (31).

For Bruschi, returning to playing football was "living his life his way." He has used his experience to raise awareness about stroke through the American Heart Association and his ongoing association with Spaulding Rehabilitation Hospital. He has been a popular and successful spokesman both on and off the field and has inspired many stroke survivors to return to sports and recreation of their choice.

References

1. Radomski MV. There is more to life than putting on your pants. *Am J Occup Ther* 1995; 49(6):487–490.
2. World Health Organization. International classification of functioning, disability, and health. Geneva:WHO, 2001.
3. www.un.org/esa/socdev/enable/rights/convtexte.htm. UN Convention of the Rights of Persons with Disabilities. Dec 13, 2006, adopted March 30, 2007.
4. www.paralympic.org/release/Main_Sections_Menu/News/Current_Affairs/2007_04_02_a.html. Record numbers of countries recognize right to sport.
5. Blauwet, C. Promoting the health and human rights of individuals with a disability through the paralympic movement. In: Higgs C, Vanlandewijck Y, eds. *Sport for Persons with a Disability*. ICSSPE, 2007, 21–34.
6. Blinde E, McClung L. Enhancing the physical and social self through recreational activity: Accounts of individuals with physical disabilities. *Adapted Physical Activity Quarterly*, 1997; 14,327–344.
7. Bhogal SK, Teasell RW, Foley NC, Speechley MR. Community reintegration after stroke. *Top Stroke Rehabil* 2003; 10(2):107–129.
8. Levasseur M, Desrosiers J, Noreau L. Is social participation associated with quality of life in older adults with physical disabilities? *Disability and Rehabil* 2004;20:1206–1213.
9. Labi ML, Phillips TF, Gresham GE. Psychosocial disability in physically resored long-term stroke survivors. *Arch Phys Med Rehabil* 1980; 61:561–565.
10. Kwok T, Lo RS, Wong E, et al. Quality of life of stroke survivors: a one-year follow-up study. *Arch Phys Med Rehabil* 2006; 87(9):1177–1182.
11. Rimmer JH, Braddock D. Health promotion for people with physical, cognitive and sensory disabilities: An emerging national priority. *Am J Health Promot* 2002; 16:220–224.
12. Pang MYC, Eng JJ, Dawson AS, Gylfadottir S. The use of aerobic exercise training in improving aerobic capacity in individuals with stroke: A meta-analysis. *Clin Rehabil* 2006; 20:97–111.
13. MacKay-Lyons MJ, Makrides L. Cardiovascular stress during a contemporary stroke rehabilitation program: Is intensity adequate to induce a training effect? *Arch Phys Med Rehabil* 2002; 83:1378–1383.
14. Eng JJ, Dawson AS, Chu KS. Submaximal exercise in persons with stroke: Test-retest reliability and concurrent validity with maximal oxygen consumption. *Arch Phys Med Rehabil* 2004; 85:113–118.
15. Pang MYC, Eng JJ, Dawson AS, et al. A community-based fitness and mobility exercise (FAME) program for older adults with chronic stroke: A randomized, controlled trial. *J Am Geriatr Soc* 2005; 53:167–174.

16. Duncan P, Studenski S, Richards L, et al. Randomized clinical trail of therapeutic exercise in subacute stroke. *Stroke* 2003; 34:2173–2180.

17. Katz-Leurer M, Sender I, Keren O. The influence of early cycling training on balance in stroke patients at the subacute stage. Results of a preliminary trial. *Clinical Rehabilitation* 2006; 20:398–405.

18. Merholz J, Rutte K, Pohl M. Jump training is feasible for near ambulatory patients after stroke. *Clin Rehabil* 2006; 20:406–412.

19. Horn SD, DeJong G, Smout RJ, et al. Stroke rehabilitation patients, practice and outcomes: is earlier more aggressive therapy better? *Arch Phys Med Rehabil* 2005; 86 (12 Suppl 2):S101–S114.

20. Gordon NF, Gulanick M, Costa F, et al. Physical activity and exercise recommendations for stroke survivors: An American Heart Association scientific statement from the Council on Clinical Cardiology, Subcommittee on Exercise, Cardiac Rehabilitation, and Prevention; the Council on Cardiovascular Nursing; the Council on Nutrition, Physical Activity and Metabolism; and the Stroke Council. *Stroke* 2004; 35:1230–1240.

21. Webborn ADJ. Fifty years of competitive sport for athletes with disabilities: 1948–1998. *Br J Sports Med* 1999; 33:138–139.

22. www.ndsaonline.org/history.htm

23. Joukowsky AAW, Rothstein L. *Raising the Bar. New Horizons in Disability Sports.* Umbrage Editions, 2002, 122.

24. Parker CJ, et al. The role of leisure in stroke rehabilitation. *Disabil and Rehab* 1997.

25. Mechan P. Impact of adaptive sports participation on quality and physical function. Unpublished data 2005.

26. Luft AR, Hanley DF. Stroke recovery: moving in an EXCTE-ing direction. Editorial. *JAMA* 2006; 296(17):2141–2142.

27. Dobkin BH. Strategies for stroke rehabilitation. *Lancet* 2004.

28. Barbeau H. Neurorehabilitation emerging concepts. *Neurorehabil Neural Repair* 2003.

29. Yang YR, Wang RY, Lin KH, et al. Task-oriented progressive resistive strength training improves muscle strength and functional performance in individuals with stroke. *Clin Rehabil* 2006; 20:860–870.

30. www.bphc.org/news/press_release_content.asp?id=278

31. www.usatoday.com/sports/football/nfl/patriots/2005-11-16-bruschi-return_x.htm

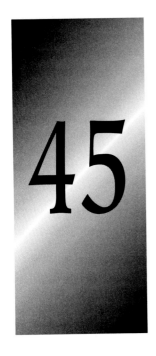

45 Sexuality after Stroke

Monika V. Shah

he importance of sexuality in the scope of human experience is profound. Sexuality is more than sexual intercourse alone. It includes a complex, multidimensional phenomenon that incorporates biologic, psychologic, interpersonal, and behavioral dimensions. The ability to form and sustain an intimate relationship is a fundamental aspect of human life. The impact of sexuality with quality of life after stroke and other neurologic diseases is even more powerful. Unfortunately, studies on quality of life in general and on sexual life specifically after stroke are relatively few. Although worldwide stroke prevalence constitutes the highest proportion of people with long-term disability, few epidemiological data are available on sexual functioning and sexual satisfaction after stroke.

The goal of this chapter on sexuality after stroke is to expose professionals in the field of stroke rehabilitation to the important complexities of sexuality and the impact of disease on sexual and psychosocial functioning as well as on issues of intimacy. Because there is a higher incidence of stroke in the elderly population, the effects of aging and medical comorbidities will also be reviewed. For the purpose of clinical practice, there is a discussion of general evaluation and management of sexuality in the post-stroke population.

PHYSIOLOGY OF SEXUAL FUNCTION

Our understanding of sexuality has its foundation in the work of Masters and Johnson published in 1966 (1). It is from their work that the sexual response cycle was categorized into four phases: excitement, orgasm, plateau, and resolution (Figure 45-1). This classification provided a means by which health care professionals could more clearly identify and treat sexual dysfunction. Later, in 1974, Kaplan simplified this into three phases: desire, excitement, and orgasm (Table 45-1) (2). Regardless of the model used, it became clearly understood that sexual function relies on a complex network of both central and peripheral neural pathways.

Sexuality involves the integration of sexual interest, physiological functioning, and sexual satisfaction (Figure 45-2). The cerebral cortex represents only one level of sexual functioning at which the brain influences human sexual arousal and response. Subcortical structures, including the limbic system and parts of the hypothalamus, also play an important role in the integration and control of reproductive and sexual functions. Sexual interest may arise from thoughts, emotions, and memories, which are all mediated through complex cerebral mechanisms. Thus, sexual arousal can occur without any sensory stimulation. Sexual satisfaction is achieved not

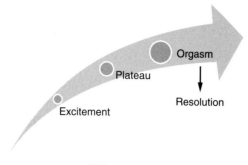

FIGURE 45-1

Classification of sexual functioning by Masters and Johnson (1966).

just by processes of physical arousal, but is also influenced by the feeling of intimacy as well as the health of one's own self-image. These additional aspects of psychological health can operate on both a conscious and subconscious level. By understanding the physiological, cognitive, and emotional aspects of sexuality, clinicians can better understand the impact of stroke-related disability on human sexuality.

Prevalence of Sexual Dysfunction

In the General Population. Sexual dysfunction is defined as any of a group of sexual disorders characterized by disturbance either of sexual desire or of the psychophysiological changes that usually characterize sexual response. Accurate estimates of prevalence are important in understanding the true burden of male and female sexual dysfunction as well as identifying risk factors for prevention efforts. Most studies of prevalence figures are quite variable as they depend on case definition, characteristics of the study population, and time frame of the prevalence estimates. The paucity of information led to a gathering of 200 multidisciplinary experts from 60 countries, including members of major urology and sexual medicine associations, who attempted to provide accurate estimates of prevalence, epidemiology, and risk factors. This international consortium described a prevalence of about 40–45% of adult women and 20–30% of adult men having at least one manifest sexual dysfunction. There was a consensus that the incidence increases as men and women age. Common risk factor categories

TABLE 45-1
Three-Phase Sexual Response Cycle
(by Helen Kaplan)

1. Desire
2. Excitement
3. Orgasm

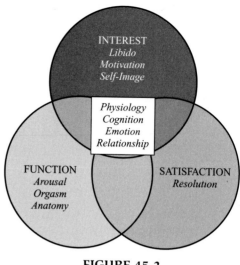

FIGURE 45-2

Concepts in sexuality and sexual functioning.

associated with sexual dysfunction include individual general health status, psychiatric and psychological disorders, and sociodemographic conditions (3). Most studies also confirm these rates of prevalence and find that, although many men and women experience sexual dysfunctions, few seek medical care to address them (4).

In the Stroke Population. Studies on the prevalence of sexual dysfunction after stroke are sparse compared with the general population. Most include a small sample size of subjects with a median age of 50 years. In general, the prevalence of sexual problems after stroke or any other neurologic disability is consistently higher than the general population with a range of 57–75% (5, 6). As the incidence of stroke itself now includes a much wider age group, it becomes even more important to include both extremes of age in studying prevalence, risk factors, and treatment of problems related to sexuality. Still, most studies focus on sexual interest and physiological aspects of sexual ability following stroke. There are few studies that address the psychosocial or intimacy issues among stroke patients and their partners.

Fortunately, some studies on sexuality after stroke do emphasize that psychological factors in addition to medical comorbidities and general health status are critical determinants of post-stroke sexual functioning. Monga and Korpelainen suggested in separate reviews that sexual problems following stroke are never a consequence of stroke alone. Rather, they may be caused by a variety of associated medical conditions and psychosocial factors (5, 6). It is general principle that sexual dysfunctions in hemiplegic individuals arise from difficulty coping with disability rather than from endocrine deficits or the side effects of antihypertensive therapy (7).

Classification of Sexual Dysfunction

As described earlier, Masters and Johnson classified their findings into a linear sexual response cycle of excitement, plateau, orgasm, and resolution (Figure 45-1). Men and women were described as having similar physiologic characteristics. More recent research suggests that women do not always fit into this model and that their sexual experience follows a more complex pattern that extends beyond having an orgasm or achieving adequate vaginal lubrication. Furthermore, studies indicate that persons with neurologic disability, such as stroke, also do not fit the linear male model whether they are female or male. Accordingly, the sexual experience in stroke survivors encompasses the impact of changes in self-esteem, body image, relationship and intimacy, pleasure, and satisfaction, in addition to the severity of disability, pain, weakness, spasticity, and many other physical variables.

Therefore, many approaches to the classification of sexual dysfunction have emerged since the time of Masters and Johnson. One modification of the Masters and Johnson model, described by Helen Kaplan Singer, is helpful in categorizing and assessing both physiological and psychological causes of sexual dysfunction (2). This model divides sexual response into three phases by combining

TABLE 45-2A
DSM-IV Female Classification of Sexual Dysfunction

1. Sexual Desire Disorder
   a. Hypoactive Sexual Desire Disorder
   b. Sexual Aversion Disorder
2. Sexual Arousal/Orgasmic Disorder
3. Sexual Pain Disorder
   a. Dysparunia
   b. Vaginismus
   c. Other Sexual Pain Disorders
4. Sexual Dysfunction Caused by General Medical Condition
5. Substance-induced Sexual Dysfunction
6. Sexual Dysfunction (not otherwise specified)

TABLE 45-2B
DSM-IV Male Classification of Sexual Dysfunction

1. Hypoactive Sexual Desire Disorder
2. Sexual Aversion Disorder
3. Erectile Dysfunction
4. Male Orgasmic Disorder
5. Premature Ejaculation

TABLE 45-3
American Foundation for Urologic Disease Classification for Female Sexual Dysfunction (Basson, 2000)

1. Hypoactive Sexual Desire Disorder
   a. Hypoactive Sexual Desire
   b. Sexual Aversion Disorder
2. Sexual Arousal Disorder
3. Sexual Orgasmic Disorder
4. Sexual Pain Disorders
   a. Dysparunia
   b. Vaginismus
   c. Other Sexual Pain Disorders

the excitement and plateau phase and then adding desire as the first stage of sexual response (Table 45-1). By adding desire as an initial response, Kaplan includes the role of subjective feeling, which involves interpersonal and psychological as well as biologic factors.

The most common classification system used by clinicians for the diagnosis and treatment of sexual dysfunction is the DSM-IV criteria, which is also adapted from older models previously described. Table 45-2 lists the classification system for both males and females. Because of the complexity of female sexual dysfunction, the American Foundation for Urologic Disease developed another system, a consensus-based classification (Table 45-3). Although these classification systems have been revised over time to include psychological causes in addition to the organic causes of sexual dysfunction, with a particular emphasis on problems in women, there remain other important limitations. For example, disease-specific issues that can affect sexuality and sexual functioning should be assessed during comprehensive evaluation, but they are not well-addressed by these classification systems.

Table 45-4 contains a new classification system to better identify, evaluate, and treat patients who have

TABLE 45-4
Proposed Classification of Sexual Dysfunction

1. Psychosocial
2. Physiological
   a. Endocrine Disorders
   b. Neuromuscular
3. Medical/Medications
4. Other
   a. Hypersexuality
   b. Age-related Changes

TABLE 45-5
Misconceptions about Sexuality

1. Sexual activity should always include intercourse.
2. All healthy couples have sexual intercourse several times per week.
3. Physical contact should always lead to sexual expression.
4. Sexual activity must be natural and spontaneous.
5. Failure to get an erection is an indication that a man in not in love.
6. Sexual activity has a fixed path that should end in a simultaneous orgasm.
7. If sex is not good, then something is wrong with the relationship.

Physiological Factors

The physiological aspects of sexual functioning not only include erection and ejaculation in men and vaginal lubrication and orgasm in women, but also adequate mobility in both partners. Achieving these goals requires a normal, functioning neuroendocrine system; however, only a minority of stroke patients has neuroendocrine changes following stroke. In contrast, neuromuscular changes that affect mobility are quite common and have a significant impact on sexual performance. These include fatigue, weakness, and spasticity. A detailed discussion on the neuroendocrine and neuromuscular changes after stroke that influence sexual function and performance follows.

Neuroendocrine Abnormalities. Any brain lesion, as occurs during stroke onset, can affect the neuroendocrine system and produce an imbalance of hormone production and release, leading to impotence and/or infertility. From a strictly physiological standpoint, normal sexual functioning involves the interaction of libido and potency. In males, erectile dysfunction is the most commonly cited complaint in able-bodied patients as well as those with disability. It is well-known that testosterone levels steadily decrease with advanced age; however, hormonal replacement has shown limited success in resolving erectile dysfunction. In females, low sexual desire and reduced coital frequency are most often reported. These symptoms tend to correlate with reduced estrogen levels. The female reproductive system and menstrual cycle are controlled by the interplay of hormones and endocrine organs. In general, other physiological changes may include decreased vaginal lubrication, anorgasmia or delayed orgasm, priapism, retarded or premature ejaculation, retrograde ejaculation, breast hyperplasia, gynecomastia, and others.

Location of Stroke. It is likely that the location of the stroke-related brain injury is related to sexual dysfunction.

A lesion located in deeper structures of the brain that regulate sexual function such as the pituitary gland or hypothalamus may result in disrupted neuroendocrine and hormonal functioning. Specifically, subarachnoid hemorrhage is commonly associated with neuroendocrine dysfunction (16). Disturbance of sexual functioning is related to severity of neurologic impairment, but no specific pattern has been detected. Early reports suggested that frontal strokes and strokes in the left hemisphere are more strongly associated with depression, which can impair sexuality, but other studies have disagreed. A systematic review by Carson and others in 2000 concluded there is no evidence for an association of left hemisphere or frontal lobe stroke with depression (17, 18).

Erectile Dysfunction (ED). Erectile dysfunction (ED) is the inability to achieve or maintain sufficient erection for satisfactory sexual functioning. ED is the most common cause of sexual dysfunction in the general male population (19). It is estimated that 50% of men over the age of 40 have experienced some degree of ED. It is likely that the incidence in male stroke survivors is even higher given the multifactorial nature of this problem. Atherosclerosis, an important risk factor for stroke, may cause reduction of blood flow that affects end organs, including genitalia. In males, this may reduce the success and effectiveness of erection. In females, there may similarly be a reduction in vulvar lubrication and engorgement. In addition, medications used to manage stroke risk factors and prevent secondary stroke may contribute further to ED. Fortunately, there are several oral medications that can be used to treat ED, that can often be used (Table 45-6), but these medications are not a panacea. It is important to identify any underlying psychological factors that may significantly contribute to ED. Table 45-7 includes alternative forms of treatment for ED.

Decreased Libido. Low sexual desire is the most prominent sexual finding in females with or without a disability. Disorders of tactile sensation and disturbed lubrication are found to have some relation to a decline in desire. Moreover, disability-related physical limitations as well as altered body image appear to be the most cited reasons for low sexual desire and reduced sexual

TABLE 45-6
Oral Medications in the Treatment of Erectile Dysfunction

1. Phosphodiesterase Inhibitors
2. Yohimbine
3. Alpha-2 Blockers
4. Trazadone
5. Topical Nitroglycerin

TABLE 45-7
Options in the Treatment of Erectile Dysfunction

---

1. Intracavernous injection therapy

2. Vacuum tumescence

3. Hormonal therapy
   a. Testosterone

4. Oral medications

5. Penile prosthesis

---

activity. Coexistent medical issues and medication side effects will also contribute to physiological changes similar to ED in men. Other reasons for low sexual drive include underlying psychological factors such as fear of rejection from a partner, anger in the relationship or other interpersonal conflicts, and passive-aggressive response to a power struggle. Treatment will depend on the underlying cause.

Fatigue. Fatigue is a common sequelae of stroke, impacting daily activities as well as psychological well-being. Fatigue can limit sexual activity and cause a reduction in libido in both men and women. As many as two-thirds of patients experience some level of post-stroke fatigue. The cause of fatigue after stroke is unclear and may be a result of multiple factors. The increase in energy output that patients with stroke require to complete usual daily activities such as transfers, walking, bathing, toileting, and dressing may cause fatigue. Fatigue may also be a consequence of altered sleep-wake cycles. Various medications that are used for secondary stroke prevention or to treat stroke-related symptoms may have sedative effects. Treatment of fatigue may include management of insomnia and the sleep-wake cycle, use of neurostimulant medications, change in medications, or change in timing of medication administration. Counseling on timing and flexibility with sexual activity is also an important strategy for managing the effects of fatigue.

Weakness. Of the various motor impairments following stroke, weakness is a constant finding (20). The pattern and severity of weakness after stroke need not prevent sexual activity if there is effective communication with partner. Alteration in usual sexual positioning will often compensate for weakness quite effectively and increase sexual satisfaction. In patients who do not have severe paralysis, there may still be some evidence of weakness in relation to post-stroke fatigue that can impact sexual performance and vary from day to day. It is important to include resistive training for both upper and lower limbs in a comprehensive rehabilitation

program, as it can produce significant strength gains for patients even after six months post-stroke. Training patients and their partners with illustrations of sex positions appropriate for patients with weakness and hemiplegia can be helpful.

Spasticity. Besides the challenges of mobility and positioning during sex, spasticity may prevent a couple from returning to sexual activity because of the unpredictability of dystonic movements and muscle spasm during sexual intercourse. Significant spasticity may preclude certain usual sexual positions when the patient assumes dystonic postures, so communication with the sexual partner is important. Discussion of sexual functioning should be included in comprehensive spasticity evaluation. In females, the presence of adductor spasms may require targeted treatment. Focal chemodenervation or motor point blocks of the hip adductors may be effective. The use of intrathecal baclofen has been studied in patients with spinal cord lesions from multiple sclerosis and spinal cord injury. Although intrathecal baclofen can reduce severe adductor spasticity, it may compromise both erection and ejaculation (21). This may be reversible, but patients should be informed of this side effect. Adjustment of the intrathecal baclofen dose may also help resolve these problems.

Post-Stroke Pain. Although stroke sequelae may often produce decreased sensation, there may be other areas of the body with heightened or even painful sensation. Areas of heightened sensation may be utilized for sexual arousal, so partners should be encouraged to experiment and recognize these areas. In the case of dysesthesia, proper diagnosis is necessary to differentiate central post-stroke pain, complex regional pain syndrome type 1, diabetic peripheral neuropathy, or other causes of tactile pain. Appropriate treatment can be provided if the correct diagnosis is made. Although rare after stroke, vaginismus and vulvodynia of muscular or noninflammatory origin can occur. Some studies suggest that botulinum toxin can be effective in treating these conditions by effectively blocking nociception (22, 23).

Neurogenic Bladder. Neurogenic bladder after stroke can include detrusor hyperreflexia, or, simply, incontinence from uninhibited bladder. This may serve as source of fear or embarrassment in those patients who wish to resume sexual activity. Avoidance of sexual activity is commonly reported in patients with urinary incontinence. Education on timed voiding and voiding before sex can minimize frequency of incontinence. For patients using a chronic indwelling catheter, it is important to provide information on its management during sexual intercourse (Table 45-8).

TABLE 45-8
Tips for Post-stroke Patients with Neurogenic Bladder

1. Empty bladder shortly before sexual activity.
2. Indwelling catheter may be temporarily removed and replaced under the direction of the physician.
3. In females, catheter may be taped to one side.
4. Reduce fluid intake four hours prior to sexual activity.
5. Plastic covering may be used on the bed to protect covering.
6. Cleaning supplies should be kept close to bedroom or bed.
7. Avoid positions that may put pressure on the bladder.

Chronic Medical Conditions and Medications

Chronic medical conditions that coexist with stroke can cause sexual difficulties either directly or indirectly. Specifically, mood disorders such as depression are commonly observed after a stroke, frequently affecting sexual relationships. Also, common risk factors for stroke, such as hypertension and diabetes, are important contributors to sexual dysfunction. For example, vascular disease associated with diabetes can impact arousal, and cardiovascular disease may inhibit intercourse because of dyspnea or fatigue. Secondary effects of stroke such as urinary incontinence may also cause sexual dysfunction or decrease sexual activity because of embarrassment and fear of having an accident. Medications used to treat many medical conditions are often associated with changes in sexual functioning. Unfortunately, the sexual side effects of chronic medical conditions and the medications used to treat them are often underreported and underdiagnosed. Therefore, it is important for the clinician to recognize and inquire about these effects and address any issues around sexuality for patients with stroke.

Post-Stroke Depression. The prevalence of major depression after stroke is reported to range from 25–40% within the first year (24, 25). Although underreported, it is well-known that sexual dysfunction is common among individuals with major depressive disorder (MDD) (26–28). In a study by Kennedy and colleagues, 40% of men and 50% of women with major depression reported decreased sexual interest and reduced arousal (29). Mood and sexual function have an interactive association such that anxiety or depression may adversely affect sexual function and sexual dysfunction may lead to depression.

The changes in mood may be related to the severity of neurologic deficit (9, 10), the dependence on partner for ADLs, fear of rejection, or performance failure. Together, these lead to a general loss of self-esteem. Although sexual dysfunction is not considered a direct symptom of MDD,

it may represent depression-related anhedonia. However, in contrast to patients with mild stroke, those with more severe physical impairments are at risk for developing emotional disorders and a consequent decrease of sexual intercourse and perceived sexual dysfunction. The treatment of post-stroke depression has been examined in several placebo-controlled, randomized clinical trials that show efficacy with drugs such as nortriptyline and citalopram (30–32). Studies also support early treatment with antidepressants can significantly increased the survival of both depressed and nondepressed patients (33). It is important to recognize that treatment of depression may improve sexual functioning, but use of antidepressant medication may also cause sexual dysfunction (34, 35). As an alternative, enhanced social support when possible may have a positive influence on post-stroke depression, improving the patient's esteem and sexual identity. With appropriate treatment, the progression of recovery following stroke can be altered, including improved recovery in ADLs and cognitive impairment.

Antidepressants. Selective serotonin reuptake inhibitors (SSRIs) are typically considered the medication of choice for the treatment of post-stroke depression. They are popular in part because of their good safety profile and relatively benign adverse effects, especially compared with the older tricyclic antidepressants and monoamine oxidase inhibitors (MAOIs). However, many of the antidepressant classes are not free of treatment-emergent adverse events. Specifically, one of the most prominent adverse effects seen with antidepressants is sexual dysfunction.

In particular, the SSRIs have been shown to cause sexual dysfunction in 30–70% of patients treated for depression (36). The clinical implication is that compliance rates of antidepressant therapy may decrease with the recognition of sexual side effects. Therefore, it is important for clinicians to monitor and recognize sexual side effects when starting empiric antidepressant therapy. Because the sexual response cycle is affected by both reproductive hormones as well as neurotransmitters, it is important to understand the effects of each of these on the sexual response cycle. Table 45-9 reviews the effects of major hormones and neurotransmitters.

Several strategies can be employed to manage antidepressant-induced sexual dysfunction. (Table 45-10). Although some patients develop a tolerance to antidepressant side effects over time, it is usually only a small number of patients. If tolerance does not occur, other strategies include reduction of dose, addition of agents that may counteract sexual side effects, direct treatment of sexual side effect, using drug holidays, or other techniques. Although antidotes such as yohimbine, amantadine, and buspirone have been suggested, they have not been shown to be effective in clinical trials. Some

TABLE 45-9
Effect of Hormones/Neurotransmitters on Sexual Response Cycle

HORMONE/ NEUROTRANSMITTER	DESIRE	AROUSAL	ORGASM
Estrogen	+	n/a	n/a
Progesterone	+	n/a	n/a
Testosterone	+	n/a	n/a
Norepinephrine	n/a	+	n/a
Dopamine	+	+	n/a
Serotonin	–	–	n/a
Prolactin	n/a	–	n/a
Oxytocin	n/a	n/a	+

practitioners continue to support the use of these agents as an option in their patients. There is significant data that shows some classes of antidepressants and certain specific agents have had success in treating depression without a severe impact on sexuality. Bupropion, mirtazapine, and nefazadone have been well-studied and have shown the

TABLE 45-10
Antidepressant Therapy: Recommendations to Reduce Sexual Dysfunction

1. Reduce dose.
   a. It may be possible to reduce dose to minimize sexual side effects while still maintaining therapeutic efficacy.
2. Schedule dose after sexual activity.
   a. The drug concentration may be at its lowest if the dose is scheduled after usual time for engaging in sexual activity.
3. Treat sexual dysfunction.
   a. There are pharmacological and nonpharmacological methods that may be useful in the case of erectile dysfunction.
4. Augment with a drug that may reduce dysfunction.
   a. Some studies suggest that there are medications that may counteract sexual dysfunction, such as dextroamphetamine, amantadine, buspirone, and so forth. These may be taken prior to sexual activity.
5. Change to another antidepressant.
   a. Certain antidepressants, such as nefazadone and bupropion, have been shown to have less effect on sexual functioning.
6. Take a drug holiday.
   a. It may be appropriate to provide a weaning schedule depending on the agent and length of treatment.

least risk of inducing sexual dysfunction (37–39). Studies have also shown lower rates of sexual dysfunction with venlafaxine, a serotonin-norepinephrine reuptake inhibitor (SNRI), compared with SSRIs (35).

Diabetes. Diabetes is a multisystem disorder that includes a high prevalence of sexual dysfunction in both men and women. Studies by Kolondy in the 1970s and McCullogh in the 1980s describe the natural history and prevalence rates of sexual dysfunction as it relates to diabetes (40, 41). Reports of dysfunction in diabetic men range from 27–75% (42–44). ED, ejaculatory dysfunction, and sometimes decreased libido are commonly cited in men with history of diabetes. It is typically the combination of neuropathy and vasculopathy rather than hormonal changes that cause impotence and dysfunction in diabetic men.

Treatment of diabetes-related sexual dysfunction is similar to treatment of ED in general (Table 45-7). Currently, there are not any prophylactic measures available to prevent diabetic ED. Tight control of blood sugar should be the initial treatment, followed by treatment of malnutrition and general physical condition. Hormonal therapy can be considered in addition to the use of medication for ED. A referral to a urologist can be made to consider intracavernous injection therapy, vacuum therapy, or penile prosthesis.

Studies of sexual dysfunction in diabetic women are limited, but have consistently reported decreased orgasmic response (45, 46). Other symptoms reported include decreased libido, reduced vaginal lubrication, dysparunia, and vaginal infections. The pathogenesis of diabetic sexual dysfunction in women is complex and multifactorial, as is its evaluation and treatment. The cornerstone of treatment begins with education of the woman and partner that decreased sexual desire and responsiveness may be caused by the diabetes and challenges in the partner's relationship. As in men, nutritional and medical status should be optimized, including a thorough review of medication use. Counseling may be appropriate if no other reversible cause is found.

Coronary Artery Disease (CAD). It is now well-documented that several of the risk factors for coronary artery disease (CAD) are risk factors for ED. These may include hypertension, diabetes, dyslipidemia, and smoking. The incidence of ED has been reported to be as high as two-thirds of patients with myocardial infarction. Recent studies suggest that ED is an early symptom of cardiovascular disease and may precede CAD by two to three years in a majority of patients. Both of these conditions, ED and CAD, have shared risk factors that contribute to endothelial dysfunction and impede the ability of the arteries to appropriately dilate in response to stimuli (47).

The Princeton Consensus Conference developed guidelines for the safe management of cardiac patients with varying degrees of coronary risk regarding sexual activity and the treatment of ED. It reports that the phosphodiesterase 5 (PDE5) inhibitors are effective in treating ED in patients with CAD. Low-risk patients can usually receive PDE5 inhibitors without additional cardiac workup. In high-risk, unstable cardiac patients, the workup for sexual dysfunction should be deferred until the cardiac problem has been corrected or stabilized. Generally, this class of medication is considered safe in patients with stable CAD and does not pose any additional risk for ischemia. On the other hand, the use of nitrate medications or alpha blockers in combination with PDE5 inhibitors is contraindicated. The American College of Cardiology/American Heart Association consensus position on medications such as sildenafil is that it is safe for patients with stable CAD who are not taking nitrates (48).

Antihypertensives. Hypertension is the major independent risk factor for stroke, so it should be treated aggressively to provide adequate blood pressure control. Unfortunately, sexual dysfunction has been associated with many of the antihypertensive medications (Table 45-11) (49, 50). It is important to understand the sexual side effect profile of various classes of antihypertensives as this will not only affect compliance, but also a patient's quality of life.

Many studies have reported ED in male subjects related to treatment with antihypertensive medications. Certain medication classes tend to show a higher prevalence of sexual dysfunction than others. In general, diuretics and beta blockers have the most negative effects on sexual performance. Beta blockers, such as propanolol, with high lipophilicity and nonselective beta

blockade are associated with ED. Thiazide diuretics are essentially devoid of central or autonomic nervous system activity, yet they are associated with ED, possibly because of fluid and zinc depletion (51), even though the definitive pathogenetic role of zinc in ED remains unclear. Spironolactone can cause ED as well as gynecomastia and a decrease in libido. As an alternative to these medications, ACE inhibitors and angiotensin II antagonists have minimal sexual side effects and are often better tolerated by patients. In fact, some studies report a positive impact on sexuality and quality of life with the use of medications such as losartan, an angiotensin II antagonist. There are several reports suggesting that drugs that inhibit the renin-angiotensin system exert favorable actions on erectile function (52–56). It is important for practitioners to communicate openly with patients and work with them closely to minimize the sexual side effects of antihypertensive agents while maintaining antihypertensive efficacy.

Seizures. Seizures are a common complication after stroke, with a reported incidence up to 10% (57–59). Some patients who experience a first seizure go on to develop epilepsy, especially those with late-onset seizures that occur beyond two weeks following stroke onset. The relationship of seizures and sexuality may be significant because sexual disorders occur in up to two-thirds of epilepsy patients. In general, patients with epilepsy have hyposexuality. In males, there may be decreased sexual desire or ED. Epileptic men have a 57% increased risk of ED versus 3–9% in the general population (60–62). In females, epilepsy is associated with menstrual irregularities or reproductive dysfunction. Estrogens lower seizure threshold so that seizure frequency may increase during menses or pregnancy.

TABLE 45-11
Sexual Side Effects Associated with Antihypertensive Classes (45, 46)

ANTIHYPERTENSIVE CLASS	ERECTILE DYSFUNCTION	DECREASED LIBIDO	IMPAIRED EJACULATION	PRIAPISM	GYNECOMASTIA
Beta blockers	+	–	–	–	+
Diuretics					
Spironolactone	+	+	–	–	+
Thiazides	+	+	+	–	–
Antiadrenergics					
Central	+	+	+	–	–
Peripheral	+	–	+	+	+
Calcium channel blockers	–	–	+	–	+
ACE inhibitors	–	–	–	–	–
Angiotensin II blockers	–	–	–	–	–
Vasodialtors	+	–	–	+	–

Sexual disorders are distinguished by a temporal relationship with seizure activity. There are two categories:

- Those directly related to the epileptic discharge period (ictal).
- Those unrelated in time to seizure occurrence (interictal).

Hyposexuality has been linked to interictal seizure activity, whereas hypersexuality has been reported in the setting of ictal seizure activity (63–65). Monga et al. described three case reports of patients who demonstrated a hypersexuality and deviant sexual behavior after stroke (66). In all three cases, there were temporal lobe lesions noted on cranial computed tomography, and all had a history of post-stroke seizure activity.

The association between sexuality and chronic anticonvulsant use is well-established. Antiseizure medications, such as phenytoin and carbamazepine, are commonly associated with sexual dysfunction. In males, they can decrease the testosterone level, which, in turn, reduces sexual desire. Antiepileptic drugs alter the serum concentrations of sex hormones and the regulatory feedback loop of the hypothalamic-pituitary-gonadal axis. Rattya et al. examined the effects of carbamazepine, oxcarbemazepine, and valproate in epileptic men and suggested that oxcarbemazepine may be the best choice of anticonvulsant in epileptic patients suffering from hyposexuality (67).

Cognitive Impairments.   Cognitive changes after stroke can cause memory problems and difficulty expressing emotions, which may influence intimacy and sexual activity. Cognitive deterioration relating to dementing disorders can include disinhibition, agitation, or depressed mood, which can cause interpersonal difficulties and have a negative impact on the couple's sexual relationship (68). Couples can manage these problems by reducing external distractions during intimacy and using verbal and nonverbal communication for sexual expression. In addition, optimizing sleep-wake cycles may minimize the cognitive impairments in patients with stroke.

Aging and Sexual Dysfunction

There is a notable sharp decline in sexual activity from 50% of couples aged 60–65 to 20% in those aged 78–83 (69). For those who care for patients with stroke, it is important to understand the normal age-related changes that impact sexual functioning in the elderly. Proper understanding of sexuality and aging can also minimize the myths and misconceptions that many clinicians have about sexuality in the elderly. This section will discuss the physiological and psychological changes commonly seen in the older adult and older stroke survivors.

Physiological Changes in Elderly.   In the aging males, the most common changes in sexual physiology include both erectile function and ejaculation. Stein et al. reported that 40% of men aged 70–79 and 60% of men over 80 experience ED (70). For example, men tend to show increased time required to produce a full erection, an increase in the time that erections can be maintained prior to ejaculation, a decrease in the force of ejaculation, and an increase in the duration of the refractory phase (68). The high prevalence of diabetes, CAD, hypertension, and depression also contribute to these changes in sexual functioning.

In older women, the physiological effects of aging on sexual function are primarily caused by decreased amounts of circulating estrogen after menopause. Lower estrogen levels not only contribute to a decline in sexual interest and coital frequency, but also reduce vaginal lubrication resulting in painful intercourse and less pleasurable sex. However, other studies have suggested that many women experience an intensification of sexual desire during menopause. In these cases, the negative effects of menopause are more than offset by the freedom to explore and enjoy sexual activity without the worry of becoming pregnant (71).

Psychological Attitudes in the Elderly.   In our modern culture, there is often still an expectation that older people are, or ought to be, asexual (71). Although sex roles have changed and there has been more freedom of sexual expression since the 1960s, the stereotypes that older people are physically unattractive, uninterested in sex, and incapable of achieving sexual arousal are still widely held (72).

Modern Western society has generally viewed sexuality in older adults in a very restrictive manner. Studies of nursing staff in extended care facilities have identified significant staff discomfort about sexual expression among the elderly residents. Older residents who display any form of sexual expression are often regarded by staff as having a behavioral problem and may even be tranquilized (73). Staff attitudes toward masturbation or sexual activity between unmarried residents are often disapproving and repressive, and adult children may complain of permissive institutional attitudes toward their parents' sexual expression (74, 75).

It is still quite common for society to consider sexual expression or activity to be unnatural or unacceptable in the aging population. Clearly, educational intervention is needed to dispel negative myths, stereotypes, and self-fulfilling attitudes in older people and to promote the perception that full sexual expression is part of the entire extent of adulthood.

Opportunity for Elderly.   Opportunities for sexual contact are greatly reduced in those with advanced age. Gender differences in life expectancy may impact the sexual experiences in older adults. For example, demographic data indicate that there are many more women than men over the age of 65. If marital status or living with a partner is a measure of increased opportunity structures for sex, elderly heterosexual women have a limited opportunity for sexual expression. In contrast, decline in sexual activity for men is less likely to be due to the lack of a partner (71). A physiological change, such as ED, is likely the reason for reduced sexual activity in men. The lack of privacy in nursing homes is a major obstacle to sexual expression. Not surprisingly, older residents report that, because of a lack of privacy and inhibiting staff attitudes, they have little opportunity to experience intimacy.

Because many types of professionals are involved in the provision of health services to older people, staff-wide education about the importance of sexuality in the promotion of mental and physical health for older adults is important and should lead to more positive attitudes. Greater knowledge and acceptance of older adult sexuality and sexual functioning are important goals for all sex educators, counselors, and therapists trying to meet the needs of older adults (76).

Management

Comprehensive medical evaluation should precede any treatment intervention for sexuality dysfunction after stroke. Early referral to the appropriate health care professional is a key strategy. Physician specialists involved in evaluation and management of sexual dysfunction include physiatrists, urologists, gynecologists, primary care practitioners, or neurologists. A thorough evaluation includes review of sexual, medical, and psychosocial history followed by medical and neurologic examination and laboratory testing. Medical risk factors for sexual dysfunction include hypertension, diabetes mellitus, depression, and cardiovascular disease. Medications should be reviewed in order to identify those that cause sexual side effects. Lab studies should include hormonal evaluation to exclude a diagnosis of hypogonadism [testosterone and prolactin levels and testing to screen for diabetes (hemoglobin A1C or glucose tolerance testing)]. Social history should be elicited to discuss other risk factors, including obesity, tobacco, alcohol, and illicit drug use. It is also important to distinguish disease processes from the normal physiologic aging process. Other specialists vital to the management of sexual dysfunction after stroke include rehabilitation nursing, physical, occupational, and speech therapists as well as social workers and psychologists. Referral to physical or occupational therapists may be appropriate in situations where positioning or energy conservation techniques would be warranted. A rehabilitation physician can provide spasticity management, including oral medications, focal chemodenervation, and other methods to reduce spastic dystonia or painful spasms that interfere with sexual functioning. Sexuality counseling is the responsibility of all involved in the care of adults with neurologic disability.

SEXUALITY COUNSELING: THE PLISSIT MODEL

In 1976, Annon described the PLISSIT model for approaching sexual dysfunction and intimacy problems. PLISSIT stands for permission, limited information, specific suggestions, and intensive therapy (Table 45-12) (77).

Permission. It is vital to give permission to both the patient as well as the partner, who often assumes a caregiver role, to discuss issues related to sexuality. Permission may involve providing the opportunity for either partner to ask questions. It may also validate the patient or partner to include healthy sexual functioning as part of the overall goals of rehabilitation. Patients may feel that sexual problems in the context of disease are not important enough to be mentioned to their physicians, and physicians may feel uncomfortable and sometimes incompetent about asking. Giving permission is generally simple and opens the door to addressing important sexual problems that may arise.

Limited Information. For many patients, this may be the first opportunity to discuss sexual issues. Premorbid sexual knowledge may be variable depending on familial, religious, or cultural backgrounds. Therefore, it is vital to provide basic information until the level of comprehension can be established. It is suggested that a clinician provide only accurate and factual information during this category of sexuality counseling. This may include basics of the neurologic disability as well as review myths or unrealistic expectations (Table 45-6). Some patients use this information to develop their own solutions to issues related to sexuality.

Specific Suggestions. Some patients may require more specific suggestions to ameliorate problems related to their sexuality. Suggestions may include specific alternatives to engaging in sexual intercourse or to ways of communicating with a partner to allow for intimacy. Specific suggestions may often involve the explanation

---

TABLE 45-12
PLISSIT Model

P = Permission
LI = Limited Information
SS = Specific Suggestions
IT = Intensive Therapy

of a medication's effect on sexual functioning or the dose adjustment of a medication to improve sexual functioning if appropriate. There will certainly be areas that fall out of realm of the clinician's expertise. In which case, referral to counselors or other clinicians is appropriate.

Intensive Therapy.   This category of the PLISSIT model usually requires referral to an appropriate specialist, such as psychologist, psychiatrist, or social worker who is qualified to provide more intense forms of therapy. Certified sexual counselors or sex therapists can also provide intensive therapy if they are available. There are two primary modalities used by therapists to provide intense therapy. The first is symptom-specific recommendations that can include homework assignments. The second deals with the fundamental issues related to the relationship and intimacy issues.

CONCLUSION

Sexual dysfunction after stroke is common and can have a significant impact on the quality of life of the affected patients and partners. Altered sexual activity after stroke may have a medical cause that is often directly or indirectly as a result of neurologic changes in libido, sexual behavior, and sexual performance. Comorbidity and general health status, together with psychological factors, are also important determinants of post-stroke sexual functioning.

Treating sexual dysfunction is part of the holistic approach to rehabilitation. Counseling should include dispelling stereotypes, myths, and misperceptions not only for the stroke survivor, but also the partners and rehabilitation staff members. Counseling stroke survivors on sexual problems is a challenging experience, but it's necessary for improving their quality of life. Education in the field of sexuality and aging is also essential for all health professionals who are in contact with older people, both in institutions and the wider community.

Studies demonstrate that disorders of sexual functions are most significantly associated with various psychosocial factors, such as patients' general attitude toward sexuality, fear of impotence, and ability to discuss sexuality as well as with the degree of post-stroke functional disability. Therefore, providing this opportunity for evaluation and management is paramount. With emerging awareness of the primary importance of quality of life as the critical indicator of good patient management and the advent of more effective treatment of sexual dysfunction, it is no longer acceptable to ignore this very important dimension of life.

References

1. Masters WH, Johnson VE. *Human Sexual Response*. Boston: Little, Brown, 1996.
2. Kaplan HS. *The Sexual Desire Disorders: Dysfunctional Regulation of Sexual Motivation*. New York: Brunner/Mazel, 1995.
3. Lewis RW, Fugl-Meyers KS, et al. Epidemiology/risk factors of sexual dysfunction. J Sex Med 2004; 1(1):35–39.
4. Dunn KM, Croft PR, Hackett GI. Sexual problems: A study of the prevalence and need for health care in the general population. *Fam Pract* 1998;15(6):519–524.
5. Korpelainen JT, Nieminen P, Myllyla VV. Sexual functioning among stroke patients and their spouses. *Stroke* 1999;30(4):715–719.
6. Monga TN, Lawson JS, Inglis J. Sexual dysfunction in stroke patients. *Arch Phys Med Rehabil* 1986:67(1):19–22.
7. Sjogren K, Damber JE, Liliequist B. Sexuality after stroke with hemiplegia. I. Aspects of sexual function. *Scand J Rehabil Med* 1983:15(2):55–61.
8. Boldrini P, Basaglia N, Calanca MC. Sexual changes in hemiparetic patients. Arch Phys Med Rehabil 1991; 72:202–207.
9. Sinyor D, Amato P, Kaloupek DG, et al. Post-stroke depression: Relationships to functional impairment, coping strategies, and rehabilitation outcome. Stroke 1986; 17(6):1102–1107.
10. Kotila M, Numminen H, Waltimo O, Kaste M. Depression after stroke. Results of the Finnstroke study. Stroke 1998; 29:368–372.
11. Sjögren K, Fugl-Meyer A. Sexual problems in hemiplegia. Int Rehabil Med 1981; 3:28–31.
12. Monga TN, Lawson JS, Inglis J. Sexual dysfunction in stroke patients. Arch Phys Med Rehibil 1986; 67:19–22.
13. Johnston BL, Fletcher GF. Dynamic electrocardiographic recording during sexual activity in recent post-myocardial infarction and revascularization patients. Am Heart J 1979; 98(6):736–741.
14. Larson JL, McNaughton MW, et al. Heart rate and blood pressure responses to sexual activity and a stair-climbing test. Heart Lung 1980; 9(6):1025–1030.
15. Muller JE. Sexual activity as a trigger for cardiovascular events: What is the risk? Am J Cardiol 1999; 9; 84(5B):2N–5N. Review.
16. Schneider HJ, Kreitschmann-Andermahr I, Ghigo E, et al. Hypothalamopituitary dysfunction following traumatic brain injury and aneurysmal subarachnoid hemorrhage: A systematic review. JAMA 2007; 298:1429–1438.
17. Carson AJ, MacHale S, Allen K, et al. Depression after stroke and lesion location: A systematic review. Lancet 2000; 356(9224):122–126.
18. Burvill PW, Johnson GA, Chakera TMH, et al. The place and site of lesion in the aetiology of post-stroke depression. Cerebrovascular Dis 1996; 6:208–215.
19. Bancroft J, Coles L. Three years experience in a sexual problems clinic. Br Med J 1976; 26; 1(6025):1575.
20. Adams RD, Maurice V. *Principles of Neurology*. New York: McGraw-Hill, 1993.
21. Denys P, Mane M, Azouvi P, et al. Side effects of chronic intrathecal baclofen on erection and ejaculation in patients with spinal cord lesions. Arch Phys Med Rehabil 1998; 79(5):494–496.
22. Ghazizadeh S, Nikzad M. Botulinum toxin in the treatment of refractory vaginismus. Obstet Gynecol 2004; 104(5 Pt 1):922–925.
23. Yoon H, Chung WS, Shim BS. Botulinum toxin A for the management of vulvodynia. Int J Impot Res 2007; 19(1):84–87. Epub 2006 May 18.
24. Robinson RG. Post-stroke depression: Prevalence, diagnosis, treatment, and disease progression. Biol Psychiatry 2003; 54(3):936–941.
25. Robinson RG. Neuropsychiatric consequences of stroke. Annu Rev Med 1997; 48:217–229.
26. Eriksson M, Asplund K, Glader EL, et al. Self-reported depression and use of antidepressants after stroke: A national survey. *Stroke* 2004;35(4):936–941.
27. Segraves RT. Psychiatric illness and sexual function. Int J Impot Res 1998; 10(suppl 2): S131–133,S138–144.
28. Casper RC, Redmond DE, Katz MM, et al. Somatic symptoms in primary affective disorder. Presence and relationship to the classification of depression. Arch Gen Psychiatry 1985; 42:1098–1104.
29. Kennedy SH, Dickens SE, Eisfeld BS, Bagby RM. Sexual dysfunction before antidepressant therapy in major depression. J Affect Disord 1999; 56(2–3):201–208.
30. Robinson RG, Schultz SK, et al. Nortriptyline versus fluoxetine in the treatment of depression and in short-term recovery after stroke: A placebo-controlled, double-blind study. Am J Psychiatry 2000; 157(3):351–359.
31. Lipsey JR, Robinson RG, Pearlson GD, et al. Nortriptyline treatment of post-stroke depression: A double-blind study. Lancet 1984; 1(8372):297–300.
32. Anderson G. Effective treatment of post-stroke depression with the selective serotonin reuptake inhibitor citalopram. Stroke 1994; 25(6):1099–1104.
33. Jorge RE, Robinson RG, Arndt S, Starkstein S. Mortality and post-stroke depression: A placebo-controlled trial of antidepressants. Am J Psych 2003; 160(10):1823–1829.
34. Balon R, Yeragani VK, Pohl R, Ramesh C. Sexual dysfunction during antidepressant treatment. J Clin Psychiatry 1993; 54:209–212.

35. Kennedy SH, Eisfeld BS, Dickens SE, et al. Antidepressant-induced sexual dysfunction during treatment with moclobemide, paroxetine, sertraline, and venlafaxine. J Clin Psychiatry 2000; 61(4):276–281.

36. Rosen RC, Lane RM, Menza M. Effects of SSRIs on sexual function: A critical review. J Clin Psychopharmacol 1999; 19:67–85.

37. Kavoussi RJ, Segraves RT, Hughes AR, et al. Double-blind comparison of bupropion sustained release and sertraline in depressed outpatients. J Clin Psychiatry 1997; 58:532–537.

38. Gelenberg AJ, McGahuey C, Laukes C, et al. Mirtazapine substitution in SSRI-induced sexual dysfunction. J Clin Psychiatry 2000; 61:356–360.

39. Ferguson JM. The effects of antidepressants on sexual functioning in depressed patients: A review. J Clin Psychiatry 2001; 62(suppl 3):22–34.

40. Kolodny RC, Kahn CB, Goldstein HH, et al. Sexual dysfunction in diabetic men. Diabetes 1974; 23:306–309.

41. McCulloch DK, Young RJ, Prescott RJ, et al. The natural history of impotence in diabetic men. Diabetologia 1984; 26:437–440.

42. Zemel P. Sexual dysfunction in the diabetic patient with hypertension. Am J Cardiol 1988; 61:27H–33H.

43. Ellenberg M. Impotence in diabetes: The neurologic factor. Ann Intern Med 1971; 75:213–219.

44. Penson DF, Wessells H. Erectile dysfunction in diabetic patients. Diabetes Spectrum 2004; 17:225–230.

45. Kolodny RC. Sexual dysfunction in diabetic females. Diabetes 1971; 20:557–559.

46. Koch PB, Young EW. Diabetes and female sexuality: A review of the literature. Health Care Women Int 1988; 9:251–262.

47. Piero M, Paolo M, Ravagnani, et al. Association between erectile dysfunction and coronary artery disease. Role of coronary clinical presentation and extent of coronary vessels involvement: The COBRA trial. *European Heart Journal* Advance Access published on July 19, 2006, DOI 10 1093/euheartj/ehl142.

48. Cheitlin MD, Hutter AM Jr, Brindis RG, et al. ACC/AHA expert consensus document. Use of sildenafil (Viagra) in patients with cardiovascular disease. American College of Cardiology/American Heart Association. J Am Coll Cardiol 1999; 33(1):273–282.

49. Burchardt M, et al. Hypertension is associated with severe erectile dysfunction. J Urol 2000; 164:1188–1191.

50. Weiss RJ. Effects of antihypertensive agents on sexual function. Am Fam Physician 1991; 44:2075–2082.

51. Khedum SM, Naicker T, Makarey B. Zinc, hydrochlorothiazide, and sexual function. Cent Alp J Med 1995; 41:312–315.

52. Fogari R, Zoppi A, Corradi L, et al. Sexual function in hypertensive males treated with lisinopril or atenolol. Am J Hypertens 1998; 11:1244–1247.

53. Fogari R, Zoppi A, Poletti L, et al. Sexual activity in hypertensive men treated with valsartan or carvedilol: A crossover study. Am J Hypertens 2001; 14:27–31.

54. Fogari R, Preti P, Derosa G, et al. Effect of antihypertensive treatment with valsartan or atenolol on sexual activity and plasma testosterone in hypertensive men. Eur J Clin Pharmacol 2002; 58:177–180.

55. Llisterri Caro JL, Vidal JL, Vicente JA, et al. Sexual dysfunction in hypertensive patients treated with losartan. Am J Med Sci 2001; 321(5):336–341.

56. Dusing R. Effect of the angiotensin II antagonist valsartan on sexual function in hypertensive men. Blood Pressure 2003; 12 (suppl 2):29–34.

57. So El, Annergers JF, Hauser WA, et al. Population-based study of seizure disorders after cerebral infarction. Neurology 1996; 46:350–355.

58. Reith J, Jorgensen HS, Nakayama H, et al. Seizures in acute stroke: The Copenhagen Stroke Study. Stroke 1997; 28:1585–1589.

59. Burn J, Dennis M, Bamford J, et al. Epileptic seizures after a first stroke: The Oxfordshire Community Project. BMJ 1997; 315:1582–1587.

60. Toone BK, Edeh J, Nanjee MN, Wheeler M. Hyposexuality and epilepsy: A community survey of hormonal and behavioural changes in male epileptics. Psychol Med 1989; 19(4):937–943.

61. Spector IP, Carey MP. Incidence and prevalence of the sexual dysfunctions: A critical review of the empirical literature. Arch Sex Behav 1990; 19(4):389–408.

62. Feldman HA, Goldstein I, Hatzichristou DG, et al. Impotence and its medical and psychosocial correlates: Results of the Massachusetts Male Aging Study. Journal of Urology 1994; 151(1):54–61.

63. Blumer D, Walker AE. Sexual behavior in temporal lobe epilepsy: A study of the effects of temporal lobectomy on sexual behavior. Arch Neurol 1967; 16(1):37–43.

64. Shukla GD, Srivastava ON, Katiyar B. Sexual disturbances in temporal lobe epilepsy: A controlled study. Br J Psychiatry 1979; 134:288–292.

65. Andy OJ, Velamati S. Temporal lobe seizures and hypersexuality: Dopaminergic effects. Appl Neurophysiol 1978; 41(1–4):13–28.

66. Monga TN, Monga M, Raina MS, Hardjasudarma M. Hypersexuality in stroke. Arch Phys Med Rehabil 1986; 67(6):415–417.

67. Rattya J, Turkka J, Pakarinen AJ, et al. Reproductive effects of valproate, carbamazepine, and oxcarbazepine in men with epilepsy. Neurology 2001; 56(1):31–36.

68. Spence SH. Psychosexual dysfunction in the elderly. Behaviour Change 1992; 9:55–64.

69. Verwoerdt A, Pfeiffer E, Wang HS. Sexual behavior in senescence-changes in sexual activity and interest of aging men and women. J Geriatric Psychiatry 1969; 2:163–180.

70. Lewis RW. Erectile dysfunction. In: Stein B, ed. *Practice of Urology*. Pennsylvania: W.W. Norton & Company, 1993:21–38.

71. Deacon S, Minichiello V, Plummer D. Sexuality and older people: Revisiting the assumptions. Educational Gerontology 1995; 21:497–513.

72. Hall A, Selby J, Vanclay FM. Sexual ageism. Australian Journal on Aging 1982; 1:29–34.

73. Brown L. Is there sexual freedom for our aging population in long-term care institutions? Journal of Gerontological Social Work 1989; 13:75–93.

74. Datan N, Rodeheaver D. Beyond generativity: Toward a sensuality of later life. In: Weg R, ed. *Sexuality in the Later Years: Roles and Behavior*. San Diego: Academic Press, 1983:279–288.

75. Robinson PK. The sociological perspective. In: Weg R, ed. *Sexuality in the Later Years: Roles and Behavior*. San Diego: Academic Press, 1983:81–103.

76. Story MD. Knowledge and attitudes about the sexuality of older adults among retirement home residents. Educational Gerontology 1989; 15:515–526.

77. Annon J. The PLISSIT model. J Sex Ed Therapy 1976; 2:1–15.

46 Vocational Rehabilitation after a Stroke

Brendan E. Conroy
Fatemeh Milani
Marion Levine
Joel Stein

F or some stroke survivors, vocational rehabilitation is a vitally important phase of recovery. Age and prior employment status play key roles in determining whether or not return to work is an important component of a stroke survivor's rehabilitation program. Although the general rate of employment among all people with disabilities is estimated at 17%, and 70% of working-age stroke survivors have some impairment of work capacity, the rate of successful return to work following a stroke is estimated at 40% among stroke survivors who were employed prior to the stroke (1). Factors that impact the likelihood of a stroke survivor returning to work include age, severity of stroke and the nature of the residual impairments, psychological factors, financial and family obligations, pre-morbid work type, socioeconomic status, and educational achievement level.

Age is a major factor in decisions for employment among the able bodied, with many individuals retiring in their 60s and 70s, and it is not surprising that stroke can be a precipitating event for a decision to cease working for someone on the cusp of retirement age. The incidence of stroke is strongly correlated with increasing age, and thus only a minority of stroke survivors will actually include return to work as one of their rehabilitation goals.

Gainful employment serves multiple roles in our society, and economic support is not necessarily the most important one for many individuals. Competence and the ability to work contribute substantially to many people's sense of self-worth. Concerns of being meaningless, of being unable to contribute, or of being a burden to one's family are common among stroke survivors.

The rehabilitation team should conduct a process of education throughout the period of recovery to provide the survivor and his/her family with realistic expectations regarding the likelihood and rate of improvement of various stroke-related impairments, and how the patient's ability to work may be affected. The process of stroke rehabilitation can require a full year in some cases before maximal functional abilities have been achieved. Motor, cognitive, and communication impairments typically improve, though the patient may not reach a level at which return to employment is feasible. Fatigue and reduced endurance may not be as prominent during the early recovery phase, but could become more evident as activity levels increase. For the stroke survivor who is otherwise well recovered, reduced activity tolerance because of fatigue can be a limiting factor in return to work.

Informing patients about the time frame of recovery helps them understand this process and provides encouragement that further progress is anticipated. Psychologically and financially, it may be beneficial for the stroke survivor to resist the temptation to retire prematurely after a stroke. There are advantages to returning to work after stroke and then ultimately retiring at the time of one's own choosing. Many people have a substantial portion of their sense of self-worth invested in the work that they do. It can be a devastating experience to abruptly enter the "what-do-I-do-now?" world of retirement directly from stroke recovery, without having planned a transition to retirement. Retirement has been described as the hardest job of all. Former United States Supreme Court Justice Sandra Day O'Connor said she wishes that she could "retire from retirement." Postponing retirement until the time feels right allows the stroke survivor to maintain a sense of control and accomplishment. Retirement should be a reward for hard work, not a punishment for illness, and the timing and circumstances of this transition play an important role in how it is viewed.

Some patients will want to wait until they are "all better" or "back to normal" before attempting to reenter the workforce. Stroke survivors with more than minor deficits rarely experience a complete recovery, and sometimes it is helpful for the survivor to return to work *in order to* feel normal, valuable, and that they are contributing again. This emotional victory can spur increased enthusiasm for rehabilitation efforts and community reintegration.

Another option a stroke survivor may wish to consider is retirement on disability with the intent to return to employment at a future date. Taking one to three years to focus on stroke rehabilitation without a specific time line can reduce the pressure to return to work prematurely in order to please an employer or avoid loss of a job altogether. This strategy allows the stroke survivor to determine the timing and circumstances of a return to work on his/her own terms once a satisfactory degree of recovery has been achieved. One drawback of this strategy is that many employers will be more inclined to make accommodations for an existing and valued employee than for a new employee. While antidiscrimination statutes should, in principle, provide protection from discrimination when seeking employment, in practice many disabled individuals have a difficult time in securing a job, despite their qualifications and experience. Thus, there is no guarantee that a stroke survivor who accepts retirement with disability from one job will be able to find another position when the time seems right.

A careful exploration of the stroke survivor's goals and objectives is essential in working with him/her toward a return to work. What does the stroke survivor really want to accomplish and why? Goal exploration must advance beyond superficial goals, such as "return to prior status." Even apparently straightforward goals, such as returning to work for financial reasons, need further analysis. What will the money be used for? Paying for food and rent, a new car, or perhaps to fund a vacation or the comfortable retirement about which the person has always dreamed? Work plays a major social role for many people. Is the stroke survivor seeking to return to work in order to avoid being home all day? Is it friendships at work he/she will miss and return to work is desired to avoid loneliness? Does he/she want/need to have money for leisure pursuits? Is there a project at work he/she feels a need to complete? Even in the cases in which the severity of impairments from a stroke make return to work impossible or impractical, understanding these motivating underlying factors in the person's makeup can facilitate the rehabilitation process.

In some cases, return to employment is feasible, but not to the exact job or work duties as previously assigned. Often this may involve using skills acquired prior to the stroke, but in a slightly different context. For example, a construction worker or an auto mechanic may not be able to return to building or repairing, but may be able to teach, manage, and/or supervise other workers.

Many stroke survivors are concerned about the impact of visible manifestations of their stroke (especially motor deficits and ambulatory aids) on their image in the workplace. An arm held in a chronically flexed posture, the use of an ankle brace, or a hemiplegic gait makes the stroke survivor visibly different from his/her colleagues. Concerns about being treated as if they are sick or crippled or needing special treatment are common. The impact of the Americans with Disabilities Act has been substantial in affording protection to workers with disabilities from losing their position without reasonable cause, but this has not erased the stigma of disability in (and out of) the workplace. Rehabilitation professionals can play an important role in overcoming these prejudices. At the most basic level, the stroke survivor can be prepared for this possibility and counseled regarding coping strategies. A review of the stroke survivor's job description (if available) can be helpful in terms of both patient education and educating the employer. With the permission and support of the stroke survivor, the rehabilitation team can help educate employers and coworkers about the ability of the stroke survivor to perform their work responsibilities. This commonly takes the form of a written letter to an employer explaining the medical safety and appropriateness of return to work. This letter usually includes a statement that the patient is medically stable, followed by an indication that the job description has been reviewed and appears within the patient's capabilities. If simple and reasonable accommodations are necessary, these should be outlined in the letter. The letter often helps the employer feel a reduced sense of risk regarding the return of the stroke survivor to the workplace. A brief and simple letter, with a minimum of technical jargon, is most effective and should not exceed a single sheet of paper.

A trial of bringing examples of typical work tasks home (or to occupational or speech therapy sessions) can be a helpful tool in assessing readiness for return to work and in developing compensatory strategies in advance. For example, an individual who is responsible for editing technical manuals at work might bring home an example of such a manual and attempt to edit it as if he/she were at work. Successful completion of this sample work task prior to actually returning to the workplace will provide confidence to both stroke survivor and employer that the stroke survivor is ready to return to work.

Certain professions require particularly high-level skills to perform at an acceptable level. For example, physicians experience demanding cognitive, social, and communication activities as part of their professional practice. Neuropsychological testing is often helpful as a means of assuring readiness to reenter the professional domain. In cases in which concerns remain regarding readiness to resume practice, having a designated colleague review and oversee their work can provide an important level of reassurance for the treating physician, the physician recovering from stroke, and for his/her patients.

Using both neuropsychological testing and a subsequent peer mentor/counselor can be very helpful for stroke survivors in other professions with demanding responsibilities and a high level of responsibility, such as lawyers, policemen, executives, other types of health care providers, scientists, etc. Neuropsychological testing can be helpful not only in order to verify that the stroke survivor has recovered sufficient capacity to resume his/her responsibilities but also to evaluate cases in which this recovery has not occurred in order to establish to the stroke survivor that he/she remains too impaired to resume their former employment. Such testing can also be used to document the disability for legal, retirement, and other benefits considerations.

Volunteer work can play an important role for stroke survivors, both for those who are unable (or choose not) to return to full-time work or for those who are seeking an interim step as preparation for return to gainful employment. Volunteer work can help the motivated stroke survivor refamiliarize him/herself with the demands of the work environment in a more flexible and forgiving atmosphere and allow him/her to rebuild their endurance and confidence. Some stroke survivors are very grateful to the rehabilitation healthcare team and seek volunteer work in a rehabilitation hospital as a means of expressing their gratitude for their recovery. Some stroke rehabilitation programs have incorporated former stroke patients as volunteers for peer visitor programs for hospitalized stroke survivors and provided specific training for this purpose (2). Other institutions commonly employing volunteers include acute care hospitals, churches, and libraries.

Many stroke survivors find it helpful to return to work on a part-time basis initially and then gradually increase to full-time. Given the high prevalence of fatigue among stroke survivors, starting with shorter days (e.g., half days) several times per week is generally advisable rather than working a fewer number of full days. Establishing success on a part-time basis will increase the confidence of both the stroke survivor and his/her employer as well as provide an opportunity to identify and address any unanticipated challenges that arise. For example if the stroke survivor finds that a familiar task takes longer to complete than in the past, the part-time status would afford more flexibility to take more time without falling behind. Note that the effort expended in commuting to work should be taken into account when planning return to work since it may significantly contribute to fatigue.

In recent years, there have been significant labor market shifts caused by technological advances, corporate restructuring, downsizing, outsourcing, and globalization. This increasingly fluid labor market has led to an increase in the availability of alternate employment arrangements including temporary, part-time, and subcontracted work. In addition to part-time work, options now may include job sharing, telecommuting, or working as an independent contractor.

Mobility aids, such as a scooter, power wheelchair, or Segway, may be useful as a means of conserving energy at the workplace. Despite the ability to complete each individual task involved in a job, some stroke survivors may find themselves limited by the cumulative effort throughout the workday, especially if the position involves prolonged standing or walking. As with other aspects of planning for return to work, a proactive plan that establishes these supports in advance is preferable to a "reactive" stance in which unanticipated problems are addressed once they have already impacted the transition back to the workplace.

DRIVING

Return to driving is important both as means of getting to and from work for many individuals as well as an actual component of the job for some individuals (e.g., a truck driver). Please refer to Chapter 43 for a full discussion of return to driving after stroke.

PROGNOSIS FOR SUCCESSFUL RETURN TO WORK

A substantial number of stroke patients achieve independence in mobility and self-care skills, but vocational outcomes are not as favorable as those for activities of daily living (ADL). Data obtained from Framingham Heart Study indicate that among stroke survivors, 78% achieve independence in mobility skills and 68% independence in daily living skills, while 63% continue to have reduced vocational function (3, 4). There are multiple factors that affect the likelihood of returning to work after stroke, including the nature of the neurologic impairments, the type of work, and the stroke survivor's age. The strongest predictor for inability to return to work is the severity of the stroke (5, 6). Other important predictive factors for successful return to work are preserved motor strength, absence of apraxia, and white-collar occupation prior to stroke (7, 8). The laterality and location of the stroke within the brain are not correlated with the likelihood of return to work (5, 6). Younger age is associated with an increased likelihood of returning to work (6). Unfortunately, many studies in this area tend to be limited by small size and selection bias since they have often focused on the subpopulation of those who successfully return to work rather than a broader population of stroke survivors. (5, 9, 10). Return to work in stroke patients should be considered one of the indicators of a successful rehabilitation since it influences self-image, well-being, and life satisfaction (5).

STRESS AND STRESS MANAGEMENT

Stress is an unavoidable and normal part of life, both in and out of the workplace. A misbehaving teenager, the death of a pet, a broken water heater, or a leaky roof is unavoidable at some point in life, as is a deadline for a work assignment, a demanding client, or an unhappy customer in the workplace. Patients and their family members are often concerned that excessive stress in the workplace could be hazardous for the stroke survivor or even lead to a recurrent stroke. While there continues to be debate on the role that chronic stress (and especially depression) might play as a chronic risk factor for stroke (11), there is no evidence that the usual stresses of the workplace represent a specific risk for stroke survivors.

WORK RESTRICTIONS

Return to work may be contingent on specific restrictions, and the rehabilitation team and physician are often asked to help establish these restrictions. The reasons for restrictions fall into the following broad categories:

1. *Risk:* When there is a risk to the general public caused by the patient engaging in specific work activity, such work must be avoided. For example, a patient with uncontrolled post-stroke seizures should not work as commercial motor vehicle driver or aircraft pilot (12).
2. *Capacity:* Refers to strength, flexibility, and endurance. A formal capacity determination should not be performed until the individual has achieved maximal functional recovery/rehabilitation. These

factors comprising capacity are measurable with a fair degree of scientific precision (12).

3. *Tolerance:* Tolerance is psycho-physiologic concept. It is the ability to tolerate sustained work or activity at a given level. A patient limited by insufficient tolerance has the ability to perform a certain task but lacks the ability to complete it comfortably secondary to discomfort or fatigue. Tolerance is not scientifically measurable or verifiable (12).

Physicians should determine work restrictions based on risk, capacity, and tolerance. Restrictions on return to work related to physical impairment (muscle weakness, spasticity, incoordination) depend on severity of disability and the type of work. If gait and coordinated activity are impaired, the individual may be at risk climbing to heights, walking on narrow surfaces, or working with hazardous materials or equipment. In the presence of severe sensory impairments of the lower extremity, prolonged standing or walking is to be avoided. Shift work and other sleep cycle alterations can exacerbate post-stroke fatigue.

IMPAIRMENTS/DISABILITY AFFECTING RETURN TO WORK

Physical functioning improves most rapidly in first three to six months after a stroke, but improvement frequently continues for a full year after stroke. Pain issues including those related to stroke such as central post-stroke pain, complex regional pain syndrome Type 1 (RSD), or other (not stroke-related) pain symptoms need to be addressed. Spasticity interfering with function or causing pain may need to be treated. Post-stroke depression is common, occurring in as many as 40% of stroke survivors and should be identified and treated (see Chapter 27).

Deficits in cognition, language, communication, and perceptual abilities all tend to improve substantially in working-age stroke survivors, though with considerable variability. Recovery from aphasia usually occurs at a slower rate and over a more prolonged time course than motor recovery (3, 13). Although most aphasia recovery occurs within the first three to six months, some patients will continue to experience meaningful recovery for a full year (3, 14). Comprehension usually returns earlier and to a greater extent than does expression (3, 15). Most improvement in perceptual recovery including hemi-spatial neglect occurs in the first 20 weeks, but some improvements may be seen up to one year post-stroke (3, 15).

VOCATIONAL REHABILITATION SERVICES

Vocational rehabilitation services are commonly coordinated by a vocational rehabilitation counselor (VRC). VRCs typically have achieved a masters degree in education or in a clinical field and then subsequently received training to become a certified rehabilitation counselor (CRC). There are no schools of "vocational therapy" as there are for physical therapists, occupational therapists, etc. VRCs often serve as the team leader for the vocational rehabilitation phase of recovery. The team may include physician, occupational therapist, speech-language pathologist, physical therapist, psychologist, and rehabilitation engineer as needed.

Vocational rehabilitation counselors help people deal with the personal, social, and vocational effects of disabilities. They evaluate the stroke survivor's strengths and limitations, provide personal and vocational counseling, and arrange for medical care, vocational training, and job placement assistance. VRCs are trained to help people with disabilities make decisions regarding work. They help people understand and accept their disabilities while emphasizing their residual strengths and capabilities.

In general, services provided by VR counselors include the following:

- Assessment of individual educational and vocational abilities, including intelligence, work-related aptitudes, vocational interests, academics, and transferable skills
- Provision of counseling services, including prevocational, individual, group, and job-seeking skills to assist individuals with vocational adjustment and community reintegration goals
- Provision of work skills training, including simulated work activities to prepare individuals for competitive employment opportunities
- Facilitation of specialized services, including employer or school consultations, school or work site evaluation and accommodations, job analysis, and selective placement options to assist individuals in returning to employment or school
- Education of prospective employers or school officials concerning the vocational and educational implications of various disabilities to assure success. This includes providing information on accessibility, accommodation, and disability-related legislation affecting employment or education and working with people with disabilities
- Following up with employer or education services to assist people with disabilities in maintaining employment or education placement

To perform these services, the VRC has to understand the needs of the employer, the demands of the job, and the capabilities of the client. One of the main tasks of the VRC is to assist individuals in meeting their goals and bridging the gap between disability and work. The VRC may be particularly helpful if an employer is resistant to providing accommodations. This resistance is often caused by a lack of information and awareness about the assistance available to make the accommodations, the specific physical limitations of a stroke survivor, and the requirements of the Americans with Disabilities Act (ADA). The VRC can provide education that helps ensure that employment is beneficial to both the client and the employer.

According to the U.S. Department of Labor, the number of people who will need rehabilitation counseling is expected to grow as advances in medical technology allow more people to survive injury or illness (16). In addition, legislation requiring equal employment rights for people with disabilities is increasing the demand for counselors because of the assistance they provide with transition back into the workforce or maintaining employment for individuals with disabilities. VRCs also play an important role in helping companies to comply with legal requirements of the ADA. VRCs are employed by state vocational rehabilitation agencies, private rehabilitation agencies, medical centers, centers for independent living, nonprofit agencies, and insurance companies. Unfortunately, at times the services of a VRC may not be available because of a lack of funding by employers or insurers or a lengthy waiting list at the state vocational rehabilitation office.

THE AMERICANS WITH DISABILITIES ACT

In 1990, President George H. W. Bush signed the Americans with Disabilities act into law. According to Title I of the ADA (www.ada.gov), it is illegal for employers with 15 or more employees to discriminate against employees with a disability. In order to qualify for protection under this act, an employee must be able to perform the essential functions of the job with or without reasonable accommodations. Essential job functions are those responsibilities that are fundamental to the particular position and can be defined using the following criteria:

- The position exists to perform the function
- There are a limited number of other employees available to perform the function
- The function is highly specialized and the person in the position is hired for special expertise or ability to perform it

The ADA defines reasonable accommodation as any change in the work environment or in the way work is managed to ensure equal opportunity. However, it is the responsibility of the employee to request the accommodation. Stroke survivors who request an accommodation as defined by this legislation need to be as informed as possible. The request should be submitted in writing and should describe the problem, identify possible solutions, and refer to resources to assist with implementing the requested changes.

Many employees hesitate to ask for assistance and may wait until their job is in jeopardy. The U.S. Department of Labor, Office of Disability Employment Policy, maintains a website entitled the Job Accommodation Network (JAN) (see Table 46-1 for URL). JAN is a free service that provides individualized worksite accommodation solutions, technical assistance regarding the ADA, and other disability related legislation, and educates consumers about self-employment options.

The Job Accommodation Process

Job accommodations generally fall into three main categories:

- Job modifications
  - exchanging job tasks with coworkers
  - flexible work hours
  - altered work schedule
  - telecommuting
  - job sharing
  - working part time
  - omitting nonessential job tasks
- Changes to the environment
  - ramps
  - reducing crowding of office furniture
  - automatic door openers
  - improved lighting
- Assistive technology
  - speaker phones or head sets
  - adjustable height work surfaces
  - wrist or arm supports
  - magnification aids

The following discusses the job accommodation process. When requesting reasonable accommodations, it is important to identify what the patient can do and where assistance is needed. A comprehensive

---

TABLE 46-1
Resources for Stroke Survivors

- Older/Disadvantaged Workers: www.rileyguide.com/diverse.html
  Lists seven senior job banks
- Seniors4Hire: Senior Job Seeker Registration: www.seniors4hire.org
  Register for job search information
- Job Accommodation Network (www.jan.wvu.edu)
  Guide to reasonable accommodations and employment for individuals with disabilities
  - ABLEDATE: www.ABLEDATA.com
    Provides information on assistive technology and rehabilitation equipment from a database of over 23,000 product listings.
  - Regional Disability and Business Technical Assistance Centers (DBTAC) at (800) 949-4232; there are ten regional DBTAC offices that provide ADA information and copies of ADA documents. They also can provide informal guidance in understanding the law. Vocational Rehabilitation Services: each state has a department that provides
  - Rehabilitation Research and Training Center on Aging with a Disability: www.agingwithdisability.org/factsheets/accom
  - Occupational Outlook Handbook; US Department of Labor; Bureau of Labor Statistics (www.bls.gov/oco)
  - O-Net (On-line occupational information sponsored by Department of Labor): http://online.onetcenter.org/
  - Dictionary of Occupational Titles (sponsored by US Department of Labor)
  - http://www.occupationalinfo.org
  - U. S. Department of Labor; Office of Disability Employment Policy (www.dol.gov/odep/pubs/ek00/hiddenemp.htm)
    Facilitating Return-to-Work for Ill or Injured Employees
  - Career Transition & Development, ERIC Digest; Career Development of Older Adults by Susan Imel, 2003 (www.vtaide.com/png/ERIC/Career-OlderAdults.htm)
  - Career Mobility: A Choice or Necessity?; ERIC Digest; by Bettina Lankard Brown, 1998 (www.vt.aide.com/png?ERIC/Career-Mobility.htm)
  - United States Small Business Administration; Starting Your Business (www.sba.gov/starting_business/index.html)
  - Directory of state vocational rehabilitation programs: http://www.workworld.org/wwwebhelp/state_vocational_rehabilitation_vr_agencies.htm
  - HIPAA Information: http://www.cms.hhs.gov/HIPAAGenInfo/Downloads/HIPAALaw.pdf
  - US Department of Labor: State Worker's Compensation Laws http://www.dol.gov/esa/regs/statutes/owcp/stwclaw/stwclaw.htm

job accommodation process includes five phases: job analysis, functional capacity evaluation, job market, job search, and reasonable accommodations.

Job Analysis. A systematic study of both the work tasks and the physical demands (ergonomic aspects) of the workplace must be reviewed. This review of the job tasks considers *how* and *when* they are accomplished and the expected outcomes. The VRC should examine job descriptions, tasks of the job, educational requirements, physical and mental demands of the environment, and employment outlook. The ergonomic job analysis is performed at the worksite by a qualified physical therapist (or occupational therapist if upper extremities are exclusively involved). The therapist measures the physical demands of the job and makes recommendations concerning ways to make the job more appropriate and ergonomically safer. When combined with the functional capacity information described below, the information from an ergonomic job analysis provides the basis for development and implementation of a successful work plan. Appropriate job tasks or workplace accommodations can then be recommended.

Functional Capacity Evaluation. An evaluation of functional capacity requires an honest and accurate assessment of abilities as they relate to specific job tasks. The evaluation is completed at a rehabilitation center, usually by an occupational therapist. Typically, this testing is not a covered benefit under insurance plans. The evaluation may include assessing capacity for handling manual materials (lifting), aerobic capacity (cardio-respiratory fitness), posture and mobility tolerance (walking, sitting, bending, stooping, climbing, twisting), and anthropometric measurements (measurements of body size, weight, and proportions). This evaluation involves measurement of actual work ability during simulated work tasks and computerized measurement of the force exerted isometrically during lifting tasks. The results of the evaluation are reviewed with the patient and the coordinating VRC. Recommendations might suggest pacing of tasks, healthy work posture, reasonable accommodations, or work redesign for safety and productivity on the job.

The functional capacity evaluation may indicate that the person is unable to return to his/her previous occupation. In that case, the VRC may suggest aptitude and interest testing to help develop alternative vocational plans. If, for example, a person can no longer physically perform nursing duties and the position cannot be accommodated, one would look at other settings in which a nursing background might be helpful—for instance, an insurance company. If the insurance company position requires additional clerical duties, the evaluation might assess that person's computer or word-processing skills and indicate additional training. Training may be required in a new setting, and a VRC would be able to assist in securing that training.

The Job Market. When considering new lines of work, the VRC's knowledge of the job market and availability of jobs is critical. Web-based resources are increasingly used (see Table 46-1). Newspaper or on-line classified ads are often the least helpful resource in seeking employment. However, they may help identify trends. Having the patient make "cold" (unsolicited) calls can reap high rewards if they are done systematically. The U.S. Department of Labor publishes *The Occupational Outlook Handbook* every few years, which identifies the future job outlook. The state department of employment offers job lists. Most jobs are found through personal contacts and networking within a field of interest.

The Job Search. Job-seeking skills are as important as the job skills themselves and can be learned through coaching by the VRC as well as through many types of publications or job clubs that are available through the state departments of employment. Job-seeking skills include identifying and following up on job leads, resume writing, application completion, and interviewing skills. The need for these skills is not unique to persons with disabilities. These skills include

1. Locating job leads
2. Selling yourself
3. Projecting self-confidence during a job search
4. Telephone techniques
5. Interviewing skills

For most patients, it is usually better to discuss disability issues at an appropriate time during a face-to-face interview and not explicitly address these issues on the application or resume. The resume is typically the first contact with employers and can be used as a means of indirectly alerting the interviewer to a disability. Disability may be referred to indirectly, i.e., "stroke support group member," "I qualify for the Affirmative Action Program under section 503 of the Rehabilitation Act," or "Am active in wheelchair sports." While it is important not to hide a disability or evade the issue, the focus of communications between patient and the potential employer should be on skills and abilities, not on disability issues.

The job applicant must be prepared to handle a wide range of interview styles and techniques. The patient should know in advance what job accommodations are likely to be needed. Role playing and/or videotaping practice interviews with a VRC are effective tools to increase interviewing confidence. It is important to avoid yes/no answers and to be able to elaborate on skills using specific examples whenever possible. The first five to ten minutes of the interview are critical since employers often make hiring decisions based on their first impressions of enthusiasm and interest.

The applicant needs to take the initiative in discussing the disability, especially if it is visible. The disability should be addressed directly, clearing up any misconceptions and speaking to any concerns or questions that the employer may have regarding the disability. A good opening statement might be "You may be wondering if I will be dependable; I have my own vehicle with hand controls, can drive independently, and pride myself on my reliability and punctuality."

Reasonable Accommodations

The ADA defines reasonable accommodations as "changes to the work environment or the way in which tasks are customarily performed to enable an individual with a disability to enjoy equal employment opportunities" (ADA, Title I, 1991). As defined by the ADA, only functional limitations that affect the essential job duties of a position are considered when making job accommodations. The reasonable accommodations concept generally applies to the job application process, work environment, and work benefits and privileges. It is interesting to note that the average accommodation cost is estimated to cost less than $100 for the employer (17).

Accessible Workplace Facilities. Ergonomic principles help fit the job to the person rather than make the person fit the job. For individuals with stroke, the job accommodations discussed below improve opportunities to succeed in the workplace.

Accessible workplace facilities are necessary if the patient has difficulty walking or climbing stairs or uses a wheelchair for mobility. Accessibility to workplace facilities is a primary consideration when contemplating employment. Often the accommodations are not costly and can be explored through appropriate resources prior to an employment interview. Depending upon the specific job, company, and work site, the VRC can assist in educating the employer. Examples of modifications that employers may make include the following:

- Reserving extra-wide parking spaces near the building entrance
- Removing walkway obstructions
- Ramping stairways
- Re-grading entranceways
- Widening entrance doorways
- Installing automatic door openers or lever doorknobs
- Installing elevators with lowered controls
- Providing accessible restrooms, lunchrooms, and training areas
- Leaving floors bare or installing low-pile carpeting

Modified Work Schedules. Modified work schedules are simple, yet often overlooked, accommodations. An employer may be able to offer a flexible work schedule by taking the following actions:

- Splitting the work position into multiple part-time jobs (also known as job sharing)
- Adjusting work hours to reduce commuting time or move commuting away from rush hour traffic
- Allowing short, frequent rest breaks to encourage muscle recovery and to refresh concentration

Job Restructuring. Job restructuring is an appropriate accommodation for almost any functional limitation. In job restructuring, nonessential functions are modified or reassigned to another employee in exchange for a task the patient can perform more easily. Examples of restructuring within a job might include the following:

- More telephone work instead of frequent travel
- Computerizing records instead of writing
- Rescheduling morning tasks to the afternoon or vice versa

A real estate agent who has difficulty writing contracts, demonstrates this job-restructuring principle when she executes property searches on a computer while her colleague completes the written contracts.

Modified Workstations. Modified workstations contribute to the conservation of energy. The workstation should be evaluated to determine the need for modification. Ask the VRC to suggest a rehabilitation engineer who may be available to make these modifications. Although some of the modifications may require the purchase of new items, many can be made with only minimal changes to existing equipment, including the following:

- Rearrange files or shelves to conserve energy
- Purchase a desktop turntable organizer to keep items within easy reach
- Organize the desk for face-to-face communication
- Relocate the desk to the most accessible area
- Raise and lower the desk to ensure proper seating posture (the desktop should be about an inch below the elbows)
- Adjust the height of computer screen to avoid neck and eye strain (the top of the computer screen should be at eye level)
- Utilize a telephone headset.

Getting the Needed Accommodations

Most employers have policies and procedures for requesting accommodations. Again, this process begins with a written request, even if the discussion has occurred beforehand. Encourage the patient to use his/her own adaptive equipment whenever possible and keep solutions as simple, inexpensive, and as cost-effective as possible. The patient can request to tour the work area, observe the job being performed, and/or review the essential job requirements with the employer. In assessing this information, the patient (with or without the assistance of a VRC) can then submit a proposal for resources. This process can even be turned into a demonstration of problem-solving skills and project management.

In negotiating for the accommodations, the patient should be sensitive to the employer's perspective. If architectural barrier changes are needed, the employer can be advised of the tax credits available for this purpose and how removal of the barriers may also potentially increase business by attracting customers with disabilities.

Another strategy in handling employer's resistance is to make a referral to the Job Accommodation Network (JAN), an international, nonprofit information and referral service providing free consultation for accommodation needs, products, and services, based in West Virginia. JAN provides information on accommodations to employers, especially on cost and resources. Employers can discuss options with the JAN staff and with other employers who have used the service. This service is provided at no cost to the employer. If a request for the provision of accommodations is denied, advocacy services can be obtained through a local center for independent living and vocational rehabilitation agencies.

Acquiring Necessary Assistive Devices

When considering equipment to purchase, remember that the assistance device should address the functional limitation in a specific task. The following equipment may be helpful:

- Telephone headsets (wired or wireless Bluetooth)
- Electric scissors and staplers
- Anti-glare computer screens
- Ergonomic arm supports for forearm and wrist support while typing
- Tape recorders
- Dictaphones
- Voice-activated computers and voice recognition technology

Job Relocation

Another option to consider is a change in the work environment. Changing to another, more accessible location may be the best possibility to pursue in the case of mobility impairments or special energy conservation needs. Documentation from the treating physician may be useful when discussing this option with human resources personnel. Some relocation options may include the following:

- Working at the company office closest to public transportation
- Working at home with a computer and internet connection to the office
- Changing the job location from the central office to a satellite office closer to home
- Changing floors or work area location at the same site

Retraining or Reassignment

Starting a new career path may be the best choice if the patient is unable to resume pre-stroke tasks, even with reasonable accommodations. As outlined in the ADA, employers are obligated to provide the necessary retraining as long as it does not cause "an undue hardship" to the business. The ADA states that "A current worker with a disability is eligible to be reassigned to those jobs for which s/he is qualified to perform. The only alternate placement positions to be considered are those that are currently vacant, or will be vacant within a reasonable amount of time."

Here are two examples of job accommodations. First, a librarian with a stroke who now must use a wheelchair is reassigned from the third floor to a similar position on the first floor. The building does not have an elevator, and it would be an "undue hardship" for the business to install one. Second, a legal secretary, who also answered phones and scheduled appointments, was unable to sustain eight hours of work at one time. A computer station was set up at home together with a change of duties involving more computer research, less typing, and no phone answering.

STATE VR AND WORKERS COMPENSATION PROGRAMS THAT PROVIDE VR ASSISTANCE

For patients who are under the age of 65 and therefore too young to receive Social Security retirement benefits, the following information provides an overview of the state VR and workers compensation programs that provide VR assistance.

State VR Programs

Under the Rehabilitation Act of 1973, each state receives federal grants to operate a comprehensive VR program. These state-operated programs are designed to assess, plan, develop, and provide VR services to eligible individuals with disabilities. An individual with a disability is defined as any individual who has a physical or mental impairment that constitutes or results in a substantial impediment to employment and can benefit from VR services to become employed. Individuals who receive SSDI or SSI benefits are presumed to be eligible. Services are available, on a sliding scale fee, depending on the individual's financial resources.

Workers Compensation

Workers Compensation (WC) replaces income that is lost because of a job-related injury or illness. It is a state-mandated insurance program that provides compensation to employees who suffer job-related injuries and illness. In most states, employers are required to purchase insurance for their employees from a workers compensation insurance company. In some states, companies with fewer than four employees are not required to carry WC insurance. In some states larger employers who are financially stable are allowed to act as their own WC insurance company (self-insured). Each state has its own laws and programs. WC provides replacement income, medical expenses, and vocational rehabilitation. Benefits are generally two-thirds of gross weekly wages and are exempt from income tax. Many states cap the maximum amounts and duration of benefits that employees may receive. The federal government also administers a worker's compensation program for federal employees.

Managing Benefits during Periods of Disability

If a stroke survivor cannot or chooses not to retain his/her job, there are programs that exist to minimize gaps in pay and health coverage. Following is a brief summary overview of these programs.

SSI/SSDI. Social Security Disability Insurance (SSDI) is an insurance program for workers who become unable to work. It is administered by the Social Security Administration and is funded by FICA tax, which is withheld from workers' pay, and by employers' contributions. Workers who have worked and paid FICA tax for at least five of the ten years prior to onset of disability will generally be covered by SSDI. Patients can apply for SSDI benefits at any Social Security Administration office or by calling toll-free at 800-772-1213.

The Supplemental Security Income (SSI) program makes cash assistance payments to aged, blind, and disabled people who have limited income and resources. The program is paid through general tax revenues.

The two programs share many concepts but are different in the rules affecting eligibility and benefit payments. Both define disability as the inability to engage in any substantial gainful activity (SGA) because of a medically determinable physical or mental impairment.

For more specific information about these programs, the Social Security Administration publishes a yearly Red Book that can be found at Social Security offices or by accessing it on the internet at http://www.socialsecurity.gov/redbook/redbook.htm.

When someone is approved for services, he/she is referred to the state VR program for assistance. For those who receive SSDI, there is an incentive program to regain income. It is called "Ticket to Work" and provides increased choice regarding obtaining employment services, vocational rehabilitation services, and other support services necessary to get or keep a job. This program is available in all 50 states and in United States territories.

Short-/Long-Term Disability. Disability insurance covers income lost because of injuries and illnesses that are not job related. A disability can mean any illness or injury that prevents working at the pre-stroke routine job for an extended period of time.

Short-term disability insurance covers possible gaps in coverage and pays a monthly benefit while a patient is disabled. It may supplement benefits from Social Security or Workers Compensation. It generally provides up to 60% of pay for a benefit period for three to six months. Preexisting conditions may not be covered. Employers may offer short-term disability insurance as part of their benefits package or it can be purchased privately, prior to illness.

In general, short-term disability plans cover employees for a maximum of three months of illness. There is normally a six-month waiting period to qualify for long-term disability benefits. Although the original period of illness covered by short-term disability plan will be counted toward the six-month waiting period for short-/long-term disability benefits, there may be a gap when no benefits are available. If a disability is expected to last longer than this period, it is important to apply for disability benefits through Social Security.

Long-term disability insurance usually begins after the short-term disability coverage period ends and covers a portion of salary in case an employee is out of work for an extended period of illness. The combination of living expenses and lack of income could bring extreme financial hardship to a family: disability insurance provides replacement income.

COBRA. The Consolidated Omnibus Budget Reconciliation Act of 1985 (COBRA) requires most employers with group health plans to offer employees the opportunity to continue temporarily their group health care coverage under their employer's plan if their coverage otherwise would cease because of termination, layoff, or other change in employment status. This coverage must be paid for by the patient.

FMLA. The Family and Medical Leave Act (FMLA) of 1993 is a federal law that protects patients and family members from being fired during an illness. It states that a person cannot be fired while they are out of work temporarily (up to 12 weeks) from an illness or while they are providing care for a sick or disabled family member. The law does not require that the person who is not working be paid, but rather protects him/her from losing his/her job. Employers commonly have their own version of a FMLA leave form, but in general it asks that a physician document provide a diagnosis and estimate how long a leave will be needed. For the family member of a stroke survivor who plans on taking leave from work, it asks what services or care will be provided, such as driving to medical appointments, supervision and assistance with daily activities, and mobility and psychological support.

The employer must maintain group health benefits than an employee was receiving at the time the leave began. FMLA leave may be taken in blocks of time less than the full 12 weeks on an intermittent or reduced leave basis.

HIPAA. The Health Insurance Portability and Accountability Act (HIPAA), signed into law by President Clinton in 1996, enhanced the portability and continuity of health insurance coverage.

The act does the following:

- Limits exclusions for preexisting medical conditions, provides credit against maximum preexisting condition exclusion periods for prior health coverage, and a process for providing certificates showing periods of prior coverage to a new group health plan or health insurance issuer
- Provides rights for individuals to enroll for health coverage when they lose other health coverage, get married, or add a new dependent
- Prohibits discrimination in enrollment and in premiums charged to employees and their dependents based on health status-related factors
- Guarantees availability of health insurance coverage for small employers and renewability of health insurance coverage for both small and large employers
- Preserves the states' role in regulating health insurance, including the states' authority to provide greater protections than those available under federal law

The law defines a preexisting condition as one for which medical advice, diagnosis, care, or treatment was recommended or received during the six-month period prior to an individual's enrollment date (which is the earlier of the first day of health coverage or the first day of any waiting period for coverage). Group health plans and issuers may not exclude an individual's preexisting medical condition from coverage for more than 12 months (18 months for late enrollees) after an individual's enrollment date. Under HIPAA, a new employer's plan must give individuals credit for the length of time they had prior continuous health coverage, without a break in coverage of 63 days or more, thereby reducing or eliminating the 12-month exclusion period (18 months for late enrollees).

Creditable coverage includes prior coverage under another group health plan, an individual health insurance policy, COBRA, Medicaid, Medicare, CHAMPUS, the Indian Health Service, a state health benefits risk pool, FEHBP, the Peace Corps Act, or a public health plan. Certificates of creditable coverage must be provided automatically and free of charge by the plan or issuer when an individual loses coverage under the plan, becomes entitled to elect COBRA continuation coverage or exhausts COBRA continuation coverage. A certificate must also be provided free of charge upon request while the individual has health coverage or anytime within 24 months after that coverage ends.

CONCLUSION AND COMMENT

There is now a wealth of information available on the career development of older adults, trends in the work force, career mobility, life and career transitions, exploring second careers, retirement, and moving from full-time to flextime work. However, limited information is available about working with a disability, aging with a disability, and the career choices available to stroke survivors or other individuals with disabilities.

In this era of job transition there are many highly trained people who are finding themselves displaced by organizational restructuring, downsizing, outsourcing, and changes in technology. Patients desiring to start a business have increasing opportunities in fields such as health, nutrition, workforce training, and technology. By identifying existing job experience, retirees and people with disabilities are finding new ways to stay productive. Forced retirements and early retirement incentives have contributed to a decline in the workforce. At the same time, inflation, increasing health care costs, and inadequate pensions are forcing older adults to reenter the work force. This is forcing employers to provide accommodations for these workers. Retirement can be described as a permanent separation from work. This is frequently being replaced with "bridge" employment, in which an older worker disengages more slowly with periods of temporary, part-time, occasional, or self-employed work.

Developments in computers and communications have made it more practical and realistic to be able to work from home. Part-time or flexible work arrangements can be equally beneficial to both the employer and the employee. Older workers have benefited directly and indirectly from recent economic changes and downturns. Flextime jobs are usually not advertised. Patients can anticipate what an employer needs and must network with business contacts, friends, and acquaintances to research opportunities.

References

1. Different Strokes Web site. Available at http://www.differentstrokes.co.uk. Accessed Nov. 2007.
2. Stein J. Personal communication.
3. Braddom RL. *Physical Medicine & Rehabilitation*. 3rd ed. Philadelphia: Saunders, 2006: 1192,1202.
4. Gresham GE, Philips TF, Wolf PA, et al. Opidemiologic profile of long-term stroke disability, the Framingham Study. *Archives PM&R* 1979; 60:487.
5. Treger SJ, Cuaquinto H. Return to work in stroke patients. *Disability and Rehabilitation* 2007; 29(17)1397–1403.
6. Wozniak MA, Kittner SJ, Price TR, et al. Stroke location is not associated with return to work after first ischemic stroke. *Stroke* 1999; 30:2568–2573.
7. Saeki S, Hachisuka K. The association between stroke location and return to work after first stroke. *J Stroke Cerebrovasc Dis*. 2004; 13(4):160–163.
8. Saeki S, Ogata H, Okubo T, et al. Return to work after stroke: A follow-up study. *Stroke* 1995; 26:399–401.
9. Joynt RJ, Return to work after stroke. *JAMA* 1985; 253(2):249.
10. Kittner SK. Stroke in the young: Coming of age. *Neurology* 2002; 59(1):6–7.
11. Carney RM. Freedland KE. Psychological distress as a risk factor for stroke-related mortality. *Stroke* 2002; 33:5–6,
12. James B, Talmage MP, Mark J, Melborn MP. *A Physician's Guide to Return to Work*. Chicago: American Medical Association, 2005. 7–12, 267–283.
13. Sarno MT, Levita E. Observations on the nature of recovery in global aphasia after a stroke. *Brain Language* 1981; 13:1–12.
14. Sarno MT, Levita E. Recovery in treated aphasia in the first year post stroke. *Stroke* 1979; 10:662–670.
15. Prins RS, Snow CE, Wagennar E. Recovery from aphasia spontaneous speech verbal language comprehension. *Brain Language* 1978; 6:192–211.
16. US Department of Labor. Job Accommodation Network. Available at http://www.jan.wvu.edu/links/adalinks.htm. Accessed Nov. 2007.
17. US Department of Labor. Available at http://online.onetcenter.org/link/summary/21-1015.00. Accessed Nov. 2007.

47 Challenges in Community Rehabilitation

Brendan E. Conroy
Richard D. Zorowitz
Fatemeh Milani

Carol Bartlett
Karen Tyner

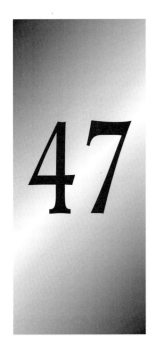

The primary challenge of community stroke rehabilitation is to maximize participation of the stroke survivor in the community. Appropriate equipment and community resources must be identified, and reimbursement from third-party payers and other sources must be secured.

CHALLENGES OF THE TRANSITION FROM INPATIENT TO COMMUNITY REHABILITATION

Stroke survivors often face very difficult transitions when being discharged from an inpatient rehabilitation or skilled nursing facility to home. During an inpatient stay, a stroke survivor has round-the-clock nursing care, daily therapy, and daily physician visits. The structured, accessible environment of an inpatient rehabilitation facility may give the stroke survivor and caregivers a false sense of security when they return to the unstructured, less accessible community setting. Once home, the stroke survivor may only have the support of a spouse, a child, or a paid third party as a primary caregiver (PCG). The patient and PCG may have only several pieces of equipment for mobility and the activities of daily living. The stroke survivor may be exhausted from the move home

and may not yet be 100% continent of bladder. On the other hand, bowel control is regained by 70% of patients by day 10 after a stroke and 90% by day 90 (1). The rehabilitation physician must anticipate these difficulties and ensure that the patient is prepared for them.

At home, patients tend to be very demanding and irritable with the PCG. They often ask for constant attendance and assistance, especially during the first few weeks at home. This may be a manifestation of their anxiety over being home without hospital support. The PCG may try to get errands done and get a little rest in between attending to the stroke survivor's needs. Nighttime may be particularly challenging. Incontinence can necessitate frequent adult diaper and bedclothes changes. The PCG may choose to sleep in a separate room from the stroke survivor in order to get some rest. This is often a good idea. Overt praise for what the PCG is doing may encourage and acknowledge that the work that the PCG is doing is hard while it is an investment in the potential recovery of the stroke survivor. It is very important to support the PCG and maintain an awareness of their health and coping status. If the PCG becomes ill or becomes discouraged that their task is unending, the stroke survivor may suffer a setback and require reinstitutionalization (2, 3).

It may be very helpful and appropriate for the PCG and the patient to agree upon limits and rules for requests for assistance. The patient may be expected to abide by a toileting schedule and not to ask for more assistance at a specific time after something is done. Often a PCG gives too much help, leading to his own imprisonment. The PCG may start doing certain activities, such as bathing or dressing, for the patient in order to reduce the amount of time spent on that activity. However, if the PCG does this, the stroke survivor will never become independent in any activity that they are not forced to practice.

There are additional challenges for the rehabilitation provider who is seeing the stroke survivor for their first outpatient visit. The inpatient setting is ideal for a rehabilitation provider to meet and start working with the stroke survivor. Resources are immediately available for the evaluation of and use by the stroke survivor. Appropriate equipment is nearby in a hallway stockroom, and teams of rehabilitation nurses and therapists can readily assess the stroke survivor's impairments and disabilities, such as responsiveness, learning capacity, and carryover. They also can observe physiologic and behavioral responses to activity, such as orthostatic hypotension, arrhythmias, or elevated blood pressure. The team also can observe the stroke survivor's and PCG's mood and general behavior, which can help to assess the strength of the stroke survivor's socioeconomic support system and to diagnose psychological issues such as depression, anxiety disorders, abulia, or overstimulation. The sooner such assessments are completed, the sooner appropriate therapeutic choices can be made to treat secondary complications or to optimize medications. These evaluations and treatments may be delayed in the outpatient setting for reasons such as bureaucratic issues, the locations of the physician and therapists, or the illegibility of handwritten documentation. In the outpatient setting, the physician also lacks the opportunity to obtain a daily assessment of the stroke survivor. Team assessment processes and information resources are much more difficult to access. Outpatient therapists often do not have time to participate in team conferences, and paper documentation does not always reliably get from the writer to the appropriate reader. The initial assessment of the new outpatient may be more disjointed and less efficient. Electronic medical records may eventually help with this inefficiency. In most health care systems, the ongoing outpatient treatment process may lack routine interdisciplinary updates and team goals.

Insurance Reimbursement Issues

When a patient is hospitalized, virtually all commercial third-party payers require periodic updates from the admitting institution. The case manager sends reports from each of the therapists to the insurance case manager and receives in return authorization for an additional period. Coverage becomes even less predictable after discharge and varies greatly, not only between insurance carriers but also from one policy to the next. Some policies may limit the number of days or sessions of therapy, and some may not have any rehabilitation or durable medical equipment benefits at all. Each situation must be evaluated on an individual basis, and stroke survivors should be educated about the restrictions and limitations of their policies.

Some HMO and PPO policies require the primary care physician to manage the stroke survivor's health care. All procedures, therapies, and follow-up appointments may require a referral from the primary care physician. Some plans permit out-of-network benefits at additional cost, but some restrict patients to the insurance company's preferred providers.

Many third-party payers use Medicare guidelines as their gold standard for authorization of home or outpatient care. Medicare pays for home or outpatient therapy as prescribed by a physician as long as measurable progress can be documented by the therapists. Home therapy is justified if a patient is deemed to be homebound. Home therapy is short term and transitional, and emphasizes progression to outpatient therapy as soon as possible. Medicare also may provide up to six hours per week of home health aide assistance if prescribed by the physician. Home health aides assist stroke survivors with personal care needs, but they may not assist with any household tasks. Medicare will also allow an RN to visit stroke survivors if they require medical care at home. Neither Medicare nor commercial third-party payers pay for transportation to and from medical appointments, but some city and county governments may provide transportation services for those who are physically challenged.

Medicaid or medical assistance plans are administered on a state-by-state basis. Coverage varies greatly, depending on the patient's home location. State Medicaid programs often provide for home care to exceed the Medicare guidelines. Some Medicaid programs provide as much as four to eight hours of personal care assistance. Some jurisdictions have a waiver program that provides for additional hours of coverage, but these programs often have lengthy waiting lists. State Medicaid will sometimes pay for transportation to and from medical appointments.

Prescription coverage also varies greatly from one insurance program to another. The new Medicare Part D prescription plans may assist patients who do not have secondary insurance. Most Medicare recipients who have other insurance coverage have opted to continue their commercial coverage for prescription medications. Stroke survivors who have both Medicare and state Medicaid are assigned a prescription plan. The stroke survivor should call the Social Security Administration to ascertain the plan to which they have been assigned and to learn the details of the terms of the prescription plan. Social Security is very careful about confidentiality and will not share any information about benefits, coverage, or personal data with anyone except the patient or the patient's power of attorney. Social Security staff will talk by telephone, but the patient must be present and give consent.

A TYPICAL OUTPATIENT REHABILITATION PHYSICIAN VISIT

History and Physical

Each visit should commence with checking vital signs, weighing the stroke survivor, asking about pain concerns, and listing current needs. The history should include the type and date of stroke, a list of comorbidities, and when they saw their primary care physician. The clinician should ask the stroke survivor about his functional status and confirm all observations with the PCG or family member if they have accompanied the stroke survivor. One should ask about any need for assistance in bathing, dressing, toileting and continence; language and cognitive dysfunction; swallowing; household and community mobility on surfaces and stairs; nutritional issues; and, if appropriate, driving and return-to-work issues. A detailed pain history should include location, frequency, intensity, and exacerbating and alleviating factors. The most common pain complaint is from the involved shoulder, usually with movement. A review of systems should include questions about falls, seizures, mood/depression, appetite, bowel regularity, sleep, and sexual function.

A physical examination should include a general review of the heart, lungs, and abdomen. It should also include some standard assessment of cognition and language capacity. Active and passive range of motion, strength, and sensation should be evaluated in the affected and unaffected limbs. Skin areas under orthoses should be inspected for pressure injury. A functional examination of transfers, ambulation, and activities of daily living should be documented.

Assessment and Talking to Patients

It is very important to provide feedback to stroke survivors. A detailed review of functional progress that has been made, further reasonable improvements that might be expected, and potential future problems that might be expected will give the stroke survivor reassurance and confidence. As time passes, stroke survivors may discover "new" impairments, such as persistent sensory impairments, minor cognitive problems, coordination problems, and an inability to concentrate on reading. As major changes caused by the stroke are understood and treated, awareness of lesser impairments grows. These problems may become less of an issue with reassurance by their "stroke doctor" that they have been present all along but were not previously recognized by the patient. It is therapeutically valuable for the patient to know that

new problems will not constantly be cropping up. However, it is also important for the stroke survivor to consult his primary care physician for treatment of comorbidities, such as diabetes mellitus and hypertension, as well as other medical issues not attributable to the stroke.

Stroke survivors will have a strong sense of trust in the rehabilitation physicians who have guided them successfully through stroke recovery and will place great value on their explanations about ongoing or new medical problems. Rehabilitation physicians, by the nature of their training and work, learn how to explain medical issues to laypeople. Consequently patients will turn to the rehabilitation physicians to get "approval" and understanding of upcoming medical procedures and treatments, such as carotid stenting or cardiac endarterectomy (CEA) (4), common coronary or cardiac procedures. Patients undergoing a procedure may suffer a temporary setback in cognition or an exacerbation of hemiparesis.

Finally, discussions with the stroke survivor may include a review of prescribed therapies as well as the goals of the therapies. A health promotion program should include medication compliance, home health monitoring of blood pressure, finger sticks, international normalized ratio (INR), and diet, and should emphasize the importance of regular aerobic exercise (5). The stroke survivor and PCG may wish to discuss various options of therapy, such as CEA or stenting. Finally, a return visit should be scheduled.

Prognostication

Prognostication of recovery from a stroke is not a science. A myriad of factors should be considered. There are general considerations that can help the rehabilitation physician make educated guesses about how much further improvement can be expected.

Generally, prognosis is good for a stroke survivor. Approximately 80% of stroke survivors walk again within a year following the stroke (6, 7). Eighty-five percent of stroke survivors recover normal swallowing (8). Forty percent of survivors who are of working age are able to return to work (9). Ninety percent are able to return to home, usually with some degree of persistent disability (9, 10). With respect to the return of arm movement, the dominant side typically recovers better than the non-dominant side. Motor recovery is better in a limb that has good sensory function than a limb that has lost a significant amount of sensation. Sensory modalities of greatest importance are light touch (LT) and proprioception, in addition to pinprick discrimination (Table 47-1) (11). The rate of recovery of arm use is inconsistent and highly dependent on personal motivation, preservation of sensation, hand dominance, mood/depression, spasticity, and location of the stroke. Stroke survivors with aphasia typically do not recover full fluency of speech but often recover functional

TABLE 47-1
Prognostic Factors (11)

Factors having good prognostic significance:
   Preserved light touch and proprioception
   Distal before proximal motor recovery
   Any early motor recovery
   Patient motivation
   Good family support
   First stroke
   Early recovery of bowel and bladder control
   Younger stroke survivors

Factors having negative prognostic significance:
   Persistently flaccid limb two weeks or more post-stroke
   Severe sensory impairment, especially of light touch
     and proprioception
   Depression
   Poor family support
   Severe mixed aphasia
   Advanced age, especially with multiple comorbidities
   Severe visuospatial neglect
   Secondary stroke

communication ability. Whatever language capacity they have may be combined with gestures, sounds, and yes or no responses. A speech-language pathologist treating a stroke survivor with aphasia may often continue long after physical therapy (PT) and occupational therapy (OT) therapies have concluded.

Stroke type and location have a powerful effect on the amount of recovery seen in stroke survivors (12). Stroke survivors with isolated lacunar strokes tend to recover better than those with big infarcts. However, lacunar strokes are seldom singular, as they may be typically one of a series of subclinical subcortical injuries that progressively and insidiously affect the degree of motor or cognitive impairment not consistent with the presenting lesion (13). Hemorrhagic strokes have a much higher early mortality rate than infarcts, but the recovery potential may be better if the patient survives. If a patient has a second hemorrhage, the prognosis is not as good. Likewise, hemorrhagic conversion of an infarct is not favorable for rehabilitation outcome because it may worsen alertness and cognitive capacity in general. The risk of having another clinical stroke after having the first one is 7–10% per year (9, 11, 14).

TYPES OF COMMUNITY REHABILITATION SETTINGS

Home Therapies

In most metropolitan and rural areas, there are very well-established systems of home care nurses and therapists that can begin providing rehabilitation services to stroke survivors on the day after the patient is discharged from the hospital if these services are given sufficient notice. It is a good practice for the rehabilitation physician to begin discussions about discharge therapies during an inpatient family conference, during which the orders for post-discharge rehabilitation therapies can be written. The principal details of the discharge plan should include equipment, follow-up therapies and medical visits, identification of the PCG and when the PCG will receive training, and the elements of the stroke survivor's health promotion plan. A social worker can assess the appropriateness of the home environment and support systems.

Home-based therapy can ease the transition from hospitalization to home living. The primary goal of home-based therapy is to improve function such that the stroke survivor can navigate in his home and eventually access the community (15, 16). It is indicated for patients who still require significant assistance for household mobility and activities of daily living. Home therapy is highly functionally oriented and time-limited. Once supervised or independent household mobility has been achieved, it is appropriate to graduate the patient to an outpatient rehabilitation therapy setting. Families tend to lack enthusiasm about this transition, because it adds another significant inconvenience to the care of the stroke survivor—transportation to and from a therapy center. However, home-based rehabilitation is a limited resource, and it must be prescribed with discretion—based on the clinical needs, not the convenience, of the stroke survivor.

Home-based nursing can be a wonderful resource for assessing a patient's medical status and reinforcing health promotion education. The nurse intermittently can monitor vital signs and teach PCGs how to take them and how to react when they obtain abnormal vital sign readings. Home care nurses also can draw blood for drug levels and for INR/anti-coagulation measurement. They can help initiate a home intravenous (IV) or tube feeding program and make sure the PCG is able to manage the process.

Outpatient Therapies

In the outpatient environment, the rehabilitation therapists continue treatment to build upon the improvements that were started in the hospital, in the rehabilitation facility, or at home. The primary goal of outpatient therapy is to maximize recovery and give the stroke survivor the tools to maintain or further facilitate functional improvement. Therapists will fine-tune the stroke survivor's gait pattern so the patient can access the community with optimal efficiency and safety. Lower-extremity orthotics can be ordered, modified, or discontinued based on the patient's evolving needs.

Outpatient therapy is not restricted to physical therapy, occupational therapy, and speech-language pathology. Outpatient rehabilitation can include a comprehensive interdisciplinary day hospital, psychological consultation, vocational rehabilitation, therapeutic recreation, access to orthotists, and rehabilitation engineering. Stroke survivors also may be considered for rehabilitation research protocols, or under certain circumstances they may work with student therapists at rehabilitation therapist training schools.

Home, No Longer in Therapy

For stroke survivors, rehabilitation therapies facilitate the natural recovery process. If the therapist judges that a "plateau" may be occurring, therapy may no longer be justified. It is often disappointing and frustrating for stroke survivors and PCGs when the stroke survivor has not achieved full recovery and still requires some level of assistance. The patient may continue to improve in spite of the discontinuation of therapies in terms of fatigue level, smoothness of gait pattern, smoothness of talking, and promptness of thinking.

Another more difficult circumstance is the stroke survivor who has not made meaningful improvement with therapy due to the severity of motor, cognitive, or communication dysfunction. The rehabilitation approach may shift to the provision of compensatory devices or adaptive equipment, as well as the use of compensatory strategies to optimize functional tasks.

SPECIFIC CHALLENGES OF COMMUNITY STROKE REHABILITATION

Pain

Pain often occurs in stroke survivors due to the underuse or overuse of joints, soft tissues, and muscles. Osteoarthritic pain may flare up in the knee, hip, or shoulder. Asymmetric weight-bearing patterns caused by weakness can cause arthritic knees and hips to become achy and sore. Gout can flare up. This pain can be treated by use of acetaminophen or non-steroidal anti-inflammatory drugs (NSAID) as indicated.

Another cause of pain in the stroke survivor is neuropathy. Stroke survivors may claim they had no problems with burning, tingling pain prior to the stroke, but the stroke or comorbid conditions may cause neuropathic symptoms to reach a perceptible level. This pain responds to a number of medications, such as tricyclic antidepressants, gabalin medications, other anti-epileptic medications, or mexiletine (17).

TABLE 47-2
Differential Diagnosis of Hemiplegic Shoulder Pain (47)

Acromio-clavicular dysfunction
Adhesive capsulitis
Central post-stroke pain syndrome
Fracture of clavicle after a fall
Heterotopic ossification
Myofascial pain syndrome—of the trapezius, supraspinatus, infraspinatus, levator scapula, rhomboids, and/or scalenes
Osteoarthritic gleno-humeral pain
Rotator cuff tendonitis
Spasticity of internal rotators with tightening
Subdeltoid bursitis
Traction/compression neuropathy

Shoulder Pain

When taking a pain history, a stroke survivor often may complain of pain in his involved shoulder (18, 19) usually with movement and occasionally associated with wrist or rarely elbow pain. The pain may awaken the survivor at night. The differential diagnosis includes osteoarthitic gleno-humeral pain, adhesive capsulitis, myofascial pain syndrome, acromio-clavicular dysfunction, rotator cuff tendonitis, subdeltoid bursitis, etc. (Table 47-2). Details of the diagnosis and treatment of shoulder pain may be found in chapter 26.

Weakness

Stroke survivors are not actually weak, as in myopathy. Their muscles have unimpaired capacity for contraction. The patient has impaired neurologic capacity to generate appropriately timed impulses in alpha motor neurons to cause muscle tissue to contract when needed. The problems caused by a stroke are twofold:

1. Impairment of the ability to generate an impulse in the anterior horn cell of the spinal cord reliably
2. Impairment of the ability to generate an impulse with the correct timing

Physical therapists and occupational therapists work with stroke survivors on positioning, tone inhibition, and motor control timing to improve functional capacity for tasks. Therapeutic approaches, such as neuro-developmental therapy (NDT), proprioceptive neuromuscular facilitation (PNF) and the motor control theory (20, 21) are based on the pioneering observations and research performed by Twitchell (22), Bobath (23), Rude, and Brunnstrom. Motor learning also may be used to decrease tone.

Speech-Language Disorders and Dysphagia

Speech-language impairments and swallowing problems often persist well into the community setting. Dysarthria often resolves spontaneously or with therapy. Dysphagia can take 9–12 months to resolve, most often for strokes involving the brain stem (8, 24). A videofluorographic swallow study should be repeated periodically to monitor the recovery and to update dietary recommendations. Lung sounds should be checked because aspiration pneumonia may occur in patients with chronic dysphagia. Chronic aphasia therapy with a speech-language pathologist or PCG is a long, slow process of rebuilding functional communication through the use of phonated output, verbal and/or written communication of words or symbols, and yes/no responses and gestures (25, 26).

Mood Disorders

Depression.   The most common mood disorder suffered by stroke survivors is depression (27, 28). The time frame to onset of depression is described as peaking at six months (29), but depression can affect self-care activities even two years after a stroke (30). Depressed mood can show up within two weeks following the stroke. Prior to the availability of serotonin-specific reuptake inhibitors (SSRIs) in the mid-1990s, tricyclic antidepressants (TCAs) and trazodone were commonly prescribed. Anticholinergic side effects of the TCAs include urinary retention and memory impairment, as well as occasional problems with confusion and agitation. However, TCAs continue to be effective antidepressant medications for stroke survivors. Lipsey showed that nortriptyline was equally effective as methylphenidate in alleviating post-stroke depression four weeks after the stroke, although methylphenidate worked much faster (29). It may take three weeks for the antidepressant effect of SSRIs to "kick in," although the medications seem to act faster when they are given in the early stages of post-stroke depressed mood. A more recent study comparing the clinical efficacy of amitryptiline to fluoxetine found that both were helpful, but that depression scores significantly improved when TCAs were used (31).

SSRIs have fewer side effects and are quite well tolerated by stroke survivors (32). Fluoxetine has a slightly enervating effect and can be selected if the patient suffers from an abulic low-energy depression (33). Paroxetine and trazodone may be sedating and can be given at night if the stroke survivor is having difficulty sleeping. Sertraline has little impact on level of alertness, but its most notorious side effect is reduction of libido (34, 35). Citalopram, escitalopram, and venlafaxine also seem to be well tolerated.

Other helpful antidepressants include mirtazepine, which has a mild appetite-stimulating and weight gain

---

| TABLE 47-3 |
| *Serotonin Syndrome Signs and Symptoms (3)* |

Agitated restlessness
Confusion
Confused talking
Diaphoresis
Diarrhea
Hyperreflexia
Hyperthermia
Insomnia
Myoclonus
Tachypnea
Seizures and coma

---

effect. Bupropion is a good choice for the patient who has anxiety or who is trying to quit smoking, but it may lower the seizure threshold. No matter which medicine is chosen, it is always appropriate to refer the patient to a psychologist for a disturbance of mood.

Anxiety.   Anxiety also may occur following a stroke. Anxiety is associated with a sense of being overwhelmed by new difficulties that lead to hyperacusis, the thought that every little twitch or bump is a sign of a new stroke. Medications that may assist with reducing anxiety include bupropion and buspirone. Sometimes buspirone can cause vivid dreams that may worsen difficulties differentiating between reality and dreamed or imagined experiences. Some SSRI medications also have an anxiolytic effect, although they take awhile to "kick in."

Benzodiazepine medications generally are not appropriate for stroke survivors. They are gamma-aminobutyric acid (GABA) inhibitors and have multiple unwanted side effects, such as sedation, depression of mood, addictiveness, amnesiogenesis, and impairment of ventilatory drive (34). The long half-life benzodiazepines, such as diazepam (Valium) and flurazepam (Dalmane), can accumulate in the slower-metabolizing bodies of the elderly and precipitate agitation and delirium (36).

Cognitive Impairment

In general, cognitive impairments of stroke survivors tend to resolve with time. Typical cognitive impairments observed in acute stroke survivors are delayed processing, impaired delayed recall, poor problem solving, poor safety awareness, impaired sequencing, reduced hemispatial awareness (e.g., neglect), poor pragmatics for activities such as turn taking in conversation, distractibility, impaired attention span/concentration capacity, and poor insight about impairments caused by the stroke. By the time a year has passed, 80–85% of the impairments caused by a stroke may resolve (37). Stroke survivors who require

24-hour supervision or assistance may be left alone at home for periods of time while a spouse returns to work or community activity. Speech-language pathologists and occupational therapists can accelerate this recovery, especially by engaging the stroke survivor in community-based exercises of problem solving or safety awareness. As a cognitive exercise, stroke survivors may practice walking on broken sidewalks, ramps, spiral staircases, crowded streets, curbs without curb cuts, and stairs without handrails. Neuropsychology also may help with outpatient cognitive retraining after a stroke, as will testing to establish baselines for interventions and to quantitatively document cognitive disability.

Stimulants such as dextroamphetamine and methylphenidate are safe (38) and can have a beneficial effect for stroke survivors complaining of impaired concentration or cognitive fatigue. Dextroamphetamines have been found to exert positive effects on mood and performance of cognitive tasks (38) but may have variable effects on motor control in humans (39, 40) and animal models (41). There also is some intriguing but inconclusive suggestion of a benefit for aphasia (42). When considering medications for use in controlling agitation and confusion in the stroke survivor, the Post-Stroke Rehabilitation Outcomes Project (PSROP) observed a positive association between use of atypical antipsychotic medications and functional outcomes during inpatient rehabilitation, whereas use of benzodiazepines had a negative association (43).

Sexuality

Stroke survivors and their partners may be hesitant, if not downright afraid, to resume sexual relations. As part of a review of systems, it is important to ask whether sex has been attempted. When the stroke survivor comes for his first outpatient visit after discharge home, it is likely that the stroke survivor and partner have not attempted sexual activity. However, there is rarely disinterest in the subject. The stroke survivor and partner should be assured that the risk of another stroke during orgasm is no worse than for a person who has not had a stroke. Anticoagulation therapy is not a contraindication for sex. If the patient has active coronary artery disease or a recent myocardial infarction, schedule an exercise/stress tolerance test prior to allowing sexual activity to resume. The patient should be able to tolerate at least five metabolic equivalents (mets) of activity, roughly the equivalent of walking up two flights of stairs without undue discomfort, to be cleared cardiologically for sexual activity.

Erectile dysfunction (ED) is often a post-stroke problem for men (44). Causes may include medications such as beta-blockers, clonidine, sertraline, or narcotics. Persistent incontinence of bladder or bowel may inhibit libido. A history of erectile dysfunction may be worsened by the impaired motor control and balance caused by the stroke. Prostate problems, hypertension, and diabetes also are common causes of erectile dysfunction.

The most common cause of ED is psychological (44). The fear of failure during love-making can and does cause dysfunction. Depression also may have a detrimental effect on sexual function. Suggest the stroke survivor may want to try masturbation prior to approaching their partner. By "trying out the plumbing" first, the stroke survivor may build confidence and not worry about being able to attain an erection or orgasm.

If a male stroke survivor is unsuccessful with masturbation or an attempt at intercourse, it is appropriate to refer the stroke survivor to a urologist. Prescriptions for erectile treatments should be given after an appropriate diagnostic evaluation is completed. The stroke survivor's primary care physician or cardiologist may wish to have the final say on these medications.

After a stroke, women may have difficulties with lubrication for ease of penetration. Use of a personal lubricant can help with this difficulty. Petroleum jelly is a desiccant of mucous membranes and should not be used. A referral to a urogynecologist for a post-menopausal woman may result in a prescription of estrogen supplementation or estrogen creams, which can have a dual benefit of improving bladder control as well as providing lubrication for sexual activity.

Education in sexual positions is essential for successful sexual intercourse. Many American couples have one position they use for sexual activity (e.g., missionary position with the man on top). It is usually more successful for the post-stroke couple to use the "spooning" position, with the man side-lying behind his partner, impaired side in decubitus. If the missionary position is preferred, the unimpaired partner should be positioned on top (45, 46). Restoration of a normal sex life to a stroke survivor and partner can be very valuable to the sense of getting back into normal life.

Vision

Vision is affected by stroke through impairment of visual acuity, ability to focus, diplopia, or loss of a portion of the visual field. Wearers of prescription glasses often may have difficulties with their pre-stroke glasses. A new prescription may be needed, but the stroke survivor should wait at least 10–12 weeks post-stroke before seeing an ophthalmologist to learn what spontaneous recovery of eye motor control, visual fields, or acuity has occurred. Brain stem strokes present more problems in this area because of the location of extraocular eye muscle control nuclei throughout the brain stem. In these cases, a referral to a neuro-ophthalmologist often is often very helpful.

The literature describing recovery of lost visual fields following an injury to the optic pathways of the

TABLE 47-4
*Stroke-Induced Impairments Disabling
to Driving Safety*

Hemispatial neglect
Delayed processing
Impaired reflexes
Impaired motor control
Impaired vision
Visual field cuts
Hemisensory impairment

supratentorial brain is quite pessimistic. However, some patients do recover a portion of the lost field of vision sufficient to qualify for a driver's license again, depending on the local state regulations for visual field.

Driving

Returning to driving probably is the second most important goal to a stroke survivor, next to being able to walk again. There are many problems caused by a stroke that are barriers to returning to safe driving (Table 47-4). Prior to clearing a stroke survivor for driving, the rehabilitation clinician should remind the stroke survivor that most people who get into car accidents are "able-bodied" and have not suffered a stroke. There may be a crushing sense of guilt if a stroke survivor is in an accident and hurts themselves or someone else. The stroke survivor will be held liable if he or she is involved in an accident without being cleared through appropriate channels.

On the other hand, stroke survivors typically are very worried that their license will be revoked. It is important that rehabilitation clinicians emphasize that license revocation is not necessarily permanent and that licenses can be reinstated with appropriate therapy and retesting. However, the rehabilitation clinician should also emphasize that driving is a privilege, not a right. If the stroke survivor is not safe on the road, he should not be driving. This explanation often is not satisfactory because a sense of personal identity and freedom can be lost when a license is revoked.

Multiple problems may impede a stroke survivor's ability to drive. First, impaired field of vision may be a major obstacle to driving. Each state has its own standards regarding the minimum field of vision required to qualify for a driver's license. Second, right hemiparesis may prevent a stroke survivor from controlling the brake and accelerator. Third, impairment of visuospatial perception may cause neglect. Fourth, marked sensory impairment of either side may cause difficulties in manipulating the foot and hand controls of a motor vehicle. Finally, delayed cognitive processing may make driving a very dangerous process.

Aphasia is not a contraindication to driving. The aphasic patient should carry a medic alert bracelet or information about themselves, should they be stopped.

To optimize a stroke survivor's chances to drive, the rehabilitation clinician should wait until the patient has become cognitively alert, prompt, appropriate, and self-aware before allowing a driving evaluation. At the earliest, this may occur several months post-stroke ictus (37). Ideally, each stroke survivor should be evaluated by a rehabilitation therapist certified in the state in which they live and work. In a pre-driver evaluation, the driving assessment therapist, usually an occupational therapist (OTR/L), tests general rules of the road, visual fields, and driving reflexes in an off-the-road simulator. The behind-wheel evaluation should be carried out in a vehicle equipped with dual steering wheel and controls.

The therapist also may recommend adaptive equipment that helps the stroke survivor compensate for impairments. A "spinner knob" attaches to the steering wheel and allows one-handed wheel control. A leftward brake or accelerator extension allows left foot control.

Once a driving evaluation is completed successfully, the stroke survivor must present himself to the local Department of Motor Vehicles (DMV) or Motor Vehicle Authority (MVA) for a full driver's test. State vehicle offices may repeat certain aspects of the pre-driver evaluation, such as visual fields. The stroke survivor's medical history is reviewed for seizures or other conditions that may cause motor or cognitive impairment. The stroke survivor will undergo another behind-wheel evaluation. Problems that may prevent a stroke survivor from passing a state behind-wheel evaluation include parallel parking or three-point turns.

Return to Work

Approximately 40% of stroke survivors under the age of 65 are able to return to work (11). The process of getting ready to work again can take at least one to two years. Barriers to returning to work are more likely to include aphasia and pain rather than than persistent hemiplegia or impaired cognition. The combined efforts of the stroke survivor, rehabilitation physician, social worker, and vocational rehabilitation (VR) therapist may be required for success. The process of vocational rehabilitation should wait until the stroke survivor has become independent at home in all areas of mobility and self-care. Ideally, preauthorization for VR is obtained from the insurer or employer, or stroke survivors may apply for aid from a state vocational rehabilitation agency. The VR will contact the stroke survivor's employer, who will provide a detailed work description of the stroke survivor's position. The VR uses the job description to develop a therapy program designed to restore the skills needed for work. In some cases, the VR may advise the stroke survivor and physician that returning to the pre-stroke job is not practical. If the stroke survivor cannot return to his premorbid employment, alternative employment opportunities and helpful therapies may be recommended (47).

Stroke survivors sometimes inquire whether they should retire from work on disability. Even if a stroke survivor applies for short-term disability, receiving this financial benefit does not mean that the patient will never be allowed to work again. Short-term disability may be just the solution that allows the stroke survivor to focus properly on the recovery process. Return to work is not a critical aspect of the early stage of stroke recovery. The stroke survivor must commit his time and energy to optimizing musculoskeletal, communicative, and cognitive capacity. Because a person young enough to return to work after stroke may have a life expectation of at least 20 or 30 more years, the few months focused on optimal recovery may pay off with many years of productivity.

Seizures

Post-stroke seizures happen more commonly in the community than in the hospital or inpatient rehabilitation facility (48, 49). The incidence of early seizures in stroke survivors is so low (<12%) that prophylaxis is not warranted in most cases. Seizures are more common in patients with cortical infarcts or hemorrhages than in patients affected in the subcortical brain matter. Cortical hemorrhages are associated with a sufficiently high incidence of seizure to justify antiseizure medication. Seizures are rare for infarcts in the infratentorial structures.

Seizure management may require a referral to a neurologist, but some familiarity with the medications is helpful. Phenytoin (Dilantin) is the most commonly prescribed antiseizure medication (50), but has several side effects. It is a common source of a pruritic maculopapular truncal rash often associated with eosinophilia, or the elevated liver enzymes alanine aminotransferase (ALT), aspartate aminotransferase (AST), and alkaline phosphatase. If it is not recognized and treated, a rash may progress to Stevens-Johnson syndrome, toxic epidermal necrolysis (TEN), or even death (34). The medication must be discontinued immediately if the rash is very pronounced as it can take several days for the rash to peak and clear. Another problem is Dilantin toxicity, characterized clinically by lateral nystagmus and "drunken" walking with loss of balance toward walls. Phenytoin levels should be monitored regularly and calculated against serum albumin. Because phenytoin is highly protein bound, a low-serum protein can hide an elevated free-serum phenytoin level. If possible, the phenytoin dosage should be tapered down prior to discontinuation, usually by reducing the dose by 100 mg every seven days, to minimize the risk of drug withdrawal seizures.

Carbamazepine and valproic acid also may be used for seizure management. Levels of both medications must be monitored. In a study of the impact of phenytoin, carbamazepine, and valproic acid on cognition in traumatic brain injury (TBI) patients, Massagli found that all had a negative impact on learning capacity, but carbamazepine caused the least problem (51). Levetiracetam (Keppra) is a newer antiseizure medication that seems to be effective and well tolerated. Blood-level monitoring is not required. Its effect on learning capacity has not been quantified nor compared against other agents.

INTERNET RESOURCES FOR THE STROKE SURVIVOR

(Adapted and updated with permission from: Zorowitz RD, Returning to life: Stroke survivor community and Internet resources. *Phys Med Rehabil Clin N Am* 1999; 10(4): 967–985.)

Smoothing the transition between the hospital and home can be accomplished through many support services and organizations that the stroke survivor finds in his community. While visiting nurse associations and outpatient facilities provide much needed care for the stroke survivor, other groups can provide the networks that the stroke survivor requires for the remainder of his life. Groups are available for both the stroke survivor and his caregivers. Some deal with the psychological issues that complicate a stroke survivor's life. Others address financial and vocational issues. This directory lists many of the organizations that assist stroke survivors in making their lives as normal as possible. Addresses, phone numbers, e-mail, and descriptions of provided services are listed so that the rehabilitation professional or stroke survivor can efficiently contact these organizations, receive answers to questions, and alleviate fears. Organizations are listed in the following categories: stroke survivor support groups (adult and pediatric); caregiver support groups; funding sources; psychological services; patient rights groups; and vocational assistance.

Adult Stroke Survivor Support Groups

American Heart Association/American Stroke Association. The American Heart Association (AHA) is home to some of the most comprehensive information on strokes both on paper and on the Internet. The AHA is a source for information on stroke risks and warning signs, patient information, medical and surgical treatments, women's issues, and rehabilitation. They serve as an advocacy group to advance issues such as federal funding of stroke research and increasing awareness of stroke in the general population.

In January 1999, the Stroke Division of the AHA was renamed the American Stroke Association (ASA). The Stroke Division was established in 1998 to coordinate and direct the AHA's increasing emphasis on stroke research and education. During fiscal year 2003–04, the ASA spent more than $162.4 million on stroke efforts. In February 2004, an alliance with the Joint Commission on Accreditation of Healthcare Organizations (JCAHO) resulted in the *Primary Stroke Center Certification Program*, which allows consumers and emergency medical service (EMS) professionals to identify those hospitals that meet nationally-recognized standards to treat acute stroke. A quality improvement program entitled "Get with the Guidelines—Stroke" provides tools for physicians to care for stroke patients according to scientific guidelines.

The ASA also created the Stroke Connection, a national outreach program comprising a grassroots network of alliances, coalitions, outreach programs, and support groups dedicated to improving quality of life for stroke survivors and caregivers. A national phone bank provides stroke survivors and their families with daily living tips, resource information, and support group referrals. The Stroke Connection also produces an award-winning magazine that covers all aspects of stroke and is distributed to medical professionals, stroke survivors, and caregivers.

National Stroke Association.   Founded in 1984, the National Stroke Association (NSA) is the only organization in the United States dedicated solely to the distribution of information about the diagnosis and treatment of stroke. The NSA is a source for information on stroke risks and warning signs, patient information, and clinical trials. They have links to products and services used by stroke survivors and caregivers, including ADL aids, assistive technology, adaptive clothing, computers and communication products, exercise equipment, food products, lifts and elevators, pharmaceuticals, reading and writing aids, therapy management, assistive devices for ambulation, and wheelchairs and scooters. Additional links include NSA chapters, U.S. government resources, university/hospital resources, international health resources, association resources, and state agencies. The Stroke Center Network (SCN) is a listing of medical centers that provide acute stroke treatment services. The Stroke Rehabilitation and Recovery Network (SRN) is a listing of medical centers that provide stroke rehabilitation services at all levels of care. A speaker's bureau is available for providing lectures on stroke-related topics to medical and lay audiences.

The NSA produces the magazine *Stroke Smart*, which provides current information about stroke prevention, diagnosis, and treatment to stroke survivors. *Stroke Smart* contains pieces by both stroke survivors

and professionals. Letters sent by stroke survivors and caregivers are answered by professionals with appropriate expertise.

American Association of Retired Persons.   The American Association of Retired Persons (AARP) is the leading organization for people aged 50 and older in the United States. It serves their needs through information and education, advocacy, and community services that are provided by a network of local chapters and experienced volunteers. The AARP offers a wide variety of benefits and services, including health insurance, drug prescription plans, and computer network access. The government information site "Across America" electronically accesses information regarding Social Security benefits, Veterans Administration forms, change of address forms, Medicare information, and comparisons of nursing homes. It publishes the magazine *Modern Maturity* and the monthly magazine *Bulletin*.

In its information and research webpage, the AARP has extensive information on the areas of health, work and economic security, independent living, consumer issues, technology, and references and resources. The health website gives members information about prescription drugs, chronic disease management, alcohol abuse, medical breakthroughs, alternative medicine, nursing home admission contracts, Medicare and Medicaid, caregiving, preventative health maintenance, managed care, and rights of nursing home residents. The work and economic security website lists such diverse issues as electronic funds transfers, food stamps, U.S. savings bonds, Social Security, home equity information, employment opportunities, managing money, funding of long-term care, investing, welfare reform, and wills and living trusts. The Independent Living section contains links to home modifications, coping with grief and loss, AARP Connections for Independent Living, safe driving, and sharing living arrangements with others. Consumer issues include fraud in Medicare, travel, credit cards, home improvement, and banking; door-to-door salesmen; funerals and burials; and energy conservation. The technology section provides members with information about computer technology and the Internet. Other references include databases on publications and Internet sites related to older adults and aging.

National Council on the Aging.   The National Council on the Aging (NCOA) is an association of organizations and individuals dedicated to promoting the dignity, self-determination, well-being, and continuing contributions of older persons through leadership and service, education, and advocacy. Members include professionals and volunteers, service providers, consumer and labor groups, businesses, government agencies, religious groups, and volunteer organizations.

NCOA accomplishes its mission through leadership, education, and training; publications; research and development; community services; employment programs; coalition building in public policy; and advocacy efforts essential in a culturally diverse society. Founded in 1950, NCOA has a long history of innovation, including the Meals on Wheels and Foster Grandparents programs, the first national guidelines for geriatric care managers, and the only accreditation program for adult day-service providers.

The website provides current newsworthy information to its viewers. Links to constituent groups include those related to health promotion, adult day care and senior centers, employment, rural issues, consumer issues, long-term care, financial issues and services, senior housing, and religious issues. Programs are available in employment opportunities, consumer advocacy, caregiver support, and research.

National Aphasia Association. The National Aphasia Association (NAA) is a nonprofit organization that promotes public education, research, rehabilitation, and support services to assist people with aphasia and their families. Facts, articles, and publications on aphasia are available to stroke survivors and their caregivers. Caregiver support can be located through various links on its website. Listings of support groups, associations, and local resource people, including the NAA Young People's Network, are readily available. Stroke survivors or caregivers may sign up as a "pen pal" to others in the network. Information on current and existing research may be accessed. Newsletters are available online.

National Association of Area Agencies on Aging. The National Association of Area Agencies on Aging (N4A) assists older Americans in allowing them to stay in their own homes and communities with maximum self-dignity and independence for as long as possible. The four principles of the N4A are:

1. Advocacy of the roles of all Area Agencies on Aging in their efforts to serve the elderly
2. Advocacy for needed resources and support services that allow older Americans to live dignified and independent lifestyles
3. Advocacy for the rights of older Americans at the national level
4. Provision of communication, training, and technical assistance to enable elderly Americans to efficiently and effectively serve and represent themselves.

The N4A also serves in other capacities. It acts as a national focal point on behalf of Area Agencies on Aging in developing and implementing a nationwide system of community-based long-term care using existing local aging networks. It facilitates cooperative relationships between the aging network and other public and private systems to expand and enhance a comprehensive system of long-term care.

The N4A operates the Eldercare Locator, a tollfree, nationwide telephone service that helps caregivers locate services for older adults in their own communities. The service is supported by a cooperative agreement with the U.S. Administration on Aging. In conjunction with the Eldercare Locator, the N4A publishes the *National Directory for Eldercare Information and Referral.*

The website includes the "Network News" and a legislative update for members containing late-breaking news on aging policies in Washington, D.C. It also contains information about its annual spring legislative briefing in Washington, D.C., and its annual conference.

Pediatric Stroke Survivor Support Groups

National Dissemination Center for Children with Disabilities. The National Dissemination Center for Children with Disabilities (NICHCY) is a national information and referral center that provides information on disabilities and disability-related issues for families, educators, and other professionals who work with children and youth from birth to age twenty-two. NICHCY provides information and makes referrals in areas including specific disabilities, early intervention, special education and related services, individualized education programs, family issues, disability organizations, professional associations, education rights, and transition to adult life.

NICHCY distributes a wide variety of publications, including fact sheets on specific disabilities, state resource sheets, parent guides, bibliographies, and our issue papers "News Digest" and "Transition Summary." Most publications can be printed off the Internet or obtained by mail. Publications are also available in alternative formats upon request.

The website has links to disability organizations, parent groups, and professional associations at the state and national level. Specialists are available to speak with survivors and their family members about specific areas of concern.

Easter Seals. The forerunner of the Easter Seals was founded in 1919 by Edgar Allen, a businessman in Elyria, Ohio, whose son was killed in a streetcar accident. The lack of adequate medical services to save his son's life motivated him to organize the building of a hospital in his community. Subsequently, he took a deep interest in children with disabilities. With the help of Rotary Clubs, he formed the Ohio Society for Crippled Children, the first organization created to help children with physical disabilities.

The movement gradually spread throughout the United States, forming the National Society for Crippled Children. In 1944, the words *and adults* were added because of the increasingly important role of the organization in serving adults. In 1967, the words *Easter Seal* were incorporated in the organization's name, reflecting the public's awareness and acceptance of the traditional campaign symbol. In 1979, the phrase *for crippled children and adults* was dropped because of its negative connotation for people with and without disabilities.

In 2007, 1.2 million Easter Seals children and adults with disabilities and their families benefited from one or more Easter Seals services: programs for children, vocational training and employment, and medical rehabilitation. Services are individualized to meet each client's needs, family-focused to meet each family member's concerns, outcome-oriented with a goal of enhanced physical and financial independence, and cost-effective because they benefit from charity support.

Easter Seals provides services in each of the 50 United States, the District of Columbia, and Puerto Rico. Easter Seals children's services include early intervention programs, preschool and day-care programs for children with and without disabilities, after-school care programs, camping programs for children with and without disabilities, and respite services that benefit disabled children and their families.

Vocational training and employment services provide physically challenged young people and adults a full spectrum of services. Job training, job placement, assistive technology, and mentoring programs help disabled clients find and keep jobs that enhance independence.

Easter Seals also continues to be one of the nation's largest networks for medical rehabilitation services. It offers physical therapy, occupational therapy, speech-language services, home health and specialized therapy, and support programs for spinal cord injuries, persons dealing with stroke and post-polio issues, and disabilities that occur as a part of aging.

Caregiver Support Groups

Family Caregiver Alliance.   The Family Caregiver Alliance (FCA) is a support organization for caregivers of adults with Alzheimer's disease, stroke, traumatic brain injury, Parkinson's disease, amyotrophic lateral sclerosis (ALS), and related brain disorders. The FCA addresses the needs of families and friends providing long-term care by developing services, advocating for public and private support, conducting research, and educating the public. Headquartered in San Francisco, the FCA has developed an array of services and a dedicated approach to working with families based on consumer needs. As a result of advocacy efforts by the FCA, specialized information and assistance, consultation on long-term care planning,

service linkage and arrangement, legal and financial consultation, respite services, and counseling and education are available throughout the state of California.

The website contains a Resource Center including an online support group, online caregiver consultation, and an expanding list of community services in the San Francisco Bay rea. More than 30 fact sheets and 11 new reading lists are available. The online News Bureau provides reporters with background materials and interviews for stories. An Interview section contains fresh perspectives on the caregiving issues of the day. The FCA accepts e-mail comments and ideas for stories or other information.

The Healthy Caregiver Community Foundation.   The *Healthy Caregiver* is a quarterly resource publication dedicated to improving the overall well-being of America's family caregivers and professional eldercare service providers. It addresses diverse social, physical, and economic issues that naturally emanate from the eldercare relationship. The publication presents high-quality information that heightens the awareness of how caregivers and care receivers can enrich each other's lives. *The Healthy Caregiver* is committed to supplying resource information that is pertinent to achieving secure and fulfilling lifestyles.

Well Spouse Association.   The Well Spouse Association is a private, nonprofit organization that provides support and information to the 7 to 9 million well spouses of the chronically ill and to educate human service professionals and the public about the needs of spousal caregivers and their families. Founded in 1988 in response to Maggie Strong's book, *Mainstay*, now a quarterly newsletter, the Well Spouse Association works collaboratively with other local and national caregiving organizations. Chapters are available in 22 states.

National Family Caregivers Association.   The National Family Caregivers Association (NFCA) is the only national charitable organization dedicated to making life better for all of America's family caregivers. More than 25 million people find themselves in a caregiving role. NFCA focuses on family caregivers of all ages, relationships, and across differing diagnoses to address the common needs of all family caregivers. Through its services in the areas of information and education, support and validation, and public awareness and advocacy, the NFCA strives to minimize the disparity between a caregiver's quality of life and that of mainstream Americans. The NFCA espouses a philosophy of empowerment and self-care that is predicated on the belief that caregivers who choose to take charge of their lives, and see caregiving as but one of its facets, are in a position to be happier and healthier individuals. They are then able to have a higher quality of life and to make a more positive contribution to the well-being of their care recipient, all of which has a positive impact on society and health care costs.

The NFCA provides several resources to the community. "Take Care! Self Care for the Family Caregiver" is a quarterly newsletter providing can-do advice, resources, and questions and answers. The Caregiver-to-Caregiver Peer Support Network helps caregiver members find a friend in similar circumstances. *The Resourceful Caregiver: Helping Family Caregivers Help Themselves* is a unique resource guide filled with the information caregivers want and need. Cards for Caregivers is a service that sends message three times a year to remind caregivers that they are not alone. The NFCA sponsors National Family Caregivers Week, which raises public awareness and caregiver consciousness from coast to coast. National Resource Referrals helps caregivers locate the help the need. Special reports and educational materials keep caregivers up-to-date on NFCA activities and issues. The Bereavement Program helps former caregivers deal with their grief and begin to look ahead. A Voice to Caregivers in our Nation's Capital is an advocacy group that speaks out on caregivers' rights.

Information Sources

Agency for Health Care Research and Quality—U.S. Department of Health and Human Services. The Agency for Health Care Research and Quality (AHRQ) was established in 1989 as the Agency for Health Care Policy and Research (AHCPR). The name changed to AHRQ in November 1999 with legislation that established AHRQ as the lead federal agency charged with supporting research designed to improve the quality of health care, reduce its cost, and broaden access to essential services. The AHRQ's broad programs of research bring practical science-based information to medical practitioners and to consumers and other health care purchasers.

The agency comprises eight major functional components, with the Office of the Director ensuring that strategic objectives are achieved. The Office of Performance Accountability, Resources, and Technology directs and coordinates agencywide program planning, evaluation activities, and administrative operations. The Office of Extramural Research, Education, and Priority Populations directs the scientific review process for grants and Small Business Innovation Research (SBIR) contracts; manages agency research training programs, evaluates the scientific contribution of proposed and ongoing research, demonstrations, and evaluations; and supports and conducts health services research on priority populations. The Office of Communications and Knowledge Transfer designs, develops, implements, and manages programs for disseminating the results of agency activities with the goal of changing audience behavior.

The Center for Outcomes and Evidence conducts and supports research and assessment of health care practices, technologies, processes, and systems. The Center for Primary Care, Prevention, and Clinical Partnerships expands the knowledge base for clinical providers and patients and ensures the translation of new knowledge and systems improvement into primary care practice. The Center for Delivery, Organization, and Markets provides a focal point of leadership and expertise for advances in health care delivery, organization, and markets through research. The Center for Financing, Access, and Cost Trends conducts, supports, and manages studies of the cost and financing of health care, access to health care services and related trends; and develops data sets to support policy and behavioral research and analyses. The Center for Quality Improvement and Patient Safety works to improve the quality and safety of health care through research and implementation of evidence.

The vision of the AHRQ is to foster health care research that helps the American health care system provide access to high-quality, cost-effective services; be accountable and responsive to consumers and purchasers; and improve health status and quality of life. Several key concepts comprise this vision. First, the vision proposes a concept for what American health care should entail. Second, it is squarely focused on all stakeholders of the health care system, including patients, providers, plans, purchasers, and policy makers, because the majority of the agency's work is centered on personal health services. Third, it asserts that improved knowledge about the outcomes and quality of care can enhance the effectiveness of decisions about health care. Finally, it links the improvement in health care through this evidence-based strategy with improvements of health status and individuals' quality of life.

National Center for Medical Rehabilitation Research. The National Center for Medical Rehabilitation Research (NCMRR) was established as a component of the National Institute of Child Health and Human Development (NICHD) within the National Institutes of Health (NIH) by P.L. 101-613, which was passed in 1990. The mission of NCMRR is to foster development of scientific knowledge needed to enhance the health, productivity, independence, and quality of life of persons with disabilities. This is accomplished by supporting research in seven areas: improving functional mobility; promoting behavioral adaptation to functional losses; assessing the efficacy and outcomes to medical rehabilitation therapies and practices; developing improved assistive technology; understanding whole body system responses to physical impairments and functional changes; developing more precise methods of measuring impairments, disabilities, and societal and functional limitations; and training research scientists in the field of rehabilitation.

National Institute of Neurological Disorders and Stroke.   The National Institute of Neurological Disorders and Stroke (NINDS), a component of the National Institutes of Health and the U.S. Public Health Service, is the leading supporter of biomedical research on disorders of the brain and nervous system. The mission of the NINDS is to conduct, foster, coordinate, and guide research on the causes, prevention, diagnosis, and treatment of neurologic disorders and stroke, and to support basic research in related scientific areas. The NINDS provides grants-in-aid to public and private institutions and individuals in fields related to its areas of interest, including research project, program project, and research center grants. It operates programs of contracts for the funding of research and research support efforts in selected areas of institute need, and provides individual and institutional fellowships to increase scientific expertise in neurologic fields. It conducts a diversified program of intramural and collaborative research in its own laboratories, branches, and clinics, and collects and disseminates research information related to neurologic disorders. Professional and patient information distributed by NINDS is listed in Table 47-5.

National Institute on Disability and Rehabilitation Research.   The National Institute on Disability and Rehabilitation Research (NIDRR) is a component of the Office of Special Education and Rehabilitative Services (OSERS), which is in turn an office within the U.S. Department of Education. The OSERS supports programs that assist in educating children with special needs, provides for the rehabilitation of children and adults with disabilities, and supports research to improve the lives of individuals with disabilities. The NIDRR provides leadership and support for a comprehensive program of research related to the rehabilitation of individuals with disabilities.

The NIDRR is composed of several components. The Interagency Committee on Disability Research (ICDR), which the director of NIDRR chairs, maintains institutional relationships with other federal agencies that conduct disability research. In addition, NIDRR cosponsors research programs with other federal government agencies and with foreign governments and international agencies. The Research Sciences Division (RSD) is responsible for national and international programs in research, training, and technical and clinical evaluation. The RSD plans, develops, implements, and manages a comprehensive national and international program of research, training, utilization, and evaluation in specific program areas. The Program, Budget and Evaluation Division (PBE) formulates budgets, coordinates policy, and plans, identifies, implements, analyzes, monitors, evaluates congressionallymandated NIDRR activities. More specifically, it ensures that NIDRR policy and guidance encompasses a broad range of the research community from regulations, statutes, and policy inquiries.

Rehabilitation Services Administration.   The Rehabilitation Services Administration (RSA) is a component of the Office of Special Education and Rehabilitative Services (OSERS), which is in turn an office within the U.S. Department of Education. The RSA oversees programs that help individuals with physical or mental challenges to obtain employment through supports, including counseling, medical and psychological services, job training, and other individualized services. The Rehabilitation Act of 1973, as amended, authorizes the allocation of federal funds on a formula basis of state and federal dollars for the administration and operation of a vocational rehabilitation (VR) program to assist individuals with disabilities in preparing for and engaging in gainful employment. The VR program provides a wide range of services and job training to people with disabilities who want to work. At present, the VR system has more than a million eligible individuals; two-thirds of them are severely disabled. Priority is given to people with the most severe disabilities.

To be eligible for VR services from a state VR agency, a person must:

1. Have a physical or mental impairment that is a substantial impediment to employment
2. Be able to benefit from VR services in terms of employment
3. Require VR services to prepare for, enter, engage in, or retain employment

---

TABLE 47-5

Publications Distributed by the National Institute of Neurological Disorders and Stroke (NINDS)

Emergency Treatment for Stroke Information on the NINDS t-PA Trial

Acute Stroke Treatment Guidelines: Proceedings of a National Symposium on Rapid Identification and Treatment of Acute Stroke

Brain Attack: Information for Professionals (information from the Brain Attack Coalition)

Brain Attack: Stroke Symptoms and Risk Factors (available in Spanish)

Brain Basics: Preventing Stroke (available in Spanish)

Stroke ("Brain Attack") (a mini-information sheet about stroke)

Stroke in Children (a mini-information sheet about stroke in children)

Information Guide on Surgery to Prevent Stroke

Recovering After a Stroke

sexual problems after a stroke. This system identifies psychological issues as being the dominant cause of sexual dysfunction in stroke patients, but it also includes the physiological and medical factors that are specific to the stroke population. A more detailed description of this novel classification system follows.

Psychosocial Factors

Korpelainen reported that psychosocial factors play a larger role in determining sexual drive, activity, and satisfaction after stroke than medical factors do. Bodrini and colleagues established that clinical factors do not seem to play a crucial role in determining changes in sexuality post-stroke, but more psychological and interpersonal factors (8). In fact, psychological factors likely are the major contributor to the sexual dysfunction after stroke. Along with common psychiatric problems seen after stroke, such as depression, anxiety, or post-traumatic stress disorder, impairment of social dimensions, such as lack of partner or loss of job, may also play a significant role in sexuality issues after stroke.

Dependency in ADLs. It has been suggested that the degree of dependence in ADLs is a strong predictor of a decrease in sex frequency (9, 10). This dependency can cause feelings of embarrassment and vulnerability as one's privacy is compromised. This may be particularly problematic when the sexual partner also provides personal care, and this is consistent with the finding that sexual dysfunction is also common in sexual partners of stroke survivors (5). This shift in role from caregiver to partner or patient to partner can have a negative effect on sexual identity. One solution is to have some aspects of care, such as toileting, carried out by a nonfamily caregiver whenever possible.

Role Shift within the Family. The profound role shift within a family after stroke may present as anger and frustration on the part of the patient and spouse. Loss of previous roles results in a serious change in the quality and style of the interpersonal relationship and requires time and patience to rediscover a loving partnership. Recognizing and anticipating such changes early after stroke and providing opportunities for counseling can allow for better adjustment to role changes in a partnership.

Altered Body Image and Self-Esteem. Across the spectrum of medical diseases and disability, changes in self-image can have a profound impact on quality of life and satisfaction. Specifically, neuromuscular changes that impact movement, the use of assistive devices or adaptive equipment, and changes in bodily function can result in feelings of decreased attractiveness and self-esteem followed by shame, frustration, and even depressed mood. There may be real or perceived fear of rejection, betrayal, and/or abandonment by the partner, resulting in loneliness or isolation and avoidance of social or sexual situations.

Lack of Sexual Partner. Because stroke survivors are often of advanced age, many have survived their sexual partner. In addition, there is high risk of abandonment by a partner following onset of neurologic disability. For those who are not in a relationship, it is often assumed that sexuality is not an issue. But lack of a sexual partner does not erase a person's concern about attractiveness, sexual functioning, and potentially finding a partner in the future. Unfortunately, social opportunities for meeting others and finding potential sexual partners are often limited after stroke, which reduces the likelihood of engaging in sexual activity. It is important to provide reassurance that sexual functioning and intimacy are still possible and to assist patients in full reintegration to the community through comprehensive rehabilitation.

Fears, Myths, and Unrealistic Expectations. There are certain fears and myths around sexuality and sexual performance that are common among stroke survivors. Most commonly, the fear of a recurrent stroke can result in reduced sexual activity, decreased libido, and sexual dissatisfaction (11). Monga and others interviewed patients with stroke and their spouses about sexuality. The most common factor identified as causing a decline in sexual activity was the fear by both partners that having sex might adversely affect blood pressure and cause another stroke (12). In reality, the cardiac response associated with sexual activity is equivalent to climbing two flights of stairs at a brisk rate. The energy expenditure during sex is also comparable to walking on a treadmill at three to four miles per hour and is equal to five to six metabolic equivalents of oxygen consumption (METS) (13–15). This level of exertion, though significant for some patients with stroke, is unlikely to overly stress cardiac function or result in a dangerous rise in blood pressure. Therefore, education, reassurance, and a focus on general physical fitness may be appropriate in certain stroke patients.

Unrealistic expectations of what constitutes a normal sex life may lay a foundation for failure. Normal sexuality is unique to each couple, as is their unique relationship. A healthy couple's perception of normalcy should align more with their personal life expectations than that of society or the media. Table 45-5 lists some myths that exist about sexuality following stroke. It may be useful to discuss these misconceptions early with both patients and their partners. The recognition of unrealistic expectations, fear, and myths can serve as an educational opportunity.

The state VR agencies assist persons with disabilities in locating employment by developing and maintaining close relationships with local businesses. They also assist persons served to become taxpaying citizens and to reduce their reliance on entitlement programs. To help unemployed persons with physical challenges join the workforce, state VR agencies must provide comprehensive rehabilitation services that go way beyond those found in routine job training programs. Services frequently include:

1. Work evaluation and adjustment services
2. Assessment for and provision of assistive technology, such as customized computer interfaces for persons with physical or sensory disabilities
3. Job counseling services
4. Medical and therapeutic services

National Rehabilitation Information Center. The National Rehabilitation Information Center (NARIC) collects and disseminates the results of federally funded research projects. The literature collection, which also includes commercially published books, journal articles, and audiovisual materials, now includes over 70,000 documents. NARIC is funded by the National Institute on Disability and Rehabilitation Research (NIDRR) to serve consumers, family members, health professionals, educators, rehabilitation counselors, students, librarians, administrators, and researchers who are interested in disability and rehabilitation. In-house services include quick information and referral, customized database searches, document delivery, and NARIC products. The website includes four searchable and browsable databases: literature, organizations, timely information, and research.

DisabilityInfo.gov. DisabilityInfo.gov is a comprehensive online resource designed to provide people with disabilities with quick and easy access on numerous disability-related subjects, including benefits, civil rights, community life, education, employment, housing, health, technology, and transportation. DisabilityInfo.gov is managed by the Office of Disability Employment Policy (ODEP) of the U.S. Department of Labor in partnership with 21 other federal agencies. It is the result of an Executive Memorandum issued on August 28, 2002, as part of the New Freedom Initiative. The New Freedom Initiative is a comprehensive plan to remove barriers to community living for people with disabilities. It is meant to increase access to assistive and universally designed technologies; expand educational opportunities; promote homeownership; integrate Americans with disabilities into the workforce; expand transportation options; and promote full access to community life.

Funding Sources

Medicare. The Centers for Medicare and Medicaid Services (CMS), a division of the Department of Health and Human Services, runs Medicare, which is the nation's largest health insurance program. Medicare provides health insurance to

1. People who are at least 65 years old
2. People who are disabled
3. People with permanent kidney failure

Medicare has two parts. Medicare Part A helps pay for inpatient hospital services, skilled nursing facility services, home health services, and hospice care. Medicare Part B helps pay for doctor services, outpatient hospital services, medical equipment and supplies, and other health services and supplies. Starting January 1, 2006, Medicare Part D helps pay for prescription drugs.

Many Medicare beneficiaries choose to enroll in managed care plans such as health maintenance organizations (HMOs) or preferred provider organizations (PPOs). Beneficiaries can get Part A, Part B, and Part D benefits in most managed care plans. People who are already getting Social Security or railroad retirement benefits are automatically enrolled when they become eligible for Medicare. Others, such as persons with acquired disabilities such as stroke, must go to their local Social Security office and apply.

The website contains vital information for Medicare recipients. Yearly costs for Medicare are listed. Satisfaction and quality performance information on managed care plans and nursing homes is available for browsing. The top 20 Medicare/Medicaid questions and answers are posted for viewing.

Medicaid. Medicaid, which is funded and administered through a state–federal partnership, is the health insurance program for certain low-income people. People who are eligible for Medicaid include certain low-income families with children; aged, blind, or disabled people on Supplemental Security Income; certain low-income pregnant women and children; and people who have very high medical bills. Although there are broad federal requirements for Medicaid, states have a wide degree of flexibility to design their programs. States have authority to:

1. Establish eligibility standards
2. Determine what benefits and services to cover
3. Set payment rates

Because states have flexibility in structuring their Medicaid programs, there are variations from state to state. However, all states must cover several basic services:

1. Inpatient and outpatient hospital services
2. Laboratory and radiology services
3. Skilled nursing and home health services
4. Doctors' services
5. Family planning
6. Periodic health checkups, including diagnosis and treatment for children

Social Security Administration. The Social Security Administration (SSA) provides benefits to stroke survivors through the Social Security Disability program. The website contains information summarizing the Social Security Retirement, Supplemental Security Income, Survivors, and Health Insurance programs. Cash benefits and eligibility requirements are discussed, and evidence needed to make a disability determination is listed. Publications and newsletters providing information on programs and their legislative changes are available online.

The SSA also can help stroke survivors get the vocational rehabilitation (VR) services they need to return to work or to go to work for the first time. They can put stroke survivors in touch with agencies that provide services such as job counseling, training, and job placement. The SSA does not provide these services but can pay for them when certain conditions are met. The SSA first refers persons to the state VR agency for consideration. If the state agency is unable to serve the stroke survivor, the stroke survivor may be referred to an alternate participant. Stroke survivors also may contact the rehabilitation agency in their state directly at any time.

Psychological Services

American Association of Suicidology. The American Association of Suicidology (AAS) is a nonprofit organization dedicated to the understanding and prevention of suicide. The organization benefits any person who is concerned about suicide, including AAS members, suicide researchers, therapists, prevention specialists, survivors of suicide, and people who are themselves in crisis. The AAS distributes suicide prevention books that are reviewed and recommended by the AAS Publications Committee, but are neither endorsed nor sanctioned by AAS. The AAS also publishes the journal *Suicide and Life-Threatening Behavior* and a quarterly newletter. The website contains possible steps people can take to receive help if they are in crisis.

National Institute of Mental Health. The National Institute of Mental Health (NIMH) supports innovative science that profoundly transforms the diagnosis, treatment, and prevention of mental disorders in the quest for finding a cure. The missions of NIMH are to reduce the burden of mental illness and behavioral disorders through research that supports and strengthens the foundation for understanding mental disorders; defining the genetic and environmental components of mental disorders; identifying more reliable, valid diagnostic tests and biomarkers for mental disorders; developing more effective, safer, and equitable treatments that have minimal side effects to reduce symptoms, and improve daily functioning; providing treatment options to deliver more effective personalized care across diverse populations and settings; and creating a more efficient pathway to disseminate scientific findings to clinicians and patients. The Outreach Partnership Program, run by the Office of Constituency Relations and Public Liaison (OCRPL), in cooperation with the Substance Abuse and Mental Health Services Administration (SAMHSA), develops partnerships with national and state organizations to disseminate scientific findings and inform the public about mental disorders in order to reduce the stigma and discrimination associated with these illnesses. The Alliance for Research Progress allows patients and families representing national voluntary organizations to advocate concerns for research initiatives with NIMH staff.

Patient Rights Groups

People's Medical Society. The People's Medical Society is recognized as a knowledgeable, effective, and relentless protector of health care consumer rights. The website contains a comprehensive reference guide to patient rights and opportunities concerning medical care, including insurance and medical tests.

Vocational Assistance

Equal Employment Opportunity Commission. The Equal Employment Opportunity Commission (EEOC) was established by Title VII of the Civil Rights Act of 1964 and began operating on July 2, 1965. The EEOC enforces the principal federal statutes prohibiting employment discrimination, including:

1. Title VII of the Civil Rights Act of 1964, as amended, which prohibits employment discrimination on the basis of race, color, religion, sex, or national origin
2. The Age Discrimination in Employment Act (ADEA) of 1967, as amended, which prohibits employment discrimination against individuals 40 years of age and older
3. The Equal Pay Act (EPA) of 1963, which prohibits discrimination on the basis of gender in compensation for substantially similar work under similar conditions
4. Title I of the Americans with Disabilities Act of 1990 (ADA), which prohibits employment discrimination on the basis of disability in both the public and private sector, excluding the federal government

5. The Civil Rights Act of 1991, which includes provisions for monetary damages in cases of intentional discrimination and clarifies provisions regarding disparate impact actions

6. Section 501 of the Rehabilitation Act of 1973, as amended, which prohibits employment discrimination against federal employees with disabilities

The website was launched in fiscal year 1997 to provide the public with greater access to an array of agency information materials and resources. The homepage consists of annual reports, addresses and phone numbers of field offices, press releases, fact sheets, and periodicals. More recently, the EEOC has added a small business information fact sheet highlighting select issues of particular interest to small businesses.

Relevant to stroke survivors is information on "Reasonable Accommodation and Undue Hardship under the Americans With Disabilities Act," revised in October 2002. This enforcement guidance clarifies the rights and responsibilities of employers and individuals with disabilities regarding reasonable accommodation and undue hardship. Title I of the ADA requires an employer to provide reasonable accommodation to qualified individuals with disabilities who are employees or applicants for employment, except when such accommodation would cause an undue hardship. The guidance sets forth an employer's legal obligations regarding reasonable accommodation. It also discusses reasonable accommodations applicable to the hiring process, the benefits and privileges of employment, and job performance. Reassignment issues include who is entitled to reassignment and the extent to which an employer must search for a vacant position. The guidance also examines issues concerning the interplay between reasonable accommodations and conduct rules and concludes with a discussion of undue hardship, including when requests for schedule modifications and leave may be denied. Questions concerning the relationship between the ADA and the Family and Medical Leave Act (FMLA) are examined as they affect leave and modified schedules.

CONCLUSION

Returning to the community can be as traumatic an experience to the stroke survivor as experiencing the stroke itself. While stroke survivors have been adjusting to his disabilities, they largely have been sheltered in the hospital and rehabilitation environments with professionals who provide a structure for therapy and emotional support. Other stroke survivors who understand the survivor's plight can form an informal network that may last well beyond discharge from the rehabilitation facility. However, once stroke survivors leave the cloister of the inpatient rehabilitation facility, they and their caregivers must negotiate a plethora of problems, sometimes with some support from the rehabilitation community, but often on their own. This chapter has sought to identify many of the issues that stroke survivors face in the community, and to offer suggestions and solutions to the issues. A number of resources can be identified on the Internet to provide support that might not be found elsewhere. With time, perseverance, and experience, stroke survivors may be guided or guide themselves through the rehabilitation "maze" and learn how to navigate the very complex system of health care that we face today. Although answers to problems may not be perfect (and, in some cases, may not be present at all), the stroke survivor and caregiver need to advocate for themselves, locate and utilize appropriate resources, and ask for help from their medical professional networks so that they can optimize and maintain an independent quality of life.

Patient Education Resources

1. American Stroke Association
   National Center
   7272 Greenville Avenue
   Dallas, TX 75231
   888-4-STROKE
   www.strokeassociation.org

2. National Stroke Association
   9707 East Easter Lane
   Centennial, CO 80112
   800-STROKES or 303-649-9299
   www.stroke.org

3. American Association of Retired Persons
   601 E Street NW
   Washington, DC 20049
   888-OUR-AARP or 888-687-2277www.aarp.org

4. The National Council on the Aging, Inc.
   1901 L Street NW
   4th Floor
   Washington, DC 20036
   202-479-1200
   www.ncoa.org

5. National Aphasia Association
   350 Seventh Avenue
   Suite 902
   New York, NY 10001
   800-922-4622
   www.aphasia.org

6. National Association of Area Agencies on Aging
   1730 Rhode Island Avenue
   Suite 1200
   Washington, DC 20036
   202-872-0888
   www.n4a.org

7. National Dissemination Center for Children with Disabilities
P.O. Box 1492
Washington, DC 20013
800-695-0285
www.nichcy.org

8. Easter Seals
230 West Monroe Street
Suite 1800
Chicago, IL 60606
800-221-6827 or 312-726-6200
www.easterseals.com

9. Family Caregiver Alliance
180 Montgomery Street
Suite 1100
San Francisco, CA 94104
415-434-3388 or 800-445-8106
www.caregiver.org

10. The Healthy Caregiver Community Foundation
12 West Willow Grove Avenue
Suite 190
Philadelphia, PA 19118
215-836-4262
www.healthycaregiver.com

11. Well Spouse Association
63 West Main Street, Suite H
Freehold, NJ 07728
732-577-8899 or 800-838-0879
www.wellspouse.org

12. National Family Caregivers Association
10400 Connecticut Avenue
Suite 500
Kensington, MD 20895-3944
301-942-6430 or 800-896-3650
www.nfacares.org

13. Agency for Healthcare Research and Quality
Office of Communications and Knowledge Transfer
540 Gaither Road
Suite 2000
Rockville, MD 20850
301-427-1364
www.ahrq.gov

14. National Center for Medical Rehabilitation Research
National Institute of Child Health and Human Development
National Institutes of Health
6100 Executive Boulevard
Room 2A03, MSC 7510
Rockville, MD 20852
301-402-4201
www.nichd.nih.gov/about/org/ncmrr/

15. National Institute of Neurological Disorders and Stroke
NIH Neurological Institute

P.O. Box 5801
Bethesda, MD 20824
301-496-5751 or 800-352-9424
www.ninds.nih.gov

16. National Institute on Disability and Rehabilitation Research
U.S. Department of Education
400 Maryland Avenue SW, Mailstop PCP-6038
Washington, DC 20202
202-245-7640
www.ed.gov/about/offices/list/osers/nidrr/index.html?src=mr/

17. Rehabilitation Services Administration
The Office of Special Education and Rehabilitative Services
U.S. Department of Education
400 Maryland Avenue SW
Washington, DC 20202-2800
202-245-7488
www.ed.gov/about/offices/list/osers/rsa/index.html

18. National Rehabilitation Information Center
8201 Corporate Drive
Suite 600
Landover, MD 20785
301-459-5900 or 800-346-2742
www.naric.com

19. DisabilityInfo.gov
U.S. Department of Labor
Frances Perkins Building
200 Constitution Avenue NW
Washington, DC 20210
800-FED-INFO
www.disabilityinfo.gov

20. Medicare
Centers for Medicare and Medicaid Services
7500 Security Boulevard
Baltimore, MD 21244-1850
410-786-3000 or 800-MEDICARE
www.medicare.gov or www.cms.hhs.gov/home/medicare.asp

21. Medicaid
Department of Health and Human Services
7500 Security Boulevard
Baltimore, MD 21244
410-786-3000
www.cms.hhs.gov/home/medicaid.asp

22. Social Security Administration
Office of Public Inquiries
Windsor Park Building
6401 Security Boulevard
Baltimore, MD 21235
800-772-1213
www.ssa.gov

23. American Association of Suicidology
5221 Wisconsin Avenue NW

Washington, DC 20015
202-237-2280
www.suicidology.org
24. National Institute of Mental Health
Science Writing, Press, and Dissemination Branch
6001 Executive Boulevard, Room 8184, MSC 9663
Bethesda, MD 20892-9663
301-443-4513 or 866-615-6464
www.nimh.nih.gov

25. People's Medical Society
P.O. Box 868
Allentown, PA 18105-0868
610-770-1670
www.peoplesmed.org
26. U.S. Equal Employment Opportunity Commission
1801 L Street NW
Washington, DC 20507
800-669-4000 or 202-663-4900www.eeoc.gov

References

1. *Harari D, Coshall C, Rudd AG, Wolfe CD.* New-onset fecal incontinence after stroke: Prevalence, natural history, risk factors, and impact. *Stroke.* 2003 Jan; 34(1):144–150

2. Lichtenberg PA, Gibbons TA. Geriatric rehabilitation and the older adult family caregiver. *Neurorehabilitation* 1992; 3:(1):62–71.

3. Schulz R, Visintainer P, Williamson G. Psychiatric and physical morbidity effects of caregiving. *J Gerontol Psych Sci* 1990; 45:181–191.

4. North American Symptomatic Carotid Endarterectomy Trial Collaborators. Beneficial effect of carotid endarterectomy in symptomatic patients with high-grade stenosis. *N Engl J Med* 1991; 325:445–453.

5. NIH MedlinePlus Medical Encyclopedia: Stroke. http://www.nlm.nih.gov/medlineplus/ency/article/000726.htm

6. Wade DT, Collen FM, Robb GF, Warlow CP. Physiotherapy intervention late after stroke and mobility. *BMJ* 1992 Mar 7; 304:(6827):609–613.

7. Wade DT, Hewer RL. Functional abilities after stroke: Measurement, natural history and prognosis. *J Neurol Neurosurg Psychiatry* 1987a Feb.; 50:(2):177–182.

8. Wade DT, Hewer RL. Motor loss and swallowing difficulty after stroke: Frequency, recovery, and prognosis. *Acta Neurol Scand* 1987b Jul.; 76:(1):50–54.

9. Gresham GE, Phillips TF, Wolf PA, et al. Epidemiologic profile of long-term stroke disability: The Framingham study. *Arch Phys Med Rehabil.* 1979 Nov; 60(11):487–491.

10. DeJong G, Branch LG. Predicting the stroke patient's ability to live independently. *Stroke* 1982 Sep-Oct.; 13:(5):648–655.

11. Gresham GE, Duncan PW, Stason WB, et al. Post stroke rehabilitation: Assessment, referral and management. Clinical Practice Guideline No. 16. Rockville, MD: US DHHS, Public Health Services, Agency for Health Care Policy and Research; 1995. AHCPR Pub. No. 95-0663. Available at http://text.nlm.nih.gov

12. Ward NS, Brown MM, Thompson AJ, Frackowiak RS. Neural correlates of outcome after stroke: A cross-sectional fMRI study. *Brain* 2003; 126(pt 6):1430–1448.

13. Guermazi A, Miaux Y, Rovira-Canellas A, et al. Neuroradiological findings in vascular dementia. *Neuroradiology* 2006 Nov 18; [Epub ahead of print].

14. Gidal BE. New and emerging treatment options for neuropathic pain. *Am J Manag Care.* 2006 Jun; 12(9 Suppl):S269–S278.

15. Portnow J, Kline T, Daly M, et al. Multidisciplinary home rehabilitation: A practical model. *Clinics in Geriatric Medicine* 1991 Nov.; 7:(4):695–706.

16. Wade DT, Langton-Hewer R, Skilbeck CE, et al. Controlled trial of a home-care service for acute stroke patients. *Lancet* 1985 Feb. 9; 1:(8424):323–326.

17. Sacco RL, Wolf PA, Kannel WB, McNamara PM. Survival and recurrence following stroke: The Framingham study. *Stroke* 1982 May–Jun.; 13:(3):290–205.

18. Roy C. Shoulder pains in hemiplegia: A literature review. *Clin Rehabil* 1988; 2:35–44.

19. Van Ouwenaller C, Laplace PM, Chantraine A. Painful shoulder in hemiplegia. *Arch Phys Med Rehabil* 1986; 67:23–26.

20. Carr J, Shepherd R. *Movement Science: Foundations for Physical Therapy in Rehabilitation,* 2nd ed. Rockville, MD: Aspen, 2000.

21. Dickstein R, Hocherman S, Pillar T, Shaham R. Stroke rehabilitation: Three exercise therapy approaches. *Phys Ther* 1986 Aug.; 66:(8):1233–1238.

22. Twitchell TE. The prognosis of motor recovery in hemiplegia. *Bull Tufts N Engl Med Cent* 1957 Jul.–Sep.; 3(3):146–149.

23. Bobath B. *Adult hemiplegia: Evaluation and treatment.* 3rd ed. London: William Hinneman Medical Books, 1990.

24. Palmer JB, DeChase AS. Rehabilitation of swallowing due to strokes. *Phys Med Rehab Clin N Amer* 1991; 2: 529–546.

25. Basso A, Capitani E, Vignolo LA. Influence of rehabilitation on language skills in aphasic patients: A controlled study. *Arch Neurol* 1979 Apr.; 36:(4):190–196.

26. Wade DT, Hewer RL, David RM, Enderby PM. Aphasia after stroke: Natural history and associated deficits. *J Neurol Neurosurg Psych* 1986 Jan.; 49:(1):11–16.

27. Depression Guideline Panel. *Detection and Diagnosis.* Volume 1: *Depression in Primary Care.* Clinical Practice Guideline No. 5. Rockville, MD: U.S. Department of Health and Human Services, Agency for Health Care Policy and Research, 1993. AHCPR Pub. No. 93-0551.

28. National Advisory Mental Health Council. Health care reform for Americans with severe mental illnesses. *Am J Psychiatry* 1993; 150(10):1447–1465.

29. Lipsey JR, Robinson RG, Pearlson GD, et al. Nortriptyline treatment of post-stroke depression: A double-blind study. *Lancet* 1984 Feb. 11; 1:(8372):297–300.

30. Parikh RM, Robinson RG, Lipsey JR, et al. The impact of post-stroke depression on recovery in activities of daily living over a two-year follow-up. *Arch Neurol* 1990; 47:785–789.

31. Robinson R, Schultz S, Castillo C, et al. Nortriptyline versus fluoxetine in the treatment of depression and in short-term recovery after stroke: A placebo-controlled, double-blind study. *Am J Psychiatry* 2000; 157:351–359.

32. Burns A, Russell E, Stratton-Powell H, et al. Sertraline in stroke-associated lability of mood. *Int J Geriatr Psychiatry* 1999; 14:681–685.

33. Wiart L, Petit H, Joseph PA, et al. Fluoxetine in early poststroke depression: A double-blind placebo-controlled study. *Stroke* 2000; 31:1829–1832.

34. ePocrates Multicheck. ePocrates Online. https://online.epocrates.com/noFrame/ Accessed September 7, 2008.

35. Gregorian RS, Golden KA, Bahce A, et al. Antidepressant-induced sexual dysfunction. *Ann Pharmacother* 2002 Oct.; 36(10):1577–1589.

36. Woo E, Proulx SM, Greenblatt DJ. Differential side effect profile of triazolam versus flurazepam in elderly patients undergoing rehabilitation therapy. *J Clin Pharmacol* 1991 Feb.; 31:(2):168–173.

37. Nouri FM, Tinson DJ, Lincoln NB. Cognitive ability and driving after stroke. *International Disability Studies* 1987; 9:110–115.

38. Martinsson L, Wahlgren NG. Safety of dexamphetamine in acute ischemic stroke: A randomized, double-blind, controlled dose-escalation trial. *Stroke* 2003 Feb.; 34(2):475–481.

39. Borucki SJ, Langberg J, Reding M. The effect of dextroamphetamine on motor recovery after stroke. *Neurology* 1992; 42:329. Abstract.

40. Sonde L, Nordstrom M, Nilsson CG, et al. A double-blind placebo-controlled study of the effects of amphetamine and physiotherapy after stroke. *Cerebrovasc Dis* 2001; 12:253–257.

41. Rasmussen RS, Overgaard K, Hildebrandt-Eriksen ES, Boysen G. D-amphetamine improves cognitive deficits and physical therapy promotes fine motor rehabilitation in a rat embolic stroke model. *Acta Neurol Scand* 2006 Mar.; 113(3):189–198.

42. Walker-Batson D, Curtis S, Natarajan R, et al. A double-blind, placebo-controlled study of the use of amphetamine in the treatment of aphasia. *Stroke* 2001; 32:2093–2098.

43. Conroy B, Zorowitz R, Horn SD, et al. An exploration of central nervous system medication use and outcomes in stroke rehabilitation. *Arch Phys Med Rehabil* 2005 Dec; 86(12 Suppl. 2):S73–S81.

44. Monga TN, Lawson JS, Inglis J. Sexual dysfunction in stroke patients. *Arch Phys Med Rehabil* 1986 Jan.; 67(1):19–22.

45. McCormick GP, Riffer DJ, Thompson MM. Coital positioning for stroke afflicted couples. *Rehabil Nurs* 1986 Mar.–Apr.; 11(2):17–19.

46. Sjogren K, Fugl-Meyer AR. Adjustment to life after stroke with special reference to sexual intercourse and leisure. *J Psychosom Res* 1982; 26(4):409–417.

47. Bates B, Choi J, Duncan PW, et al. Veterans Affairs/Department of Defense clinical practice guideline for the management of adult stroke rehabilitation care. *Stroke* 2005; 36:2049.

48. Bladin CF, Alexandrov AV, Bellavance A, et al. Seizures after stroke: A prospective multicenter study. *Arch Neurol.* 2000 Nov; 57(11):1617–1622.

49. Burn J, Dennis M, Bamford J, et al. Epileptic seizures after a first stroke: The Oxfordshire Community Stroke Project. *BMJ.* 1997 Dec. 13; 315(7122):1582–1587.

50. Ferro JM, Pinto F. Poststroke epilepsy: Epidemiology, pathophysiology and management. *Drugs Aging* 2004; 21(10):639–653.

51. Massagli TL. Neurobehavioral effects of phenytoin, carbamazepine, and valproic acid: Implications for use in traumatic brain injury. *Arch Phys Med Rehabil.* 1991 Mar; 72(3):219–226.

Index